Für lieben Kollegen
Reiner Labitzke, der
weiss wie schwer di Treppe
nach oben sind
„Es ist keine Schande auf die
Nase zu fallen. Schande ist
nicht aufzustehen und
weiter machen"

Jan 2014 Neven Olivari

Neven Olivari

Practical Plastic and Reconstructive Surgery

An Atlas of Operations and Techniques

With the Assistance of
Dirk Richter, Egon Eder, Georg Noever, Birgit Stark,
Werner Niermann, Henryk Wikarczyk, Anna Maria Olivari

KADEN

Kaden Publishing
Heidelberg, Germany

Professor Dr. med. Neven Olivari
Professor of Plastic Surgery (retired) – University of Cologne
(former Head of the Department of Plastic Surgery Dreifaltigkeits-Krankenhaus Wesseling)
Hauptstrasse 269
D-51503 Rösrath-Hoffnungsthal

Translation/Language Editing:

Tanja Bartscher
Mareike Leffler
Arash Momeni
Andreas Niederbichler
Saskia M. K. Schnabl
Alexander Stoff
Philip G. Arnold
Antony Attwood
George Lamberty
Brian D. G. Morgan
David E. Tolhurst

Photographs: Inge Goldberg
Illustrations: Neven Olivari

Bibliografische Information der Deutschen Bibliothek
Die Deutsche Bibliothek verzeichnet diese Publikation in der deutschen Nationalbibliografie; detaillierte bibliografische Daten sind im Internet unter http://www.dnb.ddb.de abrufbar.

Distribution for North America
Quality Medical Publishing, Inc.
2248 Welsch Industrial Ct.
St. Louis, MO 63146, USA
Customer Service: customerservice@qmp.com
www.qmp.com

Typesetting: Ch. Molter, Kaden Verlag, 69115 Heidelberg, Germany
Printing: Grosch Druckzentrum, 69214 Eppelheim, Germany
Binding: Buchbinderei Schaumann, 64293 Darmstadt, Germany

ISBN 978-3-922777-84-7

This book is dedicated to
my wife Anna-Maria, and
my sons Alexander and Nicolas
as well Lina Maria, Ella Brigitte and Karlo.

Foreword

Very large comprehensive books on big broad topics are undertaken by authors from time to time and successfully completed with the help of multiple co-authors and a publisher with a very capable illustrations department. Rarely, if ever, does an author address a topic as large as "plastic surgery" alone. Doctor Neven Olivari has done this and done it very well. He is a master surgeon and teacher, a tireless surgical historical researcher, and an unbelievably capable artist. This remarkable combination of abilities is memorialized in this book which has been written and illustrated by Dr. Olivari himself.

The early chapters cover the history of many flaps that we have considered under other names in the past. Bruns, Burow, Delpech and Dieffenbach are well represented. The older illustrations are the clearest and best I have ever seen. The historical accounting is very complete.

No aspect of general plastic surgery is abbreviated in his considerations and coverage of the various topics. Chapter 2 covers "general techniques" and should be required reading for all surgeons and fundamental knowledge for all plastic and reconstructive surgeons. It is truly the foundation for most of what we do and is beautifully illustrated.

The reconstructive chapters including head and neck, trunk, extremities, genitalia are unsurpassed, in my opinion. Replantation and burns are covered from their acute phase through the final reconstruction and up-to date. Aesthetic surgery of the face . eyes, and breasts as well as obesity surgery are covered very comprehensively and the author's opinions are clearly and concisely presented. Exophthalmos operation is covered very well since this is one method which Dr. Olivari developed and used since 20 years.

Problem cases are presented and the author's surgical solution along with potential problems and complications are presented. This information is based on a full surgical lifetime of having "been there and done that". Advice based on experience from an honest surgeon is priceless. Of course, there is personal preference that is present throughout this great book. That is what a book should do … give an account and defend your choices and admit the areas of weakness and when and why you change some technique. It is all here in Dr. Olivari's book. This assessment itself is also very biased.

It is not often that your heroes become your friends but that has been my good fortune over the past 3 decades and I feel particularly "blessed" by the association and friendship.

Philip G. Arnold, M.D.
Professor of Plastic Surgery
Mayo Clinic, Rochester, Minnesota, USA

Foreword

Occasionally a book appears which, on perusal, one knows is going to be a classic. Neven Olivari has produced such a book. Not only is he the author, he has also drawn all of the illustrations. Of course, this is a very significant thing, since there can be problems in communication between an author and the artist illustrating the procedure. This can result in the loss of essential details.

The first chapter is an eye-opener since Dr. Olivari has delved into the history of plastic surgery. Many interesting early publications are quoted. Firstly, there is an illustration of beautiful instruments produced in the early 1800s in a book by Bernard and Huette. Then comes the true history of many flaps. Illustrations show that Dieffenbach, Delpech, Burow, and Bruns were using flaps which have other peoples names attached to them today. These were described at a date much earlier than the book in which they appeared in 1857. In 1892, von Hagedorn was using a lip repair very similar to the Tennison. Szymanowski in 1865, illustrated a rhomboid flap. In 1967, Burian reduced a breast with a vertical mammaplasty.

Chapter 2, which is headed "General Techniques", is a very comprehensive review of grafts, local flaps involved in the face, regional flaps in the chest and limbs, tissue expansion. treatment of hemangioma und skin tumors. The diagrams are excellent and are accurate since, as mentioned above, these have been reproduced by Dr. Olivari himself.

Chapter 3 is a very important one on the face and neck area, this considers in detail reconstruction of soft und hard tissue, rhinoplasty, eyelid surgery, reconstructive and aesthetic procedures with face lift, blepharoplasty, brow lift, and dermabrasion being well-described and illustrated. Exophthalmos is covered very well since this is one of Dr. Olivari's specials. Lip und palate – primary and secondary –facial palsy, and ear reconstruction make up the remainder of the chapter.

Chapter 4, which deals with the chest, covers breast reconstruction, reduction, and augmentation. It is interesting that in 1906, Tansini presented his work on the latissimus dorsi flap. The applications of the TRAM flap, pedicled and free, are extensively described. Even hidradenitis suppurativa treatment is in this chapter.

Chapter 5 considers obesity surgery which has become so popular is presented in detail again with good illustrations.

In Chapter 6, extremity defects due to trauma are analyzed, and the appropriate reconstruction, either local or microvascular, is extensively described. In addition to this, all of the applicable local skin, muscle, and free flaps are presented.

Replantation is covered comprehensively.

The final chapter is on burns. The acute burn and post-burn reconstruction again receive the exposure required to be fully up-to-date at the present time.

This truly is a labor of love, written entirely and illustrated by a single surgeon who is a giant among giants, respected in his own country and in every other country he has visited. This book is, will become, and will continue to be a classic.

Originally this book was published in German but the publisher having realised that it is probably one of the best modern books on plastic and reconstructive surgery, has now brought out an English edition. Undoubtedly it will be a smash hit.

I congratulate my old friend on this superb production.

Ian T. Jackson, M.D.
DSc (Hon), FRCS, FACS, FRACS (Hon)
Institute for Craniofacial aud Reconstructive Surgery,
Southfield, Michigan, USA

Preface

This atlas is meant for young plastic surgeons in training. However it can be useful to aid experienced colleagues when they have problem cases. This book can be of use to general surgeons, traumatologists, ENT and maxillo-facial-surgeons as well as plastic surgeons This atlas differs from many other books as the author only describes the techniques that, in 40 years of practice, he has found most useful. It does not try to provide a comprehensive coverage of all methods and there are many techniques not described that are used by others, with success. The book is a very personal approach.

The principles that have guided the writing of this book are as follows. The best solution is the one which is, simple, low risk, gives a good functional and aesthetic result. All the methods shown have been proved clinically. I am sceptical of literature that has beautiful drawings but no evidence of clinical use. Each method shown in this book has clinical documentation, with illustrations and a short but hopefully clear text. Many well-known methods are intentionally omitted. For instance the v-y plasty for the correction of the lower lid ectropion, which one finds in many textbooks, does not work and is not included.

This atlas does not claim to describe all known methods. Most methods described are well established (see history chapter), and some have been rediscovered, given new names or improved.

Free micro-surgical flaps have changed our practice in the last 25 years however the free flaps is not a solution for every case. For instance, small defects on the face are best closed with local flaps which give better cosmetic results than free flaps. On the other hand the free flap can cover defects, where the traditional methods would have surely failed. Their use is sometimes life-saving. Initially there was an over enthusiastic development of microsurgery and search for new indications however more recently a balanced attitude of indication has prevailed.

This atlas is concerned with clinical practice and operative details. It has not been felt necessary to describe every possible methods of repairing the small to medium alar defects of the nose as the author is convinced that the cranially based flap from the nasolabial fold offers the best solution. Also for thoracic defects the Omentum plasty is not mentioned, because the Latissimus dorsi flap and the TRAM flap are the better and more reliable. On the other hand cross-leg flaps are mentioned, because there are still indications for their use (Not every hospital in the world has a microsurgical team). Cross-leg flaps are rarely used now but a plastic surgeon must have knowledge of the technique.

The clinical material for this book comes to a large extent from the Department for Plastic Surgery of the Dreifaltigkeits-Hospital Wesseling; a smaller part originates from my time at the University Hospital of Cologne. Dr. Richter, Dr. Eder, Dr. Noever, Dr. Stark and Dr. Niermann (all my former pupils and assistants) contributed to this book with valuable clinical cases and gave help and advice. I thank them sincerely. Plastic surgery, like any other kind of surgery, is not learned from books. One learns surgery from masters of the specialty. Why then write another book? There are plenty of good books about plastic surgery. It was a difficult decision. I had a large collection of material from my 40 years of surgical practice. After much consideration I decided that a "practical operative atlas" with minimum, but hopefully, clear text and many pictures and drawings would be most useful. Those who like involved extensive theoretical description will be disappointed. The decision to make every drawing by myself was not easy. Professional artist are very skilled but have little knowledge of surgery, (it also makes publishing more expensive). My intention was to place the drawings as close as possible to the clinical case. The reader should be able to easily visualise the solution to a problem. Why a single author for such a comprehensive book when the trend today is to have many contributors. Multiple contributors means spreading the burden and the editor's task is easier. On the other hand the individual chapters differ in style and quality. I sometimes regretted the decision to write this book alone. There was an enormous amount of material and it was not easy to select what should be included. It was hard work, as an amateur, drawing 400 illustrations and some had to be repeated 3–4 times until a satisfactory result was achieved. The moral support of my wife made an impossible task possible.

Hand surgery is not included in this atlas, except for some special cases (replantation and burn injury). This is because there are many excellent books published on this topic and I saw here no need to include a chapter on it. Special thanks go to my photographer, Miss Inge Goldberg, who for many years has taken outstanding quality photos of operations and patients. My wife Anna-Maria patiently corrected the very comprehensive material on the computer and gave me important moral support. Friends of mine, prominent plastic surgeons Mr. Brian Morgan, Mr. David Tolhurst, Mr. Antony Attwood, Mr. George Lamberty from London and Mr. Philip G. Arnold from the Mayo Clinic Rochester kindly corrected the English edition, which was not an easy task. I thank them most warmly.

Prof. Dr. med. Neven Olivari
Hoffnungsthal 2008

Content

3) Head and Neck

4) Chest and Chest Wall

5) Abdomen, Gluteal Region and Genitals

Abdomen

Gluteal Area

Genitalia

6) Skin and Soft Tissue Defects in the Extremities

The Lower Extremities

7) Surgical Therapy of Burn Injuries

CHAPTER 1
Short History of Plastic Surgery

Historical Development

The history of plastic surgery described here is used to illustrate the ingenious ideas of our ancestors rather than an exact anthology. Many of these ideas are still valid today; others, although ingenious, were forgotten and later again rediscovered, sometimes under other names. A classical example, of how long an ingenious method can take to be accepted by medical opinion is the "Indian Method" for reconstruction of the nose. Susruta described reconstruction of nose from the forehead 600 years B.C. More than 2000 years passed, until this method reached Europe not by medical profession, but by Mr. Urban, the publisher of the "Gentlemen's Magazine". 1794 he described this method, which was observed by two English surgeons in Bombay. It was not for a further 22 years (1816) that the English surgeon Joseph Carpue successfully performed this operation on two patients. Another example demonstrates the difficulties of discoverers of new techniques. Tagliacozzi (1597) published his book "De Curtorum Chirurgia per Insitionem" in which he described reconstruction of nose from upper arm. With this book the era of the modern plastic surgery began and one would have expected it to have caused a revolution in surgery. Far from it! First the church condemned Tagliacozzi because he interfered with the works of God. Then having been forgotten for 200 years he was ridiculed by the European medical "elite" for in 1751 Diderot published his "Enzyclopedie". One of the co-editors was the great Voltaire. He remarked that according to Tagliacozzi: "A nose is reconstructed best, if one takes skin from the hip of a slave".

In 1760 the Faculté de Medicine of Paris rejected Tagliacozzi's method. Today this sounds improbably. 163 years had nevertheless passed since the publication of Tagliacozzi. In the 15th century the Branca family from Sicily used the Indian Method of nose reconstruction, but kept it jealously secret as was the custom of that time. They did not write about it and so they remained free from pursuit by the clerics. Vesalius, in 1543, published "Fabrica", a very modern anatomical study. This should have encouraged the development of the surgery. But it was not until much later, at the beginning 19th century that surgery, including plastic surgery, made great advances.

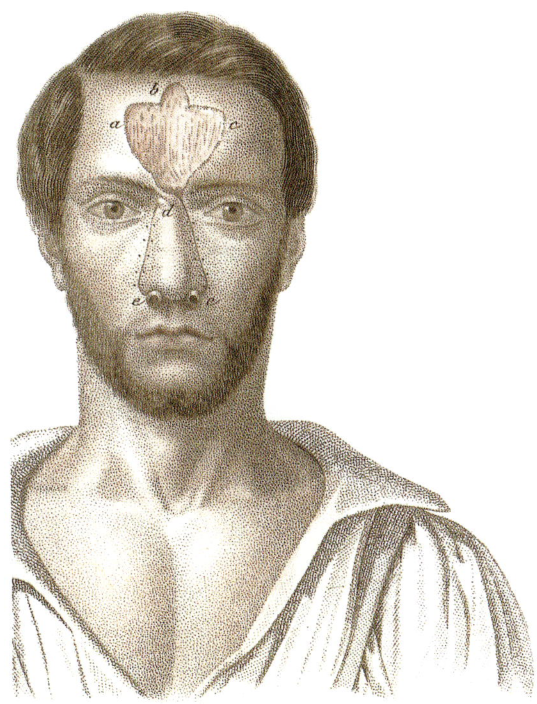

Figure 1.1 Nose reconstruction. The oldest plastic-surgical operation probably comes from Susruta Samhita (approx. 600 years B.C.). He developed the "Indian Method" of nose reconstruction using skin from the forehead. This method is still today one of best choices for covering larger nose defects.

GRAEFE, a professor of surgery in Berlin and the Prussian military surgeon general at the time of the Napoleonic war (1813–1815), performed nose reconstructions by TAGLIACOZZI's method and also used the Indian method. It was published in the book "Rhinoplastik" (1818), a very good book about plastic surgery and the first time the term "plastics" was used. It was thus 220 years after TAGLIACOZZI that with GRAEFE's publication Europe and the USA began the modern development of plastic surgery.

Delpech (1823) published his work: "Surgery clinique de Montpellier aux observations et reflection travaux de Chirurgie de cette école". He described a detailed nose and lip reconstruction by TAGLIACOZZI's method.

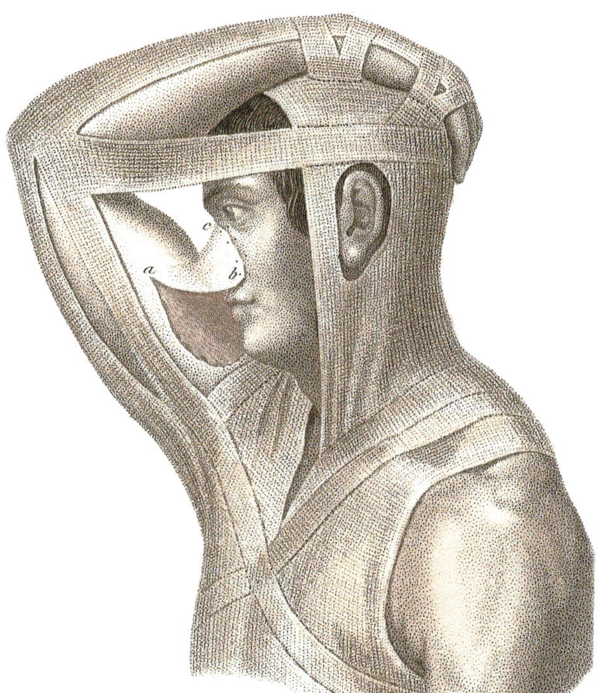

Figure 1.2 1597 the method of the nose reconstruction from the upper arm published by Tagliacozzi in his classic work "De Curtorum Chirurgia per Insitionem" was a milestone in plastic surgery. Tagliacozzi was forgotten for nearly 200 years.

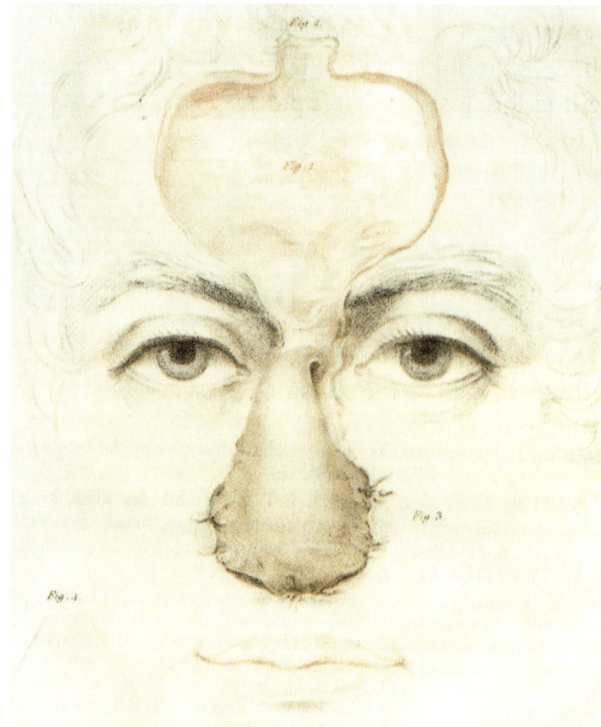

Figure 1.3 First reconstruction of nose by "Indian Method" in Europe (Carpue J.C.: An account of two successful operation for restoring a lost nose from integuments of the forehead, in the cases of two officers of his Majesty's army. London, Longman 1816).

DIEFFENBACH (1829), who succeeded GRAEFE in Berlin, was the first, to accomplish nose reconstruction as a routine with Indian and TAGLIACOZZI methods. In his monumental work "Die operative Chirurgie", Brockhaus, Leipzig (1845). He described clearly nose reconstruction, cleft lip and palate repair and many other operations.

His influence on the development of the plastic surgery was enormous. DIEFFENBACH described in detail, how second and third operations can improve the nose both aesthetically and functionally. His lower lip reconstruction is a classic. DIEFFENBACH wrote and published "Surgical experiences, particularly for the reconstruction of destroyed parts of human body with new methods". Enslin, Berlin (1829).

DUPUYTREN (1834) became known for his description and operation for "Palmar fibromatosis", which was later called DUPUYTREN's disease. But it was DUPUYTREN who first classified burns by their depth.

LANGENBECK (1810–1887) succeeded DIEFFENBACH in Berlin. He was the first to describe the

Transposition flap for lower lip defects, which he called "Cheiloplastik". He also developed new method for closure of cleft palate "Uranoplastik".

In 1838 ZEIS published the "Handbuch der plastischen Chirurgie" (manual of plastic surgery). A book that had world wide recognition. He described in detail all the plastic surgery procedures available at that time.

BRUNS (1857) published a large sized surgical atlas with excellent drawing of a nose reconstruction, cleft lip reconstruction, closure of cleft palate as well as different methods for closure of cheek defects. Many of these methods are still in use today. This atlas is a wonderful source of ideas for reconstructions.

John WOOD (1862) described the inguinal flap for covering defects of hand. This was the first axial pattern flap. The flap was rediscovered by SHAW and PAYNE as the "groin flap" in 1946. WOOD however proposed that a skin flap should have a relationship of length to width no more than 1 : 1. This rule however was harmful as it stopped the development of longer flaps for quite some time.

REVERDIN (1869) excised small pieces of skin and successfully fixed them on to a granulating surface. This was the first skin graft. THIERSCH (1874) took a larger layer of thin skin with the razor and grafted it successfully. This was a milestone for the ability to cover large skin defects. WOLF (1876) described full thickness skin for the correction of the ectropion of lower eyelid (Wolf, J.R.: "A new method of performing plastics operation". Med. Times and Gazette 1: 608, 1876).

BORGES (1904) described first Z-plasties [Borges, P. "Autoplastic pour dedoublement et echange lambeaux". Surgery Orthopedique, Paris 1904].

TANSINI (1906) was a professor of surgery in Pavia and described in 1906 a new method for covering thoracic defects after mastectomy. He used skin and latissimus dorsi muscle so it was the first myo-cutaneus flap. Unfortunately this ingenious method was overtaken by the radical Halsted mastectomy and forgotten for more than 60 years. None of the important papers of this time [Esser 1918, Lexer 1920,

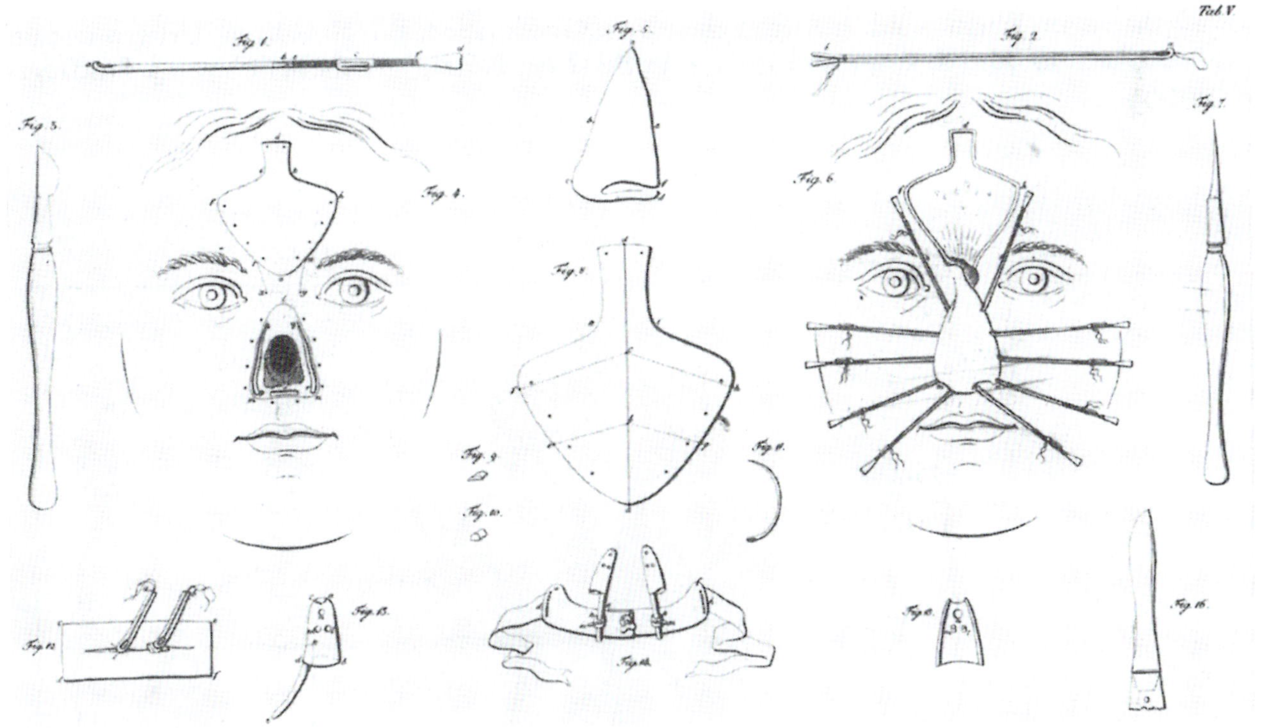

Figure 1.4 Graefe, C.F. (von): "Rhinoplasty or the art of replacing a defect of the nose by a new procedure, investigation and perfection of the technique" (1818) accurately described the "Indian method".

Gillies 1924, Morestin 1914, Filatow 1922, Kilner 1928, McIndoe 1941, Joseph 1931, Sanvenero Rosselli 1935, McGregor 1957, Limberg 1946, Converse 1964, Millard 1970, a.o.] mentioned the Tansini method.

70 years later in 1975 Olivari reported at the Winter meeting of BAPS in the Royal College of Surgeons, London, the "The Latissimus Dorsi Flap in Repair of Thoracic Defects". In January 1976 "The Latissimus Flap" was published in *British Journal of Plastic Surgery*. I had no knowledge of Tansini, his work and publication (see pages 474–475). Since then this flap has found substantial applications. The Latissimus flap as pedicle, island or free flap is one of most frequently used flap.

The First World War and the post war period was the birth time of modern plastic surgery. Many famous plastic surgeons exerted a crucial influence on development of the modern plastic surgery. There was Gilles and McIndoe in England, Morestin in France, Lexer, Ganzer and Lindemann in Germany, Esser in Holland, Pichler in Austria, Sanvenero Rosselli in Italy and many more. Morestin who was a very talented surgeon described multiple Z-plasty (1914). His contribution on the design of pedicle flaps was extremely important. He showed that skin and subcutaneous tissue can be undermined for a long distance without causing necrosis. Filatov and Gillies independently developed the tube pedicle (1917).

Filatov, V.P.: Plastie a tige ronde. Vestnik Ophtal. No. 5 (1917): This flap was very popular and useful for decades. Filatov and Gillies had no knowledge of Tansini. May be, if they had, the tube pedicle would not have achieved such importance for so long time and plastic surgery would have developed in a different way.

Esser (1918) gave the theoretical basis for the further development of flaps. He rejected the principle of length width in the ratio 1 : 1 and developed what he called the "biological flap". Esser said "A biological flap is the skin flap which contains subcutaneous tissue and muscles, which as a whole belongs to supplying area of a certain artery and its branches and which is drained by the associated vein system and lymph system."

This was the birth of axial pattern flaps. He continued to write also: "these flaps do not need to contain skin to survive." The island flap was born, long time before published by Littler (1953) and Moberg (1955).

Martin Kirschner (1920) published the island pedicled flap. The pedicle of the superficial temporal artery had no covering of skin; "skin free pedicle". Neither Esser nor Kirschner, knew about Tansini's work.

Blair developed "The delayed transfer of long pedical flaps in plastics surgery" (1921). He also developed a dermatome for the harvest of larger split skin grafts. Carl Nylen introduced the operating microscope in ENT surgery in 1921. For the first time a microscope was used for operations. In 1931 Erich Lexer wrote a book, "Complete reconstructive surgery", which was for many years an enormous help for plastic surgeons. Jacques Joseph published his book "Rhinoplasty and other plasties of the face

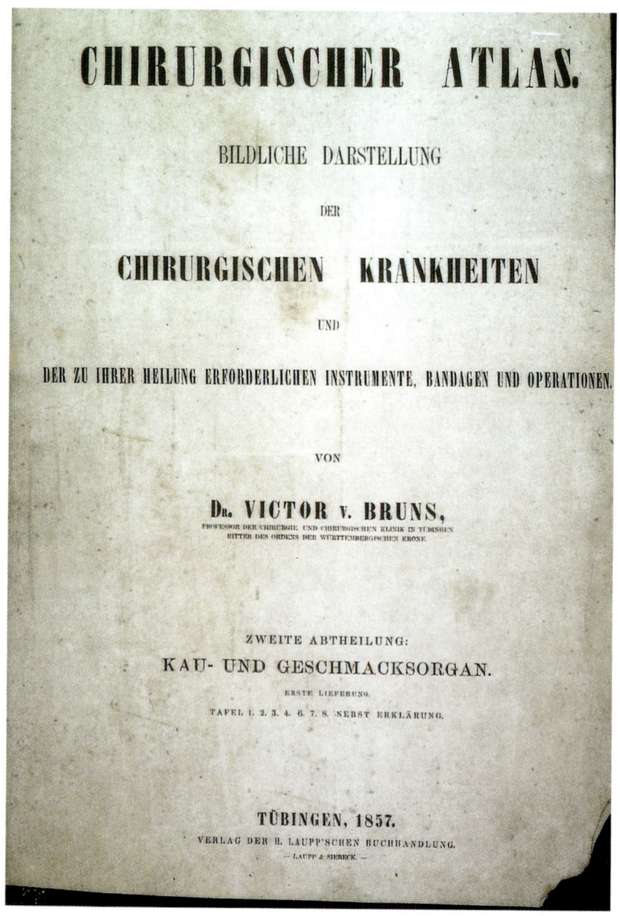
CHIRURGISCHER ATLAS.

BILDLICHE DARSTELLUNG

DER

CHIRURGISCHEN KRANKHEITEN

UND

DER ZU IHRER HEILUNG ERFORDERLICHEN INSTRUMENTE, BANDAGEN UND OPERATIONEN.

VON

Dr. VICTOR v. BRUNS,

PROFESSOR DER CHIRURGIE UND CHIRURGISCHEN KLINIK IN TÜBINGEN

RITTER DES ORDENS DER WÜRTTEMBERGISCHEN KRONE

ZWEITE ABTHEILUNG:

KAU- UND GESCHMACKSORGAN.

ERSTE LIEFERUNG.

TAFEL 1. 2. 3. 4. 6. 7. 8. NEBST ERKLÄRUNG.

TÜBINGEN, 1857.

VERLAG DER H. LAUPP'SCHEN BUCHHANDLUNG.

— LAUPP & SIEBECK. —

Figure 1.5 Bruns, V.: Surgical Atlas (Chirurgischer Atlas). Tübingen 1857 (size 50 × 35 cm)

together with mammaplasty" in 1931. This extensive book helped to the spreading the art plastic surgery is still valuable today particularly for rhinoplasty.

Joseph improved the intranasal approach for the correction of the nose. He is a really the father of modern rhinoplasty. His young colleague, Aufricht, left Germany in 1934 and remained for the rest of his life in New York, where he greatly influence the development of surgery for the nose in USA.

Manchot (1889) from Leipzig described: "Skin arteries of the human body". Unfortunately generations of surgeons did not read his work. Salmon (1936) published a book on skin arteries "Les Arteries de la peau"; perfect a work, which is still valid today. This excellent book was also completely forgotten for decades. Both books were used in the seventies and eighties as sources for the development of axial pattern flaps. In 1939 Padgett developed the drum dermatome which took somewhat thicker split skin grafts but need glue to attach the instrument to the donor area. Despite the spread of plastic surgery there was little development from 1940 to 1960 and the tube pedicle of Filatov and Gillies remained an important method of reconstruction. Jacobson and Suarez (1960) experimented with micro-surgical techniques using the binocular microscope and they achieved 100 percent success with 26 arterial anastomoses in rats.

Tessier 1967 presented a new concept of cranio-facial surgery for dealing with gross cranio-facial deformities. Janzekovic's 1968 developed a new therapy for burns. She developed tangential excision of the burned skin in the first three to five days after the burn injury and covered excised surface immediately with split skin grafts. Janzekovic technique made a dramatic improvement in the treatment of the burn injury.

A new era in plastic surgery was introduced by microsurgery. Following Jacobson and Suarez (1960) successes with micro-anastomosis on rats, Cobbet performed the first microsurgical transplantation in humans using the big toe for reconstruction of the thumb. In 1972 Ackland, Buncke and McLean due to their extensive experimental laboratory work created the basis for the rapidly development of microsurgery.

1972 saw the first free flap. Daniel and Taylor developed the free "groin flap". The first free Dorsalis pedis flaps were performed in 1975. In the same year Taylor introduced the free fibula transfer. In 1976 the *Latissimus dorsi myocutaneus flap* was rediscovered by Olivari. Godina presented the first free latissimus dorsi flaps in 1978. Godina showed with many cases that primary closure of defects of lower leg using free flaps (mostly latissimus dorsi flaps) gave substantially better results than could be obtained with secondary cover. The infection rate was dramatically reduced, the therapy time shortened and the functional results improved. In 1978 Nahai presented the tensor fascia lata flap.

Mantkelov published the gracilis flap in 1979 and Aryan the pectoralis flap. The Scapular flap was described by Santo in 1980 and in 1982 the forearm flap came from Chang in China, with an immediate wide application. In 1983 Shaw described the free

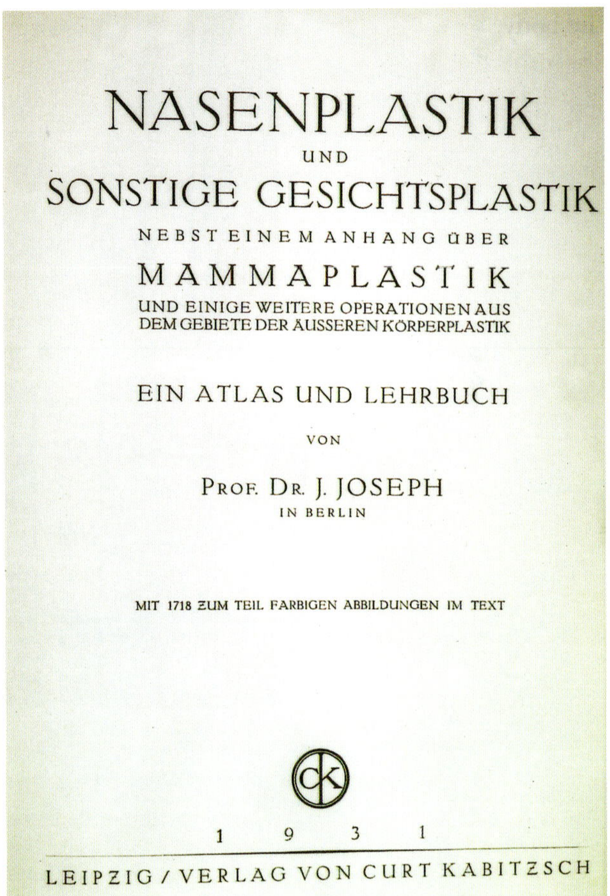
NASENPLASTIK

UND

SONSTIGE GESICHTSPLASTIK

NEBST EINEM ANHANG ÜBER

MAMMAPLASTIK

UND EINIGE WEITERE OPERATIONEN AUS DEM GEBIETE DER AUSSEREN KÖRPERPLASTIK

EIN ATLAS UND LEHRBUCH

VON

PROF. DR. J. JOSEPH

IN BERLIN

MIT 1718 ZUM TEIL FARBIGEN ABBILDUNGEN IM TEXT

1931

LEIPZIG / VERLAG VON CURT KABITZSCH

Figure 1.6 Joseph, J.: Rhinoplasty and other face plasties together with an appendix on mammaplasties. Published [in German] by Curt Kabitzsch, Leipzig (1931).

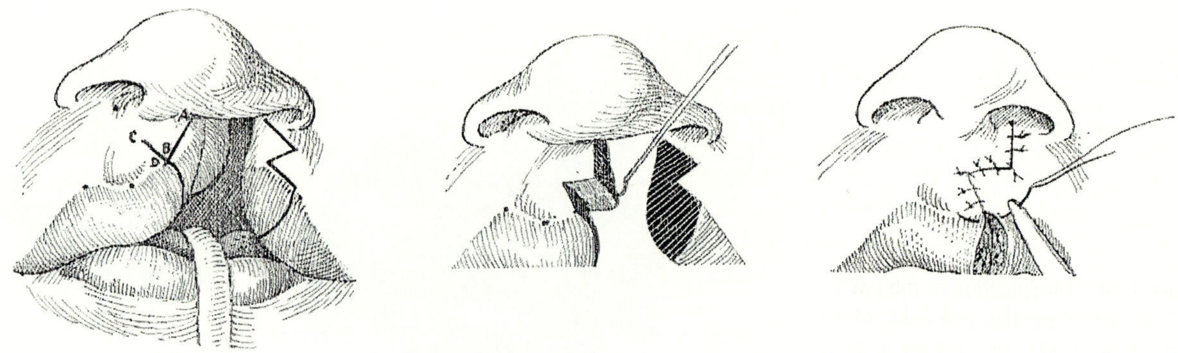

Figure 1.27 Tennison, C.W.: The repair of unilateral cleft lip by stencil method. Plast. Reconstr. Surg. 9: 115 (1952). From the author's point of view the Tennison method is still today the best operation for cleft lip. Tennison's method in fact is an improvement on the operative method of Hagedorn and Le Mesurier.

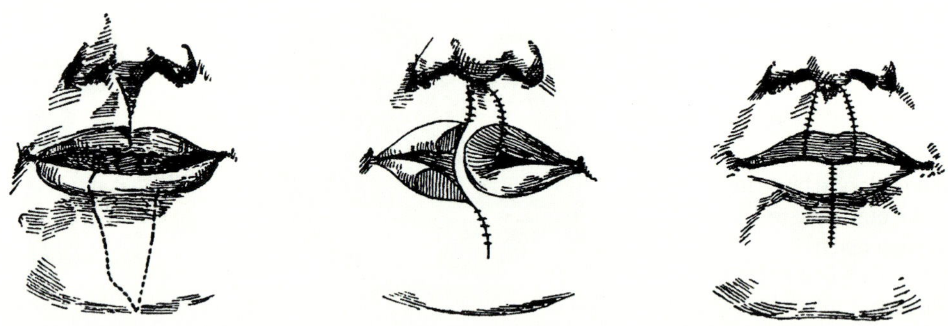

Figure 1.28 Plastic operation for correction of cleft upper lip deformity after Abbe. From: Medical Record (1898). The Abbe-Plasty is still as up-to-date as in 1898.

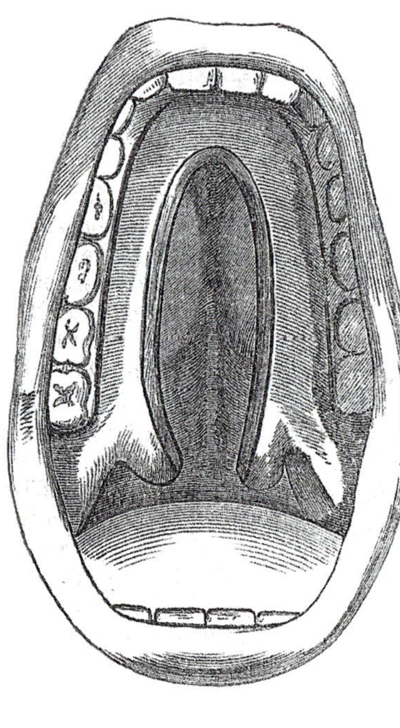

Figure 1.29 Closure of the palate after Langenbeck, which was called "Uranoplastik" by him. Langenbeck: "The uranoplasty by mobilization of the mucosa-s periostal palate flaps ". Archiv f. Klin. Chir. (1861). A typical double bridge-flap plasty.

together with mammaplasty" in 1931. This extensive book helped to the spreading the art plastic surgery is still valuable today particularly for rhinoplasty.

Joseph improved the intranasal approach for the correction of the nose. He is a really the father of modern rhinoplasty. His young colleague, Aufricht, left Germany in 1934 and remained for the rest of his life in New York, where he greatly influence the development of surgery for the nose in USA.

Manchot (1889) from Leipzig described: "Skin arteries of the human body". Unfortunately generations of surgeons did not read his work. Salmon (1936) published a book on skin arteries "Les Arteries de la peau"; perfect a work, which is still valid today. This excellent book was also completely forgotten for decades. Both books were used in the seventies and eighties as sources for the development of axial pattern flaps. In 1939 Padgett developed the drum dermatome which took somewhat thicker split skin grafts but need glue to attach the instrument to the donor area. Despite the spread of plastic surgery there was little development from 1940 to 1960 and the tube pedicle of Filatov and Gillies remained an important method of reconstruction. Jacobson and Suarez (1960) experimented with micro-surgical techniques using the binocular microscope and they achieved 100 percent success with 26 arterial anastomoses in rats.

Tessier 1967 presented a new concept of cranio-facial surgery for dealing with gross cranio-facial deformities. Janzekovic's 1968 developed a new therapy for burns. She developed tangential excision of the burned skin in the first three to five days after the burn injury and covered excised surface immediately with split skin grafts. Janzekovic technique made a dramatic improvement in the treatment of the burn injury.

A new era in plastic surgery was introduced by microsurgery. Following Jacobson and Suarez (1960) successes with micro-anastomosis on rats, Cobbet performed the first microsurgical transplantation in humans using the big toe for reconstruction of the thumb. In 1972 Ackland, Buncke and McLean due to their extensive experimental laboratory work created the basis for the rapidly development of microsurgery.

1972 saw the first free flap. Daniel and Taylor developed the free "groin flap". The first free Dorsalis pedis flaps were performed in 1975. In the same year Taylor introduced the free fibula transfer. In 1976 the *Latissimus dorsi myocutaneus flap* was rediscovered by Olivari. Godina presented the first free latissimus dorsi flaps in 1978. Godina showed with many cases that primary closure of defects of lower leg using free flaps (mostly latissimus dorsi flaps) gave substantially better results than could be obtained with secondary cover. The infection rate was dramatically reduced, the therapy time shortened and the functional results improved. In 1978 Nahai presented the tensor fascia lata flap.

Mantkelov published the gracilis flap in 1979 and Aryan the pectoralis flap. The Scapular flap was described by Santo in 1980 and in 1982 the forearm flap came from Chang in China, with an immediate wide application. In 1983 Shaw described the free

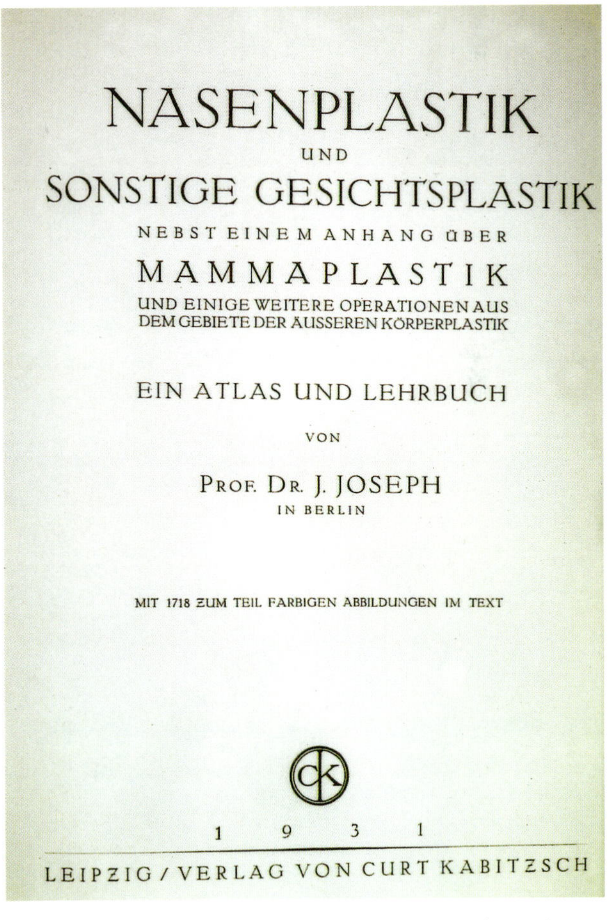
NASENPLASTIK
UND
SONSTIGE GESICHTSPLASTIK
NEBST EINEM ANHANG ÜBER
MAMMAPLASTIK
UND EINIGE WEITERE OPERATIONEN AUS DEM GEBIETE DER AUSSEREN KÖRPERPLASTIK

EIN ATLAS UND LEHRBUCH
VON
PROF. DR. J. JOSEPH
IN BERLIN

MIT 1718 ZUM TEIL FARBIGEN ABBILDUNGEN IM TEXT

1 9 3 1
LEIPZIG / VERLAG VON CURT KABITZSCH

Figure 1.6 Joseph, J.: Rhinoplasty and other face plasties together with an appendix on mammaplasties. Published [in German] by Curt Kabitzsch, Leipzig (1931).

gluteal flap for breast reconstruction. Matlaub presented the lateral upper arm flap in 1984. The development of microsurgery in Germany (1977) was the responsibility of Biemer, Duspiva and Brüser. The development of the microsurgery made it possible to close nearly every defect with free flaps. Microsurgical reconstruction is today routine and important part of plastic surgery. There are a vast number of free flaps described. At the time of writing the most frequently used free flaps are: Latissimus dorsi flap, forearm (radialis) flap, scapular flap, upper arm flap etc.

Since the rediscovery of the Latissimus dorsi flap in 1976 a large number of myocutaneous flaps have been described. Nahai, McGraw and P.G. Arnold systematically described the myocutaneous flaps 1978.

Radovan developed the expander in 1982 primarily for breast reconstruction, but after short time the indication was successfully extended to other parts of the body.

A new method for the breast reduction was developed by Strömbeck in 1960 and this made operation easier and safer. One of most important contribution in modern plastic surgery was made by Holmström "The free abdominoplasty flap and its use for breast reconstruction" [Scand. J. Plast. Reconstr. Surg. 13: 423–432 (1979)]. It was in reality the first free TRAM flap and three years before Hartrampf and Sheflan (1982) described the less reliable unilateral pedicled TRAM flap for the breast reconstruction. There is no doubt today that Holmström's free TRAM is superior to the pedicled TRAM of Carl Hartrampf, but Hartrampf popularized his flap. Pennington also used the free TRAM (1980) two years before Hartrampf [Pennington D.G. „The rectus abdominis myocutaneous free flap". Br. J. Plast. Surg. 33: 277 (1980)]. Thus breast reconstruction with the bodies own tissue become possible. Holmström and Pennington published their work in Europe, so in the USA, the TRAM is called even today the Hartrampf flap. Koshima (1989) developed the free TRAM flap, avoiding the use of rectus abdominis muscle (DIAP flap).

Suture Techniques and Instruments

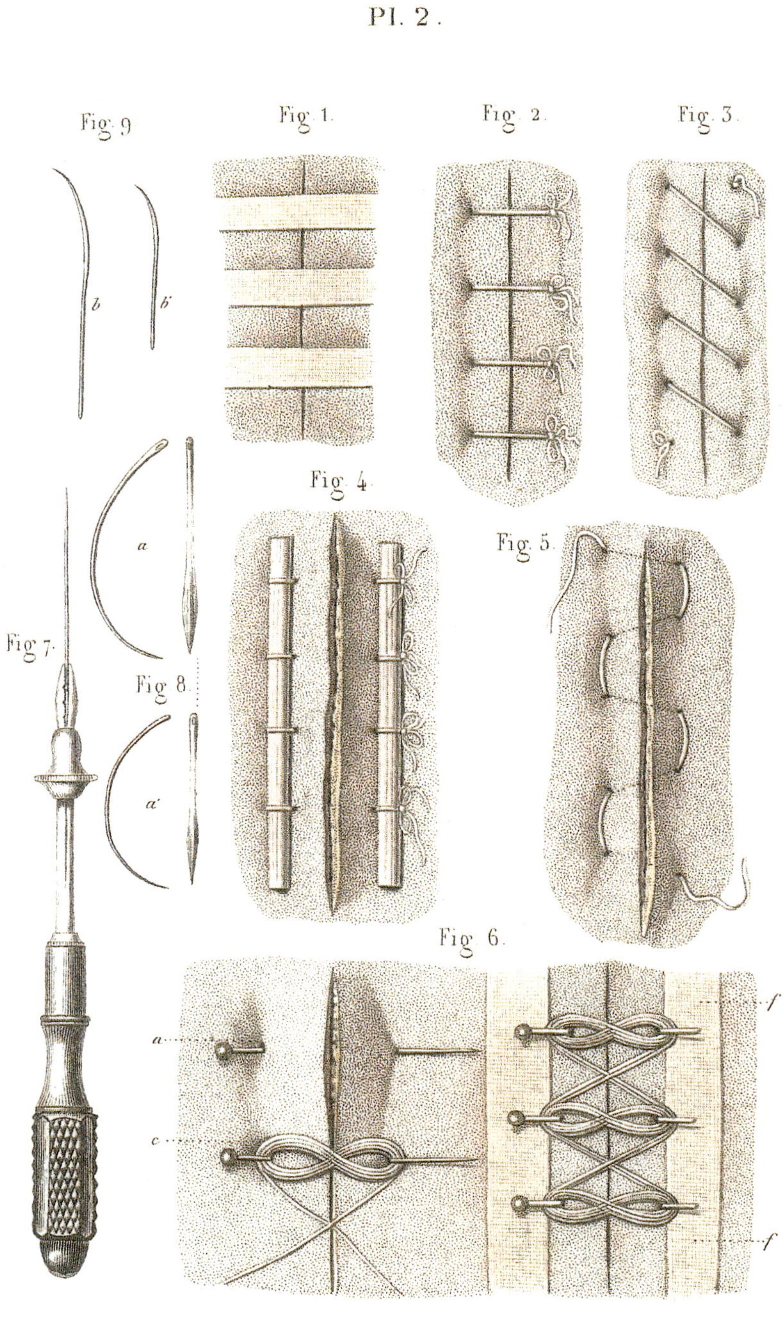

Figure 1.7 Different suture techniques. Bernard, Cl., Huette, Ch.: "Precis Iconographique de Medicine Operatoire et d'Anatomie Chirurgicale". Mequignon Marvis Fils, Paris (1848). Fig. 1 is interesting, as it shows that the wound can be approximated with tapes, rather like "steri strips". The sutures in Fig. 2.3 and Fig. 5 are also still used today.

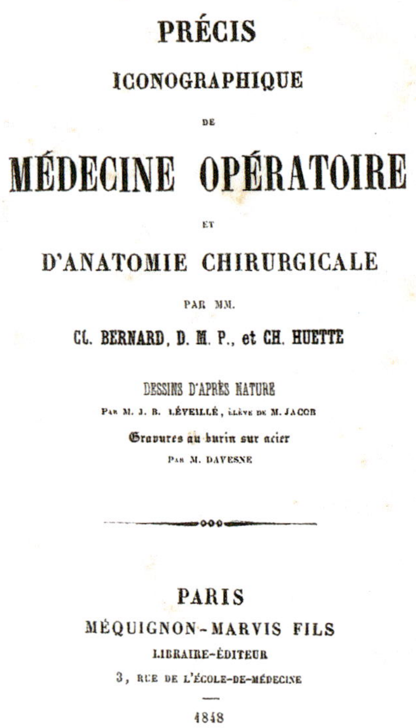

PRÉCIS

ICONOGRAPHIQUE

DE

MÉDECINE OPÉRATOIRE

ET

D'ANATOMIE CHIRURGICALE

PAR MM.

CL. BERNARD, D. M. P., et CH. HUETTE

DESSINS D'APRÈS NATURE

PAR M. J. B. LÉVEILLÉ, ÉLÈVE DE M. JACOB

Gravures au burin sur acier

PAR M. DAVESNE

PARIS

MÉQUIGNON-MARVIS FILS

LIBRAIRE-ÉDITEUR

3, RUE DE L'ÉCOLE-DE-MÉDECINE

1848

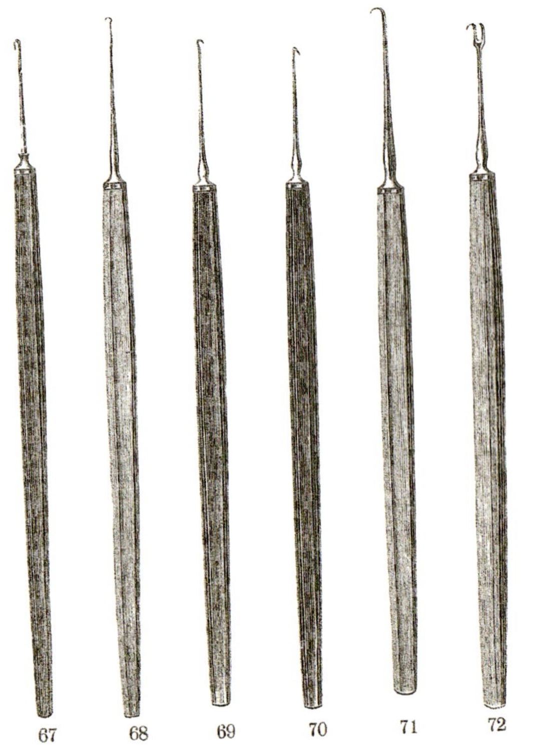

Figure 1.8c Different hooks from Haab, O.: "Operationslehre" (1904). Nearly identical to those in the book of Bernard and Huette.

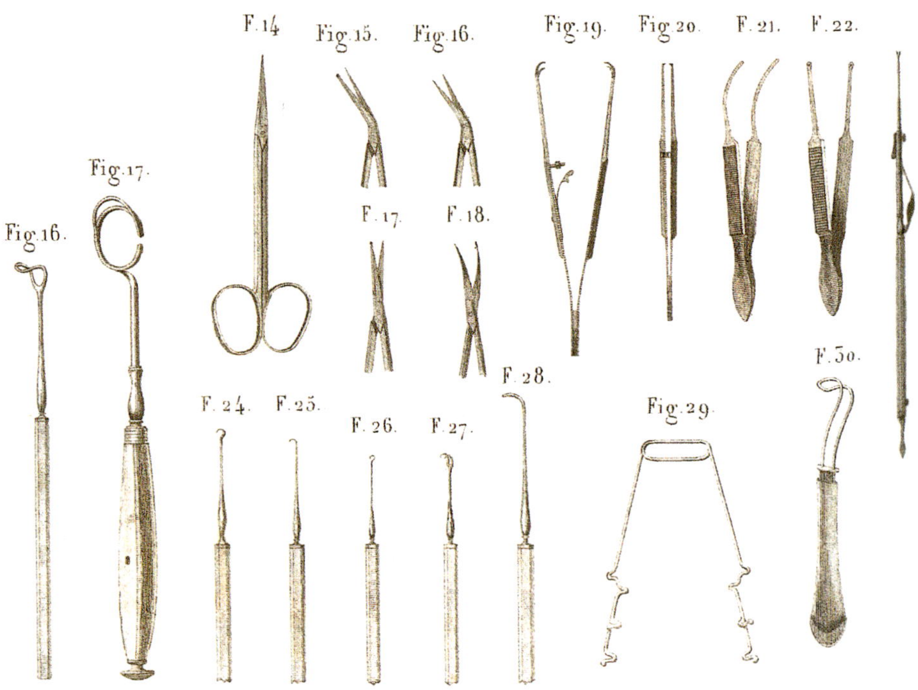

Figure 1.8 a,b Some of these instruments appear later under other names for instance, the a hook Fig. 26 (at the time Beer's hook) or the instruments Figs. 16, 24, 25,15. (Original pictures from Bernard and Huette: "Precis Iconographique de Medicine Operatoire et d'Anatomie Chirurgicale". Mequignon Marvis Fils, Paris 1848)

Historical Operations and Techniques

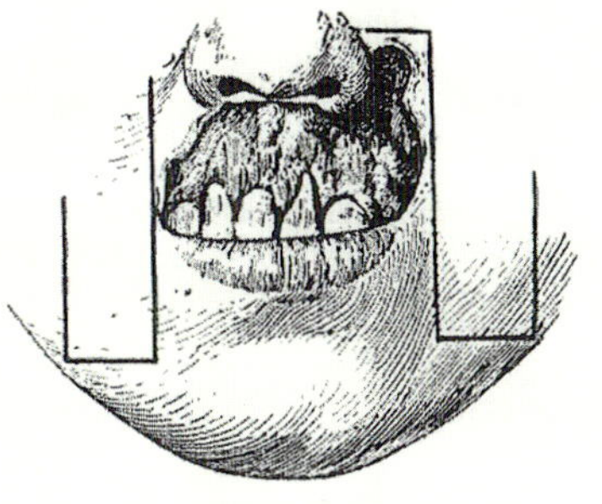

Figure 1.9a "Buccal method" for reconstruction of upper lip (Sédillot 1846)

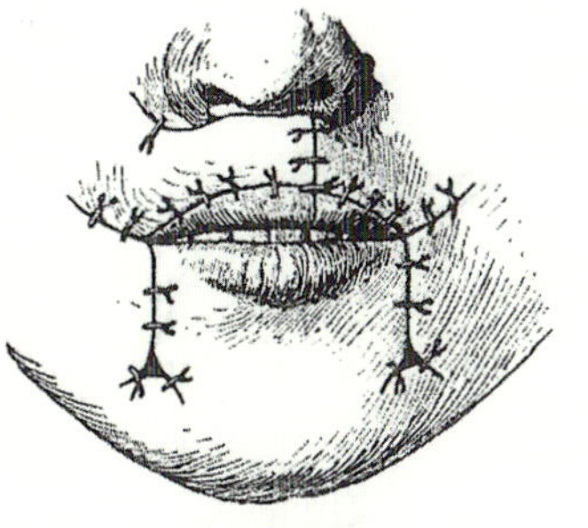

Figure 1.9b Sédillot "Traite de medicine operatoire". P. 650 (1846).

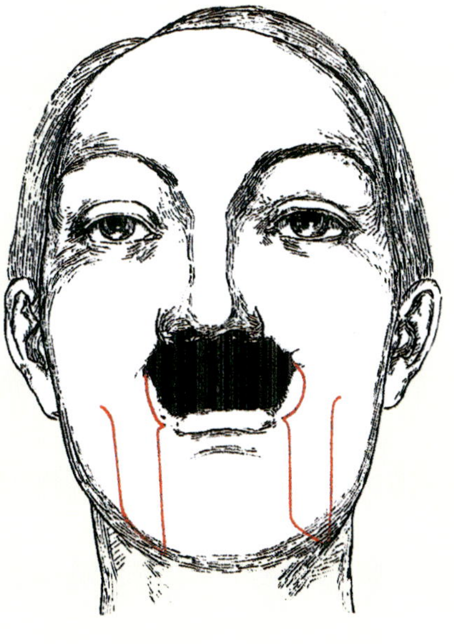

Figure 1.10a Total lip replacement after Joseph (buccal method of upper lip plasty). Published in Joseph, J.: „Nasenplastik und sonstige Gesichtplastik nebst einen Anhang über Mammaplastik" (1931) [cf. Figure 1.6]

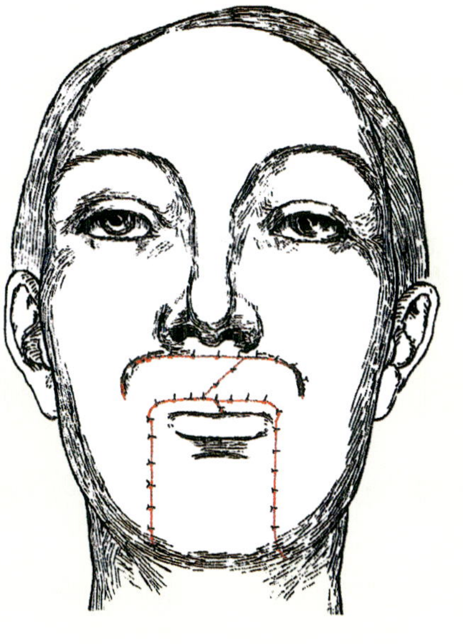

Figure 1.10b One can see Joseph was influenced by Sédillot, 83 years later.

Reconstruction of the Upper Lip after Joseph and Senn

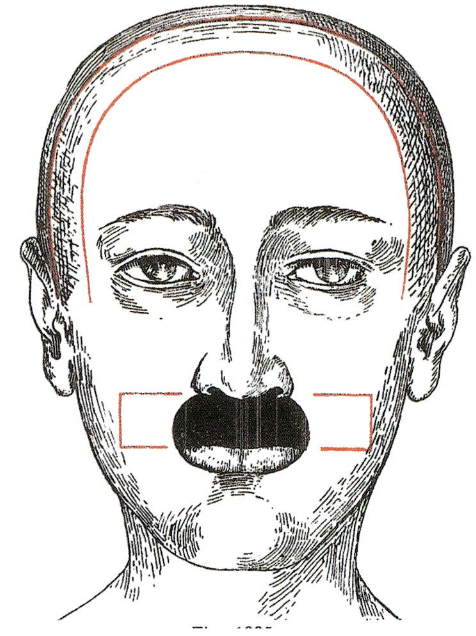

Figure 1.11a Two cheek medical pedicled flaps for the inner lining

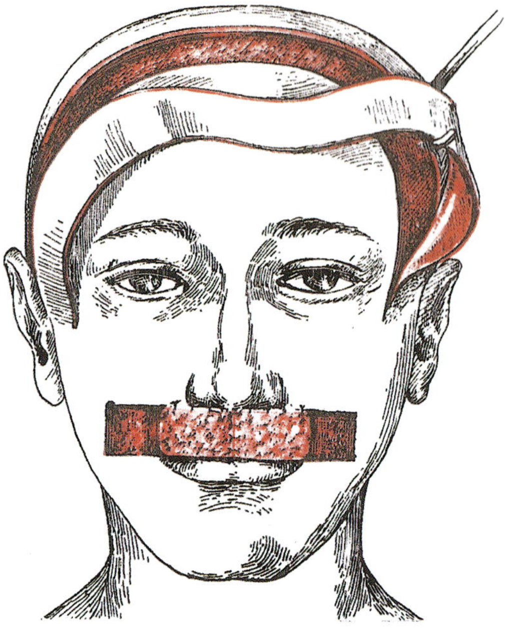

Figure 1.11b The bridge flap were vascularized bilateral by the A. temporalis superficialis.

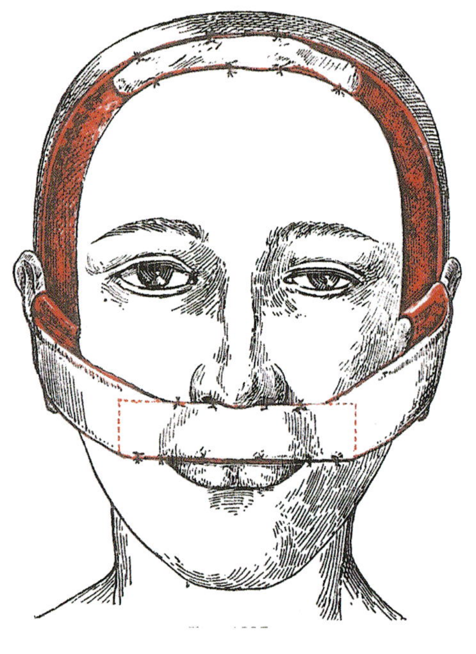

Figure 1.11c Upper lip reconstruction by a bridge head skin flap and small cheek flaps after Senn and Joseph.

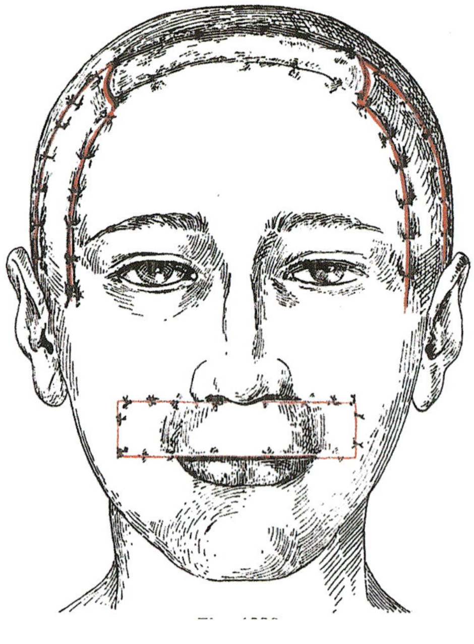

Figure 1.11d Published in: Joseph, J.: "Nasenplastik und sonstige Gesichtplastik nebst einen Anhang über Mammaplastik (1931)." [cf. Figure 1.6]

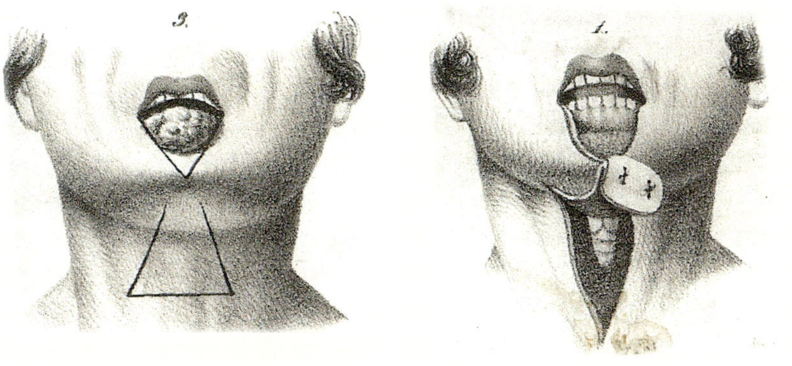

Figure 1.12 "Organic replacement of the lower lip by neck skin". Delpech: Chirurgie clinique de Montpellier aux observations et reflexions des traveaux de chirurgie de cette ecole (1823). It is an interesting two-layer reconstruction of lower lip. Published in: Bruns' Chirurgischer Atlas (1857).

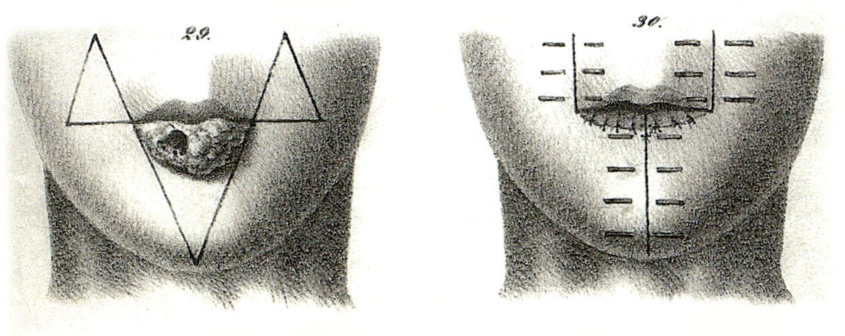

Figure 1.13 Burow: Replacement of lower lip. Published in: Bruns' Chirurgischer Atlas (1857). This method is still useful today. Here the tongue is used for the reconstruction of mucosa of the lip.

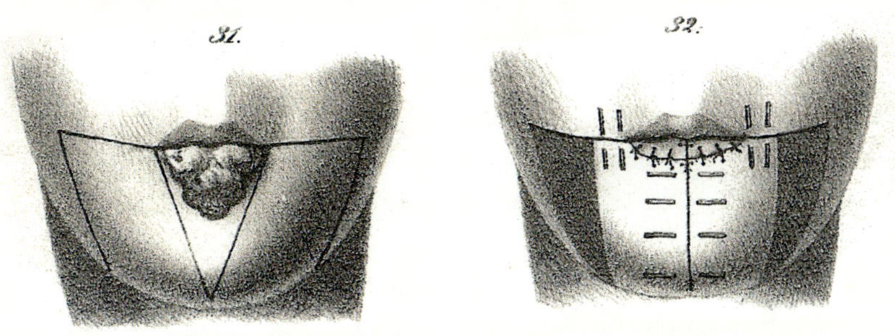

Figure 1.14 Dieffenbach: Replacement of the lower lip by sliding bilateral flaps. Operative Chirurgie, Volume 1: 419 (1836). Published in: Bruns' Chirurgischer Atlas (1857).

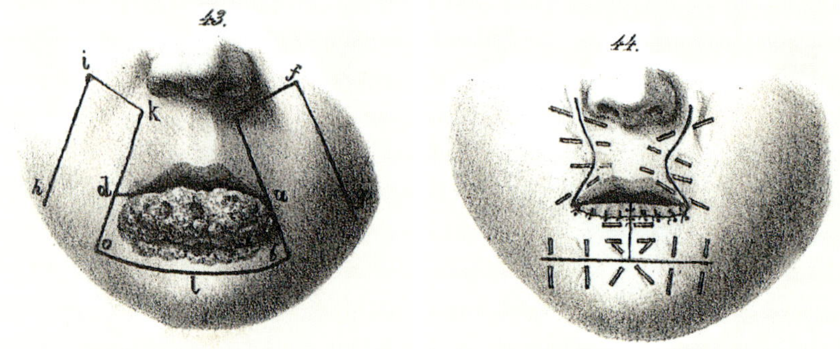

Figure 1.15 Bruns: Lower lip reconstruction with two caudallly pedicled cheek flaps (1834). Published in: Bruns' Chirurgischer Atlas (1857).

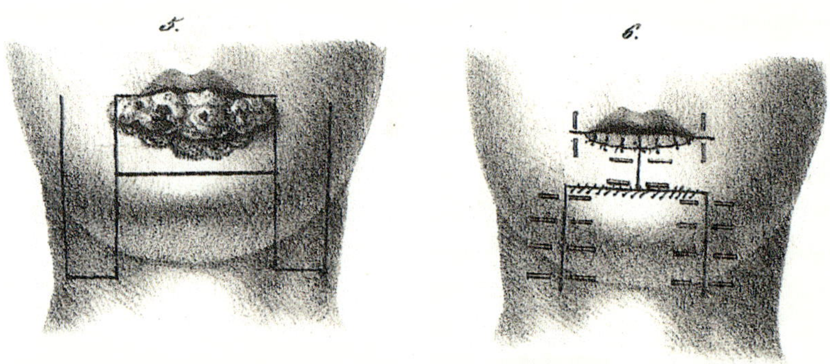

Figure 1.16 Sédillot: "Traite de medicine operatoire" (1846). From Bruns' Chirurgischer Atlas (1857). Sédillot elegantly used two cranial pedicled flaps from the cheek to reconstruct the lower lip.

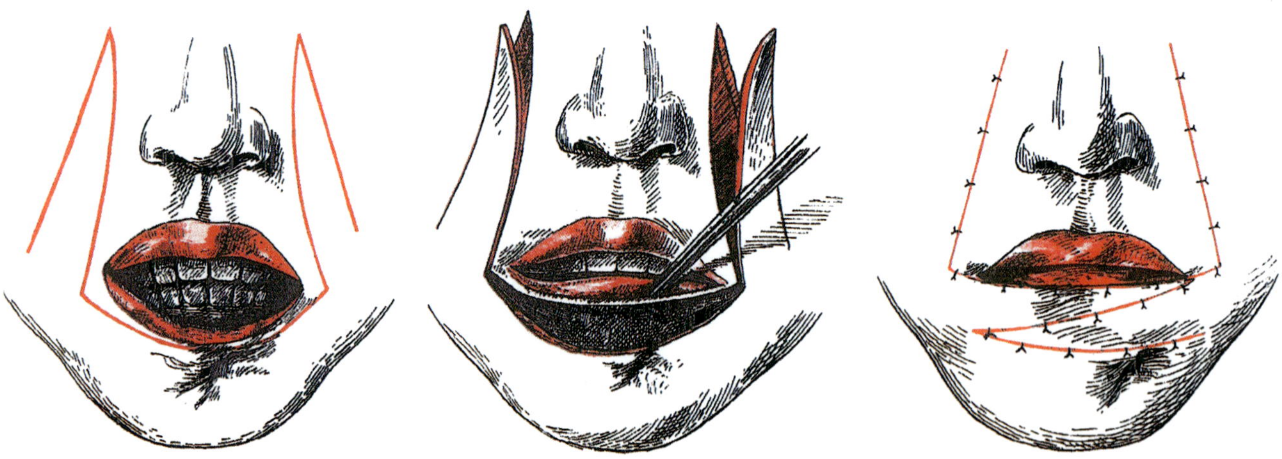

Figure 1.17 Lower lip reconstruction after Bruns, modified by Joseph. Published in: Joseph, J.: Nasenplastik und sonstige Gesichtsplastik nebst einen Anhang über Mammaplastik (1931). [cf. Figure 1.6]

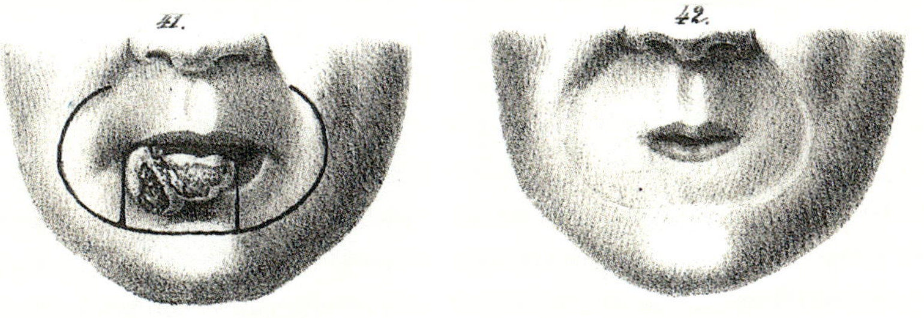

Figure 1.18 Bruns: Reconstruction of lower lip with rotations flaps from cranial. Published in: Bruns' Chirurgischer Atlas (1857). An excellent idea of Bruns. A microstoma is however possible.

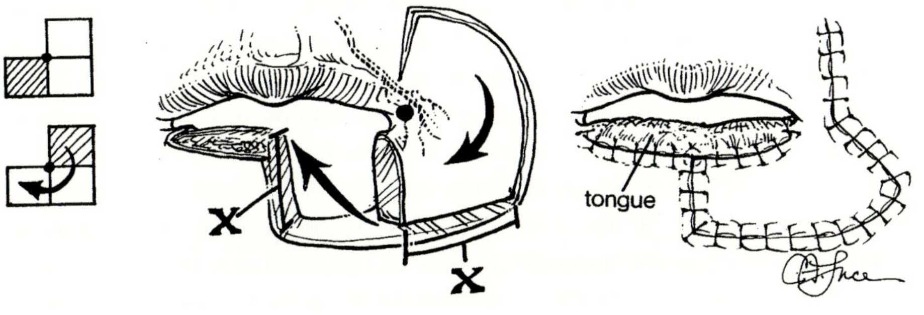

Figure 1.19 McGregor, I.A.: The tongue flaps in lip surgery. Br. J. Plast. Surg. 19: 252 (1966). McGregor made an elegantly twisting of the flap by preserving the vascularization. The mucosa is reconstructed from the tongue.

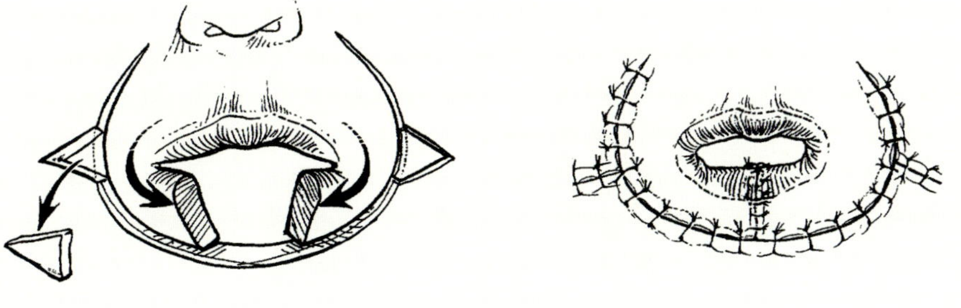

Figure 1.20 Karapandzic, M.: Reconstruction of lip defects by local rotation arterial flaps. Br. J. Plast. Surg. 27: 93 (1974). The similarity with the method of Bruns cannot be denied. There is a possibility of a microstoma by Karapandzic, as well. Through this method vascularization of the lip is preserved like in McGregor's method.

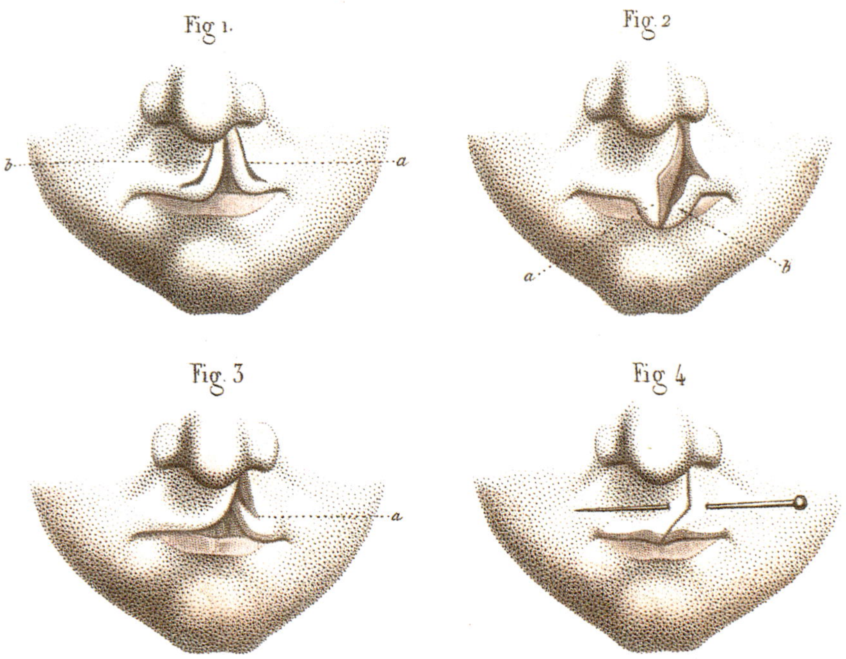

Figure 1.21 Malgaigne, M., d'Angers, M.: Operation du bec de lievre. In: Medicine operatoire (1848). Malgaigne achieved by intelligent incision an lengthening of the cleft lip.

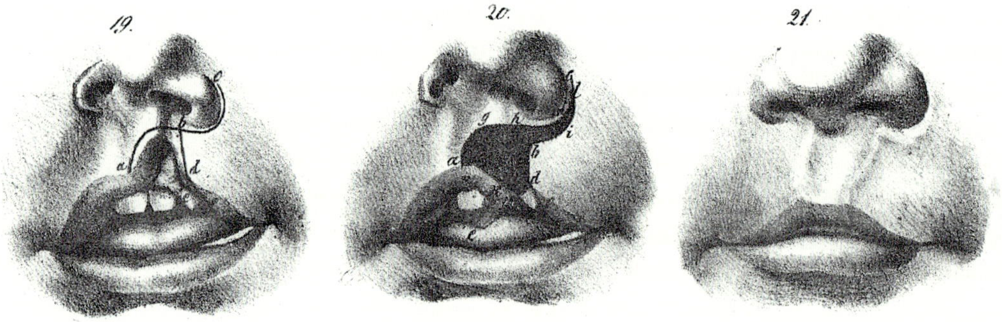

Figure 1.22 The Bruns' method of a closure of the cleft lip. From: Bruns' Chirurgischer Atlas (1857). A very accurate method of the closure of a cleft lip.

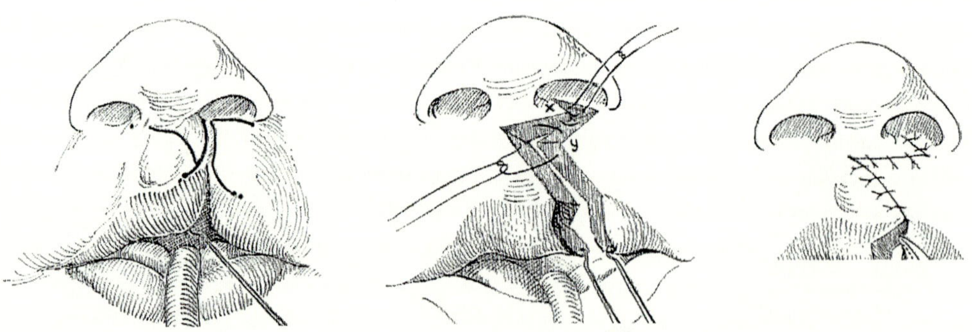

Figure 1.23 Millard, D.R.: "A radical rotation in single hare lip". Am. J. Surg. 95: 1318 (1958). A certain similarity with the Bruns' method cannot be denied. In the USA this is the most popular method today.

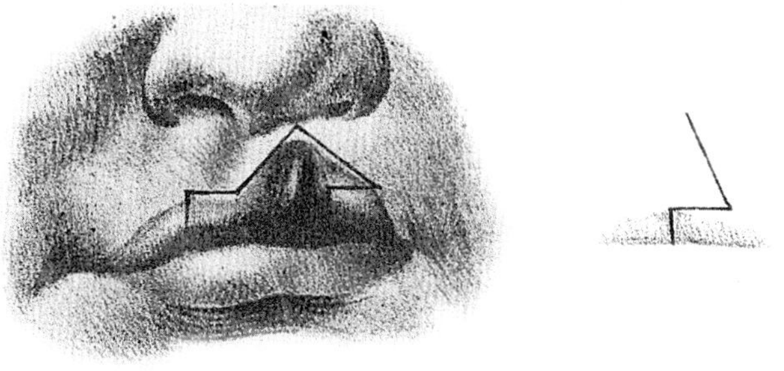

Figure 1.24 "Modification of the unilateral incision of the flap and union of the wound rims" ("Modifikation des einseitigen Läppchenschnittes und Vereinigung der Wundspalte"). From: Bruns' Chirurgischer Atlas (1857). A very logical design of the incision.

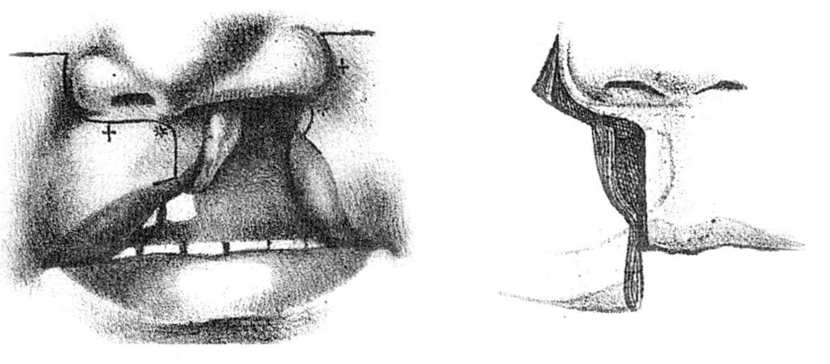

Figure 1.25 "Wound closure by a curved incision from the outer and upper part" ("Wundmachung durch Wellenschnitt nach aussen und oben"). From Bruns' Chirurgischer Atlas (1857). An interesting rotation flap to gain a lengthening of the lip.

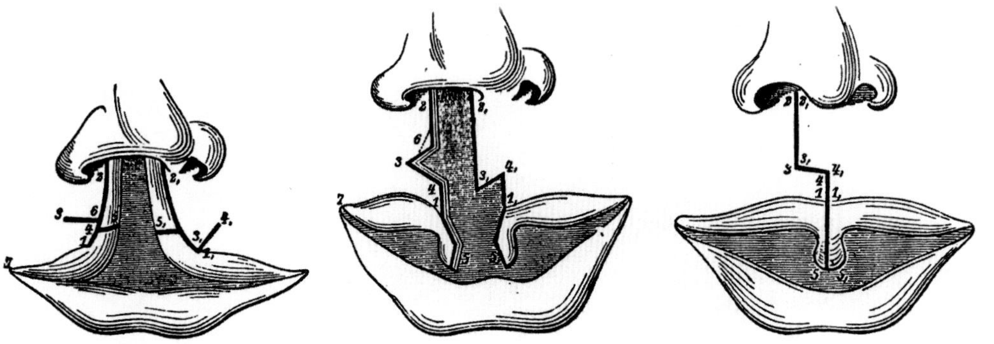

Figure 1.26 Method of Hagedorn. From: Zentralblatt für Chirurgie No. 14 (1892). First of all Hagedorn used the triangular-shaped flap to gain sufficient lengthening of the lip on the side of the cleft. The triangular method is decisive for the lip design.

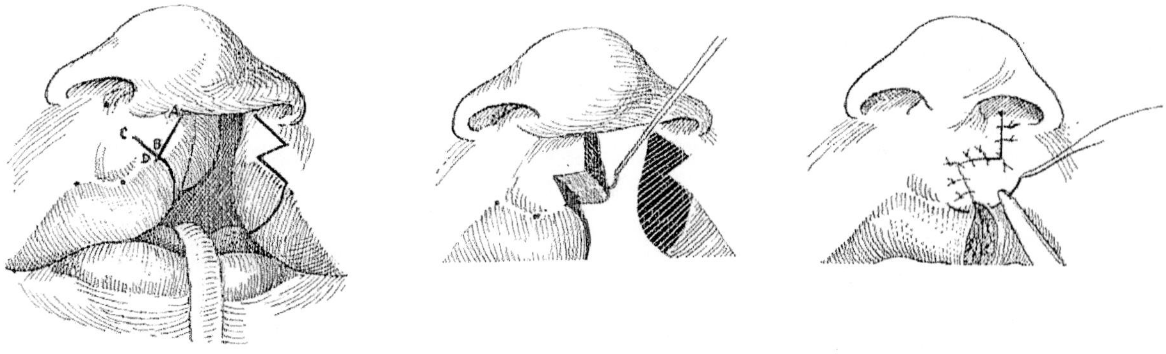

Figure 1.27 Tennison, C.W.: The repair of unilateral cleft lip by stencil method. Plast. Reconstr. Surg. 9: 115 (1952). From the author's point of view the Tennison method is still today the best operation for cleft lip. Tennison's method in fact is an improvement on the operative method of Hagedorn and Le Mesurier.

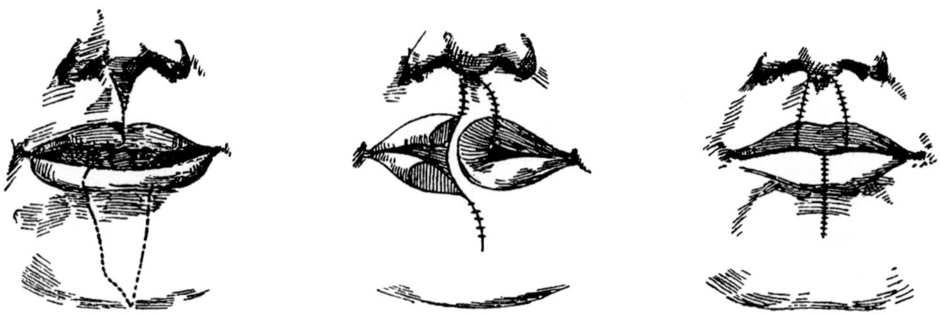

Figure 1.28 Plastic operation for correction of cleft upper lip deformity after Abbe. From: Medical Record (1898). The Abbe-Plasty is still as up-to-date as in 1898.

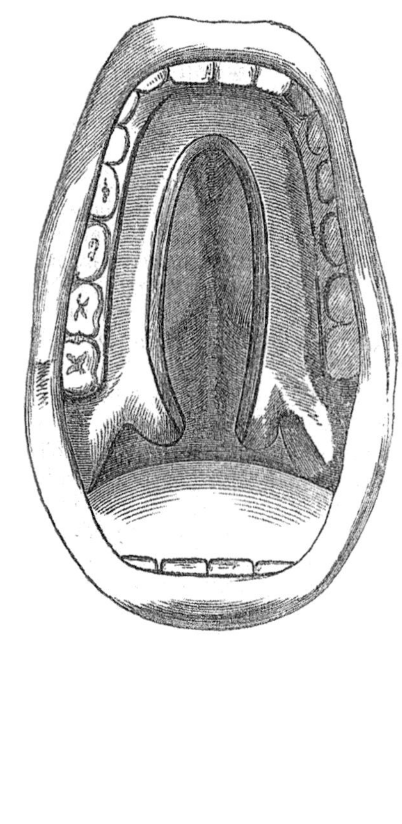

Figure 1.29 Closure of the palate after Langenbeck, which was called "Uranoplastik" by him. Langenbeck: "The uranoplasty by mobilization of the mucosa-s periostal palate flaps ". Archiv f. Klin. Chir. (1861). A typical double bridge-flap plasty.

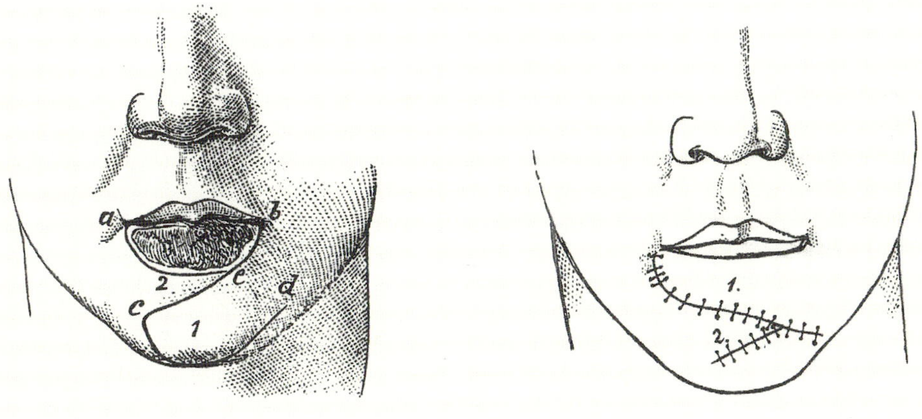

Figure 1.30 Cheiloplasty after Langenbeck. From: Langenbeck in Deutsche Klinik (German Clinic), p. 2 (1855). This beautiful transposition flap was called "cheiloplasty" by Langenbeck in 1855!

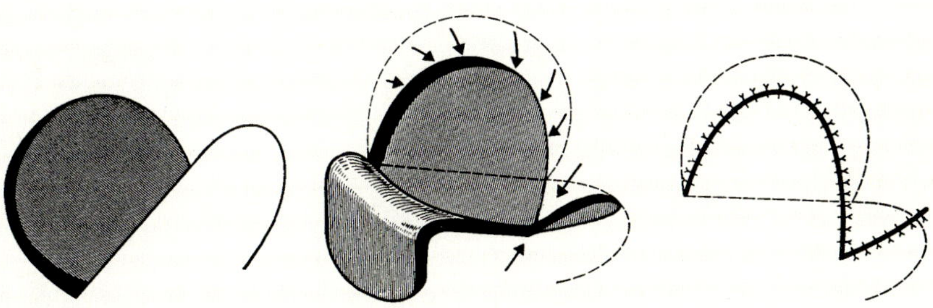

Figure 1.31 Transposition-rotation-Flap after Schrudde (1963). The merit of Schrudde is the ability of the flap for, the systemically use and the routine method in nearly all parts of the body.

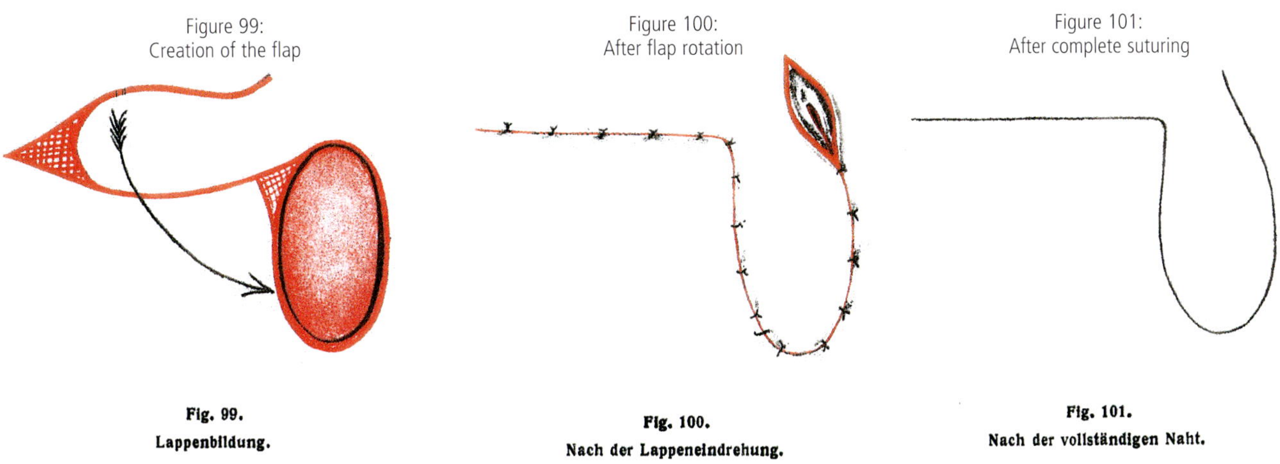

Figure 1.32 Transposition flap after Joseph. From: Joseph 1931.

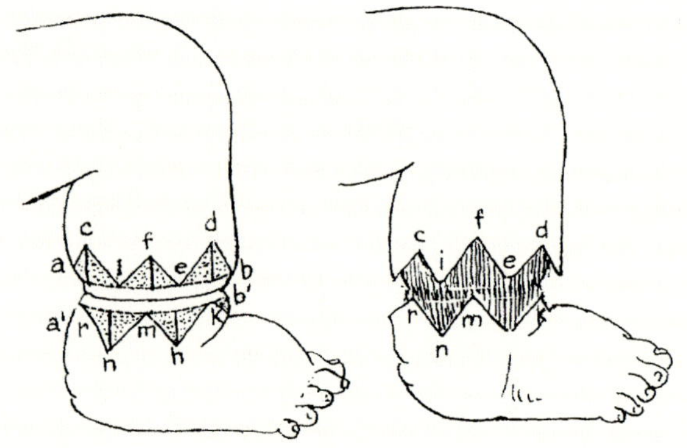

Figure 1.33 Technique after Ombrédanne to correct amniotic band of the lower extremity (1937). This method was later described as "running w-plasty".

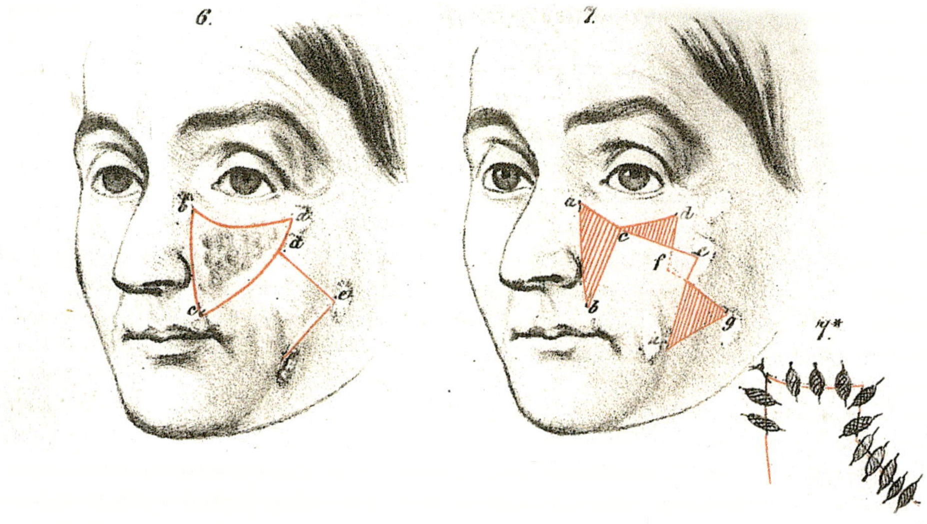

Figure 1.34 Mideldorpf's rotation flap: In: Bruns' Chirurgischer Atlas (Surgical Atlas) from 1857. The precision of the operation could be derived from Limberg. The donor-site is closed primarily.

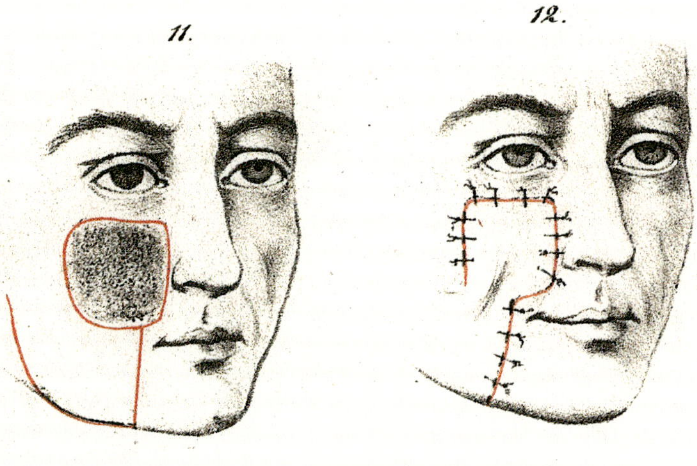

Figure 1.35 Latenneur: "Extirpation of a malignant tumour. The defect is closed with a flap which is rotated at its base". In: Bruns' Chirurgischer Atlas (1857). It is a risky flap, which, however, can be successful in the face. Today we rather prefer a rotation flap.

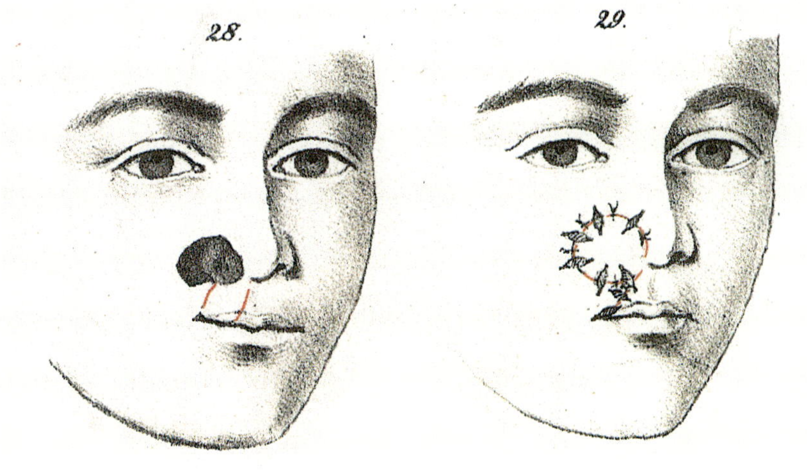

Figure 1.36 Dieffenbach: "Closure of a cheek defect with a flap from the upper lip". Published in: Bruns' Chirurgischer Atlas (1857). A transposition-rotation flap with a narrow base.

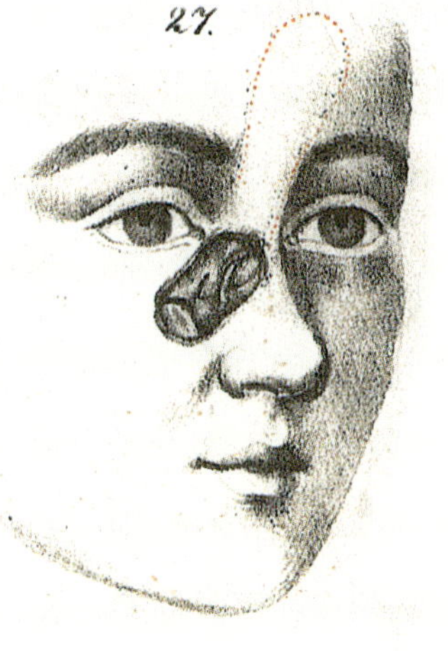

Figure 1.37 "Closure of a cheek defect with a flap from forehead skin". Graefe: "Rhinoplasty or the ability to reconstruct a nasal defect with organic tissue" ("Rhinoplastik oder die Kunst, den Verlust der Nase organisch zu ersetzen"). Berlin (1818). In fact, this is the Indian method, i.e. an axial pedicled flap. From: Bruns' Chirurgischer Atlas (1857).

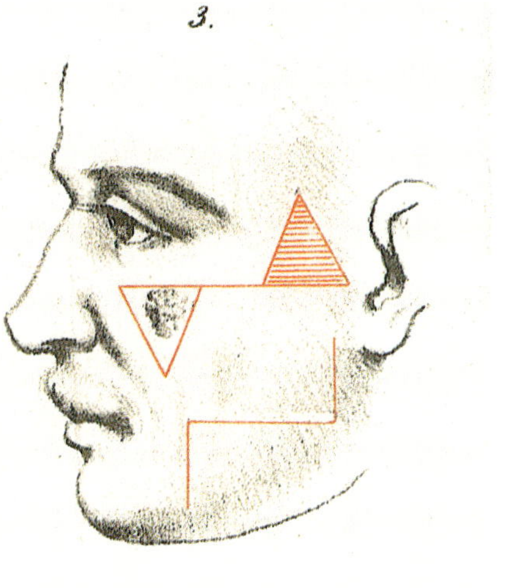

Figure 1.38 Closure of defect by the method of lateral triangles after Burow: Description of a new method of transplantation (1856).

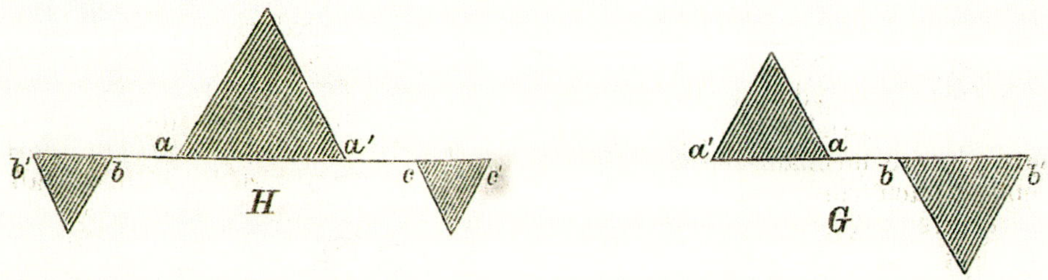

Figure 1.39 Two modifications of the Burow method for an elegant closure of defects. From: Billroth: Chirurgie, Bd. III, 1. Abt., 2. Heft (1866). Original: Burow: Description of a new method of transplantation. (Beschreibung einer neuen Transplantationsmethode). Berlin 1856.

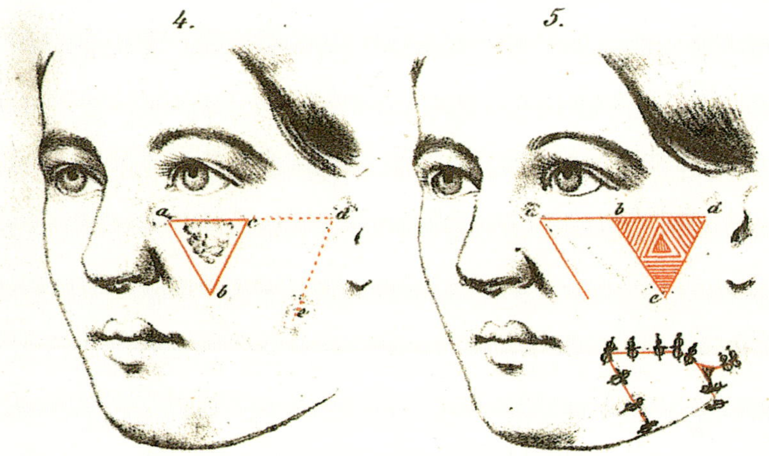

Figure 1.40 Dieffenbach: Plasty in defects of the face (1845). The donor site is closed primarily. From: Bruns' Chirurgischer Atlas (1857).

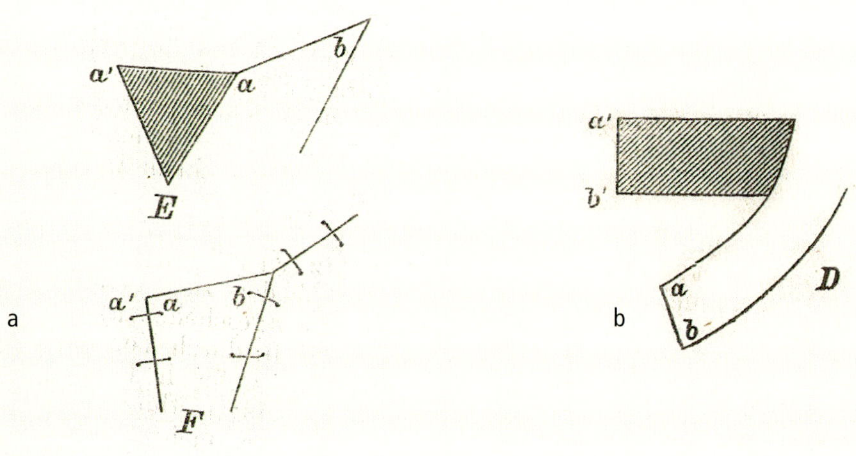

Figure 1.41 **a** Modification of the Dieffenbach flap by Szymanowsky. The secondary defect can be closed primarily. Szymanowsky: "Die Operationen an der Oberfläche des menschlichen Körpers". Kiew (1865). **b** Transposition flap after Szymanowsky (1865): The secondary defect is primarily closed. From: Billroth: Chirurgie, Bd. III, 1. Abt., 2. Heft (1866).

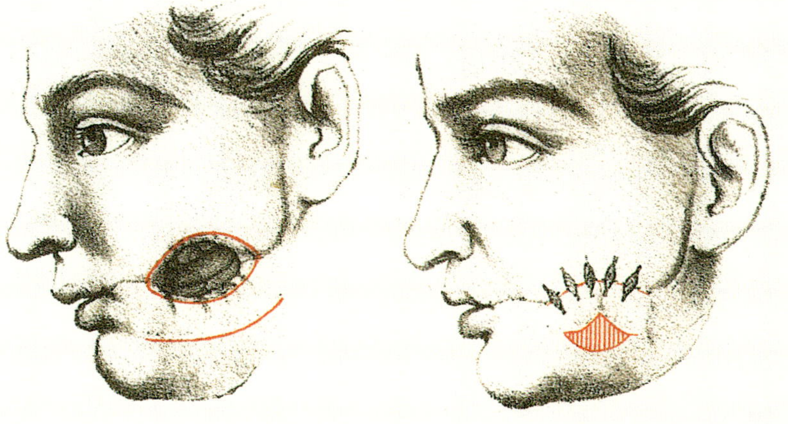

Figure 1.42 Bruns: "Closure of a defect of the cheek by a simple bridge-shaped flap" ("Schliessung eines Wangenlochs durch einen einfachen brückenförmigen Lappen". Published in: Bruns' Chirurgischer Atlas" (1857). This is the first bridge-flap the author could find.

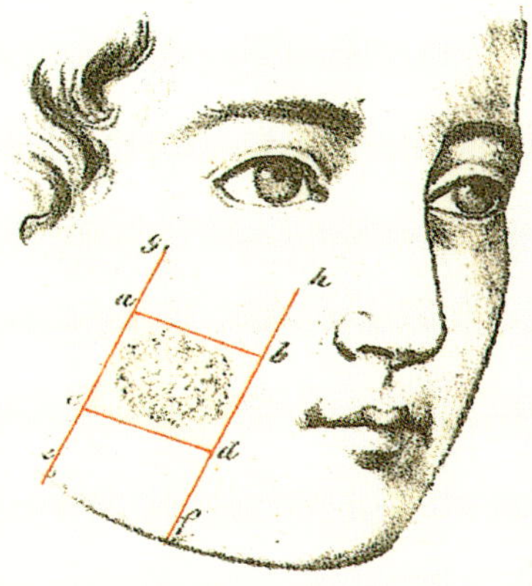

Figure 1.43 Bruns: "Viereckschnitt mit doppelter Lappenbildung". From Bruns' Chirurgischer Atlas (1857). This method was probably already used by Celsus (25 BC–25 AC). Don't try it!

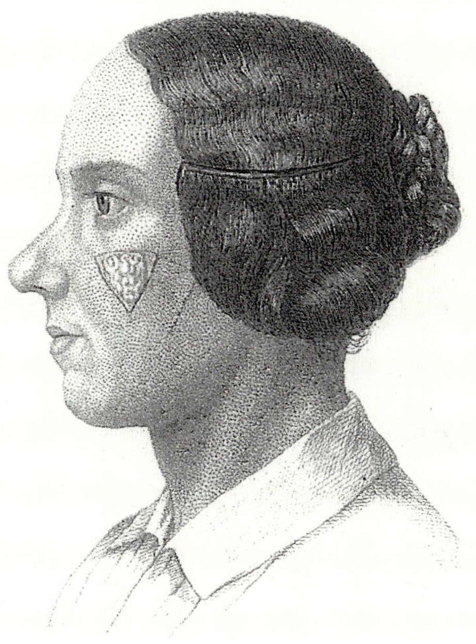

Figure 1.44 Transposition flap for closure of facial defects. From Billroth: "Handbuch der allgemeinen und speziellen Chirurgie". Erlangen (1865).

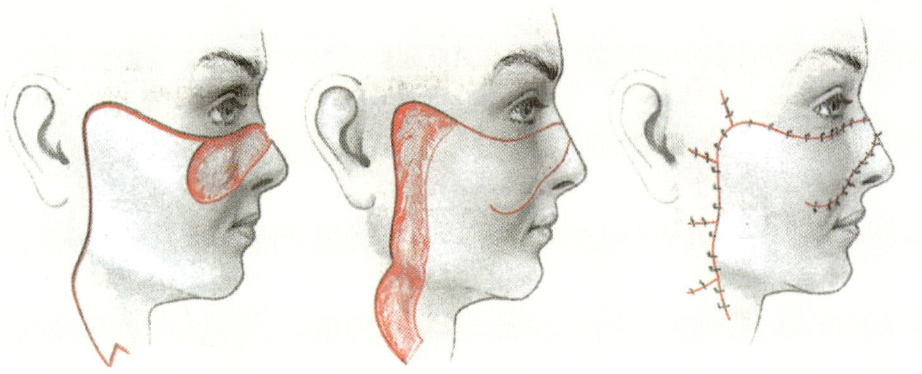

Figure 1.45 Rotation-plasty after Esser (1918). Esser, J.F.: "Rotation of the cheek". In: Denecke/Mayer: Rhinoplasty ("Nasoplastik"). This rotation plasty of the cheek was later often modified.

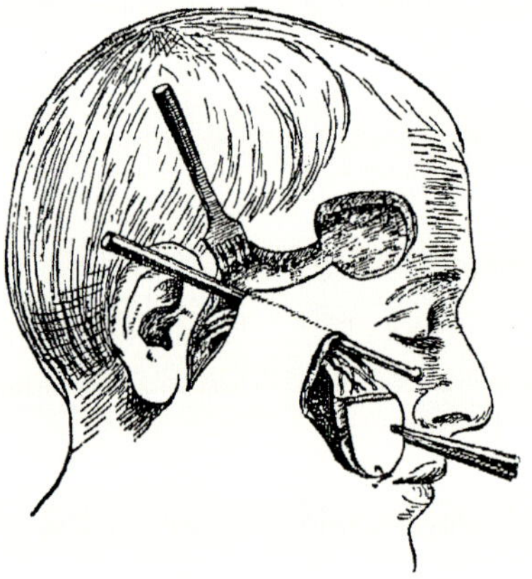

Figure 1.46 Axial pattern island flap after M. Kirschner (1920). One can clearly recognize the marked arterial and venous supply as well as the pedicle. It is not commonly known, if Kirschner knew Esser´s (1918) works.

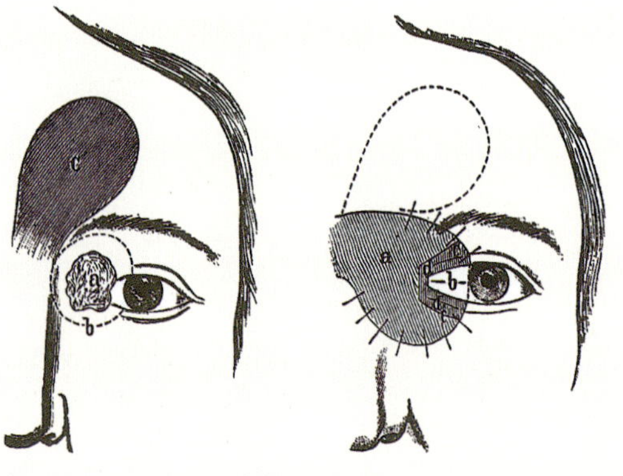

Figure 1.47 Partial reconstruction of the upper and lower lid after Jordan. He used the classical forehead flap. Jordan: "Über den plastischen Ersatz der Augenlider". Dtsch. Med. Wochenschr. No. 45: 477 (1895).

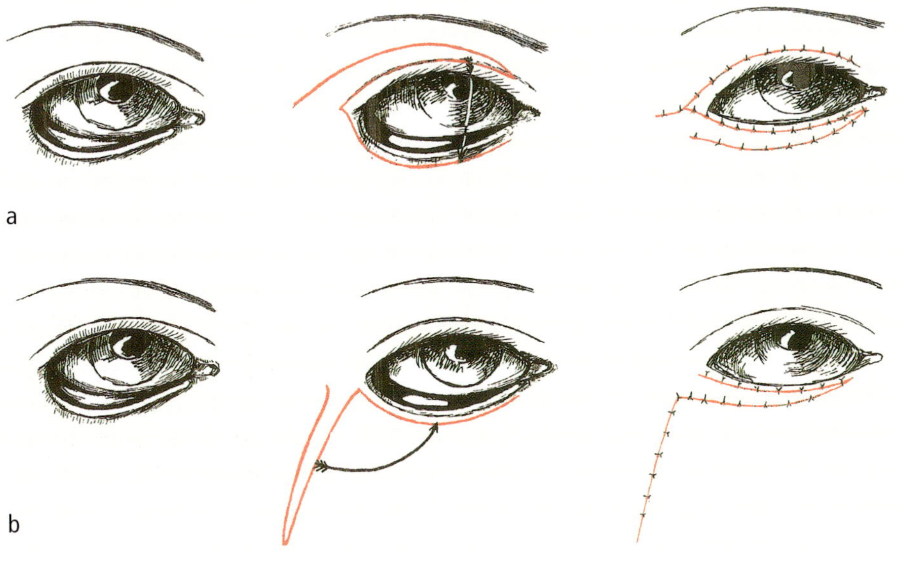

Figure 1.48 **a** Correction of ectropion of the lower lid by the use of an upper lid flap. **b** Correction of ectropion of the lower lid by cheek flap. Published in: Joseph, J.: "Nasenplastik und sonstige Gesichtsplastik nebst einem Anhang über Mammplastik" (1931). [cf. Figure 1.6]

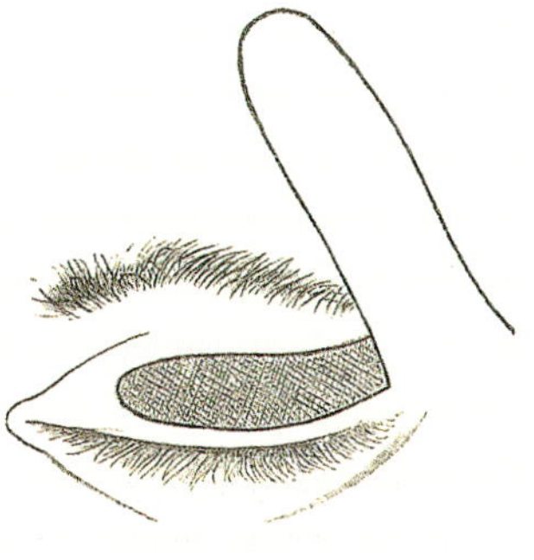

Figure 1.49 Blepharoplasty after Fricke (1829): A good transposition-flap. The donor site is closed primarily. From: Fritze and Reich: "Die plastische Chirurgie" (1845).

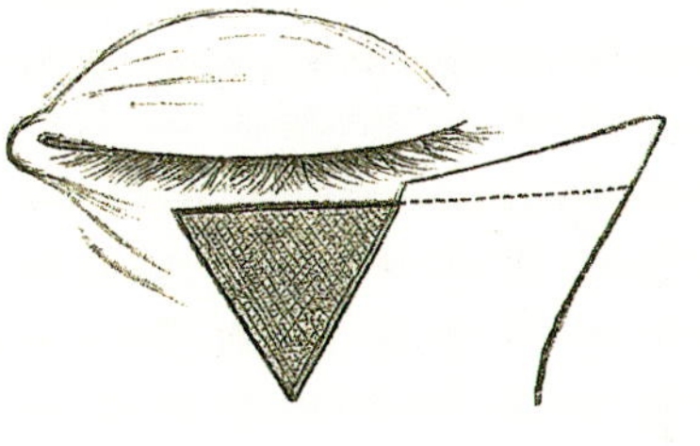

Figure 1.50 Blepharoplasty after Dieffenbach (1835): From: Fritze and Reich: "Die plastische Chirurgie" (1845). Original illustrations from: Haab, O.: "Atlas and teachings of eye operations" ("Atlas und Lehre der Augenoperationen") (1910).

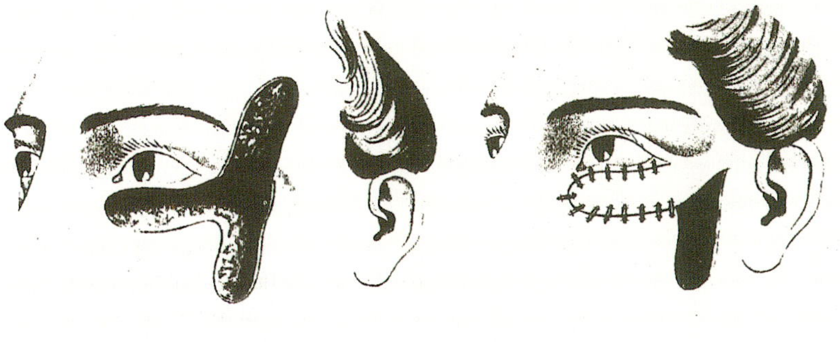

Figure 1.51 Reconstruction of the lower lid after Frick and Ammon. The donor site is directly closed. From: Fritze and Reich: "Die plastische Chirurgie" (1845).

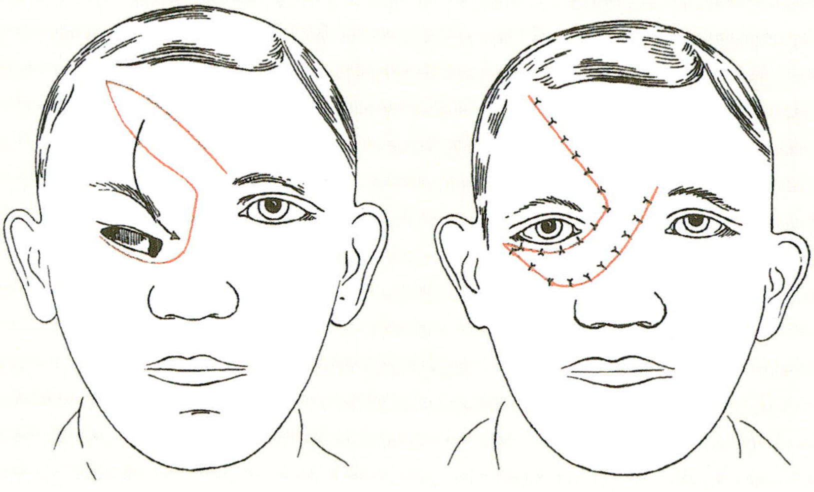

Figure 1.52 Reconstruction of lower lid by forehead flap. ("Schema der frontalen Methode der Blepharoplastik"). Joseph cleverly used the Indian flap for the lower lid reconstruction. From: Joseph, J. „Nasenplastik und sonstige Gesichtsplastik nebst einem Anhang über Mammplastik" (1931). [cf. Figure 1.6]

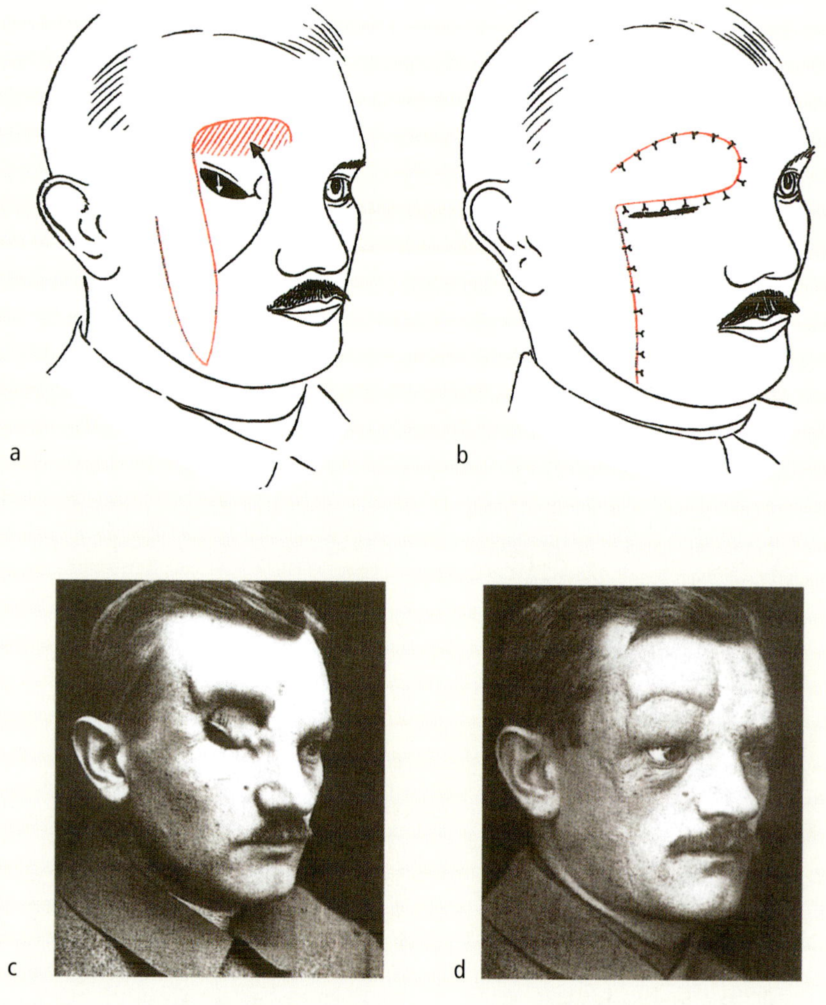

Figure 1.53 a,b Forehead skin and bony defect corrected by a cheek flap. The method of lid plasty of Fricke and Ammon is extended. **c, d** Case report of the method described above. The reconstruction is ingenious and as one can see it works well. From: Joseph, J.: "Nasenplastik und sonstige Gesichtsplastik nebst einem Anhang über Mammplastik" (1931).

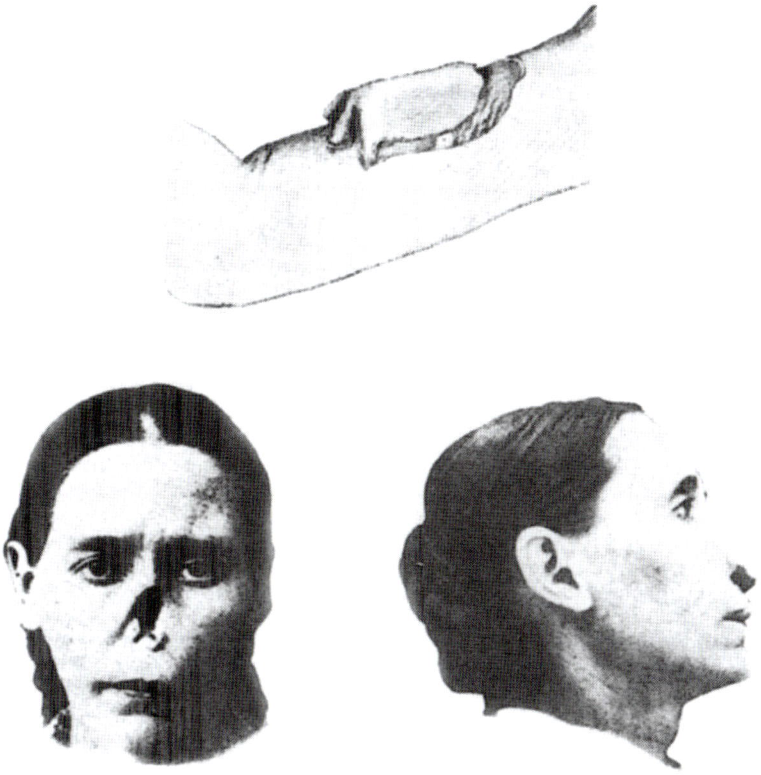

Figure 1.54 „Sterno-costal substitute of the nasal framework" (case of Fritz König). König: "About rhinoplasties" ("Über Nasenplastiken"). Bruns' Beitr. Klein. Chir. Vol. 94 (1914). Preconditioned nose at the forearm with bone transplant. 1914! With documented success. Original illustrations: Joseph, J.: "Nasenplastik und sonstige Gesichtsplastik nebst einem Anhang über Mammplastik" (1931).

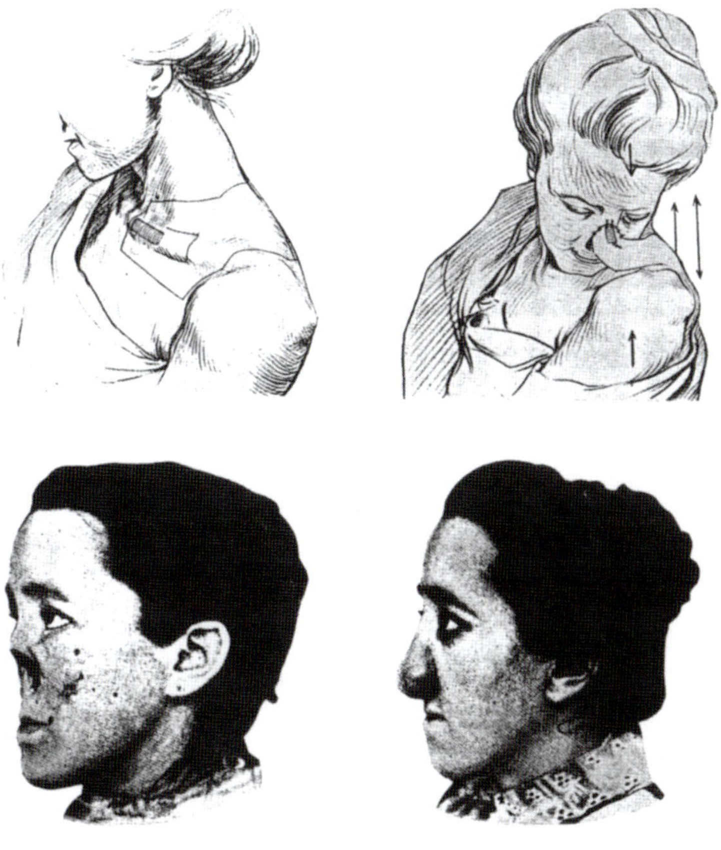

Figure 1.55 Rhinoplasty from the clavicular area after Mandry. A fabulous idea of 1908! Documented in a picture. Mandry: "Rhinoplasty with direct implantation of a skin-periostal-bone flap from the clavicular shoulder region" ("Rhinoplastik mit direkter Einpflanzung eines Hautperiostknochenlappens aus der Schlüsselbein-Schulterregion") Beitr. Klin. Chir. Vol. 77 (1908).

Double Layer Nose Reconstruction after Joseph

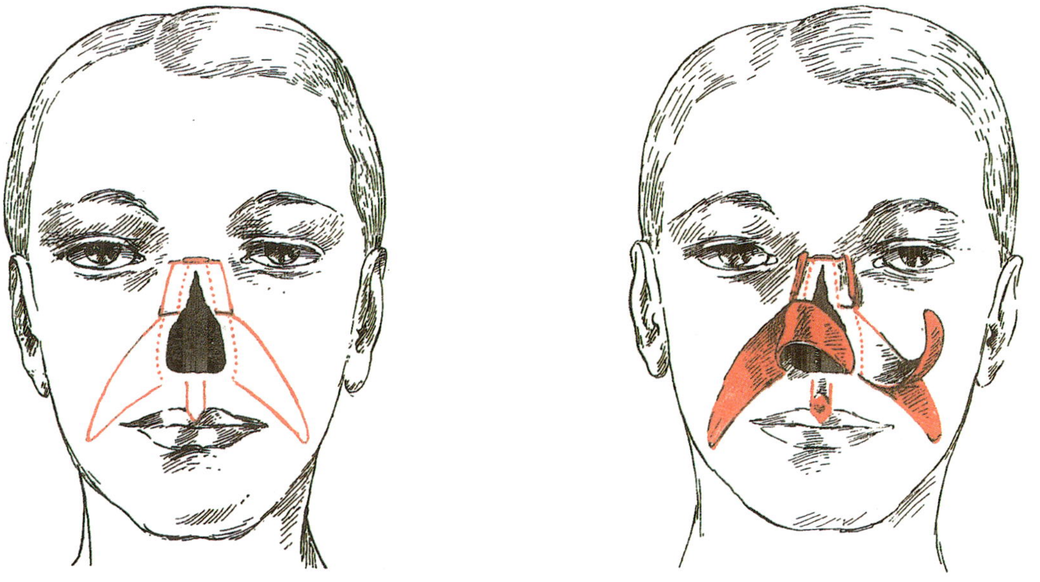

The inner lining is achieved by the use of two nasolabial flaps.

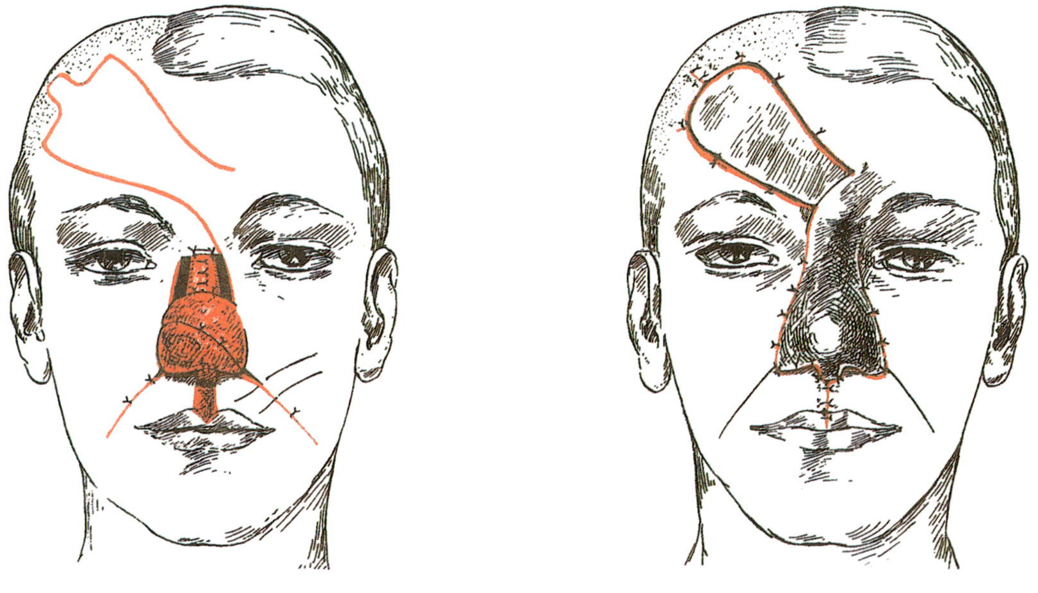

The outer defect is reconstructed by a forehead flap with additionally an L-shaped bone graft.

Figure 1.56 Bucco-nasal mucosal reconstruction from both cheeks.
Original illustrations: Joseph, J.: ("Nasenplastik und sonstige Gesichtsplastik nebst einem Anhang über Mammaplastik") Curt Kabitzsch, Leipzig (1931).
[cf. Figure 1.6]

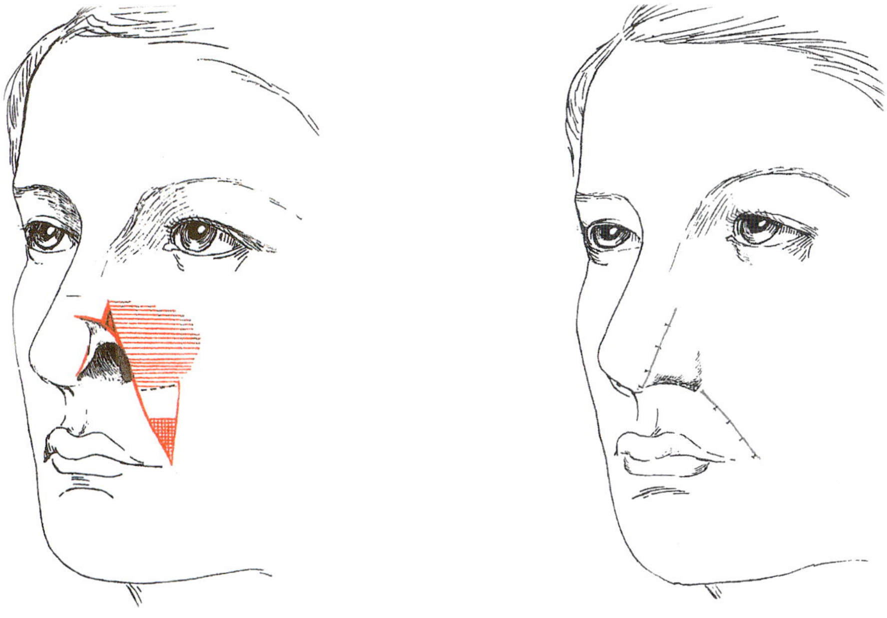

Figure 1.57 Reconstruction of the nostril after Nelaton (modification by Joseph). Original illustrations from: Joseph, J.: "Nasenplastik und sonstige Gesichtsplastik nebst einem Anhang über Mammplastik" (1931).

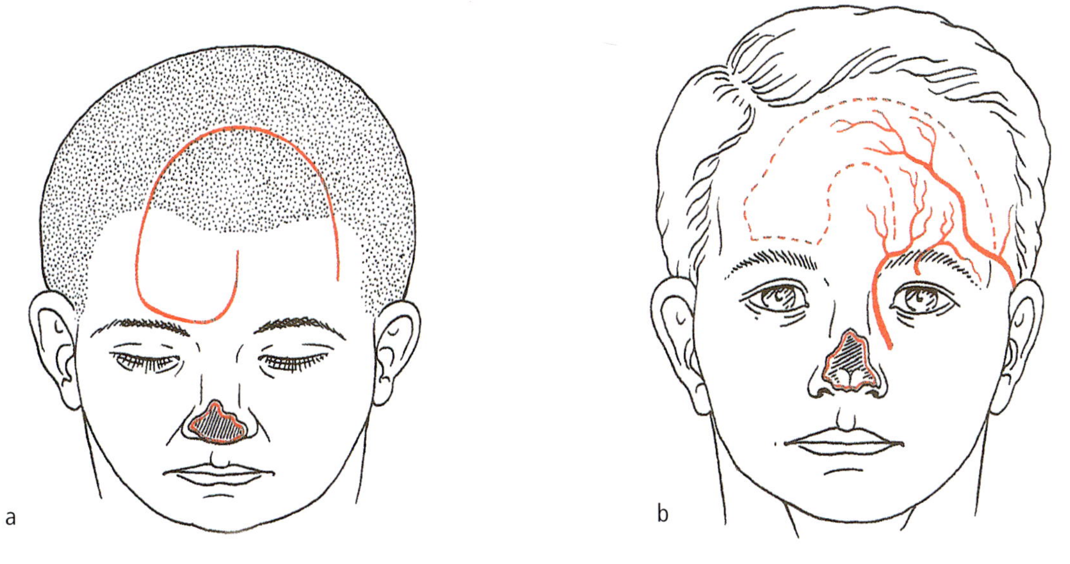

Figure 1.58 **a** "Up and down flap" after Gillies. Original illustrations from: Gillies, H.D.: Up and Down flap. Vol. 3, p. 762, New York, D. Appleton and Co. (1937). **b** Forehead flap after Kilner with arterial supply by the frontal branch of the temporal superficial artery and the supratrochlear artery and supraorbital artery.

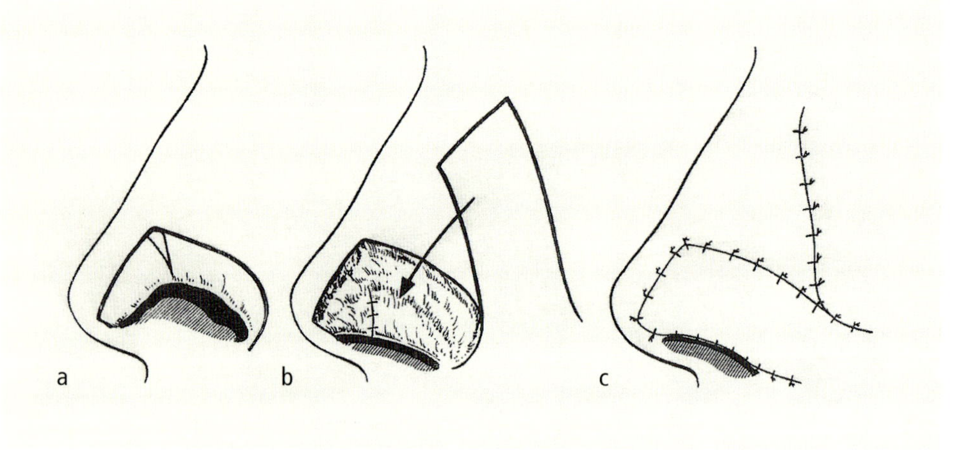

Figure 1.59 Reconstruction of nostril after Sanvenero-Rosselli. Sanvenero-Rosselli, G.: Chirurgica plastica del naso. p.148, Pozzi (1931).

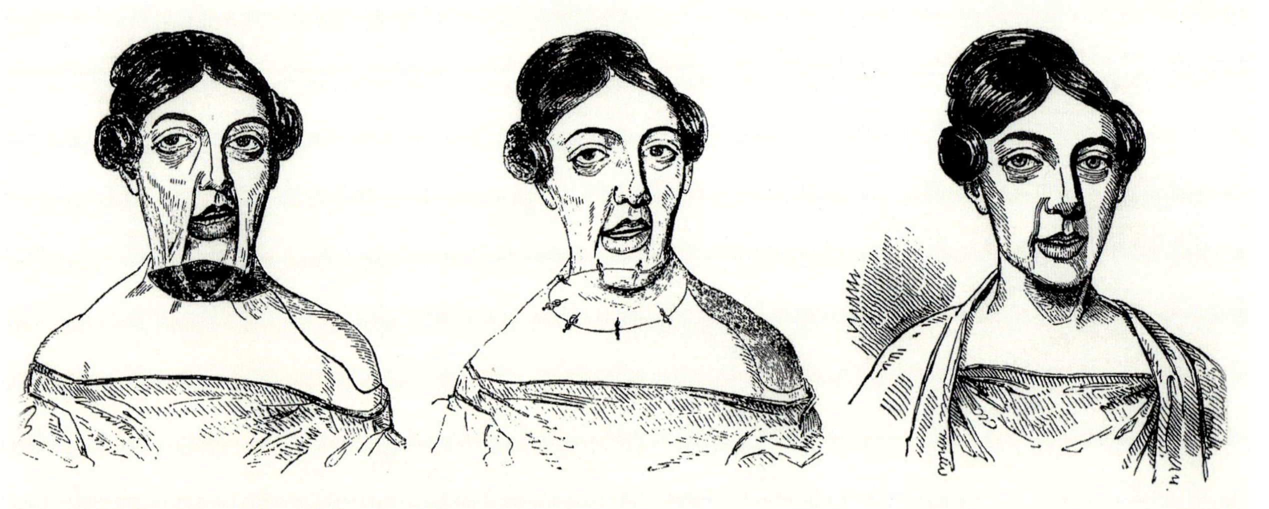

Figure 1.60 Interesting demonstration of a shoulder flap to correct a neck contracture after burn injury. Mutter, T.D.: Cases of deformity from burns, relived by operation. Am. J. Med. Sci. 4: 66–80 (1842)! One can not deny a similarity to the Acromio-cervical flap described by Kirschbaum, S.: Plast. Reconstr. Surg. 21: 131 (1958).

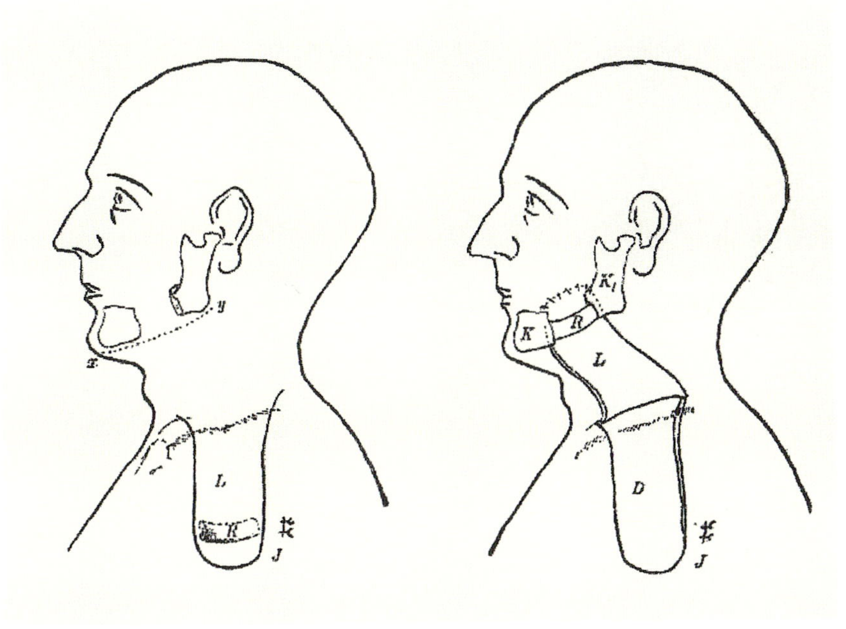

Figure 1.61 Payr: Osteoplasty by a flap of the chest wall containing a piece of a rib. Zentralblatt für Chirurgie (1908).

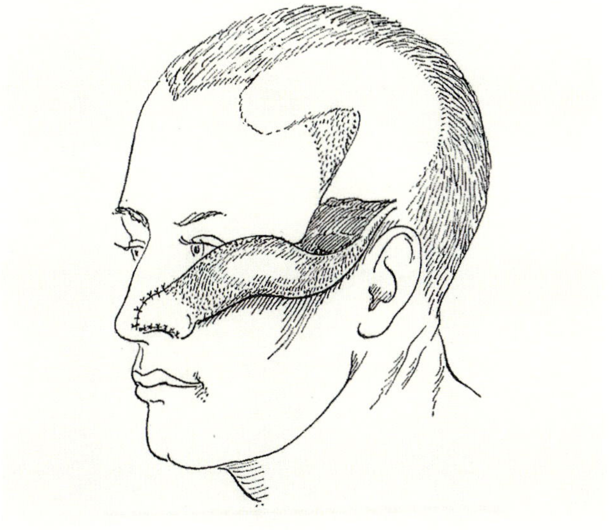

Figure 1.62 New described the "sickle flap" in 1928: an axial pedicled flap for nose reconstruction. This ingenious method was adversely criticised by Converse and was wrongly buried in oblivion. We have proved that the method after New is excellent (see Chapter on Nose Defects, pp.115–119).

Digital Reconstruction of Nose (Russian Method)

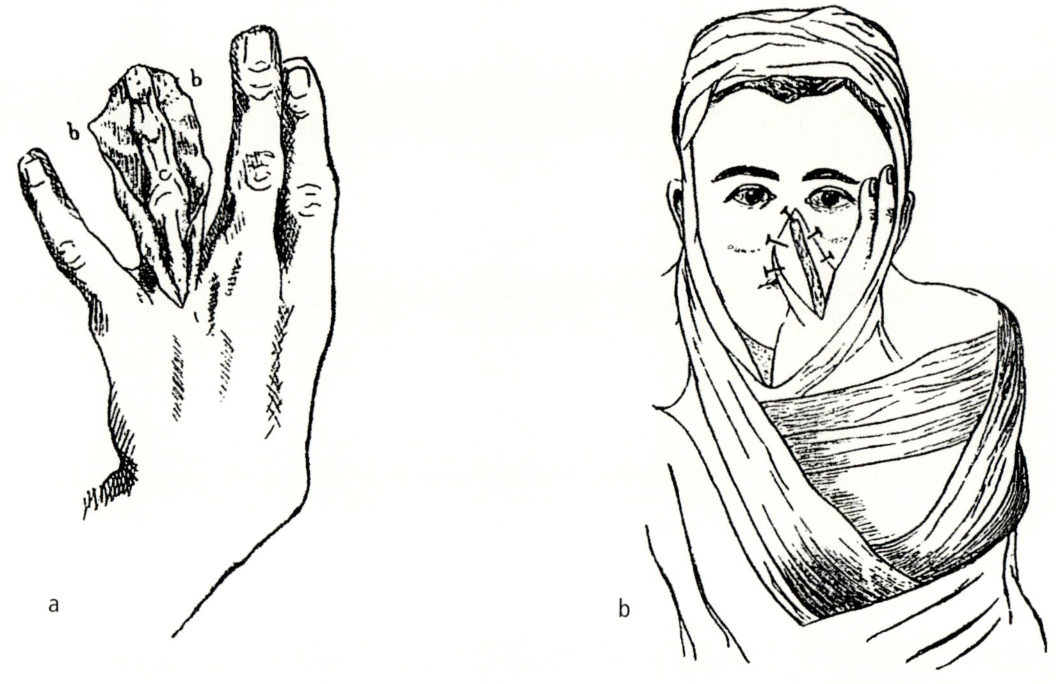

Figure 1.63 **a** Preparation of the ring finger. **b** Fixation of arm and finger

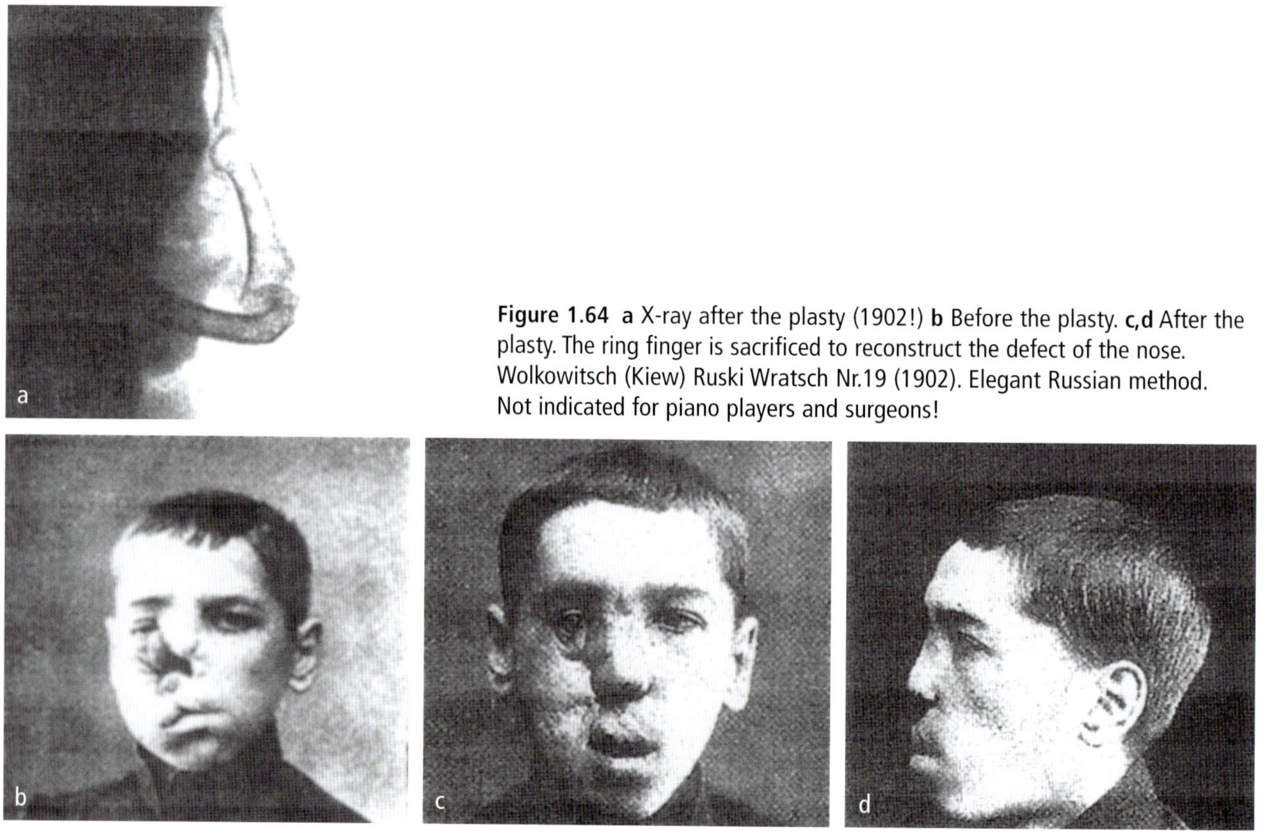

Figure 1.64 **a** X-ray after the plasty (1902!) **b** Before the plasty. **c,d** After the plasty. The ring finger is sacrificed to reconstruct the defect of the nose. Wolkowitsch (Kiew) Ruski Wratsch Nr.19 (1902). Elegant Russian method. Not indicated for piano players and surgeons!

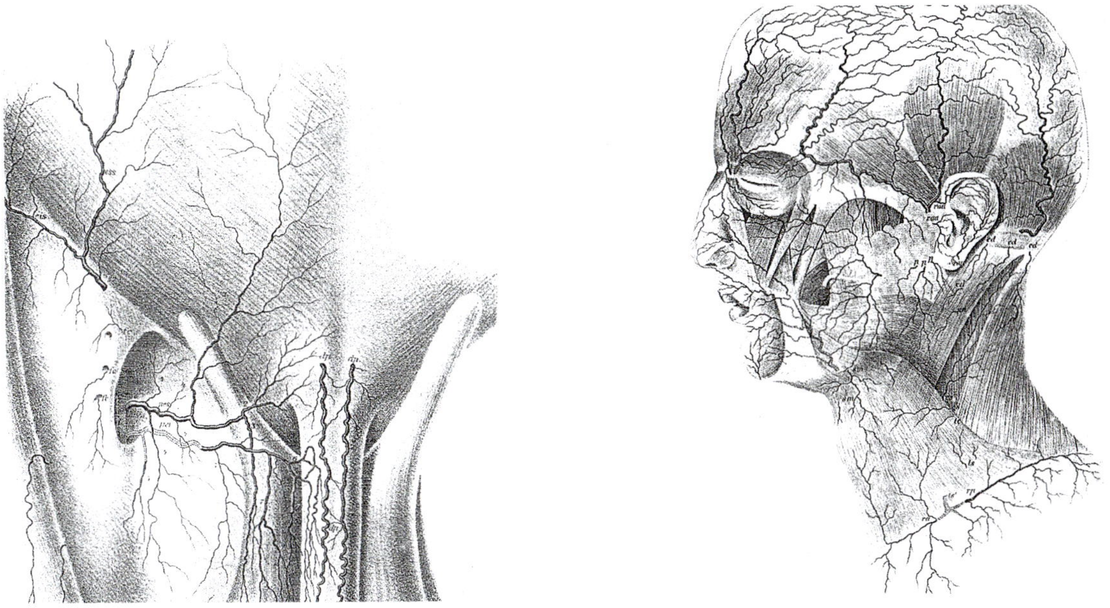

Figure 1.65 Manchot described the skin arteries in 1889. His book did not attract much interest. Simultaneously with the discovery of the axial pedicled flap his work was rediscovered.

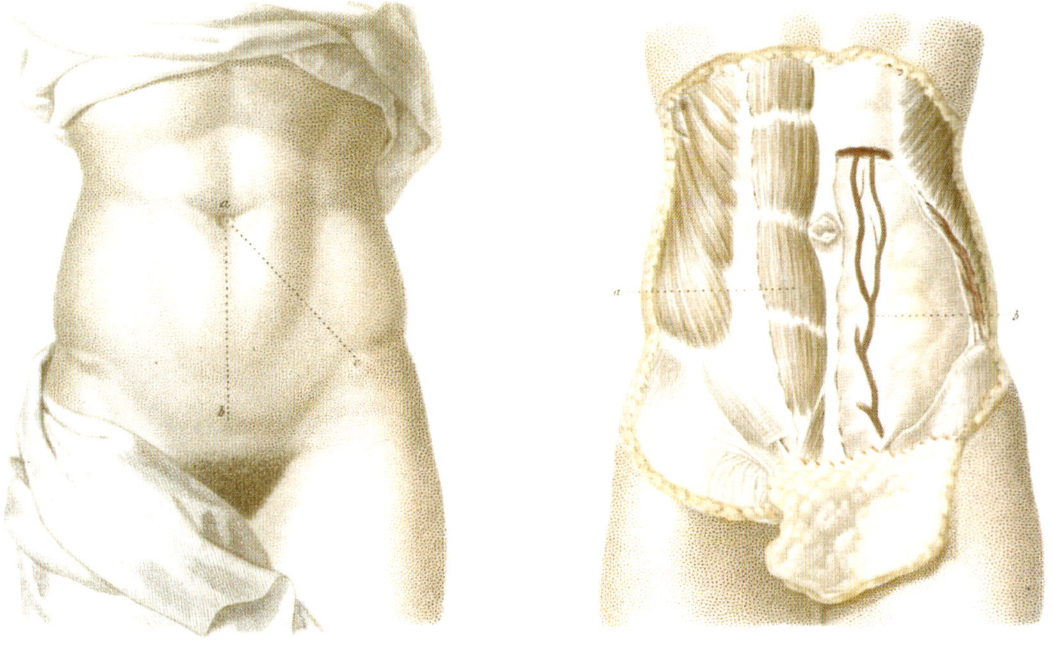

Figure 1.66 Interesting surgical-anatomical study (1848!). From: Bernard, Cl., Huette, Ch.: Précis iconographiqe de médicine opératoire et d´anatomie chirurgicale. Méquignon Marvis Fils, Paris (1848). Something for TRAM-"freaks".

Vertical Mastopexy (Burian 1967)

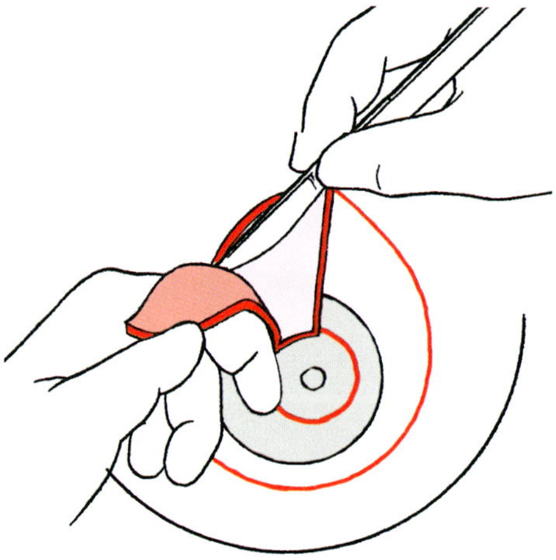

Figure 1.67a Mastopexy with vertical scar. Deepithelialization and reduction of the areola in mastopexy with vertical scar after Burian (1967). Original from: Burian: The plastic surgery atlas (1967).

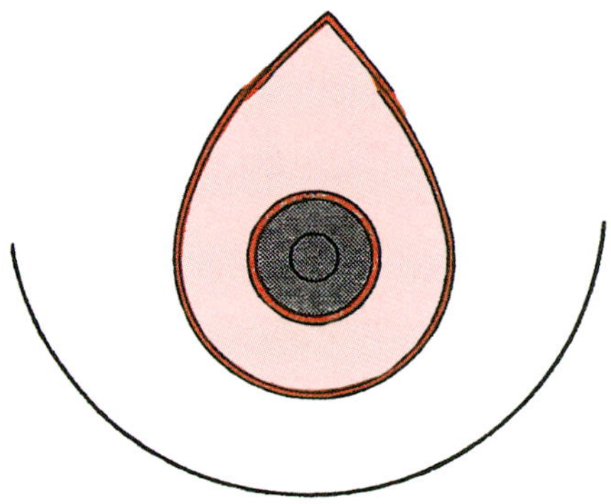

Figure 1.67b Result after deepithelialization.

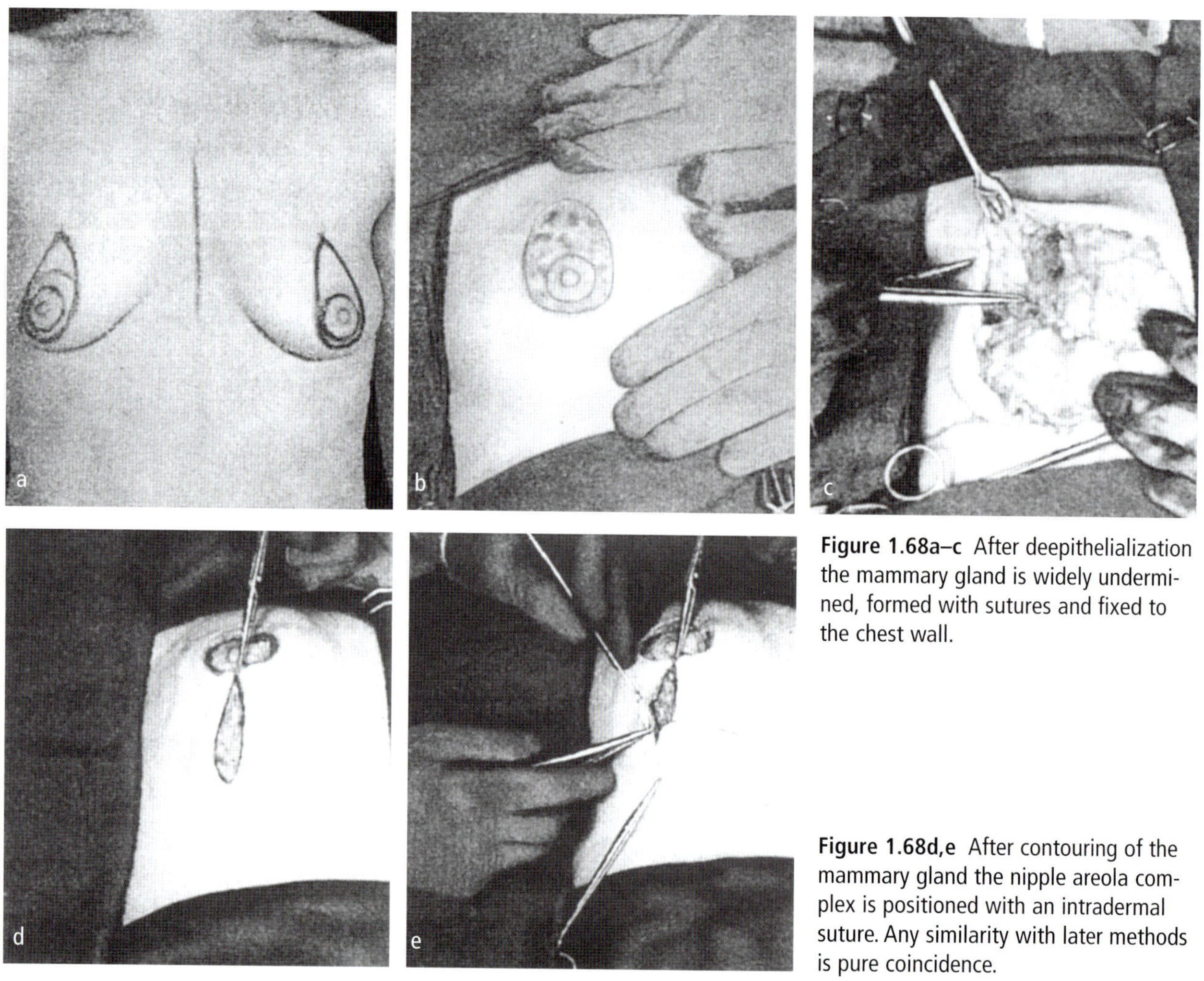

Figure 1.68a–c After deepithelialization the mammary gland is widely undermined, formed with sutures and fixed to the chest wall.

Figure 1.68d,e After contouring of the mammary gland the nipple areola complex is positioned with an intradermal suture. Any similarity with later methods is pure coincidence.

CHAPTER 2
General Principles

Classification of Flaps

a) Random Pattern Flap

The random pattern flap is supplied by a random vascular plexus which lies above the fascia. The vessels derive from the muscles and fascia and give their perforating rami in the subcutaneous tissue. These rami build a subdermal plexus which is responsible for the circulation (Figure 2.1).

Due to the lack of a dominant vessel a random pattern flap requires a sufficiently wide base. As a general rule a relation of width to length of at least 1 to 3 is advocated. However, in the face the base can sometimes be narrower. In the lower leg, one has to be more careful, so that the base is created wider or, for preference, a fasciocutaneous flap is performed. An island flap in the way of a random pattern flap is very risky and should only be used in exceptional cases by experts.

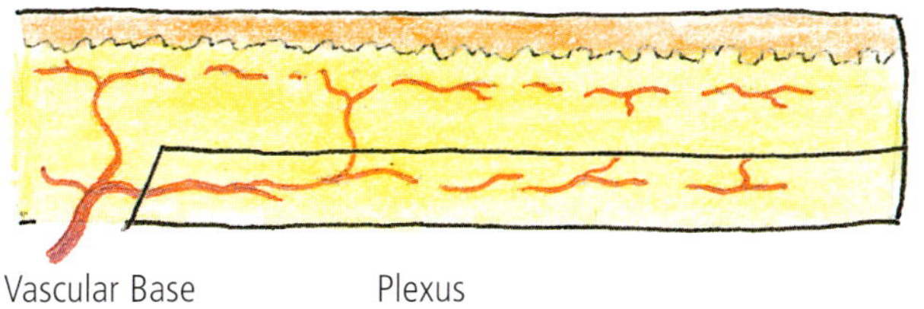

Figure 2.1 Blood supply of random pattern flap

b) Axial Pattern Flap (Arterial Flap)

The "axial pattern flap" is supplied by a dominant artery and vein. The vessels originate from a supramuscular tissue layer and are located in the deep layer of the subcutis or in the superficial fascia. The dominant artery and vein spread directly in the dermal and subdermal plexus or in the superficial fascia of the skin flap (Figure 2.2).

The *axial pattern flap* is considerably better vascularized than the random pattern flap and can be planned in greater length to breadth ratios. The base of the flap can be narrower or used as an island flap.

The axial pattern flap can be employed as a microsurgical graft. A typical arterial flap is the groin flap.

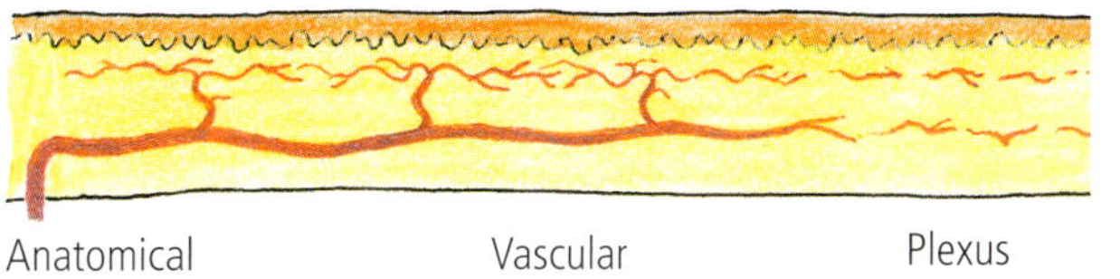

Figure 2.2 Blood supply of the "axial pattern flap"

c) Fasciocutaneous Flap

The fasciocutaneous flap includes skin, subcutaneous tissue and fascia and has a long vascular pedicle of anastomosing arterial territories. The supplying subcutaneous vessel perforates from the deep fascia and spreads via the deep fascial network into the subcutaneous tissue. This skin vessel supplies the cutaneous plexus (Figure 2.3).

Basicallly the fasciocutaneous flap is safer than the random pattern flap, but this depends on the localisation. The vascular anatomy is variable in different regions. In extremities the vascular axis lies longitudinally. Typical fasciocutaneous flaps are for example the forearm flap, the scapular flap and the fasciocutaneous foreleg flap.

Before operating on fasciocutaneous or local flaps the autor recommends reading the book "The arterial anatomy of skin flaps" by G.C. Cormack and B.G.H. Lamberty. Churchill Livingstone (1994).

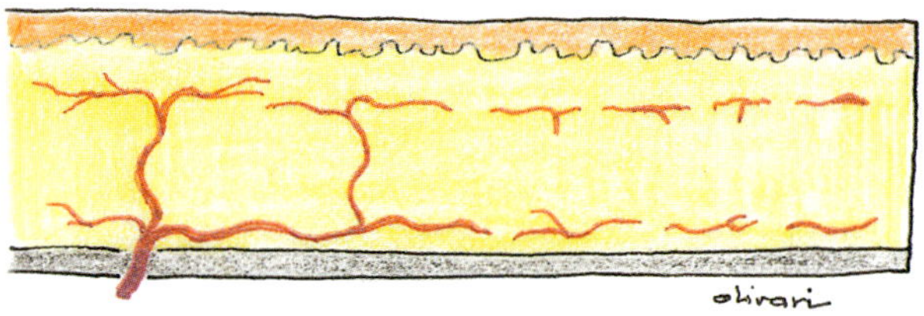

Figure 2.3 Blood supply of the fasciocutaneous flaps

d) Myocutaneous Flap

The myocutaneous flap consists of muscle, fascia, subcutaneous tissue and skin. In most cases this flap has an axial pedicle. Subcutaneous tissue and skin are well supplied by multiple perforating vessels which originate from the muscle and reach the skin (Figure 2.4). The length of the flap is limited by the course of the vessel. The myocutaneous flap can be used as pedicled transposition flap, as an island flap or as a microsurgical graft. A typic myocutaneous flap is the latissimus dorsi flap. The blood circulation of the skin area at the peripherals parts of the flap depends to its localisation.

Normally one can utilize a skin area which extends the rim of the muscle. This is maximum possible in TRAM flaps. The authors experience attests that 10 cm of skin and subcutaneous tissue beyond the rim of the latissimus muscle are well circulated.

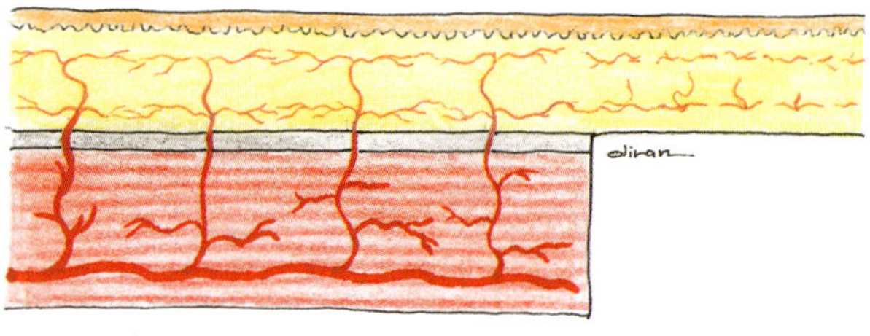

Figure 2.4 Blood supply of the myocutaneous flaps

e) Microsurgical Flap

The microsurgical flap is an axial pedicled flap which can be used either as skin flap, fasciocutaneous flap, myocutaneous flap, osteomyocutaneous flap or as a free muscle flap and so on. Microsurgical flap have revolutionized plastic surgery. The cover of defects no longer depends on the size and localisation of the defect. A typical free myocutaneous flap is the latissimus dorsi flap (Figures 2.5, 2.6). The vessels of the free flap are anastomosed with corresponding vessels in the area of the defect.

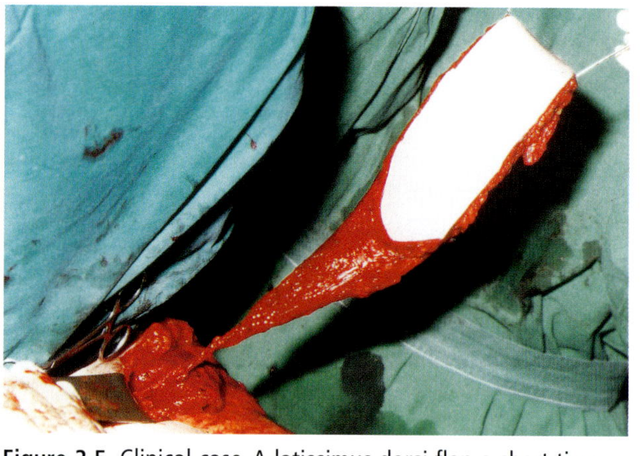

Figure 2.5 Clinical case. A latissimus dorsi flap a short time before division of the A. and V. thoracodorsalis.

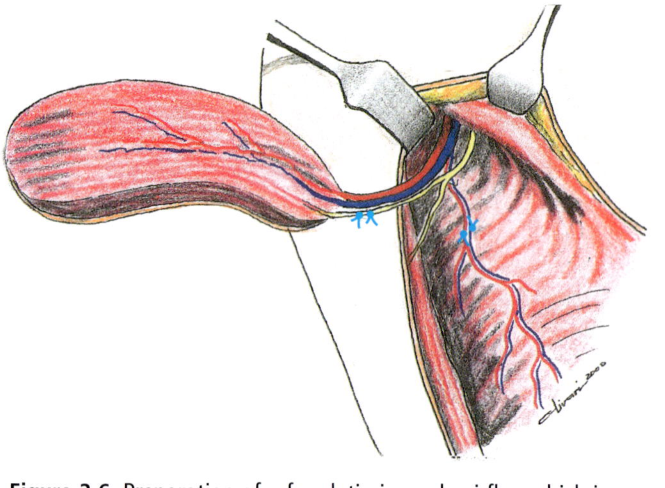

Figure 2.6 Preparation of a free latissimus dorsi flap which is pedicled at the A. and V. thoracodorsalis.

Suture Technique

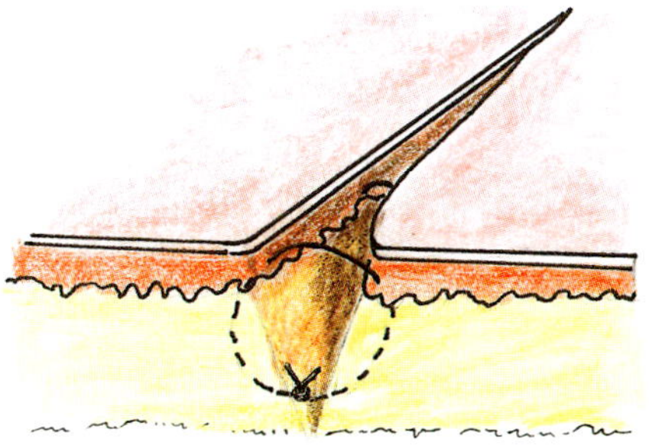

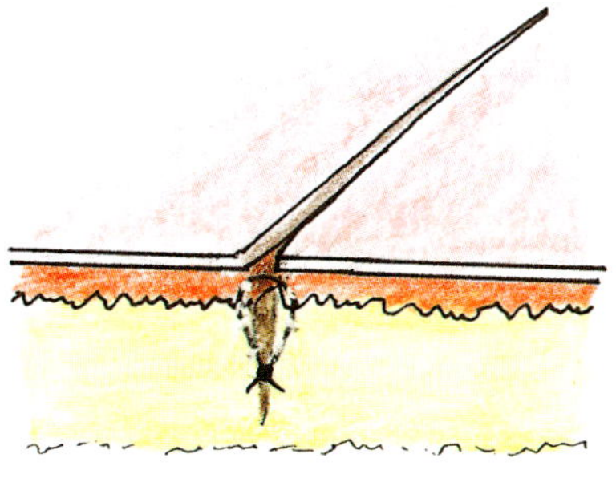

Figure 2.7a,b Subcutaneous suture with absorbable material (e.g. Vicryl)
The knot must be buried deeply, because otherwise it will protrude through the wound and disturb healing. In the face 5 × 0 or 6 × 0 is sufficient as suture thickness. In the trunk depending on the tension stronger sutures should be used.

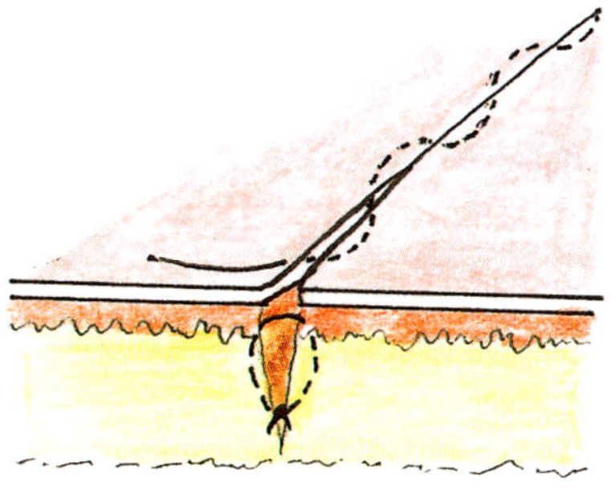

Figure 2.7c Intradermal suture
In the face 6 × 0 nylon (e.g. Trofilene) sutures are appropriate, after wound edge adaptation with subcutaneous stitches. In the eye lid an intracutaneous suture with 6 × 0 without subcutaneous stitches is sufficient. In the trunk one uses strong sutures (3 × 0) such as nylon or resorbable material as well for intracutaneous sutures.

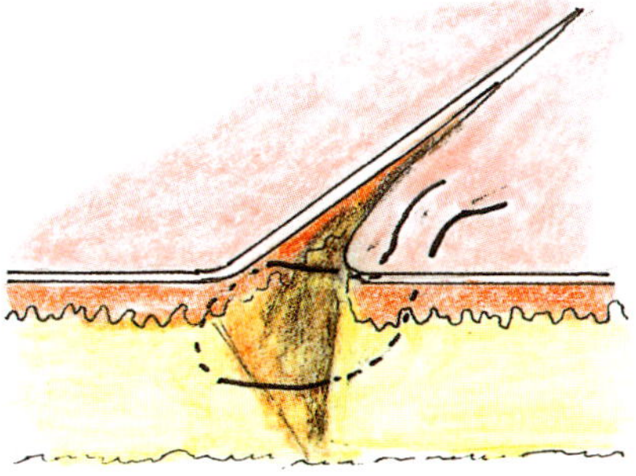

Figure 2.7d Suture in flap-adaptations
The skin of the flap is not perforated to prevent disruption of the microcirculation at the edge of the flap.

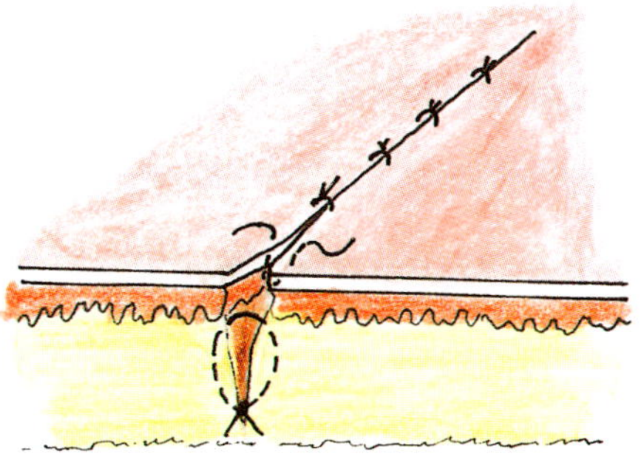

Figure 2.7e Typical suture in defects of the face
The adaptation is reached with 5 × 0 Vicryl. The knot is located deep. For the skin suture 6 × 0 nylon is used. The stitches should be located only one millimetre away from the wound rim. As an alternative one could also use an intracutaneous suture with 6 × 0 nylon.

Different Flap Types

a) Random Pattern Flap

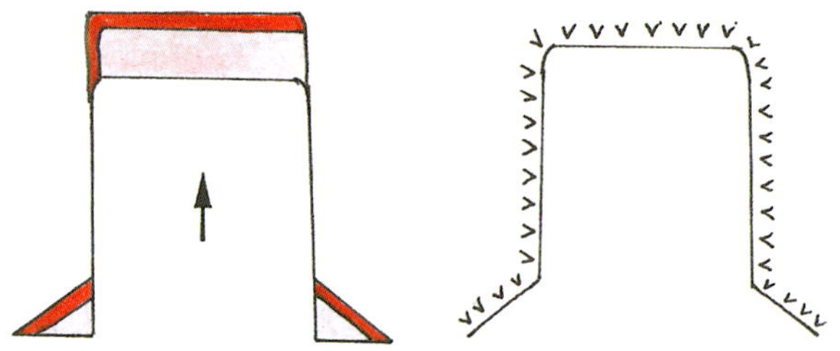

Figure 2.8 Transposition flap with two Burow triangles (advancement flap) is today a rarely used flap. A typical indication is the Rintala plasty of the dorsum nasi.

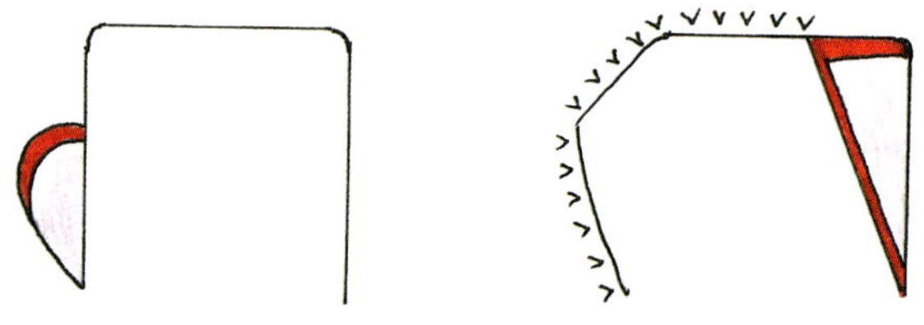

Figure 2.9 This is a transposition-flap technique, in which a large flap is needed for a small defect, and a secondary defect is created. This method is seldom used in this book. Indications would be defects of the hairy scalp.

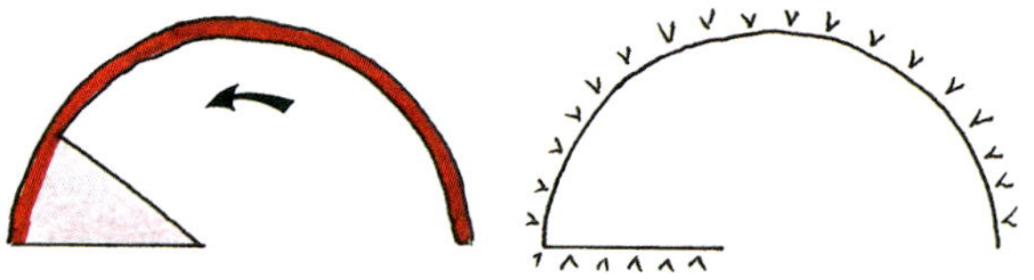

Figure 2.10 The rotation flap is used for covering of small to medium defects. In this method no donor site defect occurs. This technique is performed mainly in the face, but sometimes also on the trunk.

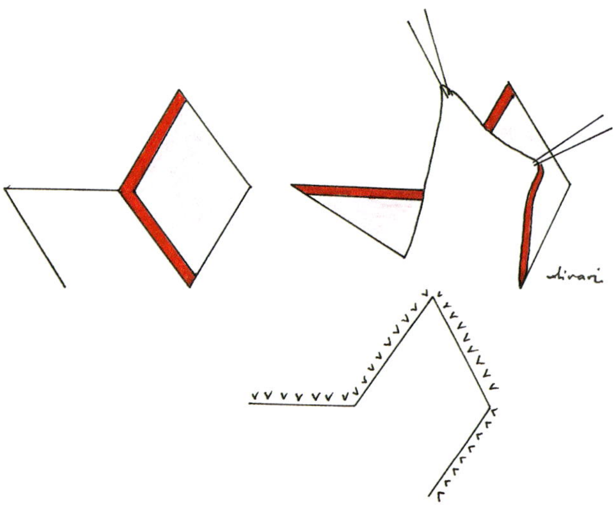

Figure 2.11 Limberg flap (1946)
This is a geometrically exact flap with acrid edges which can lead to minor circulation problems if the flap is under tension. The author favours a rounded flap. In most cases the Limberg flap is a good choice in the face.

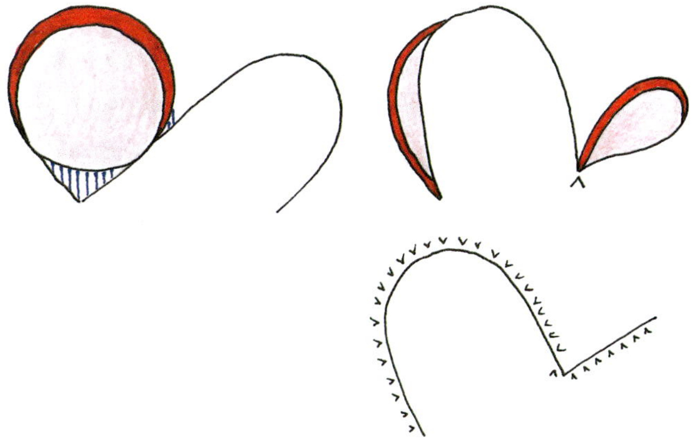

Figure 2.12 Transposition flap type I – transposition-rotation flap (Schrudde)
In round defects the secondary defect is primarily closed. Tension occurs around the donor site and it is important to elevate the flap in an area with elastic soft tissue.

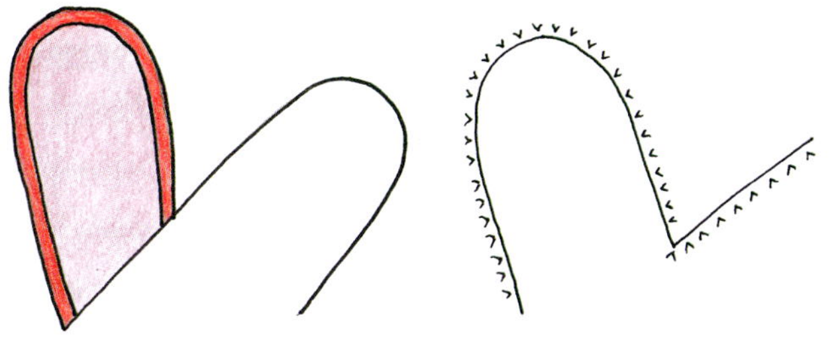

Figure 2.13 Transposition flap type II
The transposition flap type II is similar to type I, but is used in longer defects. Both types of flap (I and II) were commonly used by the author for face and trunk defects.

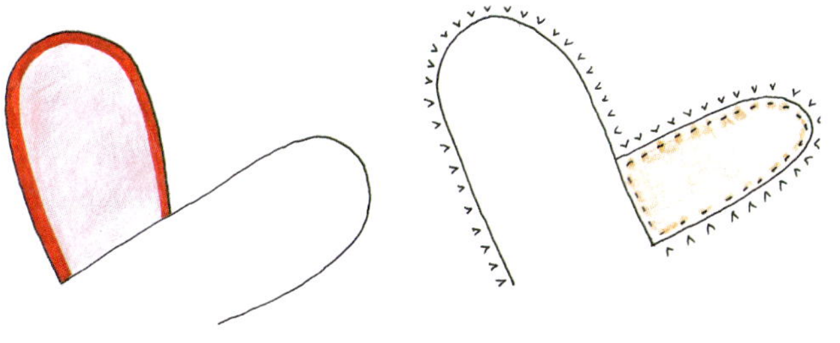

Figure 2.14 Transposition flap type III
Here the donor site is covered with split-thickness-skin graft. The secondary defect cannot be closed directly due to tension.

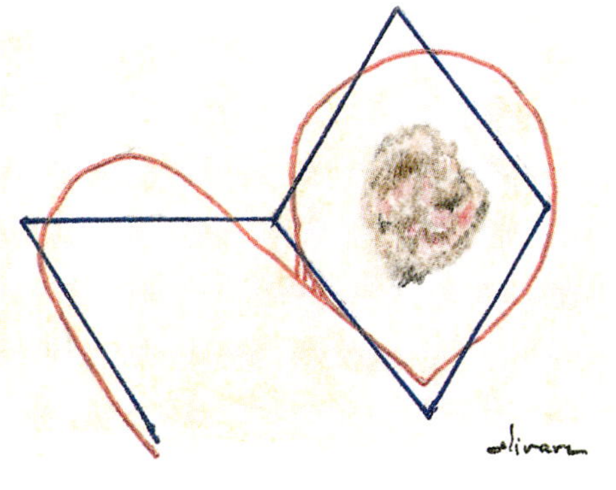

Figure 2.15 Comparison of a Limberg flap with a transposition-rotation flap. Both flaps accomplish the same function. The author has proved the transposition-rotation flap as successful as the Limberg flap, but with less problem with the tips of the flaps.

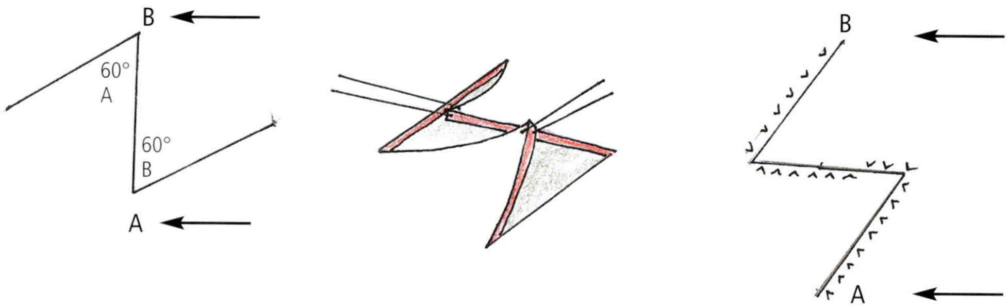

Figure 2.16a The Z-plasty is used for the purpose of lengthening of distance. In plastic surgery it is mostly exercised for correcting contractures. A Z-plasty with an angle of 60 degrees lengthens the contracted skin by about 60 percent. The technique may be used as either single or multiple Z-plasty.

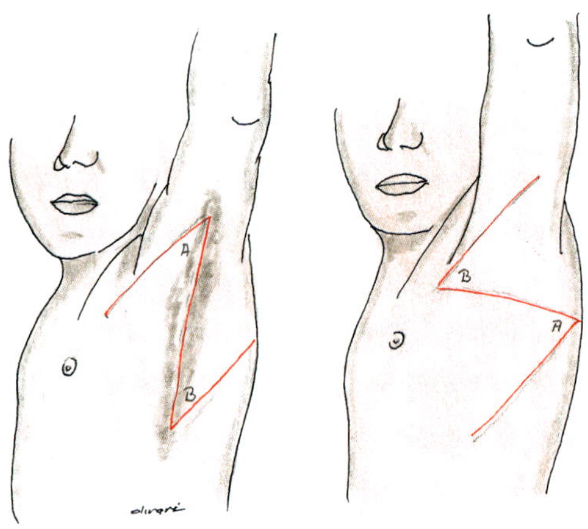

Figure 2.16b Contracture in the axilla after burn injury. The arm could only be abducted to an angle of 100 degrees. After the Z-plasty the range of motion is increased up to 180 degrees.

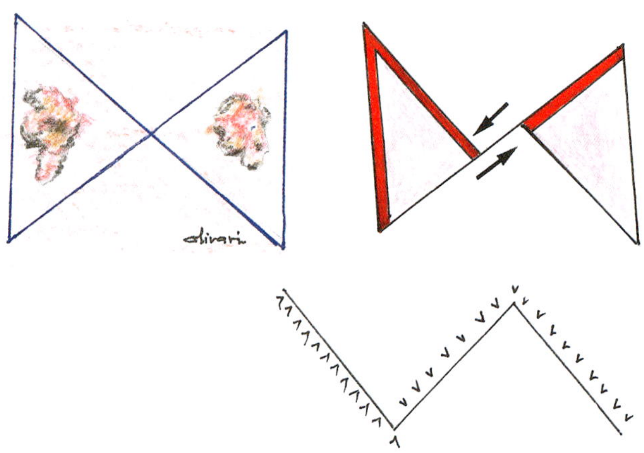

Figure 2.17 Double triangle-flap (Olivari)
In this case we have a double triangle-flap. It is very advantageous if two tumors of similar shape are located in adjacent locations.

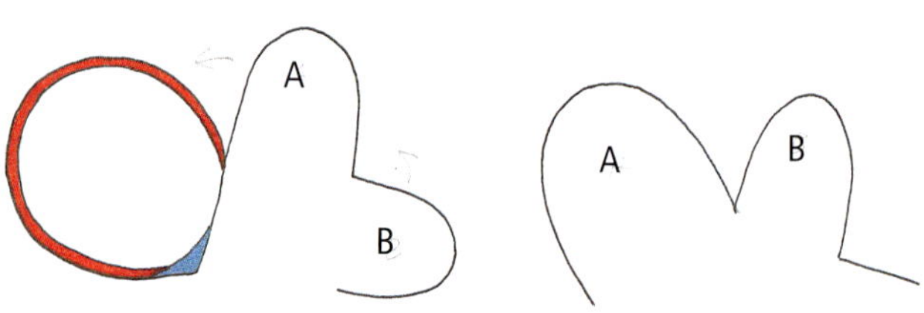

Figure 2.18 Bilobed flap (Esser 1918)
The bilobed flap allows cover of relative large defects with a larger (A) transposition flap. The secondary defect is closed with a smaller (B) flap. The donor site of flap B is primarily closed.

Rotation Flap after Esser

The father of facial rotation plasty is Esser (1918). He recommended an extensive mobilization, transposed the incision in front of the concha and lengthened the incision caudally. Mustardé has considerably improved this method.

Rotation Flap after Mustardé

In Mustardé type I the incision runs diagonally in a craniolateral direction. In the area of the ear lobe a small triangle is excised, so that rotation of the flap is possible without any tension. Extensive mobilization of the flap is important.

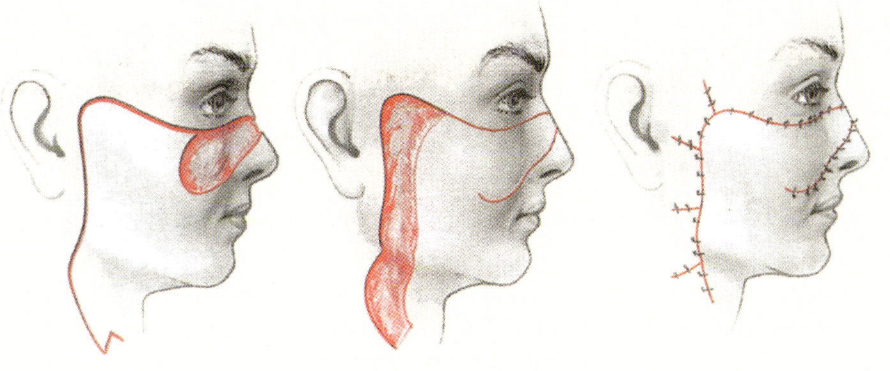

Figure 2.19 Cover of a partial defect of the lateral nose and the adjacent cheek with a cheek-rotation flap after Esser (1918).

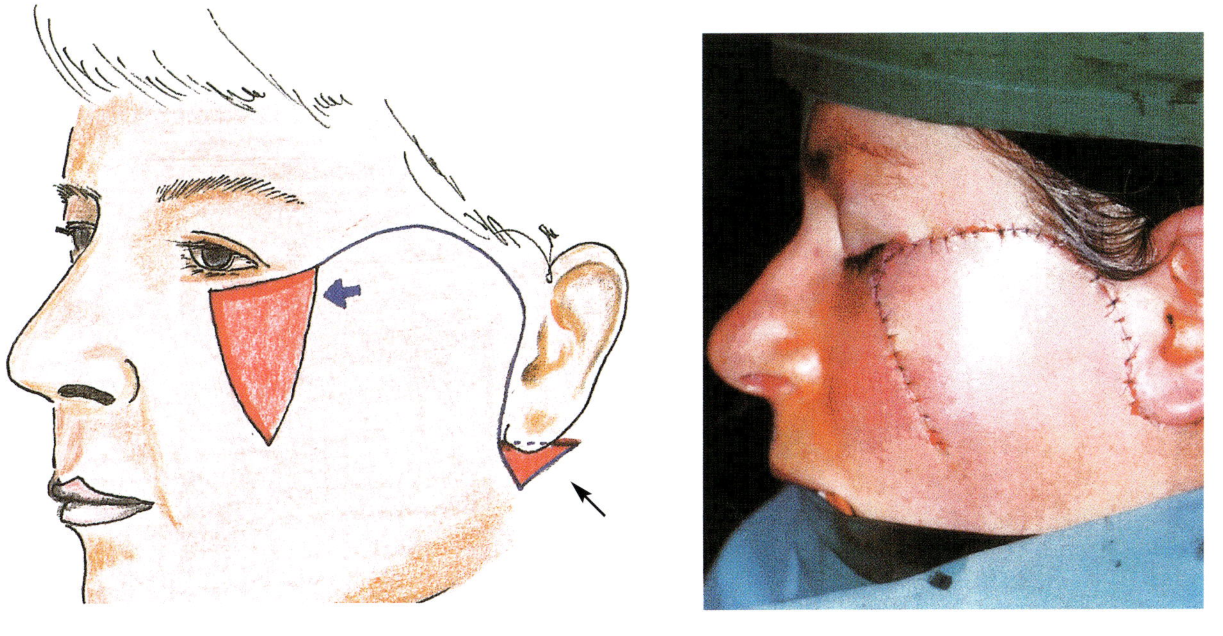

Figure 2.20 a Rotation flap after Mustardé. **b** Clinical case at the end of the operation

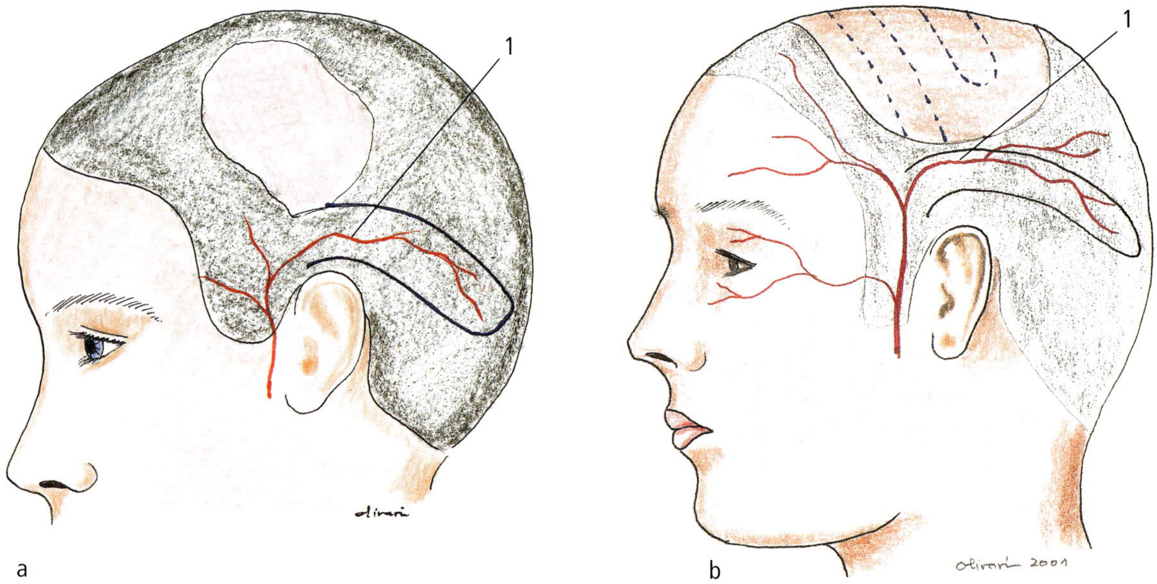

Figure 2.27 Juri flap. a Arterial (axial) flap in hairy skin (Juri flap). This flap can be up to 15 cm long, but only 2 to 3 cm in width. In Juri flaps the donor site is primarily closed. The blood supply is derived from the parietal branch of the temporal superficial artery (1). **b** Arterial flap (temporal superficial artery) in hairy skin. For cover of larger defects bilateral Juri flaps are used.

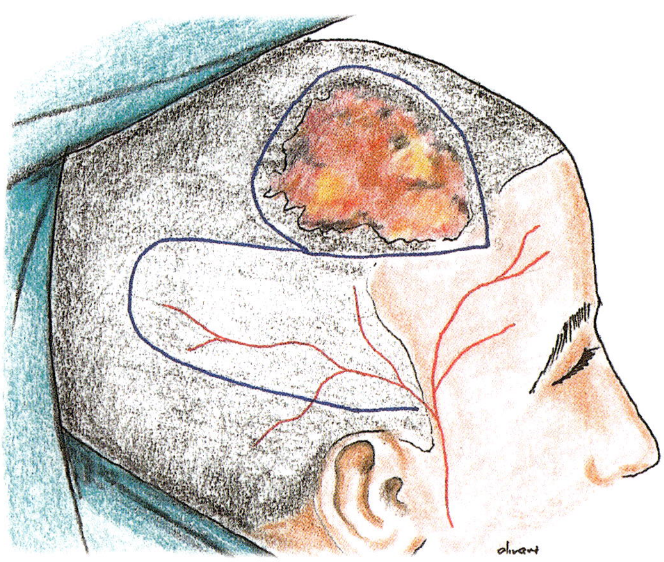

Figure 2.28 Transposition flap
In this wide arterial flap the donor site is closed with split-thickness-skin graft because of its width.

Rotation Flap after Esser

The father of facial rotation plasty is Esser (1918). He recommended an extensive mobilization, transposed the incision in front of the concha and lengthened the incision caudally. Mustardé has considerably improved this method.

Rotation Flap after Mustardé

In Mustardé type I the incision runs diagonally in a craniolateral direction. In the area of the ear lobe a small triangle is excised, so that rotation of the flap is possible without any tension. Extensive mobilization of the flap is important.

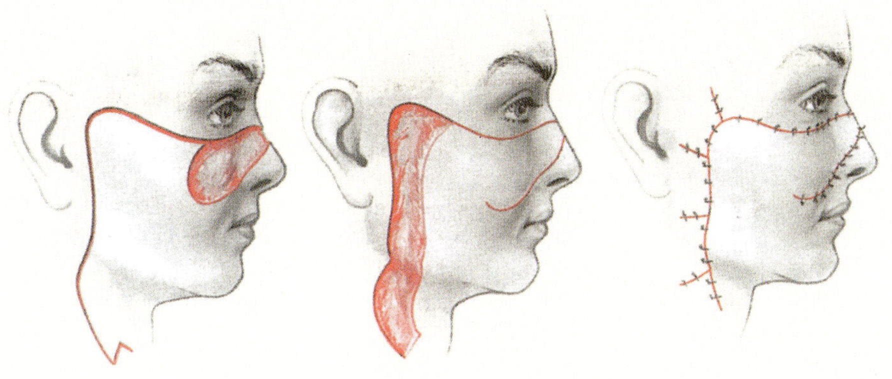

Figure 2.19 Cover of a partial defect of the lateral nose and the adjacent cheek with a cheek-rotation flap after Esser (1918).

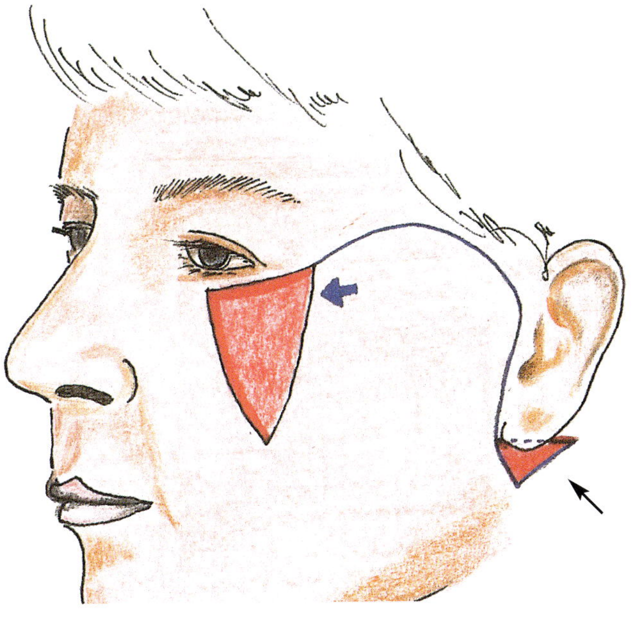

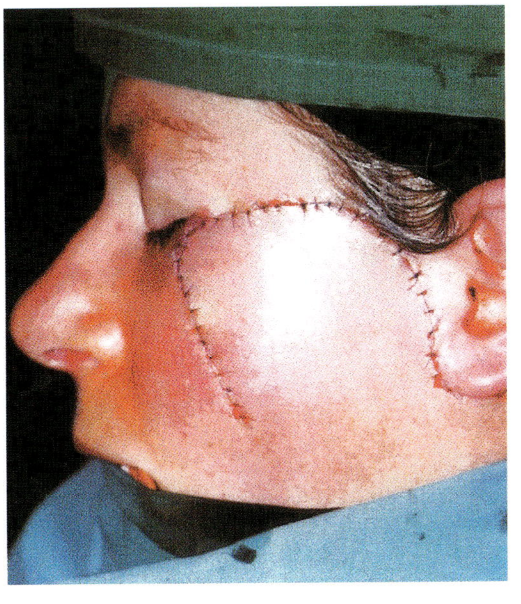

Figure 2.20 **a** Rotation flap after Mustardé. **b** Clinical case at the end of the operation

b) Arterial (Axial) Flaps

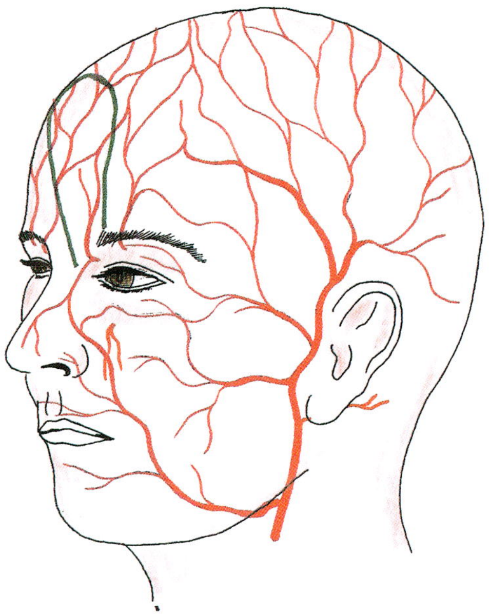

Figure 2.21 Vessel pattern in the axial forehead flap. "Indian method" (supplied by the supratrochlear artery)

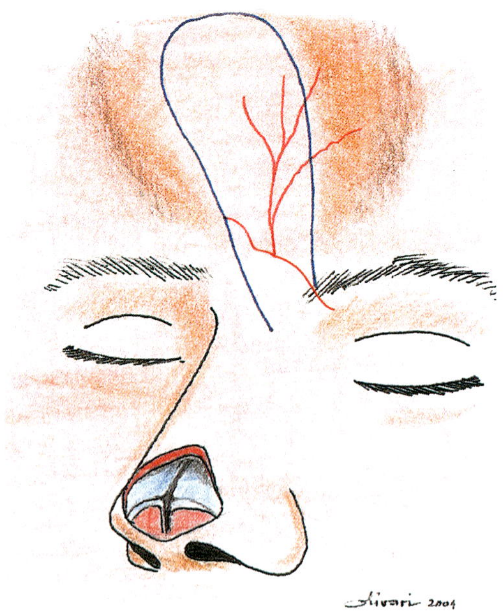

Figure 2.22 Axial forehead flap "Indian method" with expander. The tip of the flap is located at the contralateral side of the base.

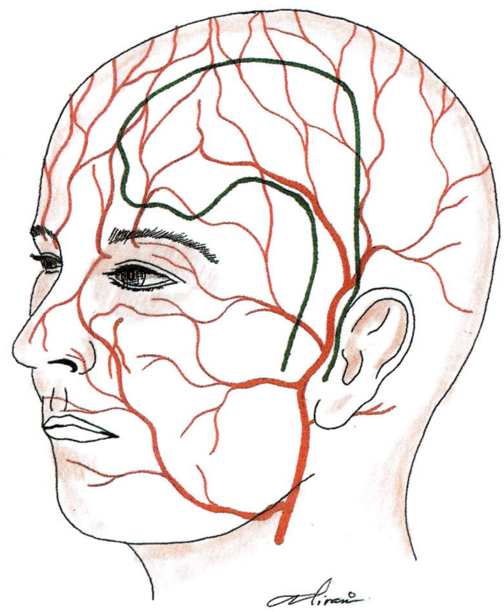

Figure 2.23 Temporo-frontal flap "sickle flap". This axial (arterial) flap is supplied by the A. temporalis superficialis and its frontal branch. This flap is convenient for cover of larger defects in the nasal area and also of the cheek area.

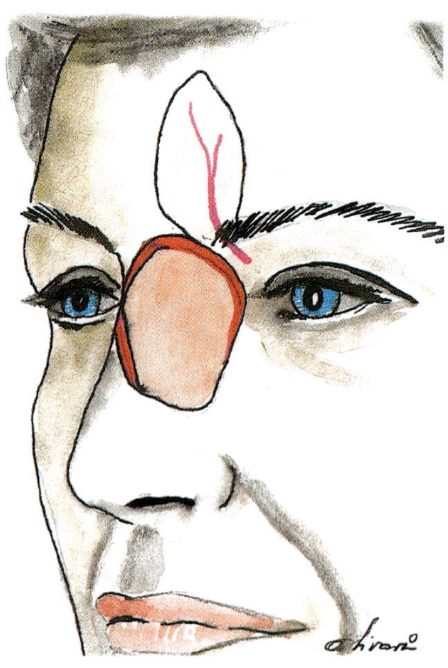

Figure 2.24 Small forehead flap (supratrochlearis flap). This technique is very suitable for defects in the upper nasal area and occasionally for defects in the area of the lower lid.

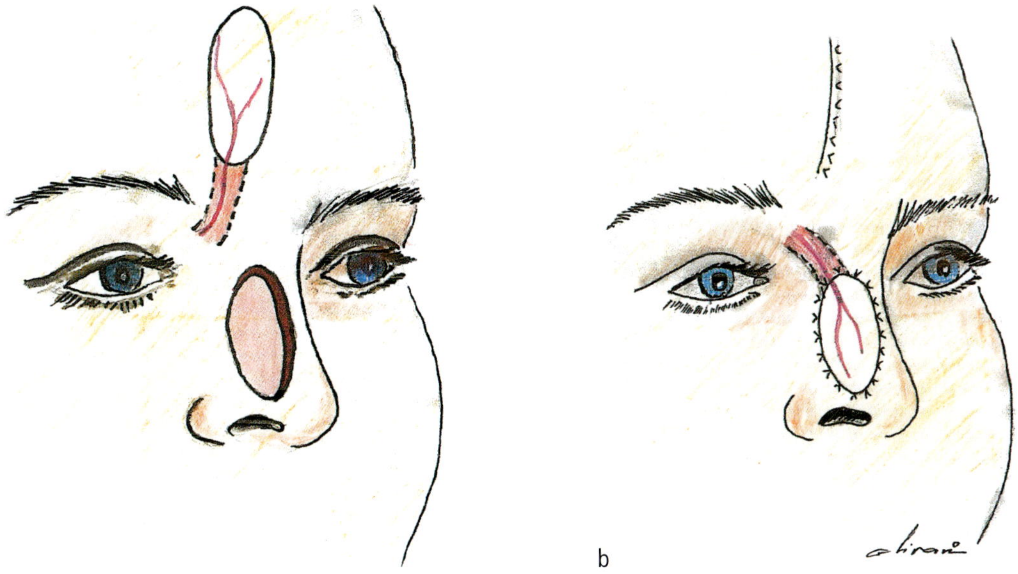

a b

Figure 2.25 **a** Arterial island flap (trochlearis island flap) for cover of defects in the nasal region. **b** During the transposition of the island flap through the tunnel the A. supratrochlearis must be protected; also, the pedicle must not be distorted because the blood supply could be endangered. Due to insufficient lymphatic drainage of the island flap temporary lymphedema is to be expected.

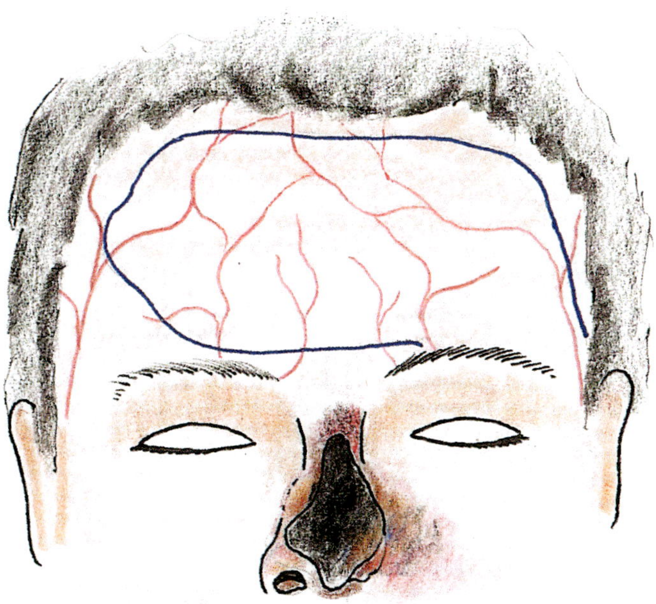

Figure 2.26 Transverse forehead flap (Converse) (scalping forehead flap) for cover of larger defects in the nose and cheek area. The Converse flap is advantageous for covering large defects. A disadvantage of this flap is the more extensive scar on the forehead. The motility of the forehead is abolished. Today one would use a free flap (forearm) or the Indian flap after expander distension.

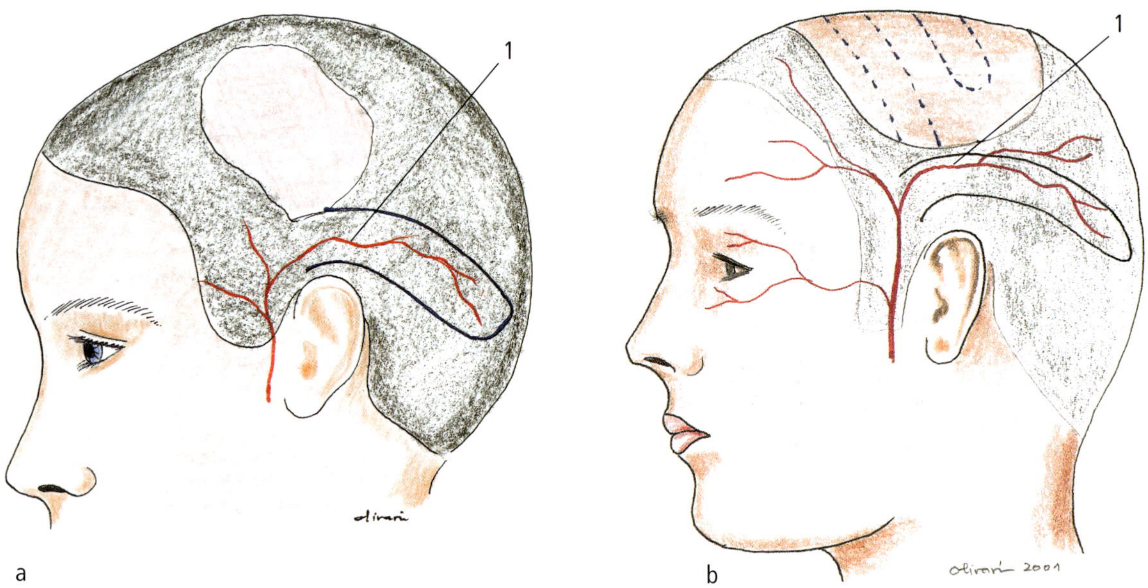

Figure 2.27 Juri flap. a Arterial (axial) flap in hairy skin (Juri flap). This flap can be up to 15 cm long, but only 2 to 3 cm in width. In Juri flaps the donor site is primarily closed. The blood supply is derived from the parietal branch of the temporal superficial artery (1). **b** Arterial flap (temporal superficial artery) in hairy skin. For cover of larger defects bilateral Juri flaps are used.

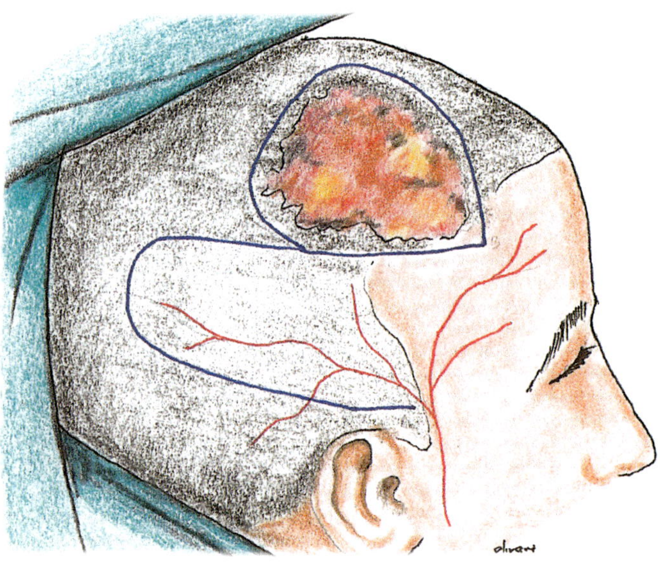

Figure 2.28 Transposition flap
In this wide arterial flap the donor site is closed with split-thickness-skin graft because of its width.

Scapular and Parascapular (Fasciocutaneous) Flap

Blood supply: The blood supply is derived from the circumflex scapular artery, of which the horizontal branch supplies the scapular flap and the inferior branch is responsible for the parascapular flap.

Indication: It is used as an island flap for cover of defects in the area of the axilla and shoulder. As a free flap it can be employed in any hairless head and neck area, in the hand, foreleg and foot.

Advantages: Relative easy operative access. The skin is of good color and hairless. The secondary defect is primarily closed. There is no known motor dysfunction. If the scapular and parascapular flap are prepared as one single flap (boomerang flap) larger defects can be closed. The scapular flap (A) and the parascapular flap (B) are very well suited for cover of medium size defects as free flaps, but also as island flaps for cover of defects in the axillary region.

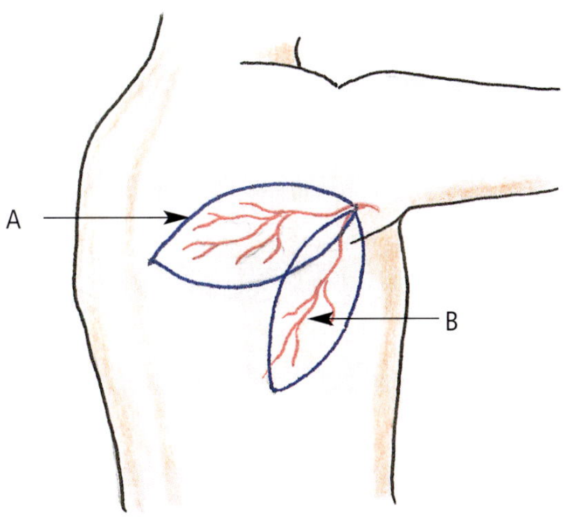

Figure 2.29 Circumflex scapular artery with horizontal and vertical cutaneous branch: Scapular flap (A), parascapular flap (B)

Epigastric Flap

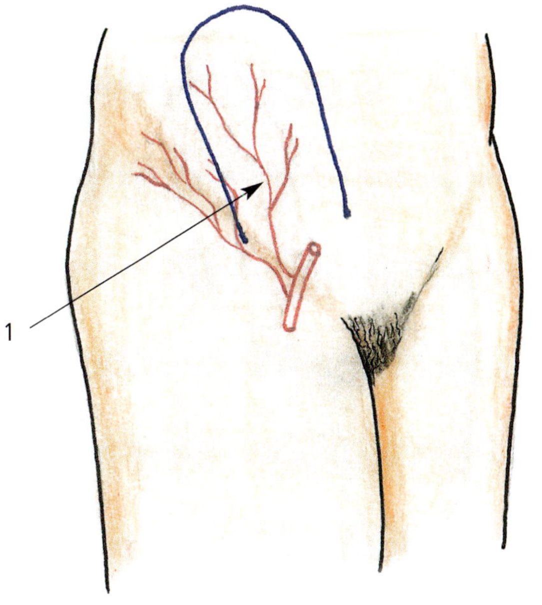

Figure 2.30a Epigastric flap with epigastric superficial inferior artery (1)

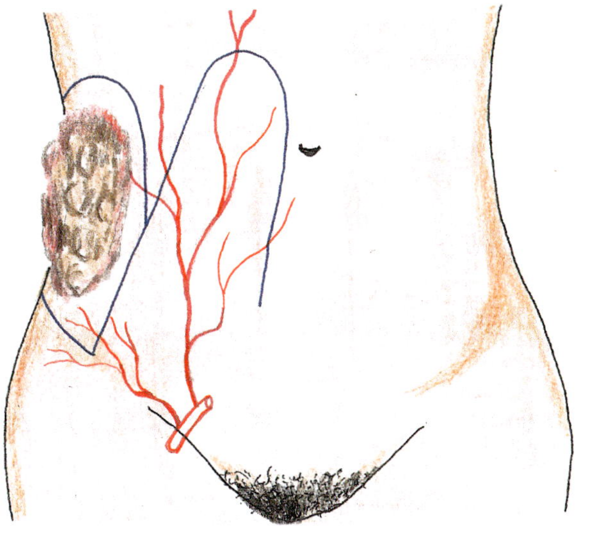

Figure 2.30b Epigastric flap. The flap is well suited as a pedicled flap for covering local defects. It is as well used as a free flap.

Groin Flap

The groin flap was one of the first and frequently used flaps in the cover of defects, especially in hand surgery; initially as a pedicled flap, tube pedicle flap and later on as free flap. The groin flap is historically the first free flap and was replaced later by other free flaps (latissimus, radialis, scapularis).

Blood supply: The flap is supplied by the circumflex iliac superficial artery. Because A. and V. communicantes run a long distance, this flap is defined as an arterial axial flap. The flap can be raised up to 30 cm long and 10 to 15 cm wide.

Indication: As pedicled flap for defects in the hand and forearm area; as free flap everywhere.

Advantage: In hand surgery this flap – if raised with a long pedicle – allows a comfortable position of the hand and early physiotherapy. The donor site is cosmetically inconspicuous; the skin in most cases is hairless.

Mind: As in all arterial flaps Doppler should be employed to examine the course of the vessels exactly.

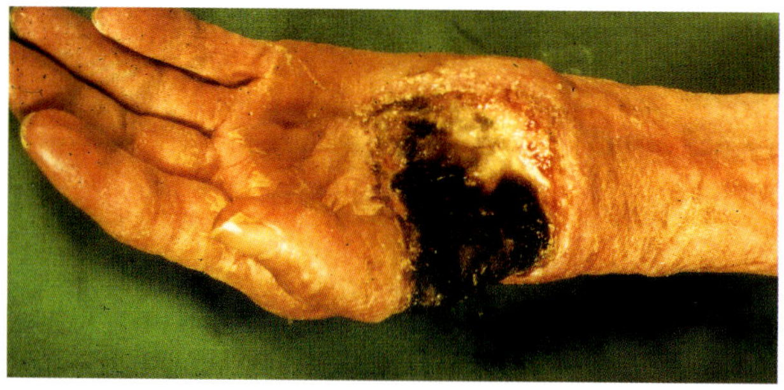

Figure 2.32a 84-year old woman with contact burn injury and diabetes.

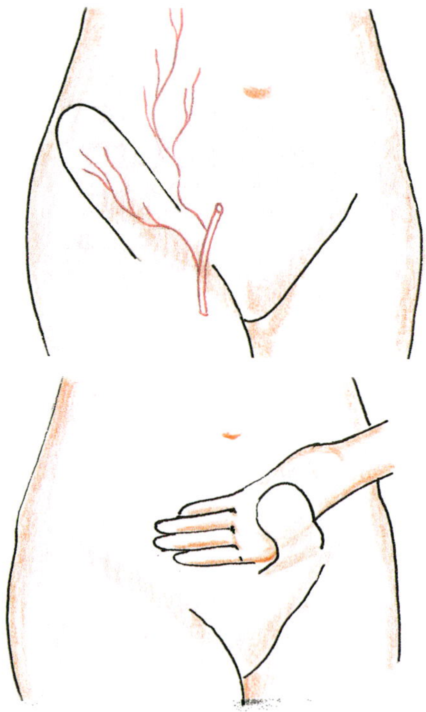

Figure 2.32b Planning of the operation.

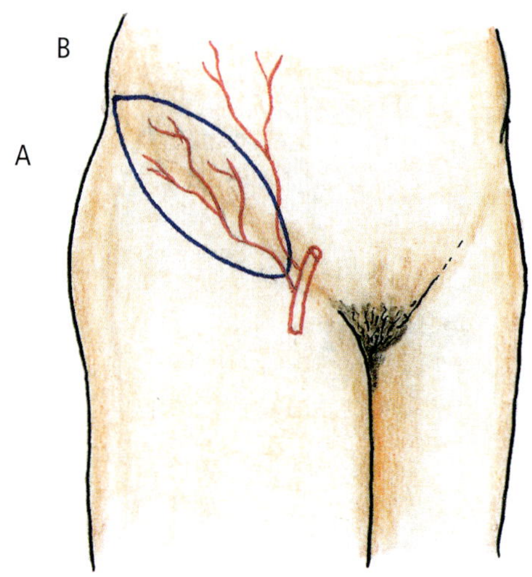

Figure 2.31 Circumflex superficial artery (A). Epigastric superficial inferior artery (B).

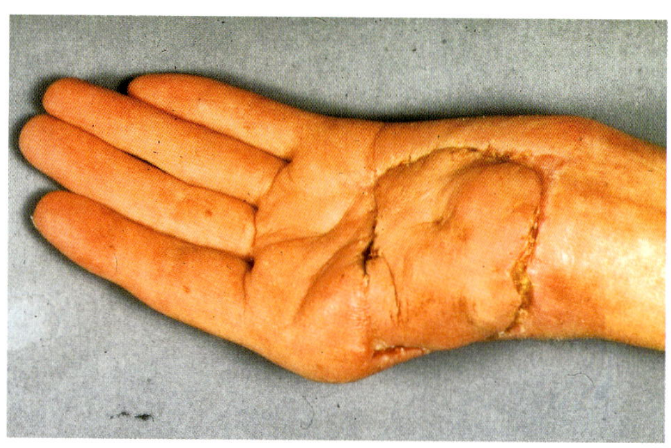

Figure 2.32c Operation: Necrectomy and amputation of the thumb, in which tendons, vessels and the metacarpophalangeal joint were destroyed. Cover of the defect with a groin flap.

Radialis Forearm Flap (Axial, Fasciocutaneous Flap)

The radialis forearm flap was developed by the Chinese and it was described a long time before the Europeans adopted the technique in the eighties. The radialis forearm flap is a versatile and safe fasciocutaneous flap, which can be used as free flap, but also as a distally pedicled island flap for defects in the hand. It is also suitable for coverage of defects in the elbow region as a proximally pedicled flap.

Anatomy: The flap is supplied by the radial artery which is the origin for many small branches which perforate the fascia antebrachii and nourish the skin. These perforating vessels are more numerous in the distal third than in the proximal third. The venous drainage is ensured by comitant veins and the superficial subcutaneous veins. Sensitivity is conducted by the N. cutaneus antebrachii, which is quite weak. So a free forearm flap as a neurovascular flap is only theoretically possible. In practice it is of little importance.

Indication: As a proximally pedicled flap it is well suited for defects in the elbow area. As a distally pedicled flap it can be used for covering defects in the hand and finger area. As a free flap it has multiple applications:

- Head and neck area
- Foreleg and foot area
- Genital area
- Combined with the radius as osteocutaneous flap or with involved tendons for the reconstruction of the Archilles tendon

Disadvantage: The sacrifice of the radial artery can lead to slight loss of power in the forearm muscles. Also cold intolerance in the hand area is described. Cosmetic disadvantages are the donor site. Before the operation an Allens test must be undertaken to check whether the A. ulnaris is sufficient for the blood supply of the Arcus palmaris.

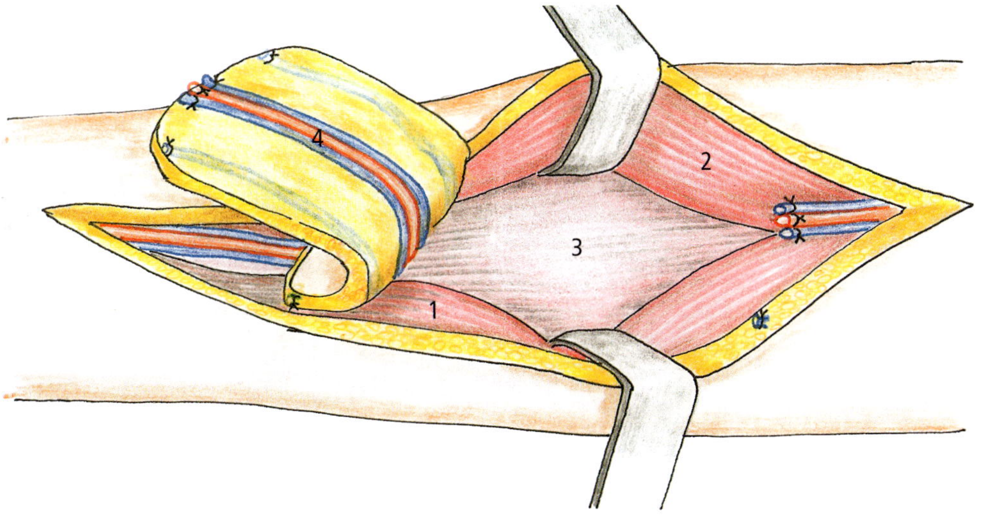

Figure 2.33 Elevation of the radialis forearm flap (distally pedicled). This flap is suitable for defects in the hand area. The radial artery and the comitant veins are compressed to test the blood supply of the flap and the hand. The blood supply is then released and the vessels are proximally ligated and cut through. The flap and the vessels can be prepared in a distal direction. 1) M. flexor digitorum superficialis, 2) M. flexor carpi radialis, 3) M. brachioradialis, 4) A. radialis, Vv. comitantes.

Distally Pedicled Radialis Island Flap

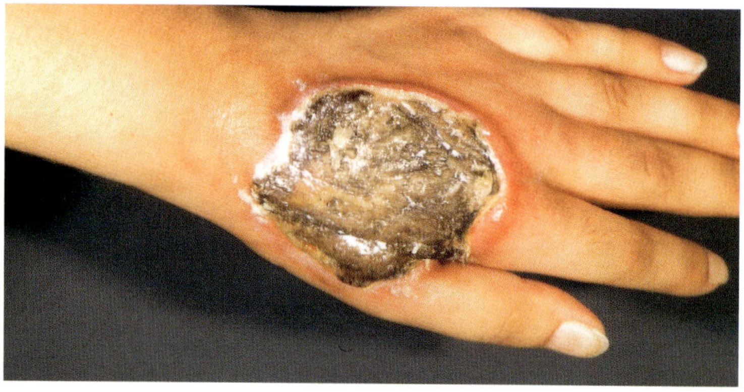

Figure 2.34a Necrosis on the back of the hand due to extravasation of chemotherapeutic agents.

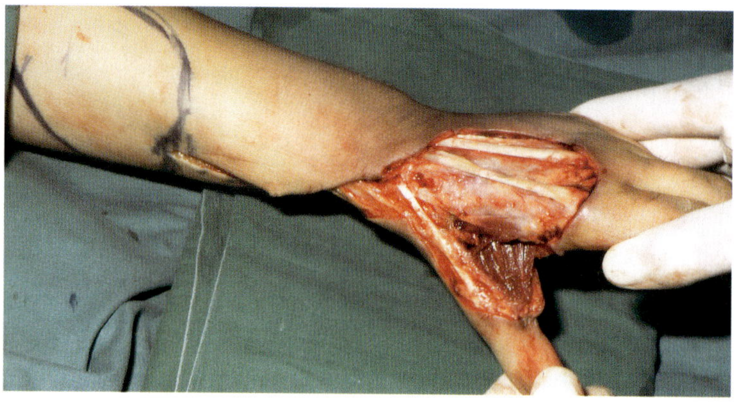

Figure 2.34b Thorough debridement of the necrotic tissue including the muscles.

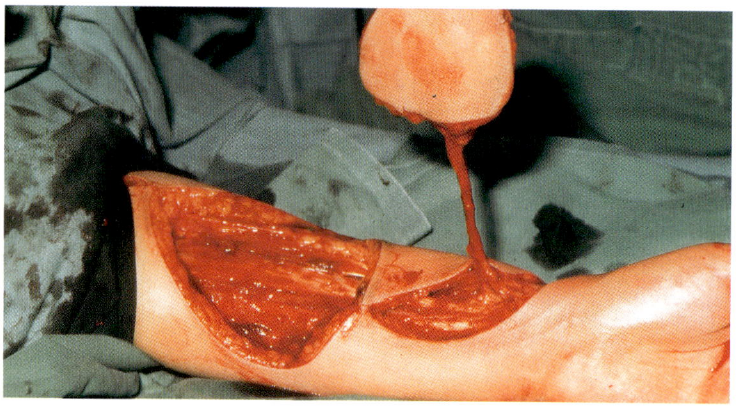

Figure 2.34c A distally pedicled radialis forearm flap is mobilized. It is important to plan carefully to avoid too short a pedicle.

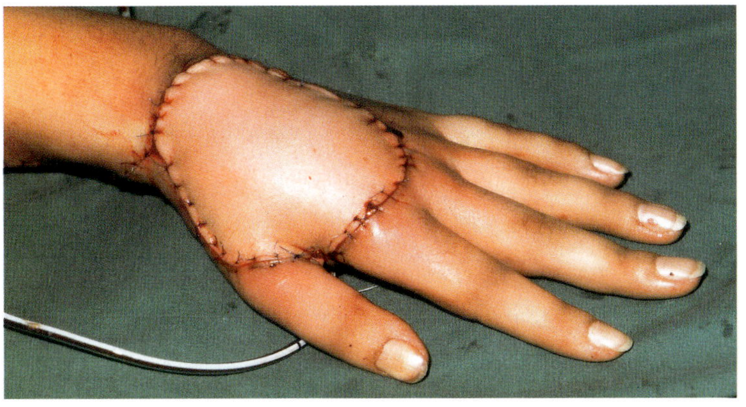

Figure 2.34d Result at the end of the operation.

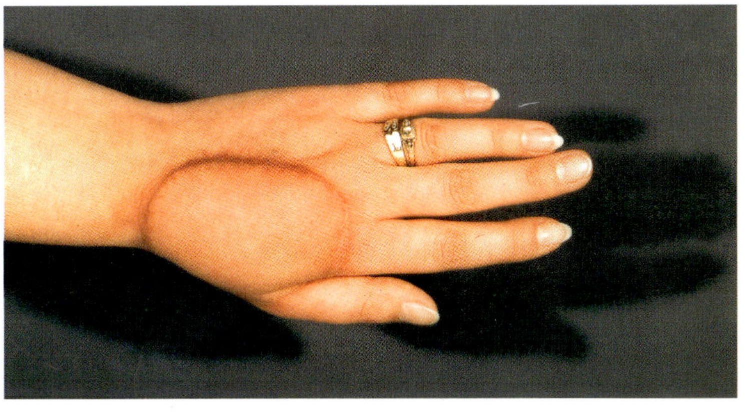

Figure 2.34e Result one year postoperatively.

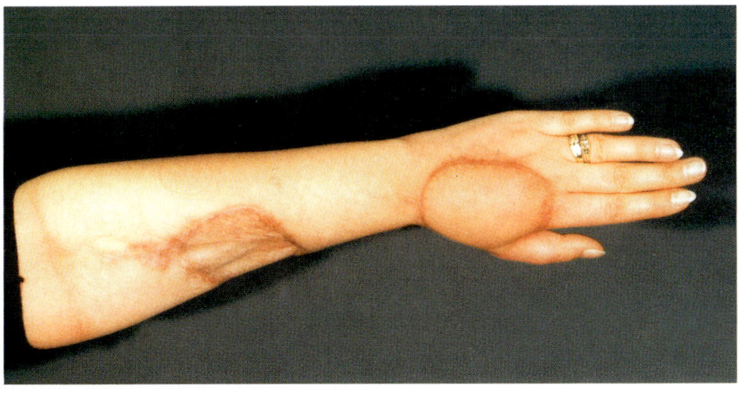

Figure 2.34f Radialis island flap and donor site.

Free Radialis Forearm Flap

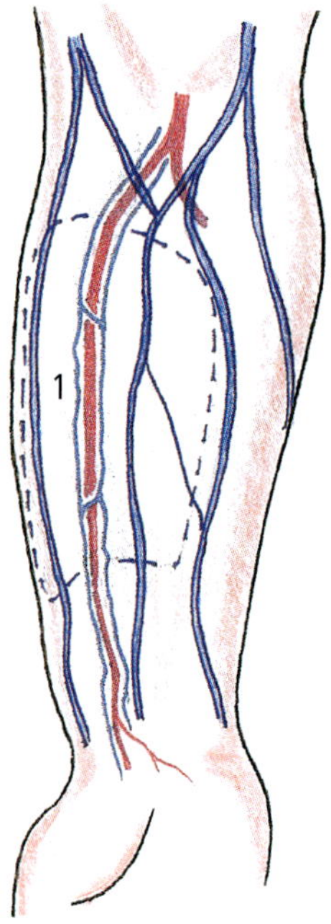

Figure 2.35 Radial artery with comitant veins (1) and superficial subcutaneous veins.

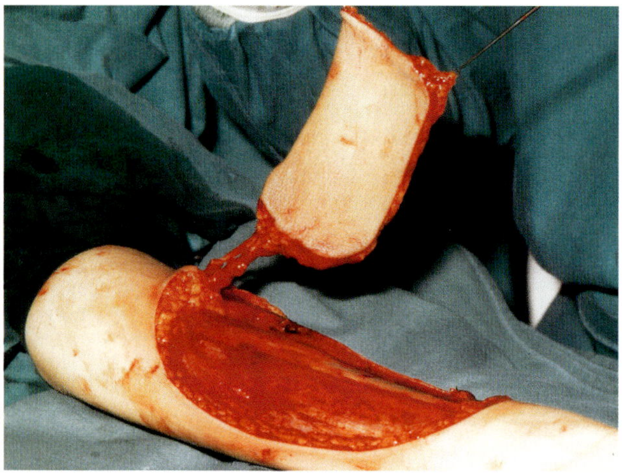

Figure 2.36 Mobilization of the flap with its vascular pedicle (proximal).

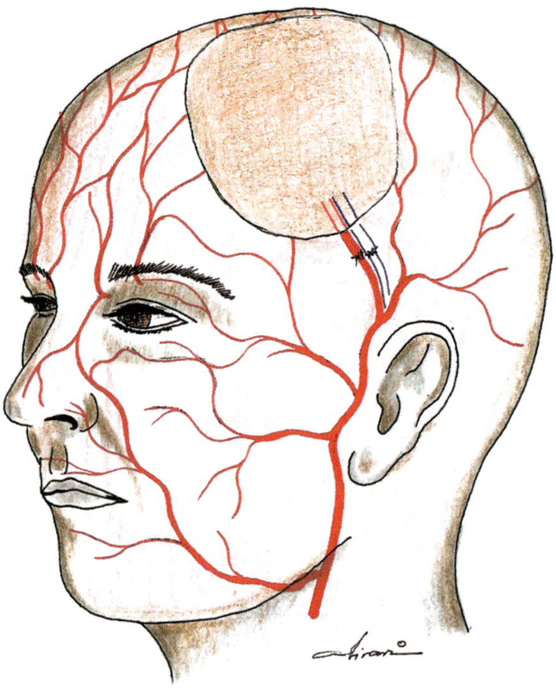

Figure 2.37 Free microsurgical radialis forearm flap for coverage of a defect on the head. The anastomosis is performed between the radial vessels and the system of the temporal-superficial artery.

The Plantaris Medialis Flap

This is a flap with a good blood supply, which is innervated by the N. plantaris medialis. The island flap is pedicled at the plantar medial artery and vein. It is a fasciocutaneous flap which is well suited for closure of defects of the heel, foot and Achilles tendon region. The secondary defect is covered with mesh-graft and is located in non weight bearing area.

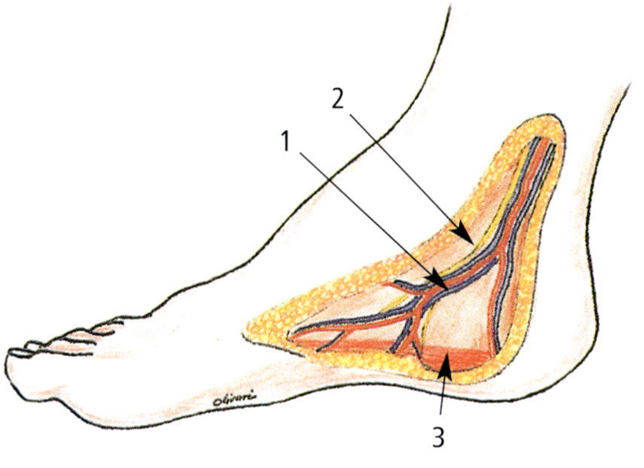

Figure 2.38 Anatomical situation:
1 A.V. plantaris medialis
2 N. plantaris medialis
3 M. abductor hallucis

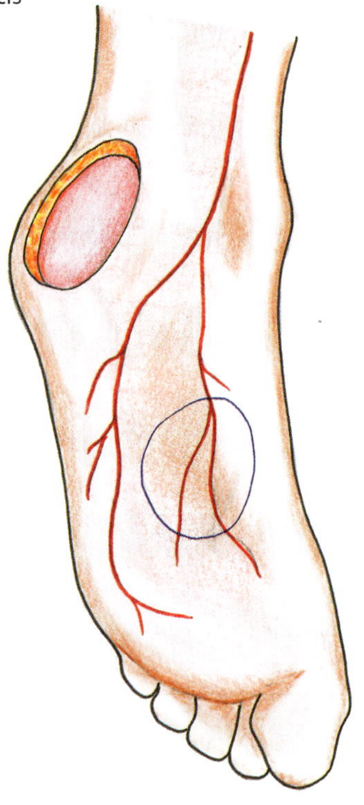

Figure 2.39 Schematic demonstration of the plantaris medialis flap.

The Lateral Calcaneal Flap

The lateral calcaneal flap is a fasciocutaneous flap which can be used as a pedicled or island flap. It is suitable for cover of defects in the lower part of the Archilles tendon. It is not adequate for the lower part of the heel because its skin is not very robust. Inferiorly, the medial plantaris flap is more suitable. The blood supply is derived from the peroneal artery, malleolar lateral anterior artery and the lateral calcaneal artery. The venous drainage is conducted by the V. saphena parva. If the N. suralis is incorporated in the pedicle of the flap, it can be used as a sensate flap (Figure 2.40).

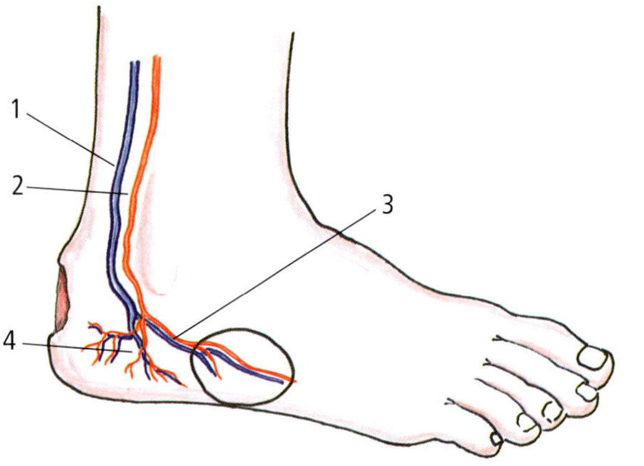

Figure 2.40 Lateral calcaneal fasciocutaneous arterial flap (island flap). V. saphena parva (1), A. peronea (2), A. calcanea lateralis (3), A. malleolaris lateralis anterior (4).

c) Musculocutaneous Flap

Pedicled Latissimus Dorsi Flap

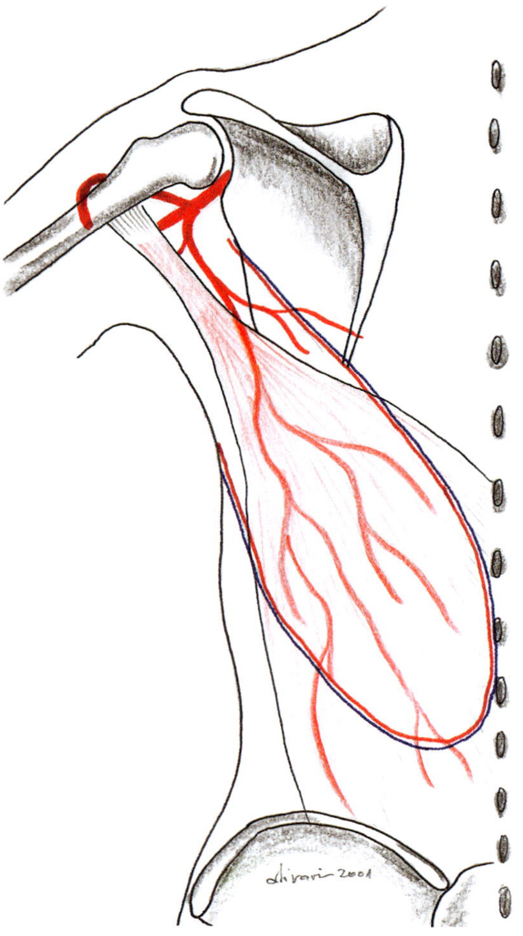

Figure 2.41 Pedicled latissimus dorsi flap for coverage of thoracic defects. The latissimus dorsi flap is an axial musculocutaneous flap. It is vascularized by the thoracodorsal artery and vein and receives innervation from the thoracodorsal nerve. This pedicled or island flap is appropriate to cover defects in the frontal part of the chest and the lower part of the face, neck and shoulder. Moreover this kind of muscular flap can be used as compensatory biceps or triceps muscle. The microvascular latissimus dorsi flap is the most common flap for many locations of the body.

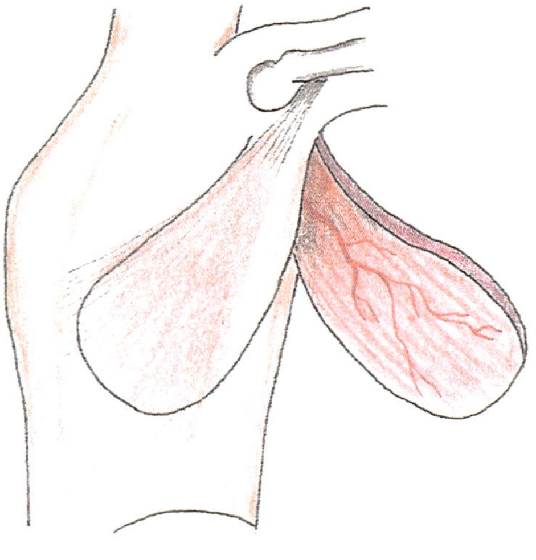

Figure 2.42a Pedicled latissimus dorsi flap for coverage of frontal thoracic defects

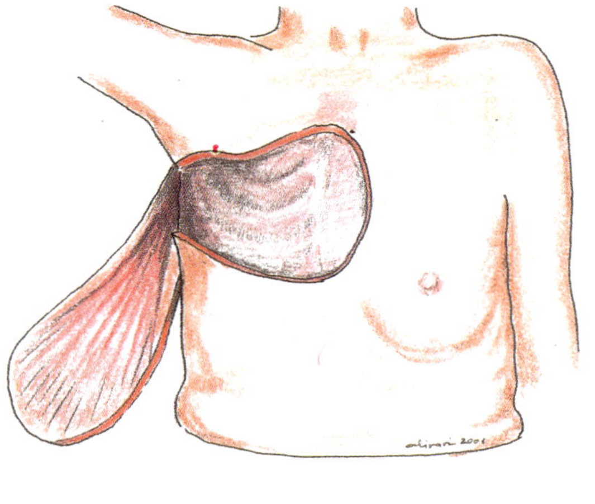

Figure 2.42b Attend to the great mobility of the flap. Thereby it is possible to adapt different forms and sizes of the flap according to the defects. Its range of coverage widely overlaps the midline.

Extreme Large Pedicled Latissimus Dorsi Flap

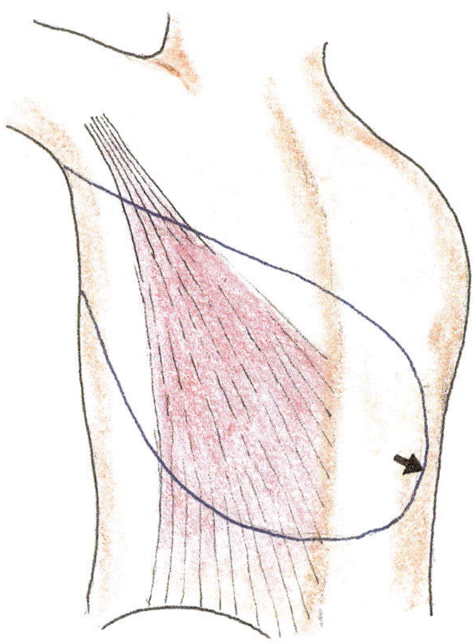

Figure 2.43a Extending the flap across the spinal column to the contralateral side is possible.

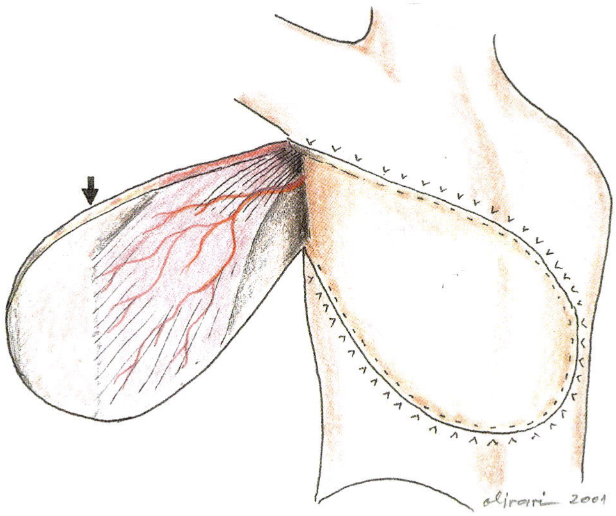

Figure 2.43b Vascular supply of the distal third is not anymore "musculocutaneous", it is random pattern. Nevertheless the perfusion is safe (approx. 10 cm above the muscle frame). In case of a very large flap the secondary defect should be covered with mesh graft.

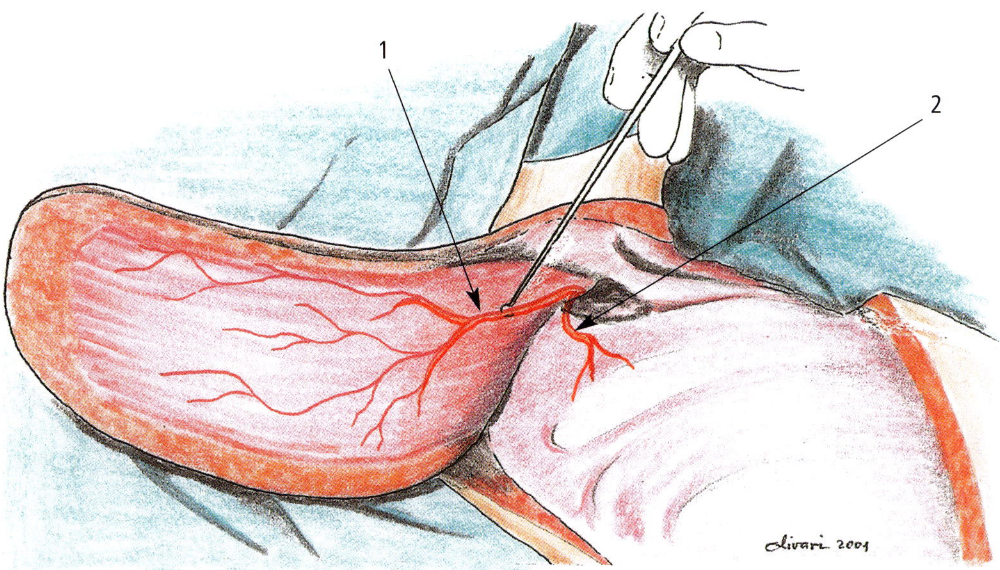

Figure 2.44 The dominant blood supply of the latissimus dorsi muscle is derived from the thoracodorsal artery (1) with numerous perforating vessels to the skin. One branch leads to the serratus anterior muscle (2).

Open Defect of the Thorax With Rib Excision

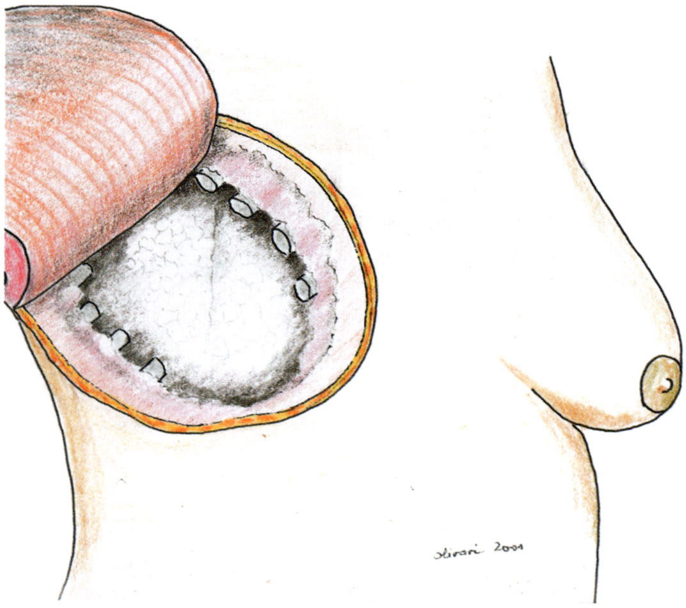

Figure 2.45a Status after resection of the thoracic wall caused by recurrence of a carcinoma, resection of four ribs, the visceral pleura stays intact.

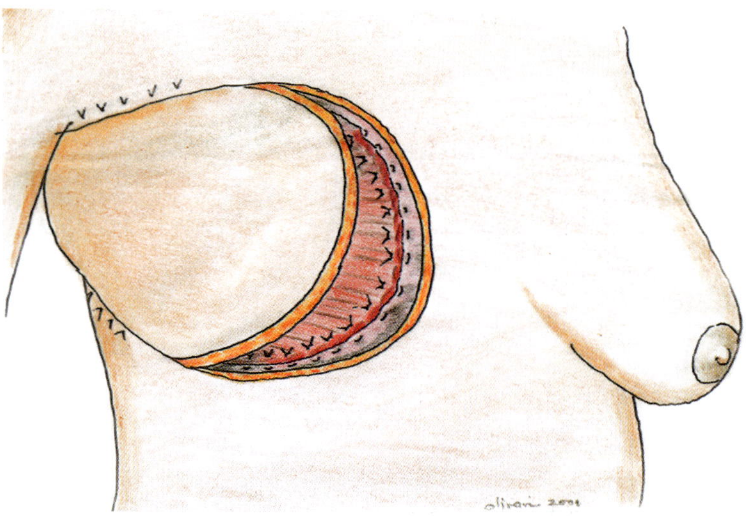

Figure 2.45b Before covering the defect with a latissimus dorsi flap the muscle should be fixed to the intercostal muscles to seal up the thoracic space. Then follows the dermal suture.

Latissimus Dorsi Island Flap

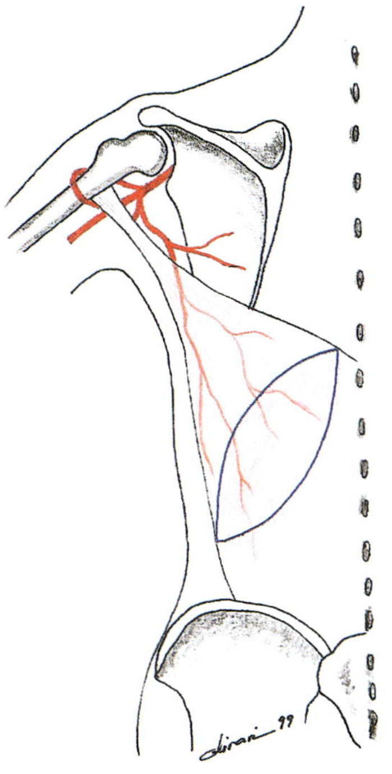

Figure 2.46a Position of the island flap: This direction allows to perform larger flaps and leave lesser visible scars.

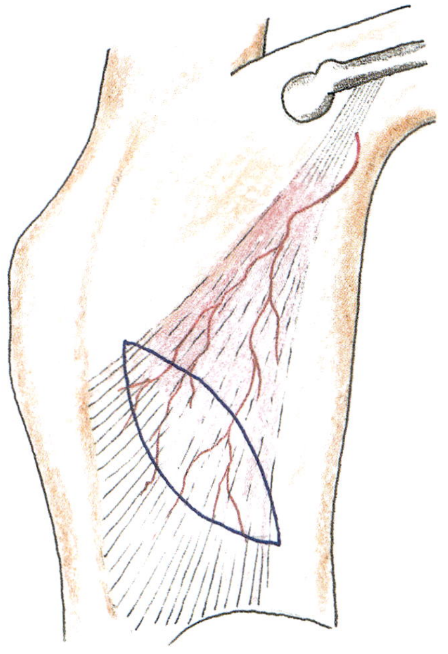

Figure 2.46b The course of latissimus dorsi island flap takes preferentially place from cranio-medial to latero-caudal.

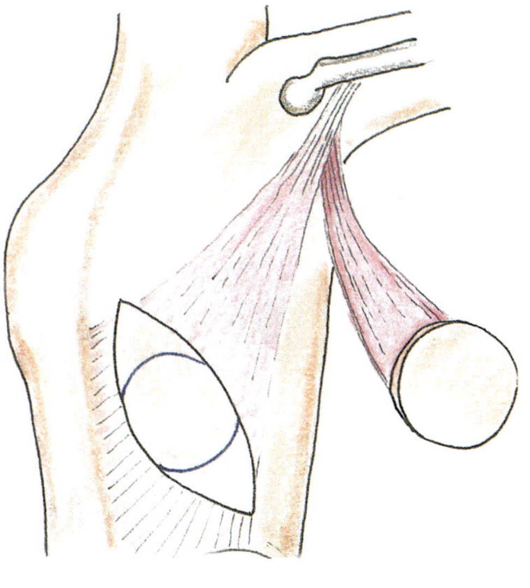

Figure 2.47a In the case of a more circular defect, a spindle-shaped island flap should be taken and fit into the form of the defect.

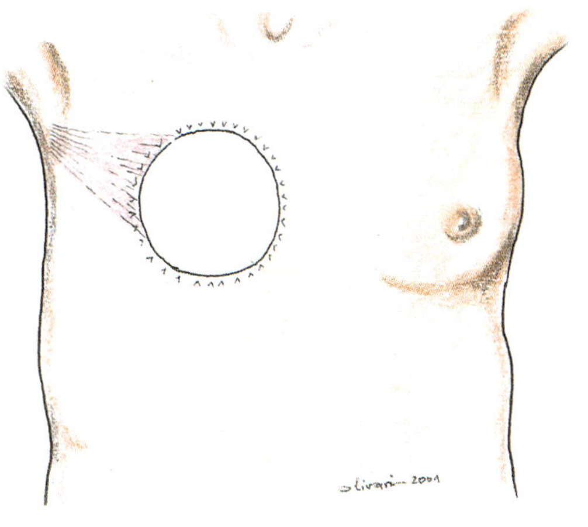

Figure 2.47b Situation at the end of the operation.

Pedicled Musculocutaneous TRAM Flap (Hartrampf)

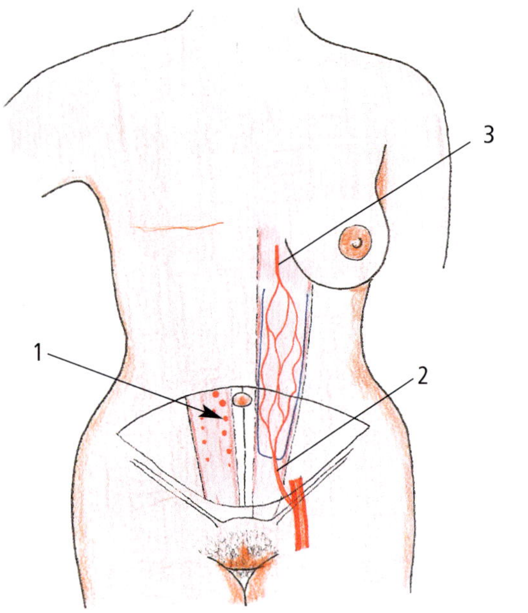

Figure 2.48a Unilaterally pedicled TRAM flap from the opposite site. The perforators are shown on the right side (1) (if necessary: duplex sonography).
The two or three strongest perforators are latero-caudal of the umbilicus. Profound epigastric inferior artery (2).

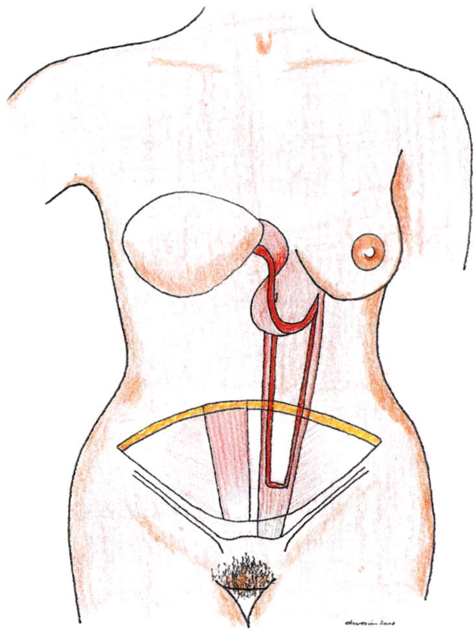

Figure 2.48b For a unilateral TRAM flap the perforators of the opposite side have to be identified first. They are almost always symmetric. The vascularization is now based on the less dominat superior epigastric artery (3).

Turbo-TRAM

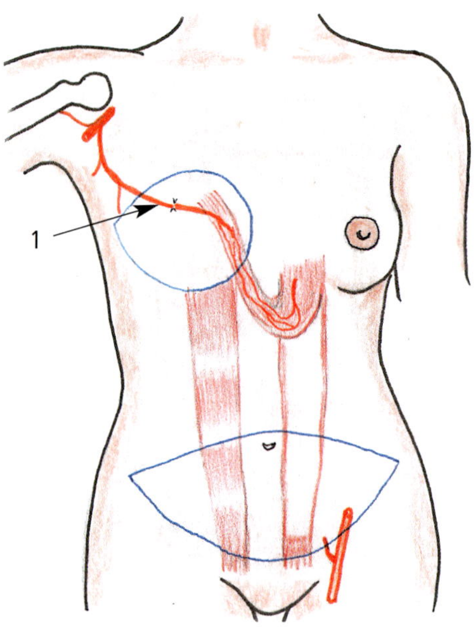

Figure 2.49a The operation is similar to the pedicled TRAM flap, but the pedicle of the deep epigastric inferior artery is dissected as long as possible. The epigastric artery is anastomosed with the thoracodorsal artery (1).

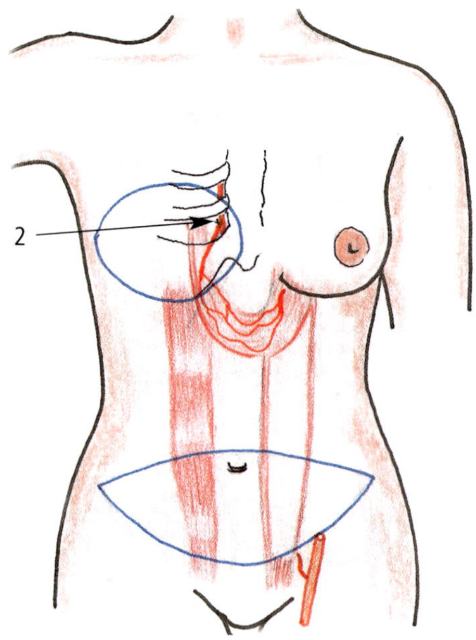

Figure 2.49b Here is the anastomosis of the epigastric artery with the mammaria interna artery (2). The Turbo-TRAM is considerable to be better perfused than a standard pedicled TRAM flap. In fact this is the best vascularized TRAM flap.

Free TRAM Flap (Holmström 1979)

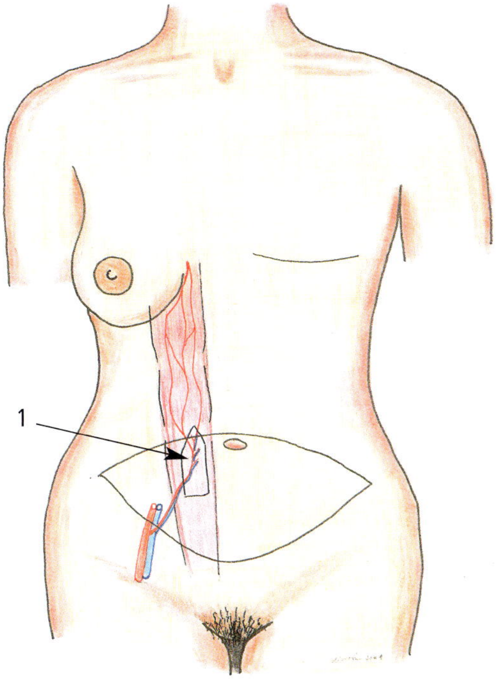

Figure 2.50a Status after mastectomy of the left breast. A free TRAM flap of the right side will be planned. Marking of the perforators the epigastric artery and vein after identification will be dissected and prepared towards caudal to keep the pedicle as long as possible. A small part of rectus abdominis muscle (1) will be taken.

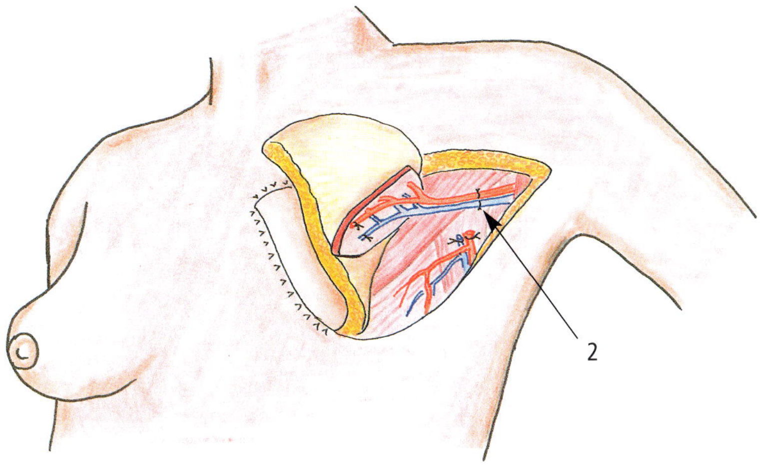

Figure 2.50c The free TRAM flap is anastomosed to the thoracodorsal artery.

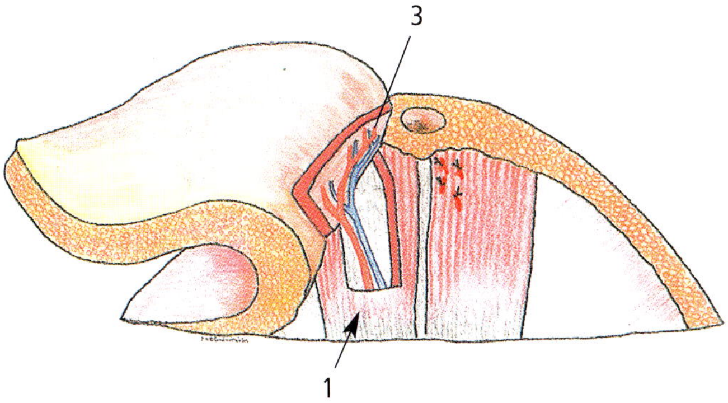

Figure 2.50b Just a small part of the rectus abdominis muscle will be taken along with the TRAM flap (3). On both sides the muscle strips are kept adequately broad. This allows an easier closing of the defect and avoids possible hernia development.

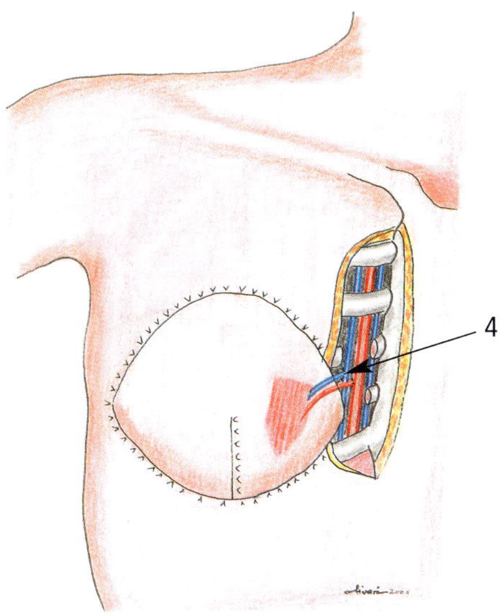

Figure 2.50d The free TRAM flap is preferably anastomosed to the A. and V. mammaria interna (4). This makes it easier to form the chest; the thoracodorsal artery stays intact. Of course not in case of irradiated thorax.

Trapezius Flap

The trapezius flap is a myocutaneous flap. The trapezius muscle is supplied by the rami cutanei of the transversa colli artery (1), one part of the occipital artery (2) and by paravertebral perforators. It is only used as a pedicled flap and hence with a mediocranial (mostly) or a mediocaucal basis. The trapezius flap serves for coverage of defects in the area of neck and shoulder. The secondary defect is covered with split thickness skin graft most times, a primary closure is rarely possible (see Chapter Torso).

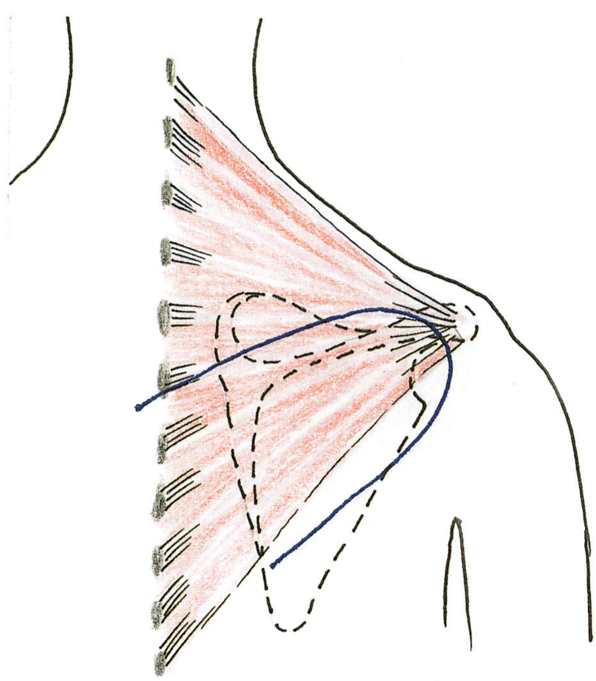

Figure 2.51a Trapezius flap with medio-caudal pedicle

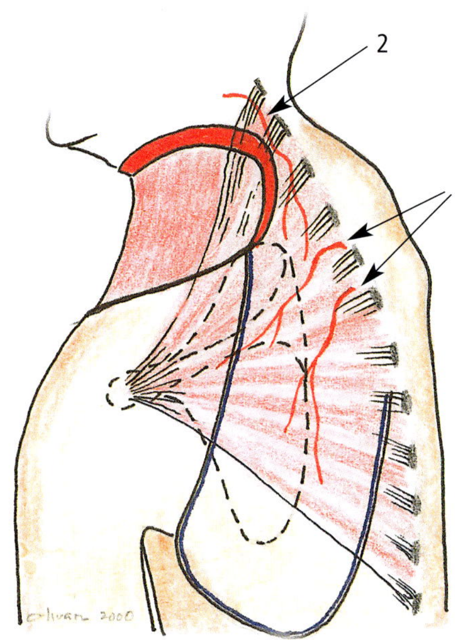

Figure 2.51b Trapezius flap with medio-cranial pedicle

d) Cross-Leg Flap

The cross-leg flap is the traditional procedure for covering defects of lower leg and feet. Today, however, this procedure is used only very rarely because free flaps are frequently used. Nevertheless there are indications for this technical easy operation. Microsurgery service is not provided all over the world. Planning is extremely important for this kind of flap. Basically it should be a fasciocutaneous flap, because of safe perfusion. The immobilization (with cast or better with an external fixator) should last 3 to 4 weeks. 14 days after operation one can apply temporary compression of the flap base with a soft gut clamp to test if the perfusion is sufficient. In doubt the immobilization should be extended for one week. We recommend a donor area beneath popliteal space for defects in the area of Achilles tendon. The secondary defect can easily be covered with local flaps.

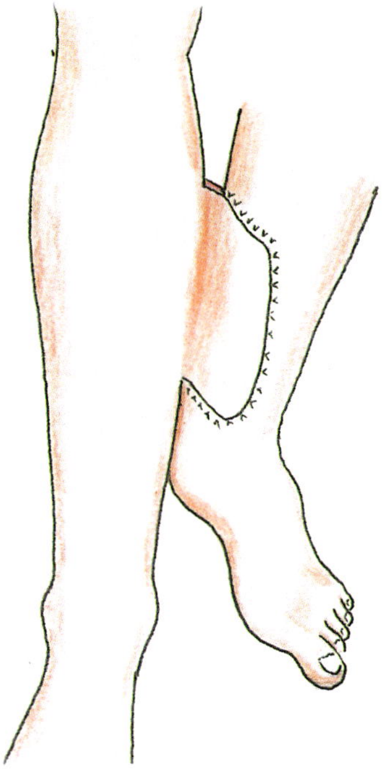

Figure 2.52c Defect closure at the lower leg (large)

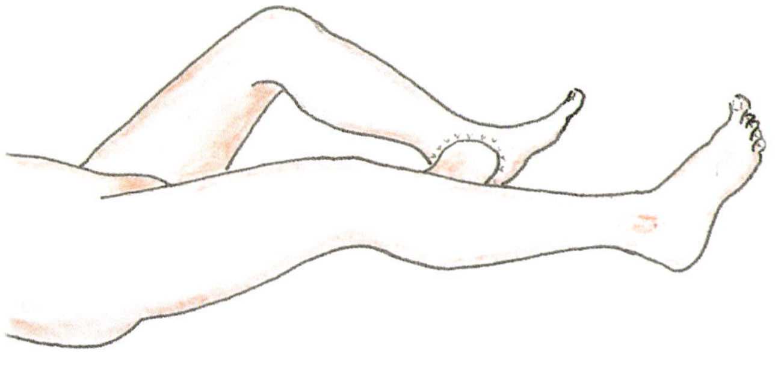

Figure 2.52a Defect occlusion in the area of Achilles tendon

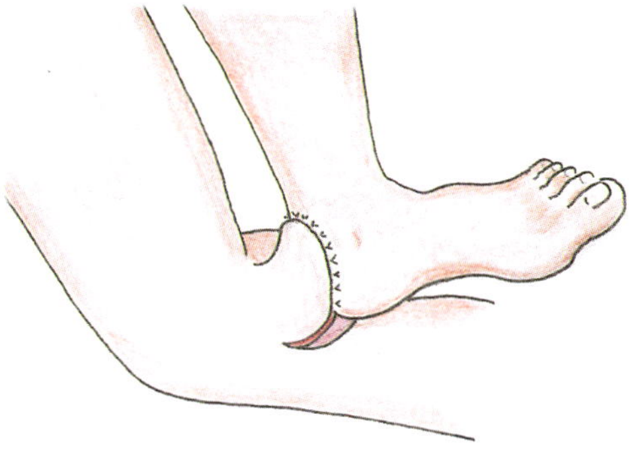

Figure 2.52b Defect closure in the area of the heel

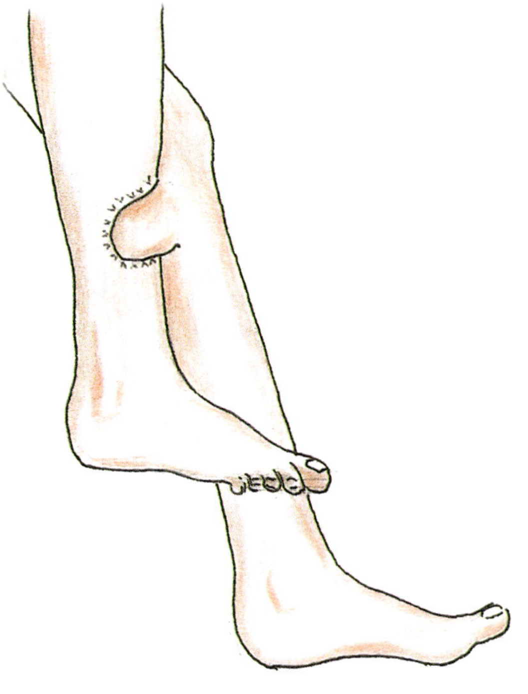

Figure 2.52d Defect closure at the lower leg (small)

e) Tube Flap

The tube flap is one of the oldest methods in plastic surgery and gain fame through Filatov and Gillies. This method became popular in First World War for treatment of many injured people and was used frequently up to the seventies when the free flaps were introduced.

Principle:
Firstly a bipedicled flap is performed, which is formed as a tube in the middle area to prevent an open wound. After three to four weeks one end will be separated and fixed into the defect. The other end will stay in the original place for another three weeks. After that the proximal end will be separate and the flap will be used to cover the defect.

The most common donor site is around the groin, but there are also cervical and abdominal donor areas. Tube flaps are used rarely, because free flaps are more common now.

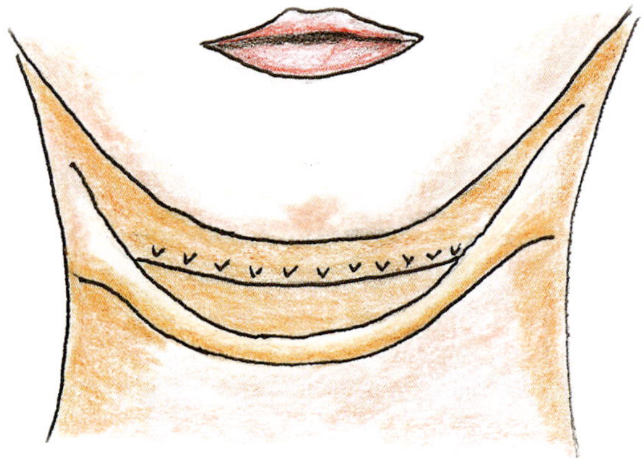

Figure 2.54a Preparation of a tube flap of the neck for front defect coverage.

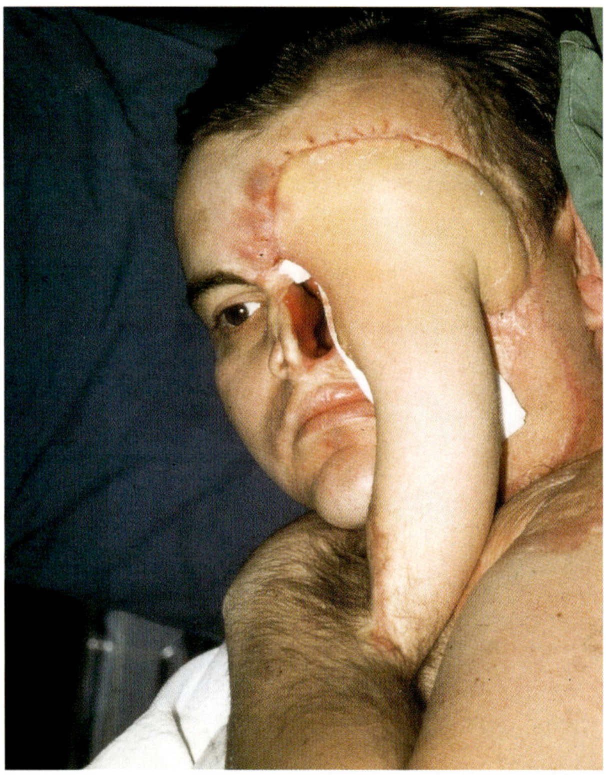

Figure 2.53 Tube flap of the groin and lower abdominal wall, which was transported over the forearm to the face to cover a large defect of the face. It is necessary to do three, four or more operations to finally cover the defect ("moving flap") (cf. p. 363).

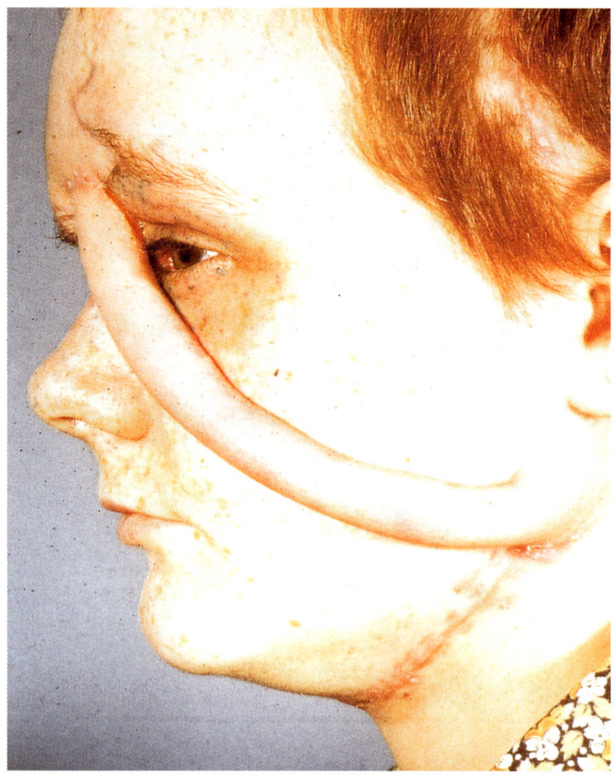

Figure 2.54b First the flap is performed in the neck area. After three to four weeks one end of the flap will be fixed in the defect and after further three to four weeks the flap will be separated (cf. p. 368).

Expander and Defect Coverage

Initially Radovan developed the expander to reconstruct the breast after mastectomy. Since that time more and more indications were found.

Principle:
The healthy skin will be stretched through stepwise filling of a silicone balloon with saline. After two to six weeks stretching there will be more healthy skin for defect coverage.

The surplus of healthy skin is the ability to close the defect or a part of it with sensitive, stable skin of very good quality and color. In certain cases several expanders are indicated coexistent or one after another to manage covering of large defects.

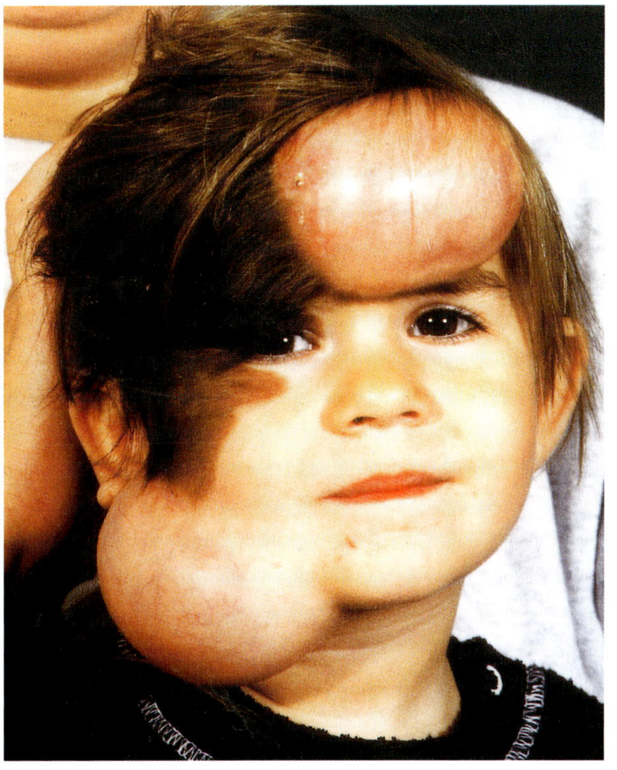

Figure 2.55 Expansion of healthy skin in the area of the forehead and neck to cover a defect after excision of a hairy nevus (cf. p. 356)

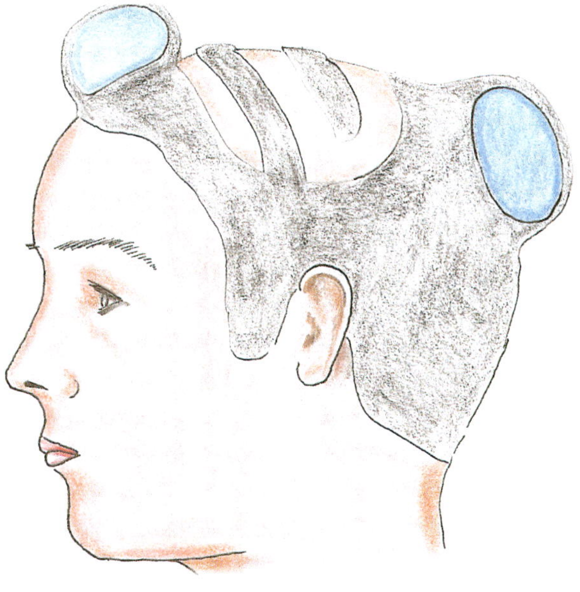

Figure 2.56a Two expanders expand the haired skin of the head to correct a traumatically induced alopecia.

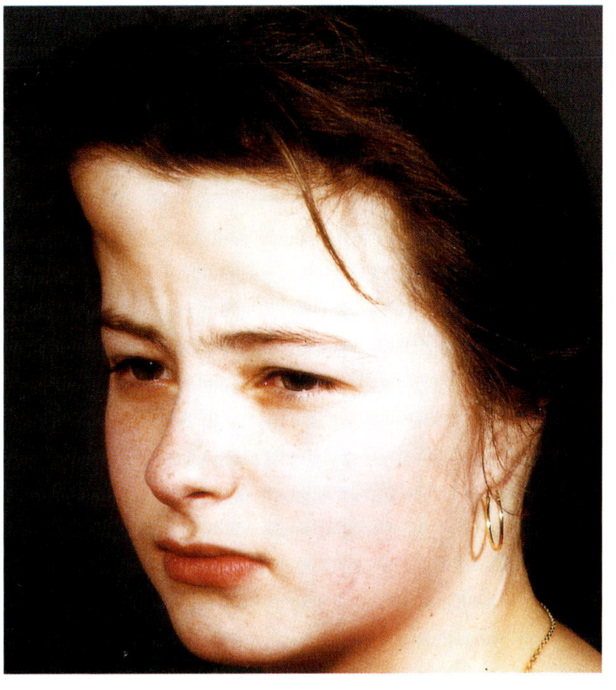

Figure 2.56b Expansion of the haired skin (cf. p. 438)

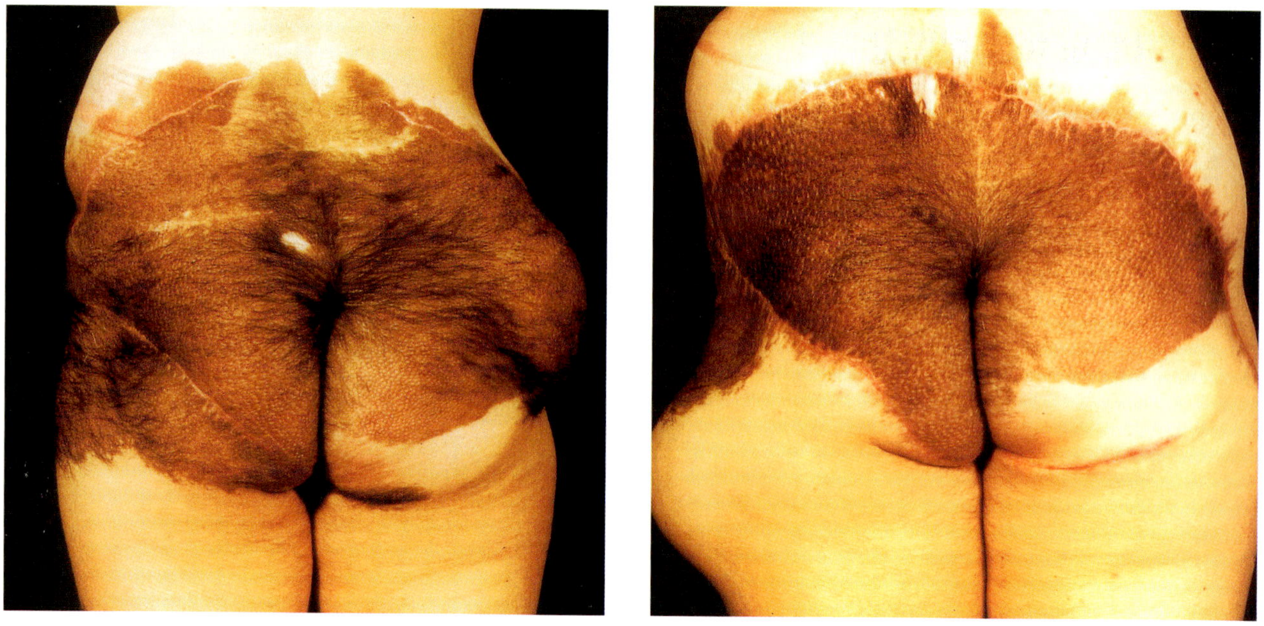

Figure2.57a,b Several expanders have been used in seven operations during three years to fractionally remove a hairy nevus. The residual parts have been replaced by local flaps (cf. p. 740).

Dermatome for Split-Skin Graft Removal

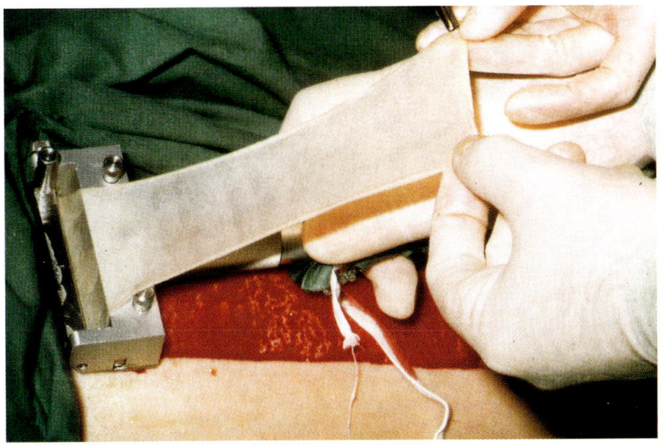

Figure 2.58a Air-driven dermatome (e.g. Davies). Advantage: Safe usage, constant skin thickness, unruffled margins, fast removal. Disadvantage: The split-skin broadness is limited on 7 cm.

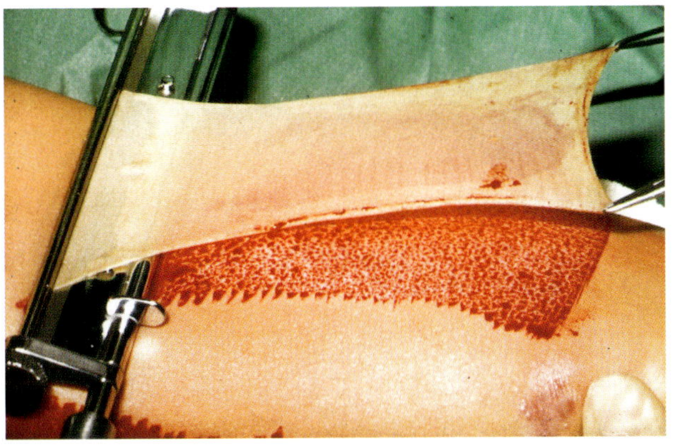

Figure 2.58b Hand dermatome (e.g. Watson). Advantage: Possibility of graft removal with broadness until 15 cm.
Disadvantage: Experience in handling is very important (the best is to practice with cadavers), otherwise ruffled margins, too thick grafts if there are wrong calibrations (until subcutaneous tissue).

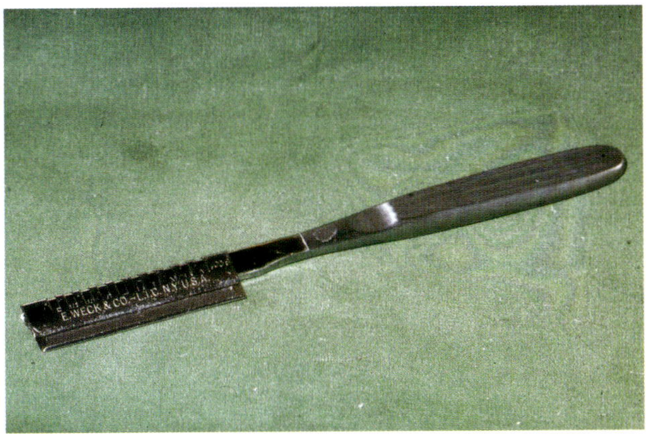

Figure 2.58c The practical and cheap Weck knife is used for removals of small split-skin grafts or escharotomy: Easy handling.

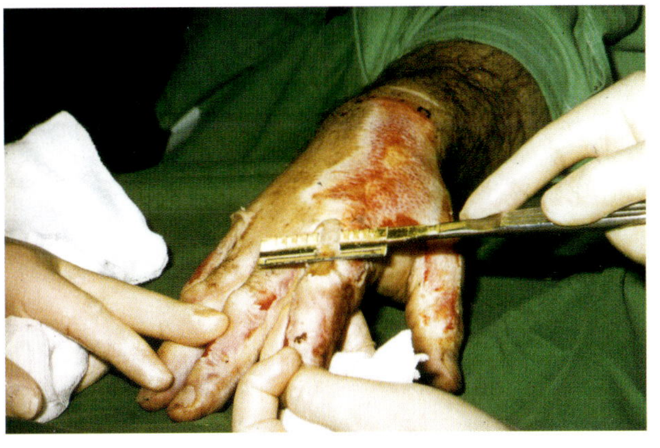

Figure 2.58d The Weck knife is an excellent instrument for tangential excision of burned skin.

Full-Thickness Skin Grafts

Full-thickness skin grafts are taken from the retro-auricular, supraclavicular or groin region.

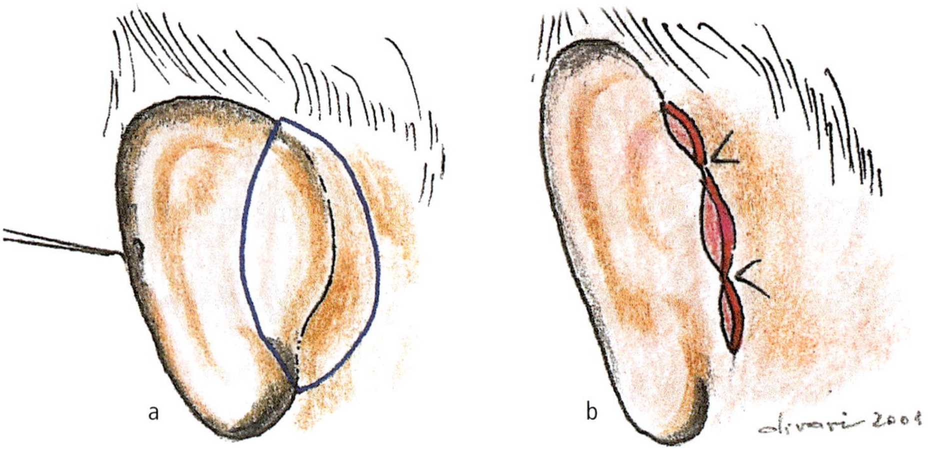

Figure 2.59 a Removal of a full-thickness skin graft. To use the graft it should be completely defatted. **b** The secondary defect is closed primary.

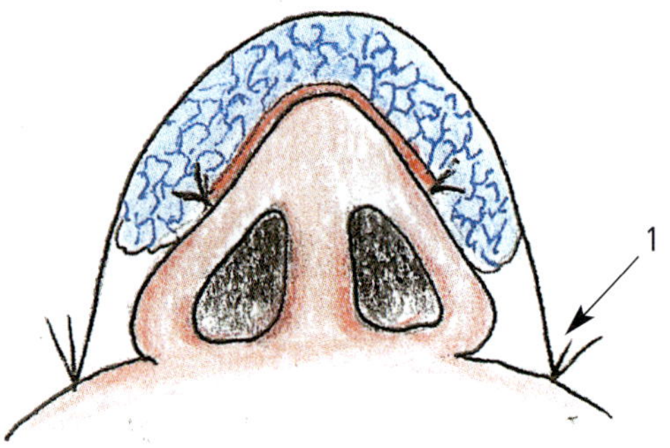

Figure 2.60 Fixation of a full-thickness skin graft on the bridge of the nose.
The compression dressing should not be fixed at the margin of the graft, but with extra sutures at the cheek tissue (1). This makes a much better scarring.

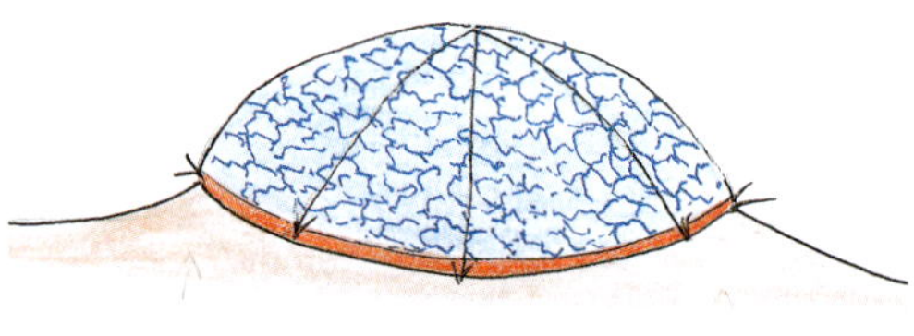

Figure 2.61a Wrong fixation of the graft
Fixation of the compression dressing with the same sutures as used for fixation the full-thickness skin graft at the defect margin. The wound margins are raised. Small parts of the graft cannot heal consequently. This way of compression dressing delivers no favourable results.

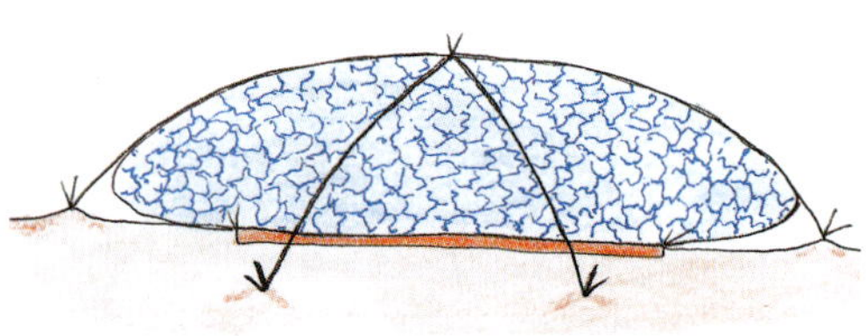

Figure 2.61b Right fixation
The full-thickness skin graft will be fixed without tension with atraumatic 6×0 nylon (e.g. Trofilene). The compression dressing, which should be larger than the defect will be fixed with some strong sutures, in approx. 3 cm distance of the wound margin. The graft keeps plain and the scarring diminish considerably.

Composite Graft

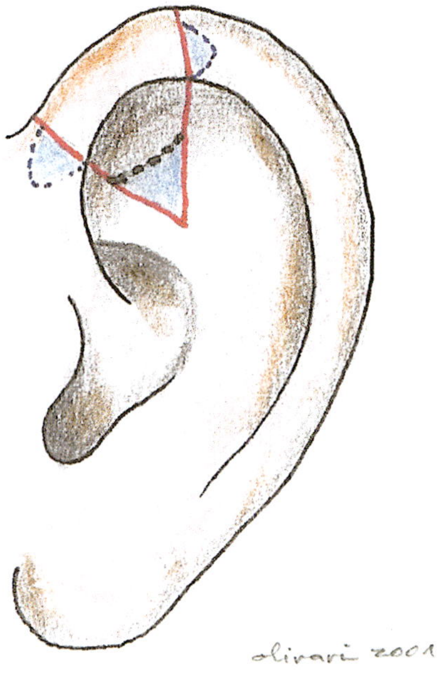

Figure 2.62a Typical donor site of the auricle, whereas more cartilage than skin should be taken.

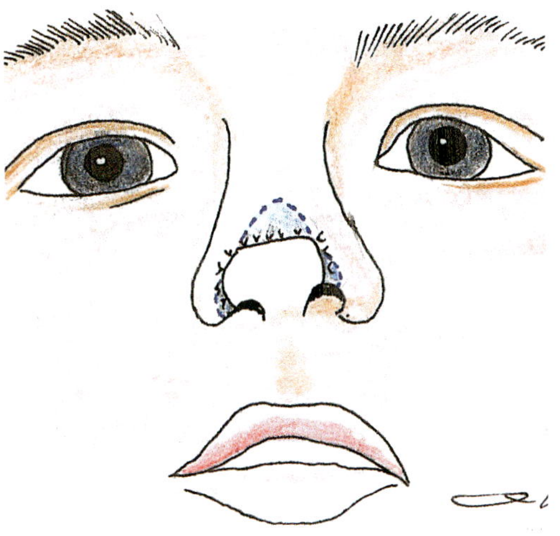

Figure 2.62b The cartilage will be fixed below the rosy skin and nourished per diffusionem. In the first 24 hours the composite graft is cooled down (cf. p. 136).

Composite graft means a graft consisting of skin, subcutis and cartilage. The first chondrocutaneous graft was performed by König (1902) in cases with nose defects. Because of its unsteadiness (loss of more than 50 %), this method was disclaimed by Lexer and Joseph. Today, in cases with good indications and special attention to technical details the healing rate is more than 85 %.

The results are considerably better, if following rules are kept in mind:

1. The graft should not be to large.
2. The cartilaginous parts should be well covered with good perfused healthy tissue. The cartilage is nourished per diffusionem.
3. One part of the graft's skin should be in contact to the refreshed skin of the nose.
4. Atraumatic treatment of the graft. No squeezing with the forceps, use only Gillies hook.
5. Postoperative cooling of the graft for 24 hours. A blue graft is considered as good sign, a white graft as suspect.

Bone Grafts

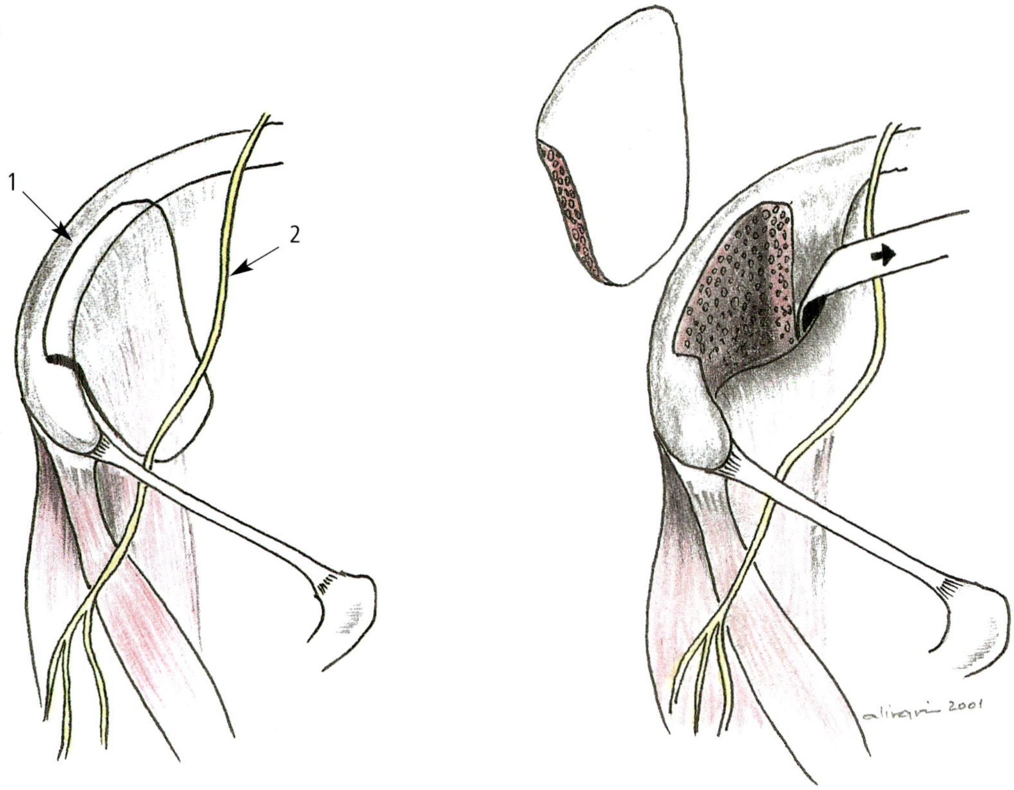

Figure 2.63a,b Bone harvest of the iliac crest (1)
The position of cutaneus femoralis lateralis nerve should be remembered (2). It should be kept on the medial side. The subperiostal access is inside of the iliac crest.
Grafts up to 10 × 8 cm can be harvested easily by chisel. Bone wax is used to stop hemorrhage. No Redon drainage is placed in the area of spongiosa; only a subcutaneous drain.

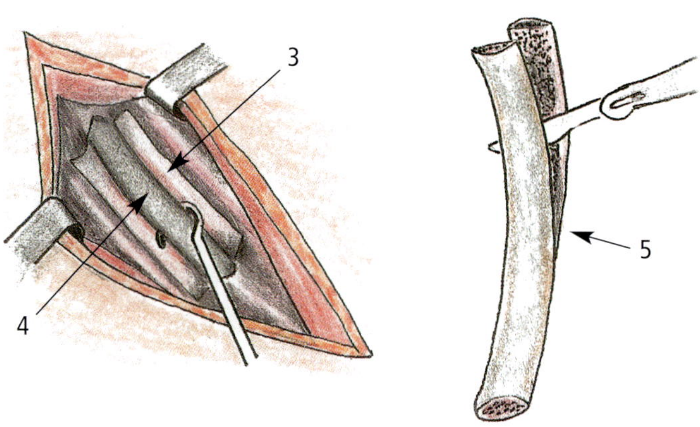

Figure 2.64a,b Bone extraction of a rib after longitudinal split of the periosteum (3). The part of the rip is extracted subperiostal (4). The periost is adapted in its original location with 5 × 0 Vicryl. A new rib develops in children within six weeks, in adults after three to four months. The rib graft is splitted (5).

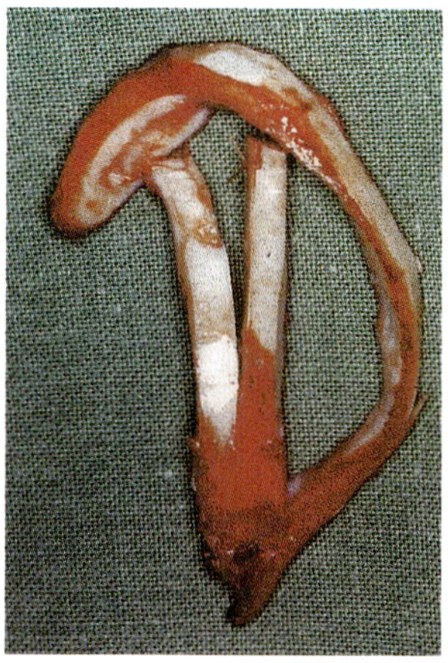

Figure 2.64c Cartilaginous graft of the rib for reconstruction of the ear after modelling

Skin Tumors

In this chapter skin tumors are described, which are most common in the clinical practice of plastic surgeons. Dermatological and oncological basic knowledge are a sine qua non for the surgeon.

Nevus Cell Nevus

The pigment nevus is the most common benign pigmented skin tumor. The nevus is classified into three categories:

- Junctions – nevus
- Compound – nevus
- Intradermal – nevus

Clinically these three variations are not differentiated easily. In the histology the nevi show predominantly an accumulation of nevus cells in the deeper layers of epidermis. Rarely there are cells in the dermis. Intradermal types show pigment cells within the cutis.

The potential for malignant alteration is small. The data of Kerl (1992) that show a risk of 5 % to develop a melanoma are controversial; probably the incidence is lower. It is only suspected, when form and colour change or when bleeding appears in a short time period:

Malignity Criteria

1. Asymmetric form: Normal nevi are round and symmetric: Asymmetry: Suspicious
2. Anomalous limitation towards the normal skin: Nevi show a sharp margin
3. Inconsistent colour: Variations of brown, black, grey and red are suspicious for malignant alteration
4. Irregular surface, in parts tubercular.
5. Very important characteristic: With loupe (magnification 2.5) the normal nevus shows a normal skin grain (small wrinkles) outreached the nevi. If the surface is plain, there is the suspicion of alteration.

Therapy

Most of the nevi are eliminated because of aesthetic reasons. In the last 20 years we prefer the tangential excision. Local anesthesia is spouted directly under the nevus and a tangential excision with a 15 scalpel is done: A micro-coagulation take place. An excision of the classic way with suturing results in more ugly scars. Assumption for a tangential excision is the preoperative diagnostic. Our experience has shown that the clinical examination with loupe glasses is a simple and safe method.

If there is the smallest suspicion, the excision is done with a safety margin. Of course all tumors are confirmed histologically.

Hairy Nevus

The hairy nevus (nevus pigmentosus et pilosus) is a melanous nevus, that shows a strong hairiness.

In most cases it is an intradermal type. The therapy consists of excision and coverage of the defect with local flaps, full-thickness skin grafts, skin expansion and rarely with free flaps.

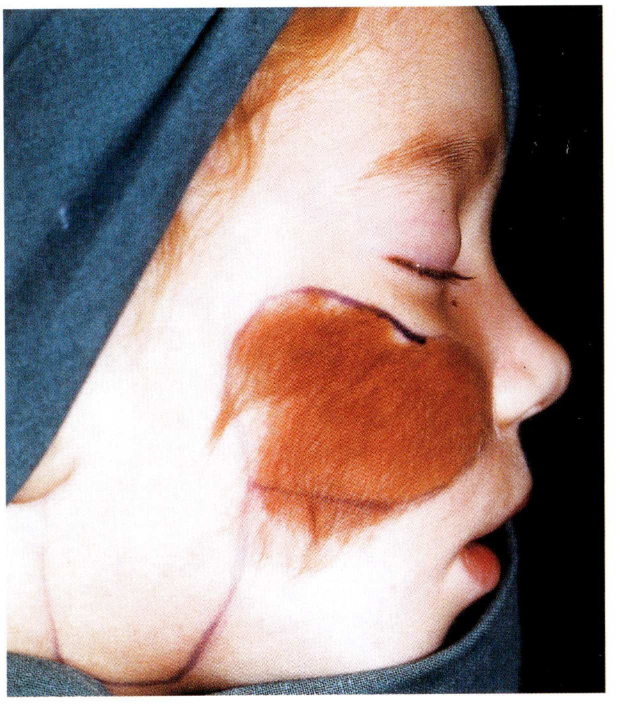

Figure 2.65 Hairy nevus in the location of the cheek (cf. p. 310)

Lipoma

Lipoma appear solitaire, but multicenter is also common. The localization is mostly subcutaneous, but could be also (more rare) intramuscular. The most common localization is the neck and the upper extremities; more rare there are lipomas abdominal and at the thigh, too. Multiple small lipomas are described with Adipositas dolorosa (Decrum's disease). The lipomas can reach an extreme size, especially at the neck and throat (Madelung's disease).

Therapy

Local anesthesia is used for operations of small lipomas. An incision of 2 mm is enough. Through this the lipoma is pulled out particular with a small mosquito clamp and pressed out with force. The method is simple, fast and results in tiny scars. Larger lipomas can be eliminated by liposuction. Madelung's disease indicates a more complex operation, which particularly necessitates a liposuction and excision.

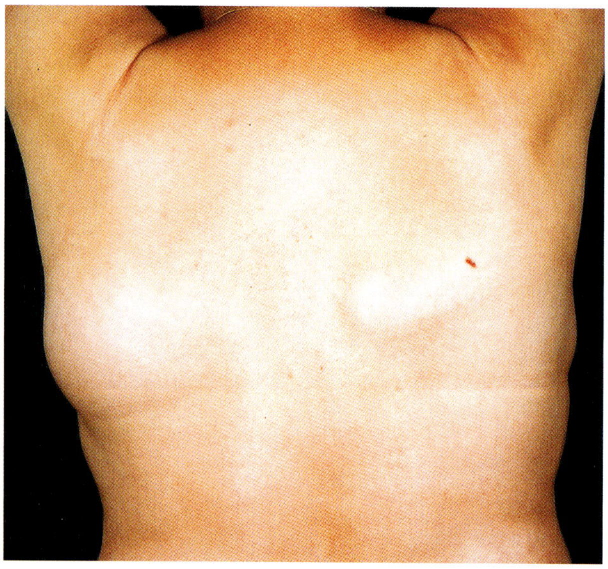

Figure 2.66a Subscapular lipoma left in the size of a fist

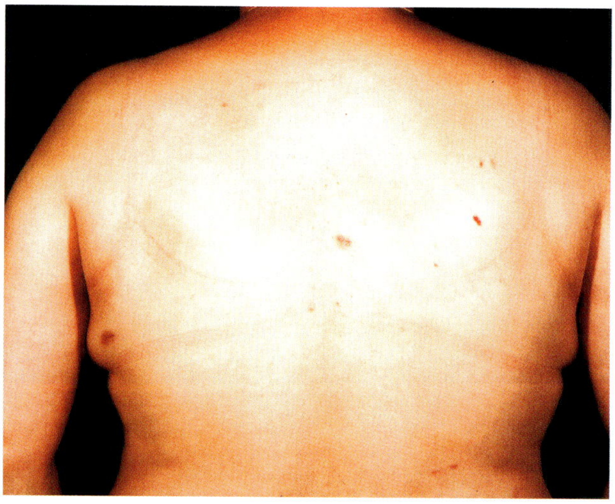

Figure 2.66c Status after six weeks postoperatively. The remained wrinkle of the skin is identical with the healthy side. The scar is minimal.

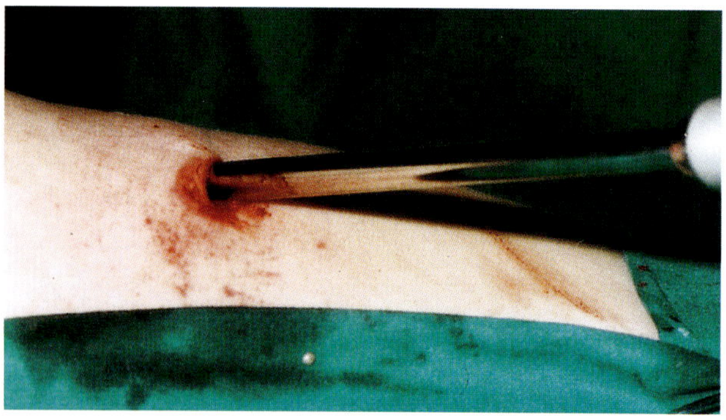

Figure 2.66b The liposuction cannula (4 mm diameter) is placed through a 0.5 cm incision. The lipoma can be sucked off.

In principle every tumor excision should follow a pathological-histological tissue examination, especially in cases with intramuscular dispersion of the lipoma or with infiltrative growing.

Hemangioma

Hemangiomas are anomalies of the vessel system with very different appearance, which results often in functional failures, and very often aesthetic problems, too. The hemangioma, especially the ones with location of the head are a heavy mental burden which can change the personality and complicate the social adjustment.

The classification of hemangioma is not uniform and sometimes depending from the fact if a clinician or a histologist performs the evaluation. Because of clinical practical reasons hemangiomas can be classified into the following groups:

1. Nevus flammeus, Port-wine stains
2. Blastomatous hemangiomas
   a) Tuberous hemangiomas
   b) Cavernous hemangiomas
   c) Tuberous-cavernous hemangiomas with arterial components and aggressive growing (A-V fistula)

1. Nevus Flammeus

The location of nevus flammeus is often in the face, more rare at the thorax and the extremities. In the face the nevus flammeus often follows unilateral the area of trigeminus nerve and can change to tuberous forms in older age. A transformation to hemangioma is described. The affected area often shows hypertrophy because of the better perfusion.

Histological a dilatation of dermal capillaries is found. The nevus flammeus do not show any spontaneous regression in contrast to tuberous and cavernous hemangiomas. Over the years the surface of the nevus flammeus develops anomalous, particular tuberous, the color changes darker and the part of the face (head), which locates the nevus flammeus shows hypertrophy.

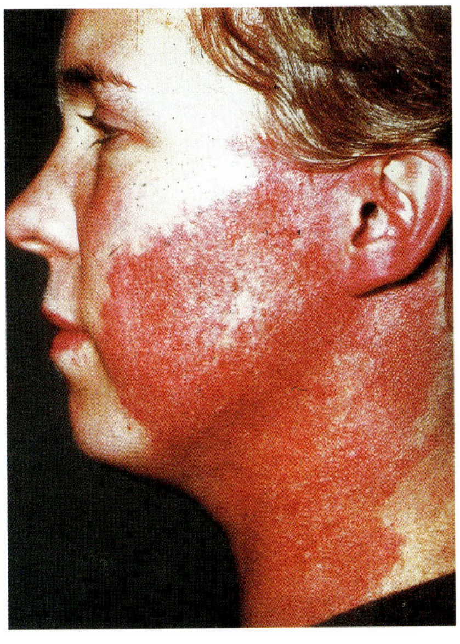

Figure 2.67 Nevus flammeus (typical spread)

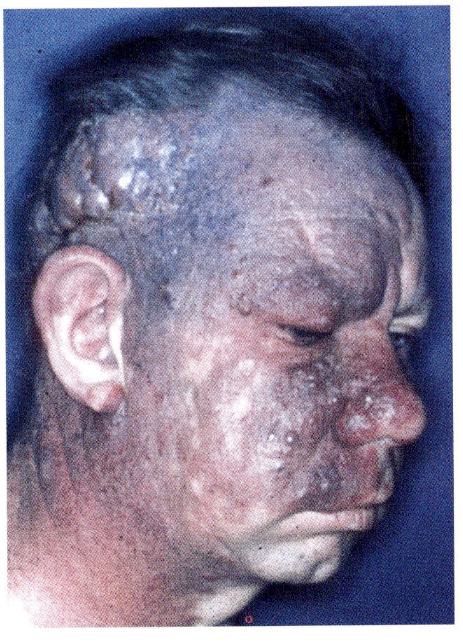

Figure 2.68a Nevus flammeus of the right head. In young age the nevus flammeus shows a plain form and lightly red colour. In older age the nevus flammeus changes to a tuberous form with increased tendency to bleed. The patient had continuously headache and suffered of disturbing (vessel) noises.

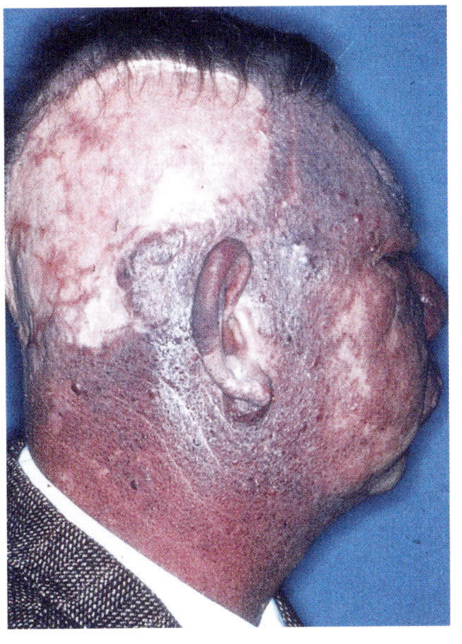

Figure 2.68b The tuberous part of nevus flammeus was eliminated. The symptoms are decreased drastically. The patient refused following operation.

Therapy

1. Excision and split-thickness skin graft
   This procedure results in cosmetic disappointing outcomes. The nevus flammeus tend to relapses at the margin of the grafts and between the graft margins. The skin color is not conform to a normal face and the expression becomes mask-like.
2. Excision and local flaps
   In cases with smaller nevi this is possible. Here the cosmetic results are better.
3. Excision and full-thickness skin flap
   Full-thickness skin grafts of the retroauricular region show excellent results.
   This method is inapplicable for larger expanse, because of the limitation of full-thickness skin graft.
4. In cases with larger nevus flammeus all three methods can be used.
5. An enormous advancement in treatment of nevus flammeus achieves laser therapy. The therapy should start early and needs several proceedings until the desired results are achieved.

2. Blastomatous Hemangiomas

Blastomatous hemangiomas (also called tuberous hemangiomas) are classified in order to their tendency of self-healing. These classifications focused on clinical aspects and for clinicians it is more important than merely histological classifications.
There are:

- Involutional forms
  They show a spontaneous regression over the course of one to four years (more than 90 %)
- Non-involutional forms
  They don't show any regression (circa 10 %)

Djindjian (1978) studied blastomatous hemangiomas with angiography and found out the following:

- Hemangiomas with slow perfusion (venous forms)
- Hemangiomas with fast perfusion (arteriovenous forms)

The first group shows an involutional development (spontaneous degenerations), the second group usually shows a continuous growth and is often a major challenge for the surgeons.

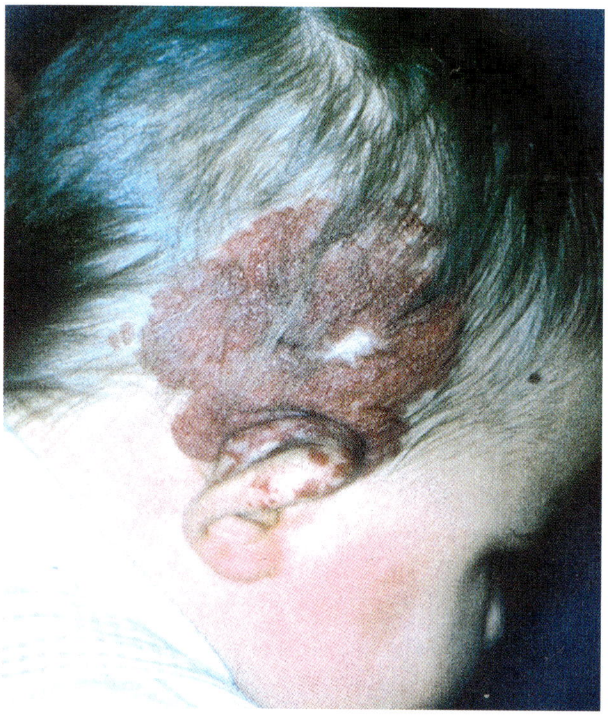

Figure 2.69a Tuberous form of the hemangioma with involutional tendency. In this case a child with the age of eight years is shown. In the middle portion of the hemangioma one can see a white spot, a sign for a beginning involution.

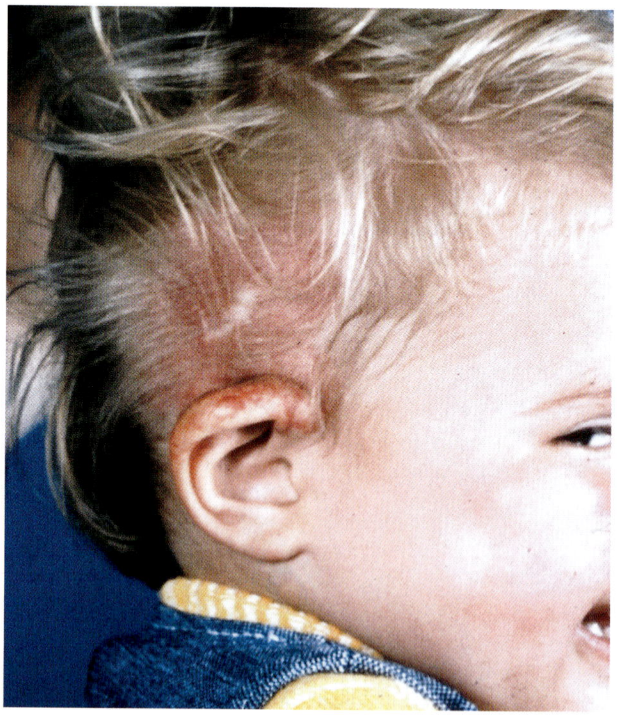

Figure 2.69b Three years later. The hemangioma had degenerated nearly completely without any therapy.

Histological in the proliferate phase hemangiomas show 30-40 times more mast cells along the hemangioma vessels than normal tissue. An involutional hemangioma normalize the number of mast cells during two to four years.

Children are more likely to have hemangiomas (5 to 10 % of newborns). It appears immediately after childbirth, is relatively plain, grows often until month 6 to 12 and results in a involution (approx. 90 %) with two to four years. At the latest in the age of 12 years the hemangioma degeneration is completed.

Petrovici (1977) differentiated in two progression forms of blastomatous hemangiomas:

- Superficial hemangiomas with fast tendency of degeneration and recovery of normal tissue
- Hemangioma of the skin and subcutis with delayed regression tendency. As a rule these forms are voluminous. They result in local deformations and leave pigmented and wrinkled skin and fibrolipomatous rest structure after regression.

Therapy

Treatment is made up of consequent wait and see tactic. 90 % of hemangiomas show a degeneration until the age of four or latest six years. The parents push the doctor for doing something from the beginning. Here the most important duty for the doctor is to clarify the facts with the parents, to control the child regular and to make pictures.

Most of the involutional hemangiomas disappear without any aesthetic problems. Sometimes wrinkled, blue colored skin persist. It should be excised. The excision lines should be done in the way of convenient aesthetic aspects. Rarely local flaps are necessary. There should be a warning for split-thickness skin grafts. They result in aesthetic worse outcomes than rests of hemangioma.

Only in some cases indications for surgical interventions are given in the early stage of hemangioma:

1. Amblyopia of disuse and following strabismus
2. Handicap of breathing and eating, because of hemangioma location
3. Recurrent spontaneous bleeding
4. High-grade anemia and thrombocytopenia

The uncommon, not involutional hemangiomas with AV fistula may create a lot of technical problems, not only because of their structure. The often difficult extirpation, optionally after previous vessel embolization, has been described as the only successful therapy. There are cases with a too high operative risk because of the high bleeding rates (cf. p. 111).

The highly praised and often performed ligation of the afferent vessels never showed mentionable results in our hospital. Radiation, in earlier times often performed, should be avoided.

Vessels are less radiosensitive – less than skin, connective tissue, cartilage and bone. The dose of radiation, which is necessary to degenerate a vessel, definitely damages healthy structures especially in periods of growth. The duration of radiation therapy is long and there are risks, which are disproportionally higher than any surgical option. Nearly 90 % of hemangiomas degenerate spontaneous and only 10 % turn out to not involutional hemangiomas in which radiation don't show any effect. Moreover irradiation consequences are not diagnosed directly; sometimes aesthetic and functional disadvantages develops after 10 to 15 years. Today's position says that irradiation of hemangiomas is an error in treatment. The injection of dexamethason in tuberous hemangioma results in a more rapid regression.

Morbus Bowen

Morbus Bowen is an intradermal precancer = carcinoma in situ.

We can see a brown-reddish lesion, which is irregularly limited. Morbus Bowen can be located at every part of the body, is the back of the hand, lower leg or body trunk are most common.

In the majority of cases it is solitary and shows superficial, squamous chronic changes. Predominantly it is round and grows very slowly. Morbus Bowen is also called spine cancer. Rarely the tumor breaks through the intradermal layer and basal level in the corium. In this manner a spinocellular cancer can develop.

Uncommonly this tumor is located in mucosal tissue and is then called erythroplasia (penis, vulva).

Therapy

Therapy includes the excision of the tumor and if necessary coverage of the defect with local flaps.

An irradiation therapy, which is often applied lasts a long time and results often in radiation defects, which make much more problems than Morbus Bowen.

Basal Cell Cancer

The basal cell cancer is a malignant tumor, which shows a slowly but progressive growing and has often destroying effects in advanced stages. Metastases are considered as a rarity. If there are any metastases a false diagnosis should be excluded.

The most common localization is the skin of the face; but the basal cell cancer is able to develop nearly everywhere. In later stages or in the sub-group "sclerodermiform lesions" the untreated basal cell cancer shows an aggressive growing ("savaged" basal cell carcinoma "ulcus rodens") and can destroy osseous structures. If for example in the area of the head the lamina externa is destroyed and the cancellous bone is infiltrated surgical treatment could be extensive and free flap is frequently indicated.

The both important factors for development of basal cell cancer are genetic and UV exposition.

Without any doubt insolation is the decisive factor. In the Australian population the appearance of basal cell cancer is three to four times higher than in Central-European people. In the colored population basal cell cancer is a rarity. Obviously melanin protect against these tumors.

Farmers, fishers, sailors, building workers are significantly more frequent sickened.

Irradiate skin develops sometimes basal and spinal cell cancer in later stages. Patients with irradiated skin should protect extra careful against insolation and a lifelong. In the literature the male/female ratio is described with 3:1. In our patients we found out a ratio of 56:44.

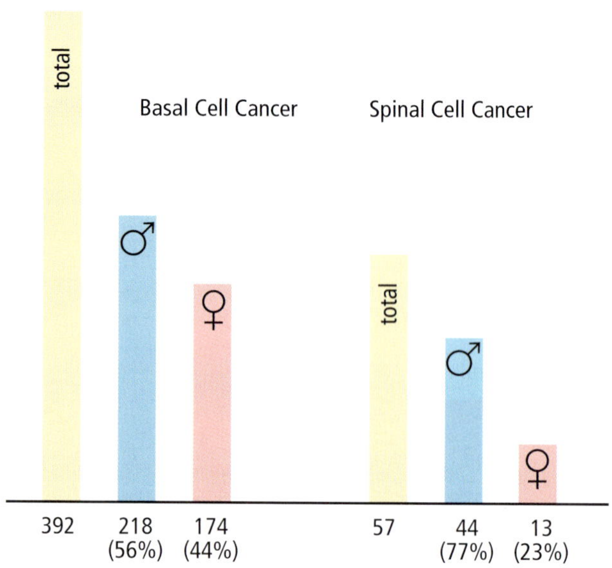

Table 2.1 Distribution of gender and histopathological differentiation in our patients

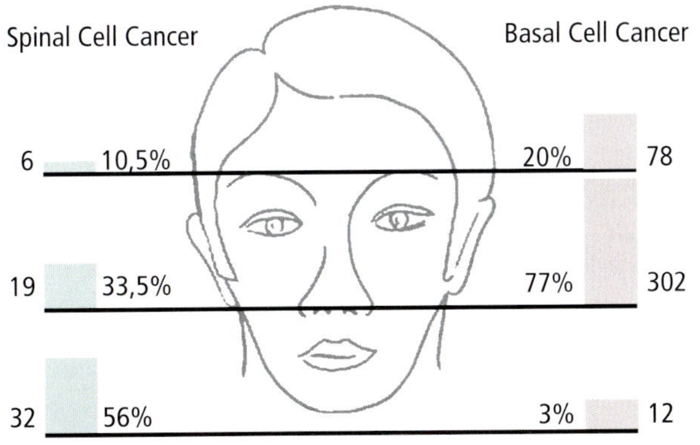

Table 2.2 Patient with basal cell and spinal cell cancer with head location (n = 392 basal cell cancer, 57 spinal cell cancer) (Olivari 1975)

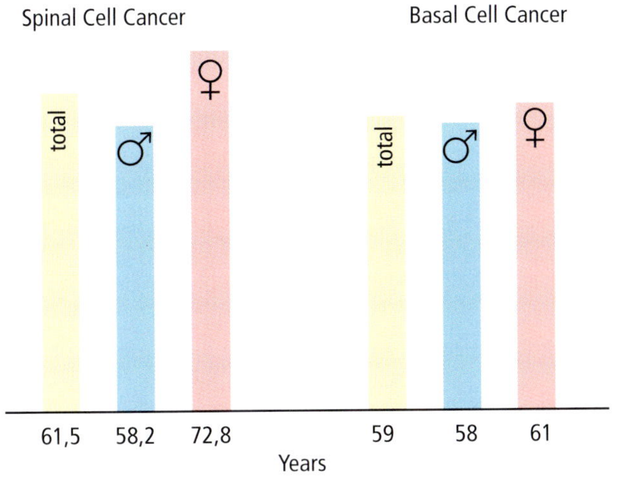

Table 2.3 Distribution of skin cancer and age (n = 392 basal cell cancer, 57 spinal cell cancer) (Olivari 1975)

Epidemiology

The data are hold for Germany and central Europe (Tables 2.4–2.6). Australian people originated from Europe e.g. Queensland have an incidence for basal cell cancer of 256/100000. This is the proof that insolation is the most important factor for development of basal cell cancer.

Therapy

Extirpation in sano. In early stage a primary closure of the wound with local flaps or more rarely with skin graft is nearly always possible. In advanced stages or in existing ulcus rodens with bone involvement a temporary coverage with mesh graft is indicated after extirpation for early identification of potential relapses. A covering with epithesis makes it easier to conceal high-grade deformations. After adequate time without relapse (approx. 2 years) the defect will be covered with local or free flaps.

Table 2.4 Frequency of malignant skin tumors in Germany

Tumor	Frequency of Tumors
Basal Cell Cancer	75/100 000/year
Spinal Cell Cancer	19/100 000/year
Melanoma	12/100 000/year

Table 2.5 Localization of basal cell cancer (1994)

Localization	Percent
Face	55.9
Head, neck	12.8
Trunk	13.4
Upper extremity	4.7
Lower extremity	3.0
Others	10.2
Total	100.0

Table 2.6 Histology of basal cell cancer

Histology	Percent
Stable basal cell cancer	76.0
Sclerodermiform basal cell cancer	3.0
Metatypical basal cell cancer	3.5
Superficial basal cell cancer	16.5
Mixed form	2.0
Total	100.0

There is no indication for irradiation in early stages because of following reasons:

- The treatment takes remarkably longer than the surgical therapy
- The aesthetic results are normally worse than with adequate surgical therapy
- The irradiated skin can develop additional, radiation induced basal cell cancer and spinal cell cancer after many years.
- Results of irradiation are not histologically controlled

We refuse abrasion of basal cell cancer as a inadequate treatment especially because of the non-specific histological control is impossible.

Spinal Cell Cancer

The spinal cell cancer develops in the skin and mucosa, firstly grows slowly and later destroying. The spinal cell cancer produce depending on literature, 8 to 15 % local metastases. The tumor results from Morbus Bowen, leukoplakia, actinic keratoderma, chronic inflamed processes, actinic and chronic cheilitis and not rare in irradiated skin areas. Sometimes the tumor develops out of a chronic scar, as a so-called scar cancer.

First the growing is slowly, hyperkeratotic nodes are build and then develops slowly thicker and solid and stays initially painless. Afterwards there are central ulcerations.

The spinal cell cancer is more seldom than basal cell cancer. A ratio of 1:4 as described in literature, we cannot confirm in our patients. We had 392 basal cell cancers and 57 spinal cell cancers, to put it in a nutshell this is a ratio of 1:7.

UV irradiation is an important etiologic factor like for basal cell carcinoma. People who work outdoors and light-skin people in equatorial areas get affected more often. On the other hand the cancer is a rarity in colored population. Localization on the lip in long-time smokers shows another noxa.

Diagnosis

In early stage the difference to basal cell cancer is clinically difficult to make. A fast growing and central ulceration are helpful in diagnosis, but the result have to be necessarily confirmed histologically.

Therapy

The extirpation in healthy tissue should be done with an increased safe distance than in cases with basal cell cancer. Local lymph nodes have to be controlled and extirpated if there is any suspicion. The defect will be closed with one of the methods of plastic surgery (local flap, split-thickness skin graft, free flap). Only if there is an unclear histological situation one should wait and cover the defect temporary with synthetic skin.

Malignant Melanoma

A malignant melanoma is an epidermogenic, malignant tumor of pigment-producing cells with a disposition to metastases formation. The tumor results from an existing nevus or establishes on the surface of normal skin.

Epidemiology

Especially affected are people with light skin, light eye color, freckles and ginger hairs.

The number of melanomas shows an increasing tendency. In Germany the incidence adds up to 12 to 14 diseases for 100000 citizens – also increasing.

The most important factor for the development of melanoma is the insolation and UV exposition. Numerous sun burns in adolescence and long time intensive sun exposure at the sea or mountains are predisposing factors. The frequent usage of solarium is an additional factor.

The Australian population with European origin suffer numerical more than European. This disease is a absolutely rarity for Aborigines and colored people (0.6/100000). Other factor which influence melanoma growing are genetic disposition and oncogenic viruses.

The melanoma appears between the ages of 20 and 70 years, the most frequent in the sixth decade. The tumor can't be exempted from children. The frequency is nearly the same at both sexes.

Risk factors are:

- Dysplastic nevus syndrome
- Melanoma disease in the family
- Red blonde hair, pale skin color, poor tanning tendency
- Number of sun burns in the teenage age
- Number of congenital and dysplastic nevi
- Hairy nevi

The back of men and the lower extremity of woman are considered to be the most frequent localization. The tumor may also appear ubiquitous, even mucosal. The malignant melanoma has a strong tendency to metastasize. A five-year survival rate can be found dependant of the stadium in about 60 to 80 %, but was at only 50 %, two decades ago. This significant improvement of the survival rate can be explained by the early diagnostic. Probably the increasing use of higher sun protection factors is also to be regarded as positive.

Diagnostics

1. Persons with elevated melanoma markers show an elevated risk of the development of melanomas (dysphasic nevus syndrome).
2. Asymmetry of the form: Normal nevi are round and symmetric. Melanomas mostly grow asymmetric.
3. Irregular border to the normal skin (nevi show a sharp border).
4. Inconsistent colorant: the color varies from brown, black, blue, grey to red. Nevi show a homogeneous color.
5. Growth of the diameter in a relatively short time
6. Irregular swell, partly tubercular.
7. Very important and simple diagnostic method: Beneath the lens (2.5 times) the normal nevi shows that the normal skin grain (small wrinkles) proceeds the the nevi. The surface of melanomas is even.

The author has found this simple diagnostic method asserted by means of histopathological checks in a plurality of cases.

Form of Appearance

- LMM (Lentigo-Maligna Melanoma)

  This is the classic melanoma older patients. In the light, exposed areas appear, particularly in the face. At first it shows itself as a superficial, pigmented lesion, which is persistent for many years. This melanoma can be found in five percent of all lesions. The lentigo maligna is presumed to be the less aggressive melanoma, but it might turn into the aggressive nodular form.

- SSM (Superficial Spreading Melanoma)

  This form represents 70 % of the melanomas. The growth is horizontal laminar. After a time period which sometimes lasts over years, the invasive depth growth begins. The surface shows an uneven border and different colors (brown, black, blue, grey, red, as well as a central white zone of regression).

- NNM (Nodular Melanoma)

  The nodular melanoma forms 10 to 15 % of all melanomas. After a short superficial growth, the growth in the depths begins. It holds a nodular surface which is stained in blue, black and red. Frequently there are ulcerations. Often metastases are formed.

- ALM (Acral Lentiginous Melanoma)

  7 % of all melanomas are acral lentiginous lesions. The attributes are the ones of the LMM and NNM with the localization of the sole of the foot, palm as well as sublingual. Diagnostic is not generally easy.

- Melanomas in Hairy Nevus

  This melanoma seldom derives. As a permanent danger lasts the hairy nevus should be removed betimes. If a malignant melanoma derives from the hairy nevus the prognoses is poor.

- Amelanotic Melanoma

  This seldom variation of the melanoma, which frequently derives on women, is accompanied by a bad prognosis, as the diagnosis is difficult and often made too late.

Distribution and Depth of the Tumor

Mehnert and Heard (1965) have demonstrated in a study with 176 patients that there is a significant connection between the depth of the tumor in the skin and the survival rate. Clark has classified the melanomas according to their penetration depth. The classification of the tumor depth has to be completed with the type of the tumor (lentigo maligna, nodular melanomas).

A study by Breslow (1970), who identified the absolute depth of the tumor including the exophytical proportion by means of an optical micrometer, added up clear correlations in the examination of 98 patients. Patients with melanomas of a depth which was less than 0.76 mm, showed a five-years survival rate of 100 percent. There were no metastases after the R0 resection and no local relapse was to be registered even when the tumor was categorized as a Clark level III.

The measurement is executed in an increasing rate as a foundation for the treatment of the melanomas. To look at it from that position, all melanomas with a greater depth than 0.76 mm get a worse prognosis. In the study of Breslow only four patients out of 18 who had a tumor depth which was greater than 3 mm have survived for five years.

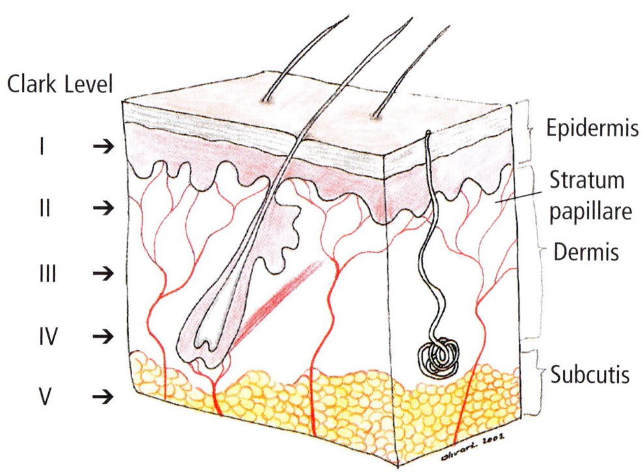

Figure 2.70 Classification according to Clark

Table 2.7 Classification according to Clark (mortality = 5 years)

Level	
I	The tumor cells are in the epidermis above the basal membrane. This level is also called melanoma in situ. The mortality is 0 percent
II	The tumor cells have penetrated the epidermis and are located in the papillary dermis. The mortality is 8 percent.
III	The tumor cells have infiltrated the papillary dermis, but have not yet reached the reticulate dermis. The mortality is 33 percent.
IV	The tumor cells are infiltrated into the reticulate dermis. The mortality is 46 percent.
V	The tumor cells are infiltrated through the reticulate dermis to the subcutaneous fat tissue. The mortality is 52 percent.

Table 2.8 Malignant melanomas and risk (modified according to Breslow)

Risk	Tumor depth	5-Years survival rate
Minimal	< 0.76 mm	98 %
Low	0.76 – 1.5 mm	90 %
Intermediate	1.5 – 4 mm	66 – 77 %
High	> 4 mm	below 50 %

Therapy

With the clinical suspicion of a malignant melanoma (even surface under the lens, irregular frame differently colored surface, central white staining) there should not be an indication for a specimen excision. The R0 excision is the right decision.

With tumors of a tumor size below 1 mm the excision should be carried out with a safety margin of 2 to 3 cm. The safety margin is not always easy to adhere to with an inappropriate localization (tip of the nose).

In the depth it has to be extirpated until the fascia. The former recommended fascia extirpation was not able to show better results. Upon operation the tumor must not be bruised with the implements and no contamination of the wound bed. *Do not touch the tumor with instruments!* The coverage of the defect has to be carried out with split thickness skin graft or a local flap.

Lymph Node Scintigraphy

Particularly with prognostic inappropriate localization (torso, upper arm, neck and scalp) the Sentinel Lymph Node identified. A radioisotope is injected (Tc99m). The scintigraphy shows this decisive first lymph node, which then will be excised.

If there is a negative histological diagnostic finding, a further lymph node extirpation is not indicated, otherwise therapeutical lymph node dissection is to be done.

The examination bases on the fact that tumors of the skin metastasize in the first lymph nodes as a rule. In case of breast cancer the first lymph nodes could be rarely jumped. A prophylactic regional extirpation of the lymph nodes is recommended to patients with "high risk" melanomas despite the fact that data is missing, which give evidence of an improvement of the prognoses.

Adjuvant Therapy

- An indication for chemotherapy of multiple skin and lymph metastases is questionable. A response rate of 20 percent has been reported.
- A hyperthermic perfusion of the extremities with cytostatics is recommended to melanomas with localization on the extremities.
- An immunotherapy with Interferon is reserved to patients with metastases. Success could be discussed
- A radiotherapy is applied to regional metastases after a palliative lymph node extirpation. The success of therapy is in doubt.

All patients with a melanoma should get presented on an oncological tumor board.

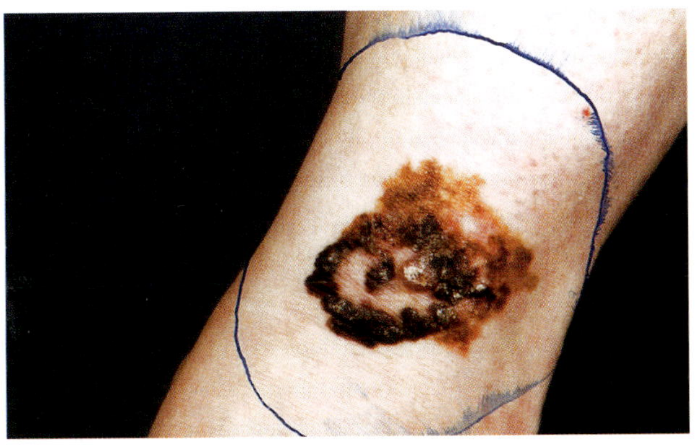

Figure 2.71a Multi-centric superficial growing melanoma in the lower third of the lower led (SSM).

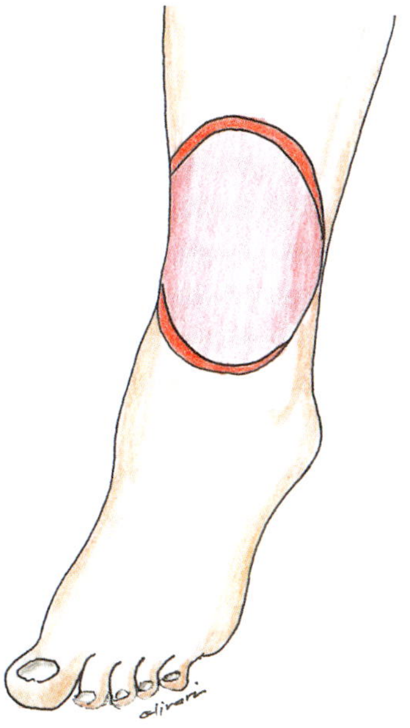

Figure 2.71b Excision en bloc until the aponeurosis. No specimen excision. In the left groin there was no lymph node lympho-scintigraphically touched.

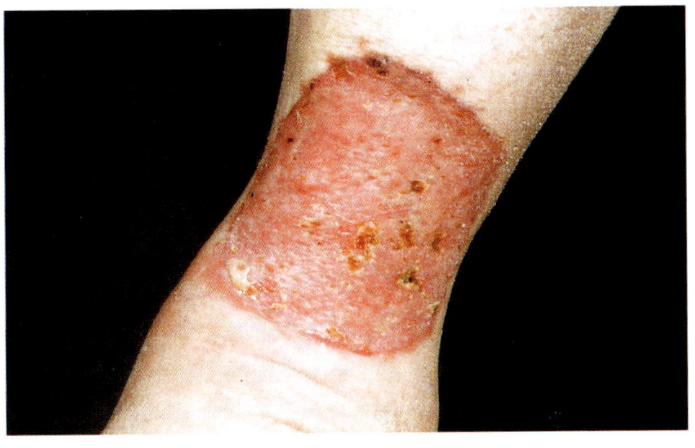

Figure 2.71c Coverage of the defect with mesh graft

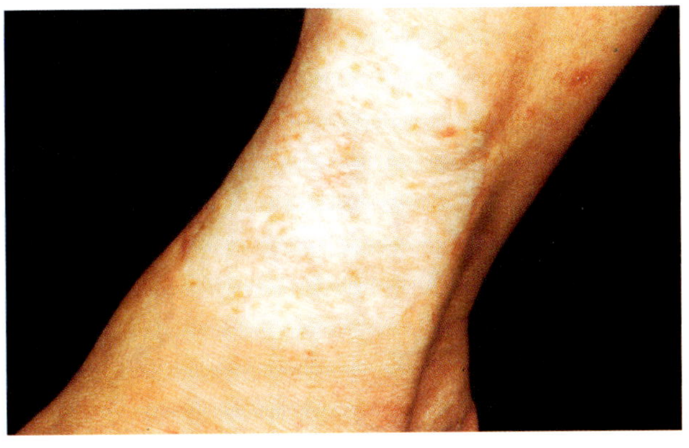

Figure 2.71d Condition nine years after the operation.

Radiation Damages of the Skin

In 1895 Roentgen discovered X-ray, which was named after him. Shortly after that Edison produced fluoroscopes which were demonstrated by his assistant Clarence Dally. He fell prey to the impact of the radiation. He died in 1897, after he had lost all his hair and suffered from heaviest burns on both hands. Elisabeth Fleischmann Aschheim was the first clinical radiologist. She began with X-ray diagnostics in 1897 and died in 1905 because of a large squamous carcinoma of the chest.

W. Markuse (1896) published the first x-ray dermatitis and alopecia. In 1896 Drury described an x-ray ulcer which showed no tendency of healing. C.A. Porter and C. J. White (1907) announced more than 11 x-ray carcinomas with lethal ending. Rowntree (1922) reported that there has not appeared an x-ray carcinoma, which has been treated by him, earlier than five years after the radiation, in two cases actually not until 17 years. Freund (1933) informed about x-ray damages which appeared 36 years after the exposure.

Growth Mechanism

Probably sulfhydril (SH)-groups change after radiation. This group is the basic element of many vital substances. It is known that radiation blocks the cell mitosis. Newly generated cell have reduced the mitotic ability or even lost it completely. The formation of radiation damages is dependent from the choice of exposure, namely alpha-, beta-, gamma rays, which have again to be distinguished into soft or hard rays, as well as from the proportioning of rays, the size of the exposure zone and the frequency of the exposure series. An ineffective underdose can lead to side-effects as well. On the other hand the damages of a often only short-term overdose are more than fatal. X-ray long-term sequelae appear particularly after exposure series with respectively high single doses.

Pathology and Clinic

The chronic x-ray dermatitis is histological labelled by atrophy and hyperkeratosis of the epithelium, by the endothelial proliferation of the vessels which leads to constriction, partly to the obliteration of the volume of the vessels. Thereby it leads to a thrombosis and pigment coating of the skin through hematin deposits. The tailback of the blood into the capillary net causes the generation of the typical teleangiectasias. Subcutaneous adipose tissue shows atrophy. By means of thc damagc of the beneath lying bone- and chondral proportions it often leads to considerable disturbances of growth in infantile. Through the progress of the mutation of the vessels and hence, the increase of the trophical disorder of the irradiated skin area, as well as by means of microtraumas it can lead to an ulcer radiologicum. The X-ray ulcer is persistent often lifelong.

The originated ulcer mostly increases slowly, but progressive in breath and depth. The ground if the ulcer is ischemic atrophic, fibroid and is always infected.

The trophical disorders in the vessel free area prevent a spontaneous healing. Sensitive proportions of nerves, which disassemble in the ground of the ulcer, lead to insufferable pain. In addition, there are the chronic losses of protein and the disturbance of foul-smelling secretion.

The X-ray carcinoma as the most dangerous complication of exposure therapy indeed tends to a late dissemination, but gets frequently detected with a delay. Does the pure ray dermatitis tend to carcinogenic degeneration in 10 percent of all causes, it is 20 to 30 percent in the radiation ulcer. The worst prognoses have ulcers which already appear in the first year after the exposure. The mortality rate in case of radiation carcinomas is by about 20 percent.

Indication Problems and Prophylaxis

Considering the heavy irreversible mutations in the irradiated skin area, there appears a exceedingly critical diagnoses to be advisable. The radiation of benign skin mutations like eczema, hemangiomas, verrucas, hairy nevi, and so on, can no longer be responsibly applied.

With regard to their sensitivity against radiation, the different parts of skin are to be damaged in the following line-up in the exposure X-ray therapy:

a) Stratum germativum of the epidermis
b) Sebaceous gland cell
c) Hair follicle-matrix cells
d) Cells of the perspiratory gland
e) Chondral cells
f) Osteoblasts
g) Endothelial cells of the blood vessels
h) Muscle cells and connective tissue cells
i) Nerves

It is important to adhere to this order as for example before blood vessels (hemangioma) are being influenced by x-rays, all the above mentioned layers are damaged prior to these structures. Under this condition even the malignant skin mutations like basaliomas and spinaliomas as far as they are reachable by an operation because of their localization, they do not belong to the domain of a radiation therapy. Hence, the surgical therapy of this damage is usually easier and mostly conductible under ambulatory conditions. The radiation therapist is familiar with mathematical formulas with whose help he can assess how strong he has to reduce the total doses, if the fraction doses has to be increased.

Despite, the results of animal experiments and clinical experience have shown that these formulas are useful for the acute radiodematitis, but underestimate the risk of chronic consequences of radiation. In the past years there has been an increase in the use of the combination of chemotherapy and radiation therapy. Above all, in the simultaneous treatment with both modalities there appears a significant fortification of acute skin reactions, which makes a reduction of the radiation dose necessary.

The chronic consequences of exposure for the skin are pathogenetical completely independent from the acute radiodermatitis. Patients with severe acute radiodermatitis frequently show no chronic consequences of exposure for the skin, give no or only a slight radiodermatitis for comment in an anamnesis. From the intensity of the acute skin reaction it is not possible to make a prognosis of the individual risk of chronic consequences of radiation, as a rule. Unless, the acute reaction of the skin has to be regarded as a consequence of an unintentional overdose.

Whilst the acute consequences of exposure are mostly very sharply defined and follow the area borders of the radiation field, the chronic mutations of radiation are not always clearly to differentiate from the healthy tissue. All attempts to prevent or to decrease this changes of exposure of the skin by medication therapy after the ending of the exposure therapy showed only very unsatisfactory results. The dependency of the frequency of hypodermic fibroses with a body size with the same dose relays on three factors.

1) The thicker a subcutaneous fat is, the more severe are the clinical consequences of a radiation induced fat tissue atrophy.
2) With the increase of the body size, it has to be given a higher skin dose to achieve the same dose in the achieved volume (i.e. in the tumor).

Personal Experience

In our hospital one group 284 patients were treated because of radiation defects. The reasons of radiation are shown in Table 2.9.

Table 2.9 Radiation defects of the skin and surgical treatment

Group	Reason of radiation	Number
1	Breast cancer	84
	Spinal cell cancer and spinal cell cancer of the skin	17
	Melanoma	9
	Sarcoma	2
	Bladder carcinoma	3
	Hypernephroma	1
2	Basal cell carcinoma and Morbus Bowen	48
3	Hemangioma	47
	Nevus, verruca, eczema, hyperkeratosis, inflammation	24
	Tuberculosis	4
	Induratio penis plastica	1
	Scars, keloids	12
4	Unknown reasons for radiation	35
Total		284

In the first group, in which we find the malignant tumors were treated, we found 116 radiation damages. We regarded these damages as a therapeutically complication which cannot be excluded. In the first group we found 48 irradiated basaliomas, i.e. Morbus Bowen. We believe that the indication for the radiation of these tumors was inadequate. At first the treatment lasted incomparably longer than the surgical one and moreover was coupled with acute reactions to the radiation. Retarded damages can never be excluded. In the third group we can find 88 radiation damages as far as benignant mutations of the skin are concerned. An amazing huge proportion form hemangioma, where according to our experience the indication for a radiation therapy was not given. It is the same with nevi, verrucas, eczemas, hyperkeratosis, inflammations, scars and keloids.

In the fourth group we have 35 radiation damages, which dated back for years and it was impossible to find out which kind of tumors were exposed.

Surgical Treatment

If a radiation damage of the skin has already appeared, the only reasonable treatment is the operation. Before the operation the patients should be brought into a good general condition. The local preoperative treatment shall be short-termed and to be conducted with saline solution and a concentrated general and local antibiotic therapy. The wish to create a completely clean wound by means of a long lasting local treatment, to achieve fresh granulations or even a complete healing is illusory.

Unfortunately the patients have been treated with different ointments over months and years and had to take high doses of pain relievers daily for months because of the disastrous pain. The goal of surgical treatment is the radical excision of the radiation damaged tissue until sufficient blood supply is warranted, that enables the healing of potential areas of tissue. The border between healthy and radiation damaged tissue is not always easy to be recognized. In order to achieve a good operation result one will in doubt rather excide a little more. Possible bone proportions in the ulcer area are debrided with a flat chisel, as they are devitalized on the one hand and on the other hand can have an impact on prominence and resulting pressure necrosis of the flap. Not only ulcer but also a chronic radiation dermatitis which shows a tendency of deterioriation should be treated in the same way. To cover defects, the following methods of operation are available:

1) Local flaps
2) Myocutaneous flaps
3) Free flaps
4) Split-thickness skin grafts are applied seldom

A Proposal for Wound Treatment

1) An operation wound is not aseptic. Shortly after the operation, blood leaks out of the operation wound, even with the best hemostasis. This forms the best nutrition for the staphylococci existent in the skin, which are part of the normal skin flora (for example coagulase-negative streptococci). The virulence is significantly less than the one of staphylococcus aureus, nevertheless they owe a great extent of variability and partly aggressiveness. The operation wound, which should not be checked for seven days according to the old rules, is therefore occasionally infected.

Personal proceeding (first day after operation): The operation wound is already to be washed with saline, afterwards treated with disinfection spray (for example Skinsept F) and greater wounds should be applied with an antibiotic ointment subsequently (Neomycin ointment).

Allergies, triggered by antibiotic ointments are very rare. In more than 20 years and several thousand patients we could only register two local allergenic reactions. The cleaning of the wound is done daily, for five days post operationem.

2) In the hairy head, the hair is to be washed on the second day after the operation at the latest, the operation wound is disinfected and treated with Neomycin ointment. Most of the infections after a facelift derive from the fact that the blood scab is not removed. This frequently happens to ambulatory operated patients who are afraid to wash their hair themselves.

3) Necroses have to be debrided. In the third week, a once emerged dry necrosis is demarcated and should be eliminated. Wet gangrene infections present a clear indication to early debridement. Dead tissue is an ideal milieu for a massive increase of bacteria. Moreover a necrosis delays each kind of spontaneous healing.

4) Granulations have to be removed before transplantation. A granulation, which is also called clean area by many authors, is always infected. Granulation tissue always shows a proliferation ecstatically infiltrates capillaries and a persistence of inflamed granulocytes. In the smear there can always be found a massive settlement of bacteria. An excision causes a strong bleeding with familiar consequences. The best method is the cleaning of the granulating area with the hand brush. Here derives a bleeding, but only of short duration. After approximately ten minutes there might possibly be transplantation under application of NaCl/adrenaline solution 1:100000. A transplantation after removing of the granulation area shows remarkable softer scarring.

5) Hematomas have to be removed as early as possible. From the third day on the hematoma begins to organize itself and to fibroid. Large hematoma formations directly after operation have to be revised operationally immediately. The earlier a hematoma is removed the better is the operational result and the smaller is the risk of an infection.

6) Blood hemostasis. At the end of an operation it is recommended to stop even the smallest bleeding with a bipolar coagulation. By means of these additionally ten minutes one is saving a lot of time and trouble which brings a possible appearing hematoma.

CHAPTER **3**
Head and Neck

Defect Coverage in the Nasal Area

History of Nasal Plastic Surgery

Between the years 2500 and 600 B.C. nasoplasties were carried out in India and Egypt. 2000 years ago Susruta Samhita described the at that time conventional method of reconstruction of the nose from forehead and cheek skin in the masterwork Ayur-Veda.

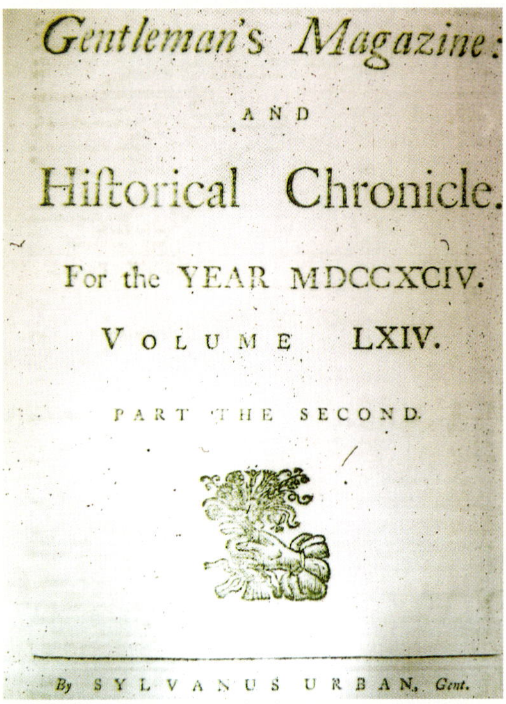
Gentleman's Magazine:
AND
Hiſtorical Chronicle.
For the YEAR MDCCXCIV.
VOLUME LXIV.
PART THE SECOND.
By SYLVANUS URBAN, Gent.

Figure 3.1a In 1794 news arrived from India about a successful nasal reconstruction. In *Gentlemen's Magazine*, i.e. not in a medical journal, a description of a nasal reconstruction carried out by an Indian surgeon from Poona appeared. The patient was an oxman who had had his nose amputated when he was convicted as a prisoner of war. During this operation two British surgeons were present. A British artist made a drawing before and after operation.

In those days it was customary to amputate noses, ears and lips for certain offenses taboo breaches, or if prisoners were captured. The reconstruction of such lost body parts was referred to the Comaas, a caste of potters who seemed predestined for this task, presumably because of their sense of form and expression and their ability to shape objects. The Indians also allegedly used free skin flaps from the buttocks for the nasal restorations. Surgeons in those days were probably very busy because the above-mentioned punishments were indeed common.

Aulus Cornelius Celsus described amazing details from the Alexandrian school about operations on the nose, lips and eyelids. Only in the 15th century did this surgical technique arrive in Greece and Italy via Persia and Arabia. In 1450 excellent reconstructions of nasal defects were carried out by father and son in the Sicilian Branca family. The family Branca used the Indian method, i.e. a forehead flap. The son Antonio Branca also began with a method employing pedicle flaps from the upper arm, a procedure that was dealt with again 100 years later by Tagliacozzi.

In the German literature the first communication about the "Italian procedure" of Heinrich came from Pfalzpaint (Pfolsprundt) from the year 1460 in his textbook on wound healing. The book was only printed in 1868 for the first time (see Sachs, Volume 3, pp. 296). Proof of this is questionable.

While the Branca family jealously guarded their method as a secret, Tagliacozzi in 1597 published the method in his famous book "De curtorum chirurgia per insitionem". It is to him that we owe our thanks

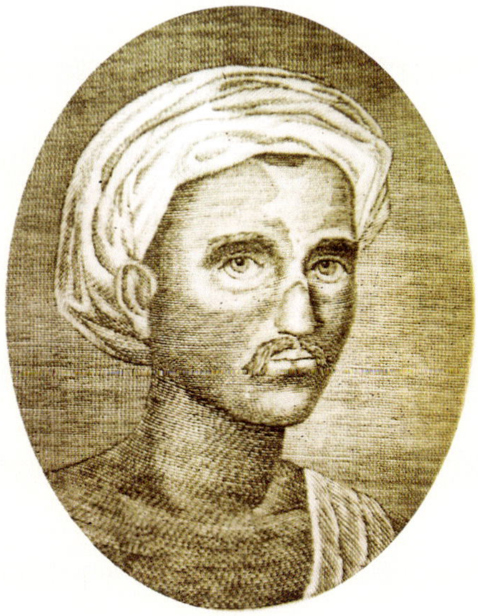

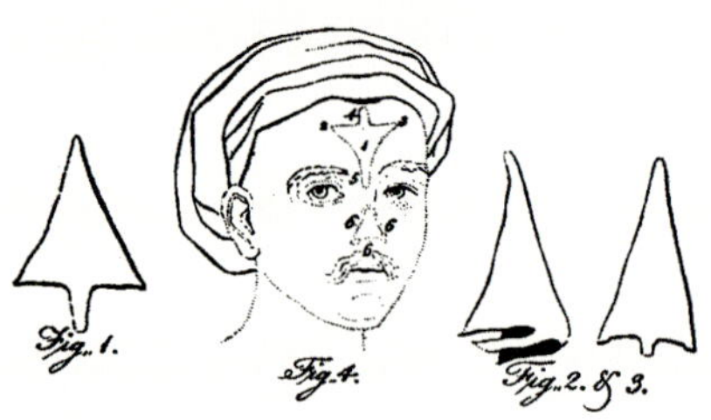

Figure 3.1b The description was accompanied by appropriate drawings. It was a forehead flap (Indian) reconstruction, a method which is still indicated today.

that this procedure became known. He himself had to fight long and hard with the church who considered that mutilation was in fact the will of god.

After the death of Tagliacozzi his soul was condemned, his body was exhumed and then buried outside of the cemetery. His work was forgotten for over 200 years.

In the year 1794 the English *Gentlemen's Journal* reported on a nasal reconstruction carried out in India using forehead flaps with appropriate drawings (Figure 3.1a, b).

In 1814 the English surgeon Joseph Constantin Carpue who had studied this procedure carried out the same operation on two officers with success.

In 1816 the Berlin surgeon Carl Ferdinand von Graefe carried out the reconstruction using an upper arm flap on a soldier whose nose had been severed by a saber blow (Tagliacozzi method). It can be assumed that he was well versed in the publications of Tagliacozzi.

Immediately after that, nasal reconstructions were reproduced in France (Dupuytren, Delpech, Lisfranc, Labat, Serre), Italy (Signoroni, Baroni, Riberi), England (Hutchison, Syme), Russia (Hoefft and Dybeck), America (Warren) and Germany (Beck, Bünger, Heidenreich and Zeis). The Berlin surgeon Dieffenbach was the most important since he mastered the Indian and Italian methods and carried out a large number of successful operations (see Chapter 1 History).

Anatomy of the Nose (Simplified)

(For Details use an Atlas of Anatomy)

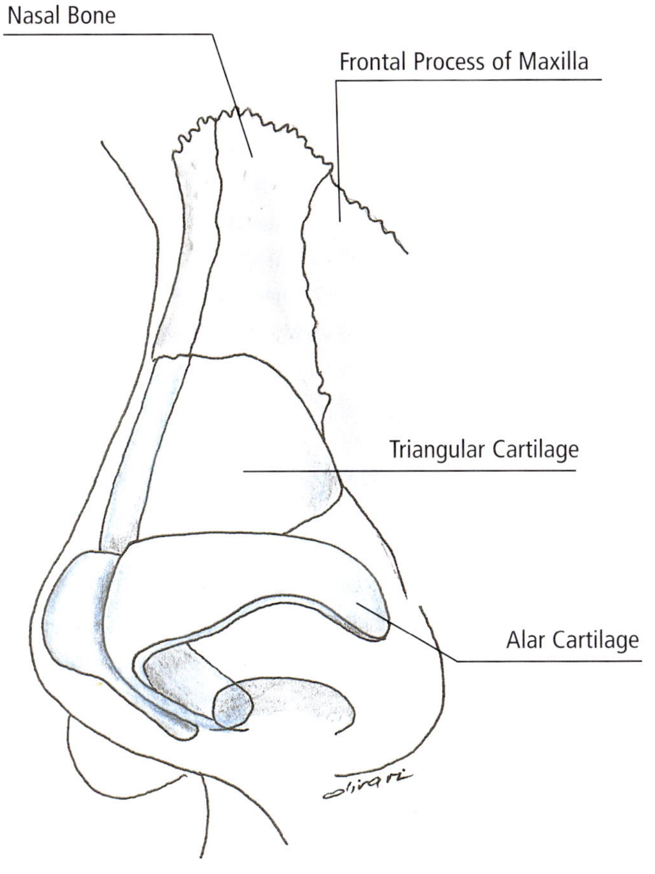

Figure 3.2a Nasal skeleton

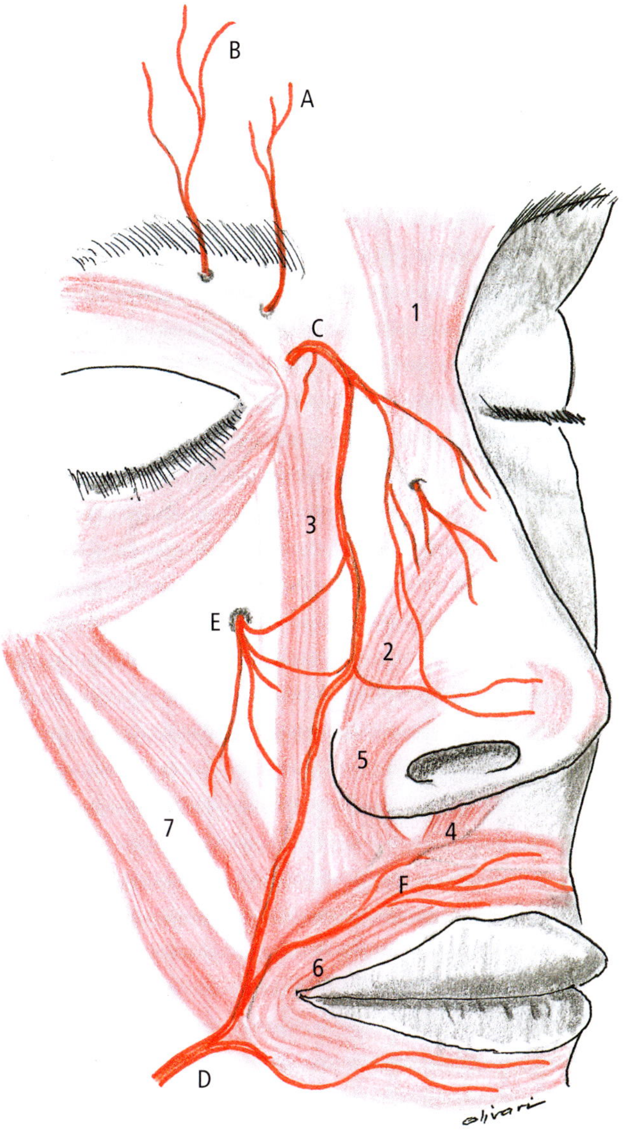

Figure 3.2b Blood supply and musculature in the oronasal area: 1) procerus muscle, 2) nasal muscle, 3) quadratus labii superior muscle, 4) depressor septi nasi muscle, 5) the alar part of the nasal muscle, 7) inferior and superior zygomatic muscle, a) supratrochlear artery, b) supraorbital artery, c) angular artery, d) facial artery, e) infraorbital artery, f) superior labial artery.

a) Nasolabial Flap Type I

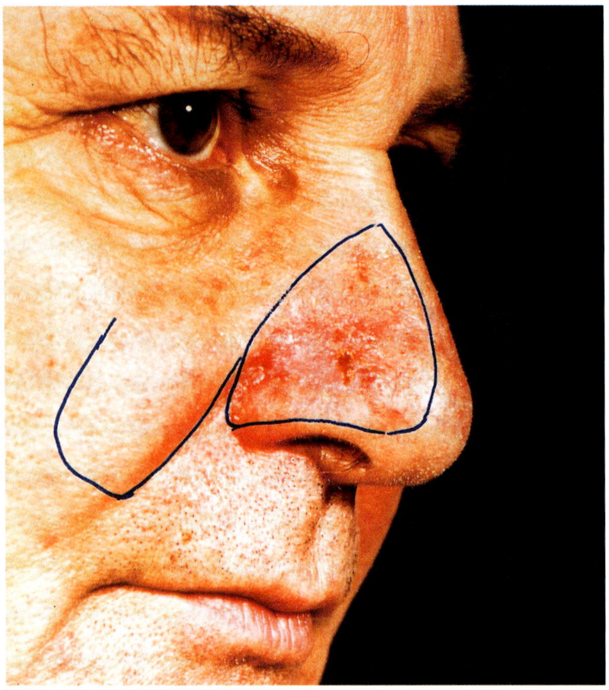

Figure 3.5a Superficial, extensive basal cell carcinoma of the right side of the nose. Cartilage or bone are not involved.

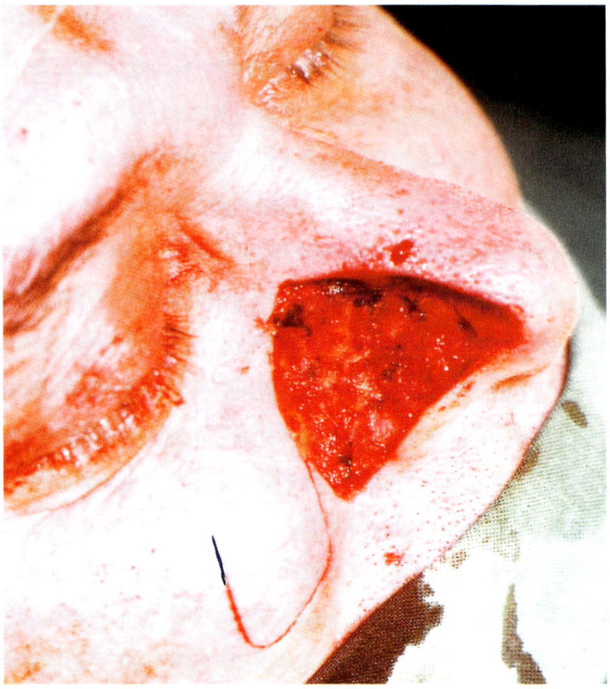

Figure 3.5b Situation after excision: The excision is carried out according to the histological findings. When planning the flap it must always be longer than required by the defect.

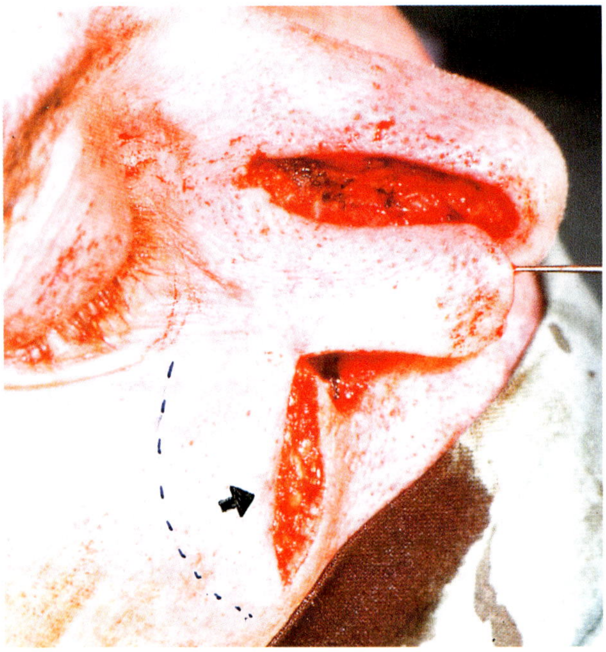

Figure 3.5c After mobilization of the cheek skin the flap is turned into the defect. The lateral mobilization in the cheek area must be carried out thoroughly. The secondary defect can be closed directly.

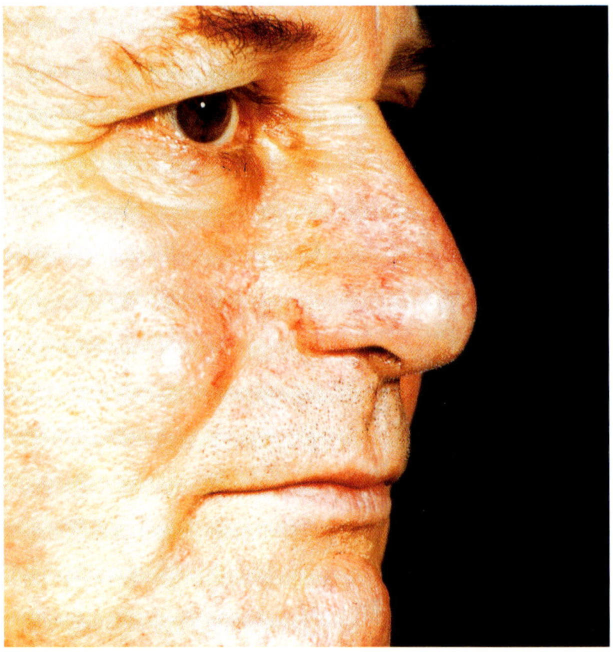

Figure 3.5d Status 18 months after the operation.

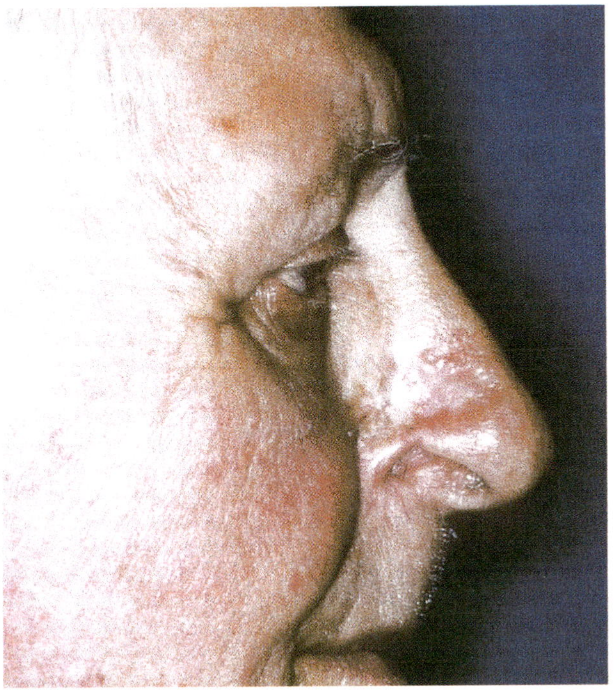

Figure 3.6a Irradiated superficial basal cell carcinoma of the right side of the nose.

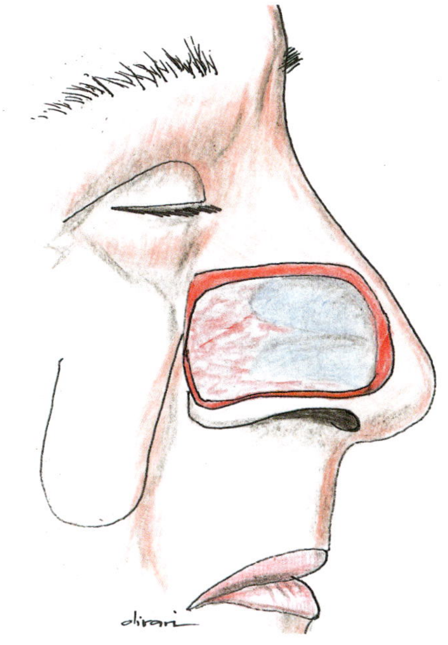

Figure 3.6b A large, but not deep defect is present after excision of the tumor. Skin, subcutaneous tissue, as well as a portion of the cartilage are excised. A correspondingly large, cranially based nasolabial pedicle flap is formed. Since an inner lining is not necessary, the flap is shorter than it is with type II and III.

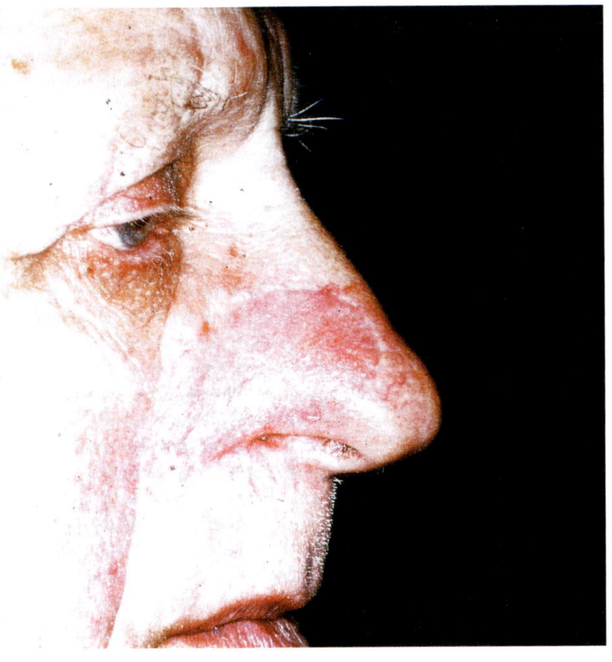

Figure 3.6c Status 18 months after the operation. Following the removal of the contracting irradiation scars, the form of the nose is clearly improved.

b) Nasolabial Flap Type II

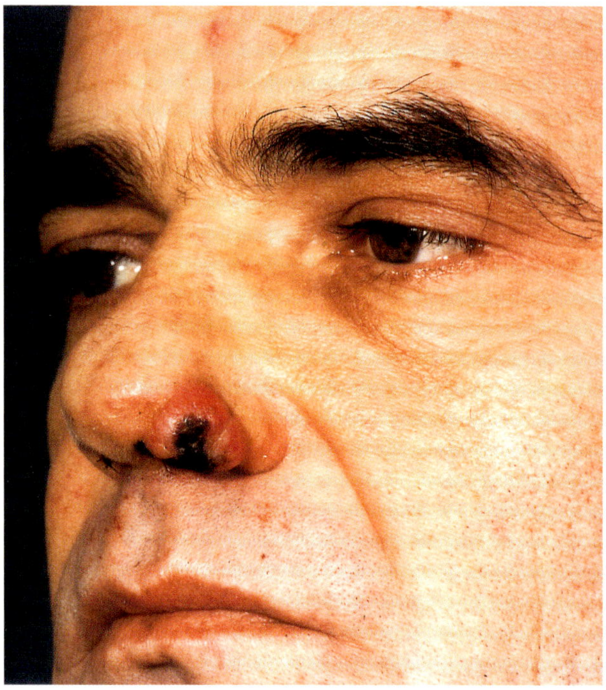

Figure 3.7a Basal cell carcinoma of the left alar area

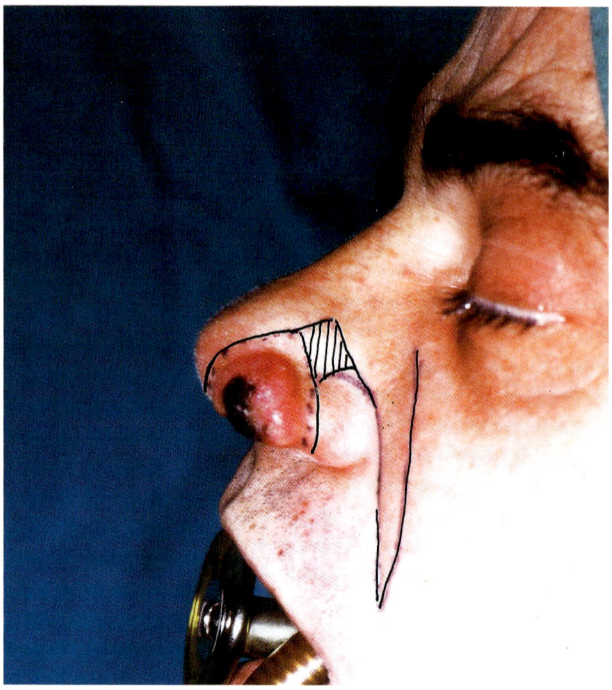

Figure 3.7b In order to ensure complete histological clearance of tumor all three layer (skin, cartilage and mucosa) must be excised.

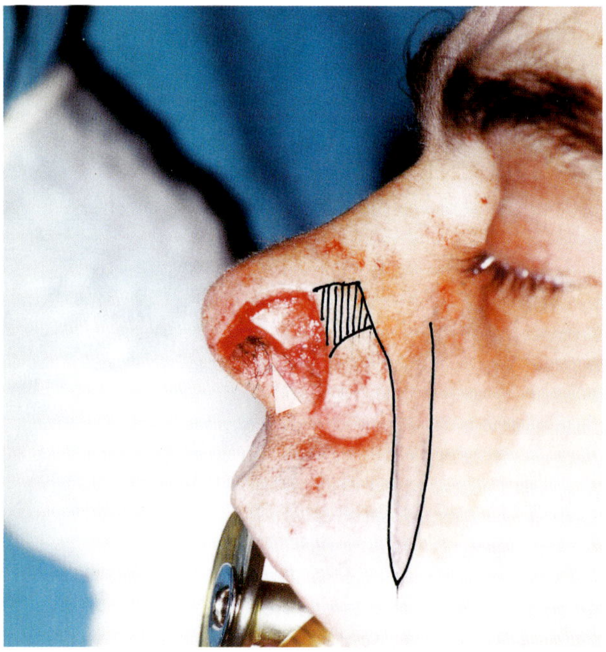

Figure 3.7c Status after tumor extirpation. The nasal wing cartilage is largely resected. In order to form a nasolabial type II flap, a portion of the healthy tissue (shaded) must also be excised.

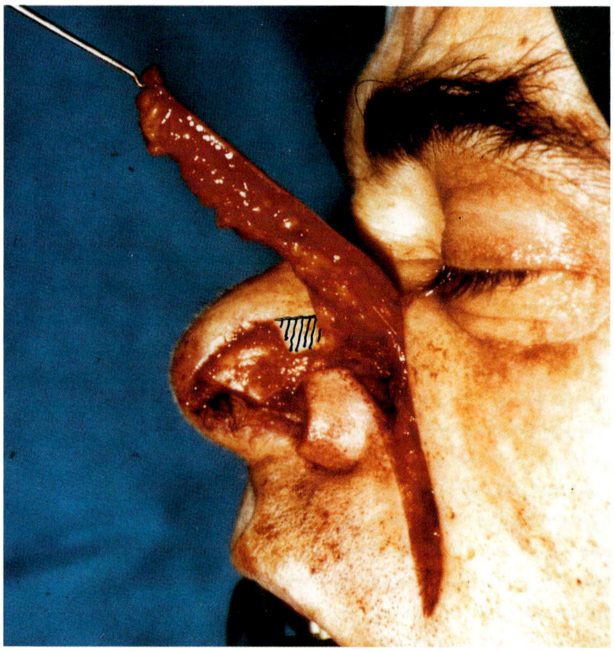

Figure 3.7d Raising of the flap. After the flap is raised the shaded part of the healthy tissue is excised.

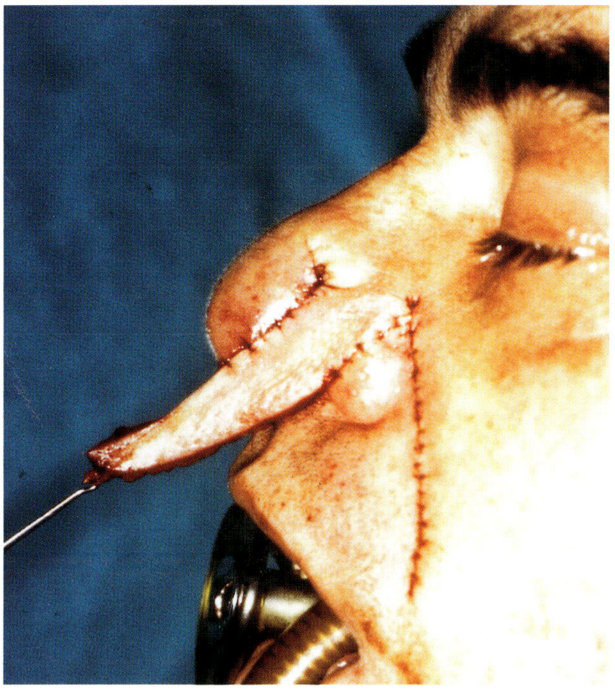

Figure 3.7e The secondary defect is sutured with 6 × 0 nylon (e.g. Trofilene). The flap is sutured on outside also with 6 × 0 nylon. The distal part of the flap is now turned into the nostril and fixed with 5 × 0 Vicryl. This part serves as the inner lining and provides adequate stability for the nasal wing.

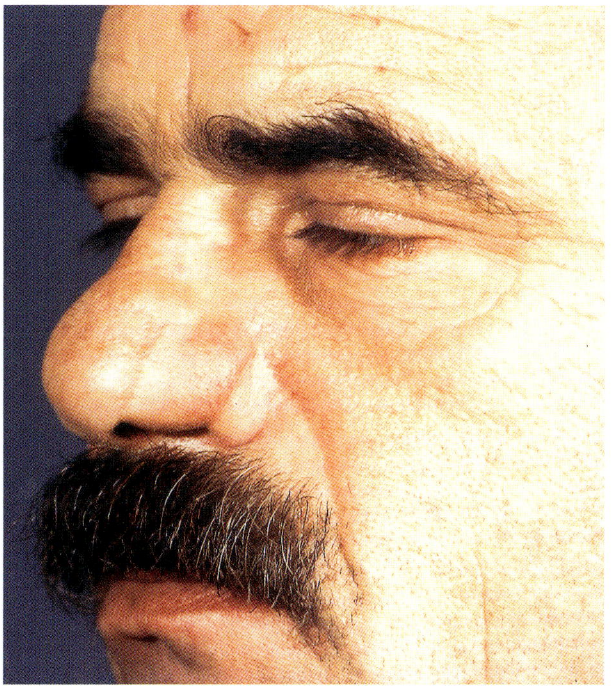

Figure 3.7f Situation two years after the surgery. There is no restriction of respiration. Scar of secondary defect is barely visible.

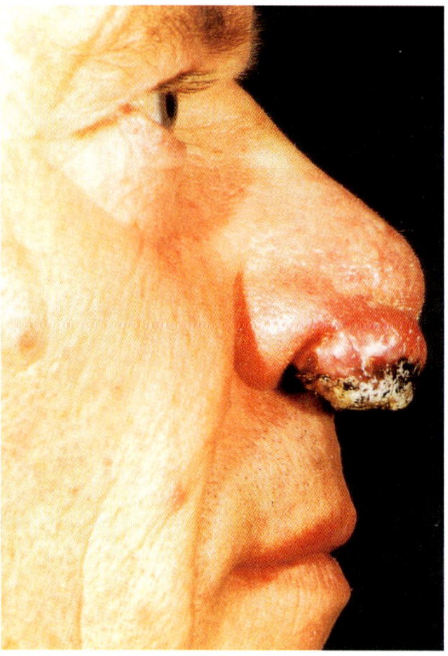

Figure 3.8a Basal cell carcinoma of the right nasal wing

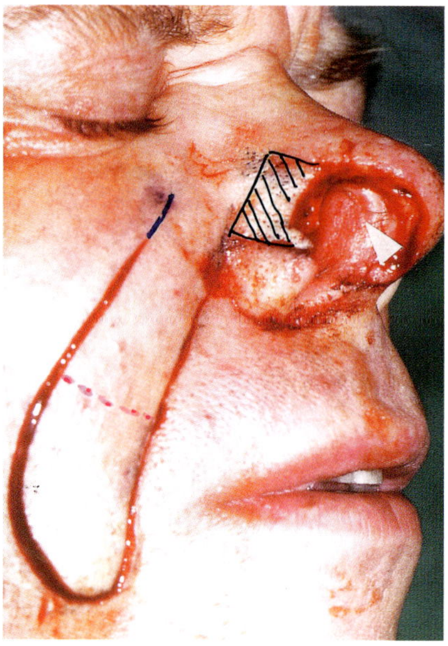

Figure 3.8b Situation after a microscopically controlled excision of the tumor (three-layer resection). The shaded part of the healthy skin must also be excised in order to achieve a better result.
Arrow = nasal septum

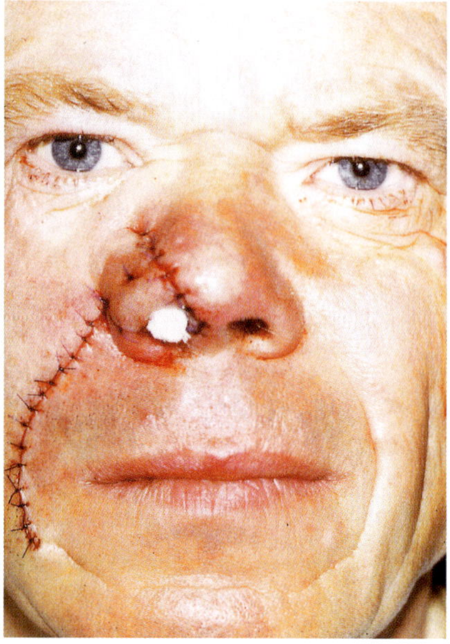

Figure 3.8c Picture at the end of the operation. It is remarkable that even larger secondary defects can be closed in the nasolabial area without any major tension.

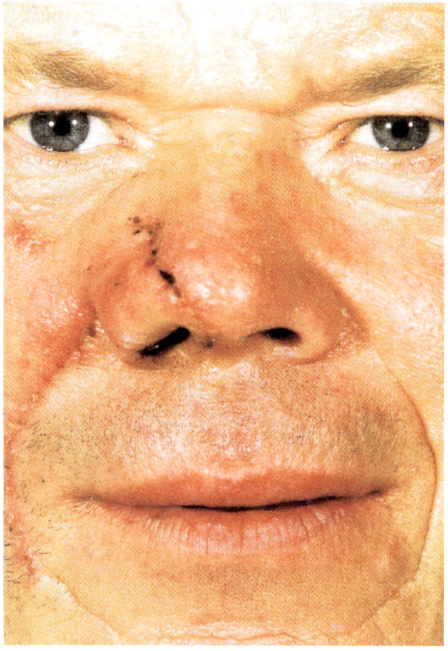

Figure 3.8d Situation 16 days after the operation

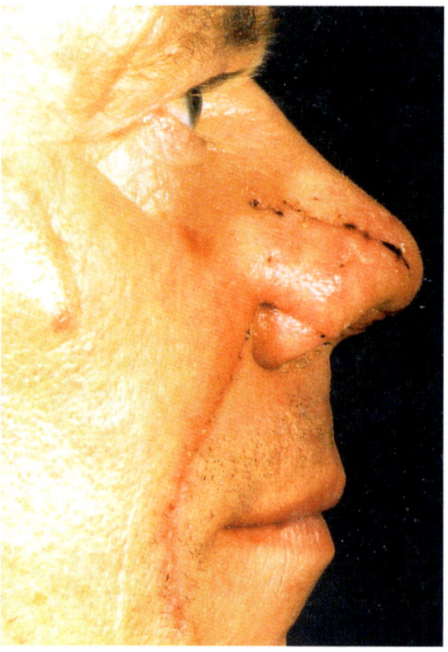

Figure 3.8e In men the distal part of the flap is often hairy. The hairs must later be cut regularly or removed by laser treatment.

c) Nasolabial Flap Type III

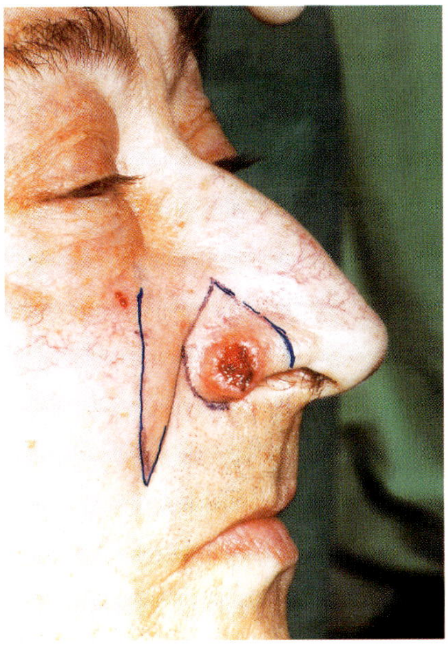

Figure 3.9a Basal cell carcinoma of the right nasal wing

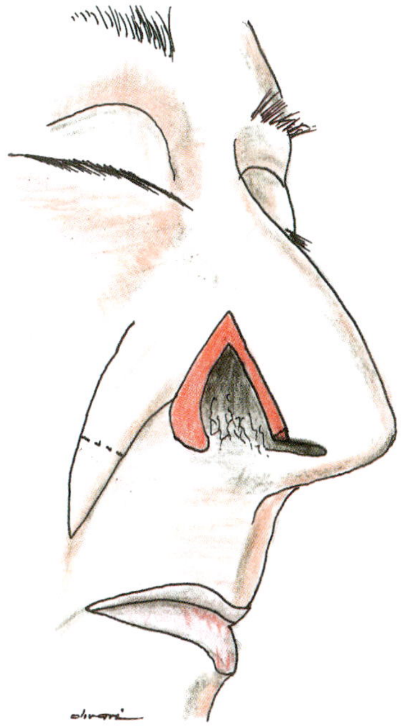

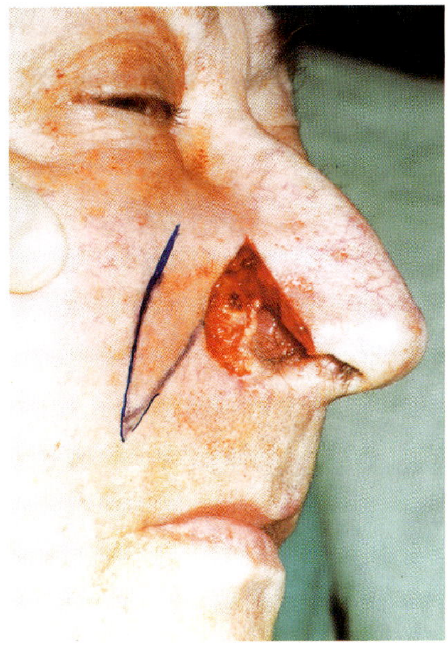

Figure 3.9b, c Excision of skin, cartilage and mucosa. Formation of a nasolabial flap type III. The lateral part of the nasal wing is excised.

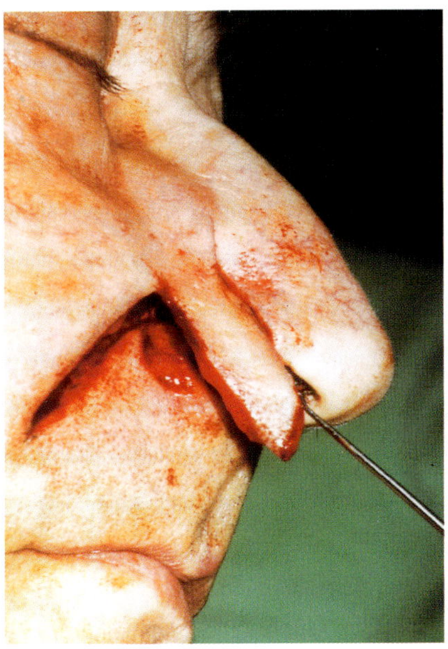

Figure 3.9d Mobilization of the flap

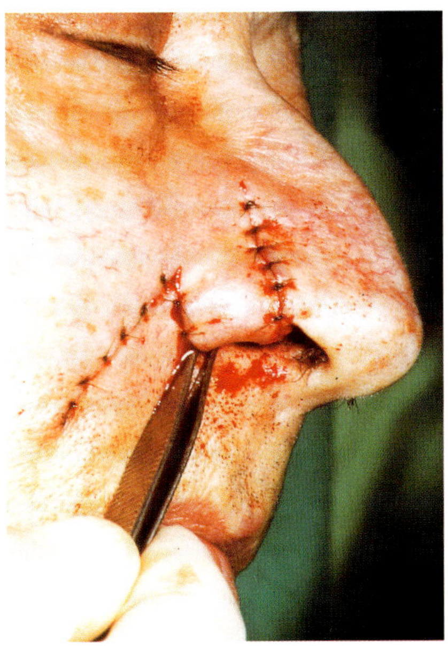

Figure 3.9e Folding of the distal flap part for the inner lining

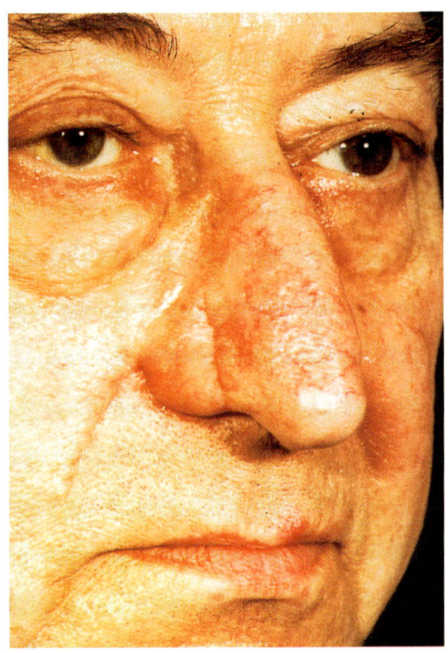

Figure 3.9f Status six months after the operation. Skin suturing with 6 × 0 nylon (Trofilene) and suturing of the inner lining carried out with 5 × 0 Vicryl.

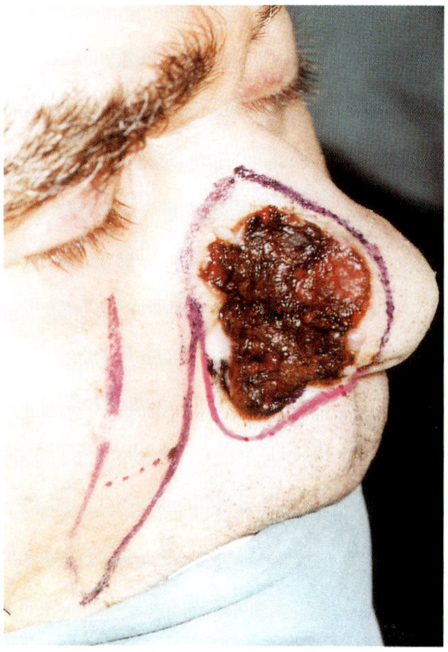

Figure 3.10a Large basal cell carcinoma of the right nasal wing and side

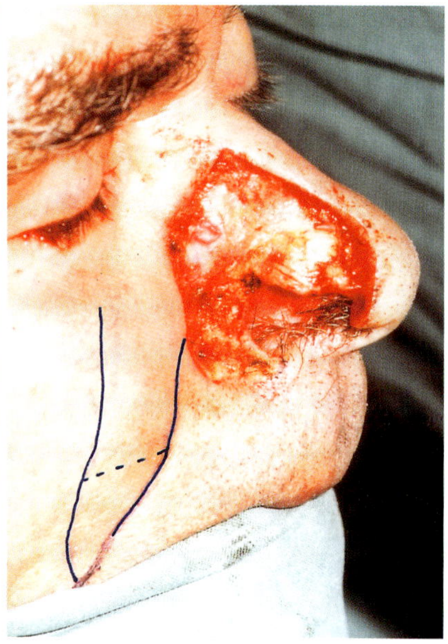

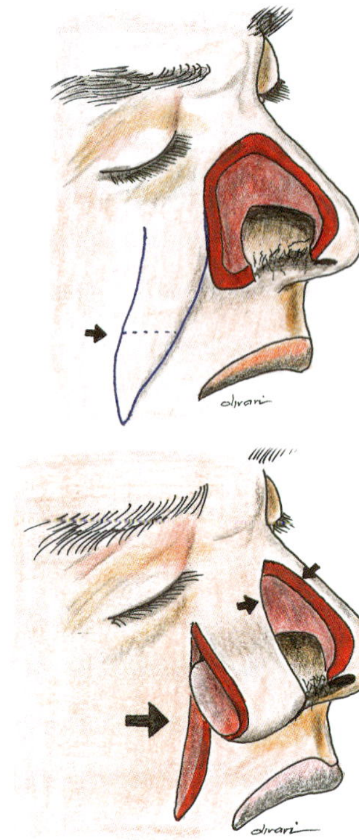

Figure 3.10b,c Planning of a type III nasolabial flap. In the lower part a three-layer resection was carried out, while in the upper part the tumor had not infiltrated the nasal bone. Here the resection was carried out up to the nasal bone. The interrupted line shows the site at which the flap should be folded.

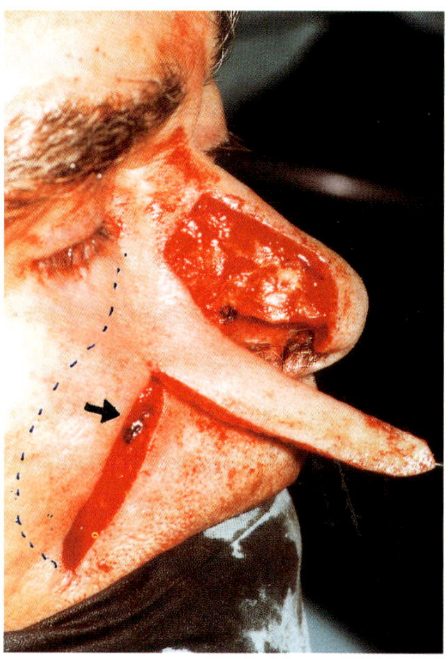

Figure 3.10d Mobilization of the flap: Because of the flap size a more extensive mobilization of the cheek skin from the lateral side is necessary. The external part of the flap is fixed with 6 × 0 non-resorbable suture, while the folded inner part is sutured with 5 × 0 Vicryl. The flap is stiff enough and does not require any additional cartilage support.

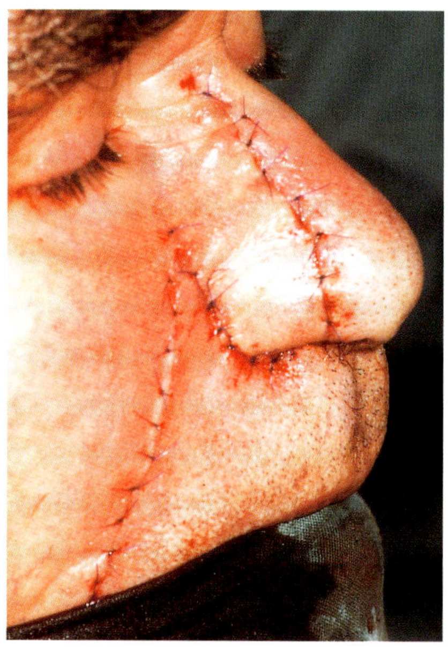

Figure 3.10e Status after the end of the operation

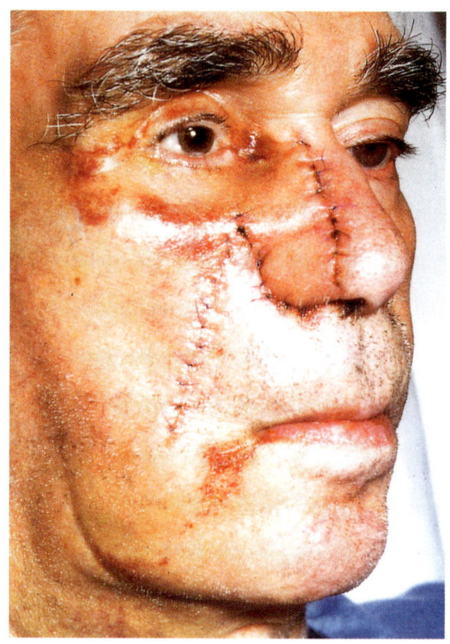

Figure 3.10f Status ten days after the operation

d) One-Stage Nasal Reconstruction With Two Nasolabial Flaps According to Olivari

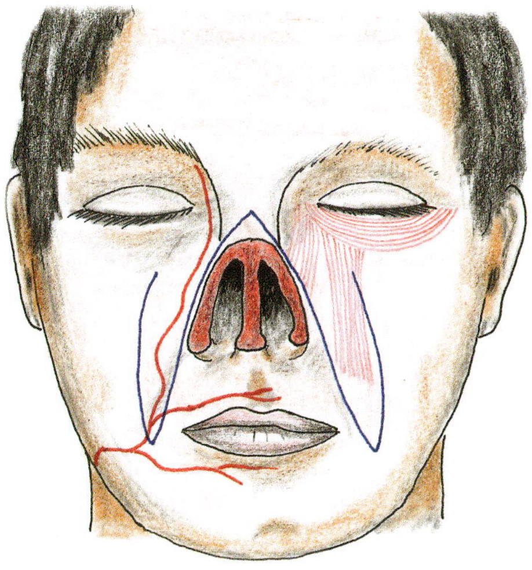

Figure 3.11a Two long, cranial pedicle flaps from the nasolabial fold were planned. In the cranial part the flaps contained parts of the nasal muscle as well as the angular head of the quadratus labii superior muscle. This cranial part is thus a myocutaneous flap. This is an axial flap supplied by angular artery.

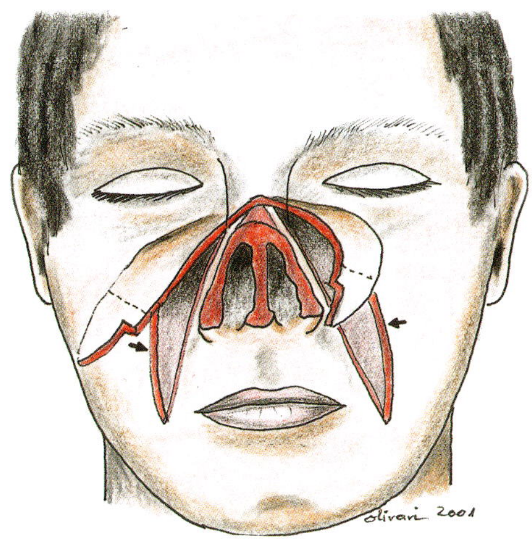

Figure 3.11b The flaps are mobilized up until the nasal root. At the tip of the flap a step is formed medially under the folding point in order to reconstruct the columella. The cheek skin is thoroughly mobilized laterally so that the secondary defect can be primarily closed. The distal part of the flap includes only skin without deeper layers so that the buccal branch of the facial nerve is not injured.

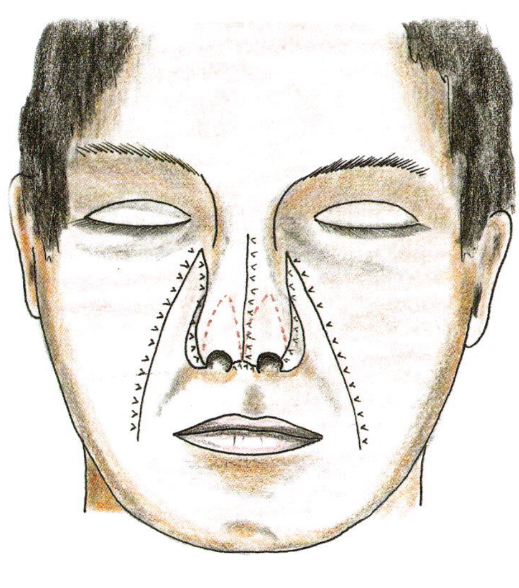

Figure 3.11c The flap is folded inside in order to form the inner lining and to provide sufficient stiffness for the nostril. Skin suture is carried out using 6 × 0 non-resorbable sutures. Intranasal lining is sutured using 5 × 0 resorbable Vicryl.

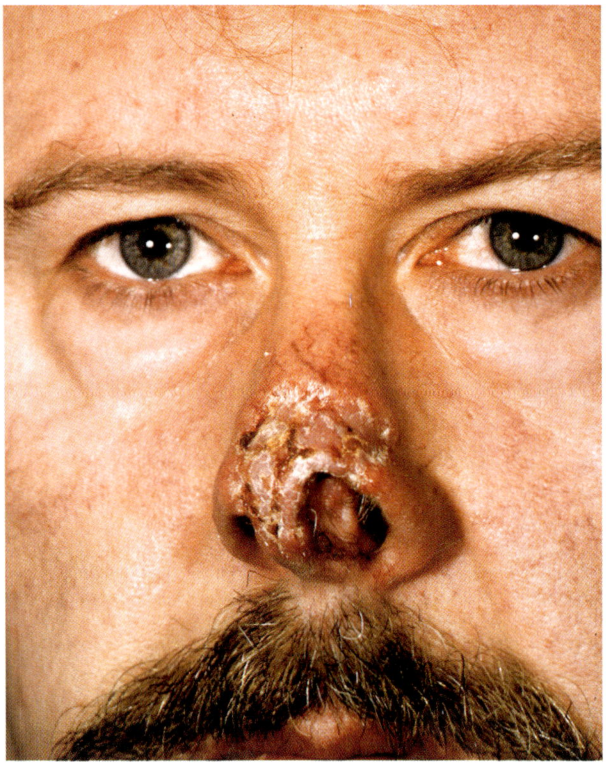

Figure 3.12a Infiltrative basal cell carcinoma of a part of the nose.

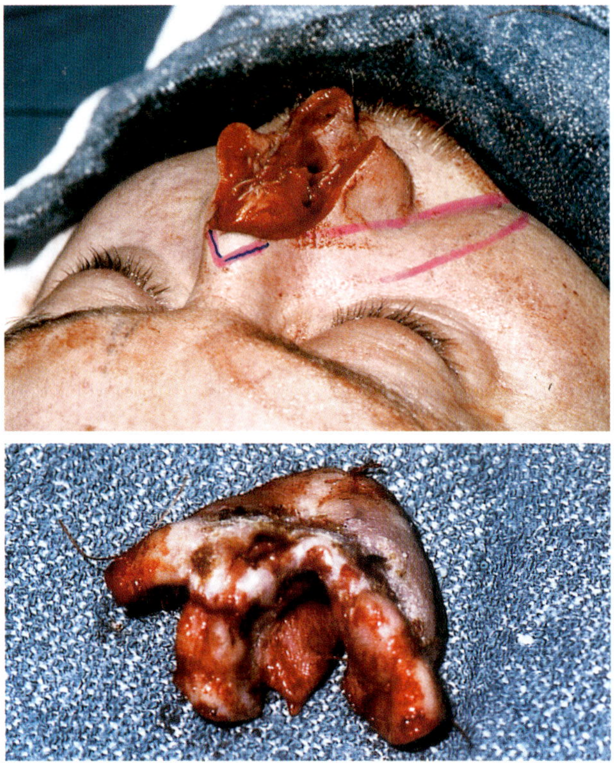

Figure 3.12b Situation after subtotal amputation of the nose, the nasal dorsum, the columella and the nasal wings.

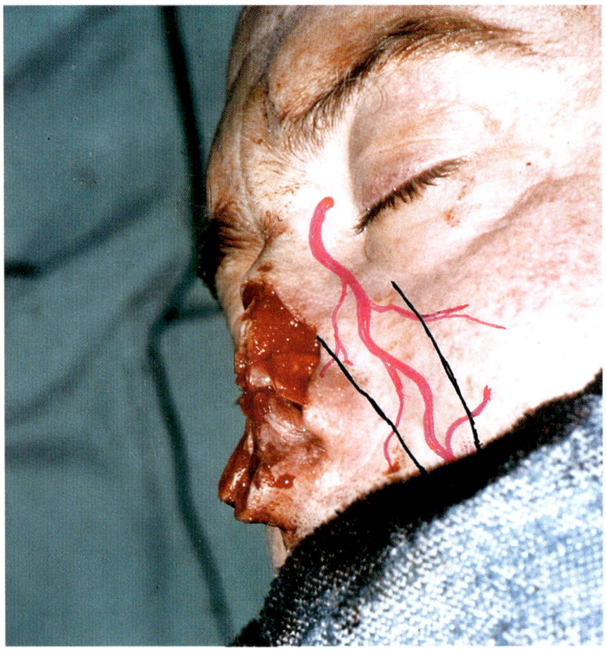

Figure 3.12c Formation of long, cranial pedicled nasolabial flaps bilaterally.

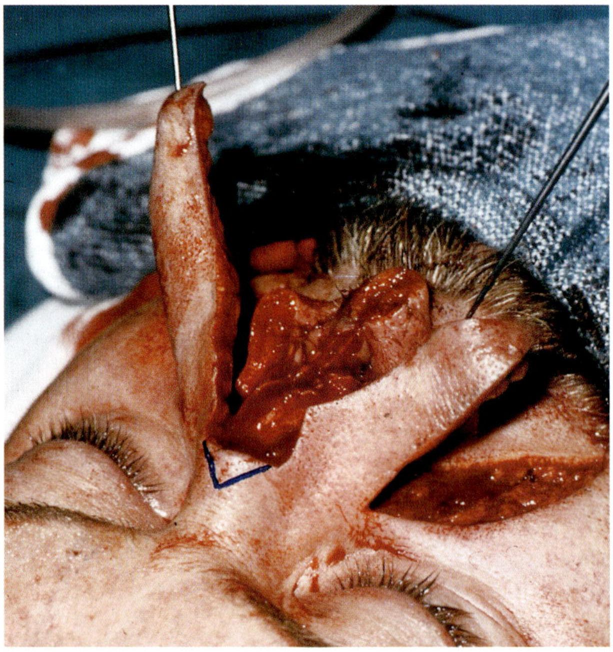

Figure 3.12d Both flaps are mobilized. The nasal muscle, the angular head of the quadratus labii superioris muscle and the angular artery are all integrated in the cranial part of the flap. In order to avoid "dog earing", a small triangle is excised at the nasal root.

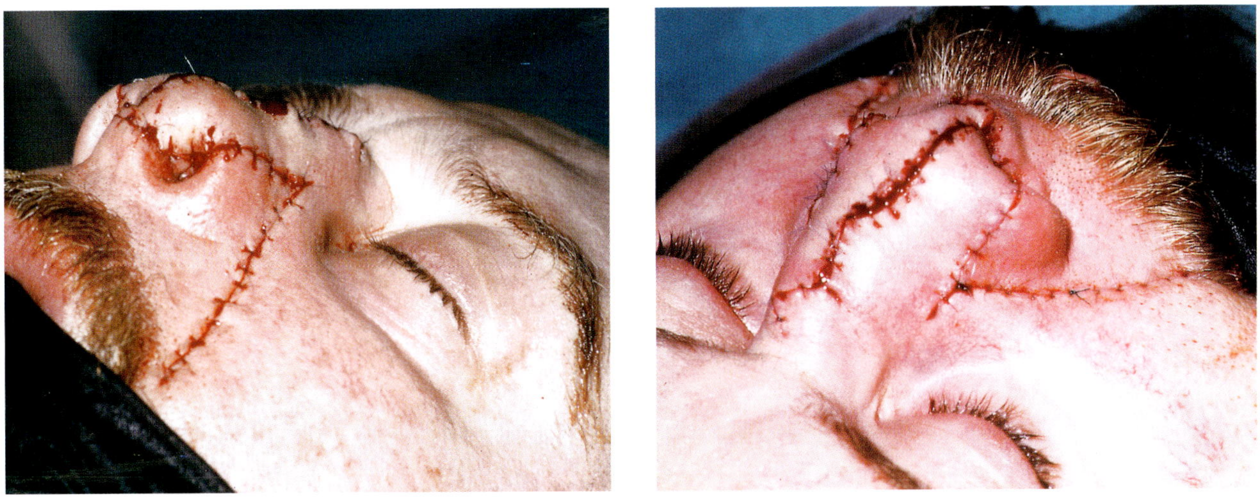

△ **Figure 3.12e,f** Both flaps are fixed in the nasal defect. The distal part of both flaps is folded inwards and used as lining. A portion of the two flap tips is required for the columella reconstruction while another part is required for the nasal wing reconstruction.

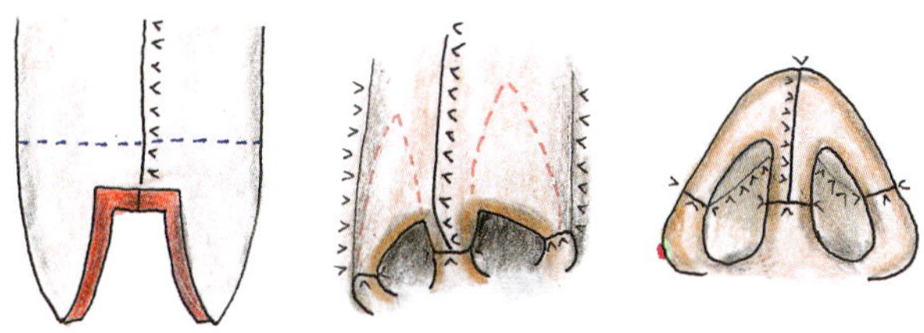

▷ **Figure 3.12g** Shaping of the nasal tip and the columella. The dotted line shows the folding point of the flap tip. The step formation is important for the reconstruction of the columella.

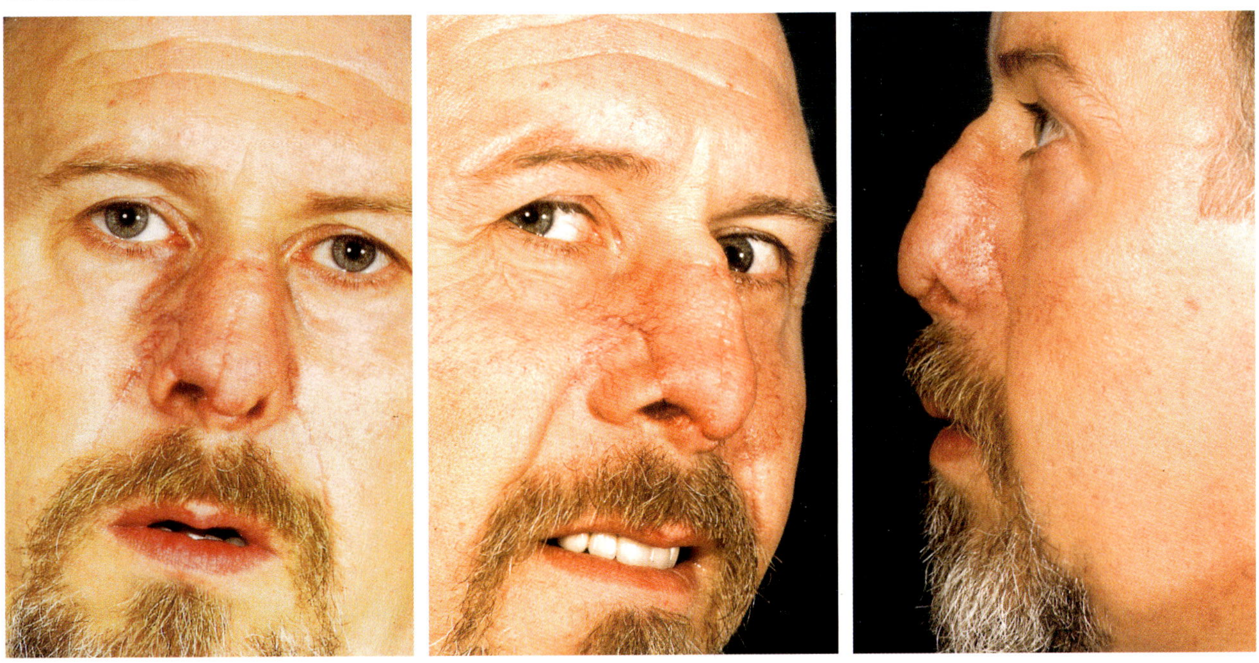

Figure 3.12h–j Situation one year after a one step nasal reconstruction according to Olivari. There is not relapse, nasal breathing is normal, the nasal form is satisfactory. The flap removal sites look inconspicuous. In the lower third the flap is only composed of skin; one should go not deeper in this area so that the buccal branch of the facial nerve is not injured. The double flap is stiff enough so that a bone or cartilage graft is not necessary. If tumor recurrence occurs, an option still remains open, for a forehead flap.

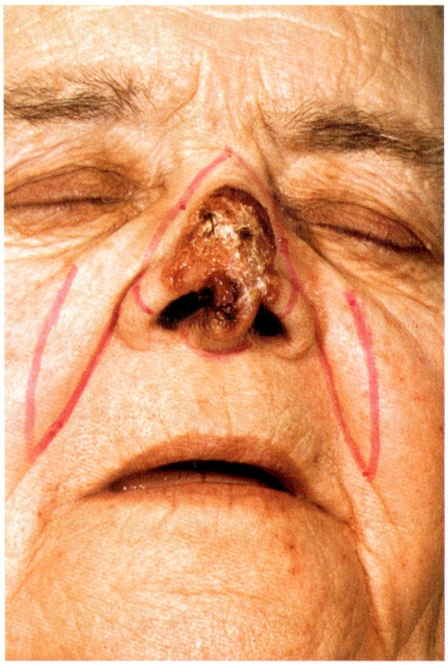

Figure 3.13a Extensive basal cell carcinoma of the nasal dorsum, the nasal tip, the nasal septum as well as the nasal wings

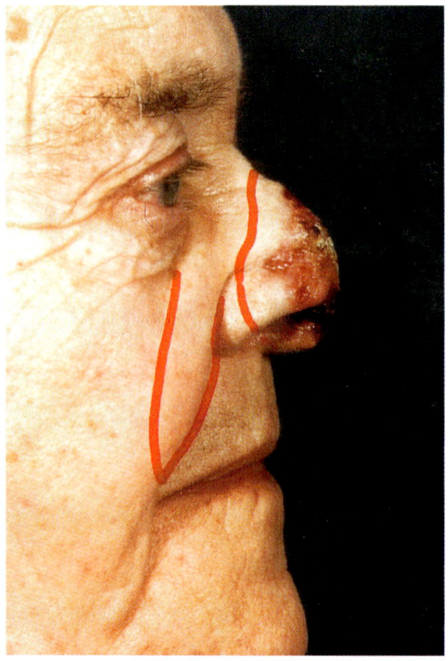

Figure 3.13b 83-year old patient who had been treated for diabetes for several years. Planning of the operation.

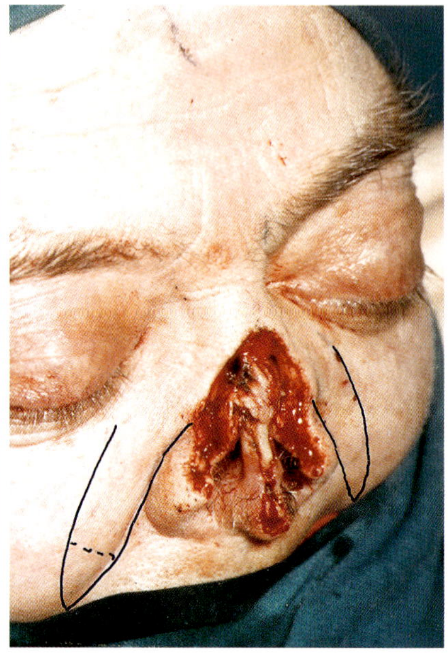

Figure 3.13c Situation after a subtotal resection of the nose

Comment

For a subtotal nasal reconstruction of the nose two cranial pedicled, very long flaps are used. The flap includes in its cranial part the nasal muscle as well as the angular head of the quadratus labii superioris muscle. The axial blood supply through the angular artery is safeguarded. As such it represents an axial pattern myocutaneous flap.

The one step reconstruction of the nose with two nasolabial flaps (Olivari method) has the following advantages:

1. The blood supply of the flap is safe. Flaps of considerable size and length can be raised.
2. Larger defects at the nasal wing as well as at the nasal septum, i.e. a subtotal nasal amputation, can be reconstructed.
3. The flap is relative slight surgical invasion particularly for older and very ill patients.
4. A forehead flap is still available should further reconstruction be needed after excision of recurrence.
5. The procedure is relatively easy from a technical point of view, requiring only a single operation.

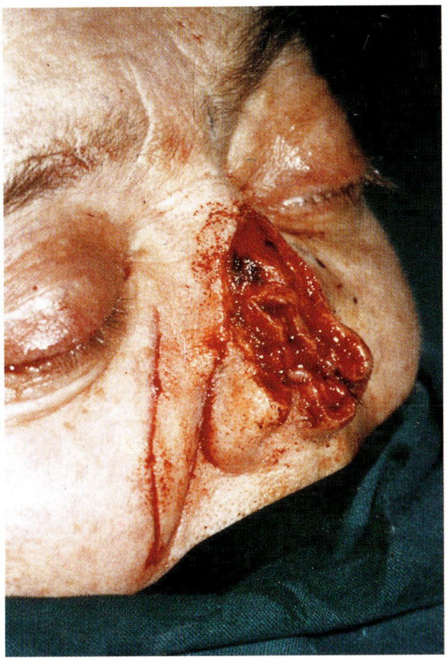

Figure 3.13d Status after microscopically controlled resection of the tumor extending into healthy tissue.

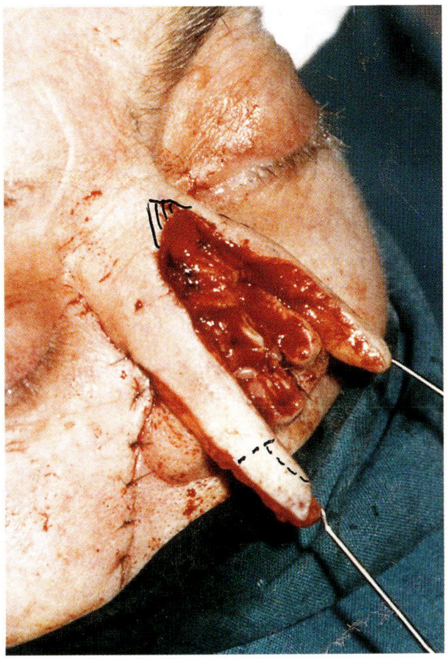

Figure 3.13e Both nasolabial flaps are formed. The flaps are long enough to ensure that the distal third can be used as an inner lining.

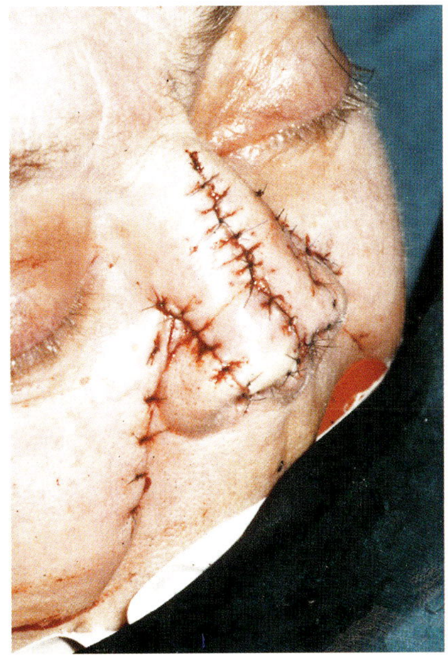

Figure 3.13f Situation at the end of the operation. The flap removal site is closed in a tension-free manner.

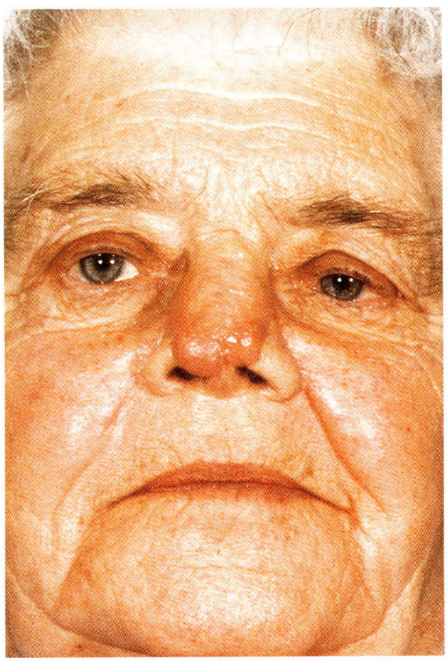

Figure 3.13g Status one year after the operation. Function and form of the nose are good.

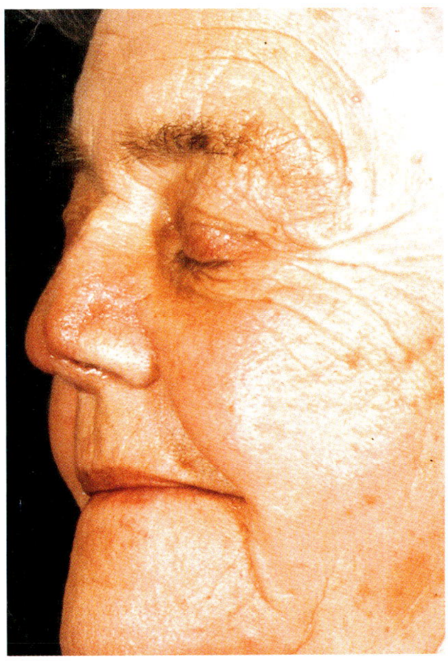

Figure 3.13h Secondary defect is almost invisible

e) Nasolabial Island Flap

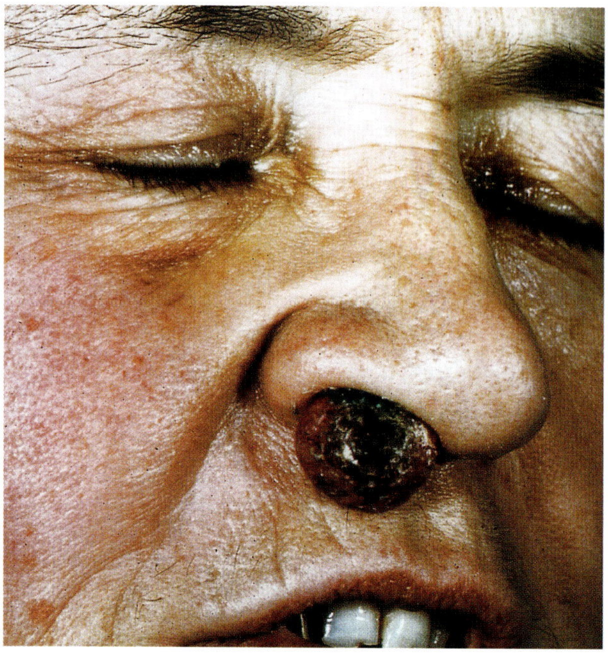

Figure 3.14a Basal cell carcinoma of the nostril

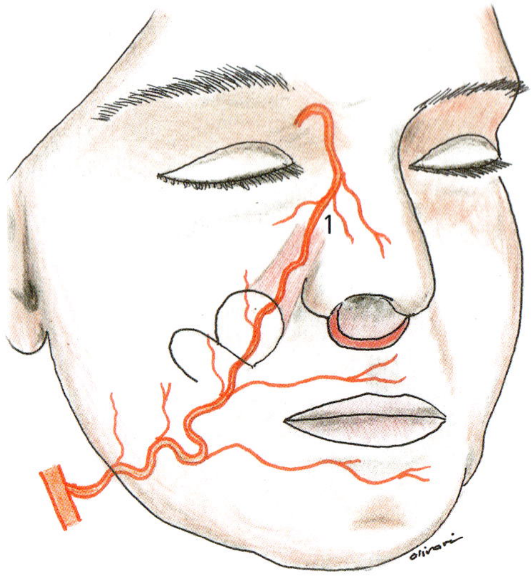

Figure 3.14b Planning of the nasolabial island flap.
The pedicle of island flap is formed from the nasolabial fold.
It is an arterial flap, supplied by the angular artery (1).
The skin flap size corresponds to the defect size.

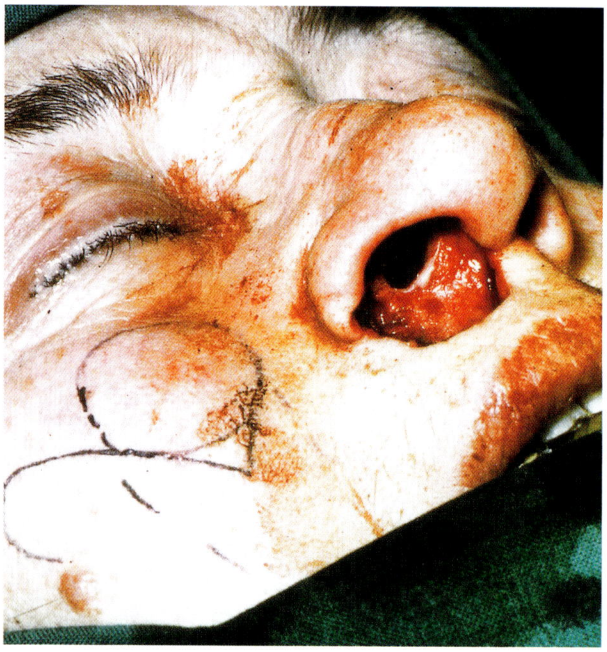

Figure 3.14c The tumor is excised.
The island flap is planned. At the same time a local transposition flap for secondary defect closure.

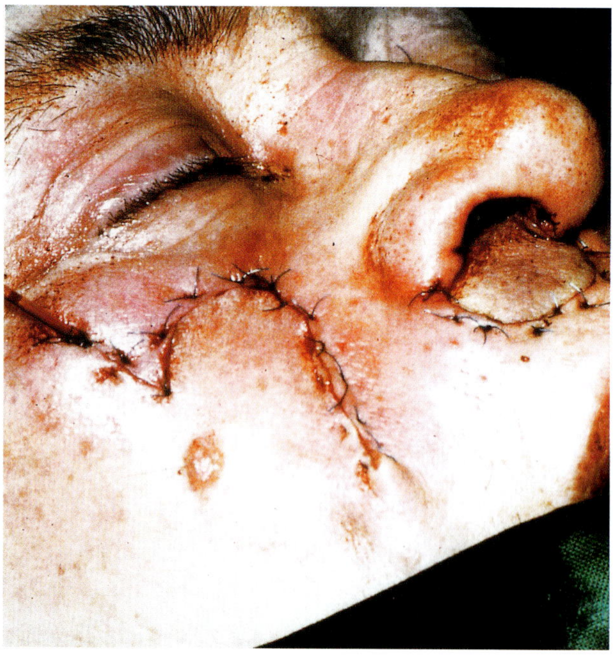

Figure 3.14d Situation at the end of the operation.
The island flap in the nostril is well vascularized with blood.
The secondary defect is closed with a local flap.

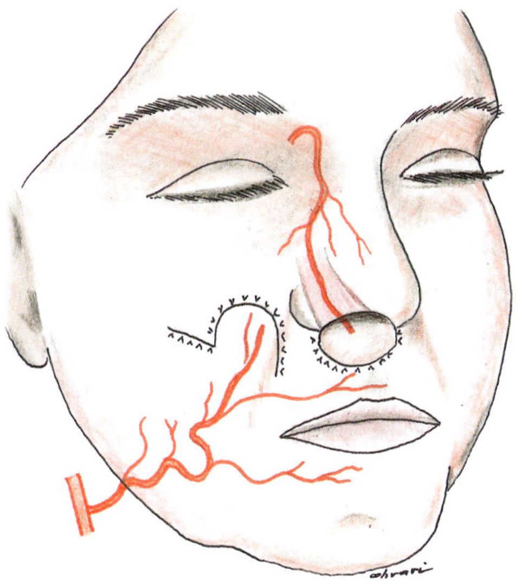

Figure3.14e Schematic picture of the artery supply of the island flap at the end of the operation.

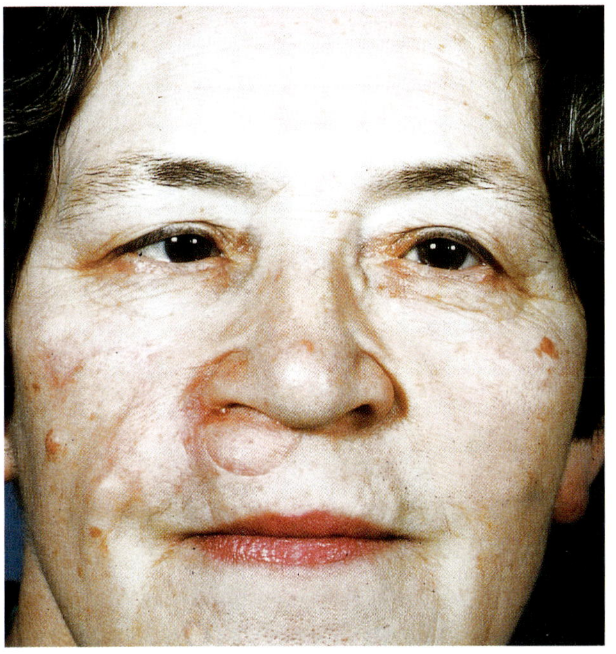

Figure 3.14f Situation one year after the operation. A mild lymphedema of the island flap exists. This is a frequent transient condition with island flaps.

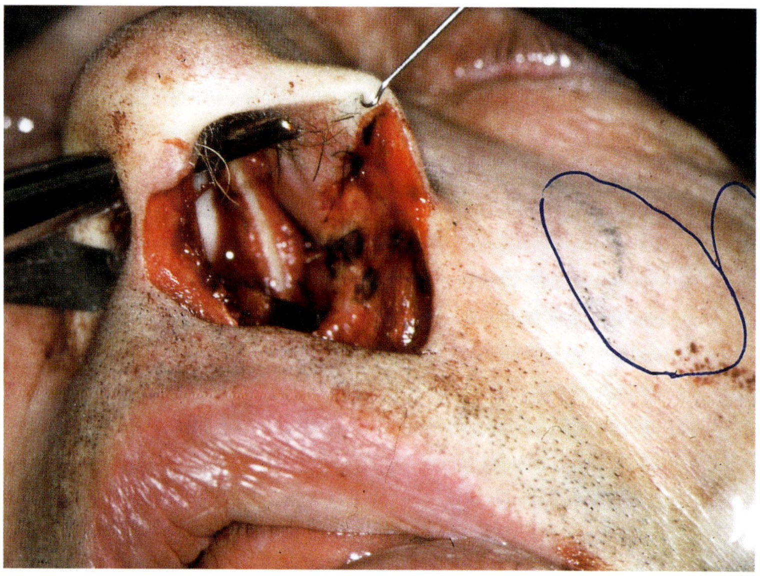

Note:

Island Flaps: Because of the interruption of lymph flow in this flaps a mild swelling can persist for a few months. The patient must be informed about this.

Figure 3.15a A basal cell carcinoma in the nostril is excised. A part of the septum is also resected.

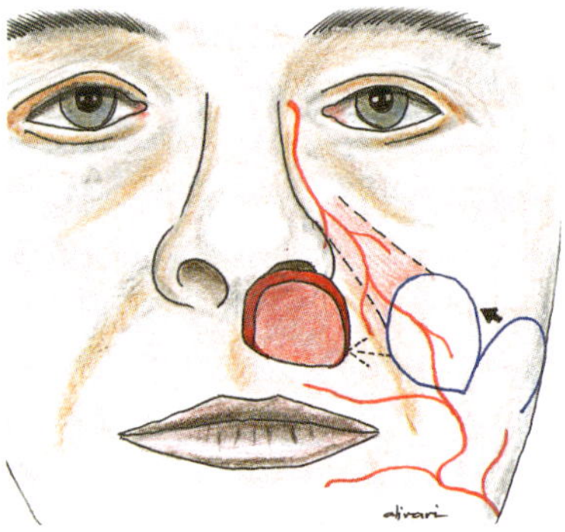

Figure 3.15b An island flap is formed from the left nasiolabal fold, which is perfused via the subcutaneous tissue axially by the anastomosis between the facial and angular artery.

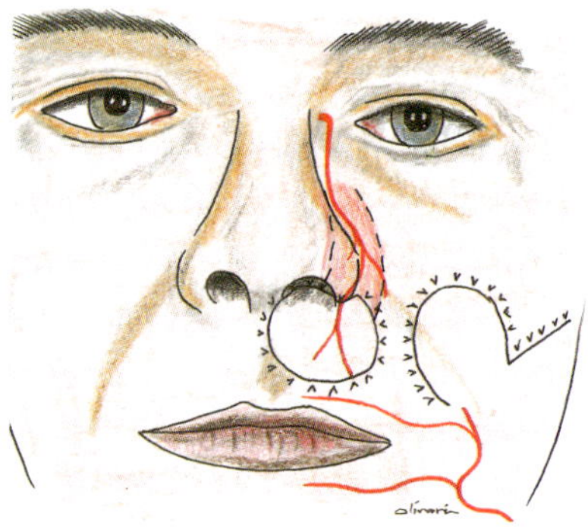

Figure 3.15c The defect was closed with an island flap and the secondary defect is closed using a local flap.

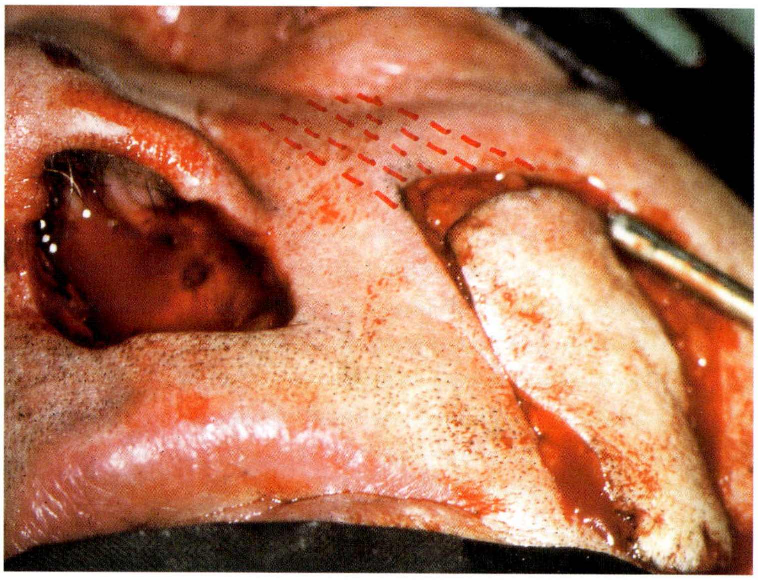

Figure 3.15d Mobilization of the island flap

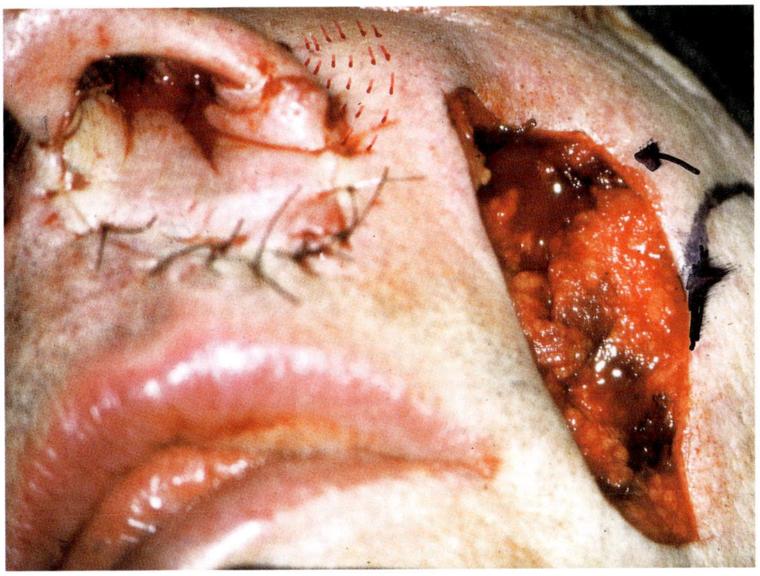

Figure 3.15e The island flap is pulled through a subcutaneous tunnel into the defect and fixed

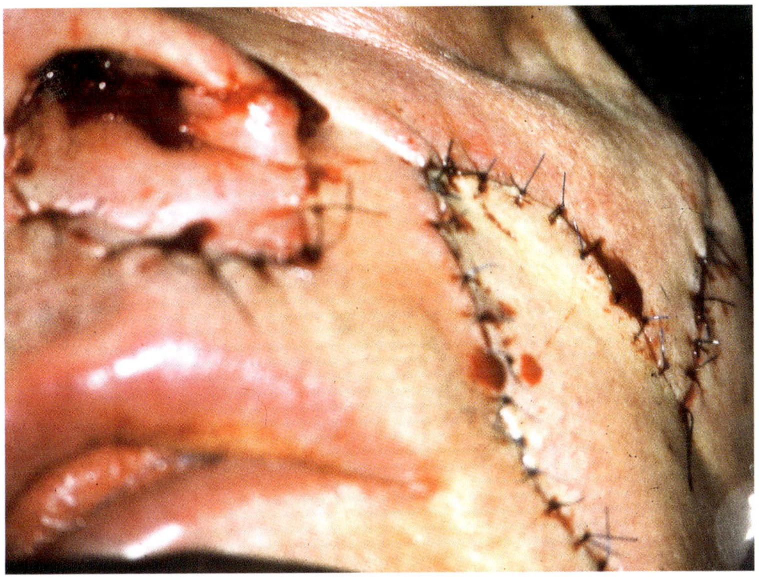

Figure 3.15f The secondary defect is closed using a local flap

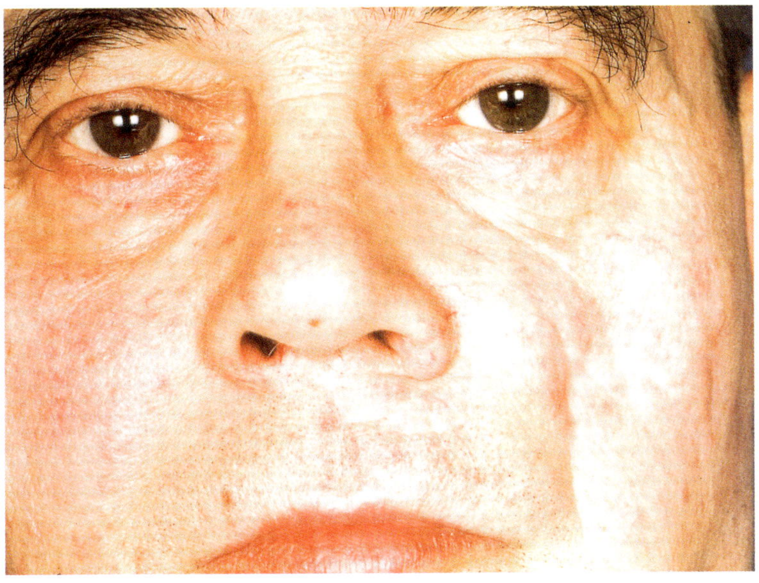

Figure 3.15g Situation two years after the operation

Defect Coverage With Forehead Flaps

a) Small Forehead Flap (Supratrochlear Flap)

The supratrochlear flap is an axial flap and as such is well supplied with blood. The flap pedicle can be very narrow. This improves flap mobility. The supratrochlear flap is suitable for covering defects in the upper part of the nose, the inner eye corner and up to the medial part of the lower eyelid. Use of the Doppler may be useful in identifying the supratrochlear artery.

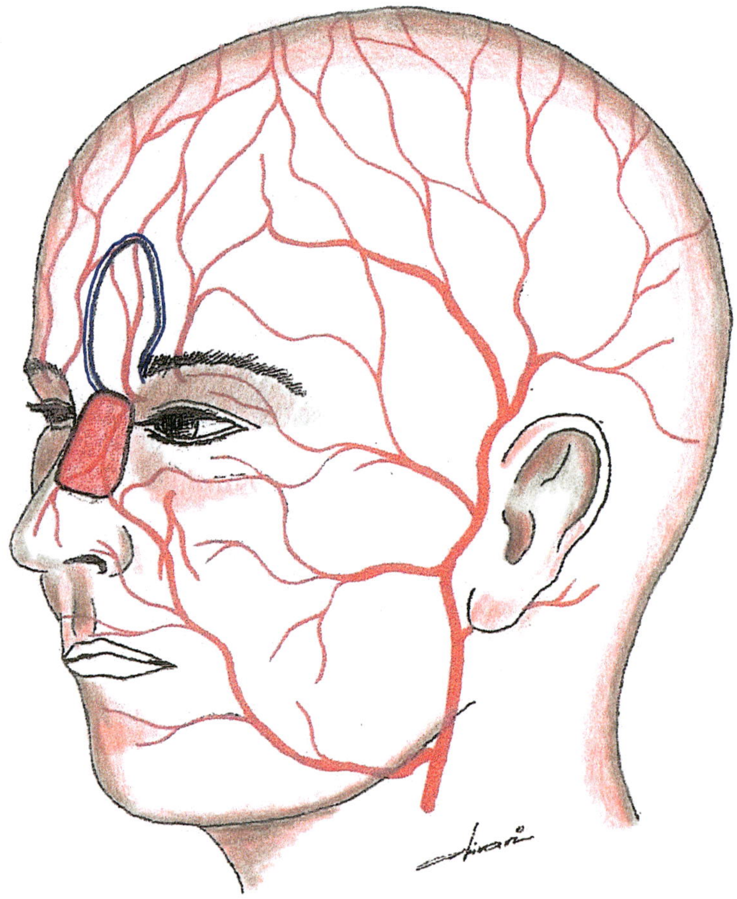

Figure 3.16 Perfusion conditions in a small forehead flap (supratrochlear flap)

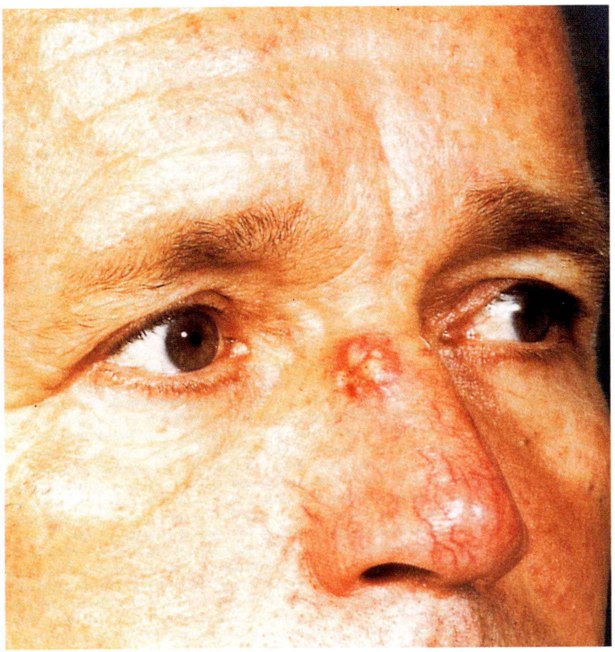

Figure 3.17a Basal cell carcinoma at the right nasal dorsum

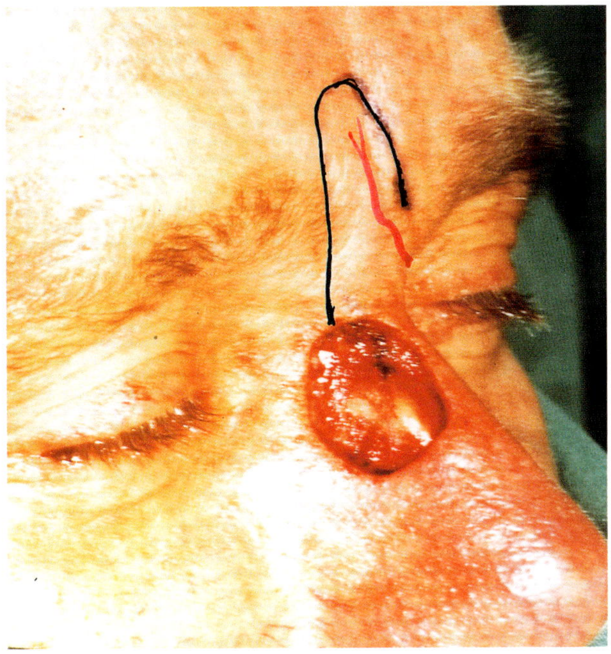

Figure 3.17b Situation after excision to the periosteum and planning of a supratrochlear flap.

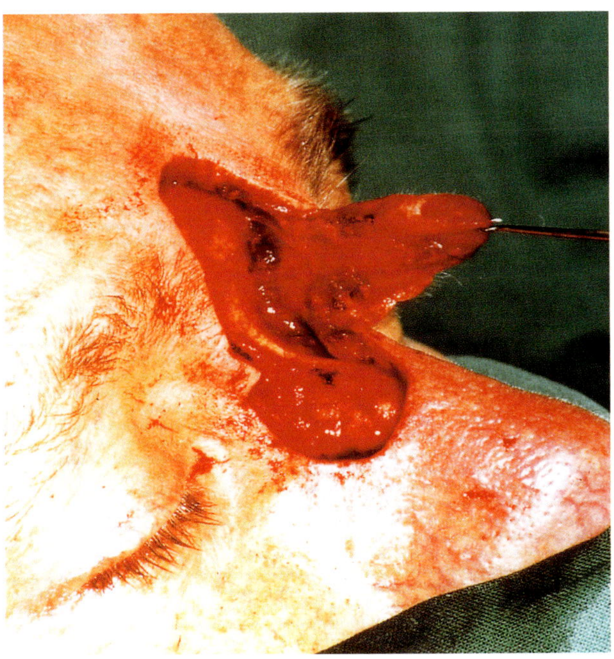

Figure 3.17c Mobilization of the flap that is fixed without tension into the defect.

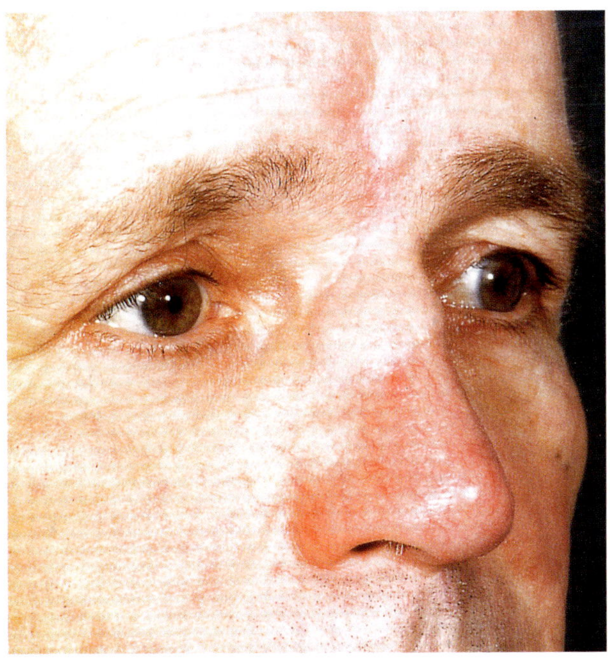

Figure 3.17d Situation one year after the operation. The secondary defect was primarily closed.

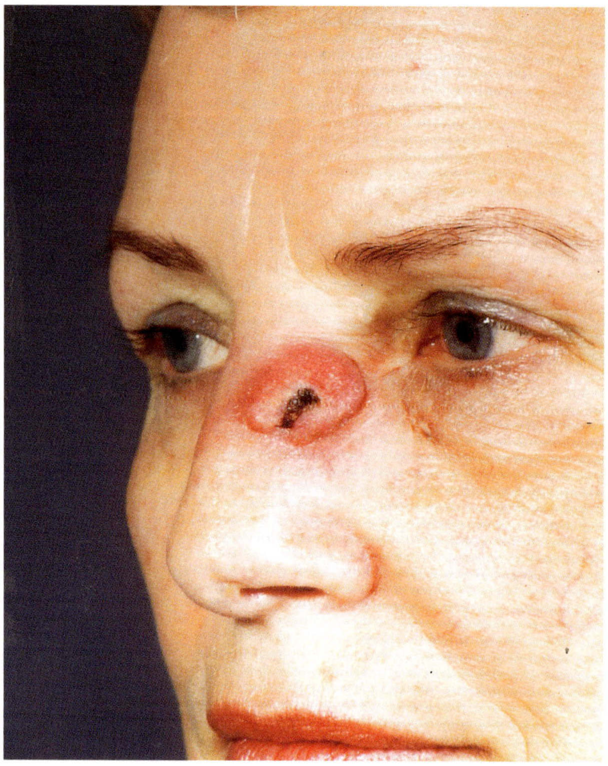

Figure 3.18a Basal cell carcinoma of the left upper part of the nose

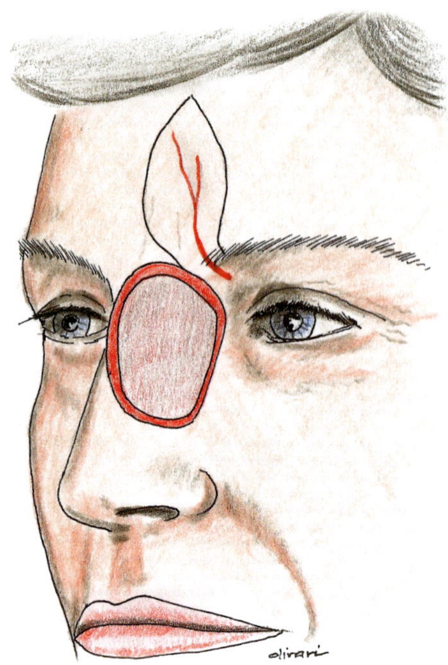

Figure 3.18b Excision occurs into healthy tissue to the periosteum which is not affected. An appropriately large forehead flap, vascularized axially by the supratrochlear artery, is formed, mobilized and fixed to the defect. Since the flap is relatively small, the secondary defect can be primarily closed. Note the narrow flap pedicle.

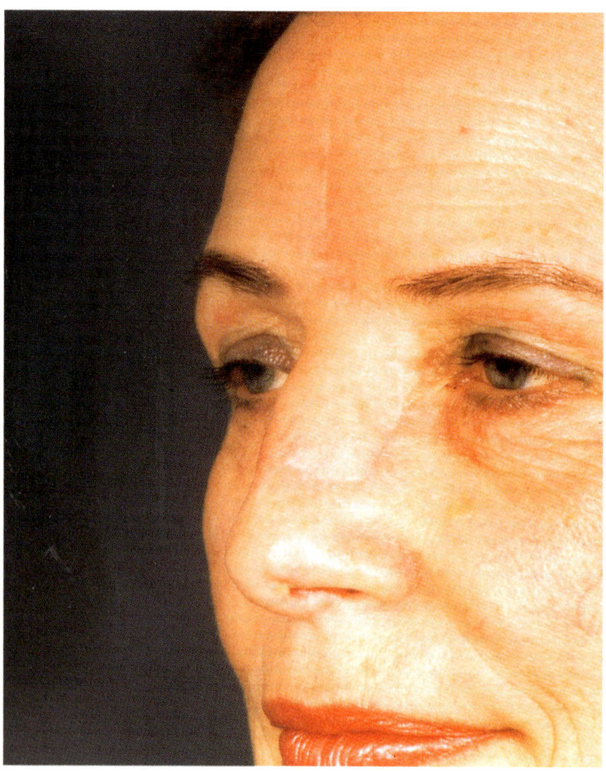

Figure 3.18c Picture one year after the operation

b) Large Forehead Flap "Indian Method" With Expander

The oldest method for nasal reconstruction is still the best method for covering large nasal defects. Preparation of the flap using an expander has increased the possibilities of this method. In this way one can normally close the secondary defect directly as well. Mesh skin grafts are still indicated in exceptional cases. The prefabrication of the nasal tip with underlying cartilage can be readily achieved. The axial blood perfusion through the supratrochlear artery is reliable. Despite this the arterial course should be visualized for safety with the Doppler device.

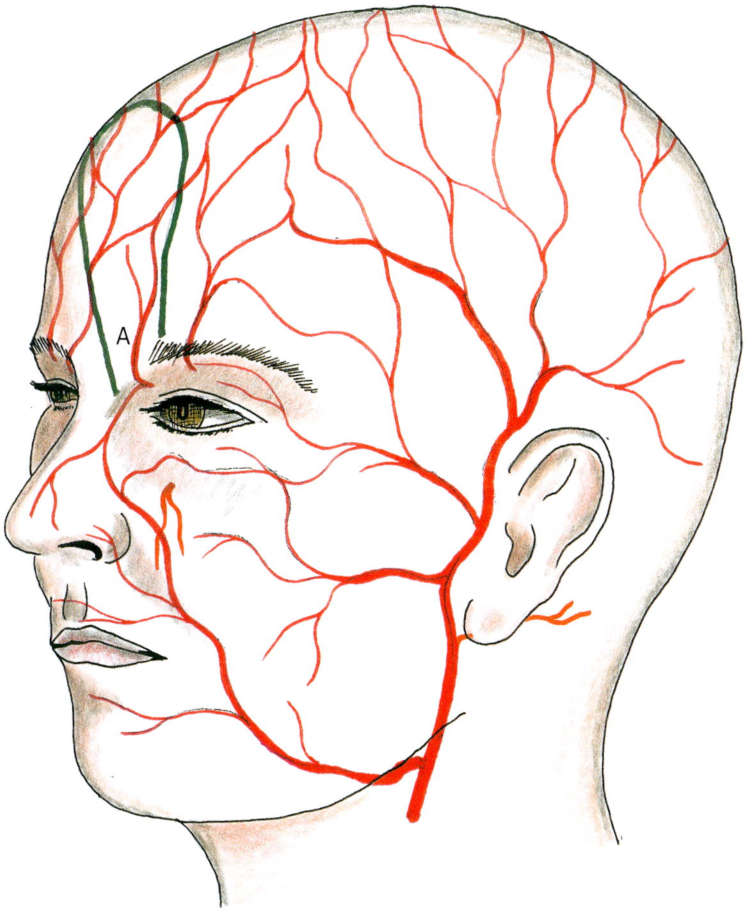

Figure 3.19 Large axial forehead flap "Indian method" (A = supratrochlear artery)

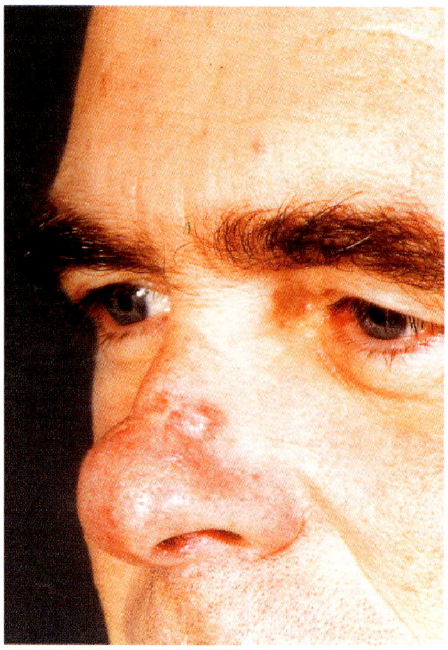

Figure 3.20a A previously excised and recurrent basal cell carcinoma on dorsum of the nose. A large forehead flap with an expander is planned.

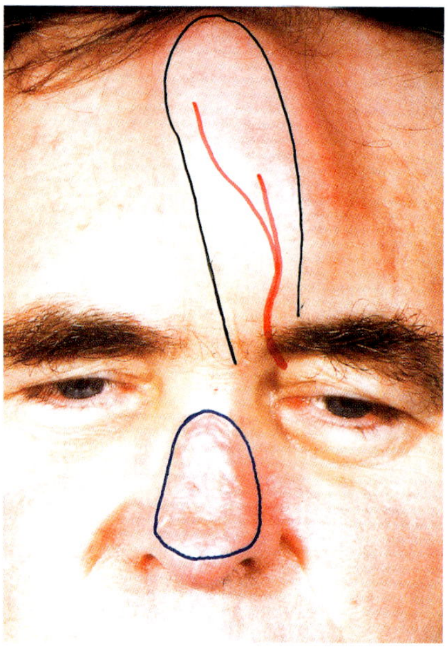

Figure 3.20b The tumor was excised and the defect covered with a mesh graft until histological clearance was confirmed.

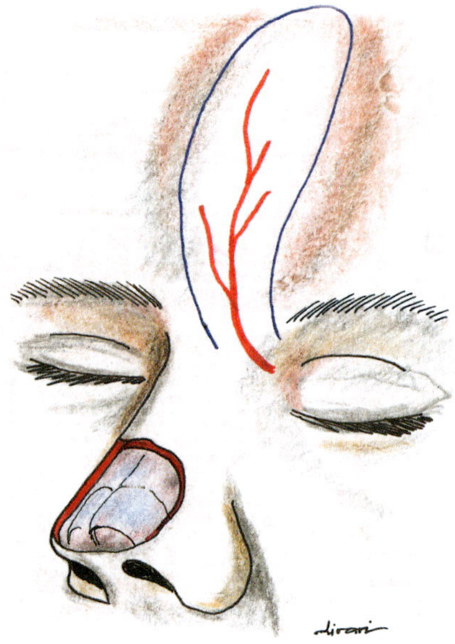

Figure 3.20c The expander was filled within three weeks

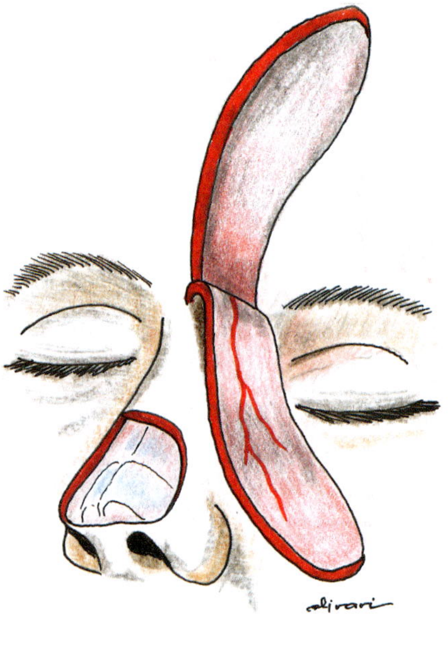

Figure 3.20d The supratrochlear artery must be identified

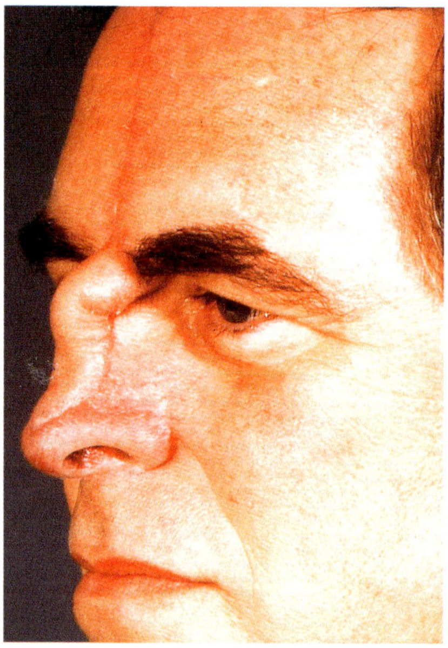

Figure 3.20e After removal of the expander the forehead flap is fixed in the defect. Secondary defect is closed primarily without tension. After three to four weeks the flap base is severed and the nasal dorsum is adjusted.

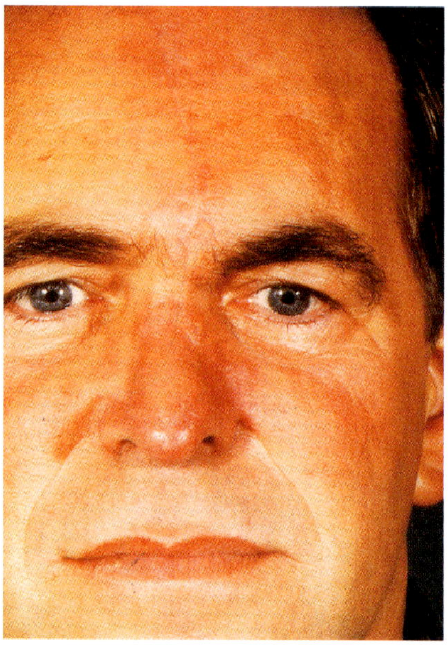

Figure 3.20f Situation nine months after the operation. The scar on the forehead at the expander site is barely visible.

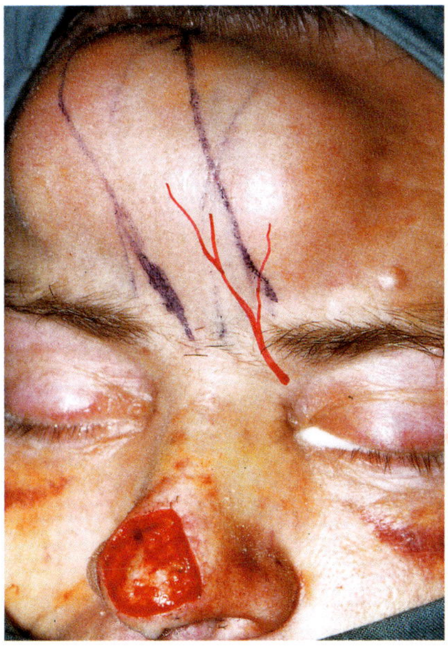

Figure 3.21a Basal cell carcinoma of the nasal tip: the tumor was excised following the insertion of a 10 ccm expander three weeks earlier.

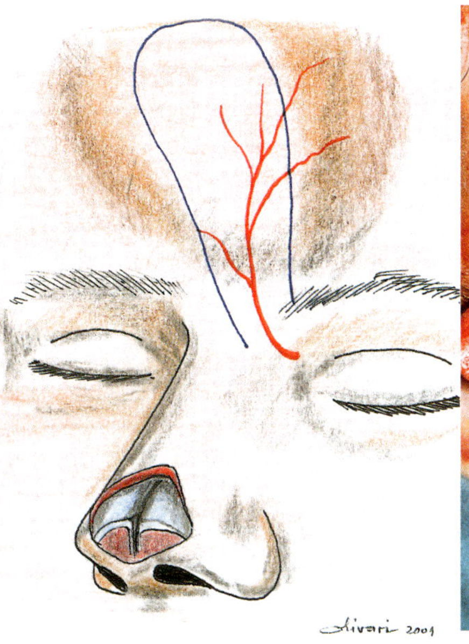

Figure 3.21b Position of the supratrochlear artery

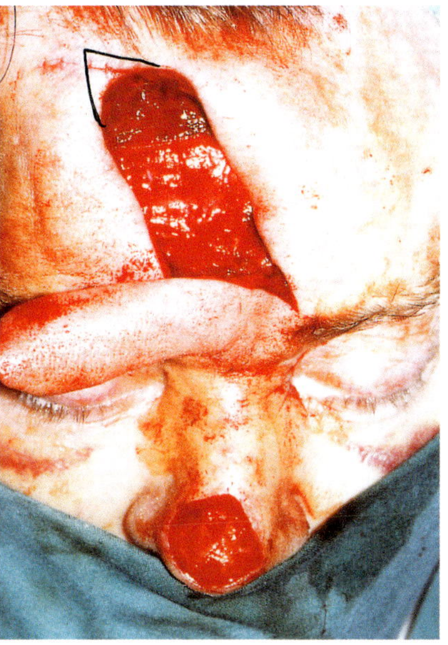

Figure 3.21c The forehead flap is mobilized after removal of the expander

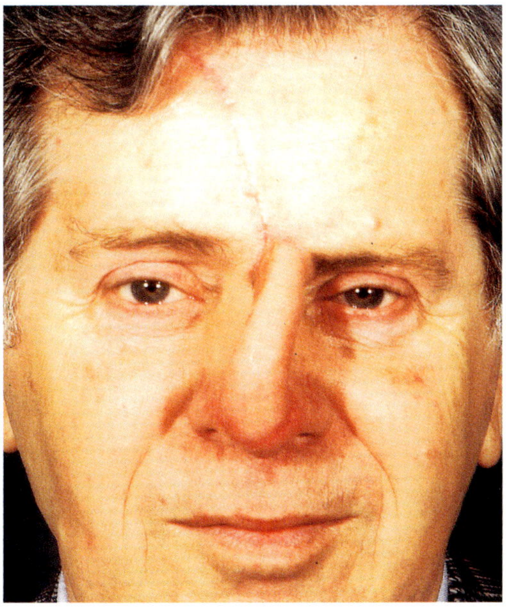

Figure 3.21d Transfer of the flap to the nasal tip. The frontal defect is closed primarily

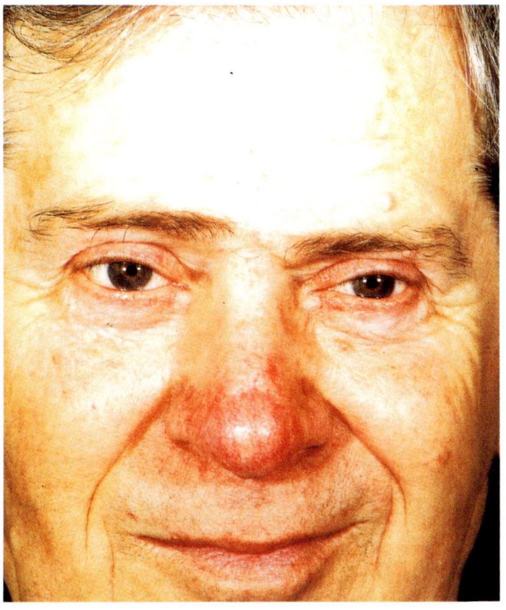

Figure 3.21e Situation one year after the operation with acceptable scaring

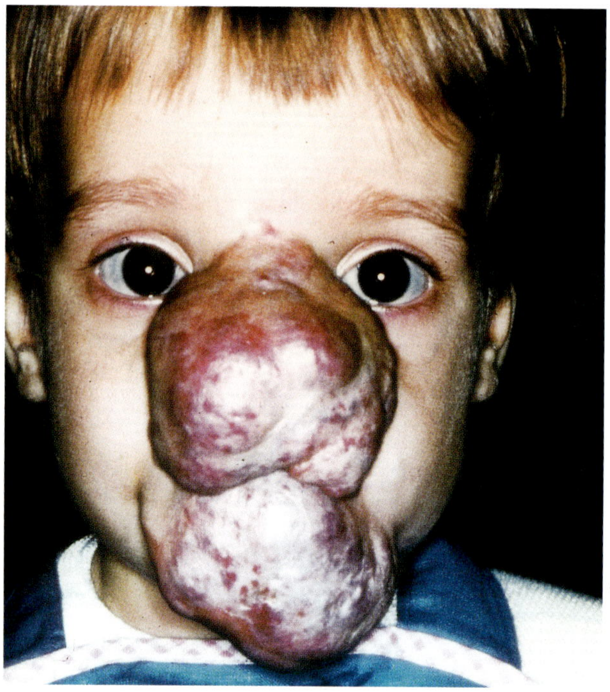

Figure 3.22a A huge tuberous hemangioma of the nose as well as the upper lip. Respiration as well as intake of food were considerably impaired and there was clear indication for surgery.

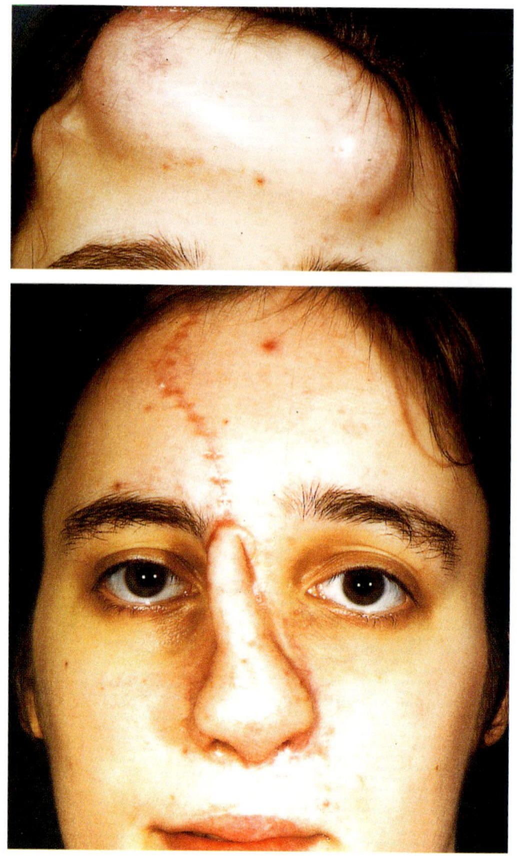

Figure 3.22c,d 19 years later the patient (now a nurse) presented herself again because as she wanted her flat nose improved. A forehead flap was prepared, after previous stretching of the forehead skin with an expander, for nasal reconstruction.

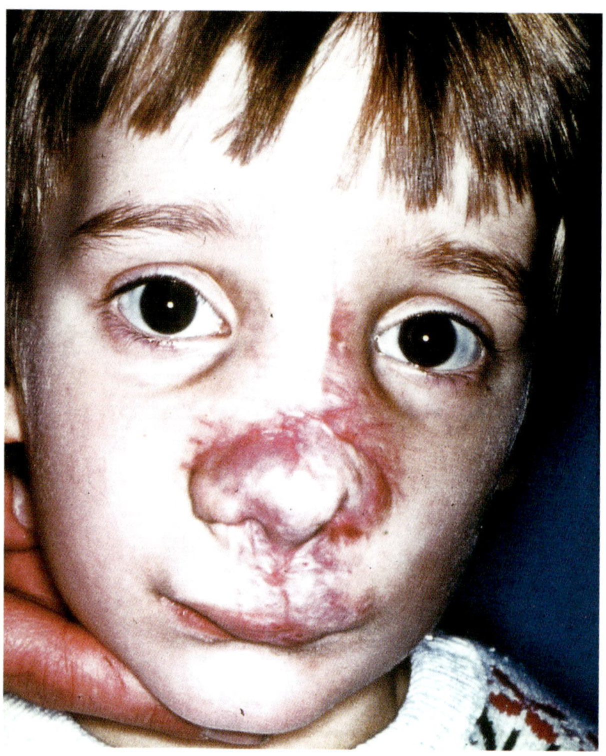

Figure 3.22b Hemangioma of nose and upper lip was as widely as possible removed. Picture shows situation four months after operation (1976).

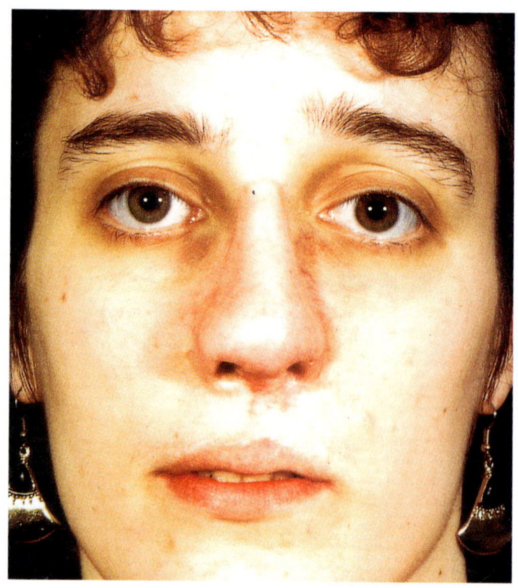

Figure 3.22e Situation one year after the application of the forehead flap (1994).

c) Supratrochlear Island Flap

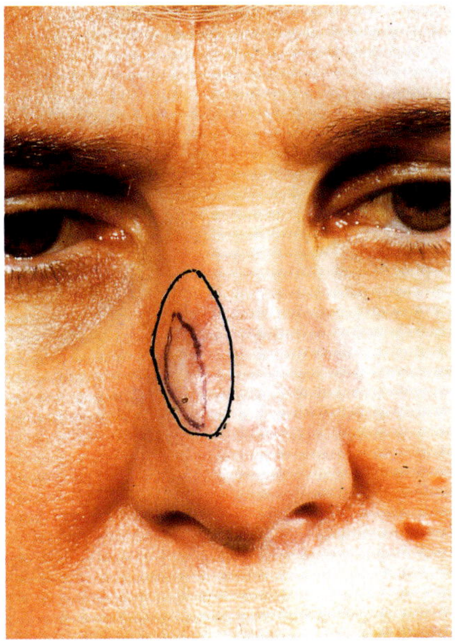

Figure 3.23a Basal cell carcinoma recurrence three years after primary operation: Planning of the excision.

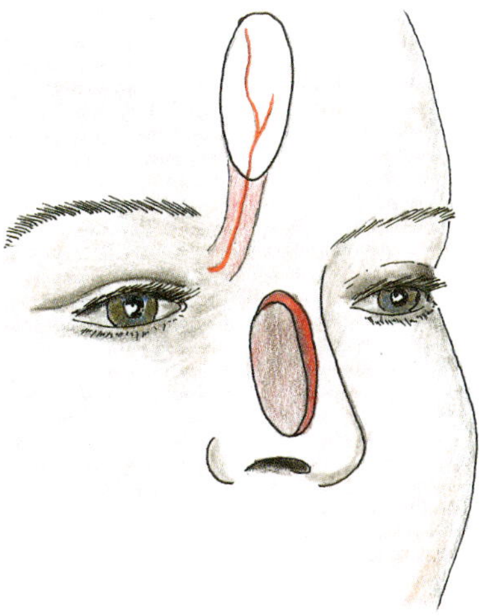

Figure 3.23b First the tumor is excised. An suitable large part of the forehead skin is raised. A subcutaneous, caudal pedicle flap is carefully prepared.

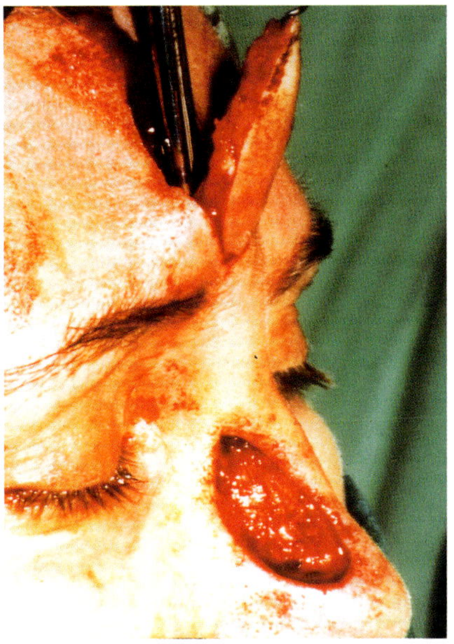

Figure 3.23c After a sufficiently large subcutaneous tunnel is formed, the island flap is now turned round and fixed into the defect. The island flap must be pulled through very carefully.

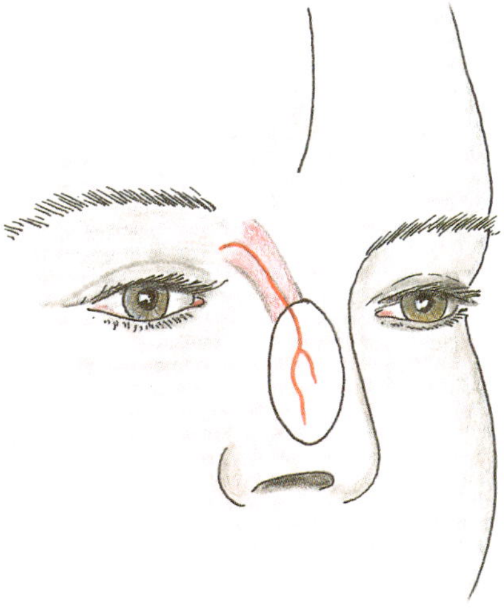

Figure 3.23d When pulling the island flap through the tunnel the supratrochlear artery must remain intact. In addition the pedicle flap must not be twisted since this may disturb the blood supply. Because of the poor lymph drainage from the island flap, temporary swelling of the flap is usually to be expected.

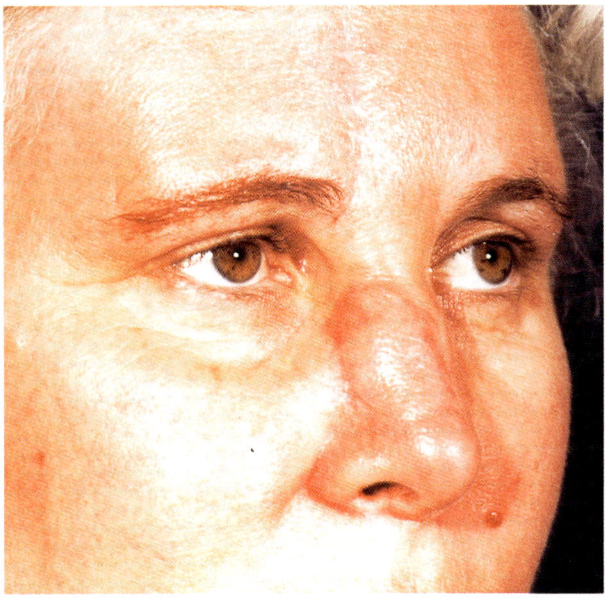

Figure 3.23e Situation four years after the operation

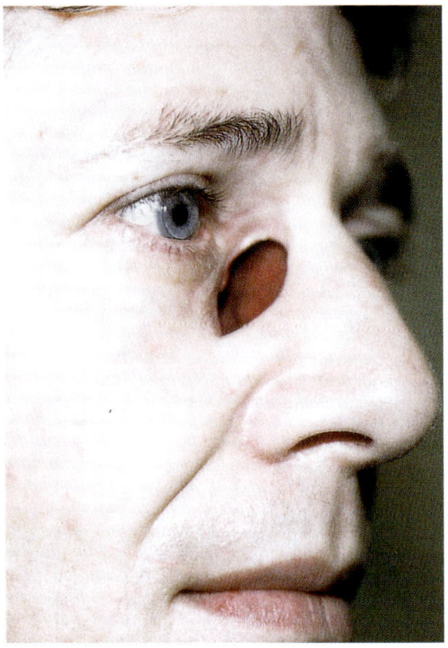

Figure 3.24a Defect of all three layers on a right side of the nose

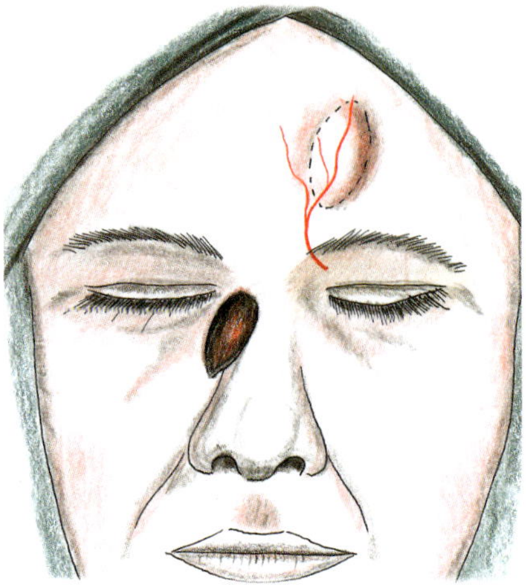

Figure 3.24b Preparation of a supratrochlear island flap. Firstly a full-thickness skin graft is transplanted under a tip of future flap for the inner lining of the nose. At the same time a small expander is implanted.

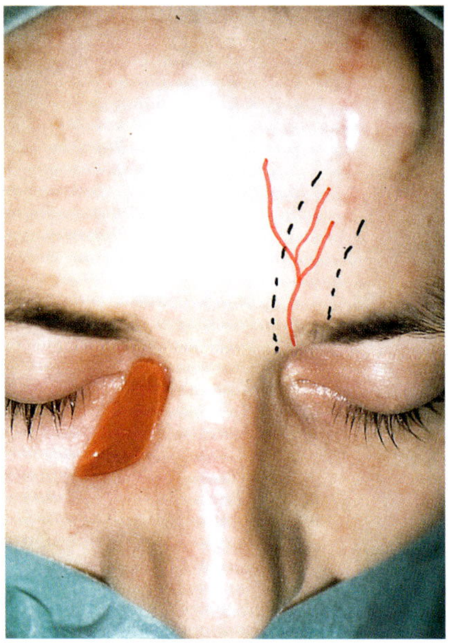

Figure 3.24c The full-skin thickness graft is taken and the expander was filled. Note the course of the supratrochlear artery.

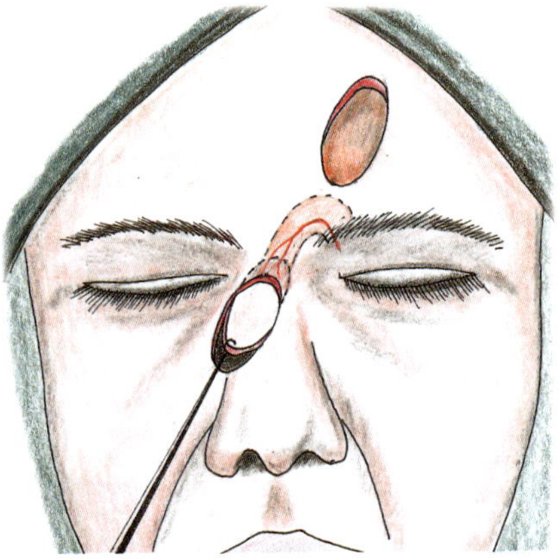

Figure 3.24d The supratrochlear island flap is passed through a subcutaneous tunnel into the defect. The flap has a subcutaneous tissue pedicle that contains the supratrochlear artery.

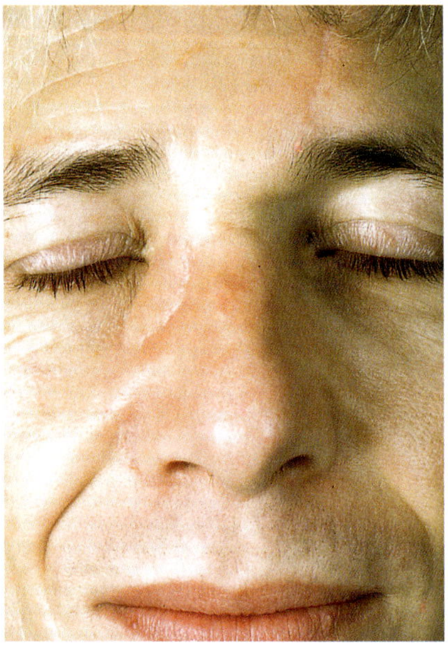

Figure 3.24e Status two years after the operation

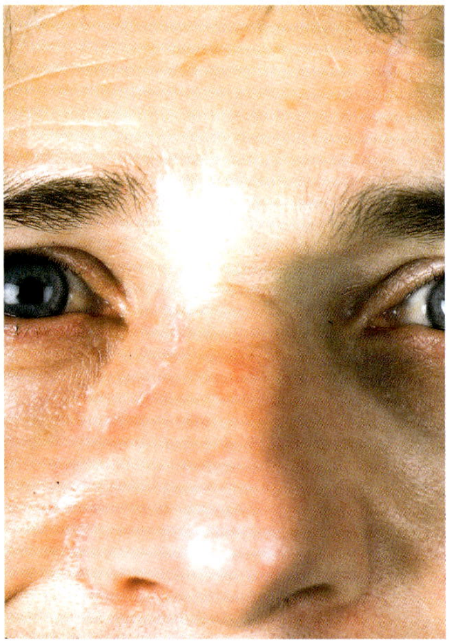

Figure 3.24f Secondary defect is well healed

d) Converse Flap (Scalping Forehead Flap)

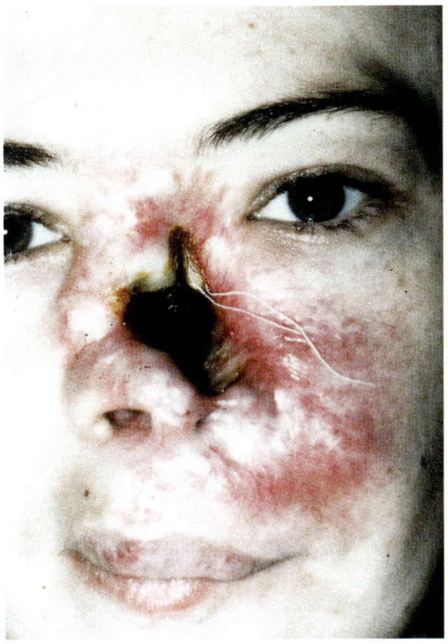

Figure 3.25a Situation after a multiple excisions of a hemangioma with an extensive arterial component. Because of repetitive life-threatening nose bleeding, the nasal septum and the nasal conchas were radically coagulated.

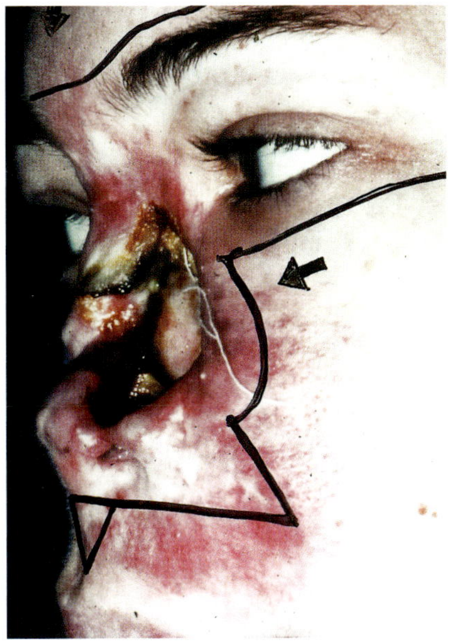

Figure 3.25b Planning the reconstruction:
1) Scalping forehead flap (Converse)
2) Rotation flap from left cheek
3) Partial resection of the upper lip

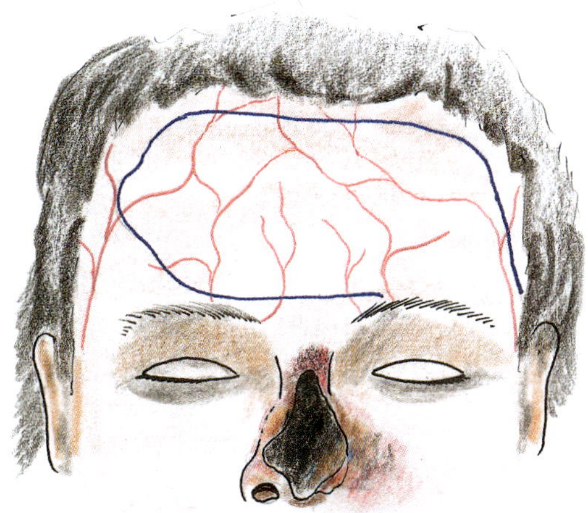

Figure 3.25c Converse flap and blood supply

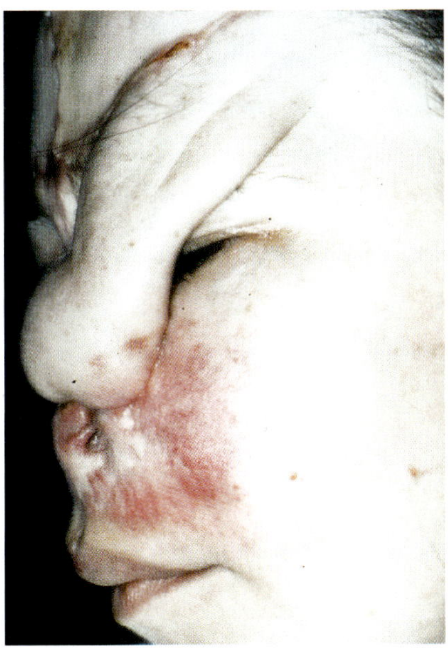

Figure 3.25d The forehead flap is fixed with the distal part in the defect. The secondary defect is covered with mesh graft. After approximately four weeks the flap pedicle is divided and the nose is roughly formed. After a further six weeks the nose tip has been formed.

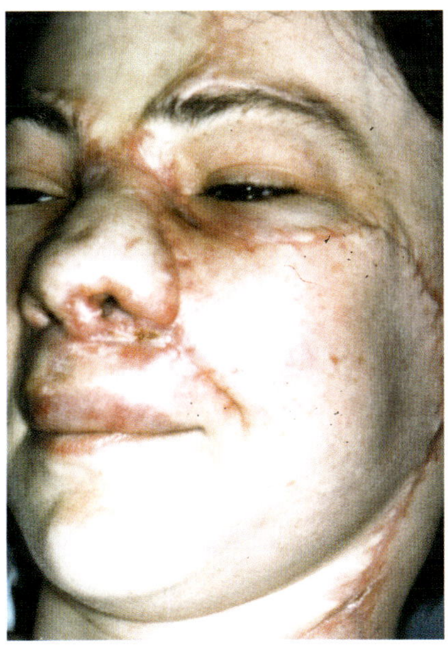

Figure 3.25e Six months after repositioning of the rest of the forehead flap and forming of the nose. Two months following this a rotation flap was performed (Mustardé) to correct the defect of the left cheek as well as the left upper lip.

A Converse flap has a benefit of being able to cover a large defect. The disadvantage of the flap is that larger scars are visible in the forehead area. The forehead mobility is abolished. These days a free flap, such as a forearm flap would be preferred.

e) Forehead Flap Combined With Two Nasolabial Flaps

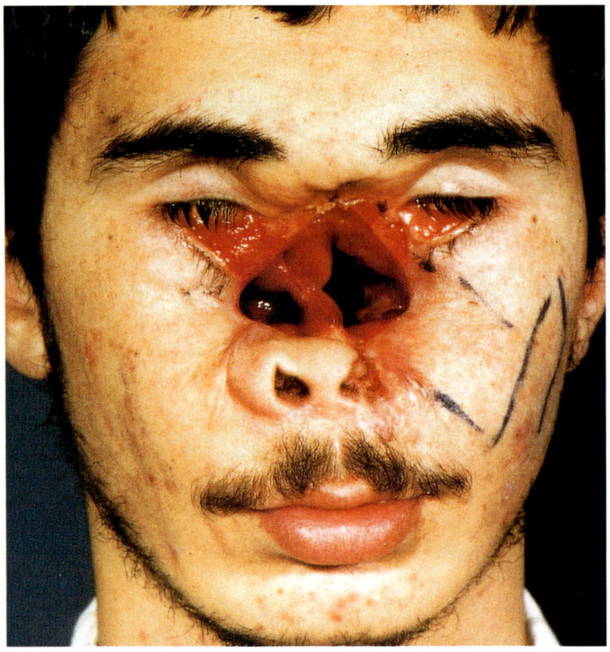

Figure 3.26a War injury (1983 Iraqi-Iranian war)
1) Loss of the nose
2) Loss of the medial parts of the maxilla bilaterally (midface defect)
3) Loss of sight with severe ectropium bilaterally

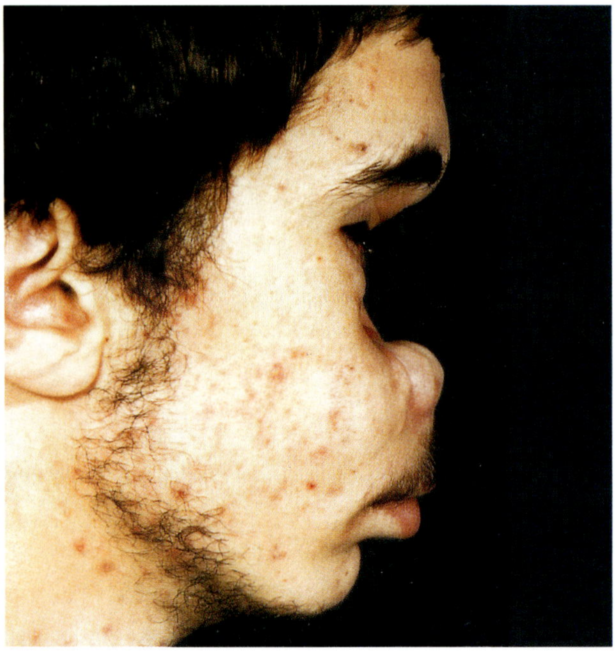

Figure 3.26b Profile with clearly visible loss of substance in the midface

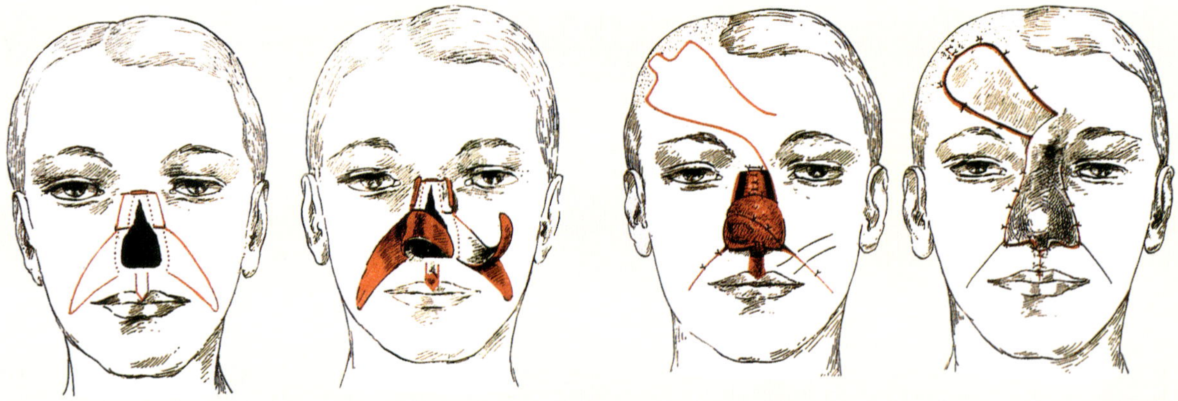

Figure 3.26c Planning of the reconstruction: Original illustrations from Joseph, J.: Nasoplastik (1931). In order to form the inner lining, two nasolabial flaps are mobilized and turned inwards. A forehead flap was planned for the nasal reconstruction.

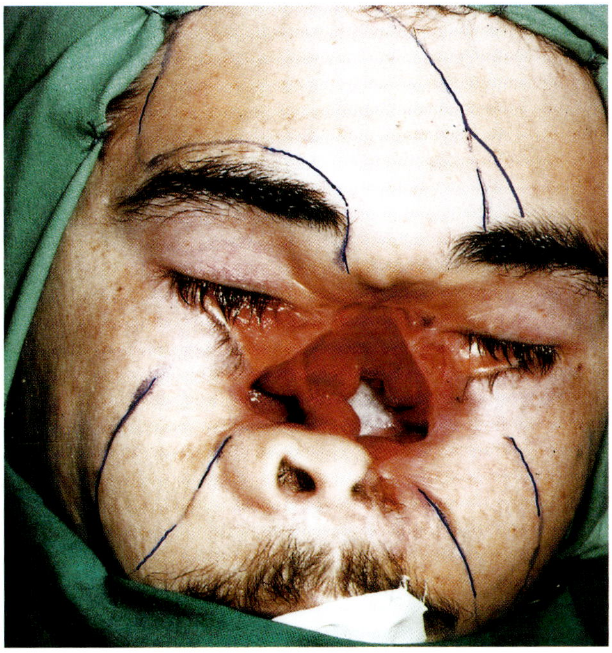

Figure 3.26d Planning of the flaps: For the outer covering of the nose a forehead flap is planned, cranio-transversally because of the very low forehead of the patient.

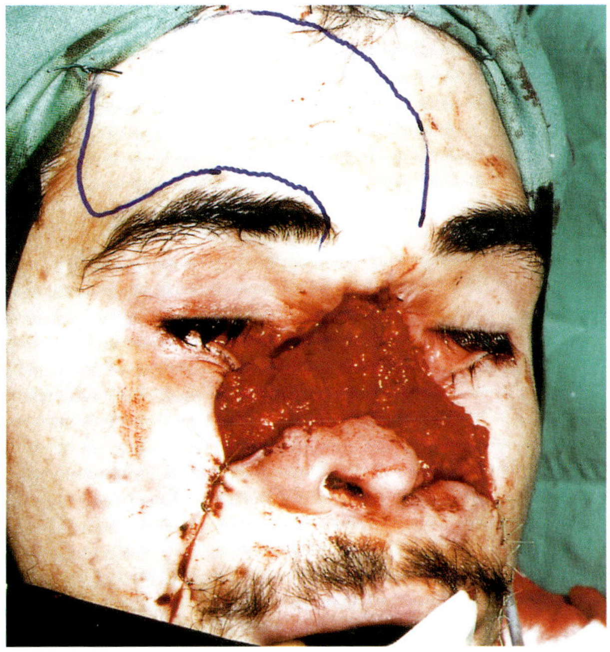

Figure 3.26e Planning of the flaps: Firstly the inner lining of the nose is constructed with two cranial nasolabial based pedicle flaps.

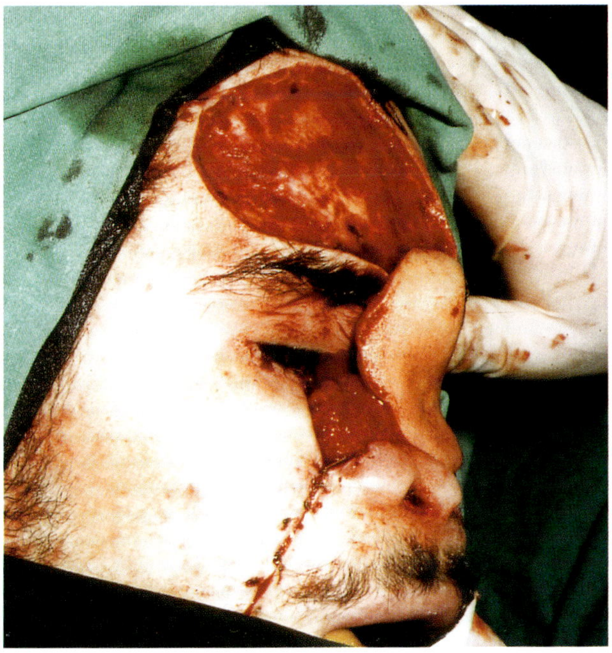

Figure 3.26f The inner side of the nose is lined with nasolabial flaps. The removal site is primarily closed following mobilization of lateral cheek. Using the forehead flap the external part of the nose is formed. At the same time the bilateral ectropium is corrected, partly by rotation from the cheek, and partly using the forehead flap.

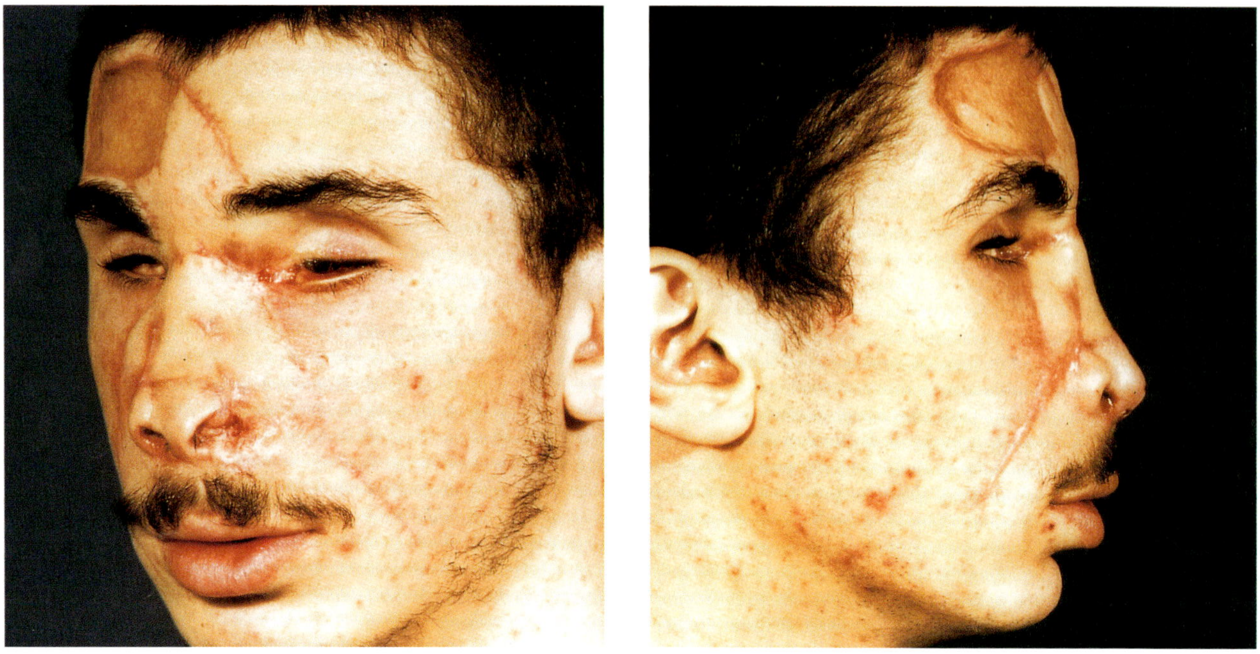

Figure 3.26g,h Result six weeks after the operation. Despite the poor initial state we were able to achieve an acceptable result. Nasal respiration was considerably impaired, and the profile was still flat. Further operations were not possible as the patient had to travel back to his homeland. One can discuss whether a free forearm flap might have achieved a better result.

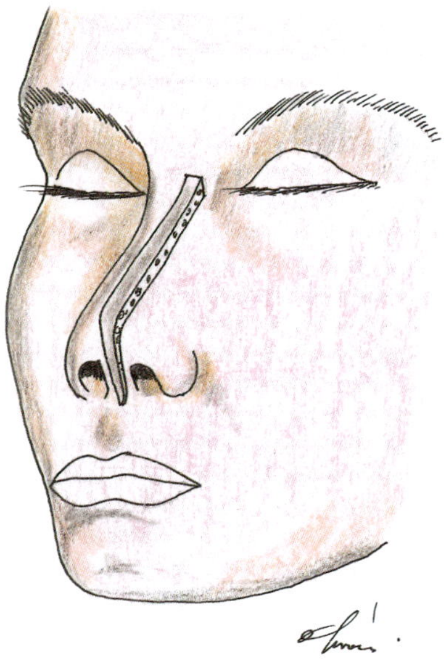

Figure 3.26i In order to support the nasal profile, an L-shaped pelvic bone graft was used.

Temporofrontal Flap (New Flap)

Defect Coverage With the Temporofrontal Flap (Sickle Flap)

In 1928 New described the temporofrontal flap (sickle flap) for nasal reconstruction. This flap, however, did not achieve much popularity for two reasons:

1) The perfusion course of the superficial temporal artery was not precisely respected, so that a delay was necessary.
2) Converse condemned the "sickle flap" as unreliable and popularized his own "scalping forehead flap" which was much more extensive surgically and left many scars.

Our experience has shown that the temporofrontal flap is completely reliable. Preconditions for its success include the preoperative identification of the branches of the superficial temporal artery using a Doppler device as well as careful planning.

A delay is not necessary. It is in fact an axial flap with which one can cover very large nasal defects. However, it is absolutely necessary to check the blood supply.

Originally, Converse stated : "New's sickle flap has two disadvantages: (1) The pedicle of the flap is long, requiring one or two preliminary delay operations, and (2) the base of the flap is kinked or twisted after transfer; this tends to interfere with the blood supply of the flap."

Our experience with 14 temporofrontal flaps has confirmed the safety and reliability of this flap. None of these 14 flaps had any circulatory problems. In two cases a lateralization of the nasal tip in the direction of the flap arose that had to be corrected later. When skin expansion is used the flap has possibilities of wider use.

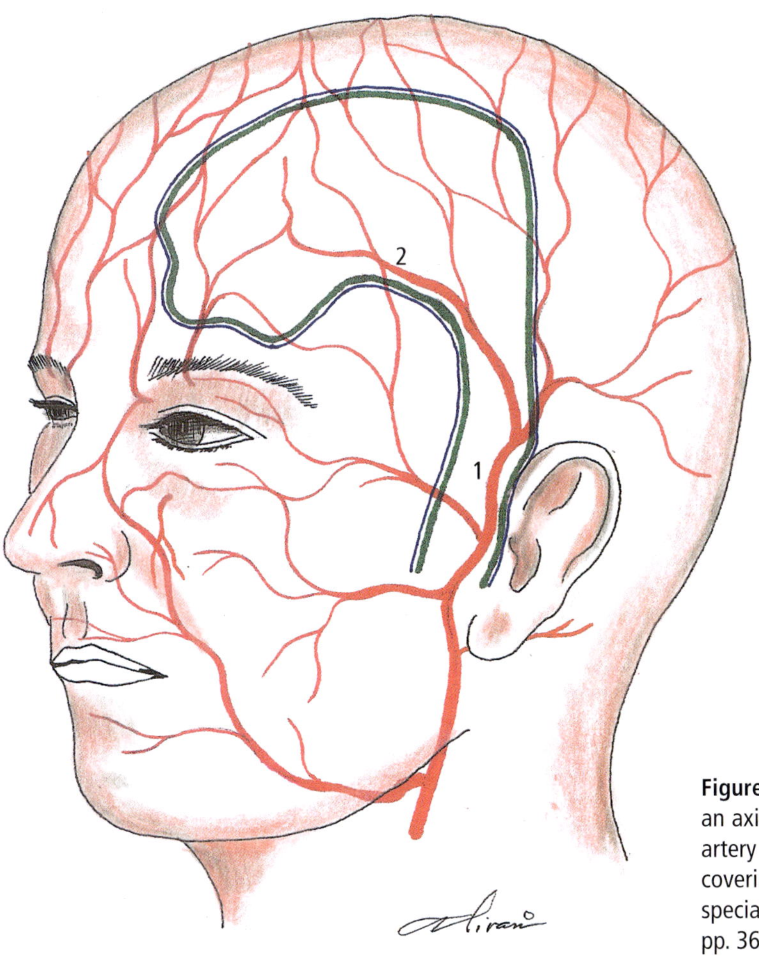

Figure 3.27 Temporofrontal flap (sickle flap): This represents an axial, arterial flap, perfused by the superficial temporal artery (1) and its frontal branch (2). The flap is suitable for covering larger defects. This flap is highly recommended for special indications (see also the Chapter on Cheek Defects, pp. 363–367)

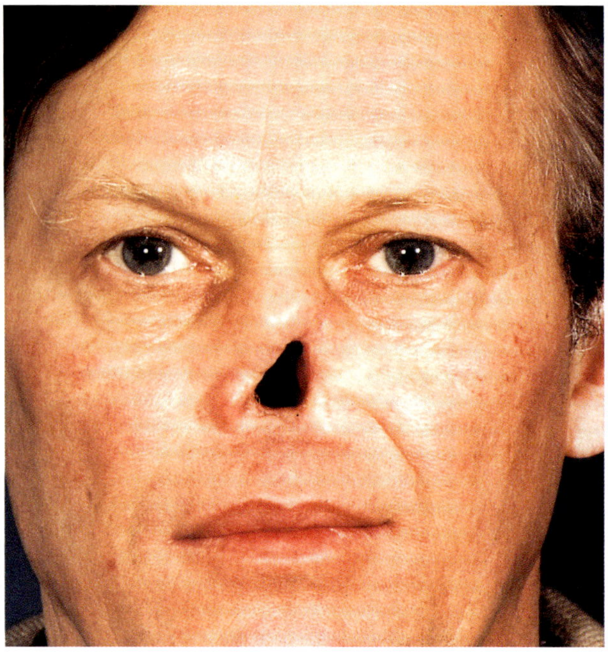

Figure 3.28a Nasal defect following earlier excision of a basal cell carcinoma

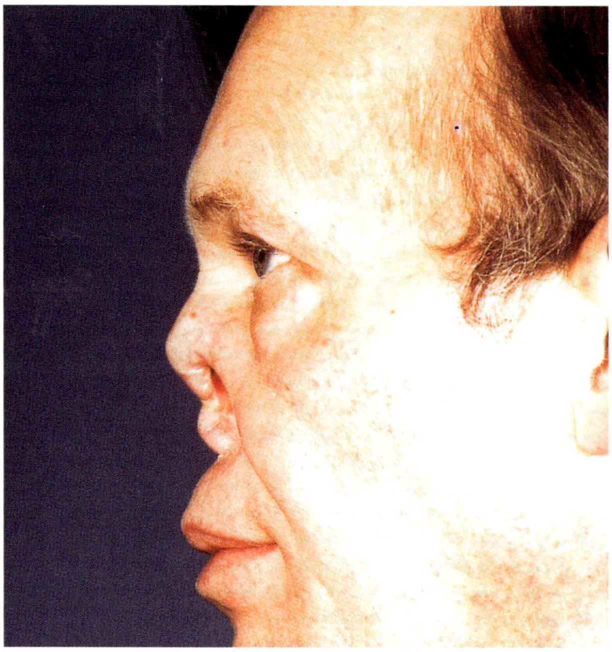

Figure 3.28b Profile view

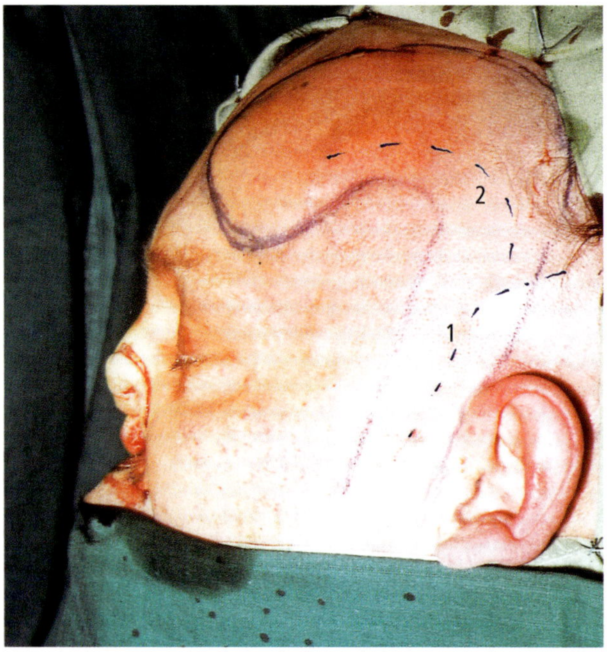

Figure 3.28c Temporo-frontal flap "sickle flap". This axial (arterial) flap is supplied by the superficial temporal artery (1) and its frontal branch (2). This flap is convenient for coverage of larger defects in the nasal area and also of the cheek area.

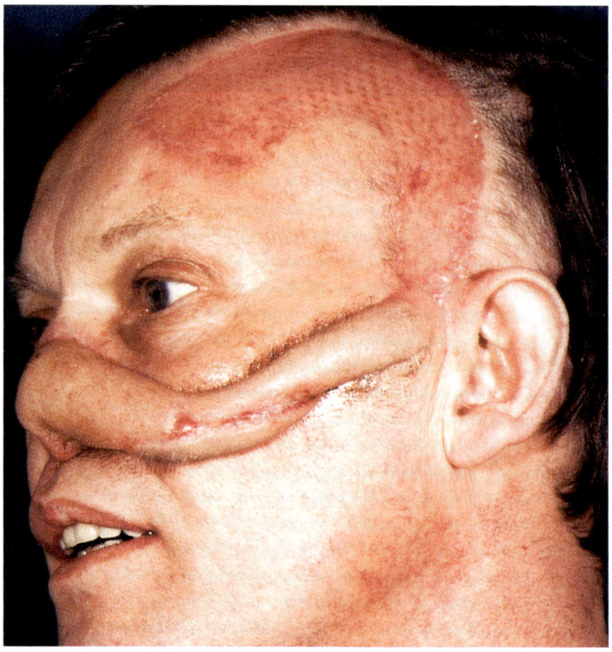

Figure 3.28e The temporo frontal flap

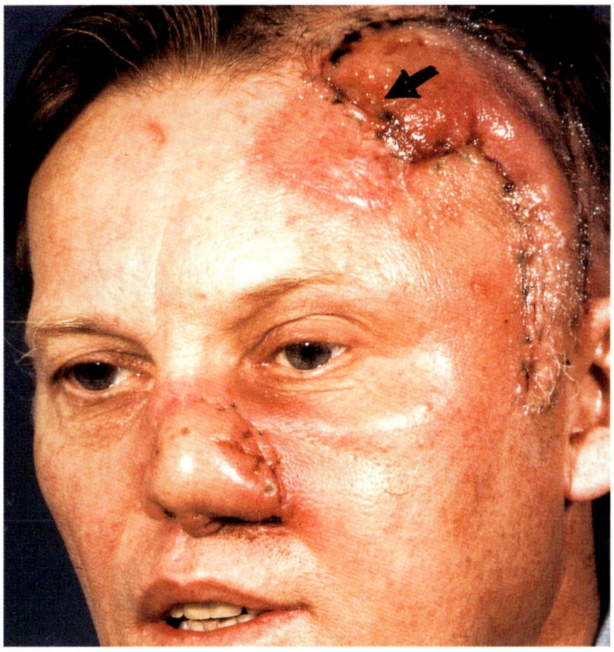

Figure 3.28f The temporo frontal flap is divided and the stump relocated in its original position. By rotating the rest of the flap ventrally the donor defect becomes considerably smaller.

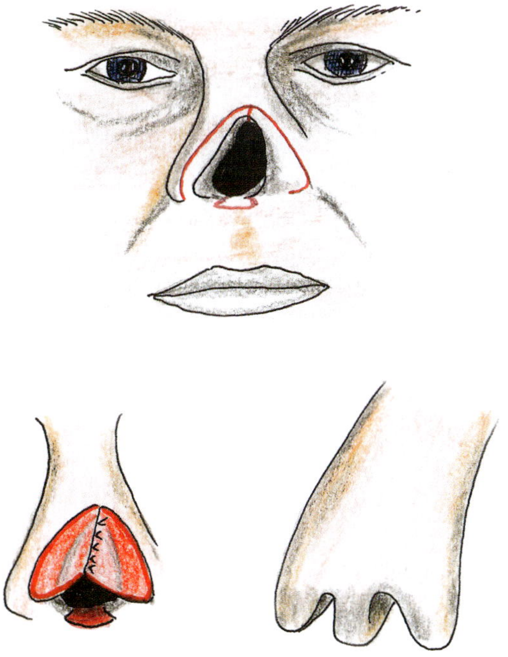

Figure 3.28g Schematic illustration showing turnover flaps for lining and shaping of the of the flaps tip as well as the columella and the nasal wings.

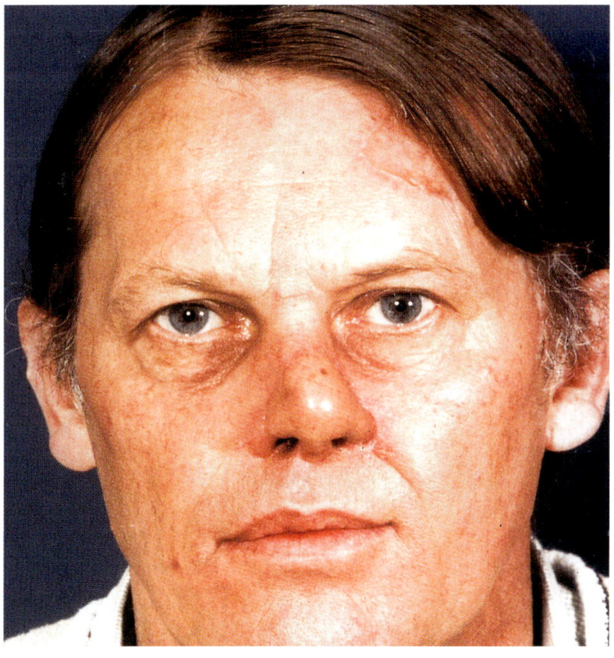

Figure 3.28h Status one year after two operations

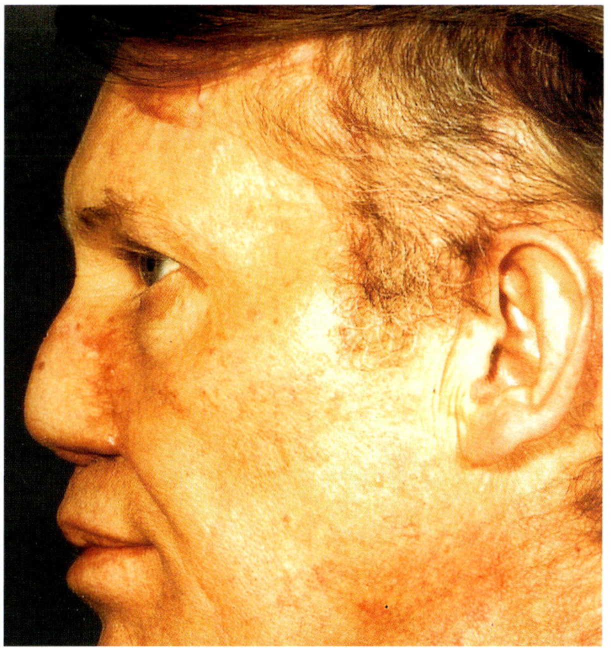

Figure 3.28i Further corrections were not necessary

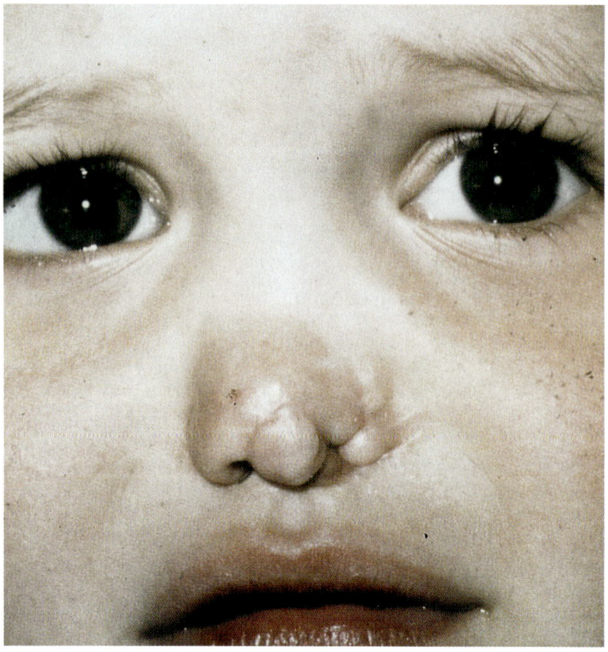

Figure 3.29a Nose deformity caused by a nasal tube which was inserted for too long, and accompanied by a local infection.

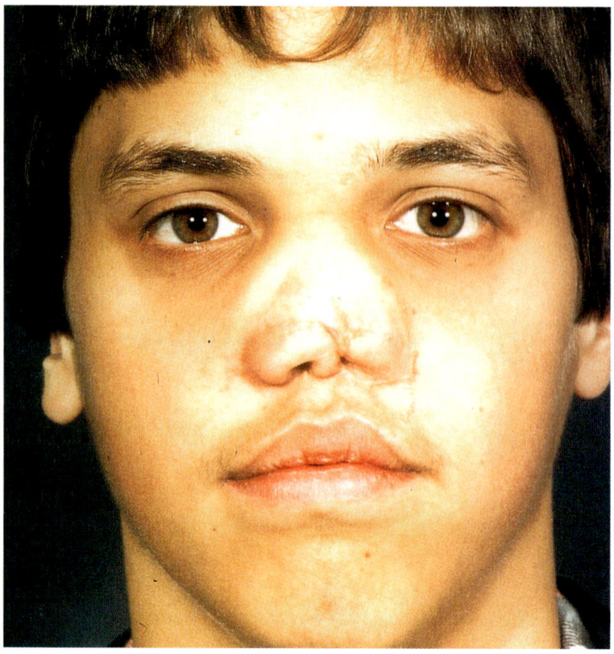

Figure 3.29b Status at the age of 14 years. The nasal tip is missing and the left nostril is obstructed. The alar cartilage, particularly on the left side, is atrophied and deformed.

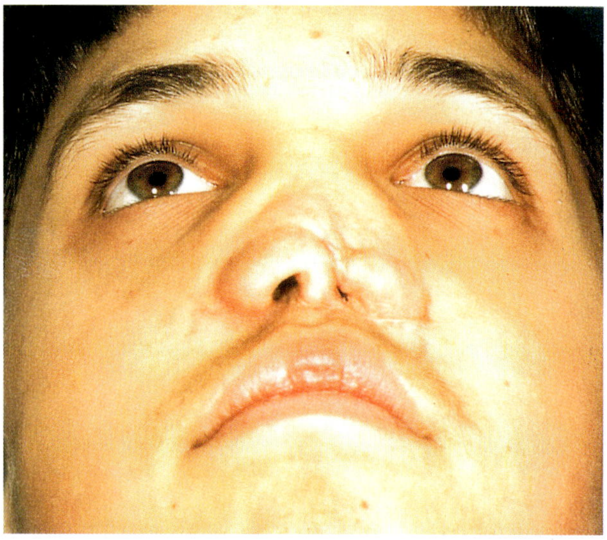

Figure 3.29c Preoperative situation

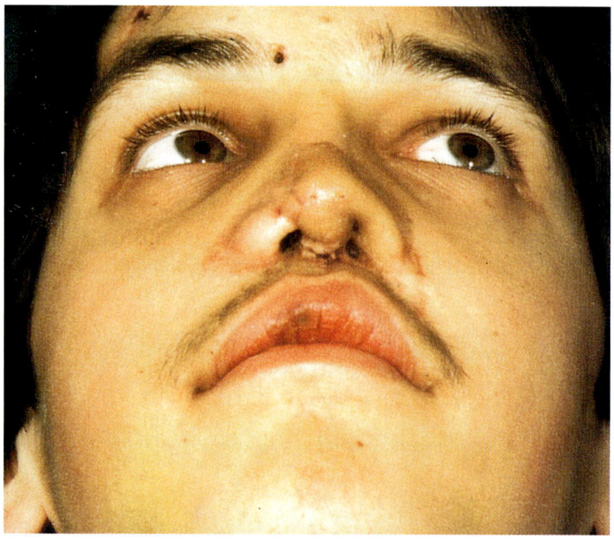

Figure 3.29d Postoperative result

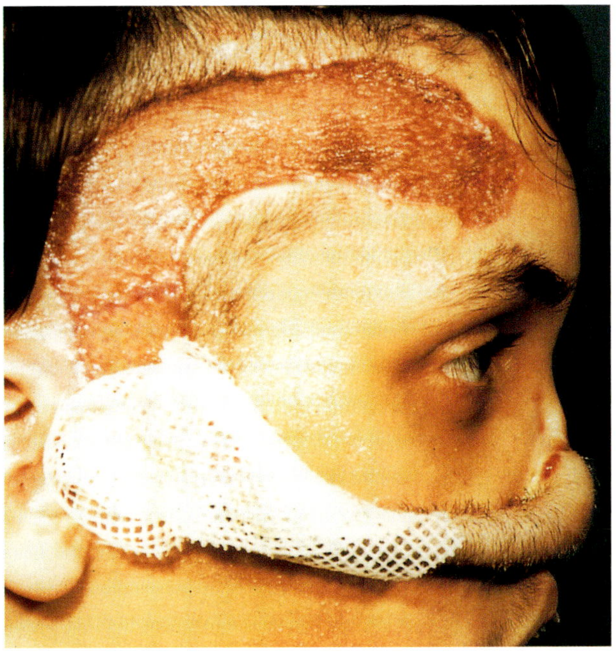

Figure 3.29e A tubed temporal frontal flap is sutured in the defect. The pedicle was divided after four weeks.

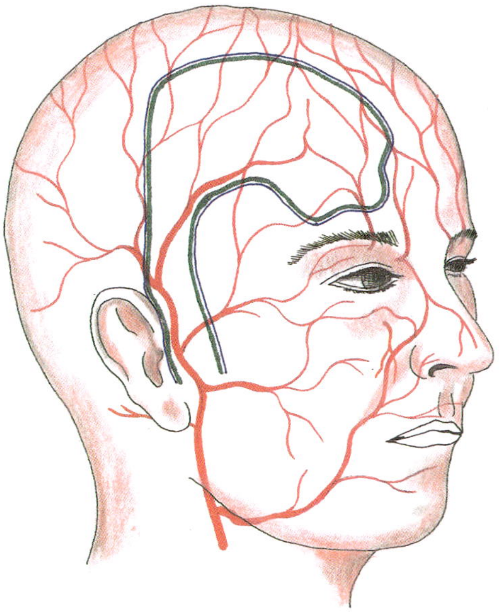

Figure 3.29f The blood supply is via frontal branch of the superficial temporal artery

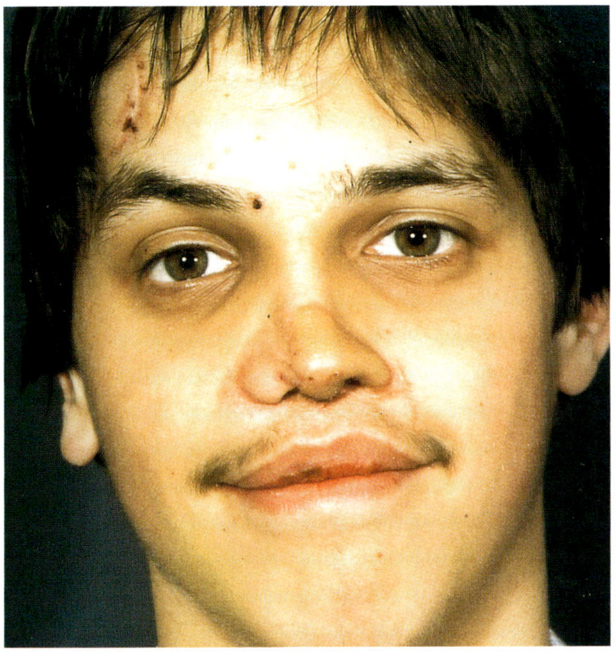

Figure 3.29g Result five months postoperatively. Donor site is completely closed by returning the remainder of the flap to its original site.

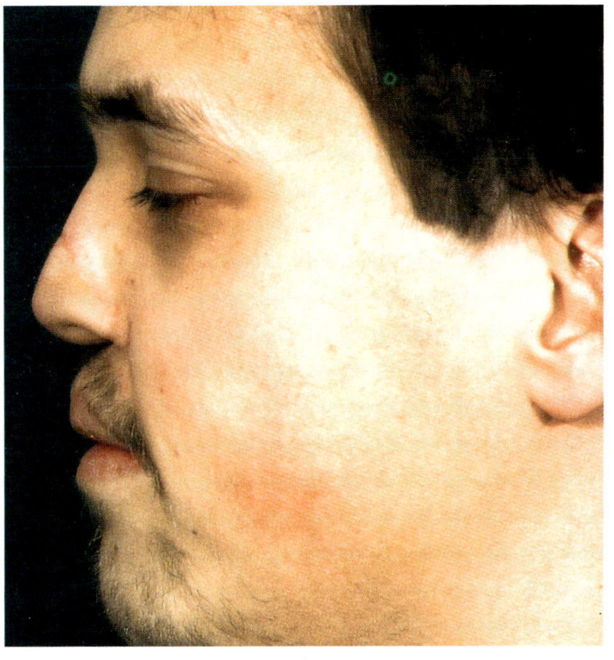

Figure 3.29h The left nostril is reconstructed and the profile is normal

Defect Coverage With the Rintala Flap

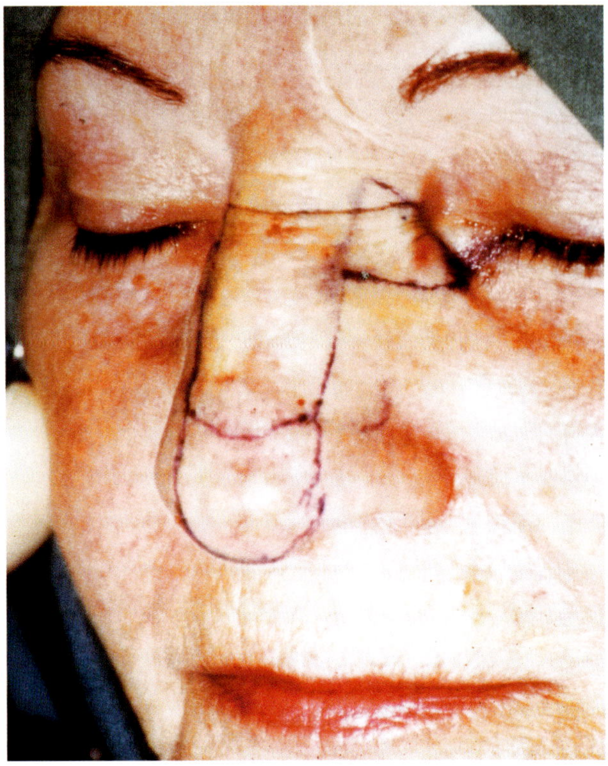

Figure 3.30a Basal cell carcinoma of the nasal tip

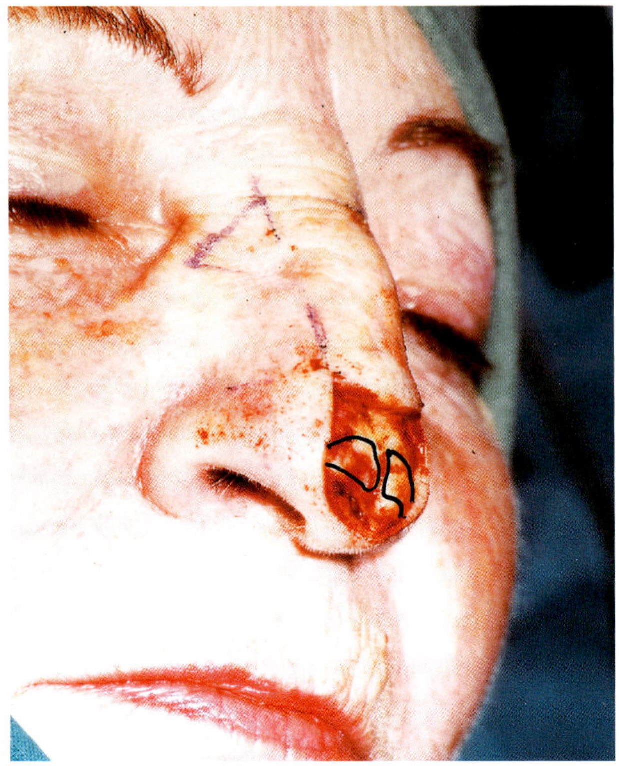

Figure 3.30b A flap with cranial pedicle is dissected down to the periostium and mobilized up to nasal root. Two relieving triangles were excised from both sides of the nose as this improved mobility of the flap in the caudal direction.

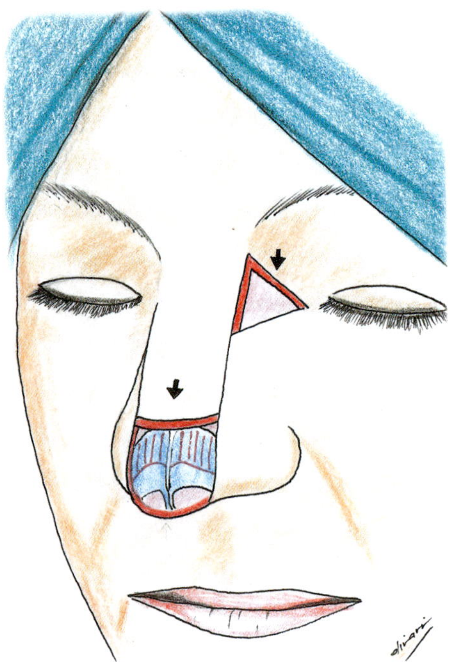

Figure 3.30c In long noses the cranial part of the alar cartilage should be resected (1). This makes the operation easier and shortens the nose.

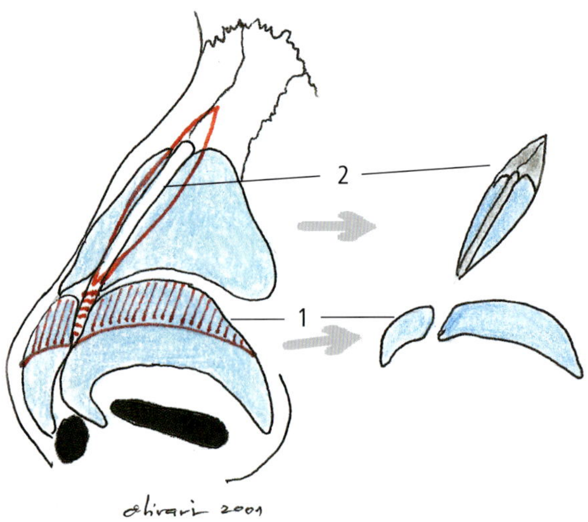

Figure 3.30d If a nasal hump is present this can be readily reduced under direct vision. This also facilitates the advancement of the flap as well as improving the appearance.

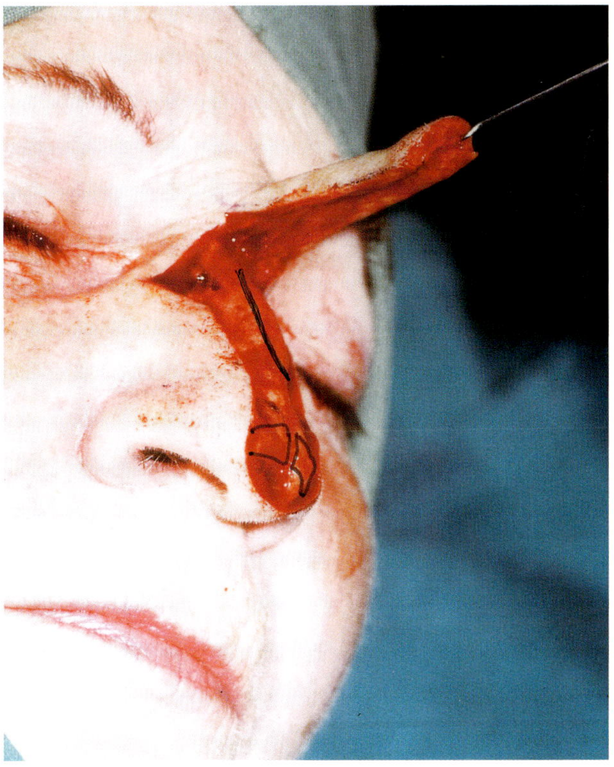

Figure 3.30e The Rintala flap is mobilized. The cranial portion of the alar cartilage as well as the nasal hump are resected under direct vision.

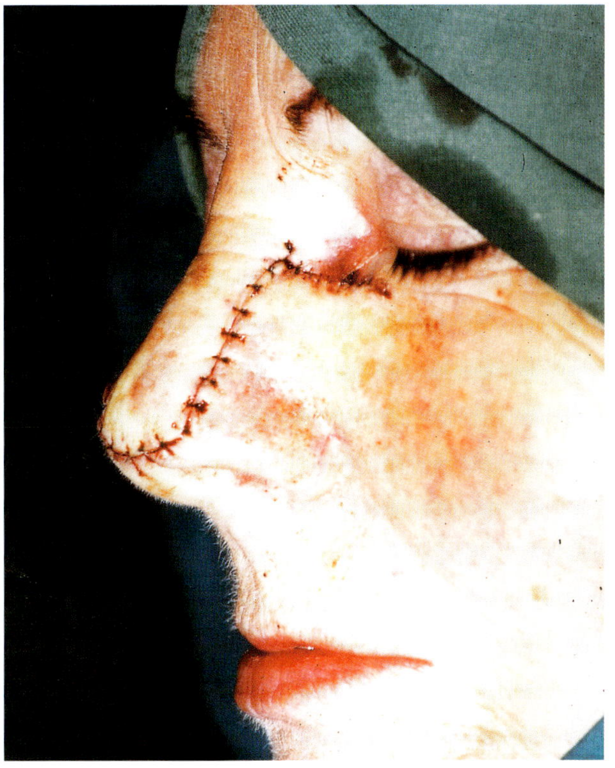

Figure 3.30f Situation at the end of the operation

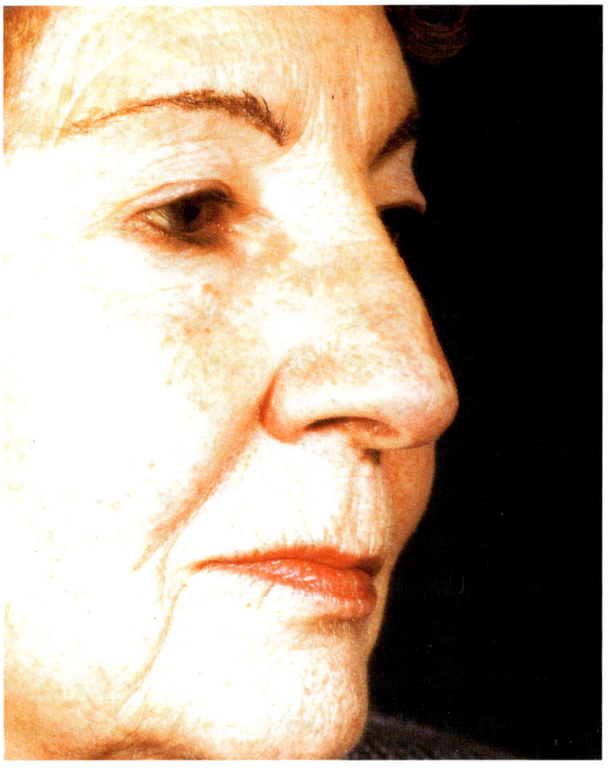

Figure 3.30g Result one year after the operation

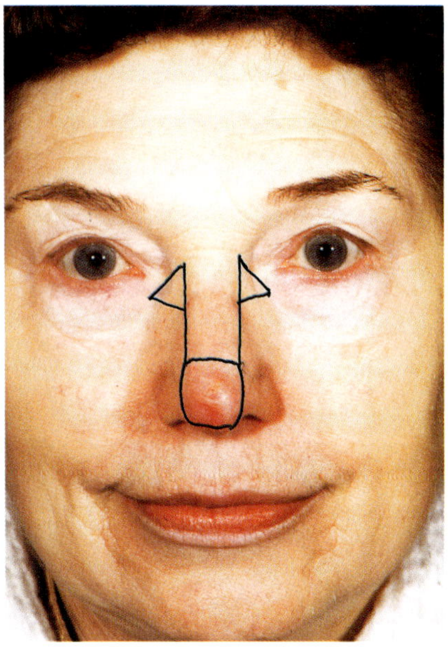

Figure 3.31a Basal cell carcinoma of the nasal tip. The excision is performed into the healthy tissue as confirmed by histology. A modified Rintala flap is planned.

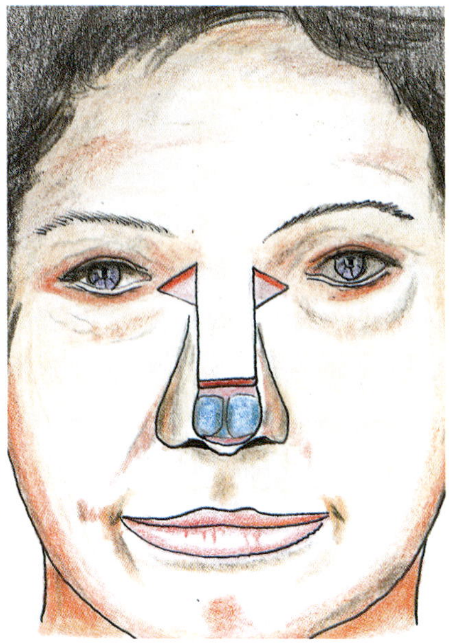

Figure 3.31b Rintala operation – modification. The flap is dissected down to the level of the cartilage and the periostium. Two triangles are excised and the flap is advanced caudally.

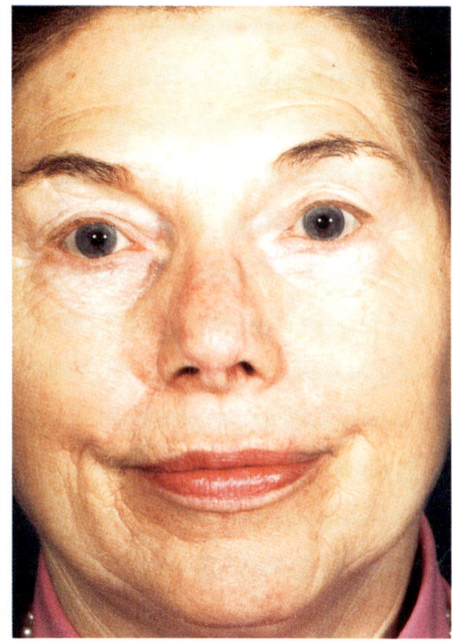

Figure 3.31c Result 18 months after the operation. There is no tumor recurrence and the nasal shape is well preserved.

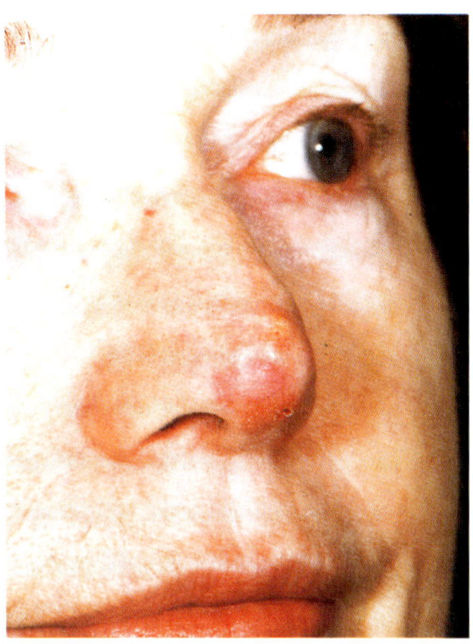

Figure 3.31d Status before the operation

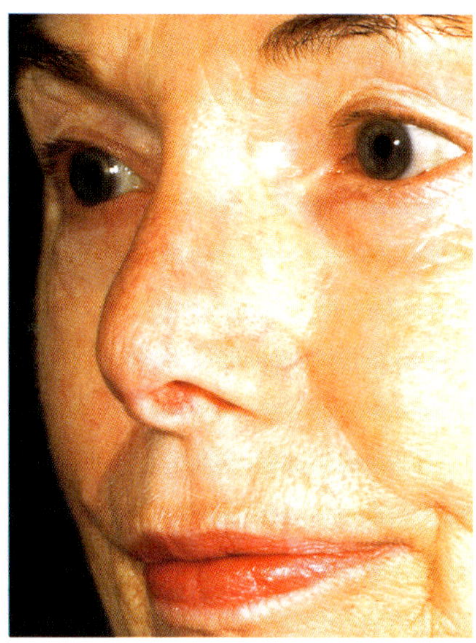

Figure 3.31e Result 18 months after the operation

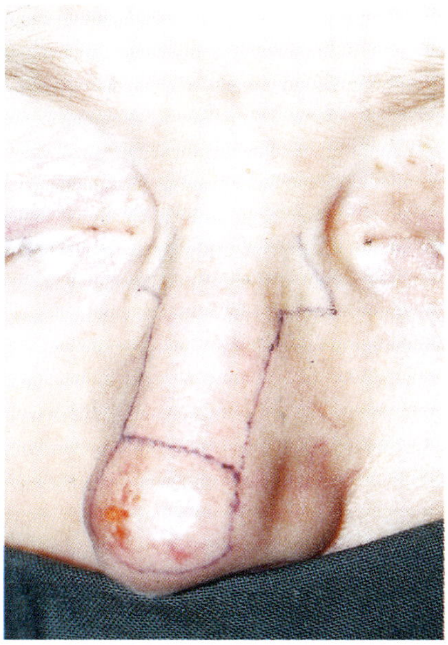

Figure 3.32a Basal cell carcinoma at the nasal tip

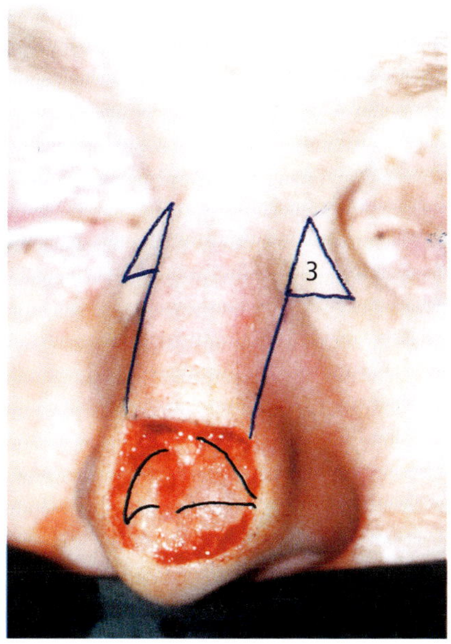

Figure 3.32b Planning of the Rintala modified operation: The tumor at the nasal tip is excised. The prominent alar cartilages are reduced.

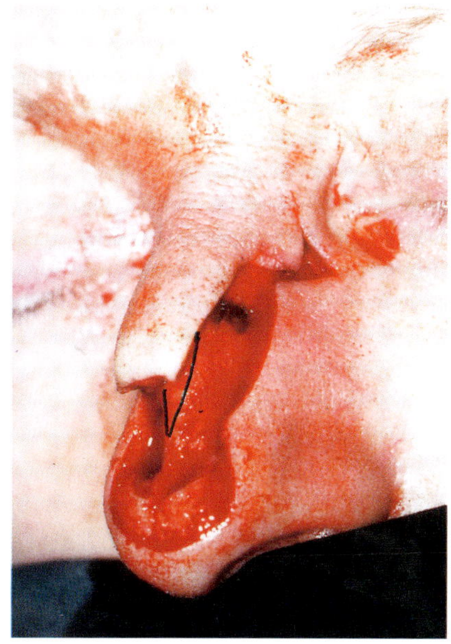

Figure 3.32c Situation following dissection of the flap. The cranial parts of the alar cartilage (1) are resected and the nasal hump is also removed (2). This decreases the tension in the flap and improved the shape of the nose.

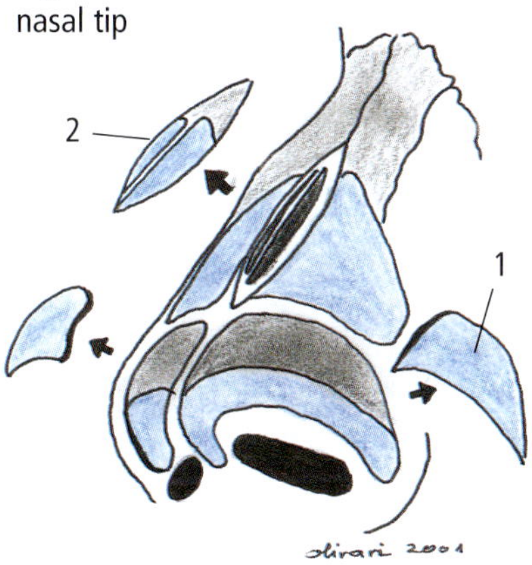

◁ **Figure 3.32d** Operation plan for a–c

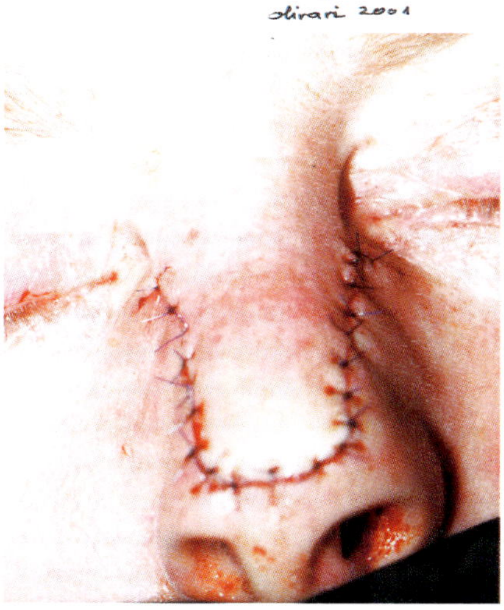

Figure 3.32e At the end of the operation flap show some tip parlor, due to the use of adrenaline, but flap remains viable.

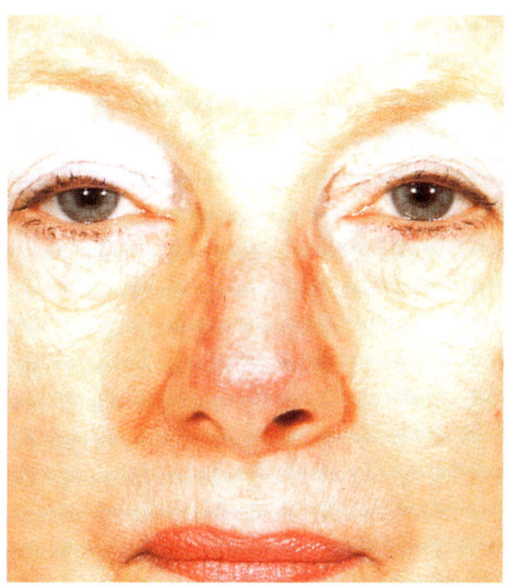

Figure 3.32f Status one year after the operation: There is still a slight reddening of the scar. The nasal shape is normal. No recurrence of tumor.

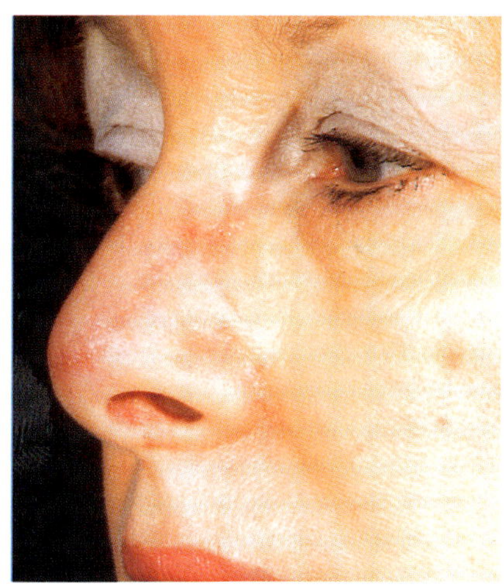

Figure 3.32g Status one year after the operation

Coverage of Nasal Defect With the Schmid Flap

This is a transversal supraorbital, transverse tube pedicle flap. Two delays are necessary in order to ensure a safe and reorientated blood supply. The flap crosses the course of the blood vessels, i.e. the supraorbital artery (2) and the supratrochlear artery (1). The operation is technically demanding and somewhat risky!

This flap is only recommended if no other options are available.

It was popularized by Schmid in the 1970s and enjoyed a limited use. There is no doubt that with the patience on the part of both surgeon and patient, a good result can be achieved.

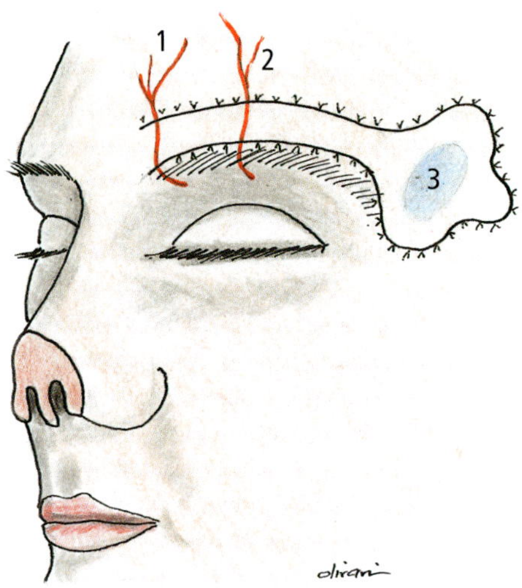

Figure 3.33a Delay of the flap. A piece of cartilage can be implanted beneath tip of flap before transposition in order to achieve a better profile (3).

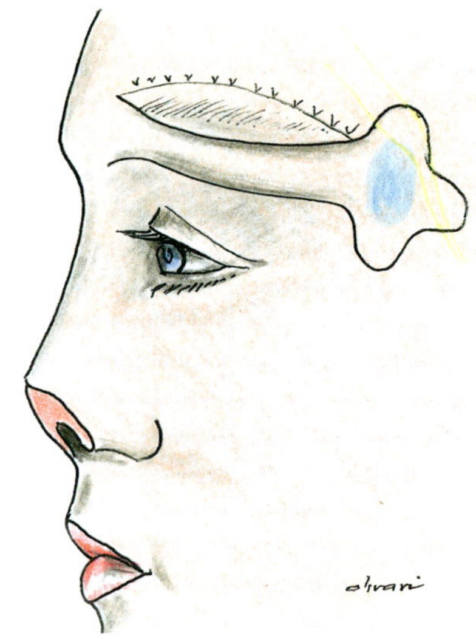

Figure 3.33b Formation of the tube pedicle flap after approximately two weeks

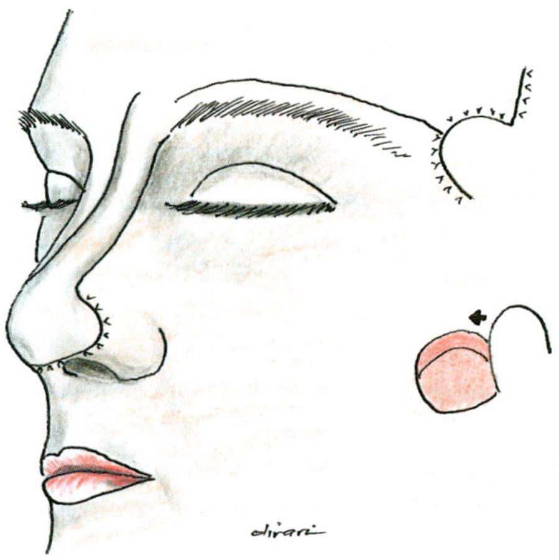

Figure 3.33c The tip of the flap is fixed to the defect at the nasal tip.

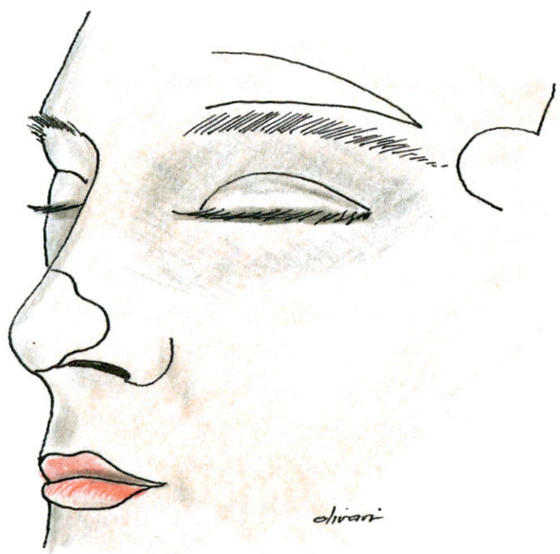

Figure 3.33d The remainder of the flap is returned to its original site three weeks later to prevent a elevation of the eyebrow. The defect in the temporal area is closed with a small local flap.

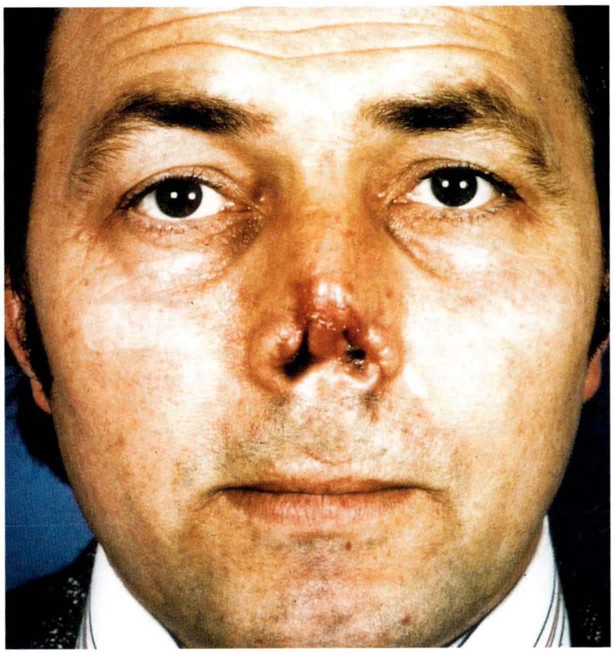

Figure 3.34a Nasal defect due to trauma

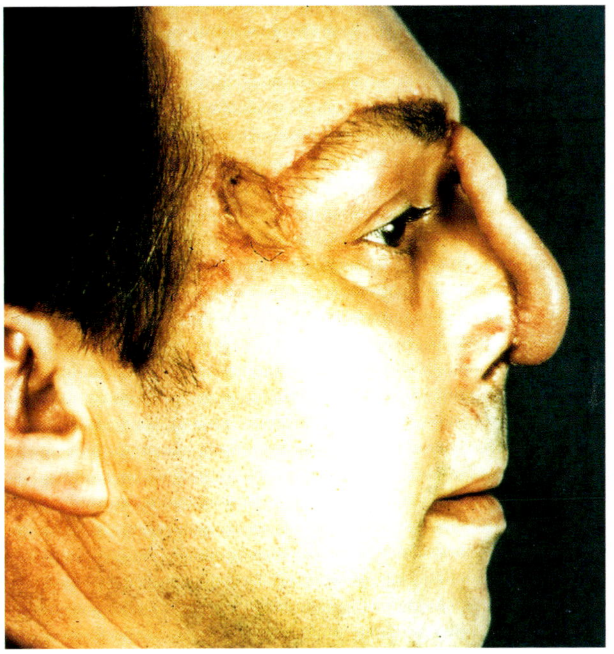

Figure 3.34b The Schmid flap is sutured after two delays at the nasal tip

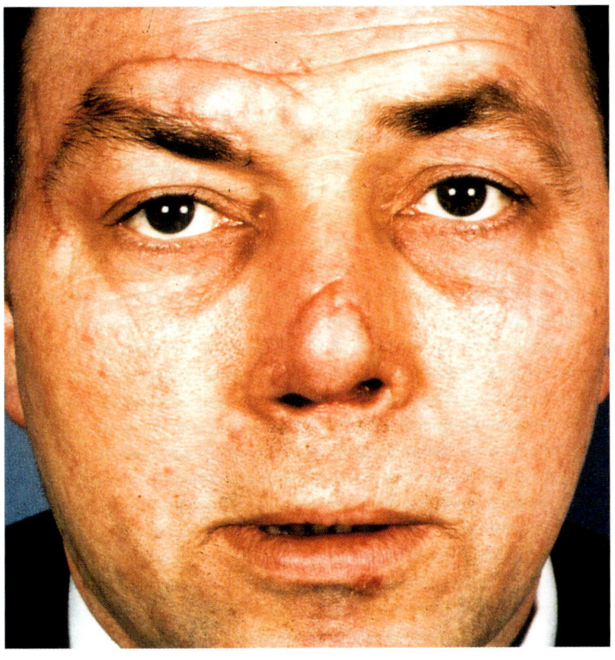

Figure 3.34c Status three months postoperatively: The nasal tip is reconstructed and the remaining flap is returned to its original site in order to avoid an elevation of the eyebrow. The defect in the temporal area is closed with a local flap. In all, four operations were required in order to correct the defect.

Summary on the Schmid Flap

This is a tube pedicle flap that traverses the vascular course of both the supraorbital and the supratrochlear artery. Thus necessity of two or three delays.

There is also risk of injury to the frontal branches of the supratrochlear and the supraorbital nerve.

This flap is only recommended in exceptional circumstances. However good results an be achieved.

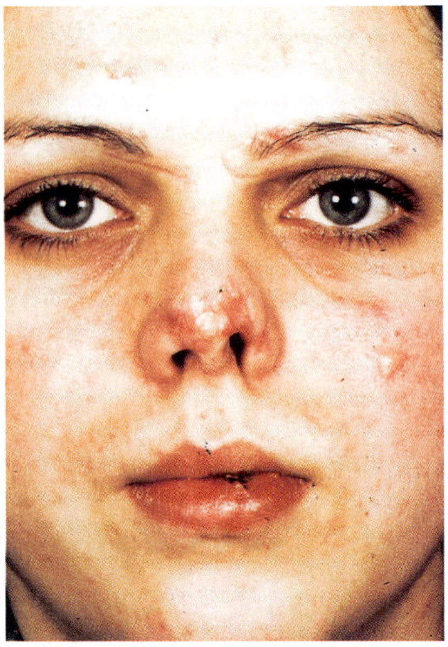

Figure 3.35a Nasal tip defect due to trauma

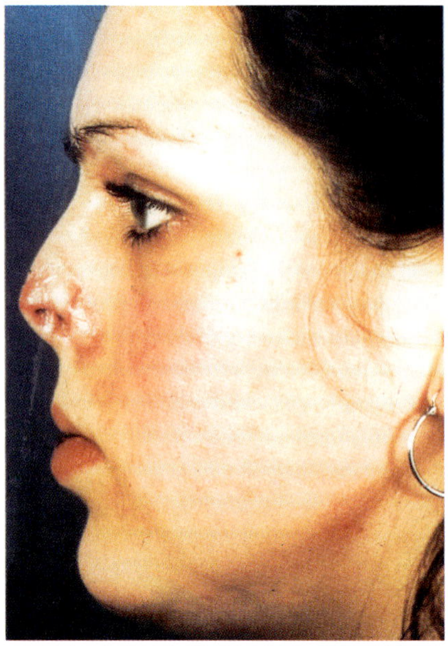

Figure 3.35b Lateral view

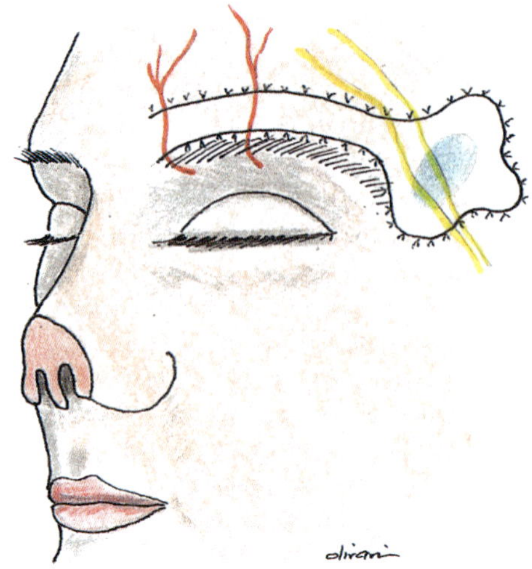

Figure 3.35c Schmid flap: Initial incision and implantation of a piece of cartilage beneath the flap tip. The cartilage must be carefully implanted subcutaneously in order to prevent injury to the frontal branch of the facial nerve.

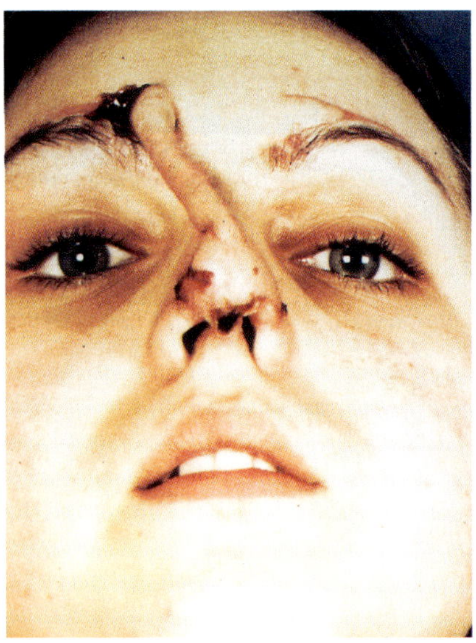

Figure 3.35d The Schmid flap is fixed to the nasal tip. The initial flap from the left side became necrotic due to vascular problems. A second flap from the right side was then delayed four weeks.

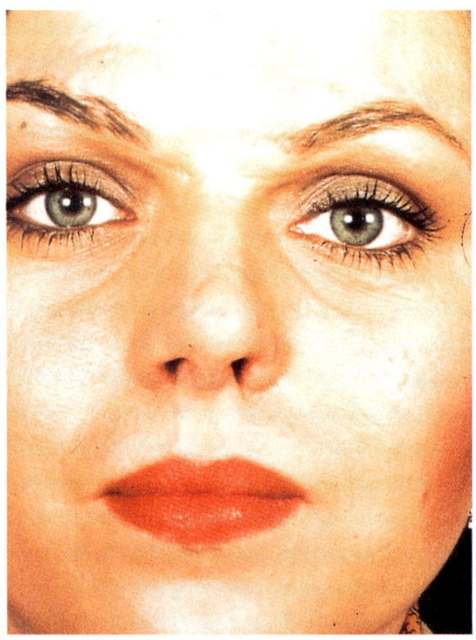

Figure 3.35e Result one year after operation

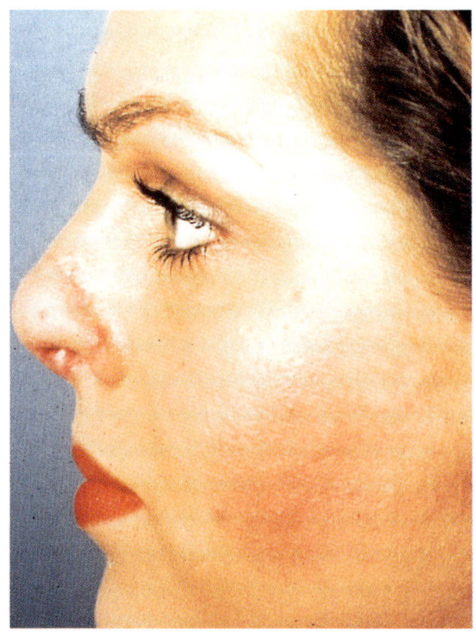

Figure 3.35f Lateral view

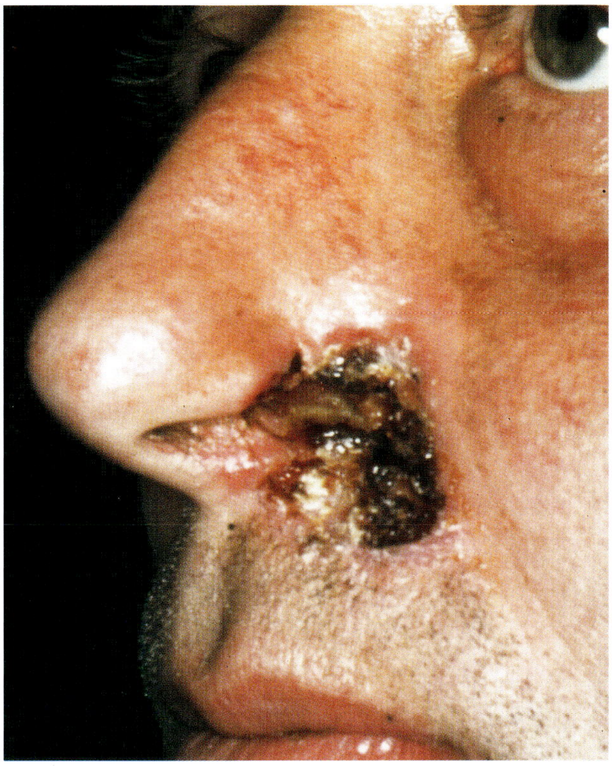

Figure 3.36a Basal cell carcinoma in the left alar area extending into the upper lip

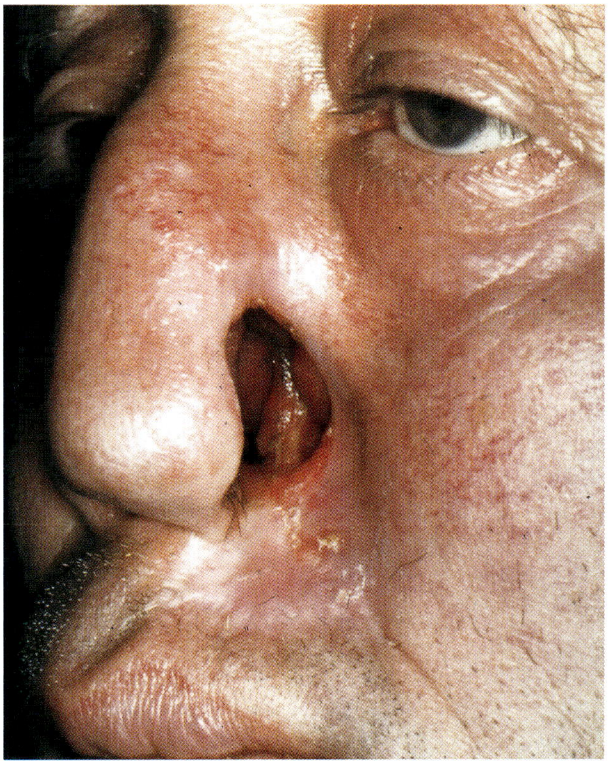

Figure 3.36b Following two excisions showing tumor-free margins histologically we waited one year to be sure there was no recurrence. This resulted in marked deformities.

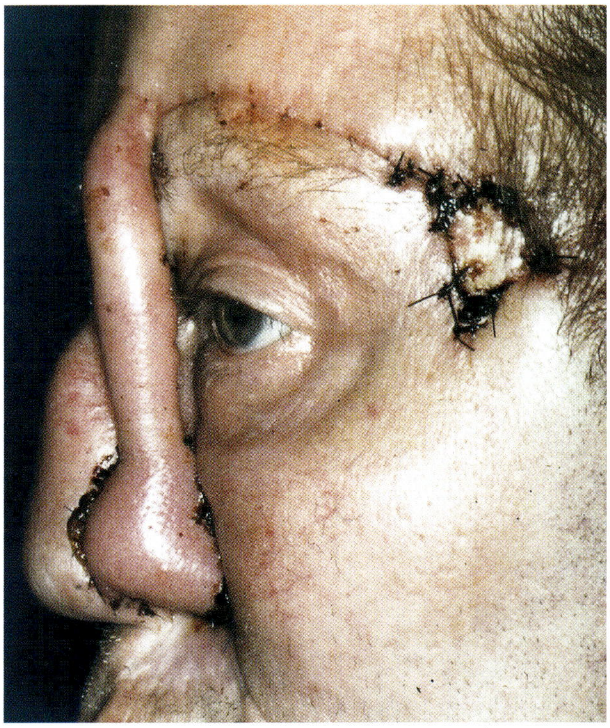

Figure 3.36c Left sided Schmid flap large enough to ensure closure of both lip and nose deformity was raised.

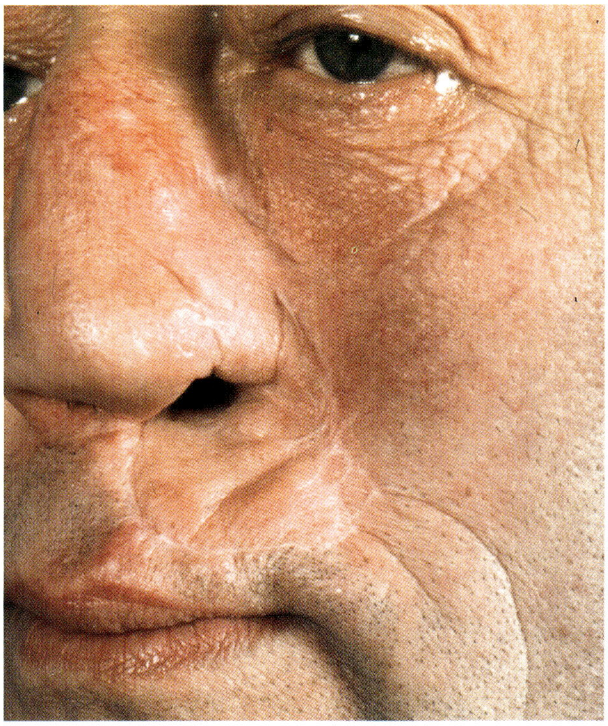

Figure 3.36d Result one year after the reconstruction of the nose as well as the upper lip showing deflection of the nose tip.

Wikarczyk Rotation Flap

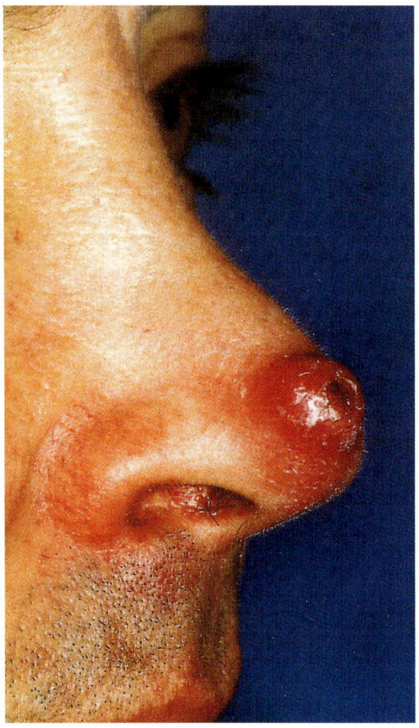

Figure 3.37a A large rotation flap dissected following excision of tumor

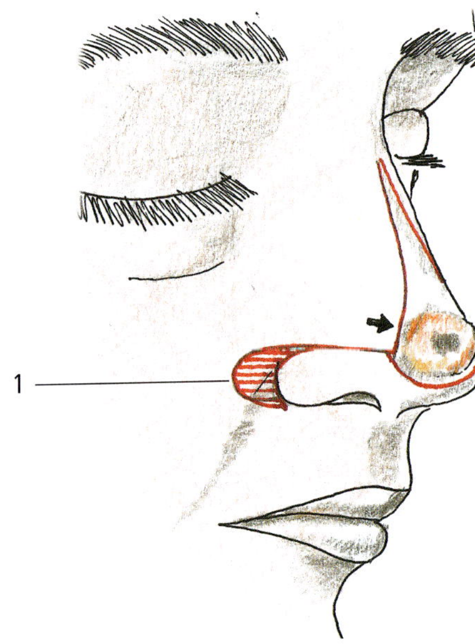

Figure 3.37b In order to facilitate flap rotation, a sickle-shaped excision of skin is carried out lateral to the alar base (1).

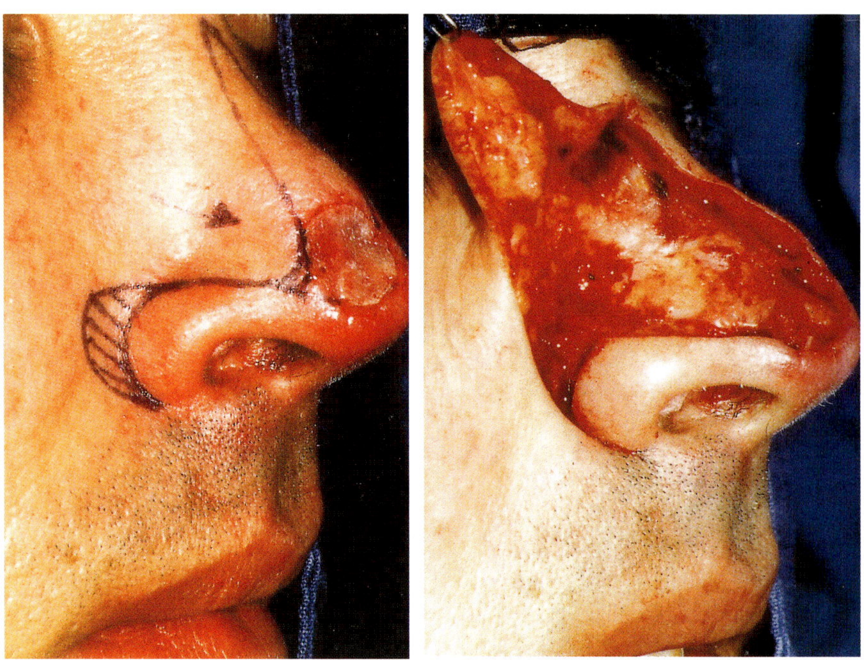

Figure 3.37c,d Rotation is only possible after extensive mobilization laterally. It is important to free the flap from the periostium of the nasal bone.

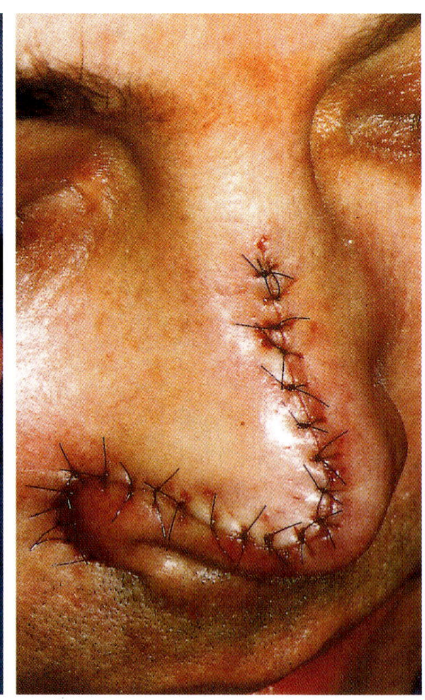

Figure 3.37e Situation at the end of the operation

Bilateral Wikarczyk Rotation Flap

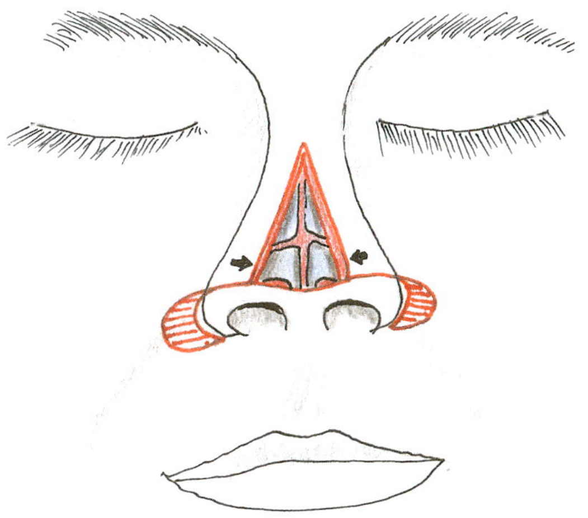

Figure 3.38a With larger defects of the nasal tip a bilateral rotation flap is employed

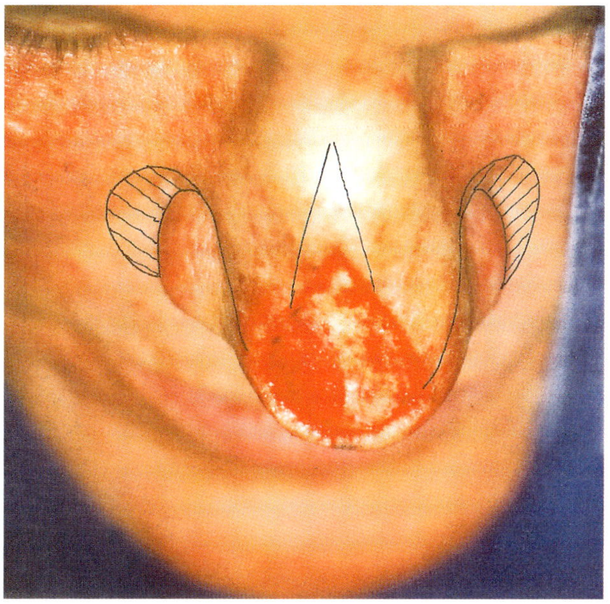

Figure 3.38b The incisions are identical to that of a unilateral rotation flap. It is important to mobilize both flaps.

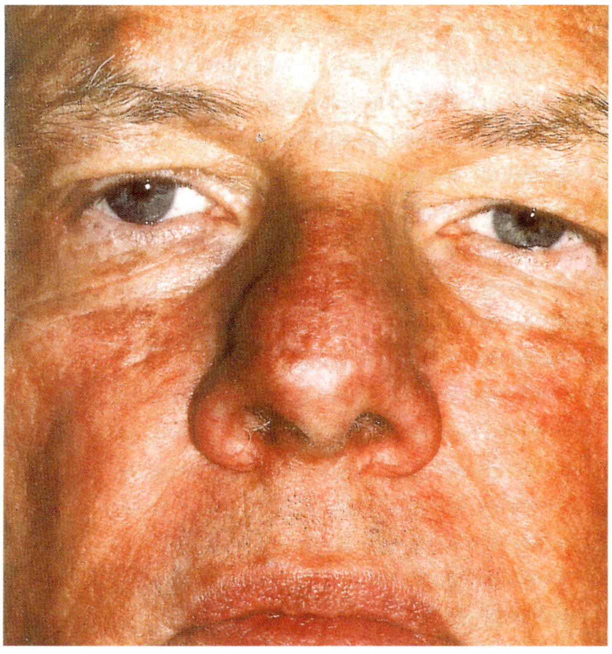

Figure 3.38c Result six months after a Wikarczyk bilateral rotation flap

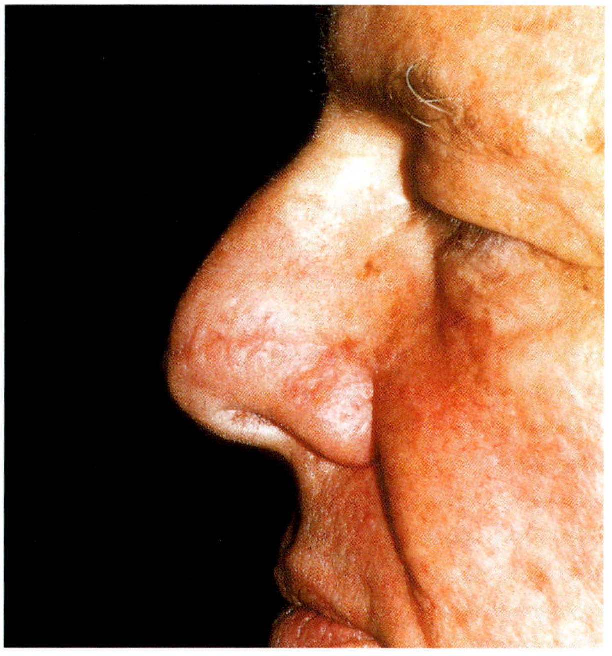

Figure 3.38d Profile six months after the operation

Sanvenero Rosselli Plasty

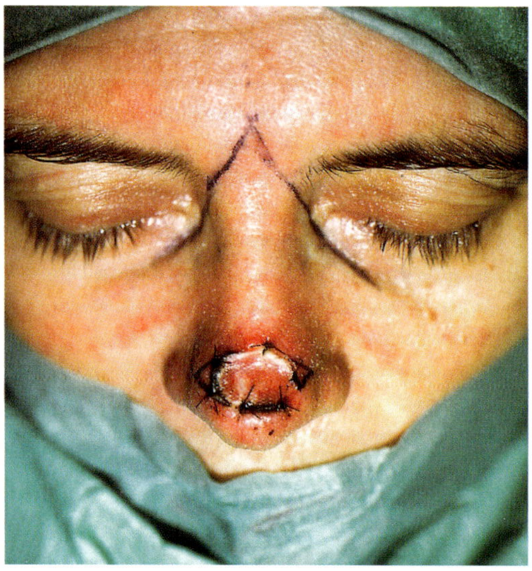

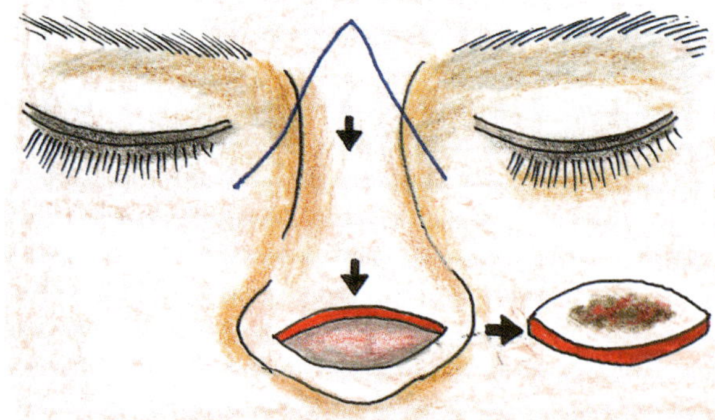

Figure 3.39a Basal cell carcinoma of the nasal tip. A transverse oriented defect has been created. The tumor is excised and covered with Epigard until histological clearance is confirmed. The skin of the nasal dorsum is then completely mobilized and a V incision is made at the nasal root and the glabella. The skin flap is then advanced caudally and upper defect closed as a VY.

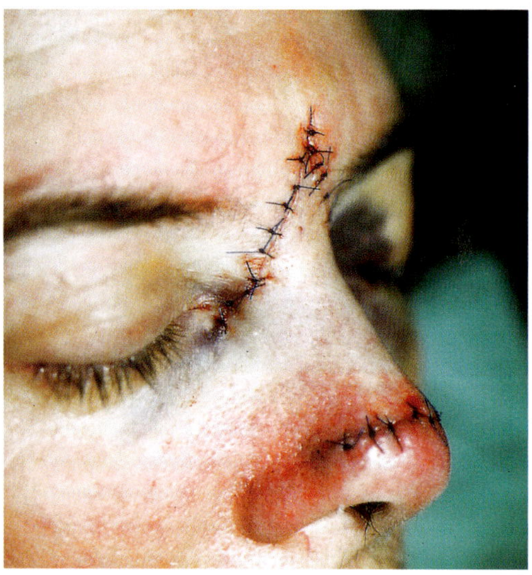

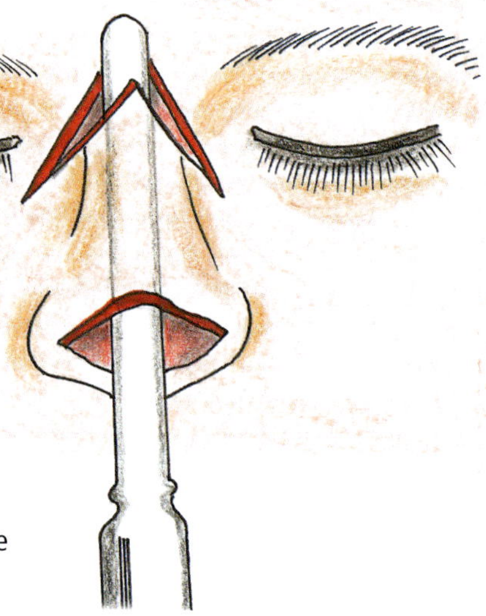

Figure 3.39b Mobilization of the nasal dorsum

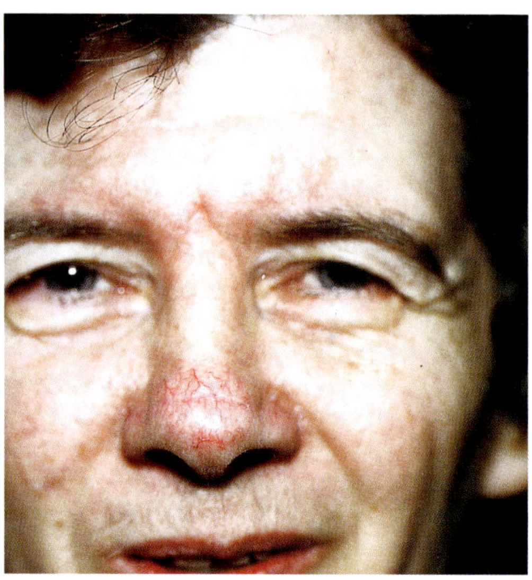

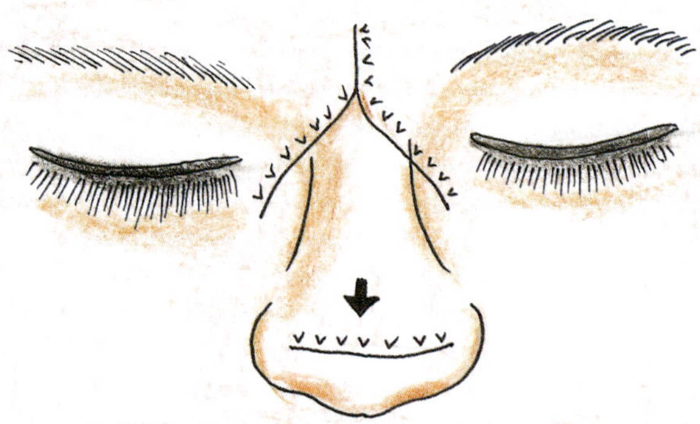

Figure3.39c Result 14 months postoperatively

Rhinophyma

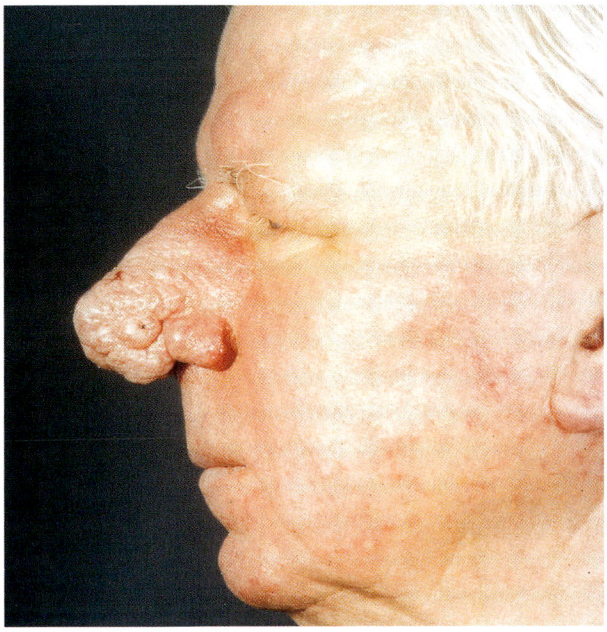

Figure 3.40a Rhinophyma

Rhinophyma is a rare disease of the skin. It is a form of *acne rosacea*. The skin of the nose becomes grostly hypertrophic. The cause is unknown although the number of sebaceous glands increased enormously. The skin of the nose becomes greatly thickened and there is accompanying increase in dermal collagen and dilatation of blood vessels. Frequently local infections occur. An association with alcohol abuse has not been verified.

Therapy

Operation under general anesthesia is preferable. After injection of local anesthetic with 1/200000 adrenaline, the rhinophymatous tissue is excised tangentially with a 22 scalpel until the nose acquires the desired form. Bleeding is controlled by coagulation and compression. Postoperatively a crust develops which separates in eight to ten days. The surface reepithelializes from the remaining sebaceous and sweat gland ducts so skin graft is not necessary.

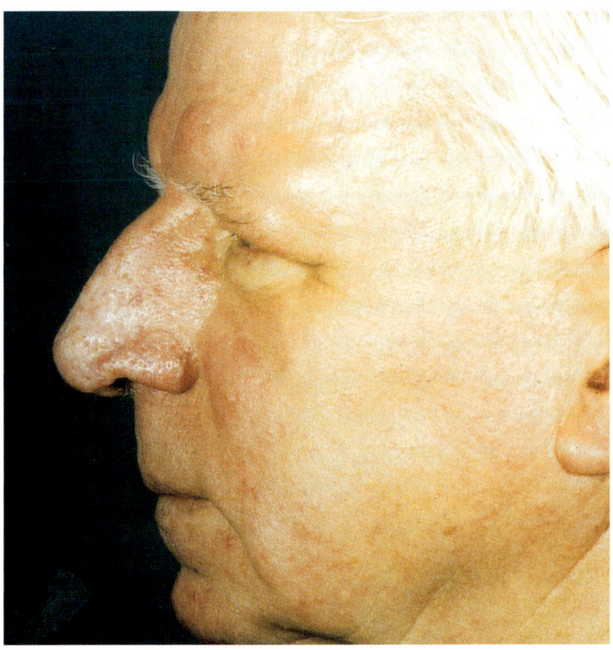

Figure 3.40b Result one year after the operation

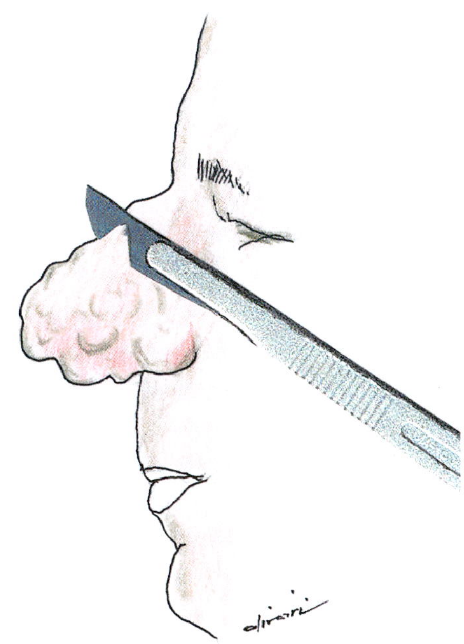

Figure 3.40c Excision of tissue in a case of rhinophyma: Bleeding is reduced by coagulation and compression. Epithelialization occurs within one to two weeks.

Defect Coverage With Full Thickness Skin Graft

Area of scar deformity of the nose, caused by trauma or burns, can be treated with full thickness skin grafts.

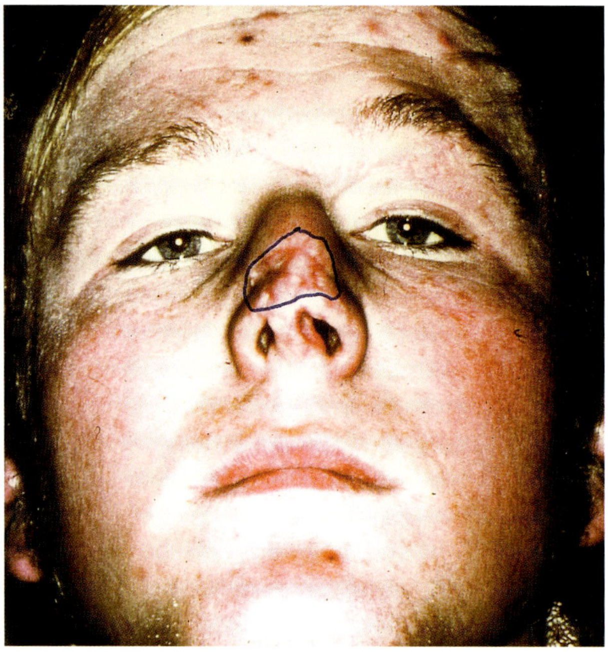

Figure 3.41a Scar deformity of the nose after burn trauma. The cartilage is intact.

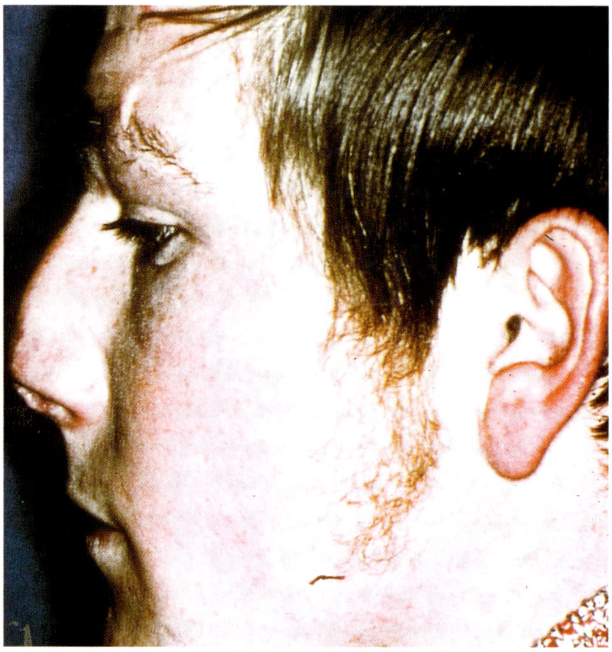

Figure 3.41b The scar is excised and the defect is covered with a full thickness skin graft from the retroauricular area.

Figure 3.41c The retroauricular area is an ideal donor site for full thickness skin graft for face and nose.

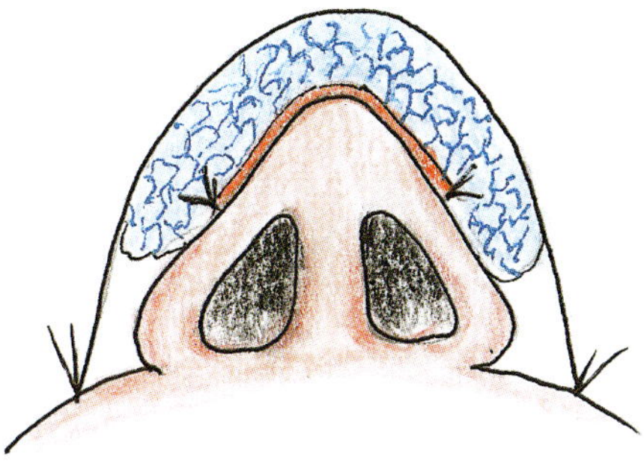

Figure 3.41d Fixation of the full thickness skin graft to the nose. The compression bandage of the full skin graft should not be fixed to the defect margin, but held with single sutures placed at a distance. The compression bandage consists of flammazine tulle gras and artificial cotton wool. As a result the graft edges remain flat and the scars are considerably flatter.

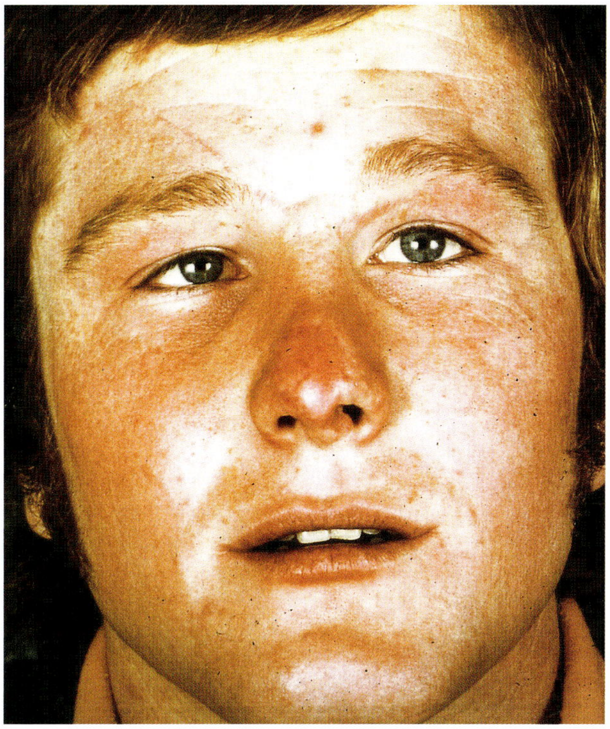

Figure3.41e Situation one year after the operation: Scar has improved. The form and color of the nose has improved. Cartilage graft is not needed.

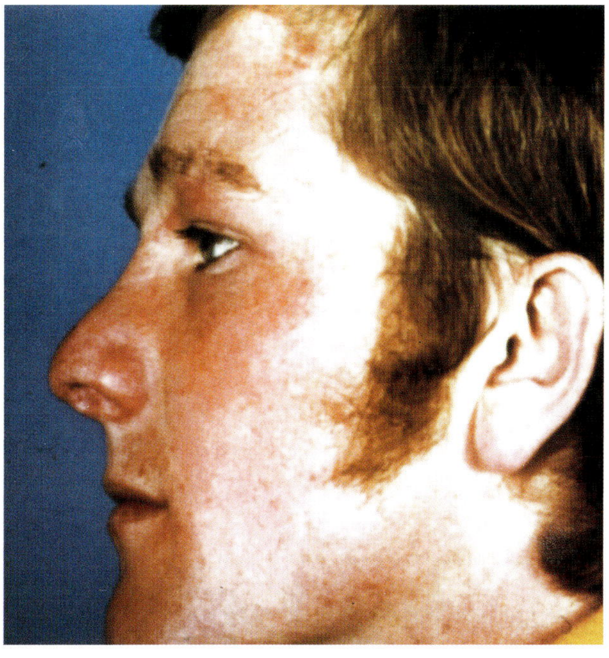

Figure 3.41f A good result can sometimes be achieved with simple surgery.

Defect Coverage With a "Composite Graft"

The "composite graft" is a composite of skin, subcutaneous tissue and cartilage. The best sites for harvesting a "composite graft" is the root of the helix and anthelix. The smaller the "composite graft", the better are the chances of success but there is a limit of the size of the graft. Some counted that only 50 % success can be expected, but we believe 80 % of composite graft succeed.

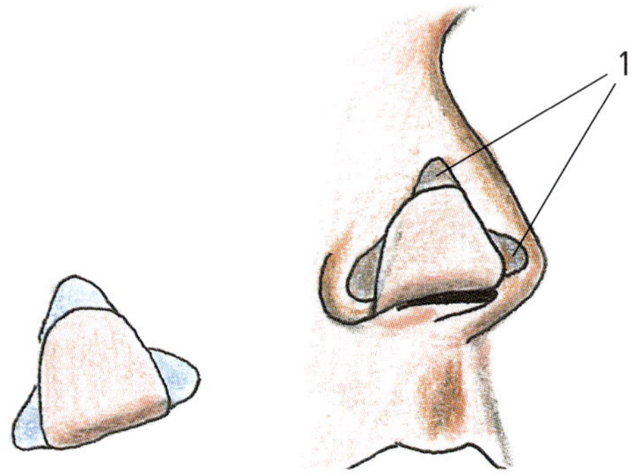

△ **Figure3.42c** Carefully measured "composite graft" is taken from the concha of the right ear. Note the cartilage incisions that are to be implanted under the healthy skin of the nose (1). The graft must be handled with delicacy and is cooled for 24 hours.

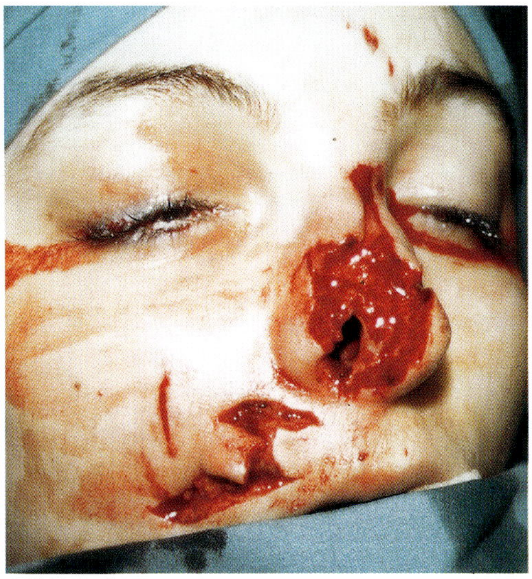

Figure 3.42a Alar defect and several wounds on the cheek on right cheek due to a dog bite

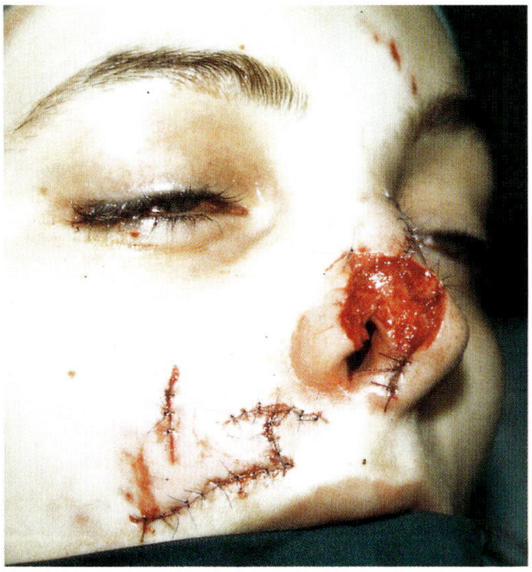

Figure 3.42b Atraumatic closure of the wound at the cheek and the columella. Preparation of the wound bed for composite graft.

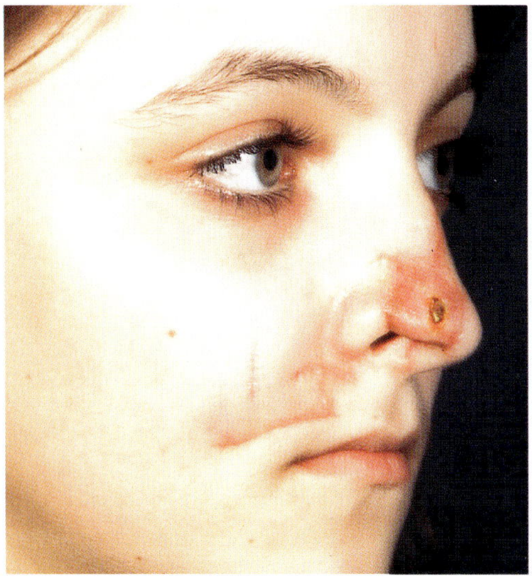

Figure3.42d Appearance three weeks postoperatively

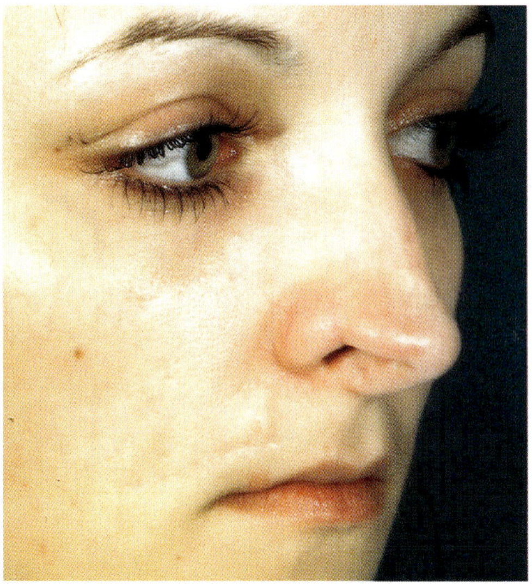

Figure 3.42e Result three years after the operation

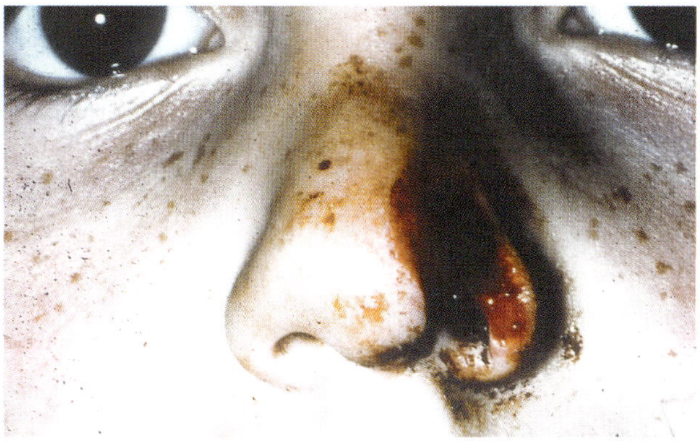

Figure 3.43a Alar defect following accident

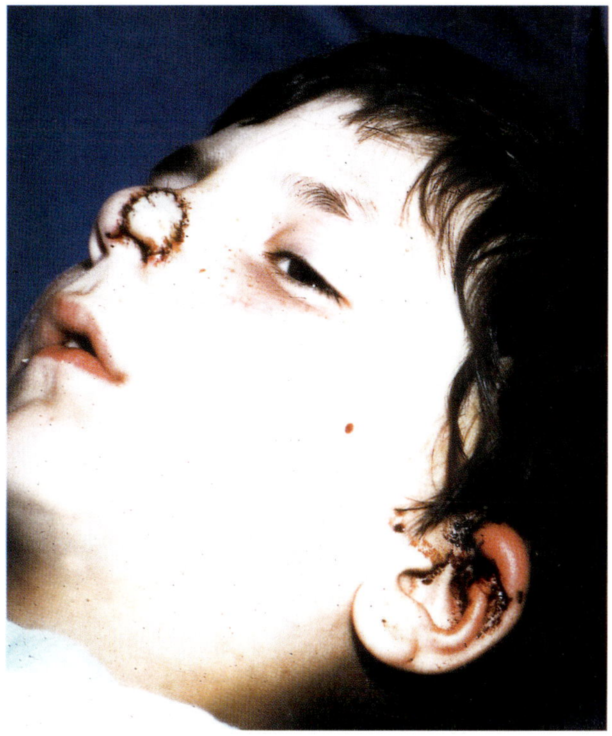

Figure 3.43b Situation three days after the operation: The transplant is slightly congested. A composite graft was taken from the left upper part of helix and concha. The transplant was cooled for 24 hours.

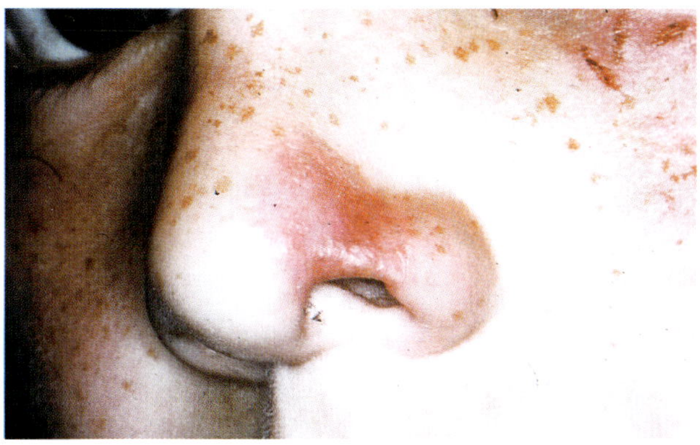

Figure 3.43c Situation six months after surgery

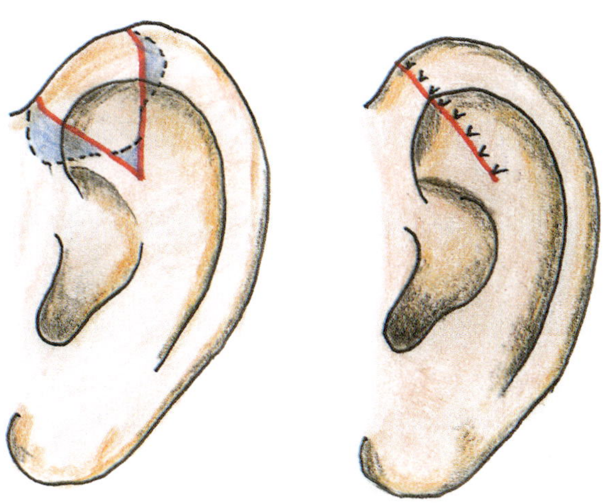

Figure 3.43d Schematic representation of the removal of a "composite graft". The amount of cartilage excised, exceeds the area of removed skin. This part of the cartilage is placed subcutaneously and as the cartilage is nourished by diffusion, the chances of healing are better.

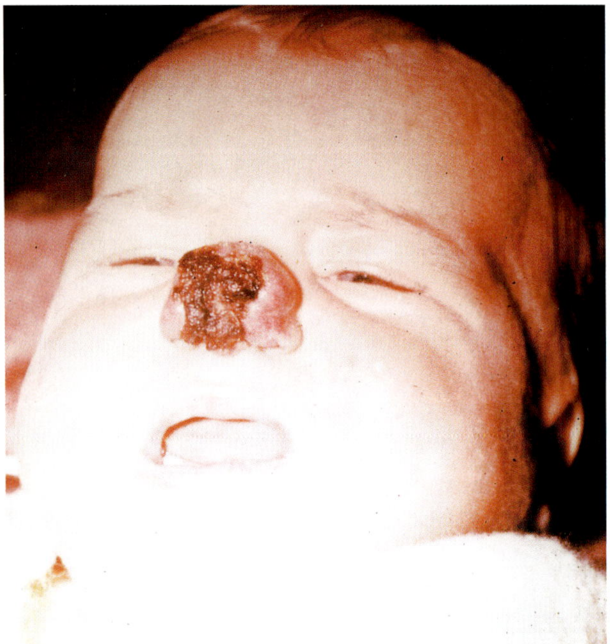

Figure 3.44a A irradiated hemangioma of the nose showing a bad result. Cartilage in children is particularly sensitive to irradiation and this treatment should never be administered.

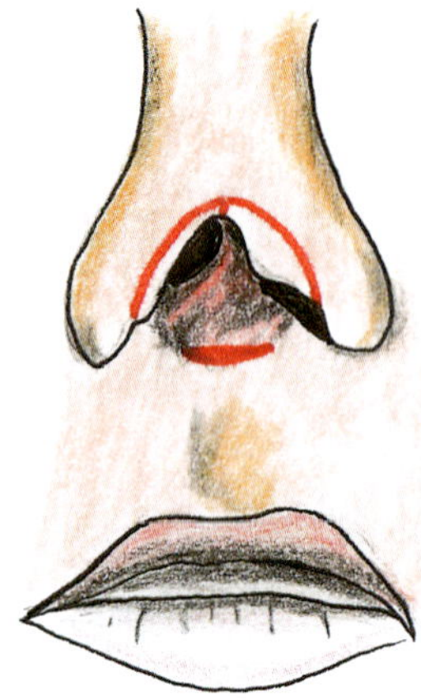

Figure 3.44b Preparation of the nasal defect for a composite graft

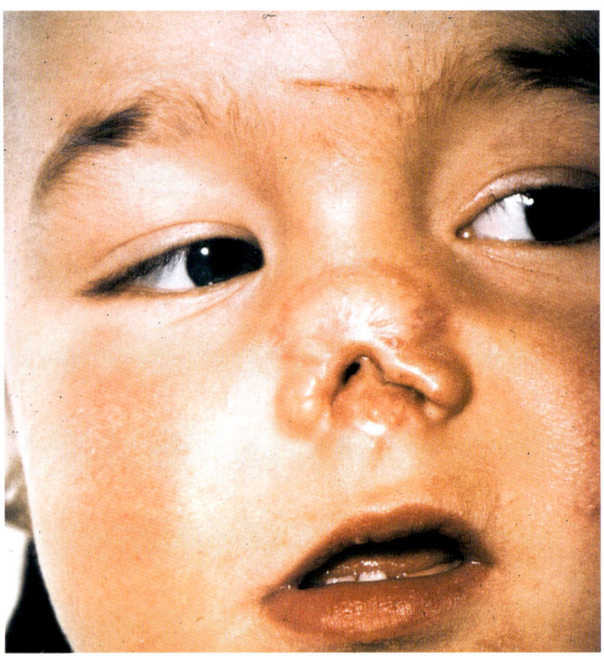

Figure 3.44c Situation three years later after spontaneous, secondary healing. The destruction caused by irradiation is evident, the nasal tip, parts of the alar wing and a part of the columella.

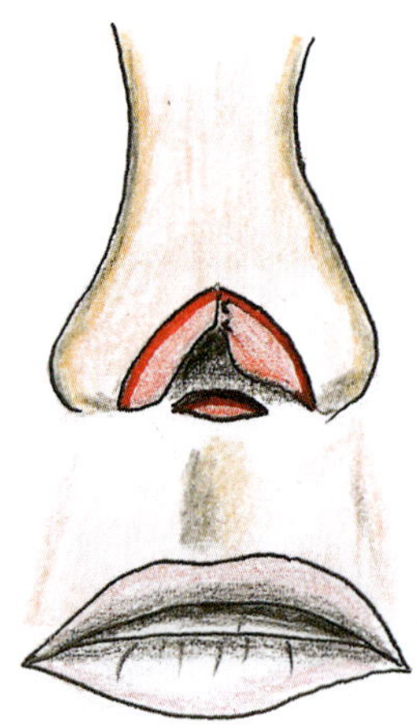

Figure 3.44d Preparation of the nose for the composite graft. The incision around the defect gives, a greater area of contact for the graft, and thus a better blood supply.

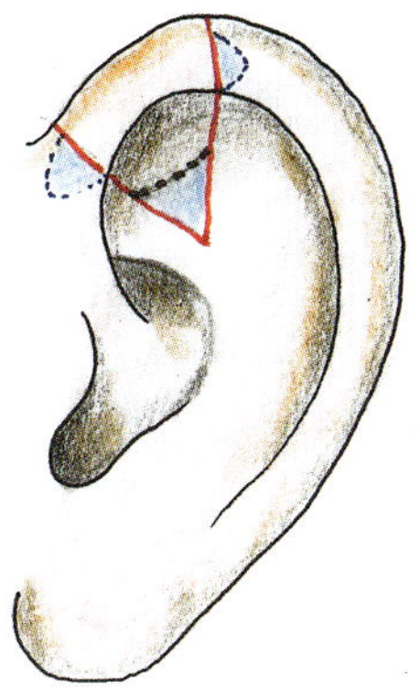

Figure 3.44e Typical harvest site for the composite graft

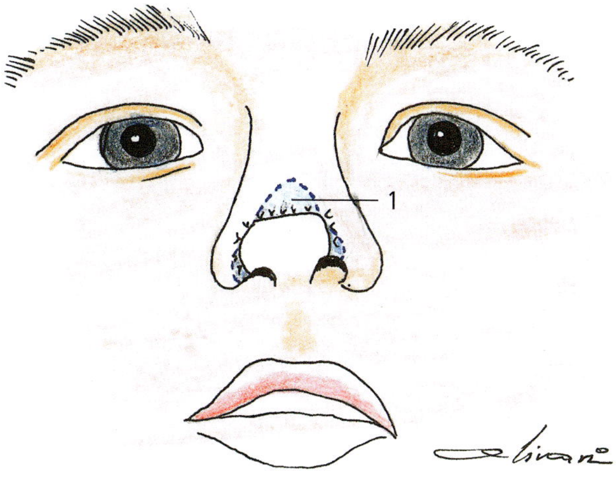

Figure 3.44f Subcutaneous positioning of the cartilage is advantageous (1).

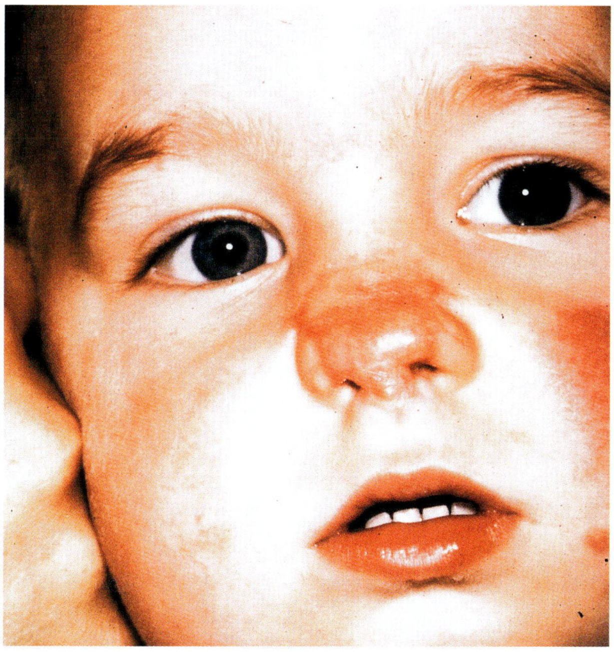

Figure 3.44g Result one year after the operation

The results are considerably better when the following rules are observed:

1. The graft should not be too large.
2. The cartilaginous parts should be covered with well vascularized tissue. The cartilage is fed by diffusion so that no new vessels formation is required.
3. A part of the skin of the graft should make contact with a freshened area of skin of the nose.
4. Completely atraumatic handling of the graft. No grasping with forceps, but only with a fine Gillies hook.
5. Postoperative cooling of the graft for 24 hours. A blue graft is good, while a white bode is ill.
6. The blood vessels invade cutaneous portion of the composite graft within 24 to 48 hours.

Defect Coverage With an Epithesis

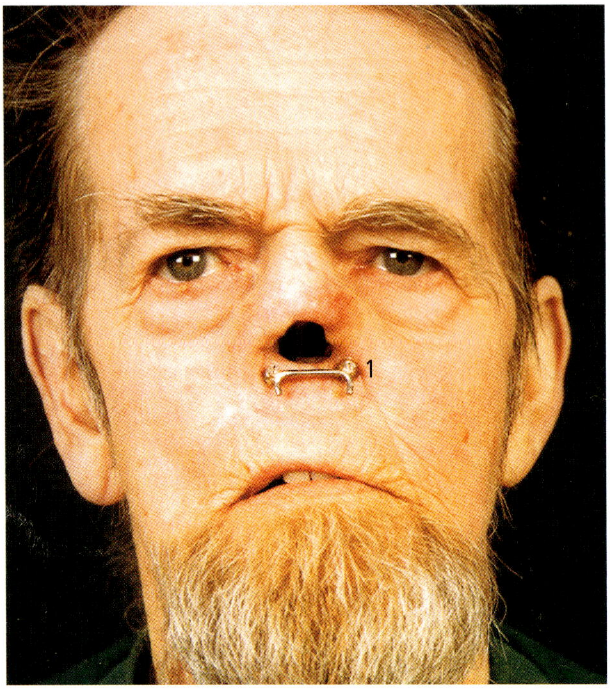

Figure 3.45a Status after partial amputation of the nose. Metal implants allow the metal frame of the prosthesis to be fixed firmly (1) to the maxilla.

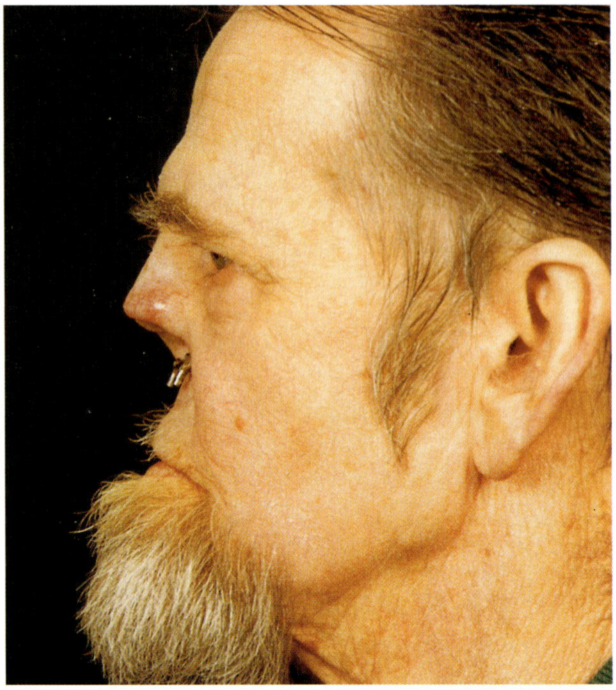

Figure 3.45b Lateral view

Sometimes a perfect epithesis is better than undistinguished reconstruction!!

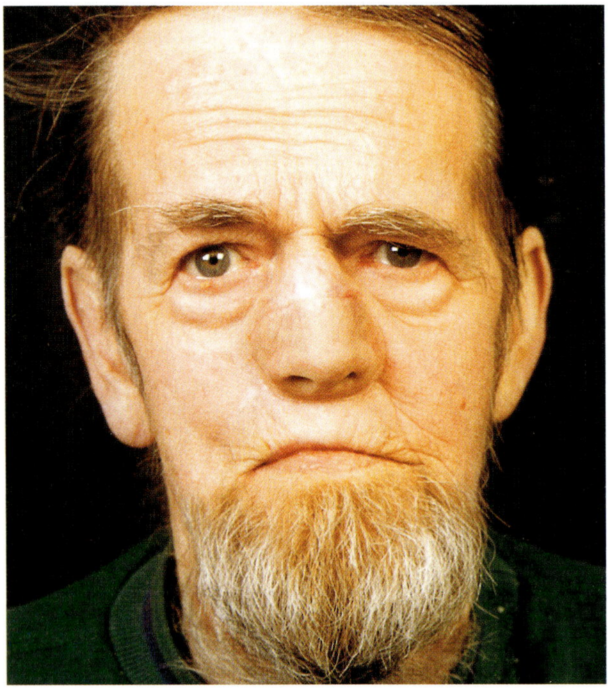

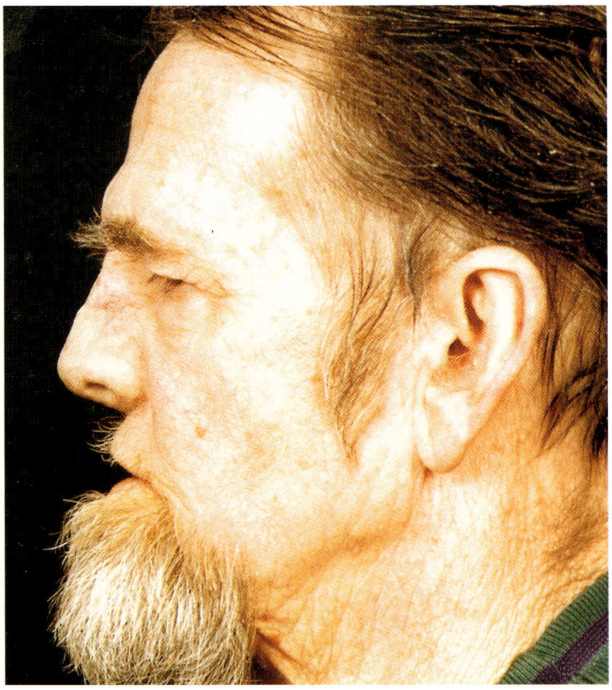

Figure 3.45c,d The well-adapted epithesis represents a perfect match in form and color with the remainder of the nose. Indications for an epithesis include:

1) Risk of a tumor recurrence (e.g. sclerodermiform basalioma).
2) As a temporary procedure before the final operation is carried out.
3) Patient aversion to a complicated reconstructive operation.
4) Considerable psychological rehabilitation.

Traumatic Saddle Nose

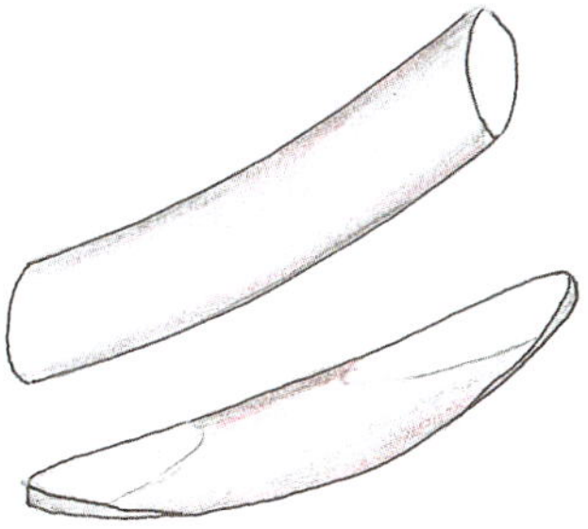

Figure 3.46a Modeling of piece of a costal cartilage for the correction of a saddle nose. Resorption of cartilage is minimal. After healing the nasal tip retrains slight mobility.

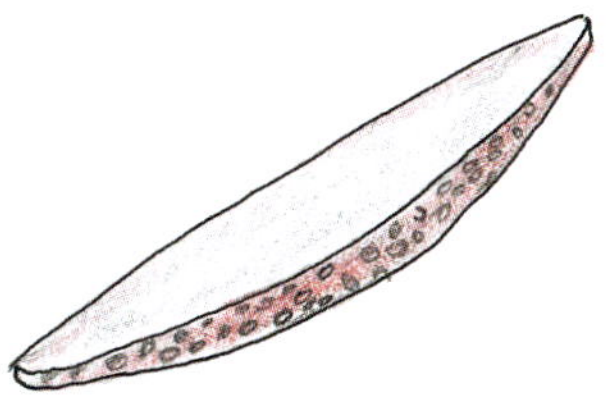

Figure 3.46b The saddle nose can be corrected using a flake of bone from a rib or the pelvic crest. However risk of resorption of bone is considerably higher and the nasal tip becomes unnaturally stiff.

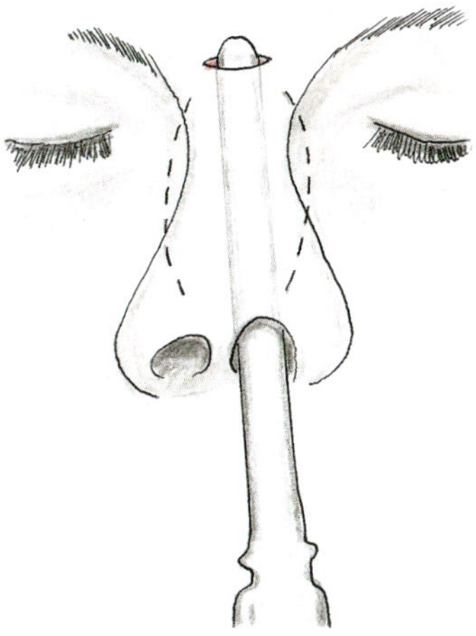

Figure 3.46c Formation of the tunnel for the transplant. A small incision in the glabella area allows the exact positioning and fixing of the bone or cartilage transplant with a mini-screw. The mobilization must be extended on both sides of the nose (shaded).

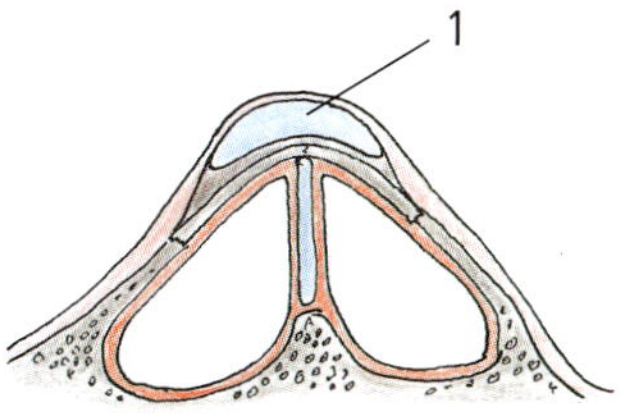

Figure 3.46d Position of the transplant, in this case a costal cartilage graft (1).

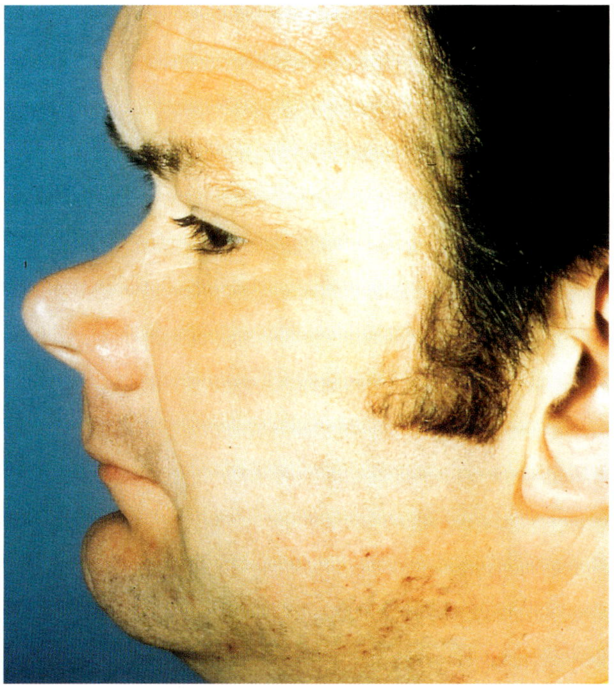

Figure 3.47a Appearance after a depression fracture due to a car accident. Operation: Access via intranasal incision. The skin is widely undermined laterally and on the dorsum of the nose. The grafts should not cause skin blanching as this may inhibit vascularization. A small incision in the glabella area allows a better positioning of the graft and the transplant is fixed with a mini-screw. **No dressing or splint is applied.**

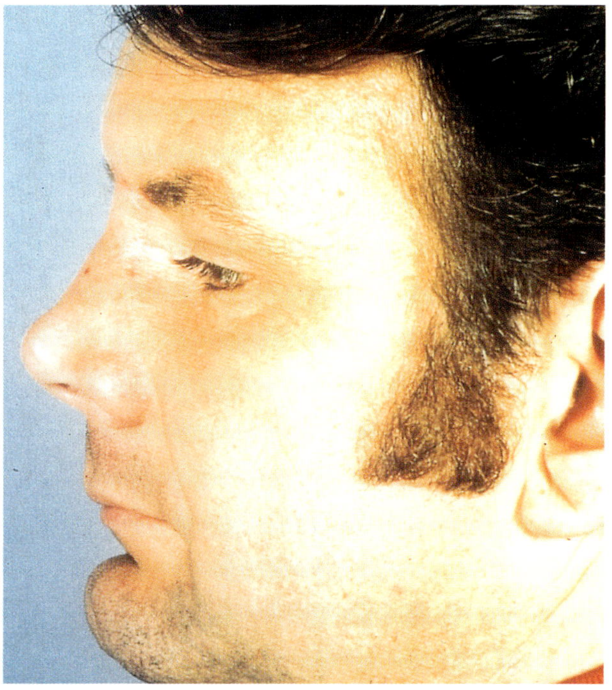

Figure 3.47b Result one year postoperatively

Aesthetic Rhinoplasty

Rhinoplasty is one of most commonly performed procedure in plastic surgery and is doubtless the most complex. To perform this operation successfully, the surgeon must have clear concept of nasal anatomy and must be able to predict the changes that will result from alterations to the shape of the bone and cartilage.

Aesthetic rhinoplasty is mostly carried out on patients with no respiratory or olfactory disturbance. Only a reasonable desire of the patient to modify nasal form can represent an indication for such an operation.

The responsibility that the surgeon assumes here is considerable. Apart from the technical competence of the surgeon, the expectations of the patient must also be questioned very thoroughly. The patients wishes frequently conflict with surgical options.

A fully informative consultation is an absolute precondition for an aesthetic nasal correction. The patient must be thoroughly informed about the operation, the postoperative course, and any possible complications *both verbally and in writing*:

a) The function of the nose will not be improved by a cosmetic operation and sometimes may even be temporarily impaired (e.g. olfaction and breathing complaints may occur due to persistent swelling).
b) After the operation the nose requires three to six months in order to achieve its final form. Nasal bones must usually be broken, and take time to heal.
c) The nose is the center of the face and is its most prominent feature. Relatives and acquaintances willl notice a change after surgery and the patient must be prepared for this.
d) A thorough explanation of the immediate postoperative course is necessary. A nasal splint is fitted for seven to 14 days and some impairment of the nasal airway is present two to three weeks, and sometimes even longer.
e) After three to six months secondary corrections may be necessary in order to achieve the desired form.

Aesthetic nasal corrections should be refused:

a) If there are major discrepancies between the outcome and suffering, e.g. a minimal change that can entail serious psychological problems for the patient
b) With noses that have already been operated on several times for cosmetic reasons, and where acceptable results have been achieved, but the patient nevertheless describes the situation as a "disaster".

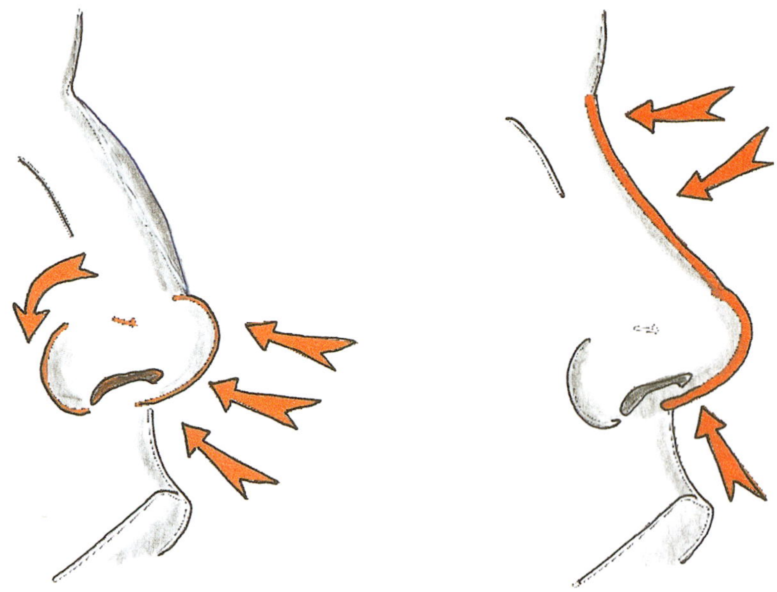

Figure 3.48 Operative sequence

First the nasal tip as well as the alar cartilage are corrected.

In the second part of the operation the hump, the septum and the columella are corrected.

c) For patients who expect that other problem can be solved by the operation (e.g. work, or merit all the difficulties, etc.)
d) When the surgeon considers the operation is too risky for anatomical or physiological reasons.

The wishes of the patients should be respected to a certain degree. However unrealistic demands and surgical impossibilities should be refused.

Operation Sequence

1) First the nasal tip as well as the alar cartilage are corrected.
2) In the second part of the operation the hump, the septum and the columella are corrected and the nose narrowed.

Nature of the Operation

As a matter of principle there are two kinds of operation.

1) **Closed rhinoplasty** via an intranasal approach. The columella remains intact. The advantage of this operation is that there is no scarring of the columella. It is suitable for moderately complicated or uncomplicated noses. For many surgeons with considerable experience this type of approach can be used for almost all types of nasal correction.
2) **Open (transcollumelar) rhinoplasty**. By incising the skin of columella, the nasal framework is exposed. The desired modifications of the cartilage, hump and septum can be carried out very precisely under direct vision. The method is becoming more popular and can be recommended especially for less experienced surgeons. The scar at the columella is usually inconspicious.

Anesthesia

General anesthesia is comfortable not just for the patient, but also for the surgeon. It does however have two disadvantages:

- the tendency to bleeding is increased
- the operation becomes more expensive

Local anesthesia is carried out using 0.5 % Scandicain and 1/200000 adrenaline.
The same solution is also infiltrated under general anesthesia to induce vasoconstriction, and also to reduce postoperative pain.
It is important to wait 15 to 20 minutes before commencing operation. This is no easy task in this day and age where time is of the essence, but waiting does pay off!

a) Operation Access With a Closed Rhinoplasty

The intranasal incision is carried out mostly in the middle of the alar cartilage and is prolonged medially in the septum.

It is advisable to place the incision in mucosa so that the alar cartilage is also incised in place at the same time. The part of the cartilage to be removed is situated cranially to the incision. The incision is prolonged medially in order to achieve a better view and if necessary to shorten the septum.

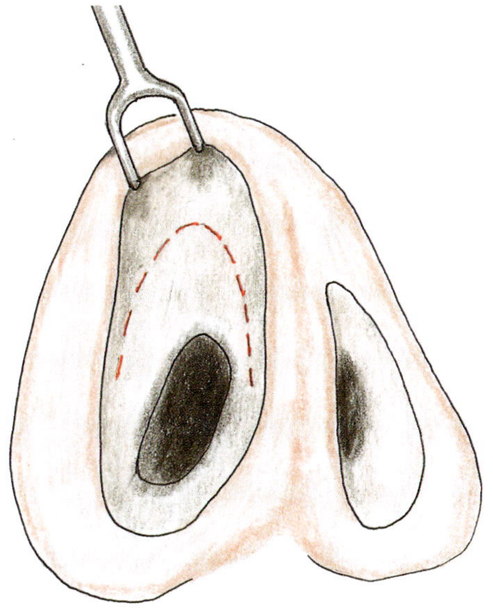

Figure 3.49 Closed rhinoplasty: Intranasal incision through the alar cartilages with prolongation medially in the septum.

Operation Technique for a Humped Nose

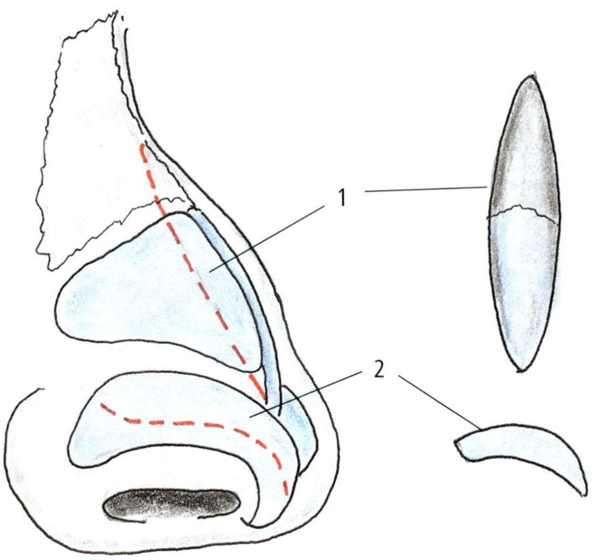

Figure 3.50a Planning of the hump removal (1) as well as the resection of the cranial parts of the alar cartilage (2).

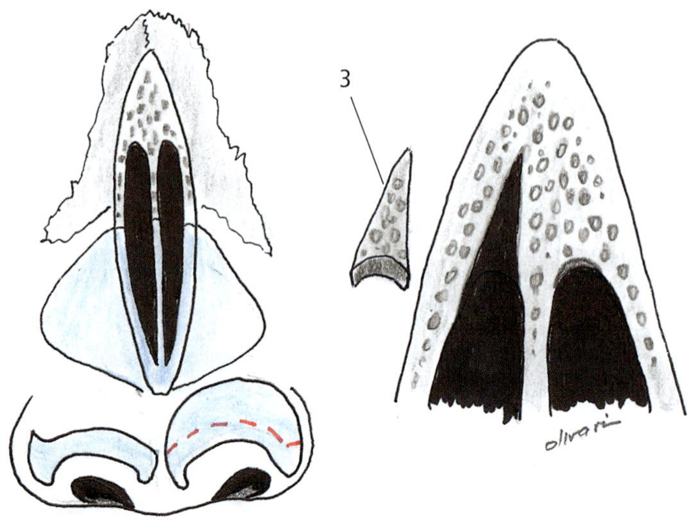

Figure 3.50b The cartilaginous part of the hump is removed with the scalpel, and the cranial part with chisel. The cranial part of alar cartilage is resected intranasally, retaining the mucosa. A bone fragment is resected bilaterally in order to facilitate the lateral osteotomy (3).

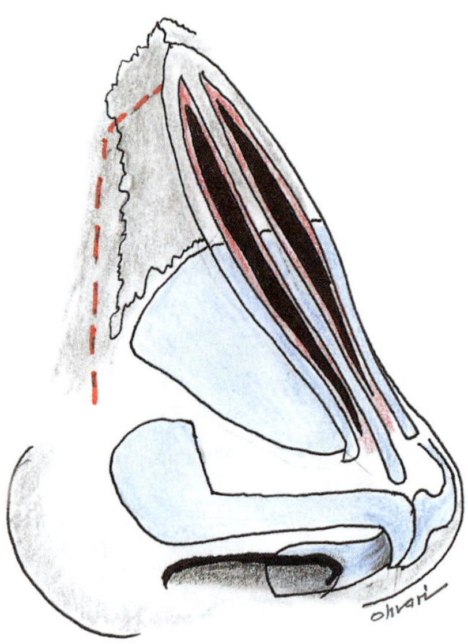

Figure 3.50c The cartilage fragment of the nasal hump is removed using a scalpel and the cranial part is removed using a chisel.

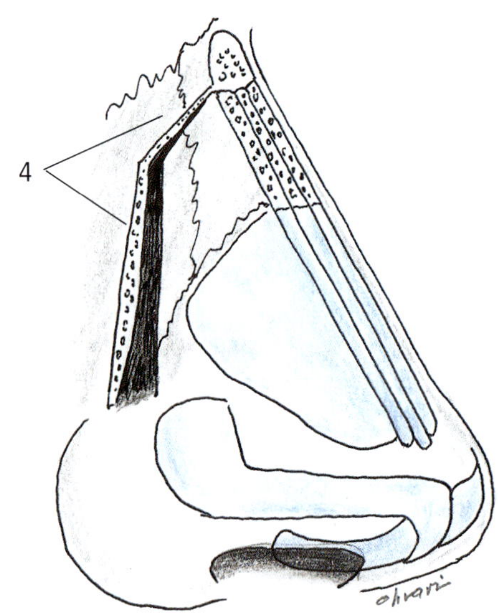

Figure 3.50d The lateral osteotomy is carried out using the chisel or an Olivari rhinotome. An infracture then narrows the nose (4).

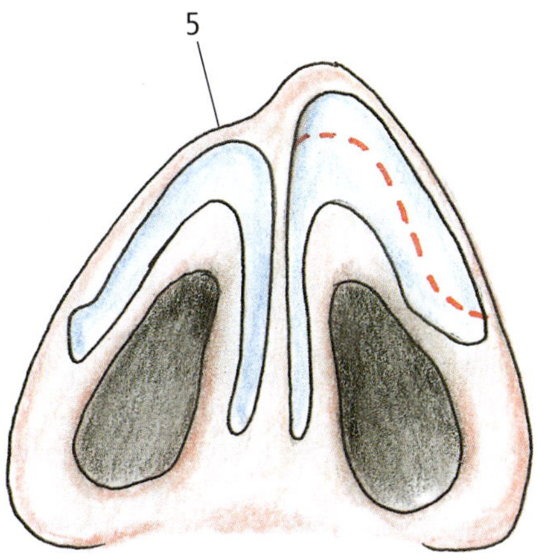

Figure 3.50e Following the resection of the upper part of alar cartilage, the nasal tip becomes narrowed and less prominent (5).

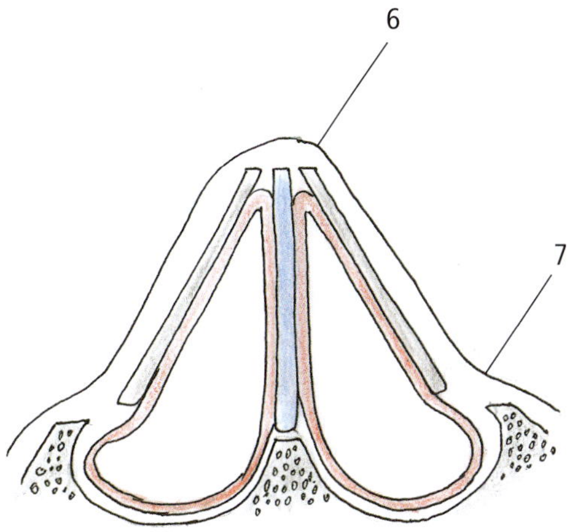

Figure 3.50f Situation after hump removal (6) and lateral osteotomy (7)

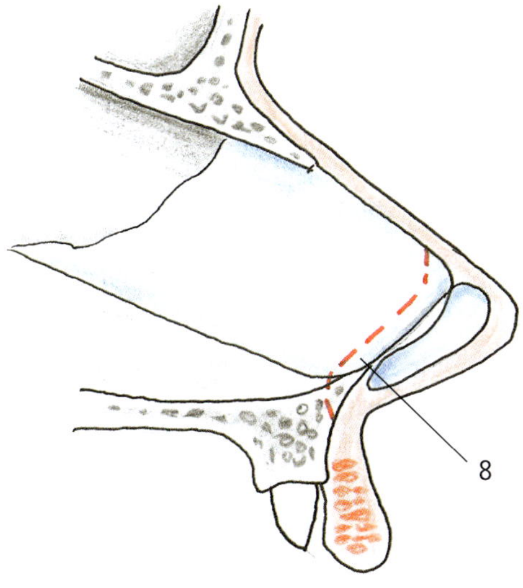

Figure 3.50g Incision of the caudal part of septum. As a rule the nasal spine should also be partly resected (8).

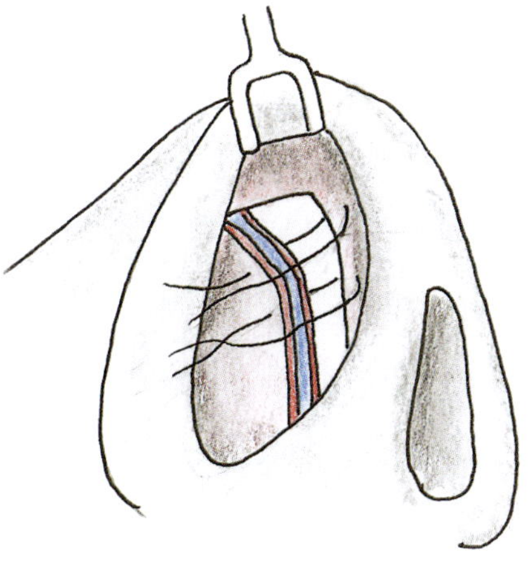

Figure 3.50h Suturing after shortening of the septum

Skoog Method for Humped Nose

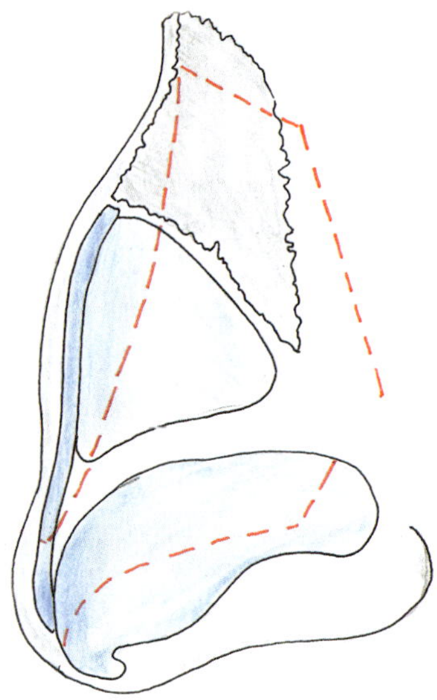

Figure 3.51a Planning of the operation on the humped nose

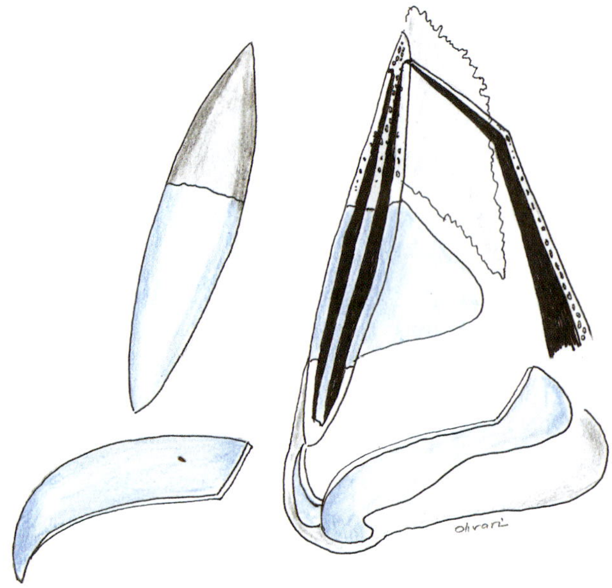

Figure 3.51b Operation of a big humped nose. The cranial parts of the alar cartilage are resected. The hump is removed and a lateral osteotomy performed.

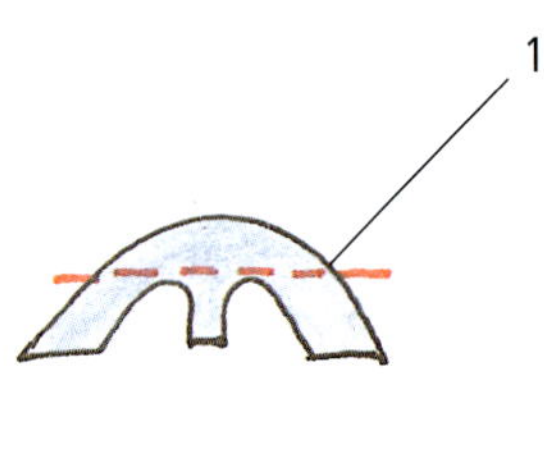

Figure 3.51c The removed nasal hump is reduced in size (1) and reinserted (Skoog).

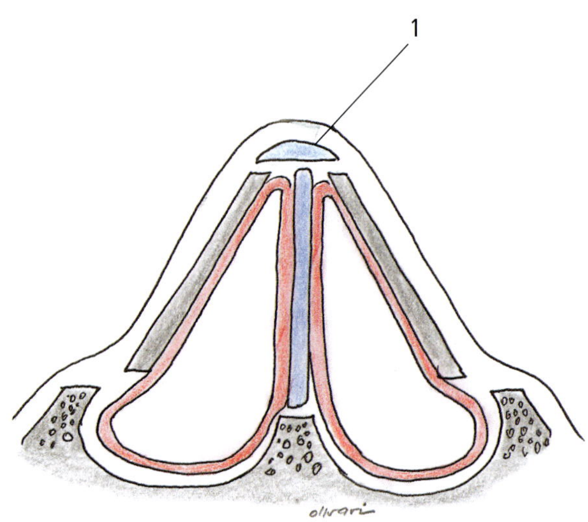

Figure 3.51d In order to prevent an excessively narrow nasal dorsum as well as an "open roof", the Skoog method is highly recommended. The removed nasal hump is flattened and reinserted. As a result of this the nasal dorsum appears more natural. It is advisable to fix the reimplanted nasal hump in order to prevent a postoperative dislocation.

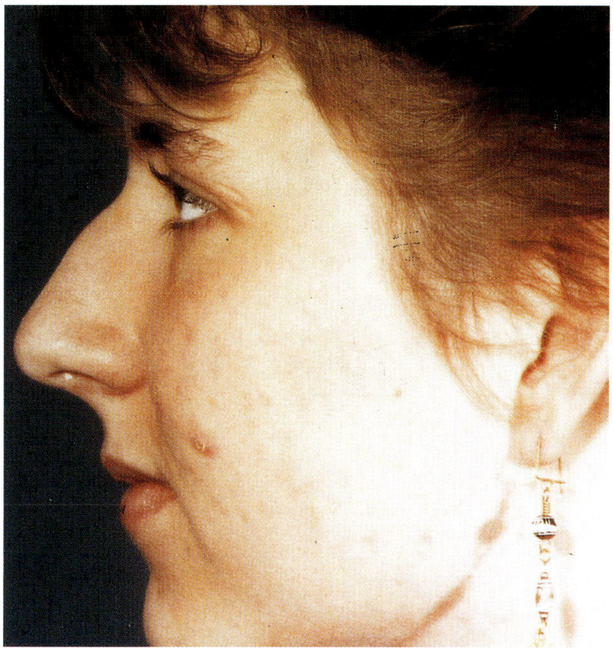

Figure 3.52a Humped nose

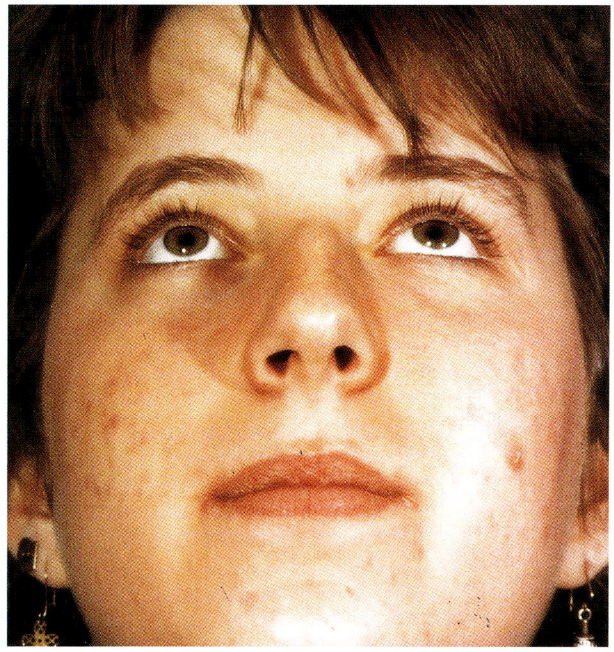

Figure 3.52b Apart from the hump the broad nasal tip is obvious.

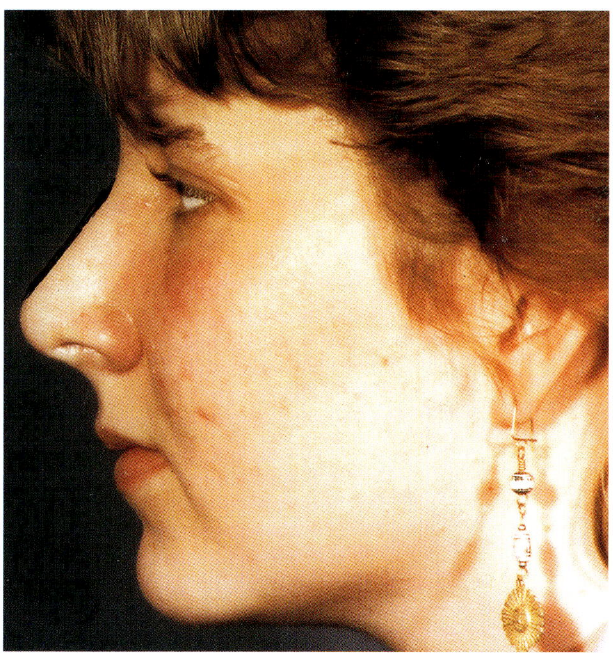

Figure 3.52c Result three months after the operation. An improvement in the profile has been achieved by removing the hump and slightly shortening the nose.

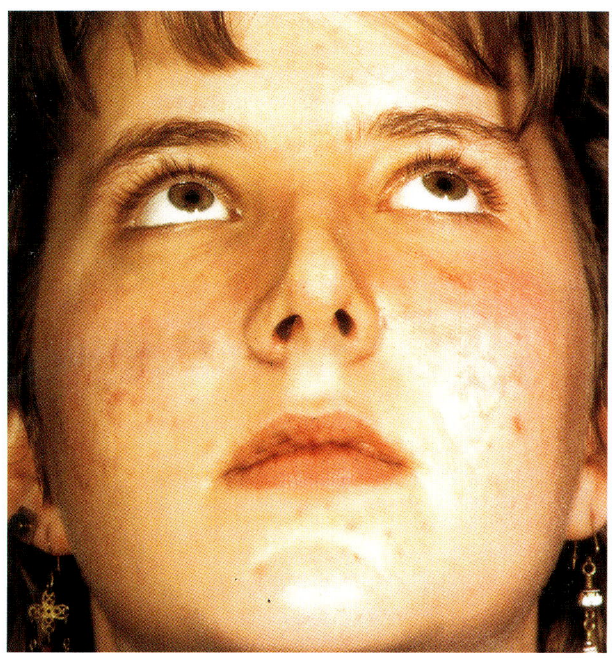

Figure 3.52d Narrowing of the nose by a lateral osteotomy as well as a partial resection of the alar cartilage. The septum was also slightly shortened. Resected hump was flattened and reimplanted (Skoog). It is a wise to fix the reimplantated hump, to prevent dislocation.

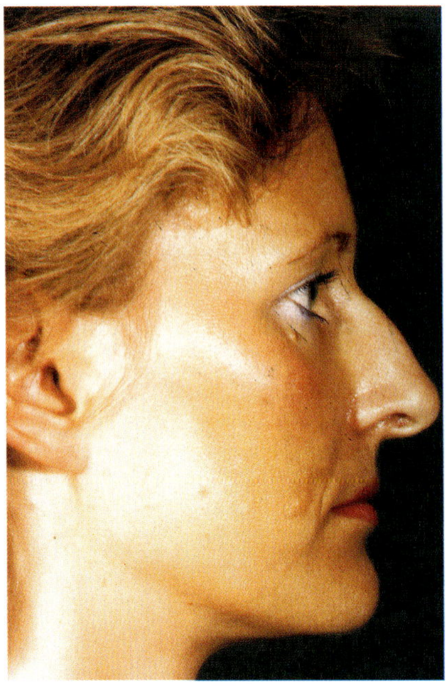

Figure 3.53a Long humped nose

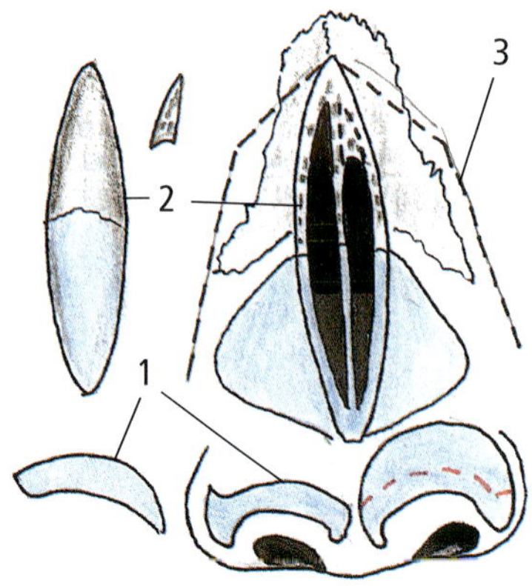

Figure 3.53b Operation – reduction of the alar cartilage (1), hump removal (2) and lateral osteotomy (3)

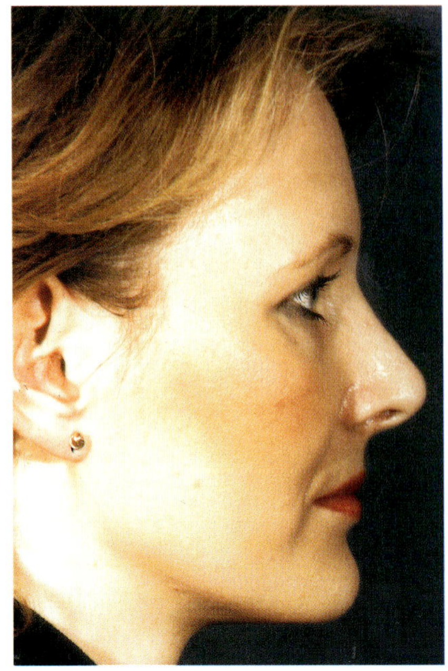

Figure 3.53c Result six months after the operation

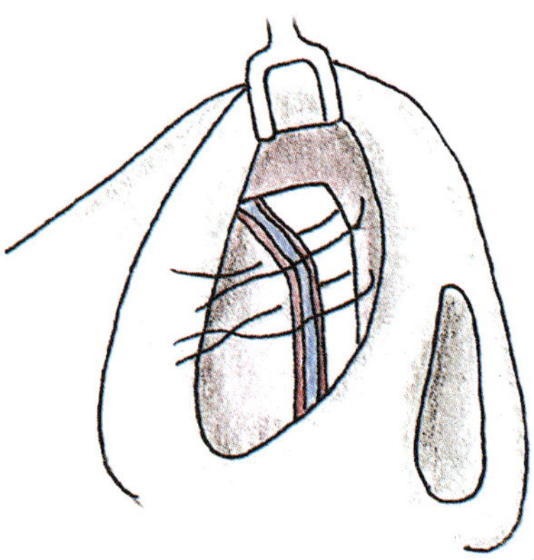

Figure 3.53d Shortening of the septum

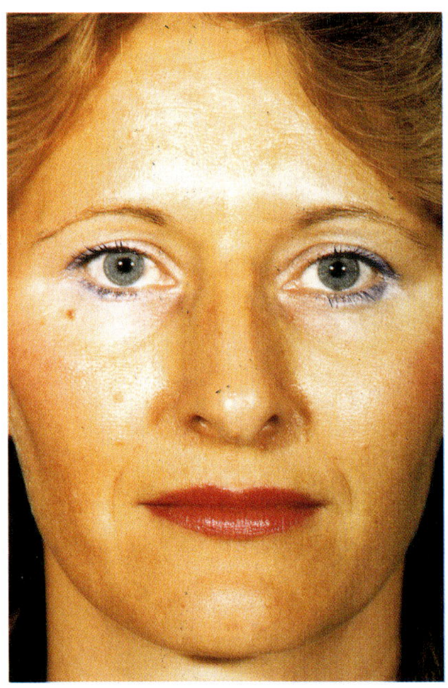

Figure 3.53e The frontal preoperative appearance of the nose is relatively unremarkable, but after the removal of hump a lateral osteotomy is essential in order to narrow the nose.

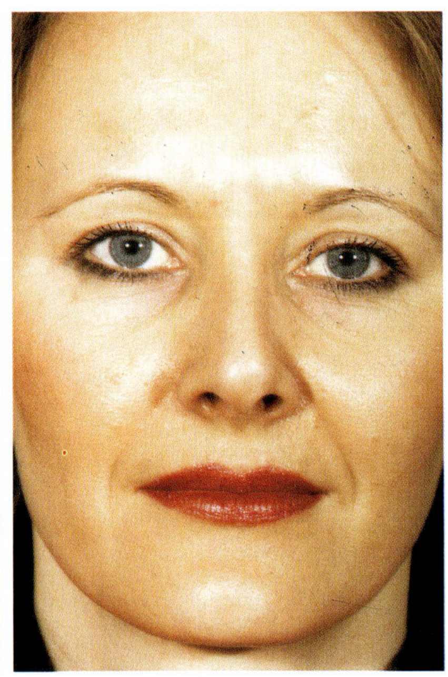

Figure 3.53f Result six months after operation.

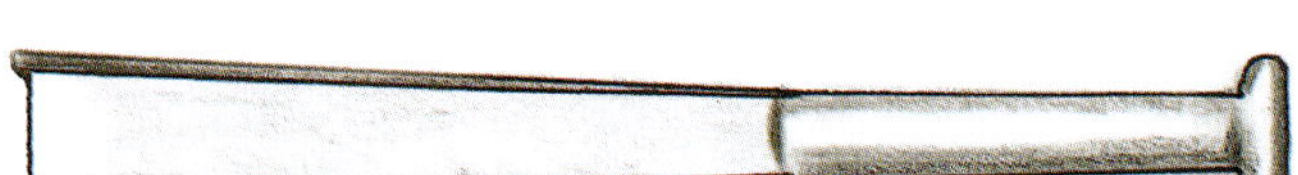

Figure 3.53g Chisel used for removal of the bony nasal hump. The lateral rounding of the chisel head prevents soft tissue injuries. Chisels are available in various sizes (Ulrich, Ulm).

Olivari Rhinotome

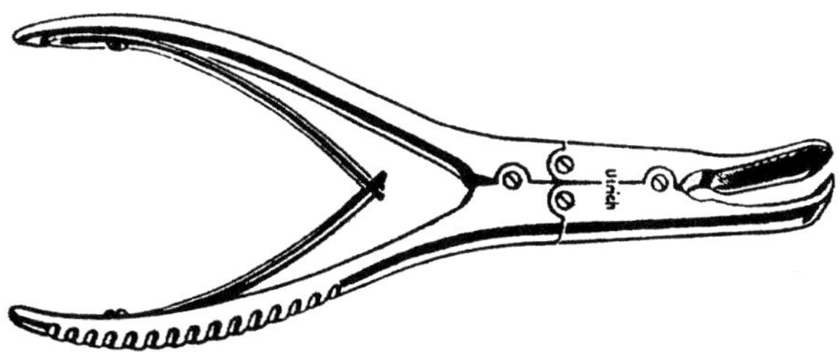

Figure 3.54a Olivari rhinotome with vertical and horizontal cutting edges (Ulrich, Ulm)

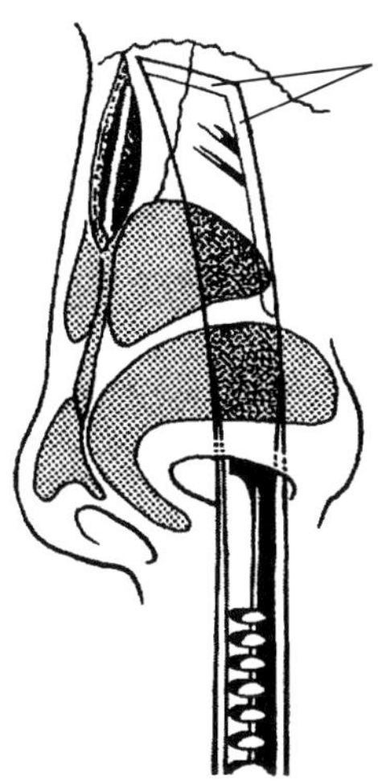

Figure 3.54b Positioning of the rhinotome for a lateral osteotomy

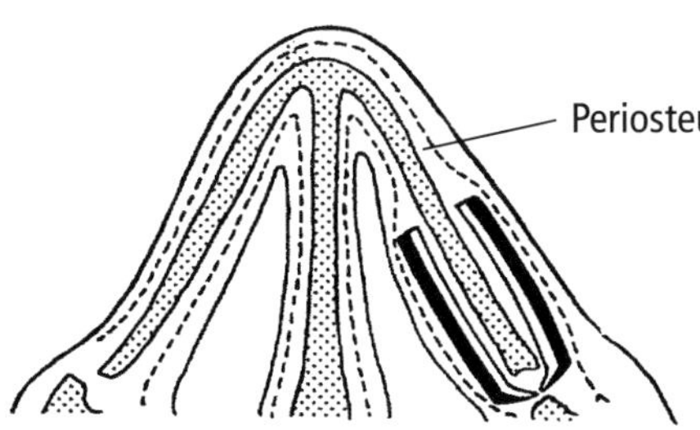

Figure 3.54c The rhinotome is positioned subperiosteally

Technique of Lateral Osteotomy Using a Rhinotome

The piriform aperture is searched for. Using an intranasal approach Scandicain (Mepivacain hydrochlorate) with 1/200 000 adrenaline is injected subperiosteally and then a small incision is made.

Using the raspatory the subperiosteal space is formed on the inner side as well as the outer side of the fronto-maxillary process.

The rhinotome is introduced. From the outside it is easy to feel where the rhinotome is positioned to carry out the vertical and horizontal osteotomies.

The osteotomy is carried out by applying strong pressure to create the fracture and the fragment is mobilized medially.

The advantage is that one is able to determine the osteotomy lines from the outside. The procedure is less traumatic than would be the case if a saw was used and more precise than if a chisel was used [Olivari, N. (1972) Lateral subperiostal osteotomy using the rhinotome. Chir Plastica (Berlin) 1: 261–264].

If you use another instrument successfully, do not change your method!

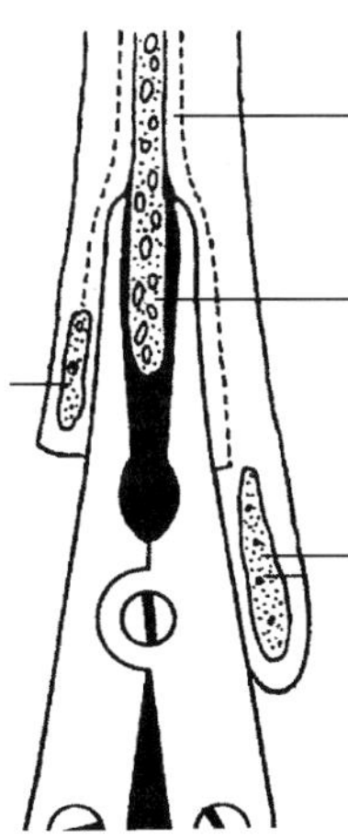

Figure 3.54d The rhinotome is placed intranasally and subperiosteally after the periostium is mobilized bilaterally using the raspatory.

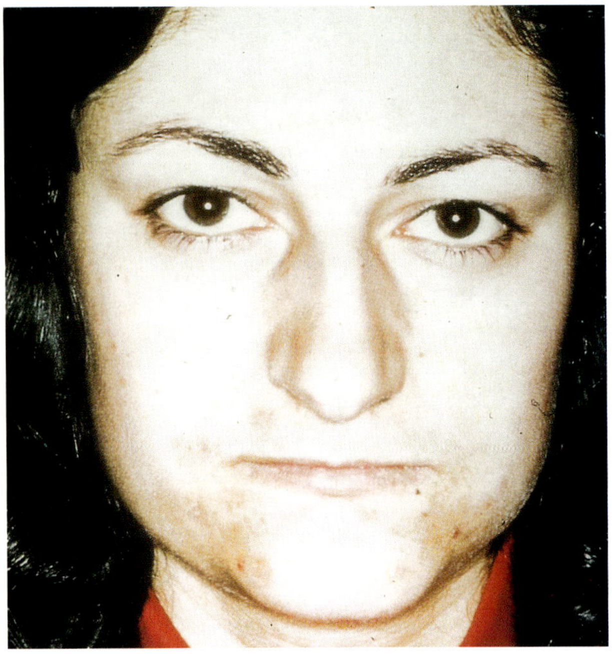

Figure 3.55a Ethnically conditioned long hump nose

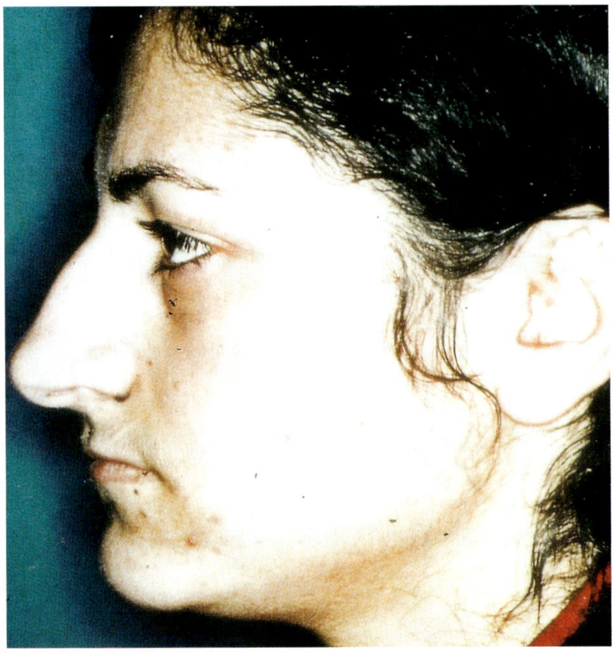

Figure 3.55b Because of the excessively long septum and the low nasal spine the upper lip looks as if it is too short.

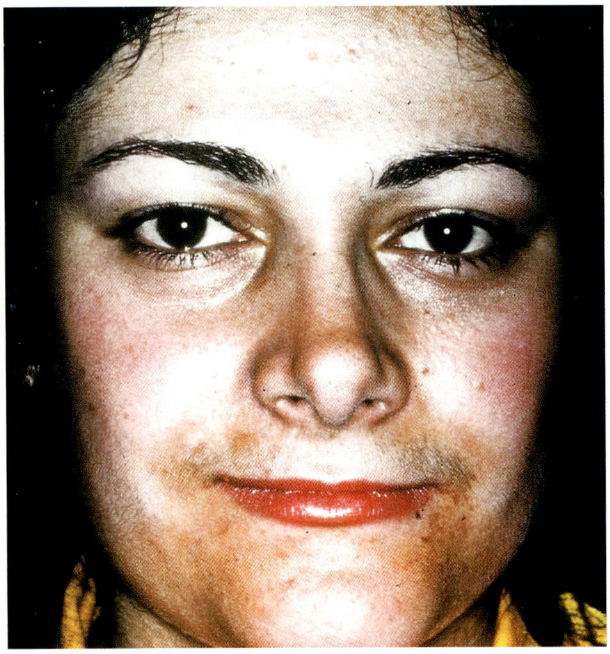

Figure 3.55c During the operation the cranial parts of the lower lateral cartilage were excised and the nasal hump was removed. At the same time a lateral osteotomy, septal shortening and resection of the nasal spine were all carried out.

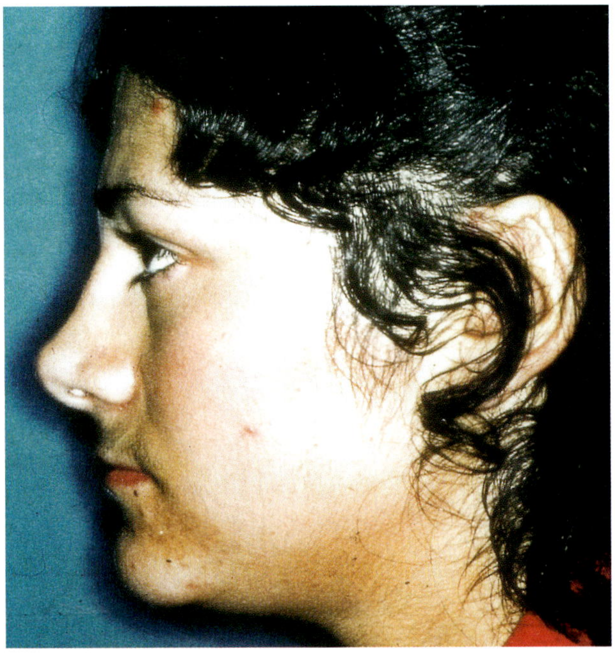

Figure 3.55d Situation one year after the operation

b) Surgical Approach With an Open Rhinoplasty

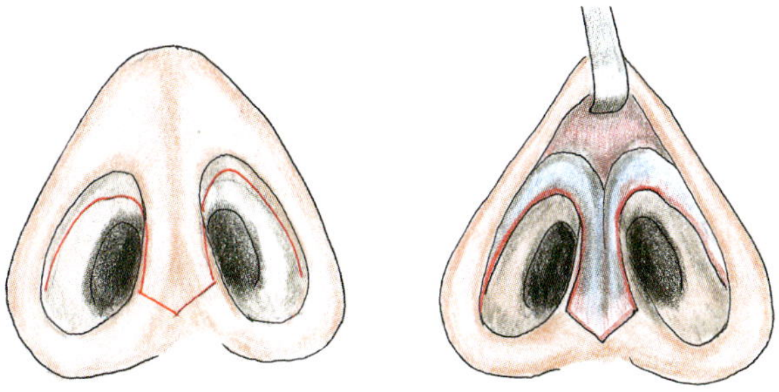

Figure 3.56a Incision line with an open rhinoplasty

An open rhinoplasty is to be recommended for problematic noses where a hump, a septal deviation and a difficult nasal tip are present at the same time. With clear visibility one can operate considerably more precisely.

For cartilage or bone grafting in to the nasal dorsum an open rhinoplasty is the method of choice. The transverse scar at the columella represents a negative aspect although the patients almost never complain about this. This method is particularly recommended for inexperienced surgeons.

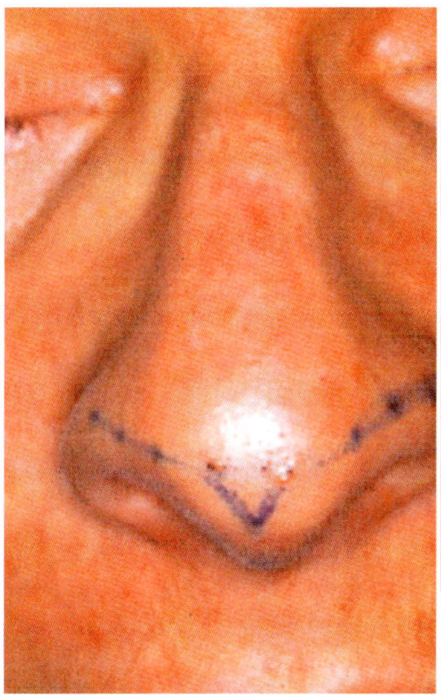

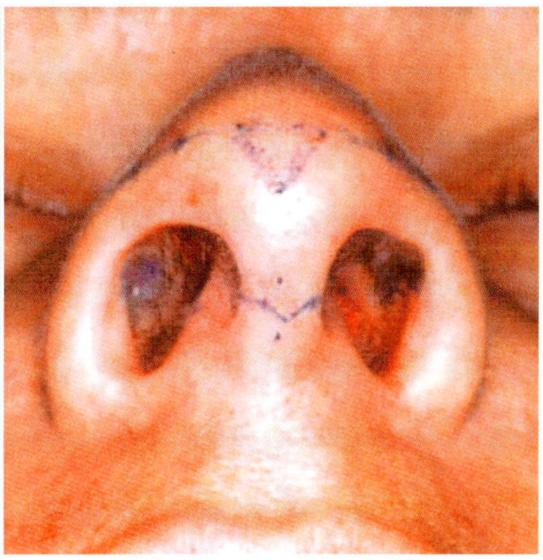

△ **Figure 3.56c** Incision line at the columella
◁ **Figure 3.56b** Planning of the nasal correction

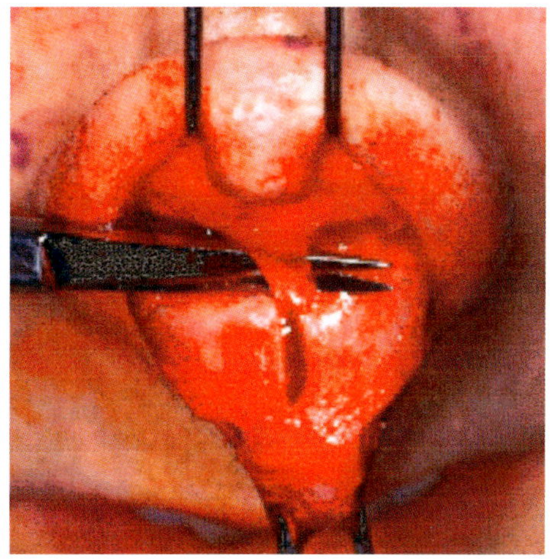

Figure 3.56d Exposure of the lower lateral cartilage and Pitanguy ligament

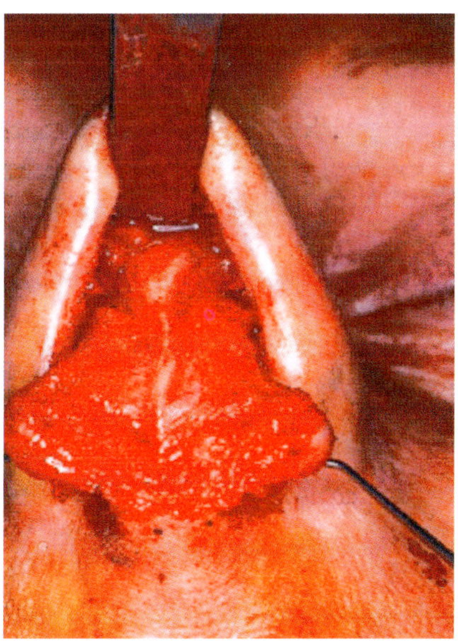

Figure 3.56e Preparation in the direction of the nasal dorsum

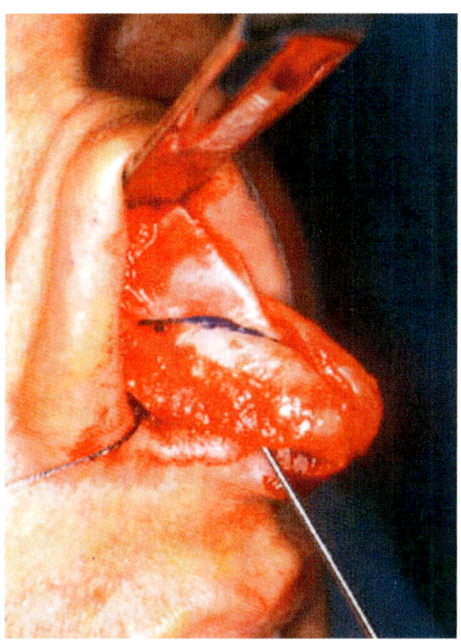

Figure 3.56f The inner structure of the nose is exposed

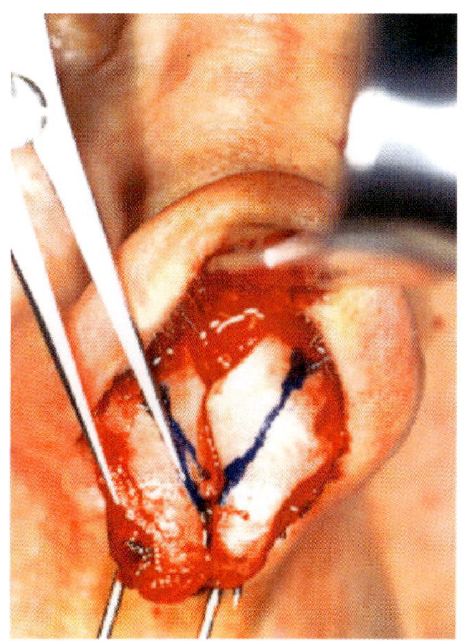

Figure 3.56g Marking the parts of the alar cartilage that are to be resected

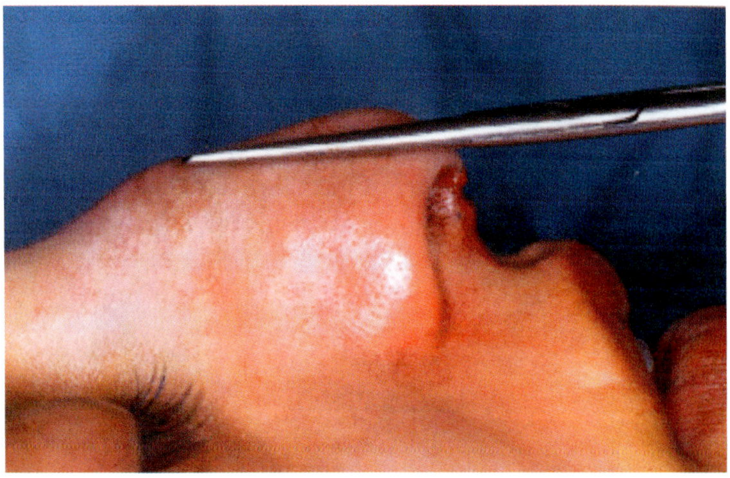

Figure 3.56h After partial resection of the lower lateral cartilage and the nasal tip adjustment, the amount of hump which has to be removed, is assessed.

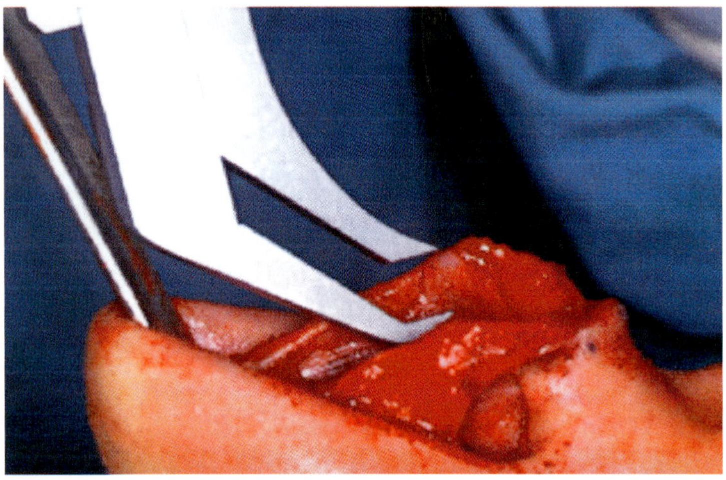

Figure 3.56i The hump is completely exposed

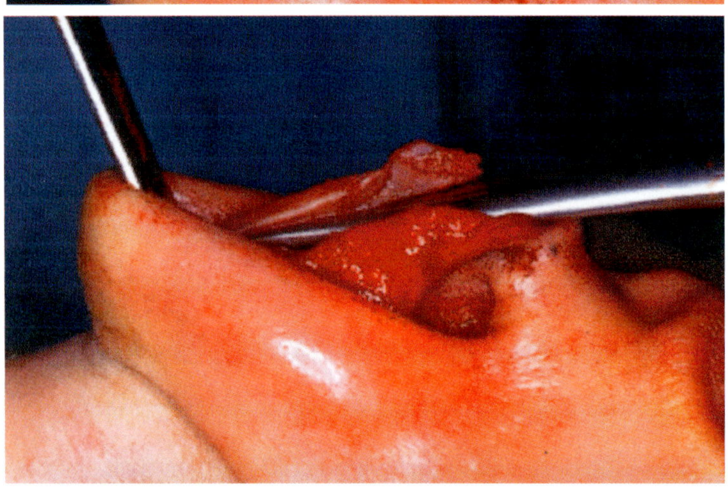

Figure 3.56j The cartilaginous part of the hump is removed with scissors (or with a scalpel), while the bony part is removed with the chisel.

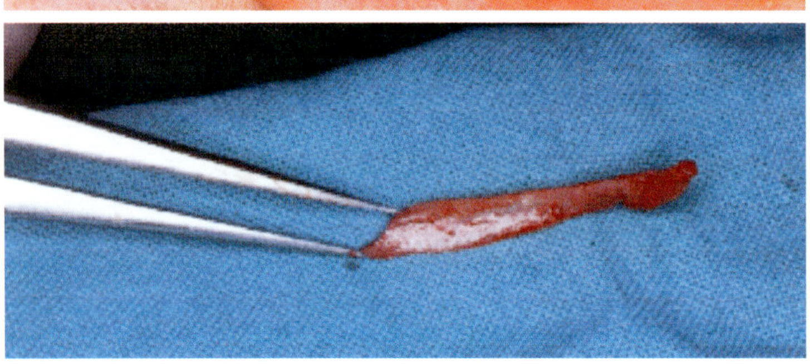

Figure 3.56k Removed hump

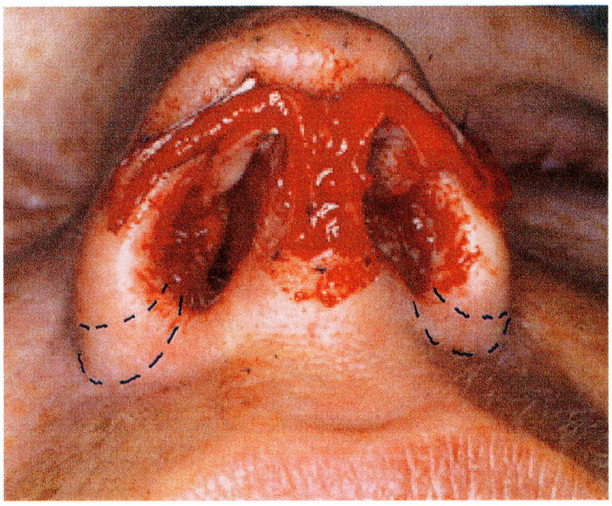

Figure 3.56l At the end of the operation the medial part of cartilages were sutured together to achieve improvement of the nasal tip. V excision of lateral part of nostril (1) for narrowing the nose.

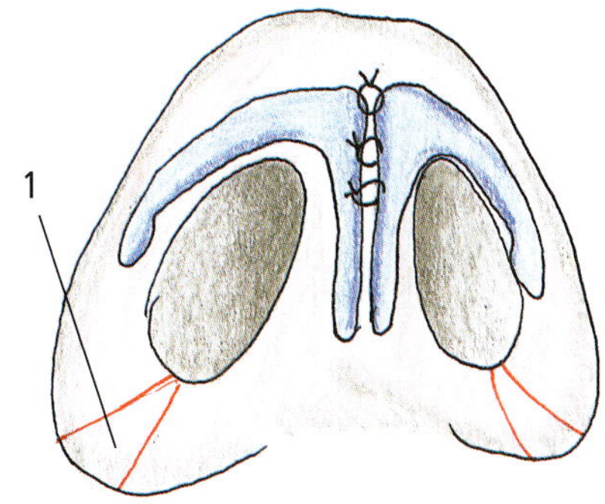

Figure 3.56m Scheme for l

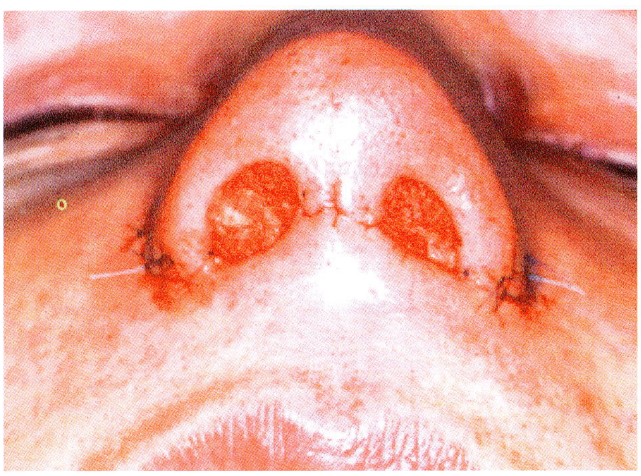

Figure 3.56n Status at the end of the open rhinoplasty. Here the nasal wings have also been reduced in size. Nasal pack of flammazine tulle is followed by a plaster cast splint.

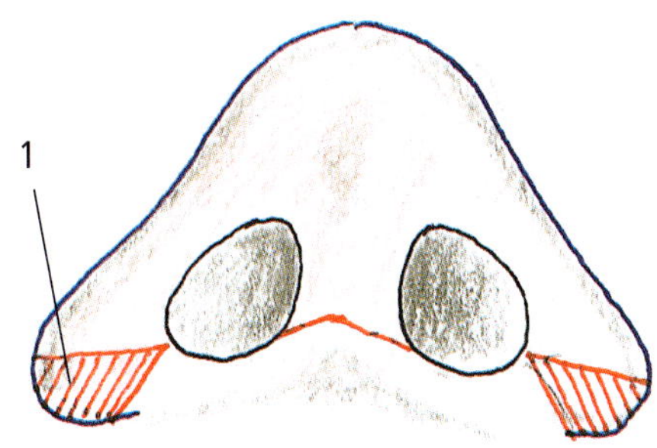

Figure 3.56o Scheme for n

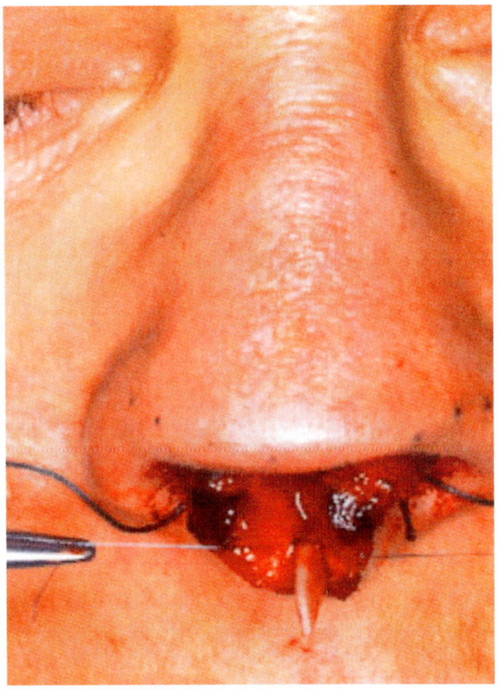

Figure 3.56p In order to shape the nasal tip, a cartilage graft is fixed between the medial crura of the lower lateral cartilages.

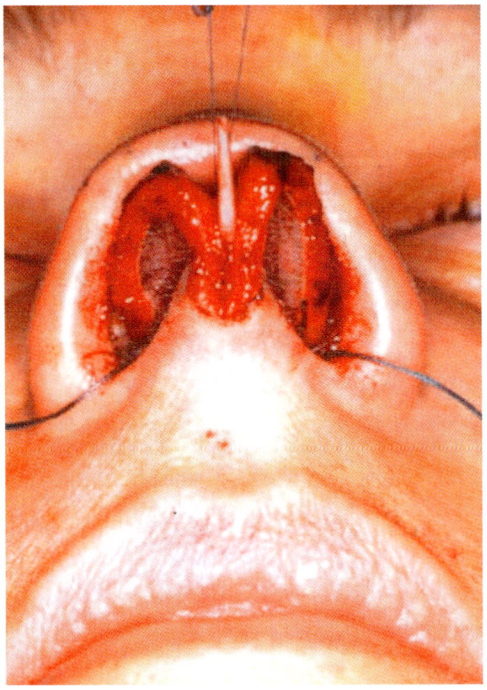

Figure 3.56q The cartilage graft used here comes from the nasal septum, alternatively a graft taken from ear cartilage may be used. When the nasal tip is reduced the intercartilaginous ligaments must be severed.

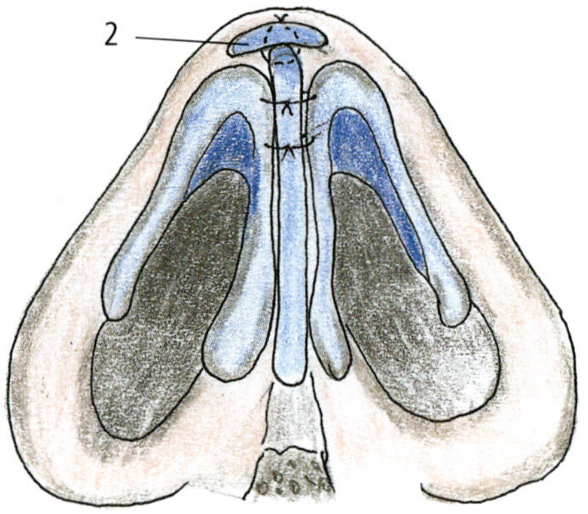

Figure 3.56r In order to give a harmonious shape to the nasal tip, a smaller T-shaped graft is sometimes fixed at the tip (2).

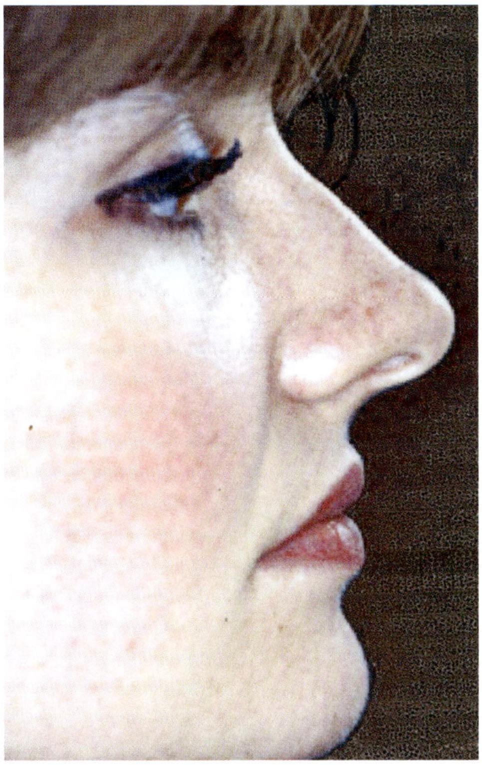

Figure 3.57a A relatively large nose with a prominent nasal tip

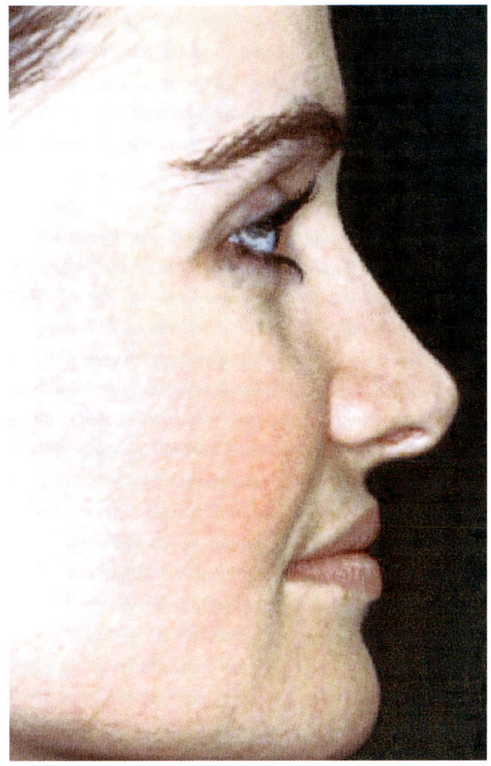

Figure 3.57b Appearance six months after the operation

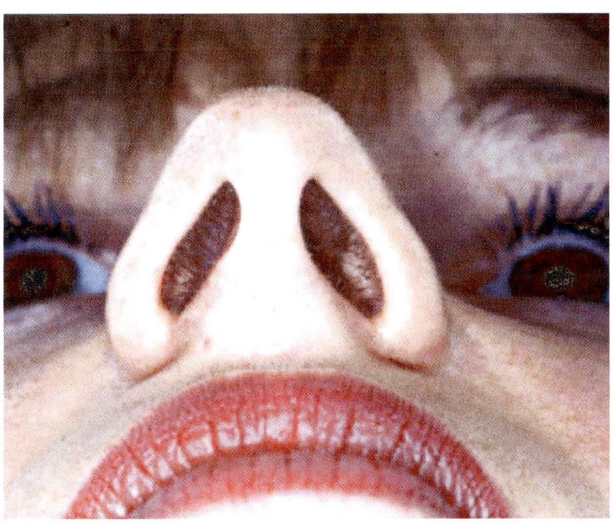

Figure 3.57c Preoperative state

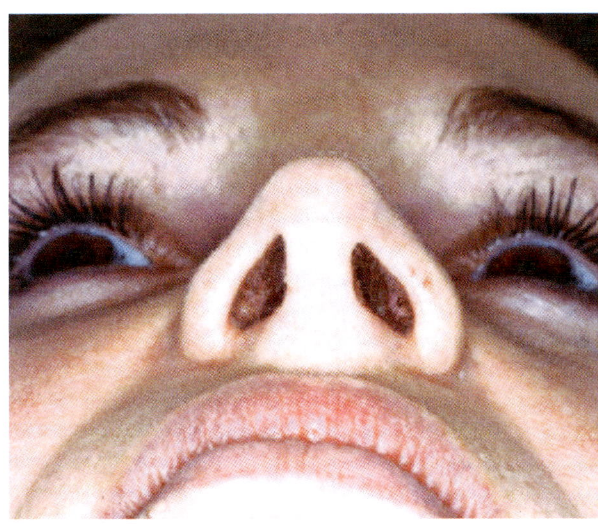

Figure 3.57d Appearance six months postoperatively. Note the naturally narrow nasal tip, and reduced height as well as the inconspicuous scar at the columella after the open rhinoplasty.

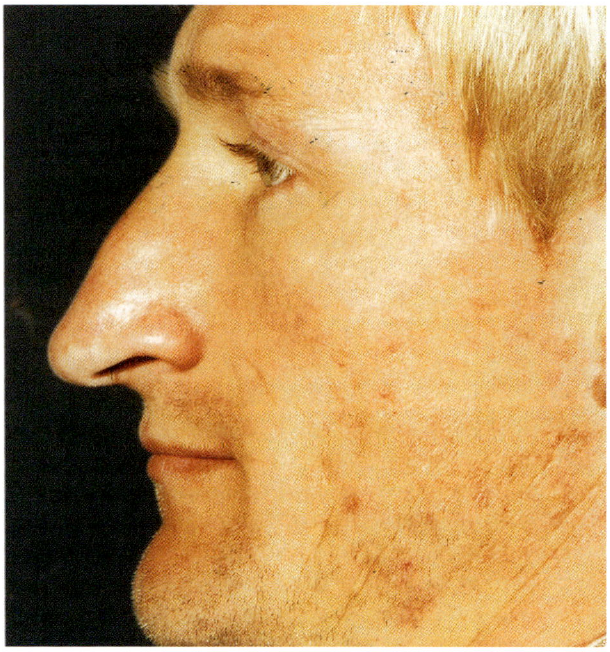

Figure 3.58a Long humped nose with septal deviation and breathing difficulties

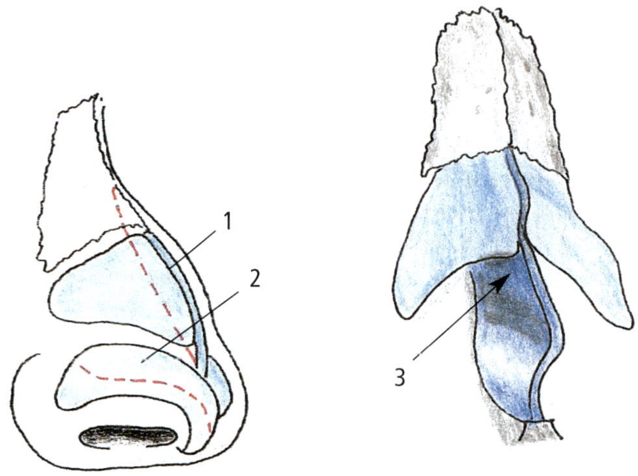

Figure 3.58b Planning of the operation: Hump removal (1), resection of the cranial parts of the lower lateral cartilages (2), straightening and shortening of the deviated septum (3).

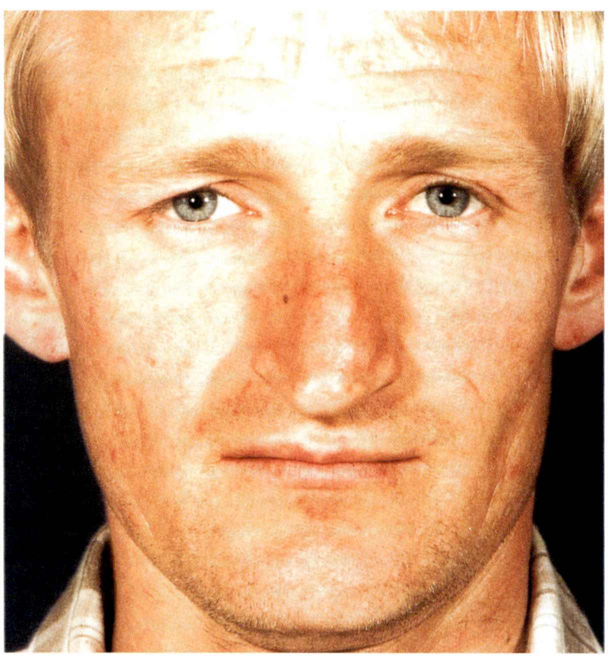

Figure 3.58c Frontal view before operation

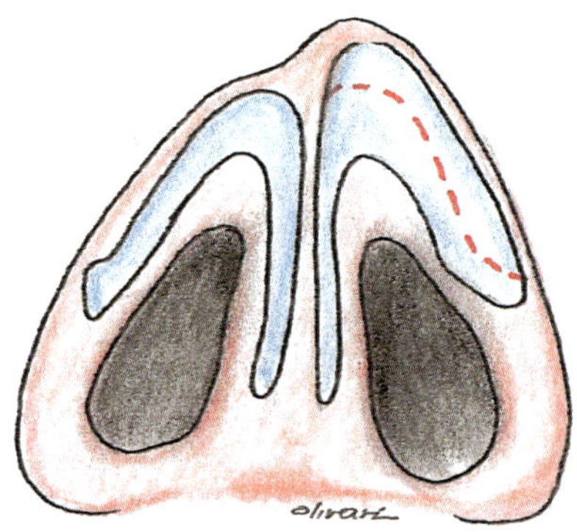

Figure 3.58d The nasal tip is reduced in size by partial resection of the lower lateral cartilage.

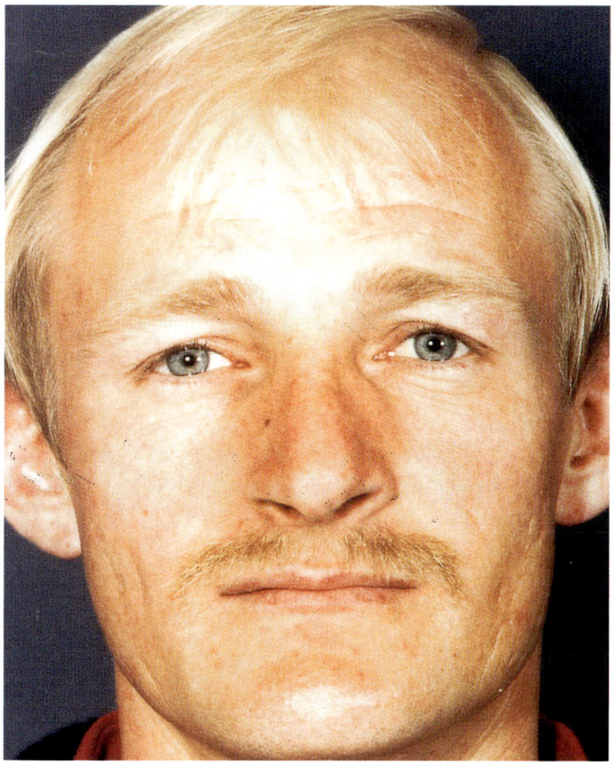

Figure 3.58e Appearance six months after the operation

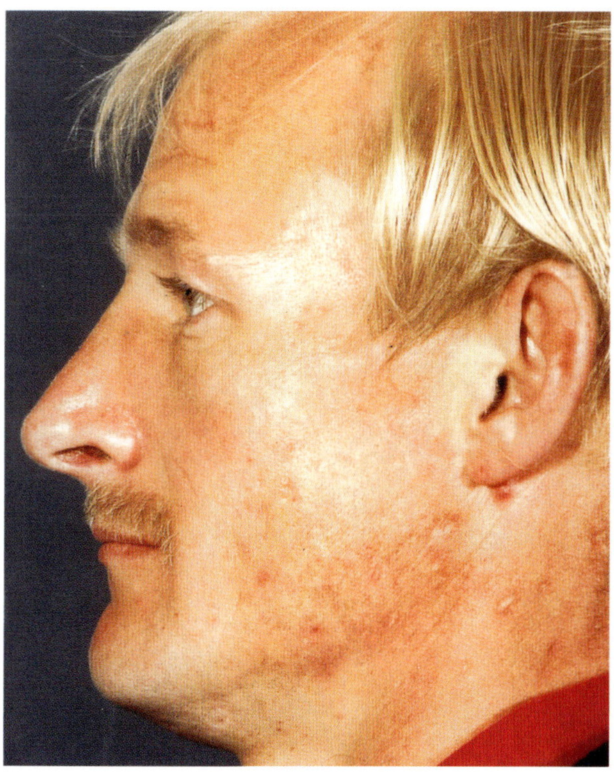

Figure 3.58f Appearance six months after the operation

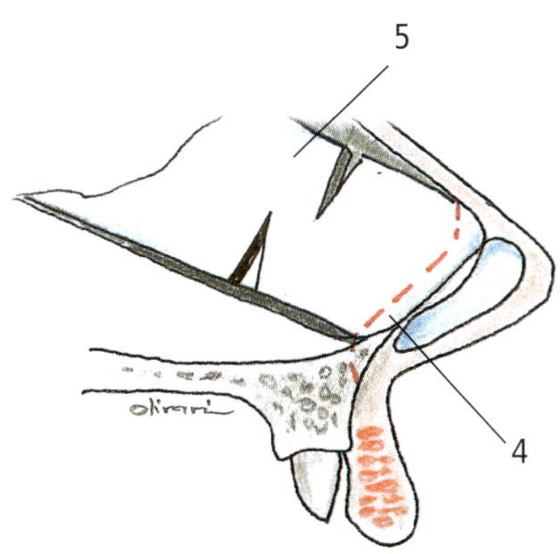

Figure 3.58g A shortening of the nose is achieved by partial resection of the septum and the nasal spine (4). The septum is straightened (5).

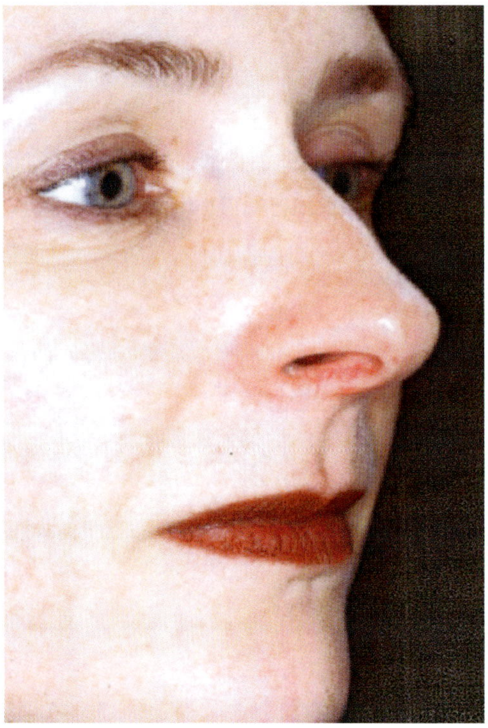

Figure 3.59a A large nose; the columella is too long; slight hump

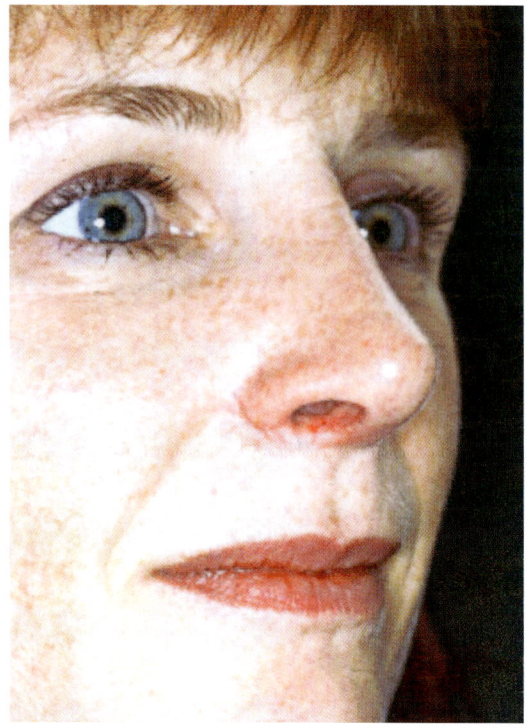

Figure 3.59b Appearance six months after the operation

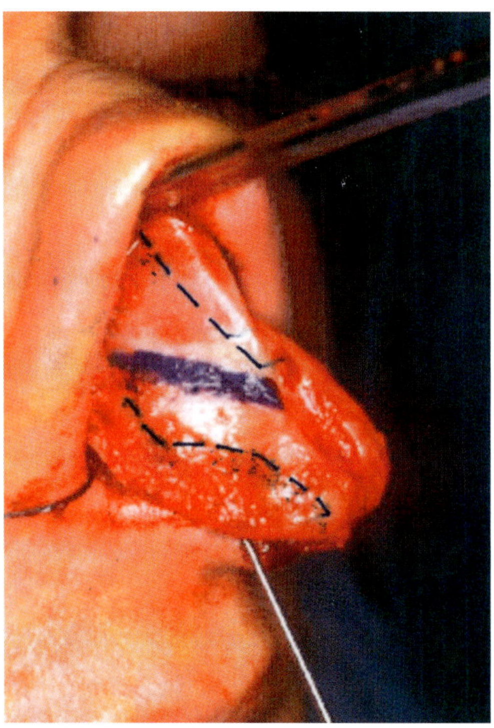

Figure 3.59c Open rhinoplasty operation

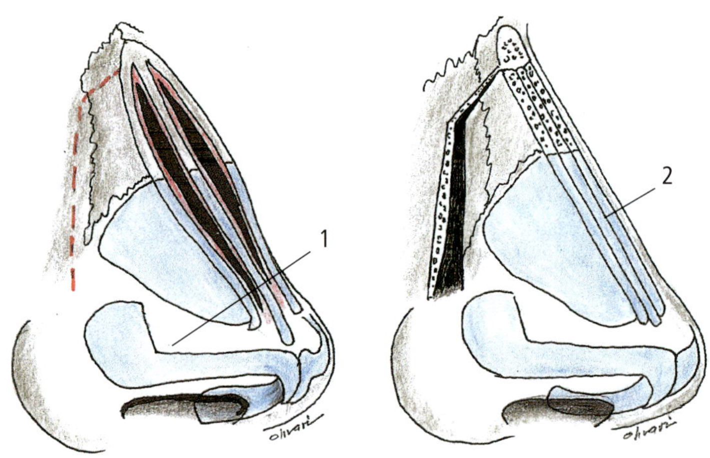

Figure 3.59d Parts of the alar cartilage are resected (1), the nasal tip is narrowed, the hump is removed (2) and the nasal septum has been shortened. The nasal spine has been partially resected.

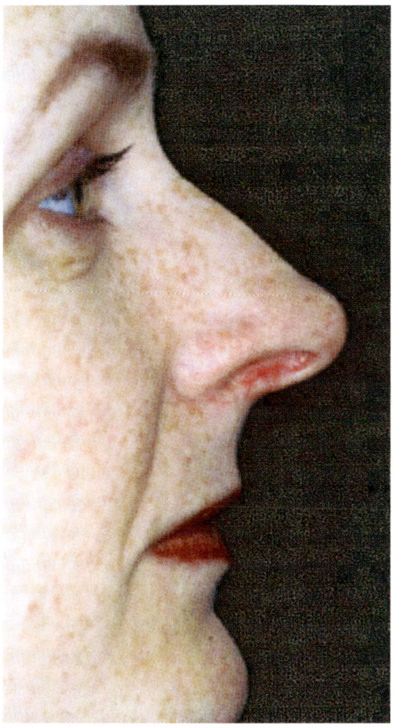

Figure 3.59e Profile before the operation

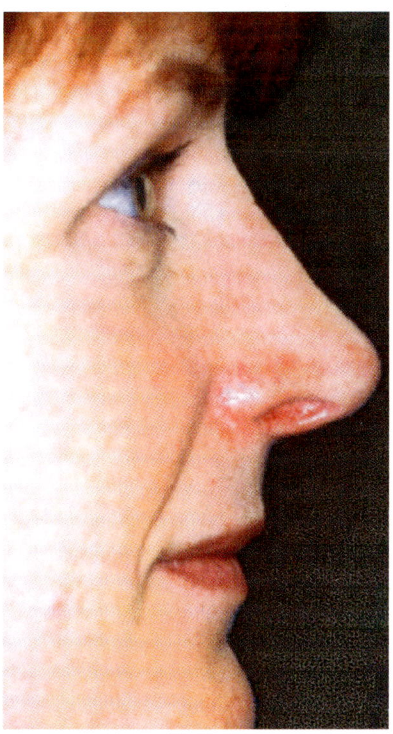

Figure 3.59f Profile six months after the operation

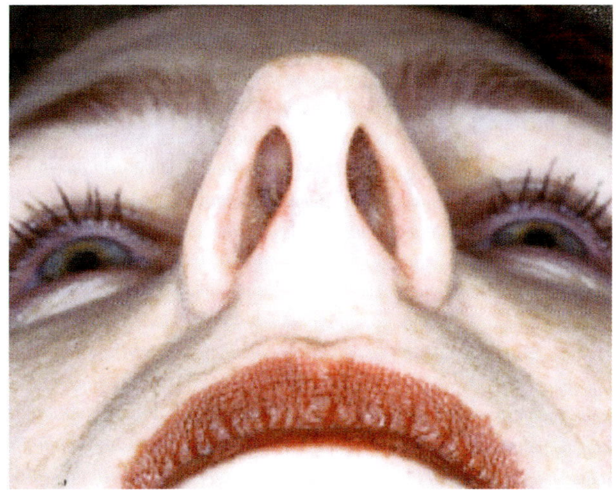

Figure 3.59g Preoperative image: Wide nasal tip, excessively high columella

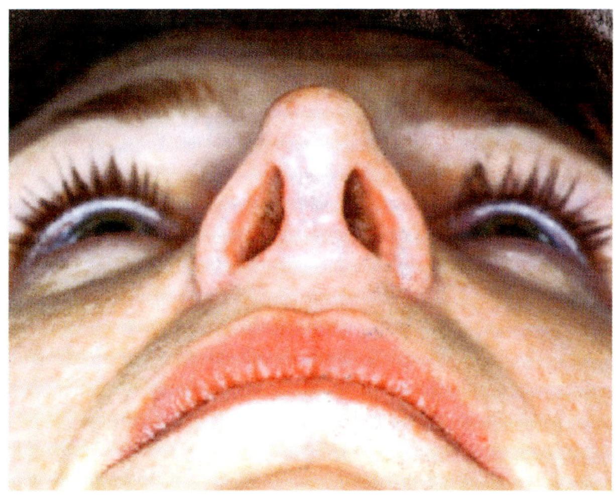

Figure 3.59h Clear improvement in the form of the nasal tip, shortening of the columella. The scar is barely visible six months after the operation.

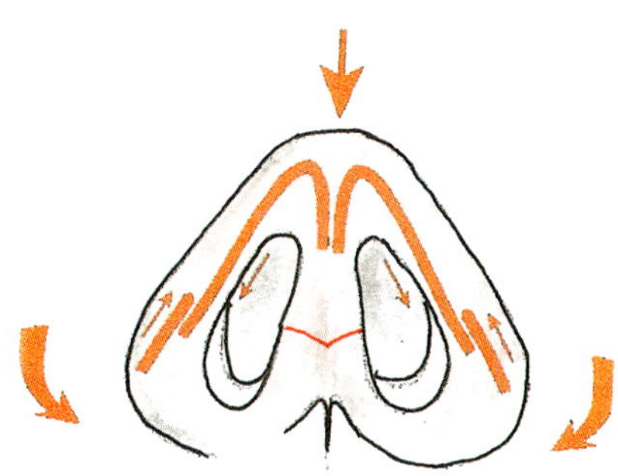

Figure 3.59i Principle of the surgical procedure

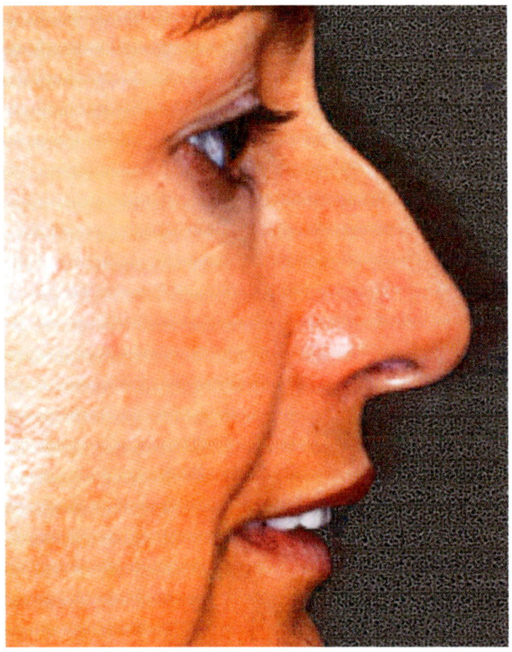

Figure 3.60a Long humped nose

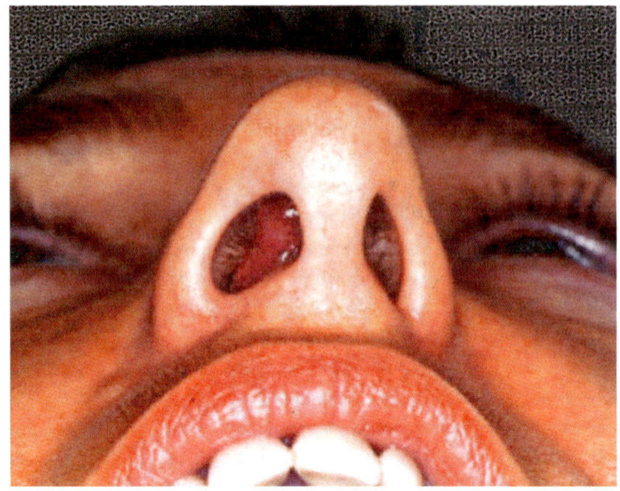

Figure 3.60b Clear septal deviation with convex deformation to the right side resulting in breathing difficulties. Operation: Partial resection of the alar cartilages, hump removal according to Skoog, lateral osteotomy, straightening of the septum.

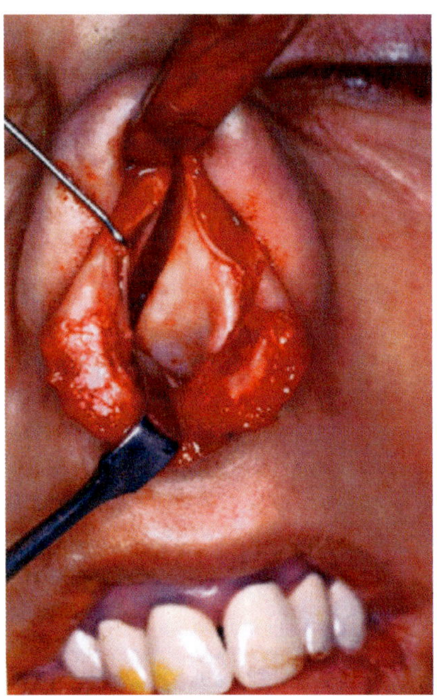

Figure 3.60c High-grade septal deviation

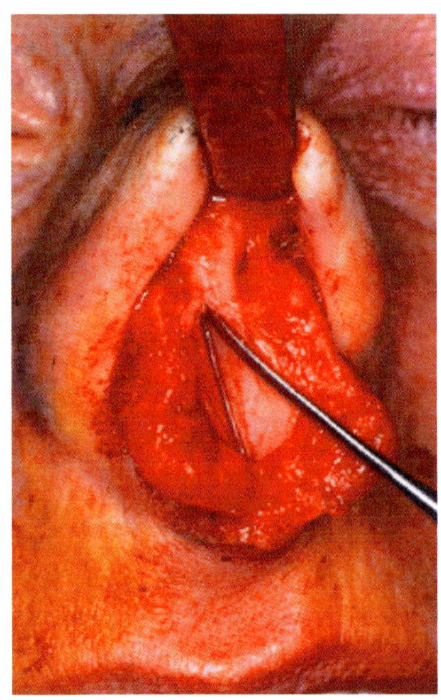

Figure 3.60d Submucosal exposure of the septum. Straightened partly by incision and partly by support of septum with two cartilage grafts. (Held in place with mattress suture).

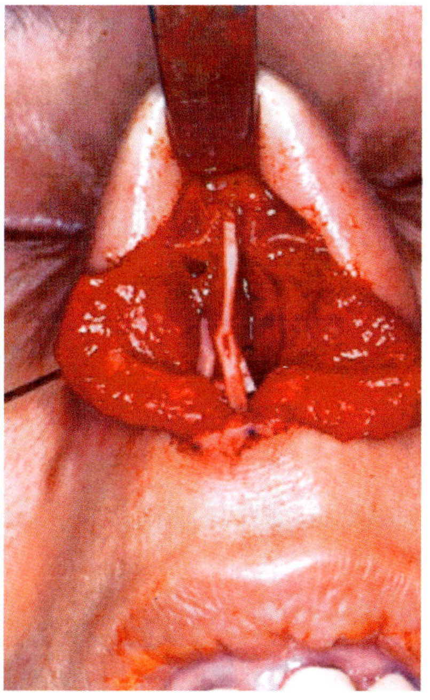

Figure 3.60e In order to fix the septum in a central position, two cartilage components are fixed bilaterally with mattress sutures.

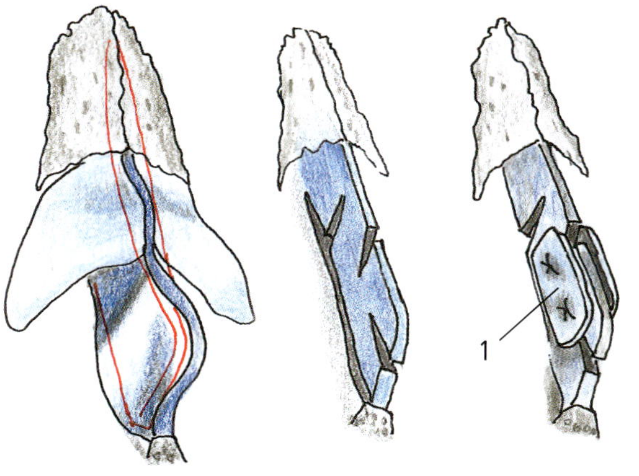

Figure 3.60f Schematic representation of the correction of the septum and fixing with two cartilage components (1) that had been removed from the septum beforehand.

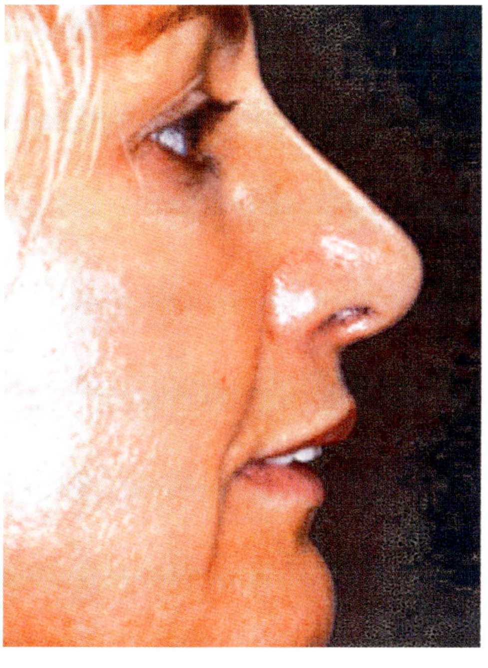

Figure 3.60g Appearance six months postoperatively

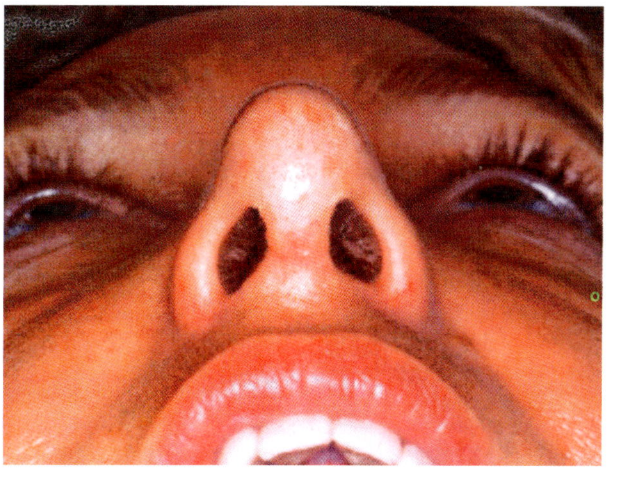

Figure 3.60h The scar on the columella is inconspicuous. Function (breathing) is considerably improved.

Defect Coverage in the Eyelid Area

For the purpose of this discussion, not all known procedures have been listed. Instead, the clinically more favorable techniques are featured. Author's principles:

The best procedure is the one that achieves the best aesthetic and functional results. Technically it should not represent the most sophisticated option. There is no doubt that another surgeon may use another method with success.

The procedures were documented clinically. We have deliberately tried to illustrate every single step.

Anatomy of the Eyelids
(please use an Atlas of Anatomy)

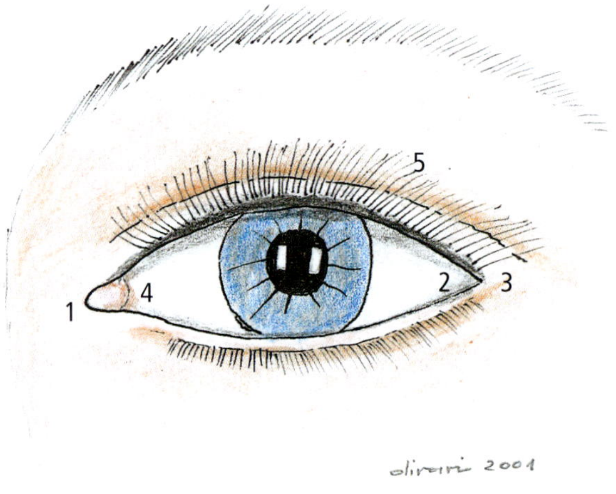

Figure 3.63
1. Medial commissure
2. Lateral canthus
3. Lateral commissure
4. Medial canthus
5. Superior palpebral sulcus

Closure Technique in the Eyelid Area for Small Defects

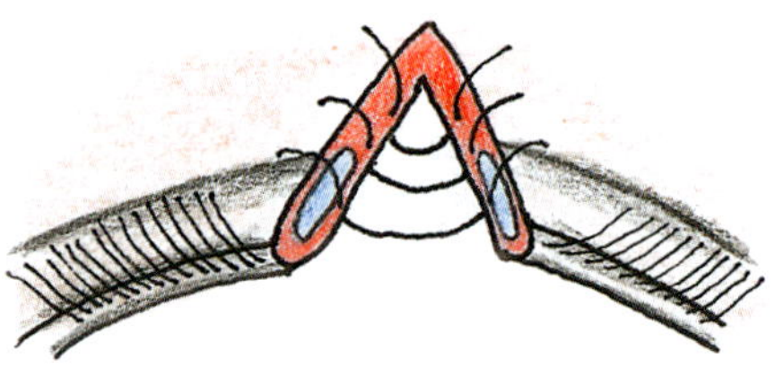

Figure 3.64a V-shaped excision.
The conjunctiva is sutured with 6 × 0 Vicryl so that the knots lie externally and do not irritate the cornea.

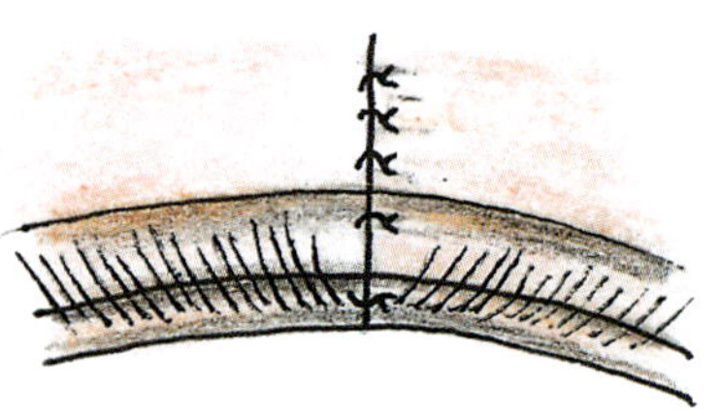

Figure 3.64b Skin suturing with 6 × 0 Trofilene (nylon)

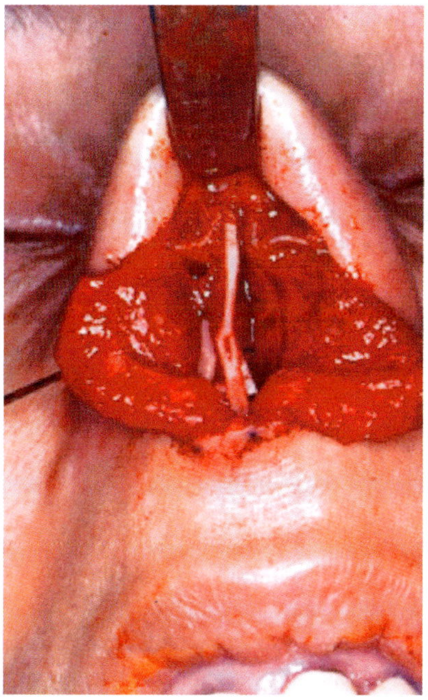

Figure 3.60e In order to fix the septum in a central position, two cartilage components are fixed bilaterally with mattress sutures.

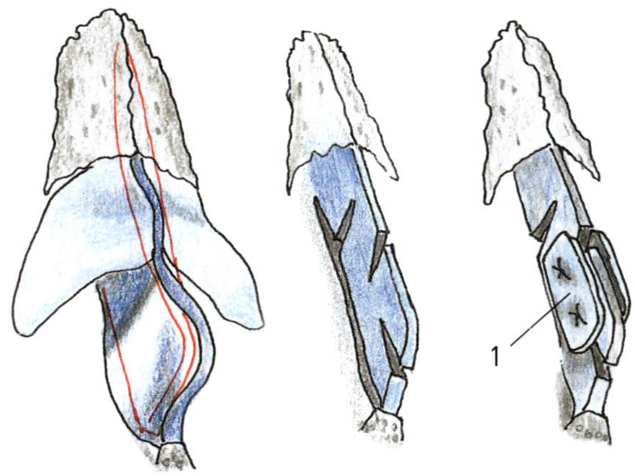

Figure 3.60f Schematic representation of the correction of the septum and fixing with two cartilage components (1) that had been removed from the septum beforehand.

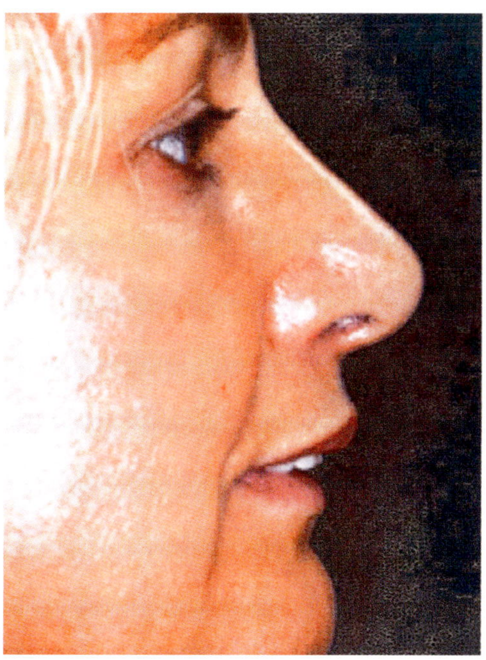

Figure 3.60g Appearance six months postoperatively

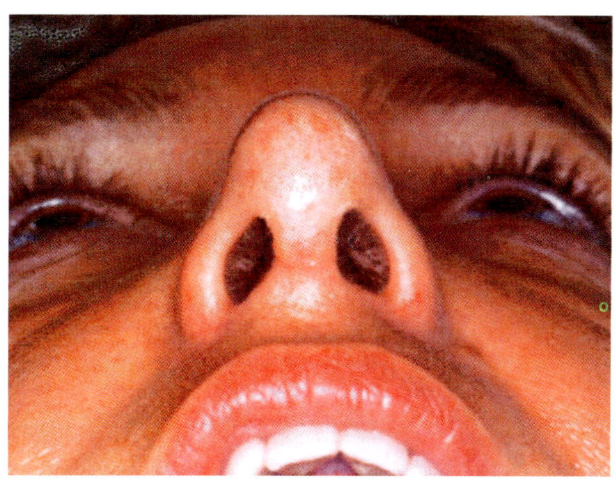

Figure 3.60h The scar on the columella is inconspicuous. Function (breathing) is considerably improved.

Secondary Rhinoplasty

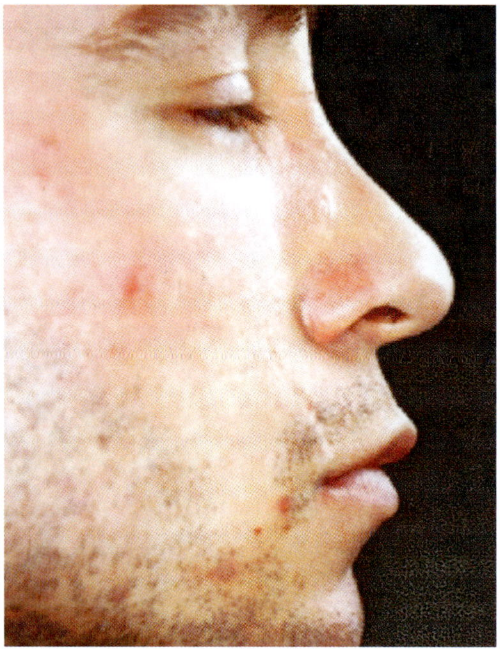

Figure 3.61a Patient had undergone rhinoplasty one year before. In the upper half the nose is flat. There is a supratip deformity as well as an excessively long nasal tip. This is a frequent postoperative complication. Too much was removed from the hump and the nasal tip had not been properly corrected.

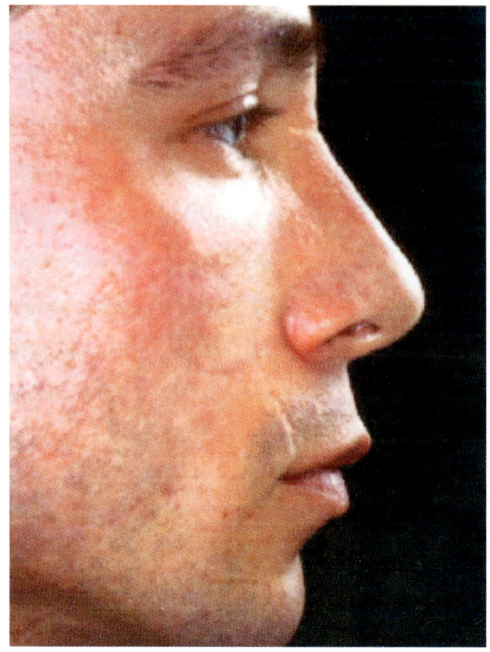

Figure 3.61b The operation consisted of correction of the nasal tip (1) (see below) and an ear cartilage graft for reconstruction of the nasal dorsum (2).

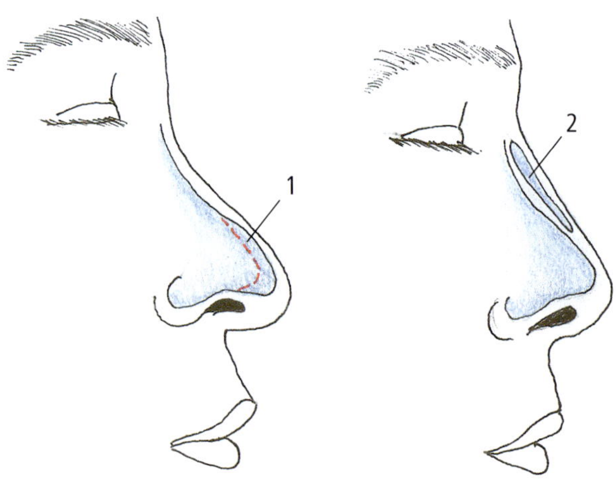

Figure 3.61c Planning of the operation (left). Appearance at the end of the operation (right). The nasal tip is reduced in size (1) and the cartilage graft has been implanted in the upper half of the nasal dorsum (2).

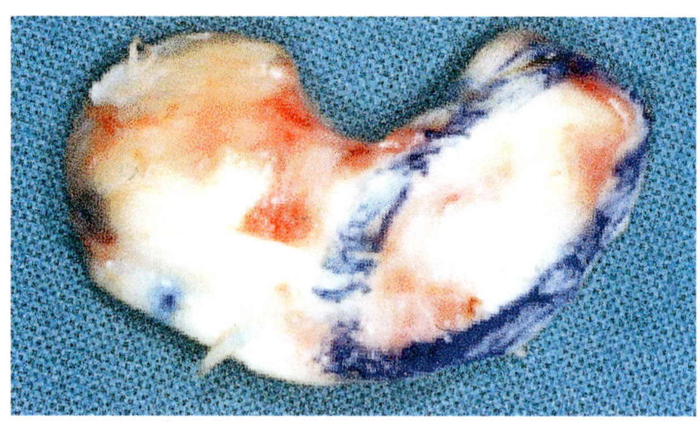

Figure 3.61d Ear cartilage graft. Planning of the graft (the blue marked part is used as an implant).

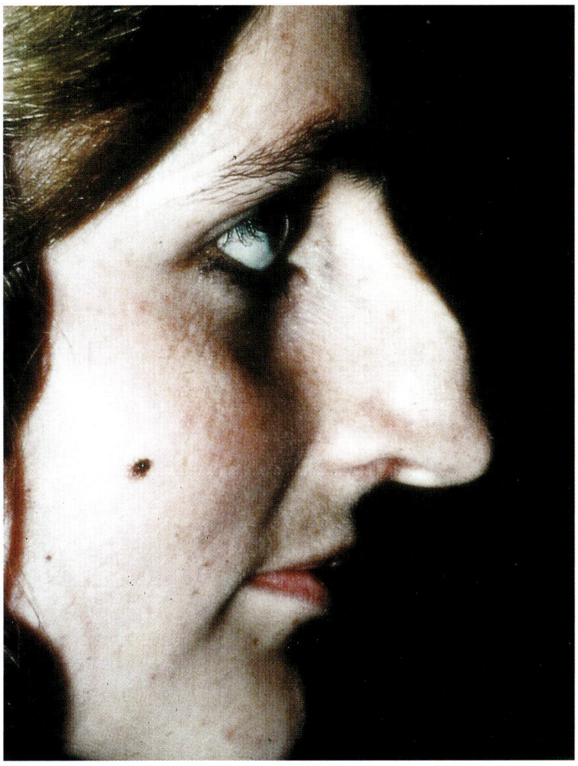

Figure 3.62a Long humped nose and severe septal deviation with breathing problems. The operation is carried out by removing the hump, performing a lateral osteotomy and shortening the nose. The deviated nasal septum was straightened.

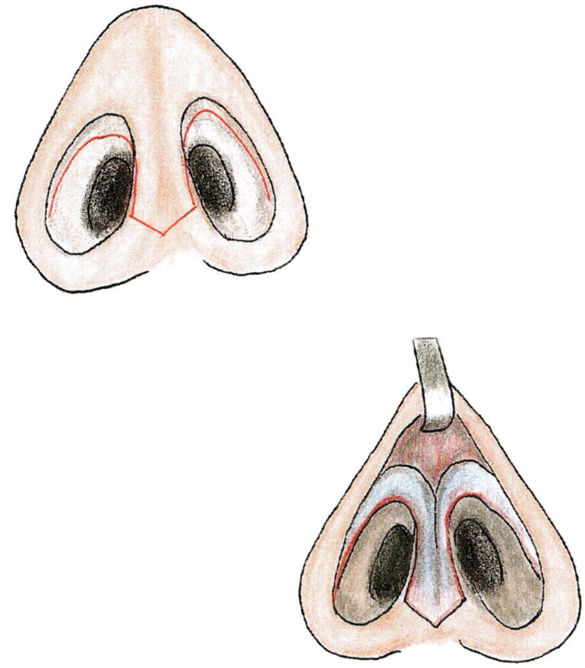

Figure 3.62b Open rhinoplasty is helpful particularly in patients with severe septal deviation.

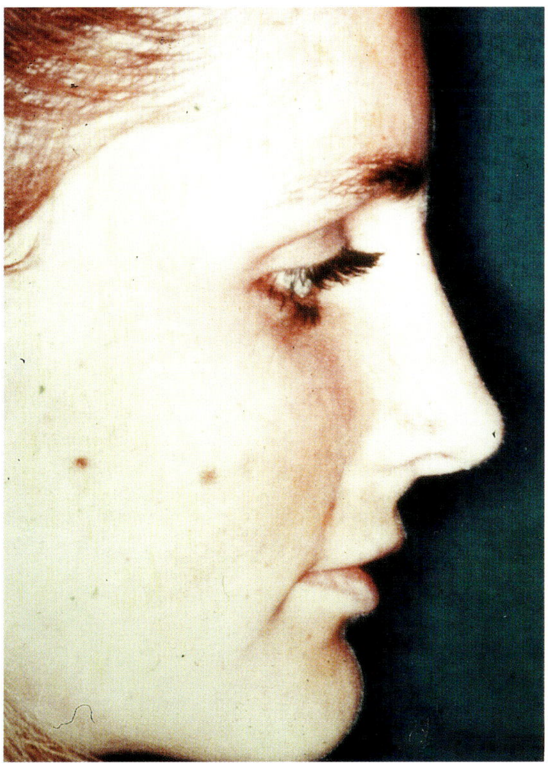

Figure 3.62c Appearance six months after the operation. The preoperative breathing problems have been eliminated.

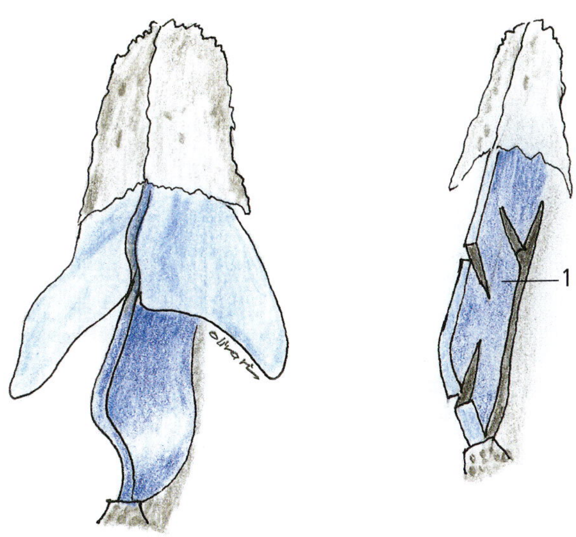

Figure 3.62d The septum must be resected submucosally so that it is totally exposed. The septum is straightened by making a longitudinal incision at the base and several transverse incisions (1). After the nasal correction and precise adaptation of the mucosa a nasal pack and plaster cast needs to be applied for approximately 7 to 14 days.

Defect Coverage in the Eyelid Area

For the purpose of this discussion, not all known procedures have been listed. Instead, the clinically more favorable techniques are featured. Author's principles:

The best procedure is the one that achieves the best aesthetic and functional results. Technically it should not represent the most sophisticated option. There is no doubt that another surgeon may use another method with success.

The procedures were documented clinically. We have deliberately tried to illustrate every single step.

Anatomy of the Eyelids
(please use an Atlas of Anatomy)

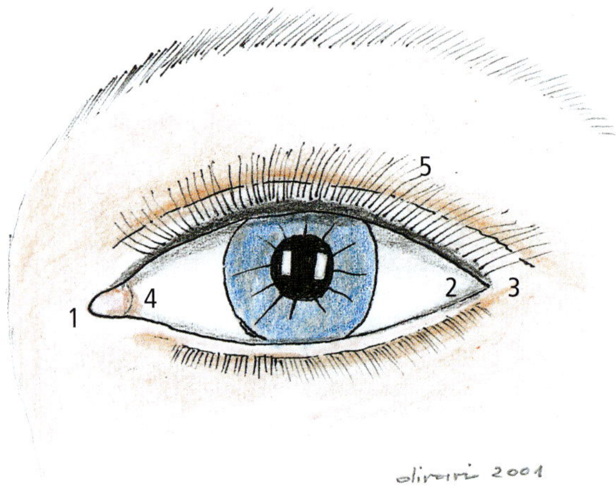

Figure 3.63
1. Medial commissure
2. Lateral canthus
3. Lateral commissure
4. Medial canthus
5. Superior palpebral sulcus

Closure Technique in the Eyelid Area for Small Defects

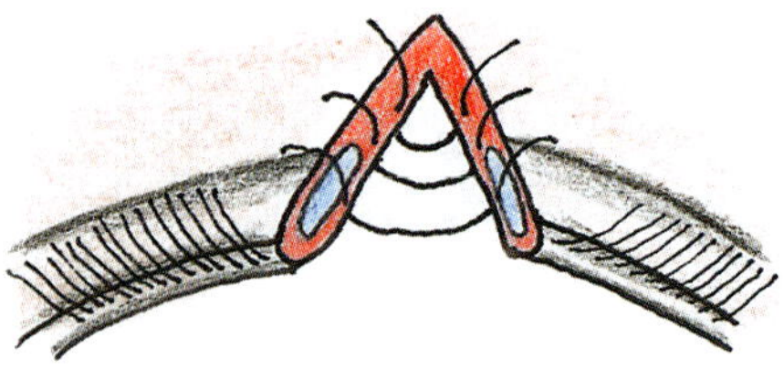

Figure 3.64a V-shaped excision.
The conjunctiva is sutured with 6 × 0 Vicryl so that the knots lie externally and do not irritate the cornea.

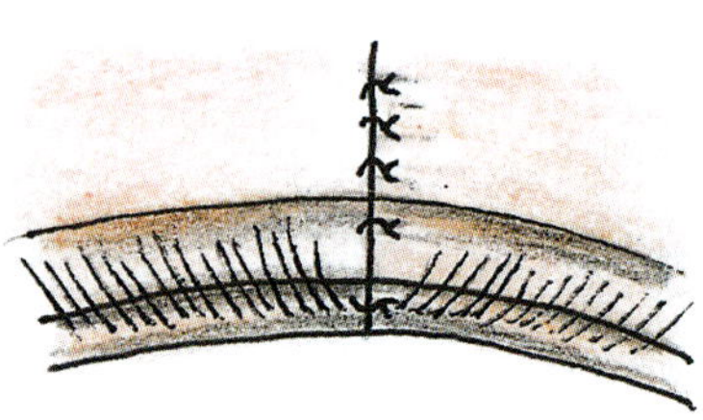

Figure 3.64b Skin suturing with 6 × 0 Trofilene (nylon)

Lower Lid Ectropion

a) Myocutaneous Upper Eyelid Flap

The myocutaneous flap from the upper eyelid is excellent for treating a lower lid ectropion and a lower lid ptosis.

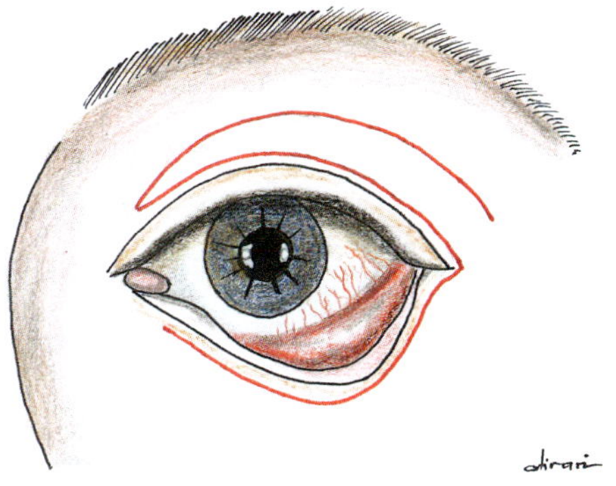

Figure 3.65a The lateral pedicle flap of the upper eyelid includes skin as well as the orbicularis oculi muscle. This ensures the blood supply is quite safe. The flap length may exceed the width by 3:1 or 4:1.

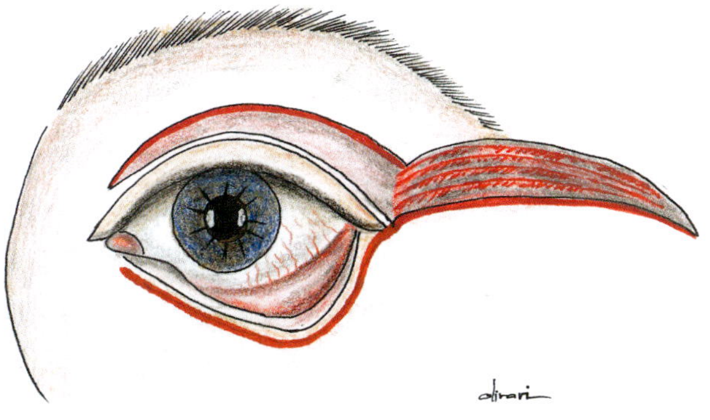

Figure 3.65b It is of great importance that the orbicularis oculi muscle is indeed included in the flap. The innervation of the muscle (which arises laterally) is preserved.

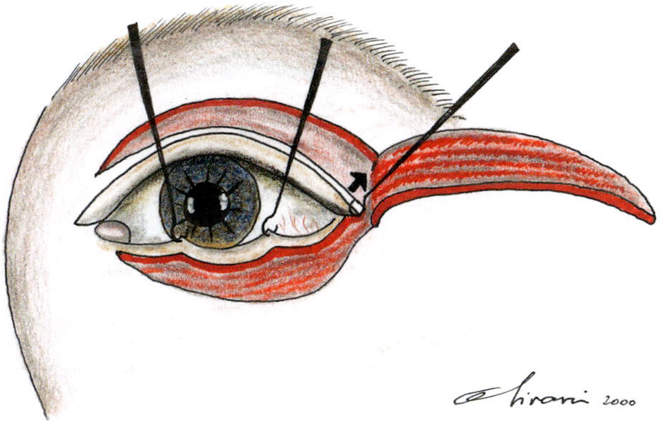

Figure 3.65c In order to correct a lower lid ectropion, the incision is made approx. 2 to 4 mm from the edge of the lower eyelid. A caudal subcutaneous mobilization then follows. The orbicularis oculi muscle is freed and divided transversely. If fibrous connections to the orbital margin are present, these must be divided. The eyelid edge must lie in its normal position without tension at the end of the preparation. Special attention must be paid to the lateral canthus. In most cases this is fixed caudally. The lateral canthus is freed of all adhesions. At the end of the preparation this must be fixed in a tension free manner in the cranial part of the flap base.

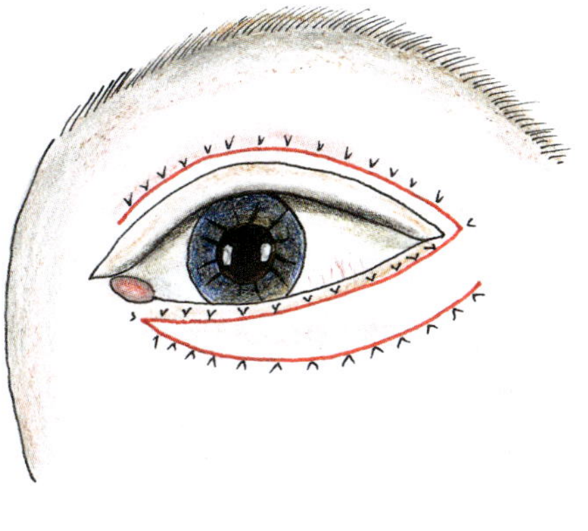

Figure 3.65d At the end of the operation the upper eyelid flap is sutured into the defect of the lower eyelid. The flap donor site is closed primarily.

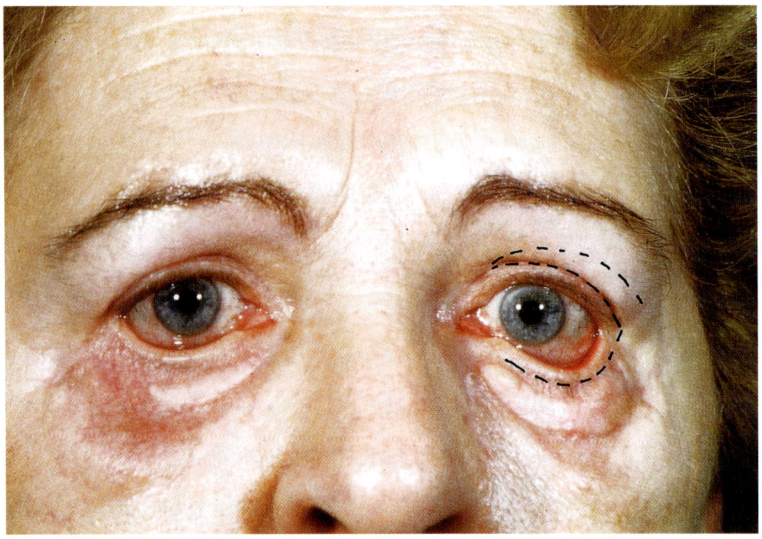

Figure 3.66a Appearance after bilateral blepharoplasty. A frequent complication of blepharoplasty of the lower eyelid is an ectropion with an associated conjunctivitis. Here, too much skin was removed from the lower eyelids. In order to correct the ectropion, a full-thickness skin graft was applied by the first surgeon. The graft was too small and also wrongly positioned. The result remained unsatisfactory.

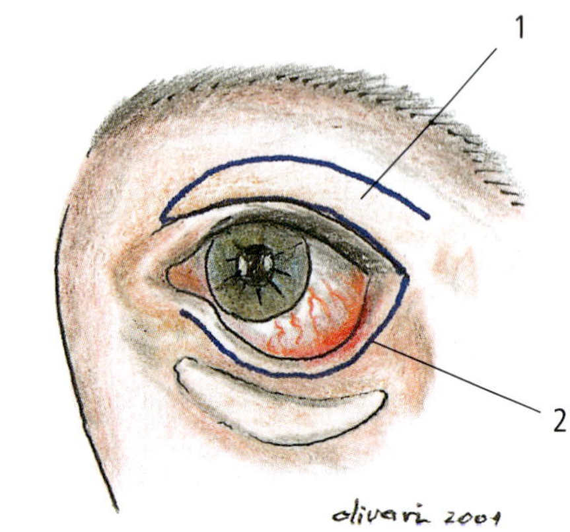

Figure 3.66b Flap formation in the upper eyelid (1), incision in the lower eyelid (2)

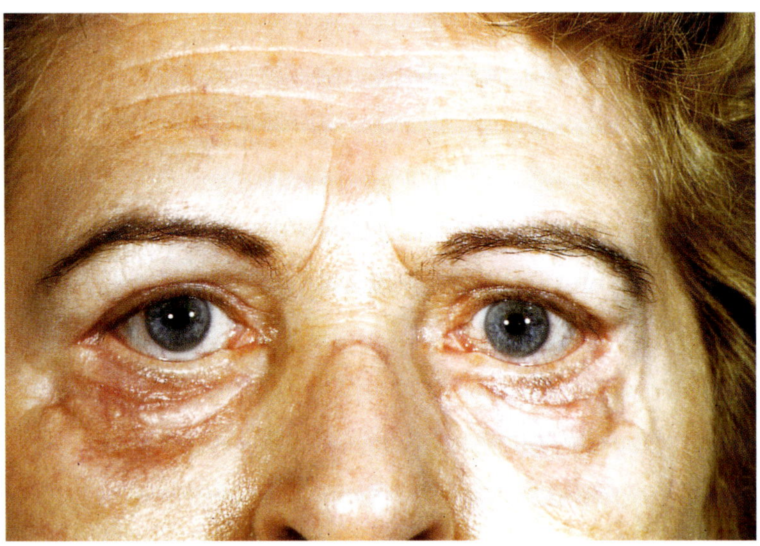

Figure 3.66c Appearance seven weeks after the operation: After mobilization of the lower eyelid a laterally pedicled myocutaneous flap from the upper eyelid was used for correction. **Although the upper lid correction was carried out only a few weeks earlier,** a sufficiently large flap could be formed to correct the ectropion completely. The mobilization of the lower eyelid and the lateral canthus in a cranial direction is very important.

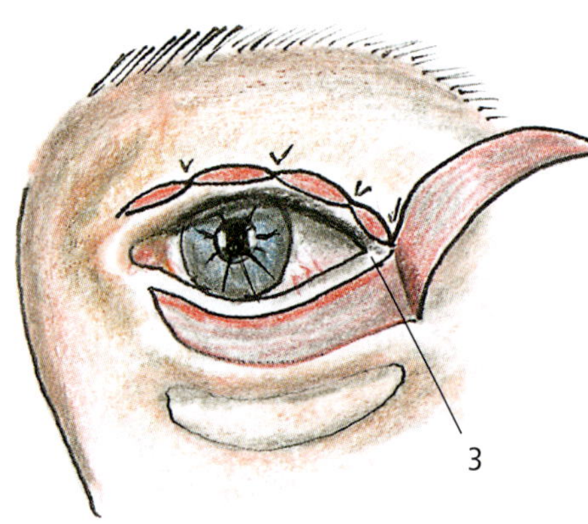

Figure 3.66d Mobilization of the lower eyelid as well as the lateral canthus (3) cranially

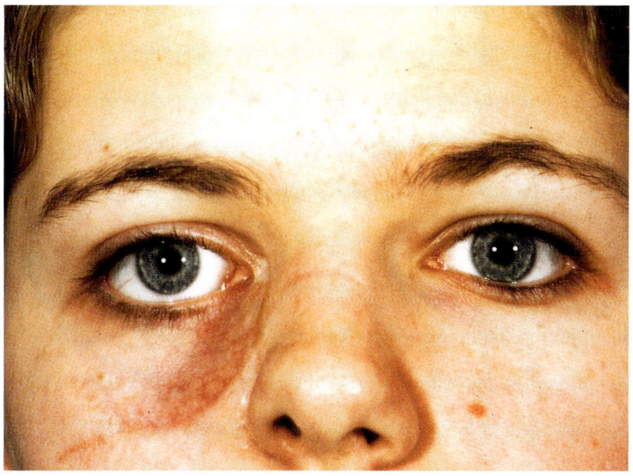

Figure 3.67a Ptosis of the right lower eyelid (scleral show) caused by a dermatological disease.

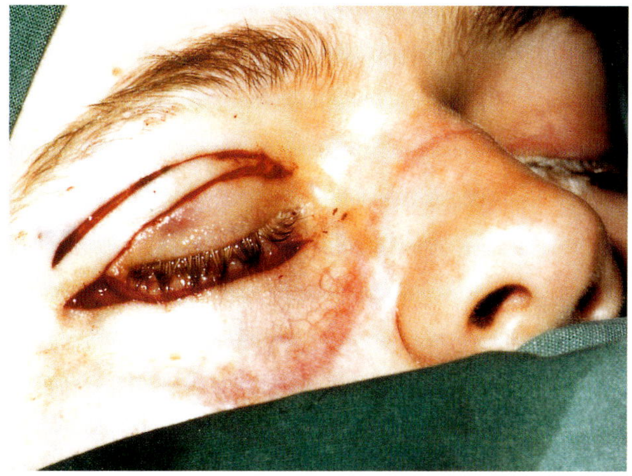

Figure 3.67b Formation of a laterally pedicled myocutaneous flap from the upper eyelid. Note the length that can be achieved.

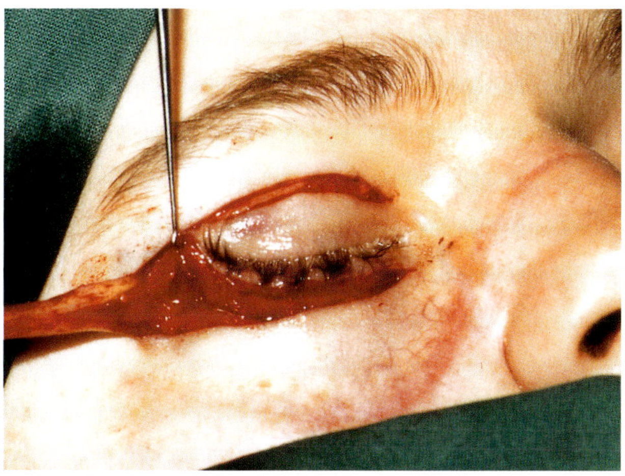

Figure 3.67c The lower eyelid is mobilized and the lateral canthus is released and then fixed cranially.

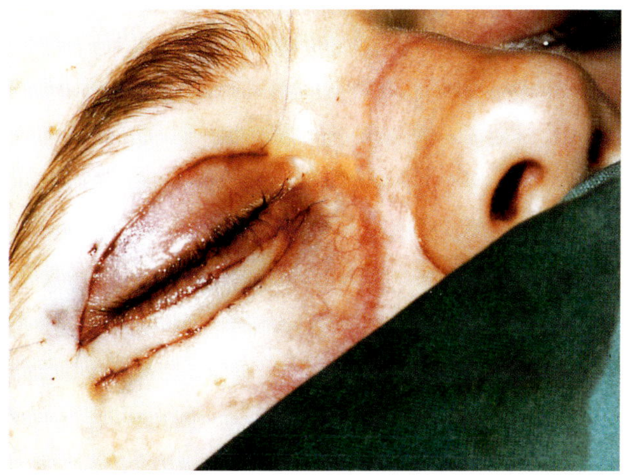

Figure 3.67d The flap is fixed in the lower eyelid using 7×0 Vicryl. The secondary defect in the upper eyelid is sutured intracutaneously using 6 x 0 Trofilene.

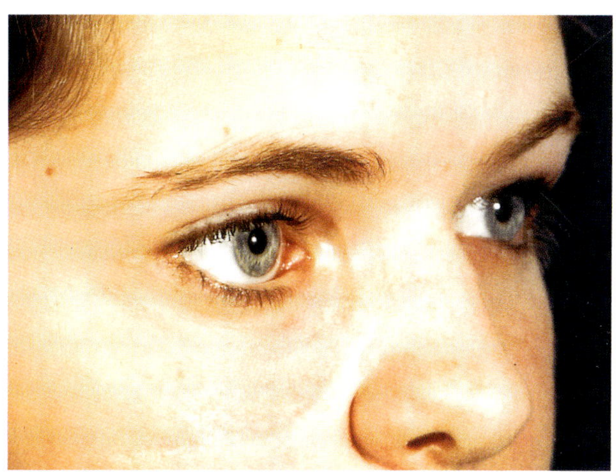

Figure 3.67e Appearance one year after the operation. Scars in the eyelid are almost always barely visible.

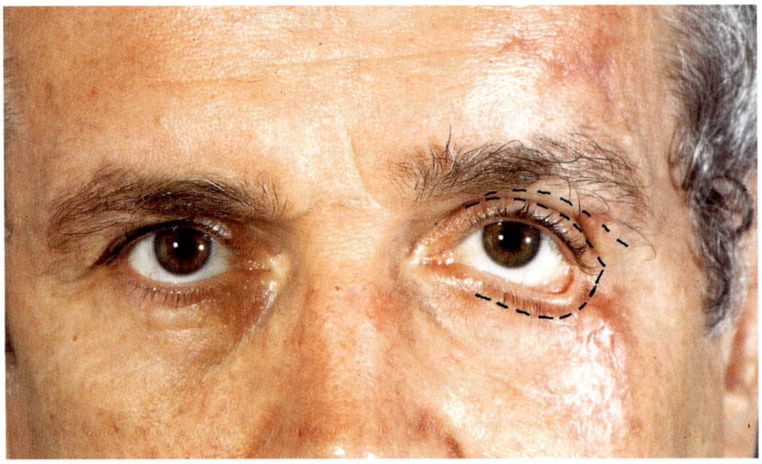

Figure 3.68a Traumatic ectropion of the left lower eyelid, particularly in the lateral part

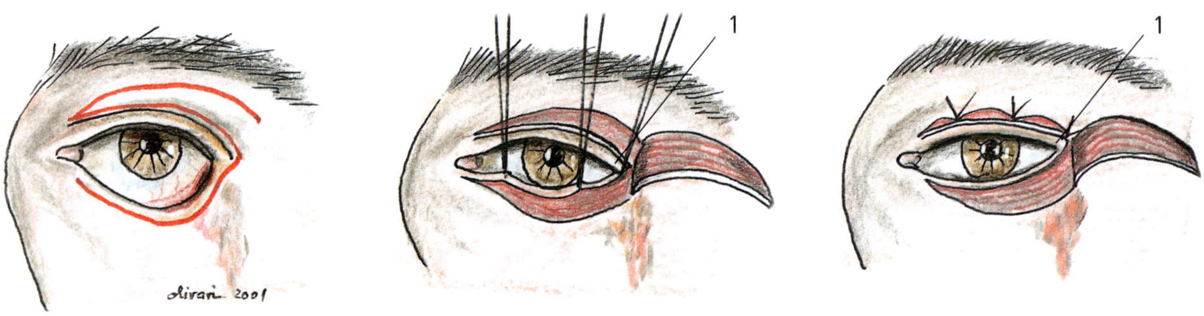

Figure 3.68b The most important part of the operation is the complete mobilization of the lower eyelid which must be freed of scars and adhesions. The lateral canthus (1) in particular must be fixed cranially without any tension.

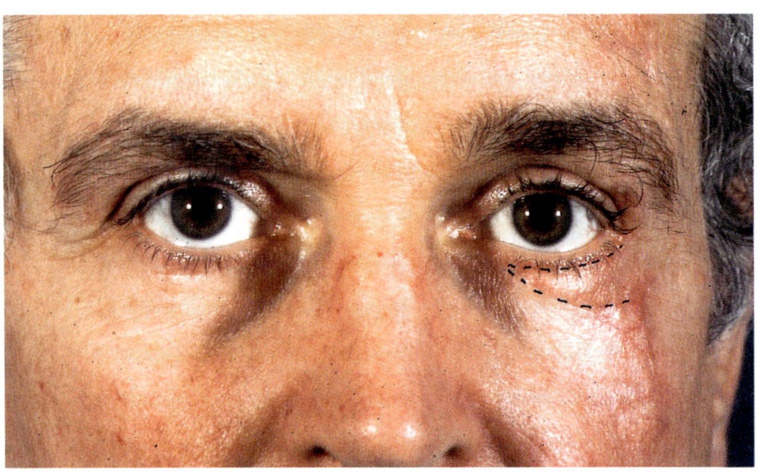

Figure 3.68c Appearance five months after the operation. In the lateral part the flap base is 10 mm wide.

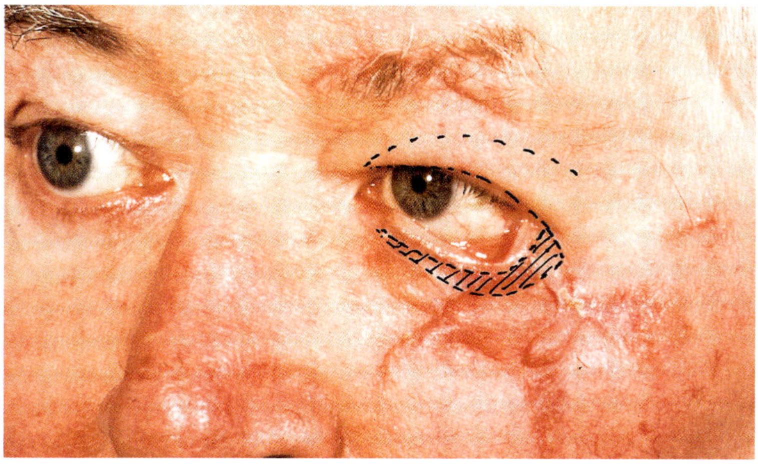

Figure 3.69a Traumatic ectropion of the left lower eyelid. The scar (shaded) will be excised.

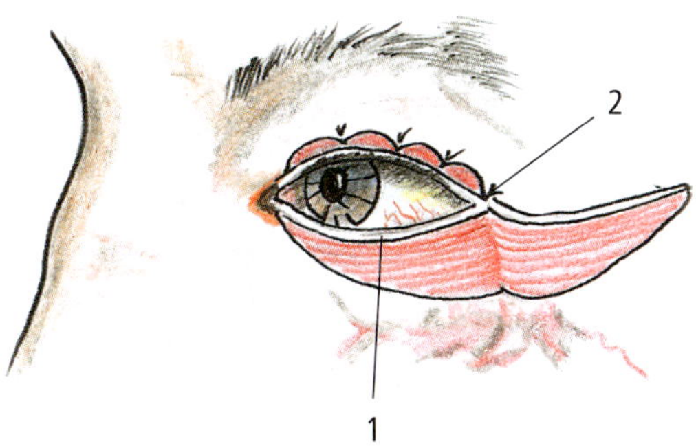

Figure 3.69b Formation of a myocutaneous flap from the upper eyelid. Mobilization of the lower eyelid (1) as well as the lateral canthus (2).

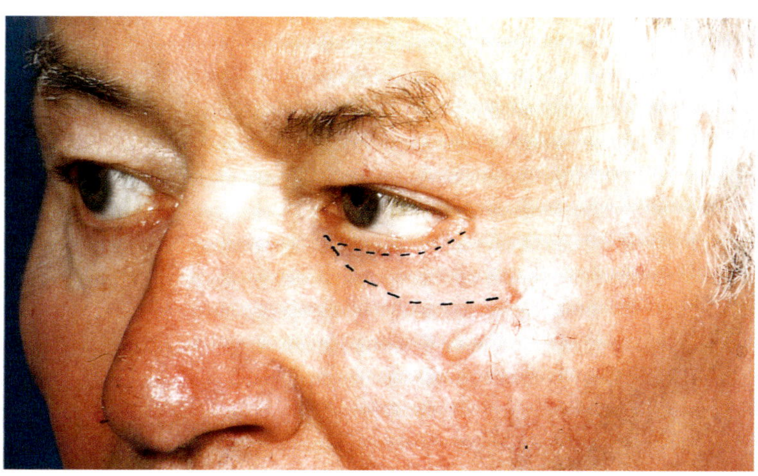

Figure 3.69c Situation six month after surgery

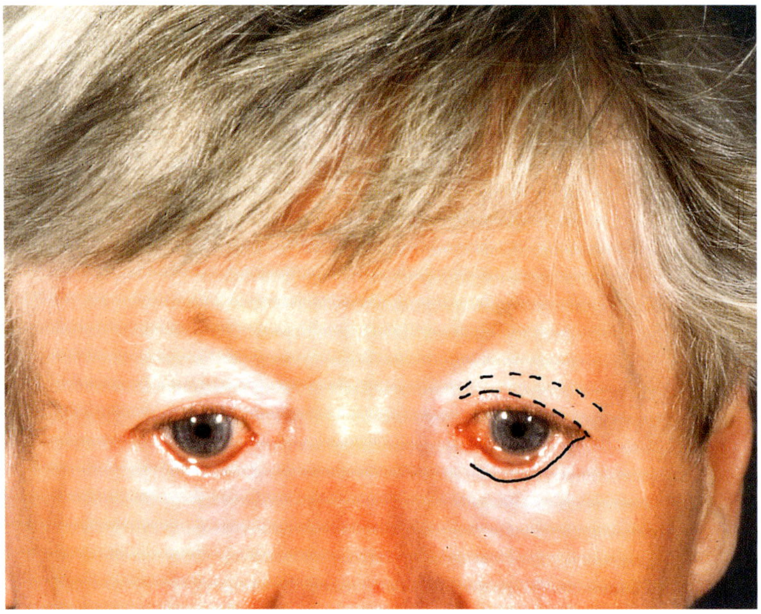

Figure 3.70a Ectropion of both lower eyelids (senile ectropion) with chronic conjunctivitis, photophobia, keratitis and tear flow. Appearance after lateral canthopexy performed elsewhere.

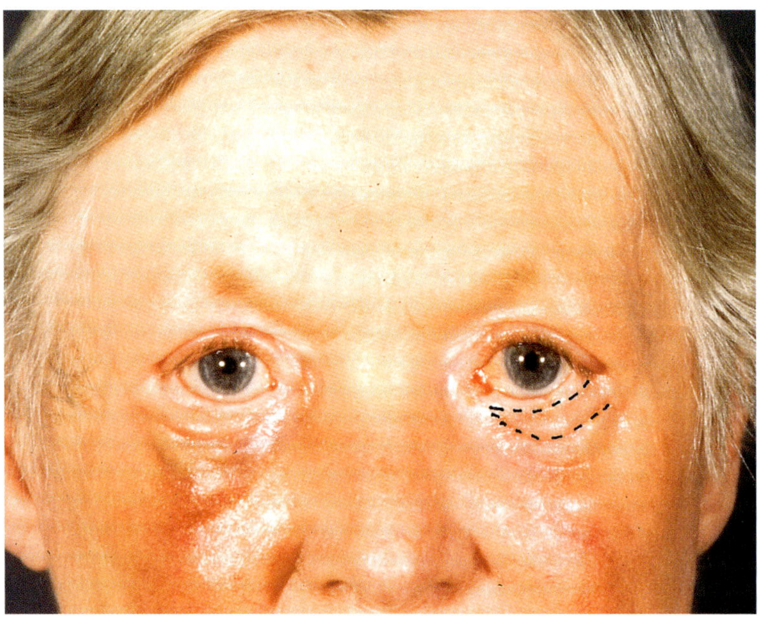

Figure 3.70b Appearance three weeks after the operation: By mobilizing the lower eyelid the elevation of the eyelid edge was corrected using a myocutaneous flap from the upper eyelid bilaterally.

Upper Eyelid Island Flap

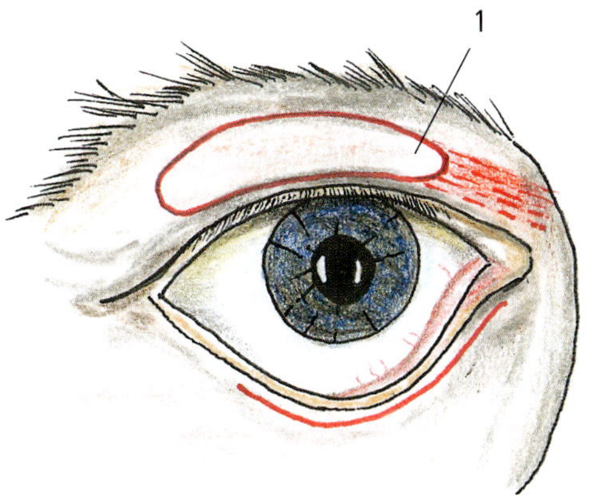

Figure 3.71a For correction the upper eyelid island flap is pedicled medially at the orbicularis oculi muscle (1).

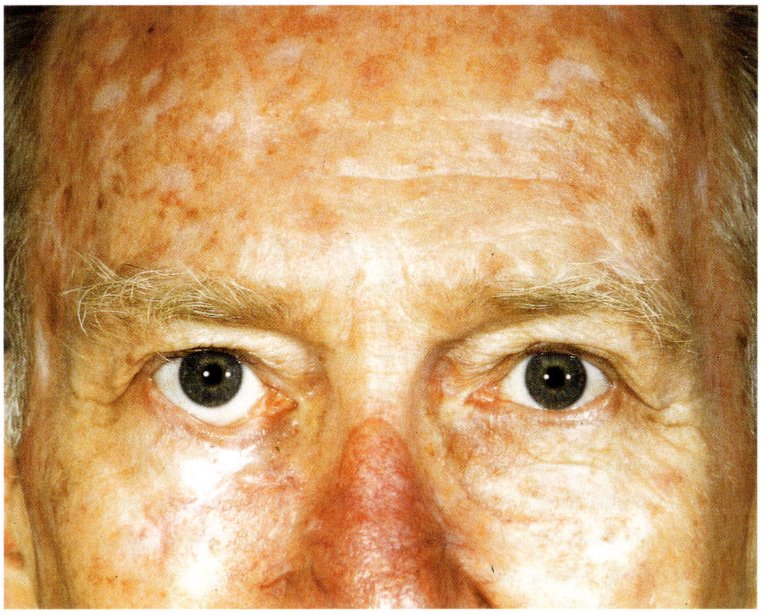

Figure 3.71b Ectropion of the right lower eyelid after removal of a basal cell carcinoma. Formation of a medial upper eyelid island flap.

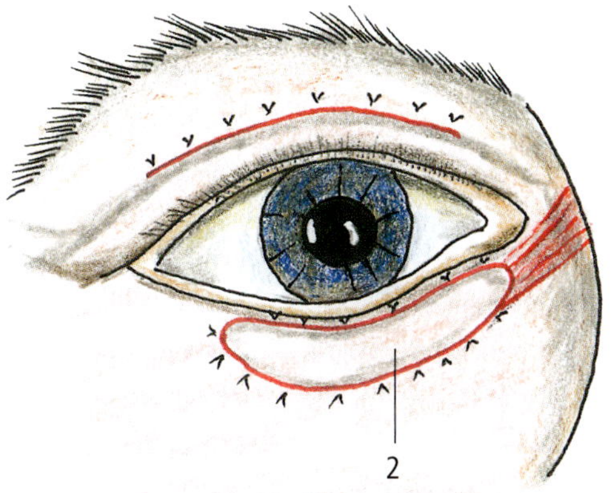

Figure 3.71c The island flap was formed from the upper eyelid skin and passed through a subcutaneous tunnel (2) into the lower eyelid.

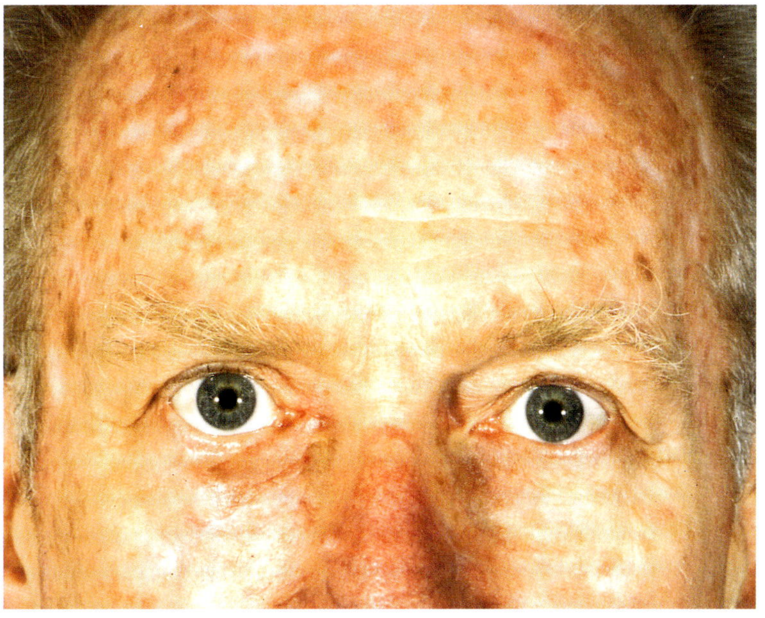

Figure 3.71d Appearance six months postoperatively

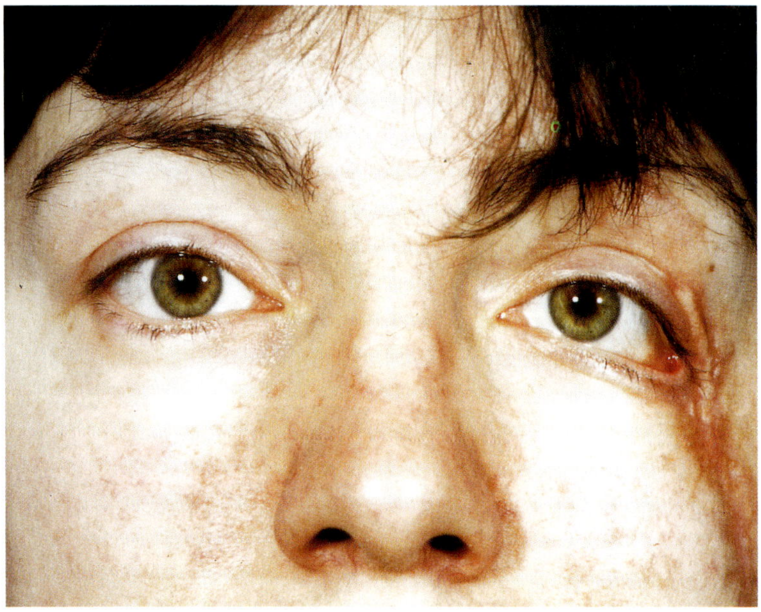

Figure 3.72a Traumatic ectropion of the left lower eyelid. The ectropion is aggravated by the vertical orientated scar contracture.

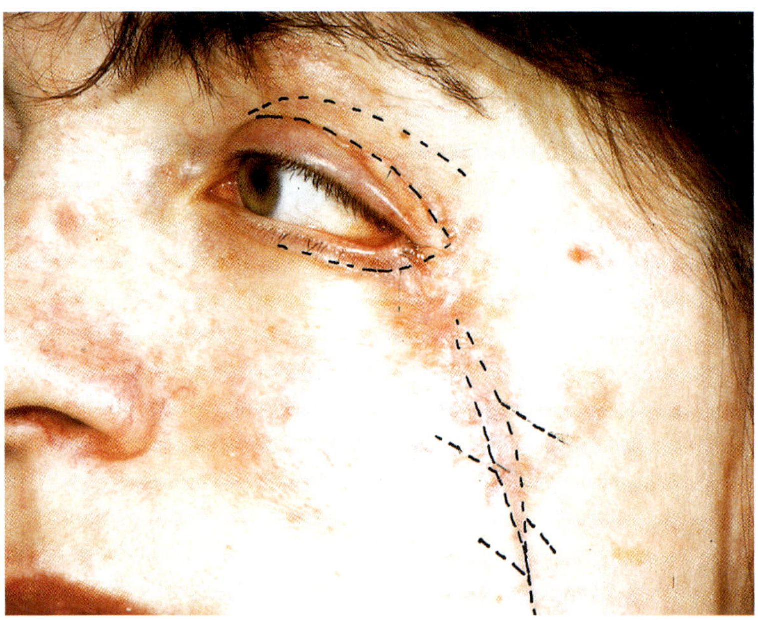

Figure 3.72b A myocutaneous triangular flap from the upper eyelid is planned for correction of the lower eyelid. After excision of the scar of the left cheek, two Z-plasties are carried out to relieve any vertical tension.

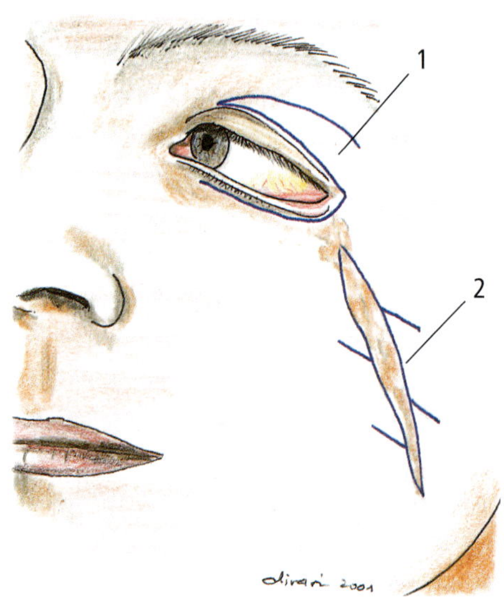

Figure 3.72c Planning of the upper eyelid flap (1) (see b) as well as a double Z-plasty (2).

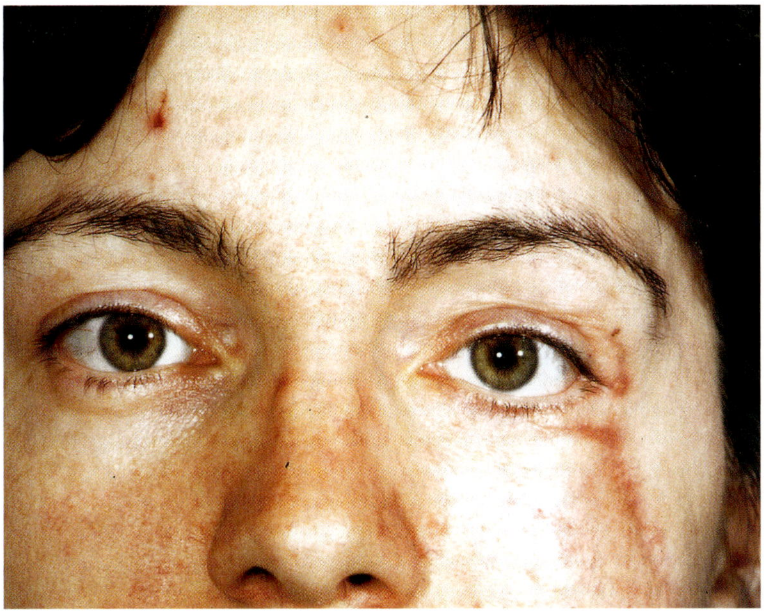

Figure 3.72d Appearance seven months after the operation.

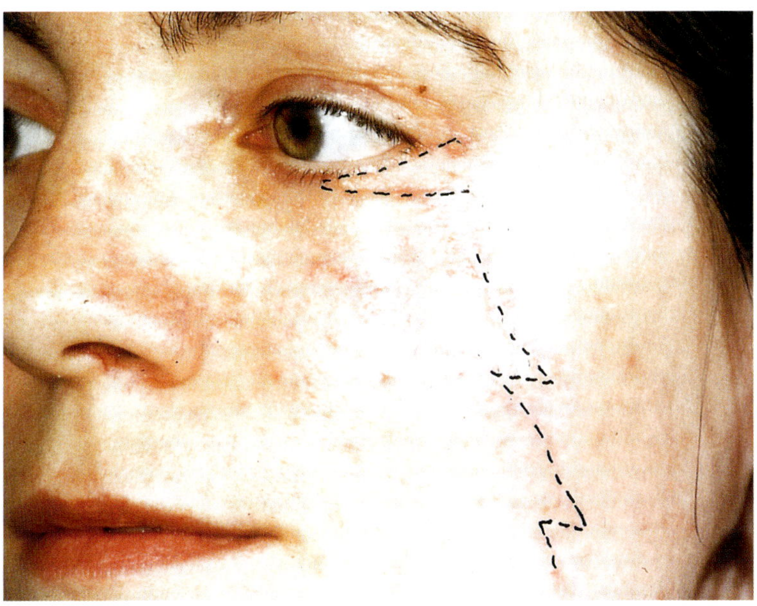

Figure 3.72e The scar on the left cheek is also corrected by the double Z-plasty.

b) Full-Thickness Skin Graft

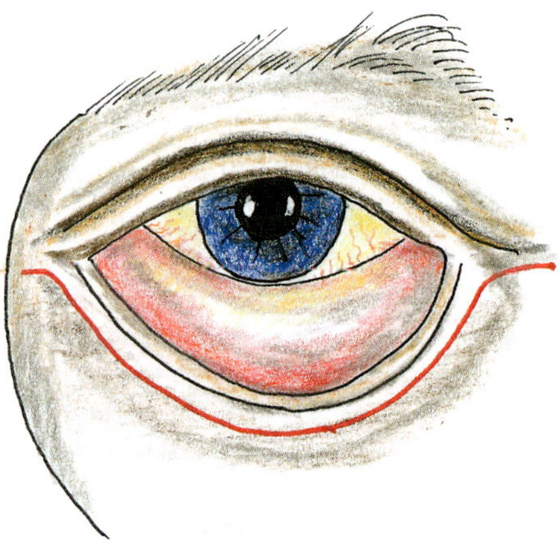

Figure 3.73a Incision in the lower eyelid extending both medially and laterally canthus (red)

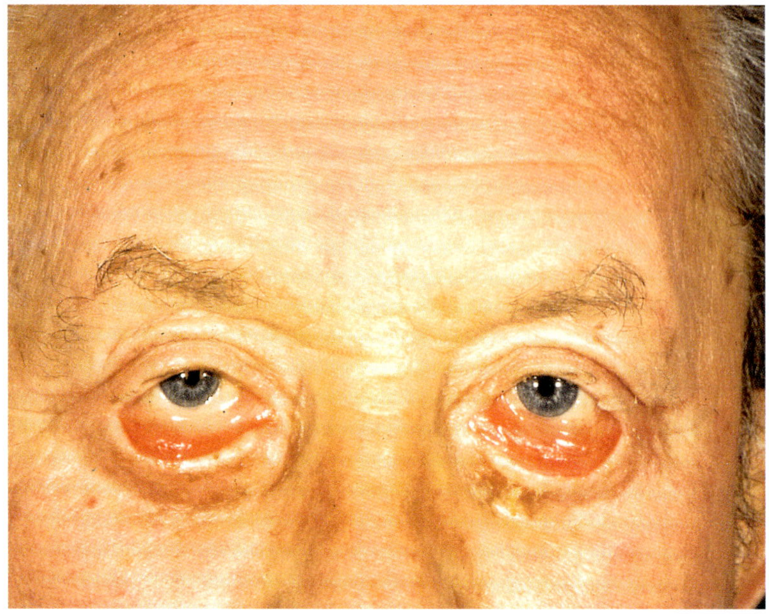

Figure 3.73b Severe ectropion after blepharoplasty with postoperative complications

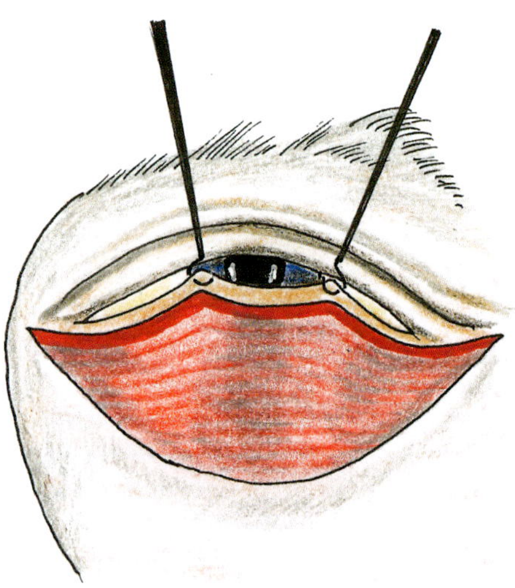

Figure 3.73c In order to correct the ectropion, the lower eyelid must first be extensively mobilized. All adhesions must be released so that the edge of the lower eyelid assumes its correct position in a relaxed manner. The incision, as well as the mobilization, should be extended beyond the medial and lateral canthus.

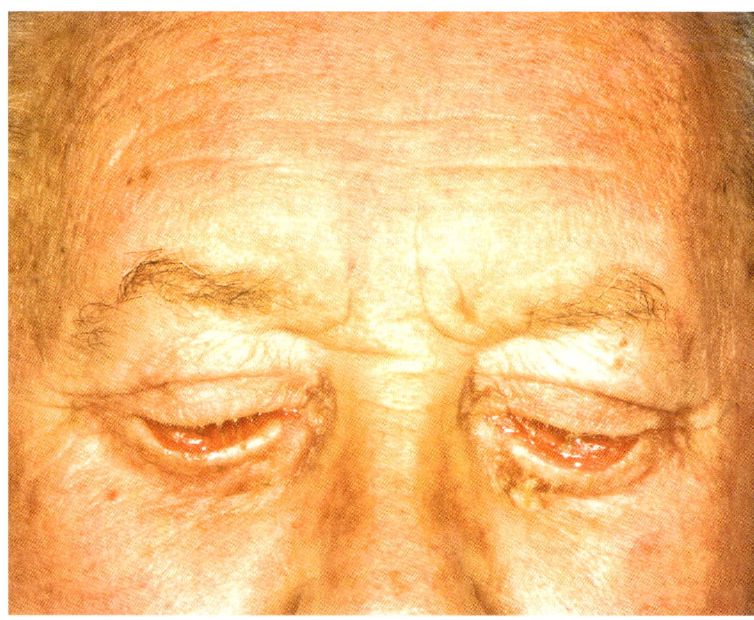

Figure 3.73d The patient is suffering from chronic conjunctivitis as well as incomplete eyelid closure.

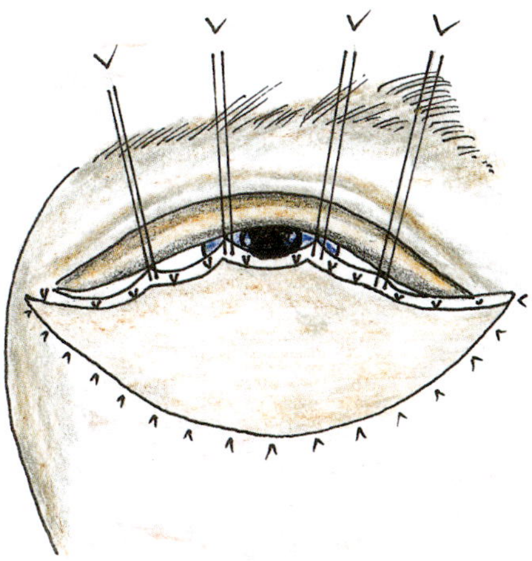

Figure 3.73e A full thickness skin graft is taken from the post auricular area. The graft must be larger than the defect. The eyelid margin is fixed with several sutures to the forehead skin so that the full-thickness skin graft can heal fully stretched out.

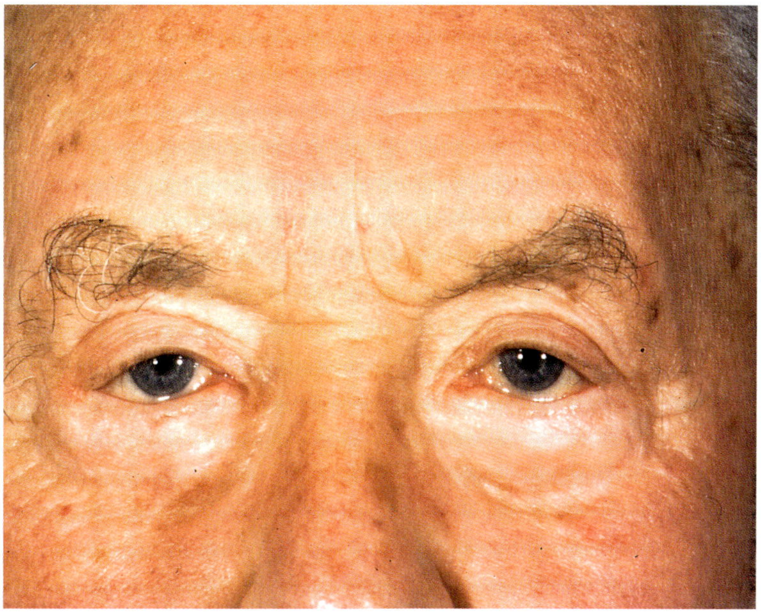

Figure 3.73f Appearance eight months postoperatively. A functionally and aesthetically acceptable result can be seen.

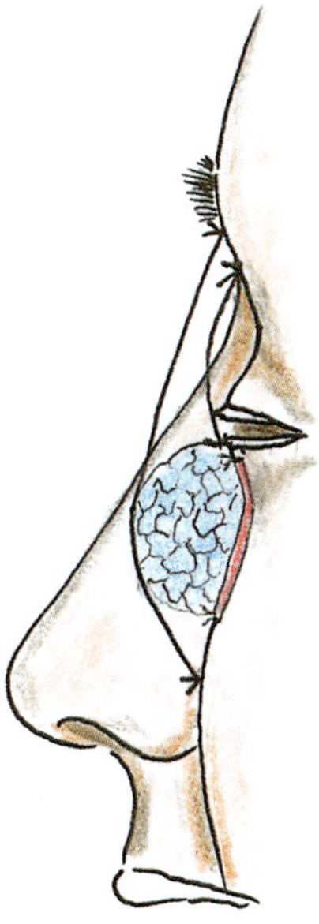

Figure 3.73g The compression bandage over the full-thickness skin graft is not attached to the graft edge, but to the forehead and the cheek.

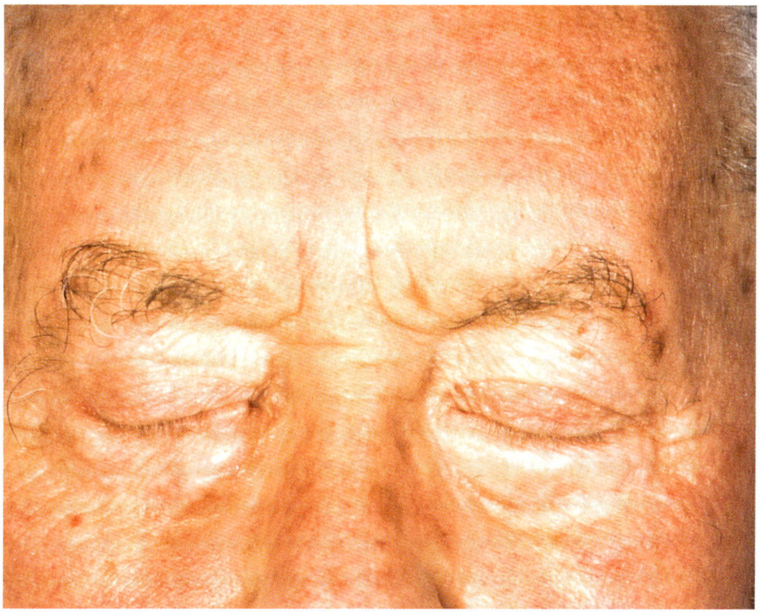

Figure 3.73h Appearance eight months postoperatively. Normal eyelid closure.

c) Combined Myocutaneous Upper Eyelid Flap With Full-Thickness Skin Graft and Island Flap

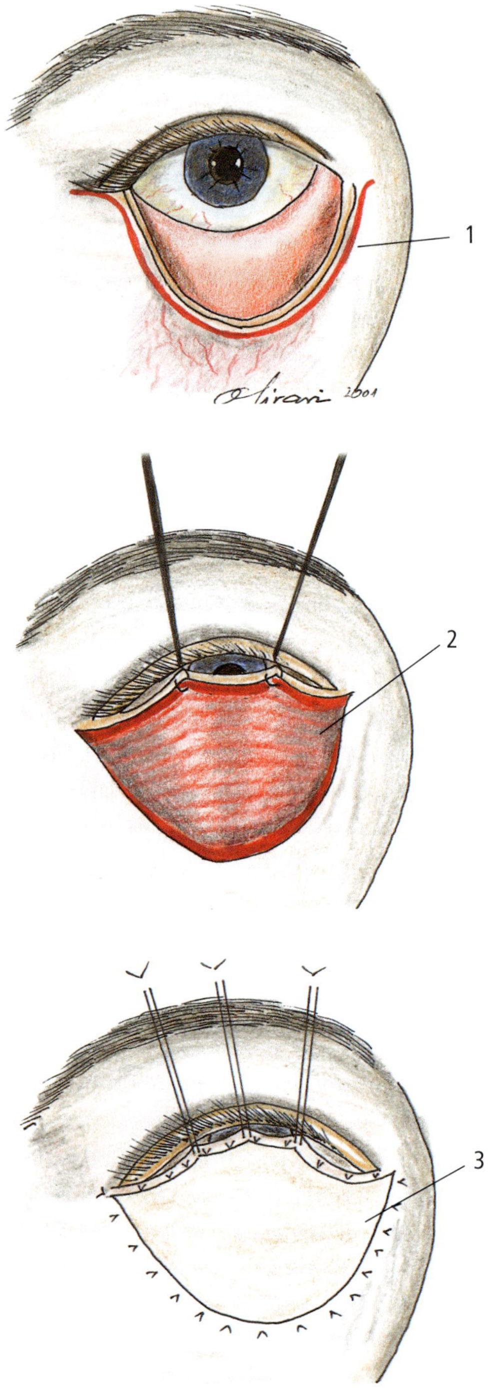

Figure 3.74a Incision at the eyelid margin (1). A very careful mobilization of the orbicularis oculi muscle (2), which is in part atrophied and in part fibrotic. The affected skin in the lower eyelid is excised. Two full thickness skin grafts (3) from the post auricular area are used to cover the defect. Measuring out for the full-thickness skin graft should be generous!

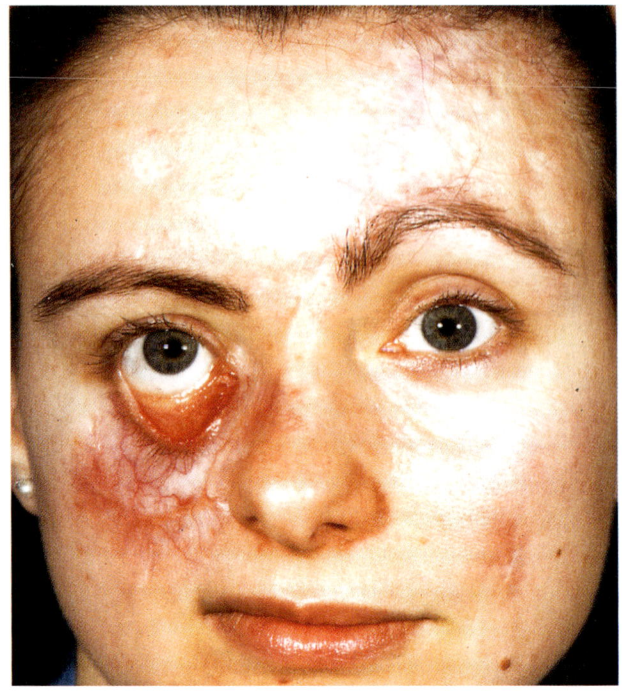

Figure 3.74b Extreme ectropion of the right lower eyelid after a year-long dermatological therapy of a skin infection. The skin on the left forehead is also affected. Following long term application of corticosteroids the skin has become atrophic, fibrotic and features ectasias. The eye is at risk because eyelid closure is not possible. Conjunctivitis, keratitis are also present.

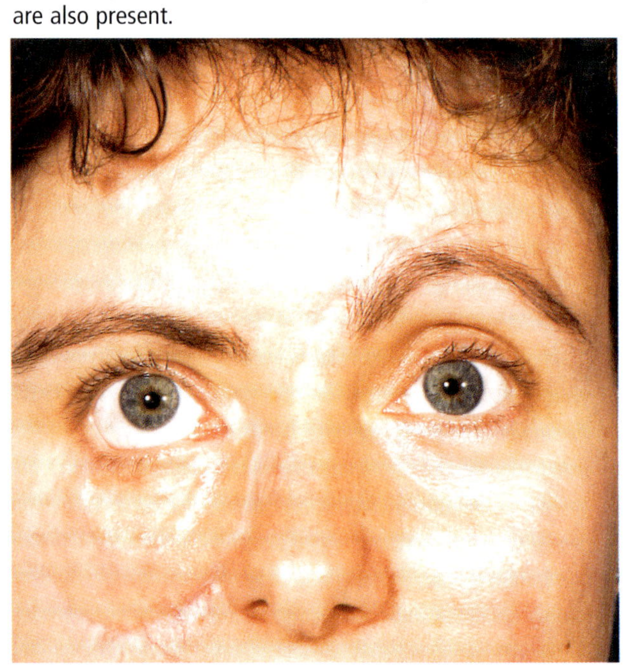

Figure 3.74c Four months after the first operation there is still a clear lower lid ptosis. Further corrective measures are planned.

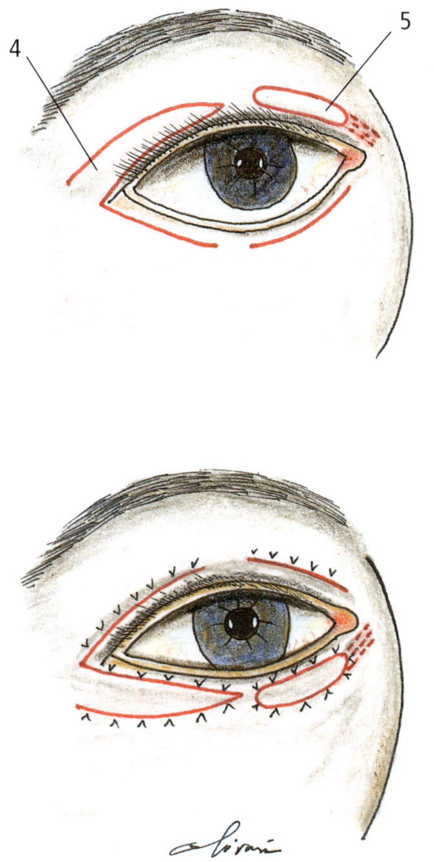

Figure 3.74d For correction of the lower lid ptosis, a myocutaneous, laterally pedicled, triangular flap from the upper eyelid is used (4). In addition, an island flap from the medial part of the upper eyelid, that is pedicled on the orbicularis oculi muscle, is brought through a subcutaneous tunnel into the lower eyelid (5).

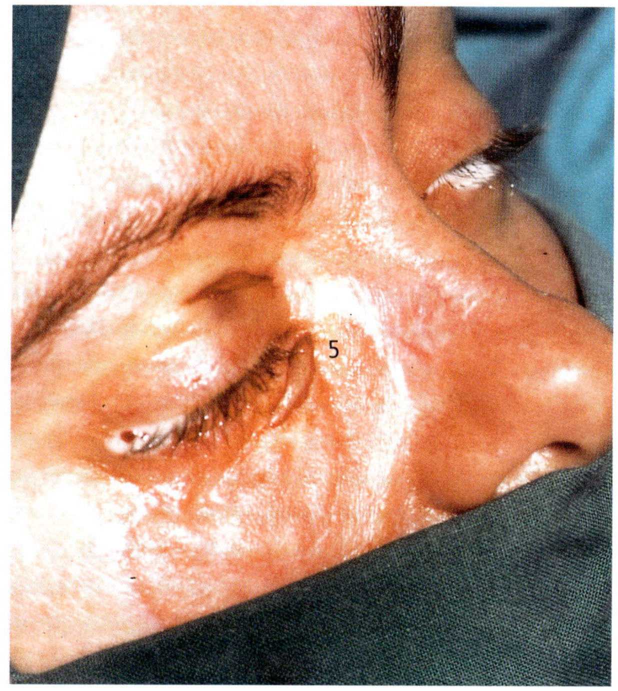

Figure 3.74e Intraoperative image: An island flap from the upper eyelid is brought into the lower eyelid (5).

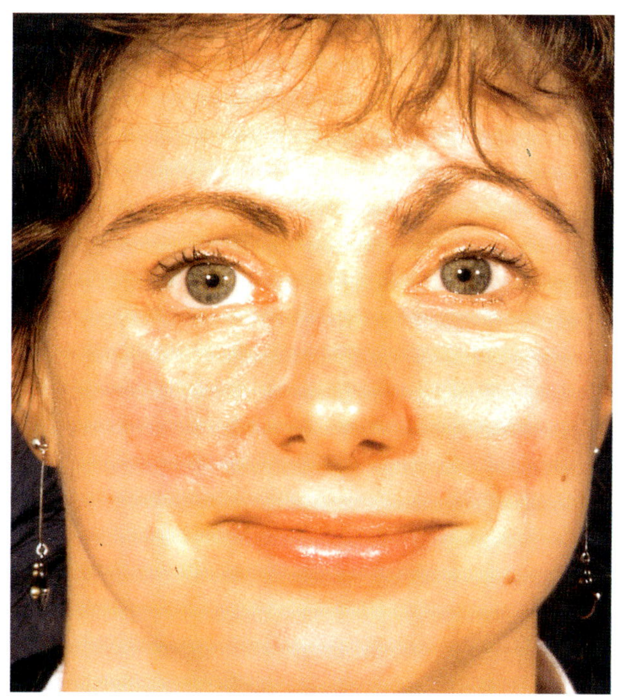

Figure 3.74f Appearance one year after two operations

d) Supratrochlear Flap

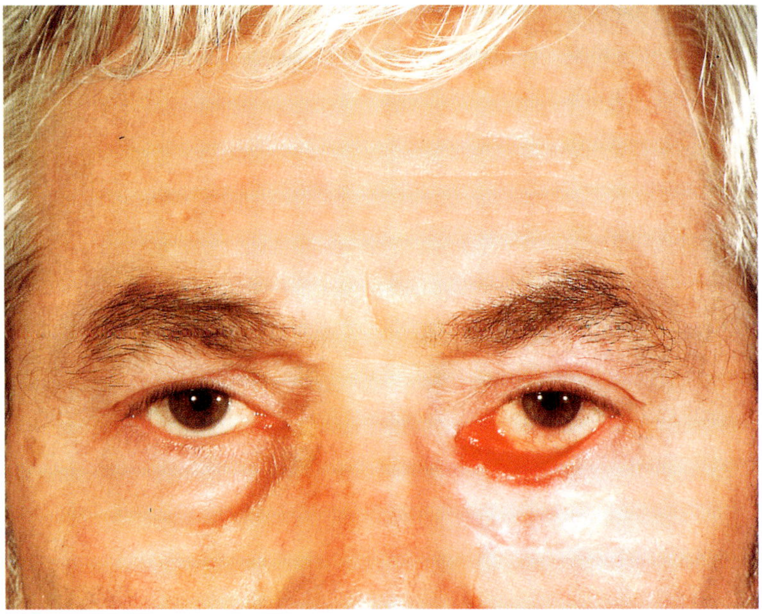

Figure 3.75a Ectropion of the lower eyelid after basal cell carcinoma excision and inadequate coverage with a meshed graft.

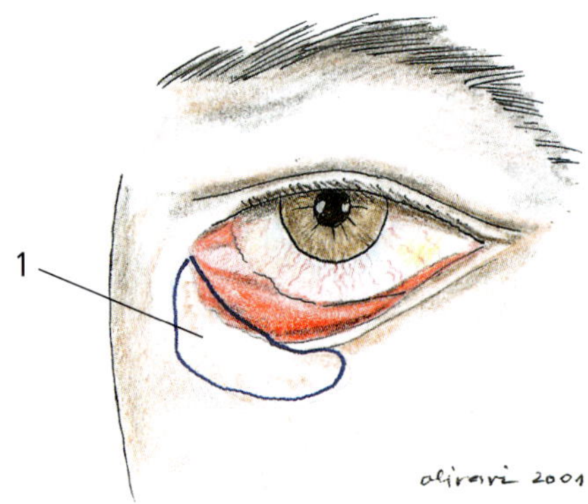

Figure 3.75b The ectropion causes a chronic conjunctivitis, keratitis and tear flow. The fibrotic region (scar) is excised (1).

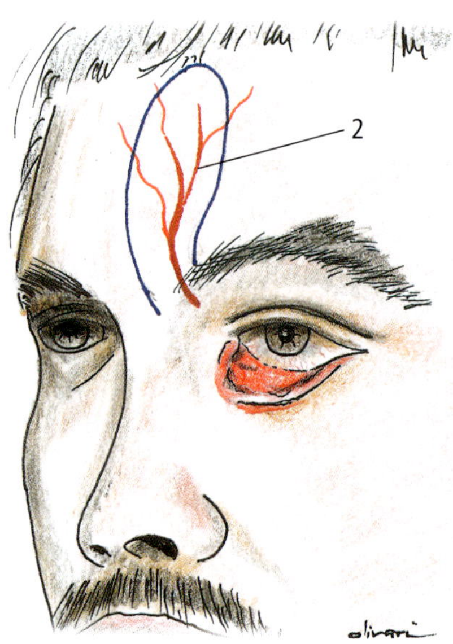

Figure 3.75c Planning of the operation. A small supratrochlear flap (forehead flap) (2) of sufficient length is planned.

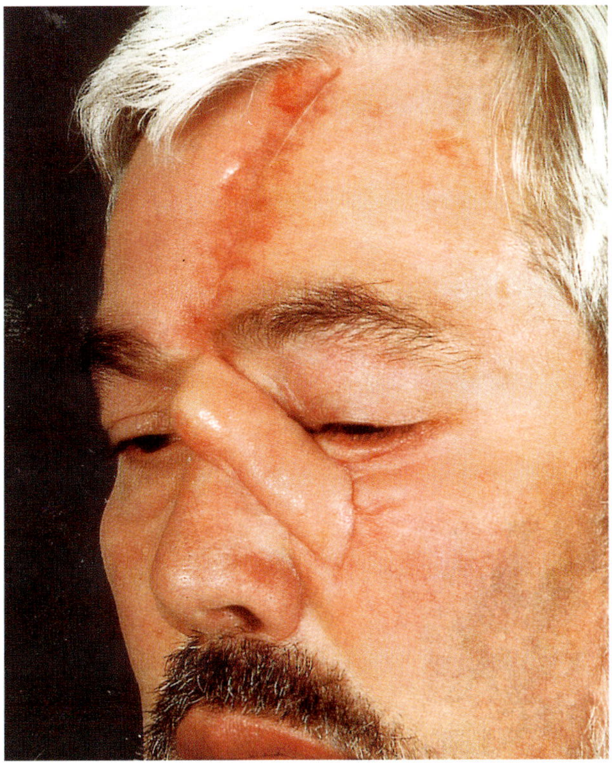

Figure 3.75d After resection of the scarred tissue, the remaining conjunctiva is mobilized for the inner lining. The forehead flap is fixed in the defect for three weeks before it is divided at the base. Two months later the modeling and thinning of the flap is carried out.

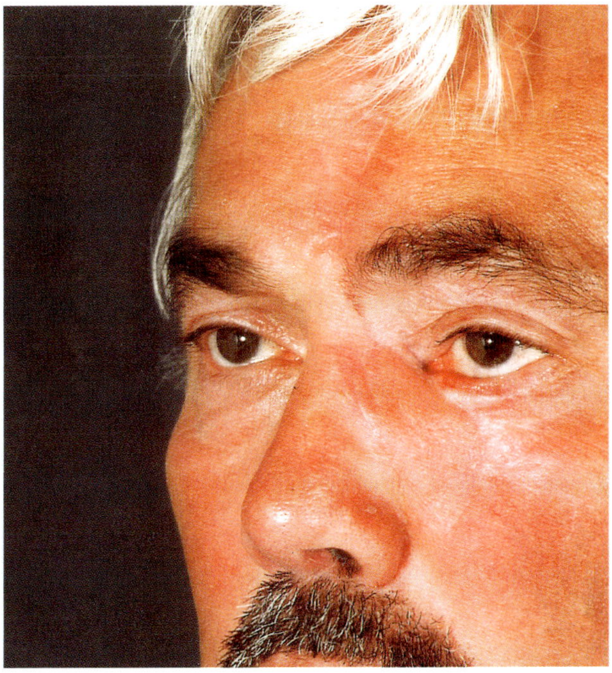

Figure 3.75e Appearance one year after the operation

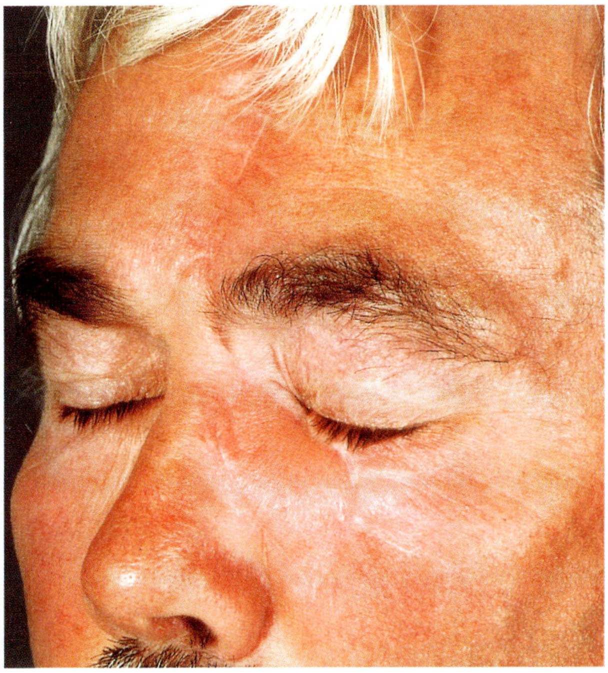

Figure 3.75f Functional result: Eyelid closure is normal

Upper Lid Retraction

a) Local Flap and Y-V Plasty

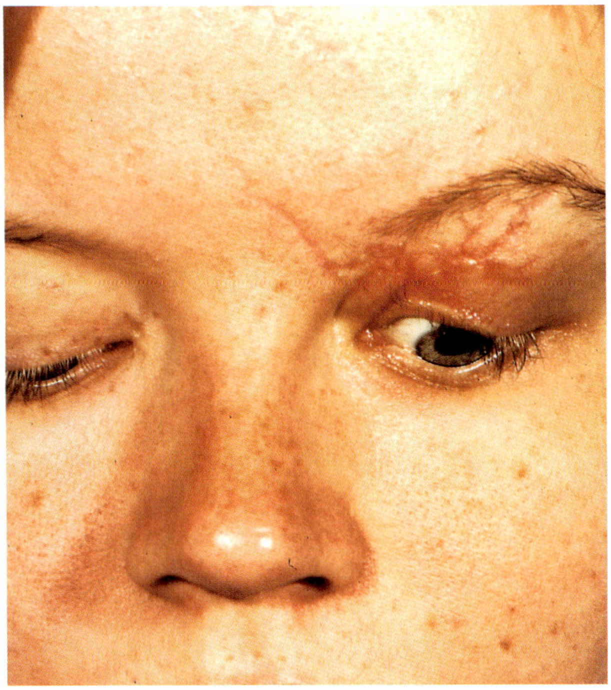

Figure 3.76a Upper lid retraction due to cicatrization after a glass splinter injury

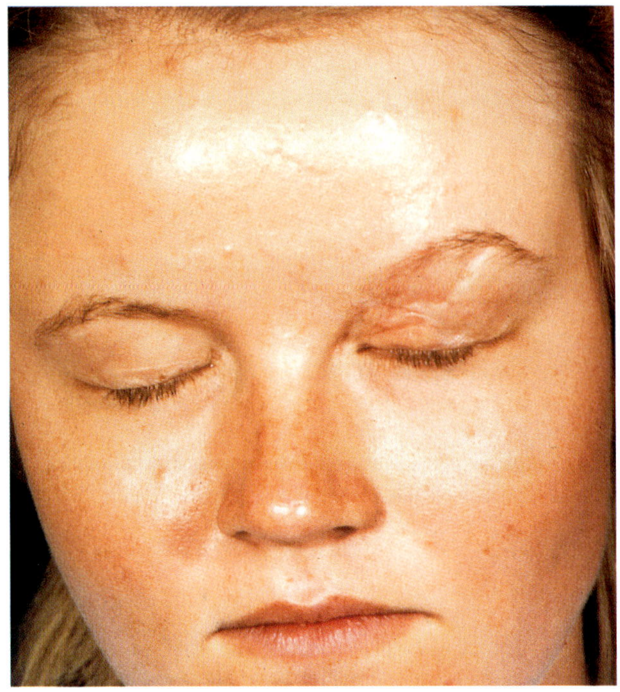

Figure 3.76c Appearance two years after the operation. Function has been restored.

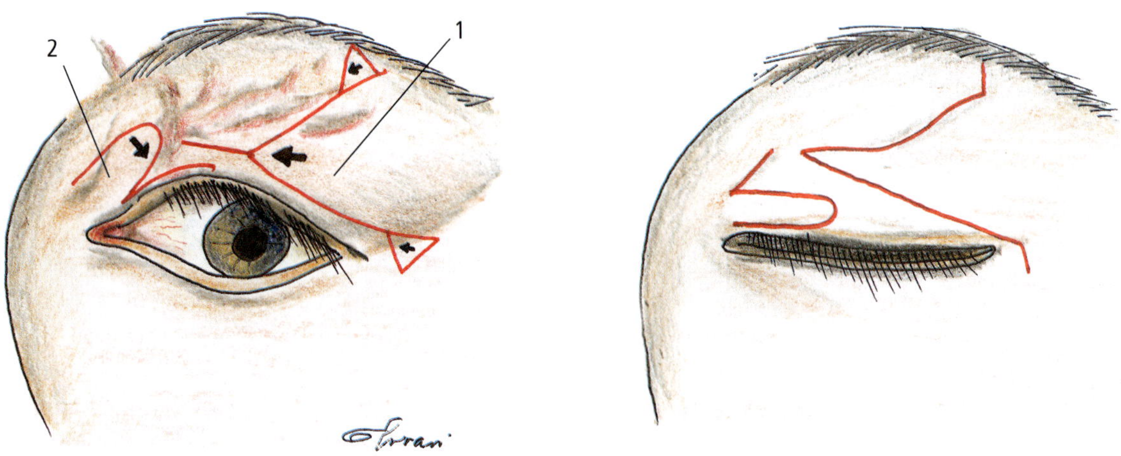

Figure 3.76b In order to correct the retraction, a myocutaneous triangular flap is formed laterally (1), mobilized and moved medially as a Y-V plasty. From a medial approach a local flap is fixed to the eyelid edge after mobilization (2). As a result of these two procedures the upper eyelid is adequately prolonged so that eyelid closure becomes possible. Of course a full thickness skin graft would be a good choice.

b) Transposition Flap From the Cheek

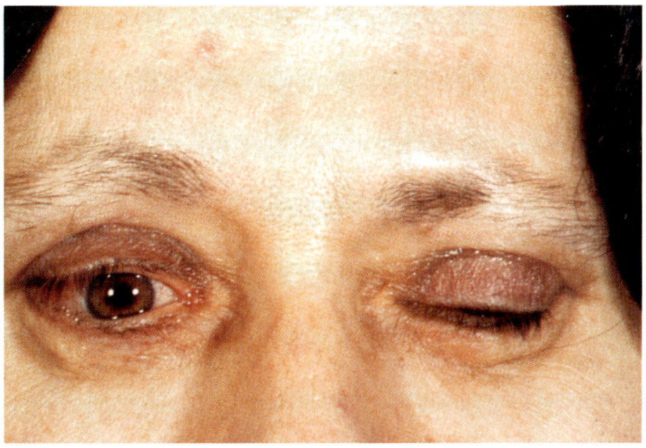

Figure 3.77a Right upper lid retraction after an exophthalmos operation. After division of the levator aponeurosis and Mueller's muscle, an interposionate consisting of GoreTex was implanted. A severe fibrosis developed resulting in retraction of the upper eyelid.

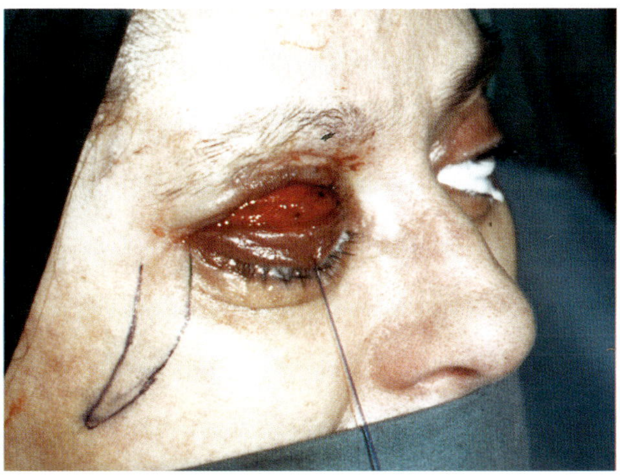

Figure 3.77b Mobilization of the upper eyelid and formation of the flap

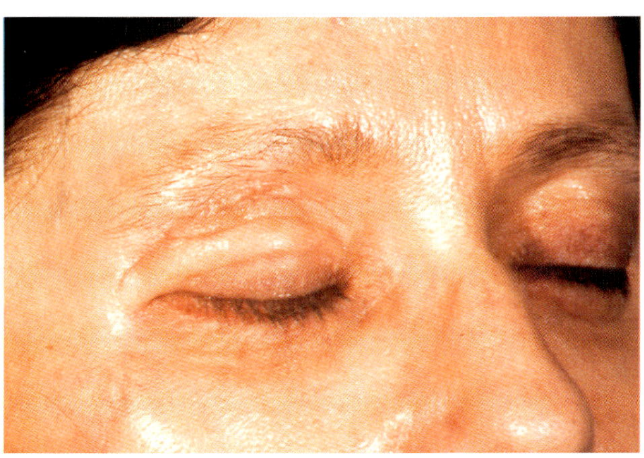

Figure 3.77d Appearance one year after the operation

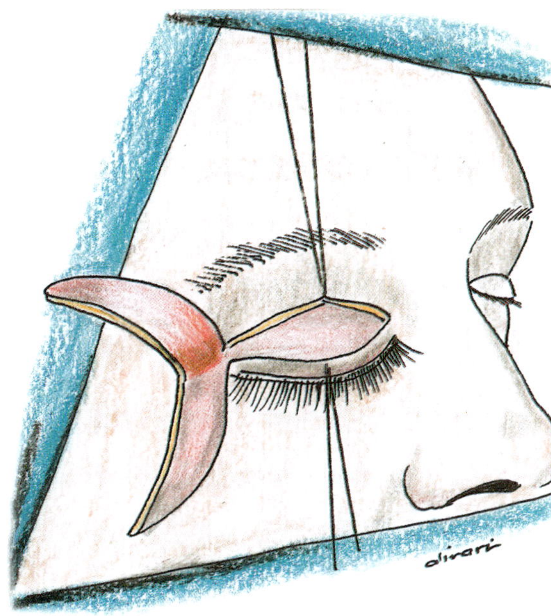

Figure 3.77c The upper eyelid is mobilized and freed of scarred adhesions and the GoreTex implant is removed. A cranially pedicled flap from the right cheek is used to cover the defect. This flap was described by Frieke (1829).

Tumors of the Eyelids

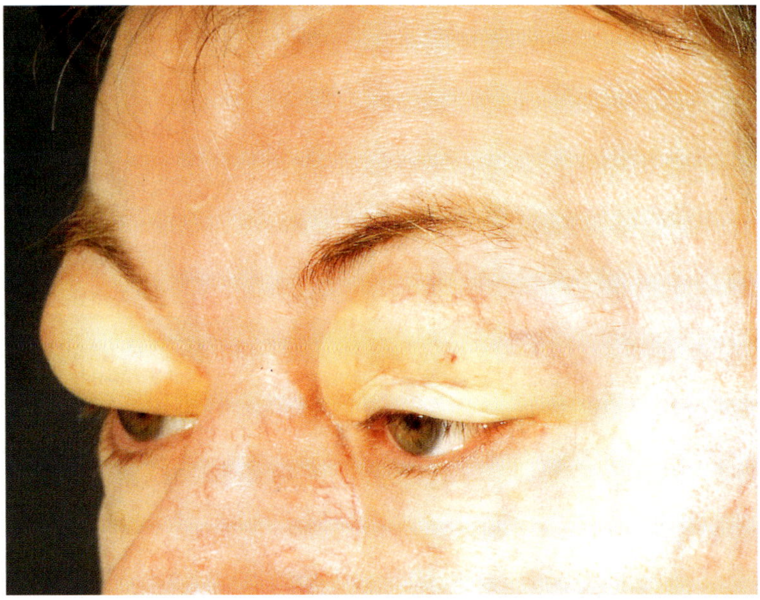

Figure 3.78a Advanced xanthelasma of both upper eyelids

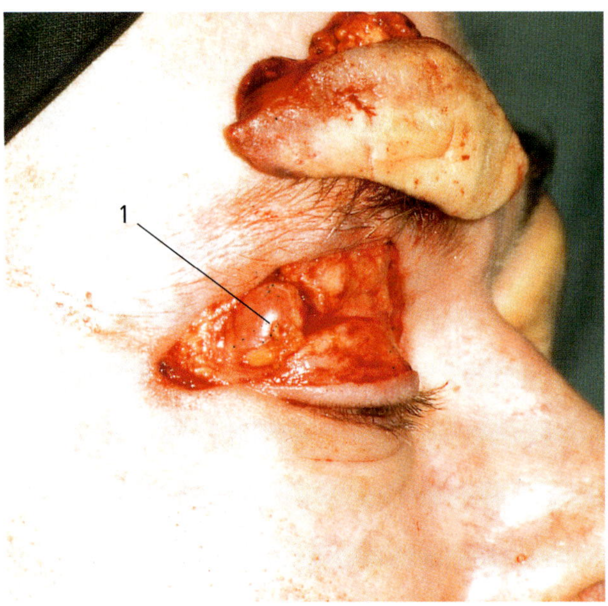

Figure 3.78b The entire area between the eyelid margin and the eyebrows is extirpated bilaterally. On the right side a severe hypertrophy of the lacrimal gland is evident. It is sunk into the orbit with 5 x 0 Vicryl sutures at the orbital septum (1).

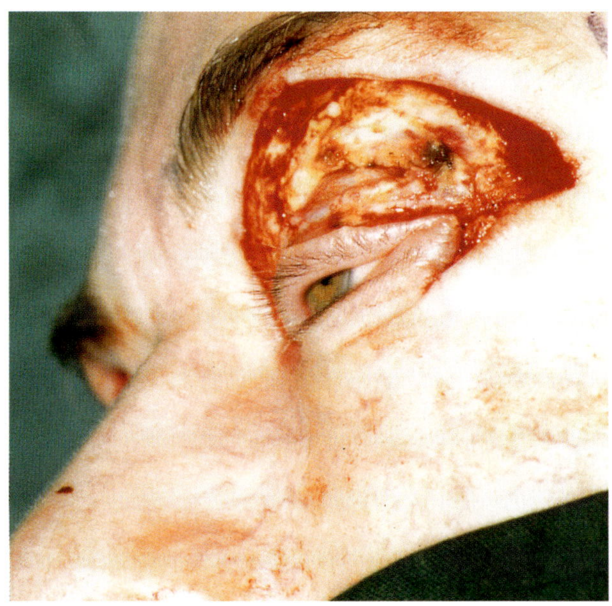

Figure 3.78c The changes are deeply subcutaneous and reach up to the orbital septum which is also partly infiltrated.

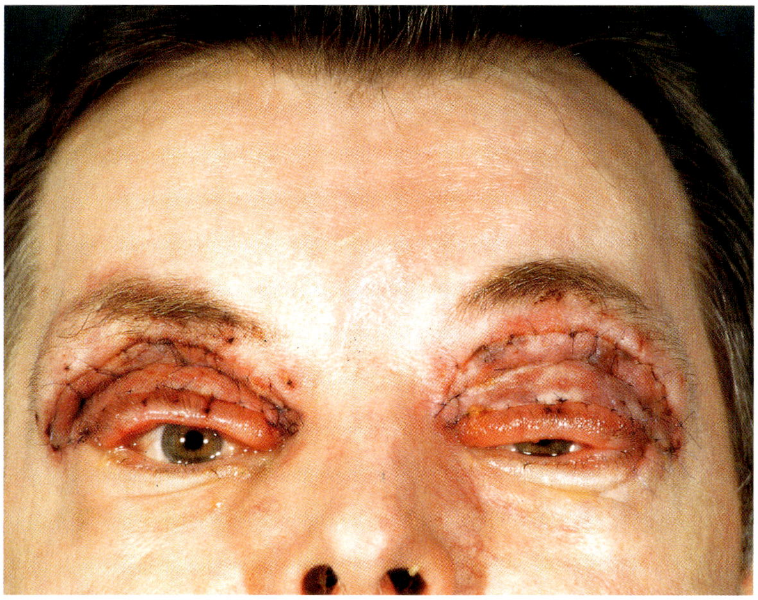

Figure 3.78d Appearance three days after the operation: The defects are covered on both sides with full thickness skin grafts from the post auricular area.

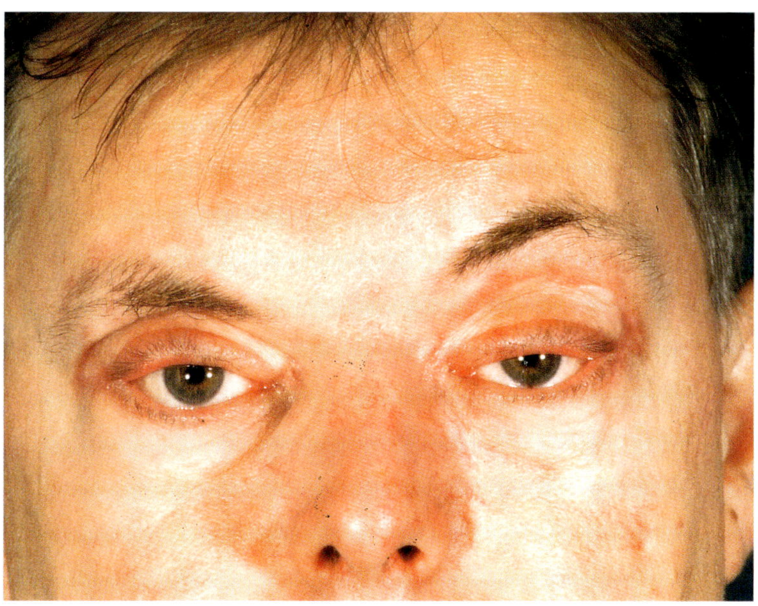

Figure 3.78e Appearance two months after the operation

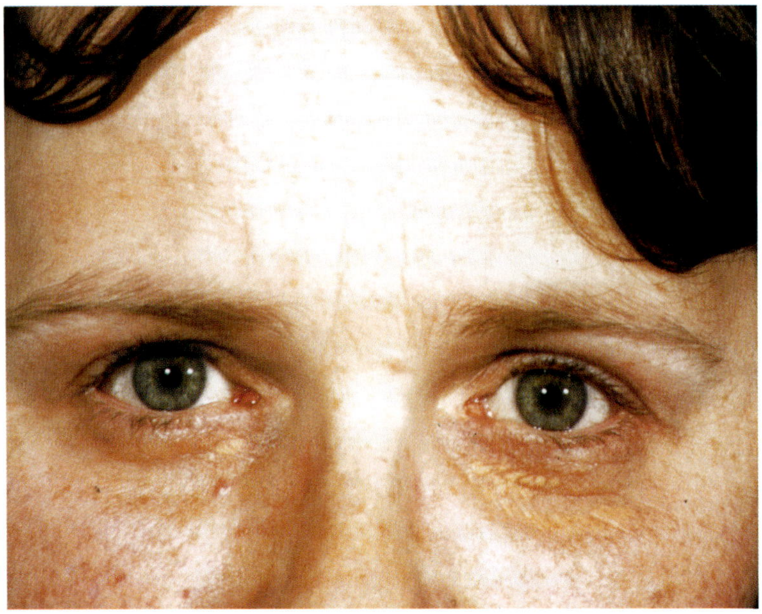

Figure 3.79a Xanthelasma of the left lower eyelid

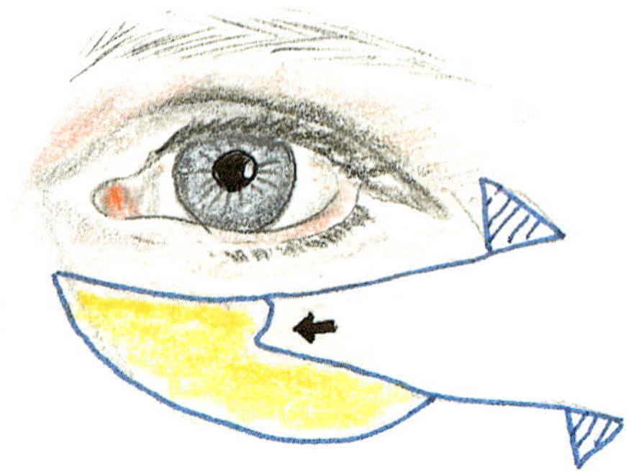

Figure 3.79b After the excision, a sliding flap carried out from a lateral approach using two Burow's triangles.

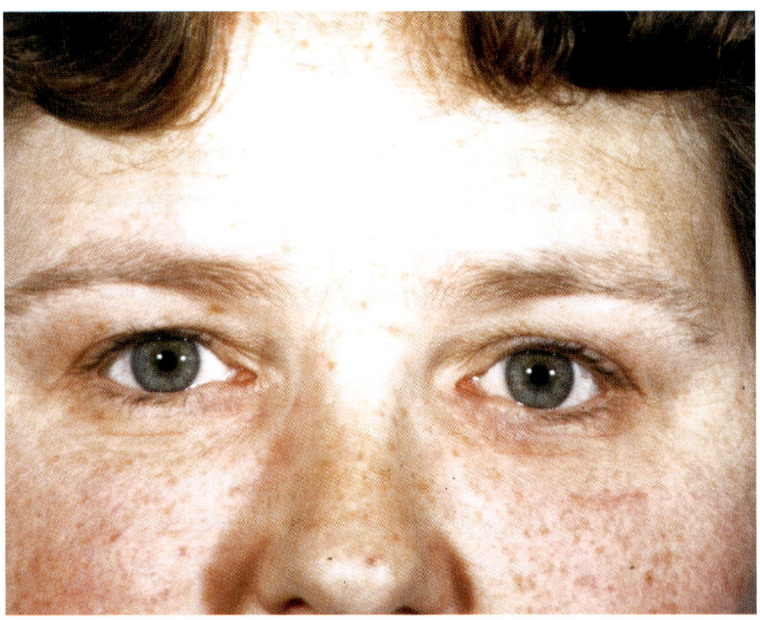

Figure 3.79c Appearance two years after the operation

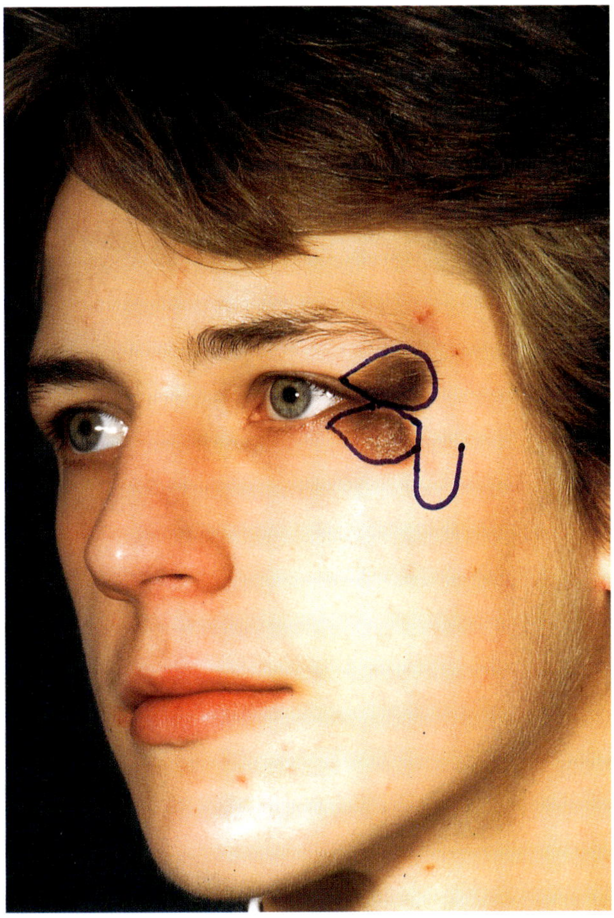

Figure 3.80a Nevus of the upper and lower eyelids. Planning of the operation: The nevus of the left lower eyelid is closed using a local, pedicled flap. The defect of the upper eyelid is treated after resection of the nevus using a full thickness skin graft from the post auricular area.

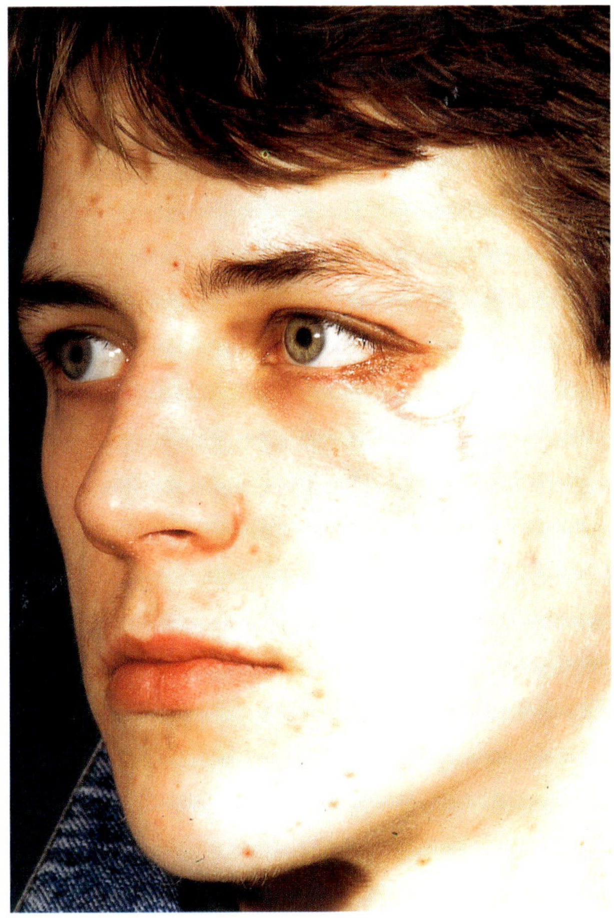

Figure 3.80b Appearance one year after the operation

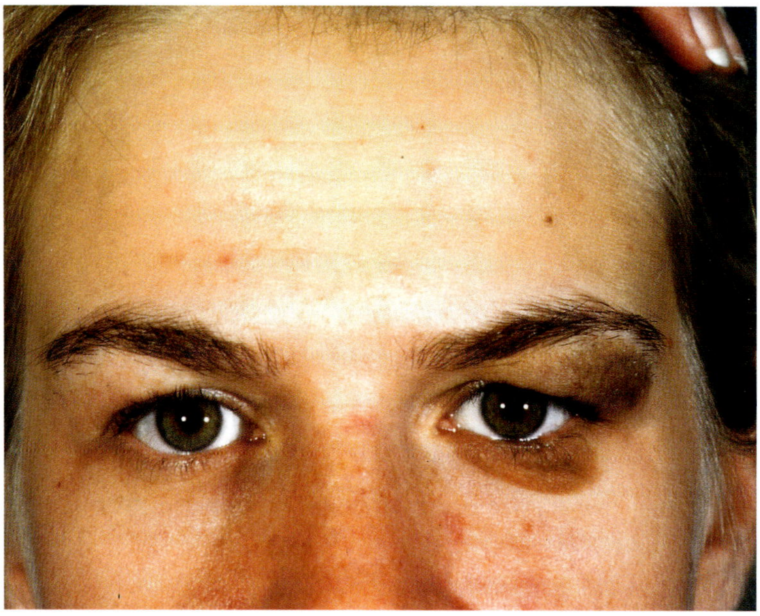

Figure 3.81a Nevus (giant nevus) of the left upper eyelid and left lower eyelid

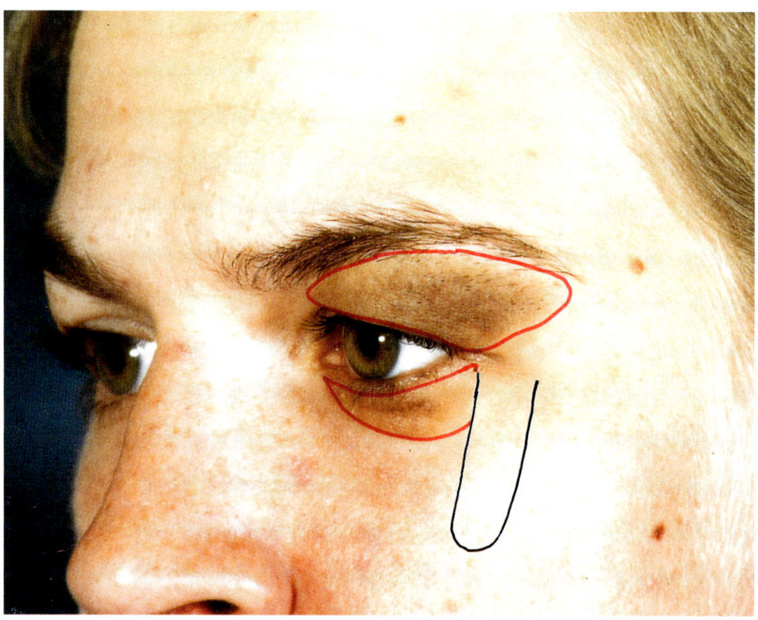

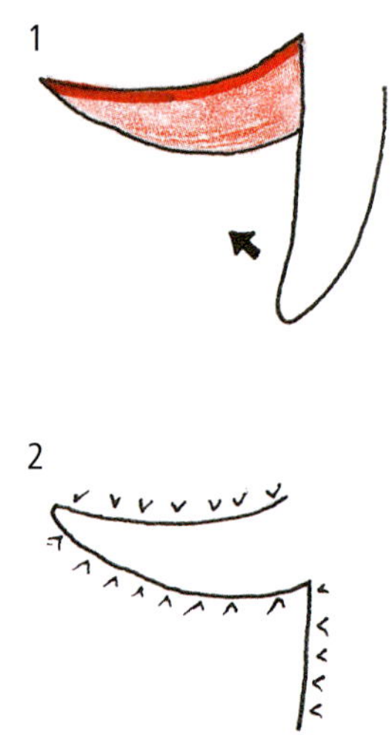

Figure 3.81b Planning of the operation: A combined procedure is planned with local flaps and a full thickness skin graft. The upper eyelid is treated with a full thickness skin graft from the post auricular area, and the lower eyelid is covered with a local flap. The flap design is chosen in such a way that tension in the donor area runs transversely and consequently does not pull on the lower eyelid (cf. scheme).

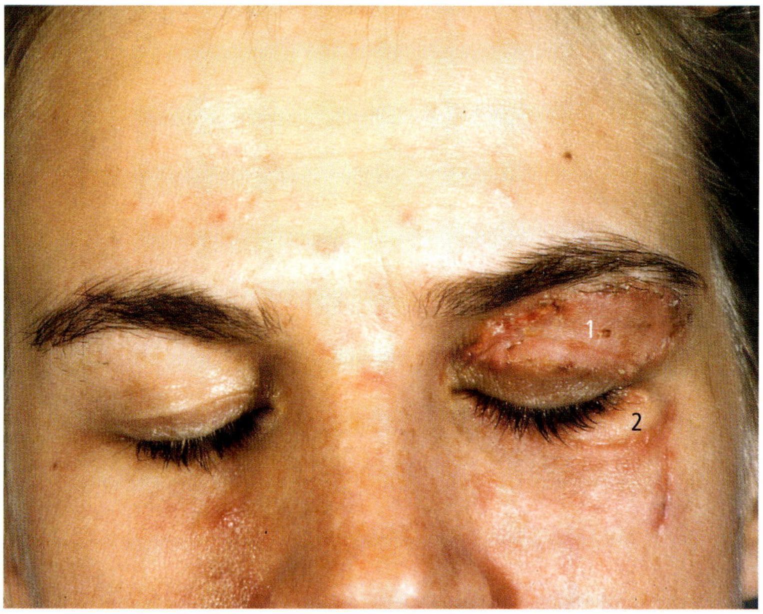

Figure 3.81d Appearance two weeks after the operation with the healed full thickness skin graft in the upper eyelid (1) as well as the healed local flap in the lower eyelid (2)

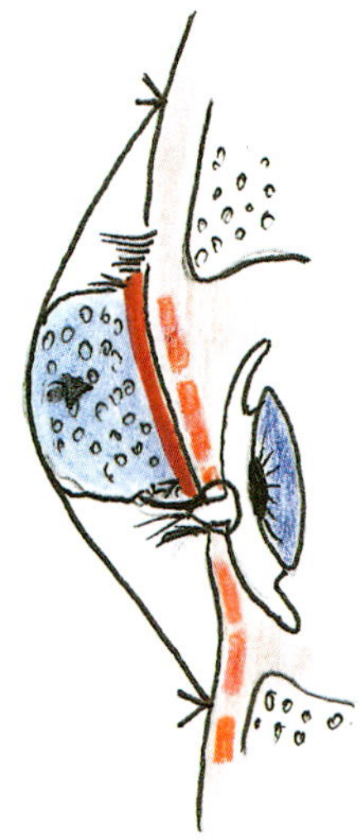

Figure 3.81e The full thickness skin graft is taken from the post-auricular area. The compression bandage is not fixed at the graft edge, but instead above the eyebrow and at the lower eyelid. Both eyelids are closed temporarily with a suture for five days. This kind of compression bandage produces better scar formation as well as better overall aesthetic results.

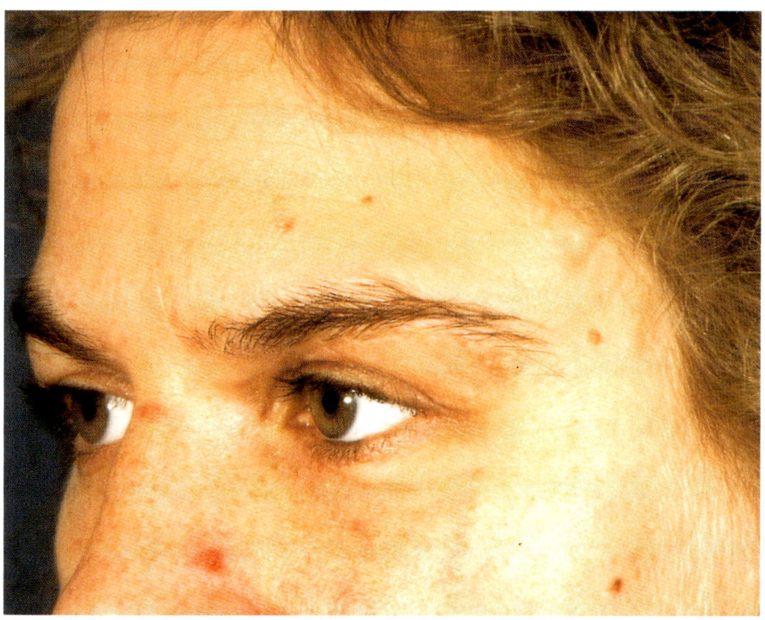

Figure 3.81f Appearance nine months after the operation

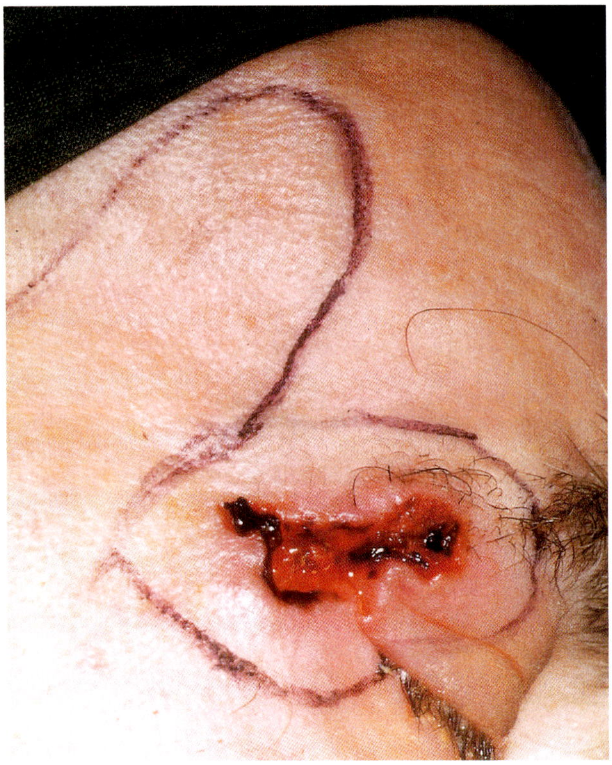

Figure 3.82a Basal cell carcinoma at the side of the orbital margin which infiltrated the lateral part of the upper eyelid, part of the lateral commissure and part of the lower eyelid.

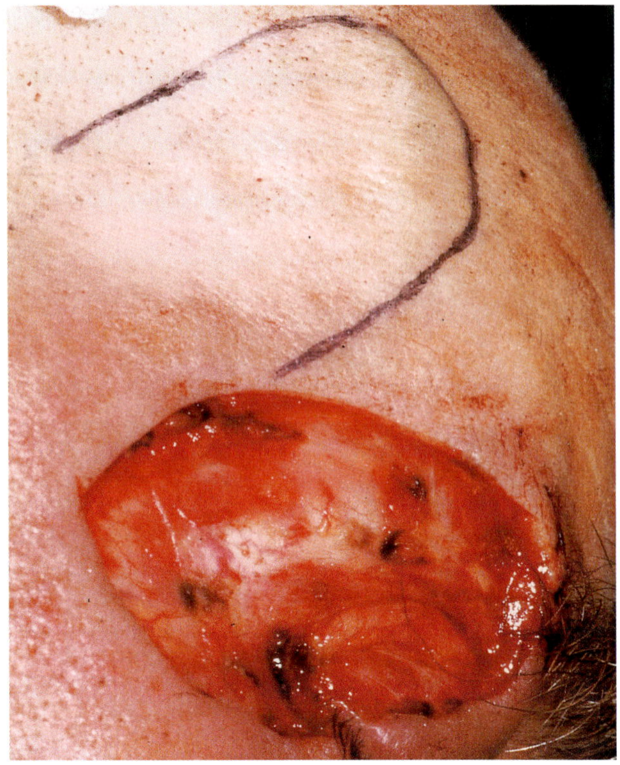

Figure 3.82b Microscopically controlled excision of the basal cell carcinoma. **Caution:** The frontal branch of the facial nerve can be injured here!

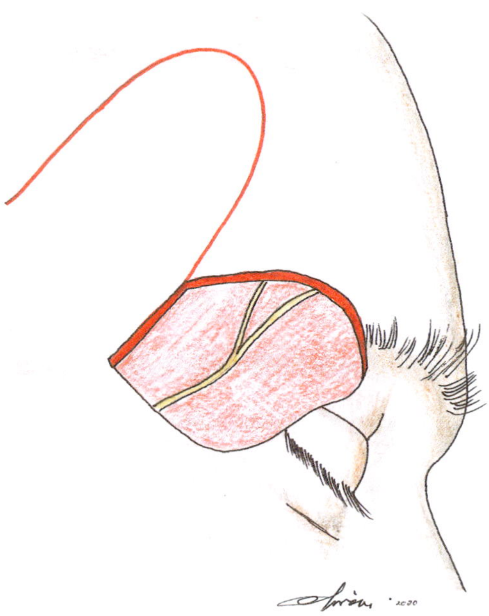

Figure 3.82b,c The excision is carried out. The lateral part of the upper eyelid is resected up to the orbital septum. The frontal branch of the facial nerve must be preserved if at all possible.

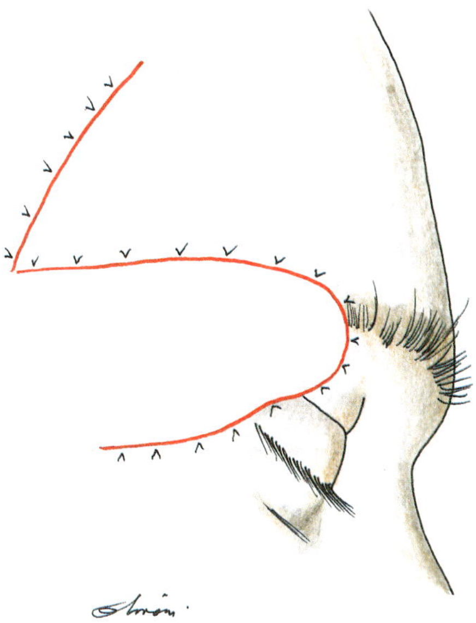

Figure 3.82d The axial temporal flap supplied by branches of the superior temporal artery is excellently supplied with blood. After mobilization the donor defect is closed primarily.

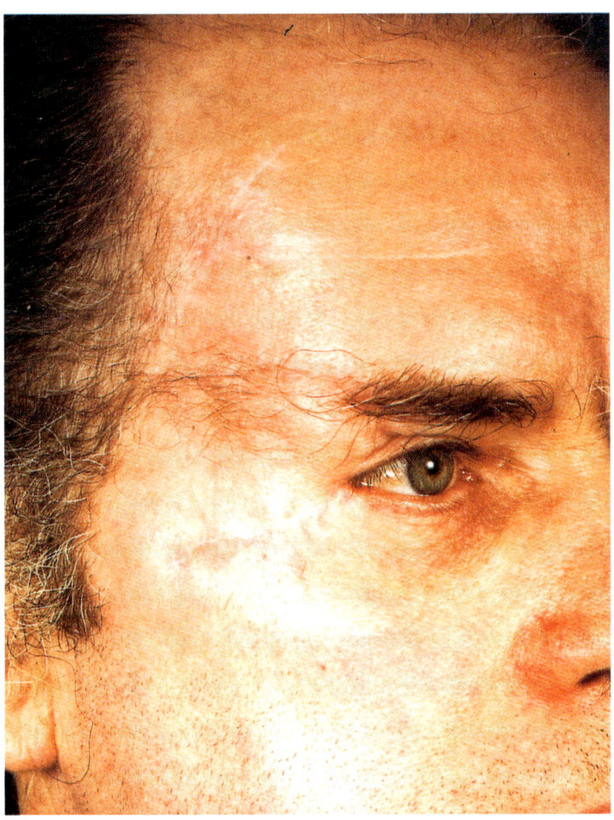

Figure 3.82e Appearance ten months postoperatively. It is not always easy to close the secondary defect primarily.

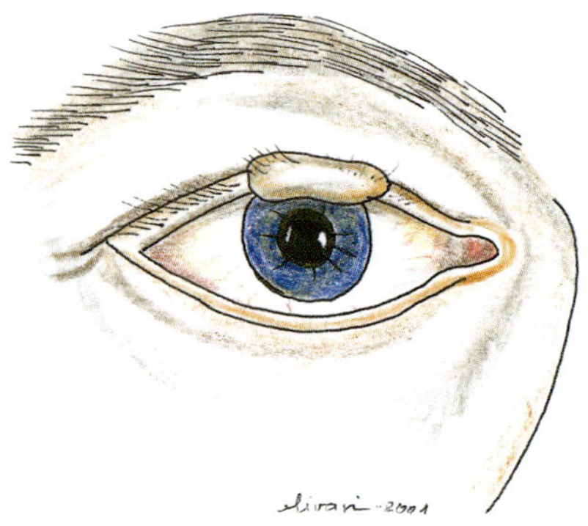

Figure 3.83a Basal cell carcinoma of the right upper eyelid

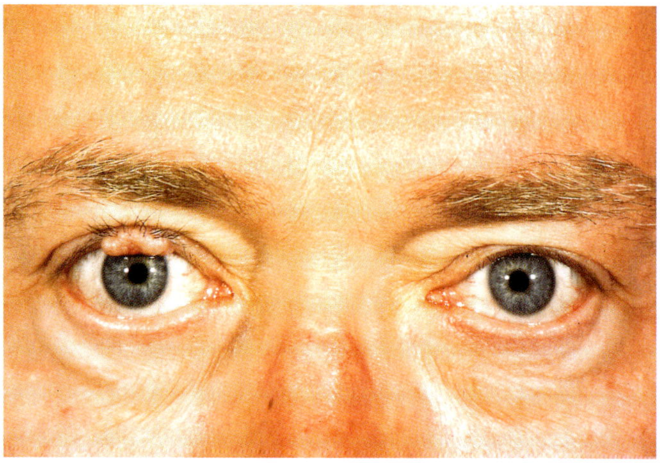

Figure 3.83b Basal cell carcinoma at the upper eyelid margin on the right site

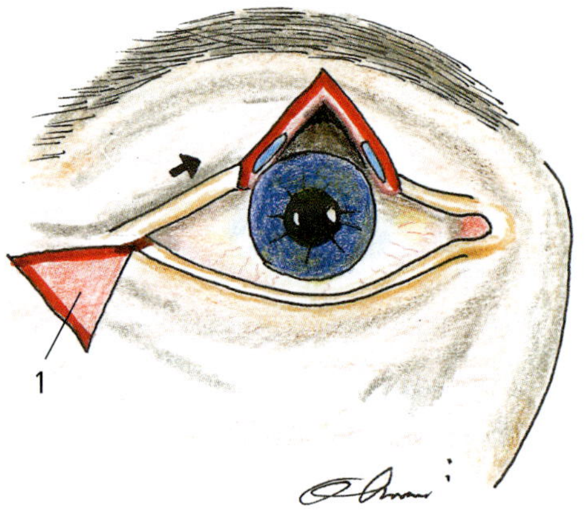

Figure 3.83c V excision is carried out. A Burow's triangle is excised laterally from the canthus (1). The lateral canthus (lateral ligament) is divided and mobilized medially.

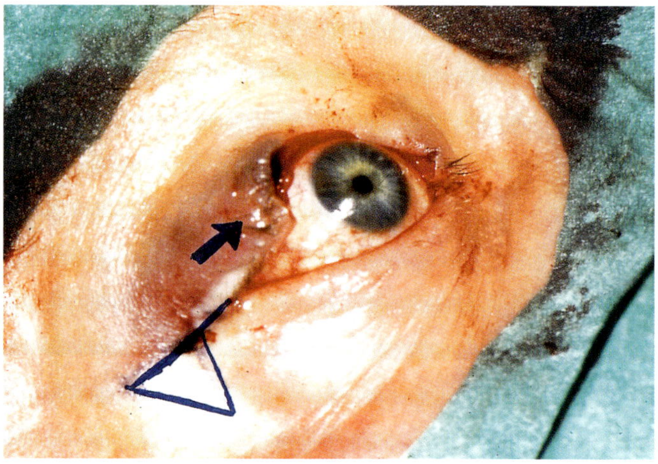

Figure 3.83d Intraoperative view

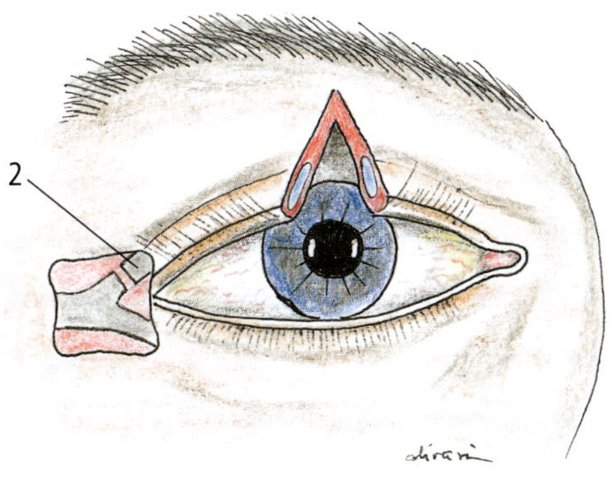

Figure 3.83e Appearance after excision of the Burow's triangle as well as dissection of the cranial flank (2) of the lateral ligament. The entire part of the upper eyelid is mobilized medially.

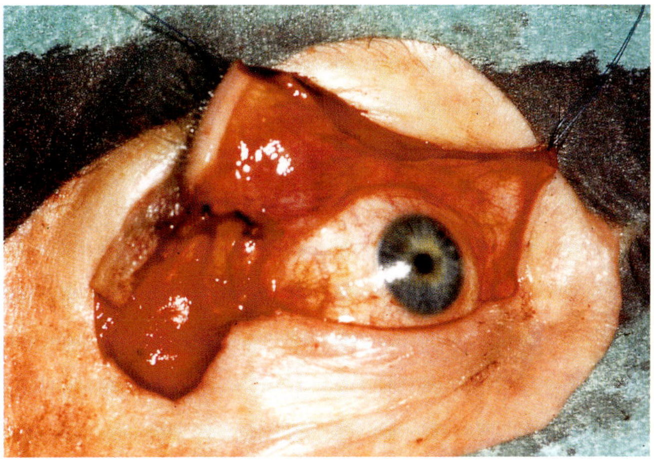

Figure 3.83f Appearance after excision of the tumor and Burow's triangle as well as complete mobilization.

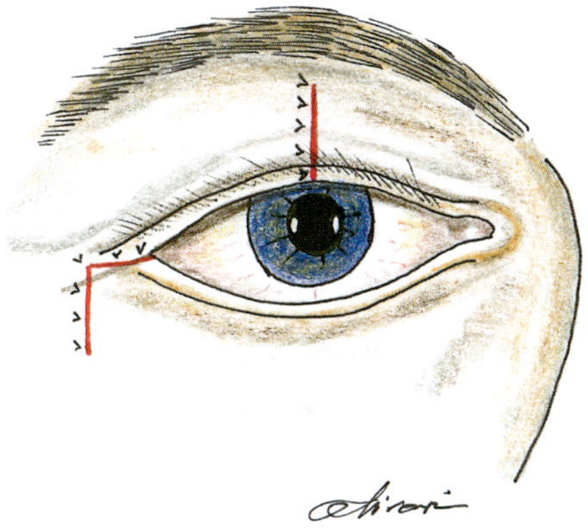

Figure 3.83g A tension-free closure of the defect and the Burow's triangle follows.

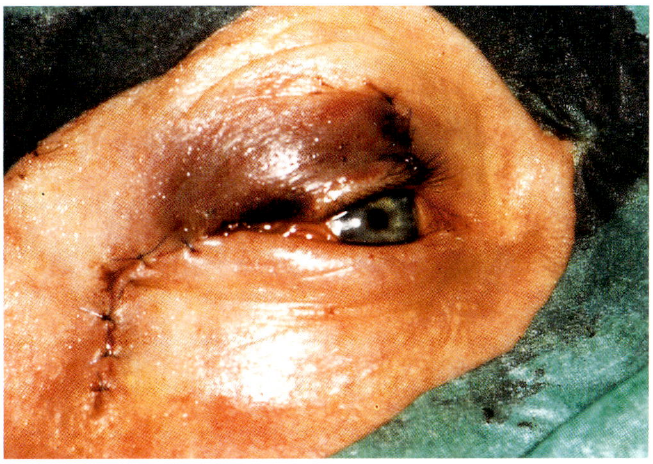

Figure 3.83h Appearance at the end of the operation

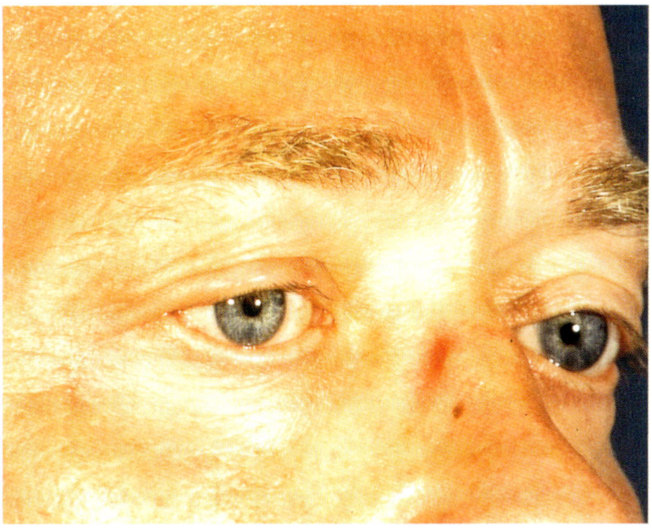

Figure 3.83i Appearance six months after the operation. More than a third of the upper eyelid could be reconstructed in this way.

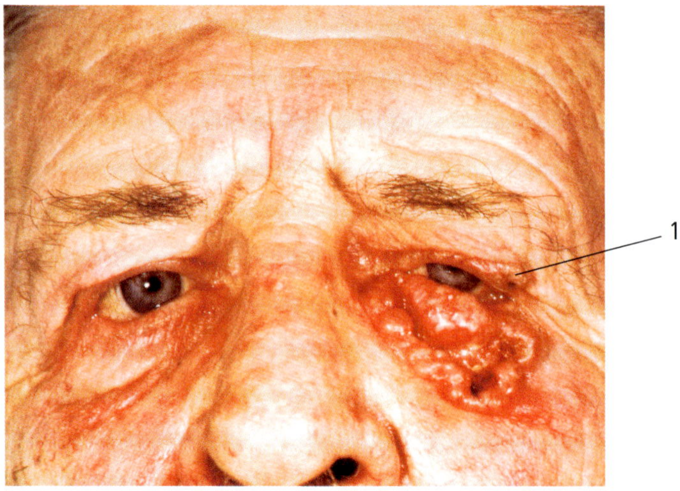

Figure 3.84a Basal cell carcinoma of the left lower eyelid: In places the tumor has infiltrated to the conjunctiva. A small basal cell carcinoma is also found at the lateral part of the left upper eyelid (1).

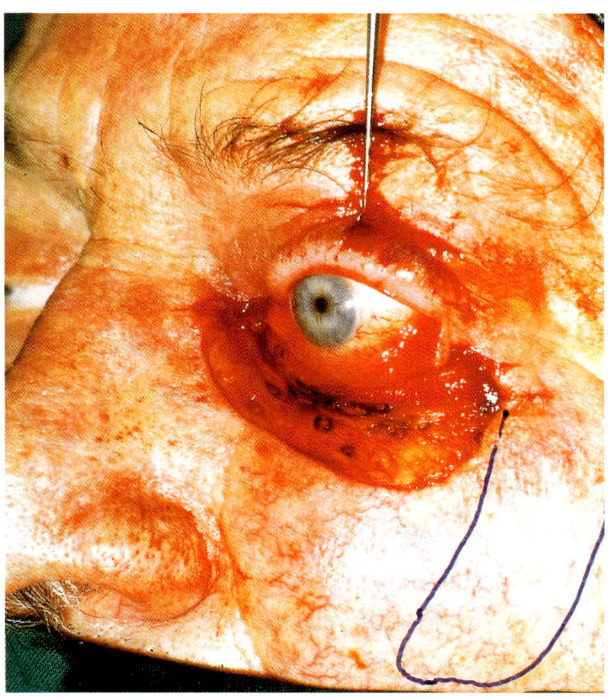

Figure 3.84b Resection of the tumor: A part of the conjunctiva could be preserved and mobilized. A cranial pedicled flap is planned from the left cheek.

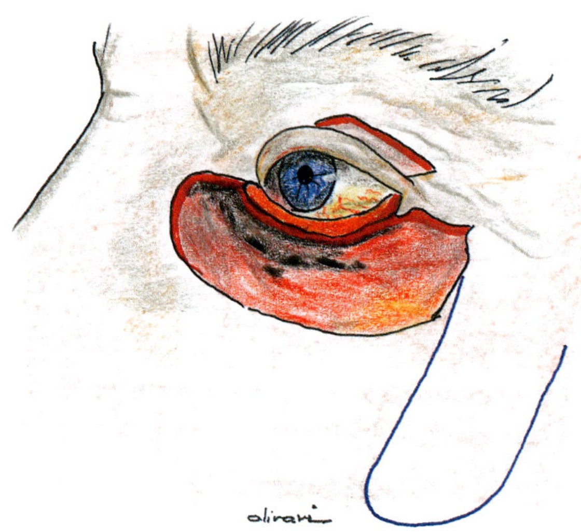

Figure 3.84c The flap must be of sufficient length. If doubts prevail, it is better to plan the flap a little longer because the coverage of the secondary defect does not present any special problems (this flap was first described in 1829 by Fricke)

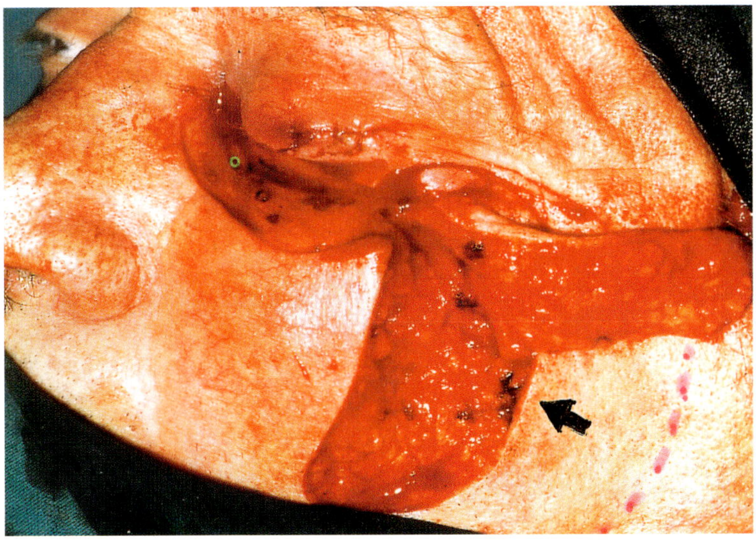

Figure 3.84d Mobilization of the flap: The cheek skin is undermined extensively in a lateral direction and the secondary defect closed. A small defect in the upper eyelid was closed primarily.

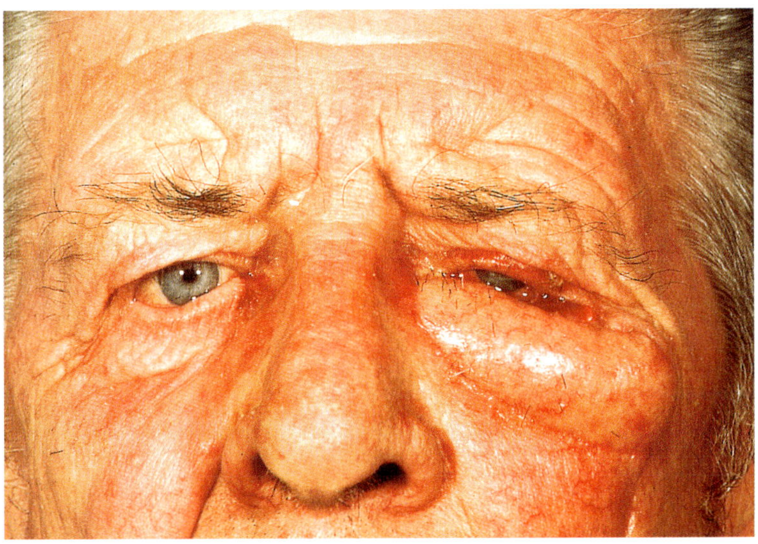

Figure 3.84e,f Appearance 15 months postoperatively

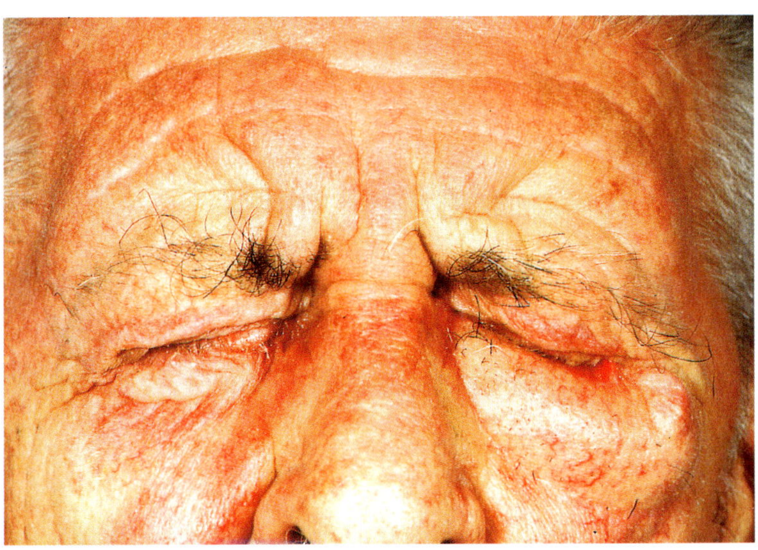

Figure 3.84f Eyelid closure was possible. The indolent patient refused any thinning of the flap.

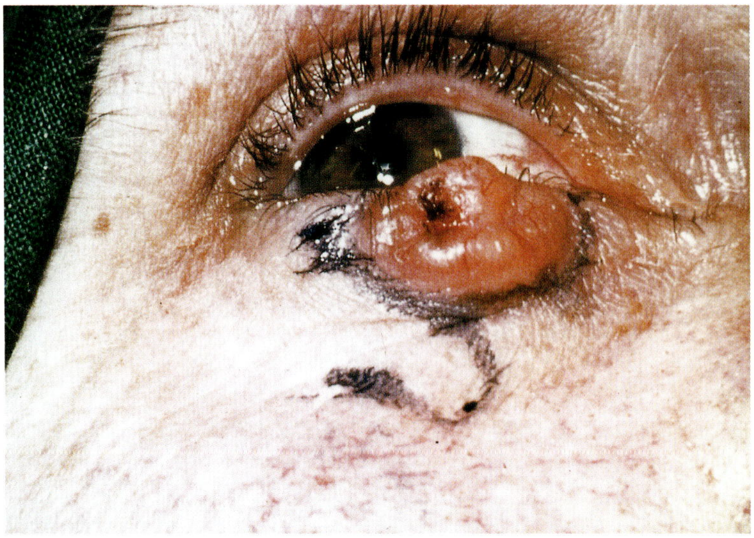

Figure 3.85a Small solid basal cell carcinoma in the lower eyelid: Planning of the operation

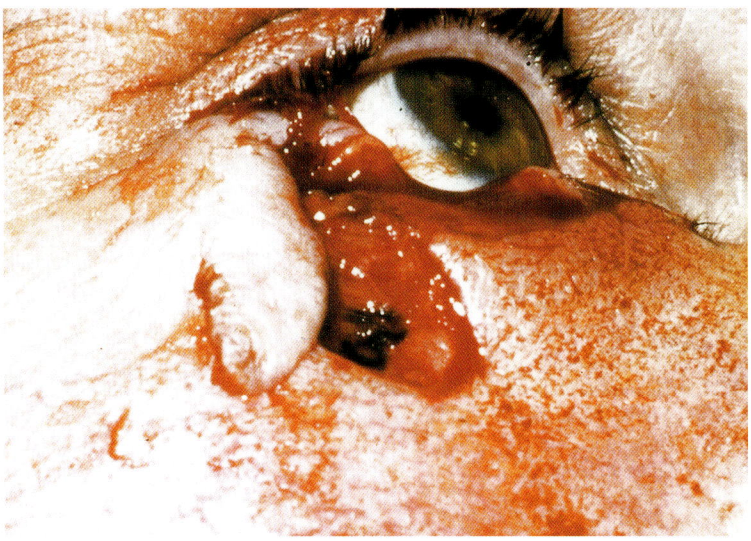

Figure 3.85b The excision was carried out. Part of the conjunctiva was also excised. A local flap is mobilized.

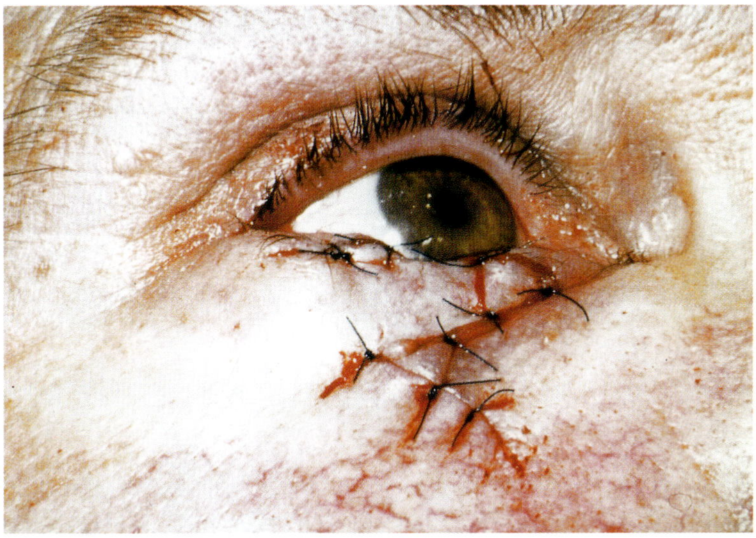

Figure 3.85c Defect closure is carried out using a local flap.

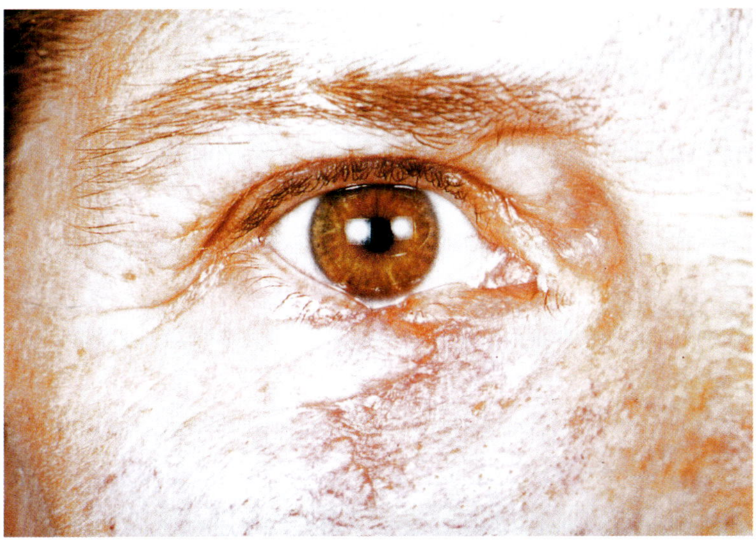

Figure 3.85d Appearance one year after the operation: Minimal "scleral show" and without functional disruption.

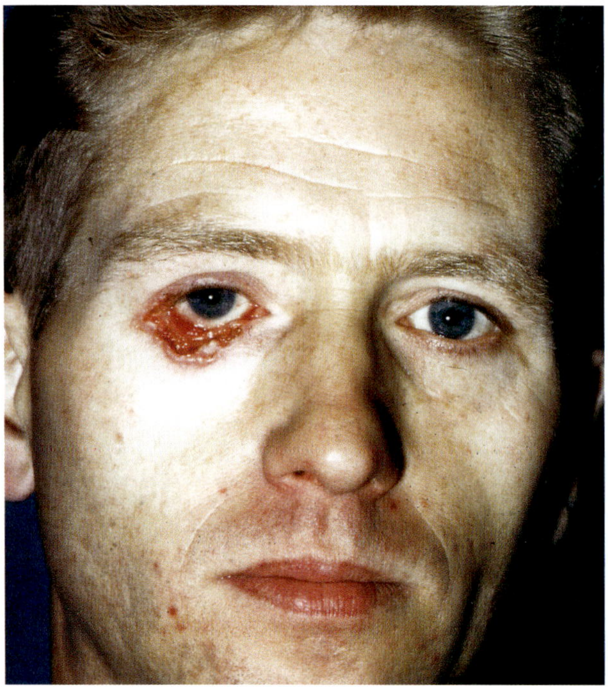

Figure 3.86a Basal cell carcinoma of the right lower eyelid as well as part of the right upper eyelid

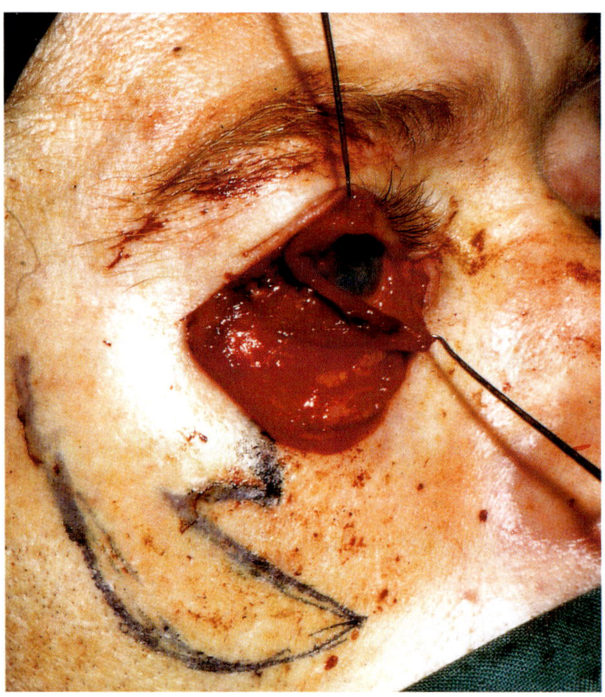

Figure 3.86b The tumor is excised far into the healthy tissue. In the lower eyelid; skin, tarsus, the orbicularis oculi muscle and part of the conjunctiva are removed. In the upper eyelid, the lateral part was excised which included skin, tarsus, the orbicularis oculi muscle and part of the conjunctiva.

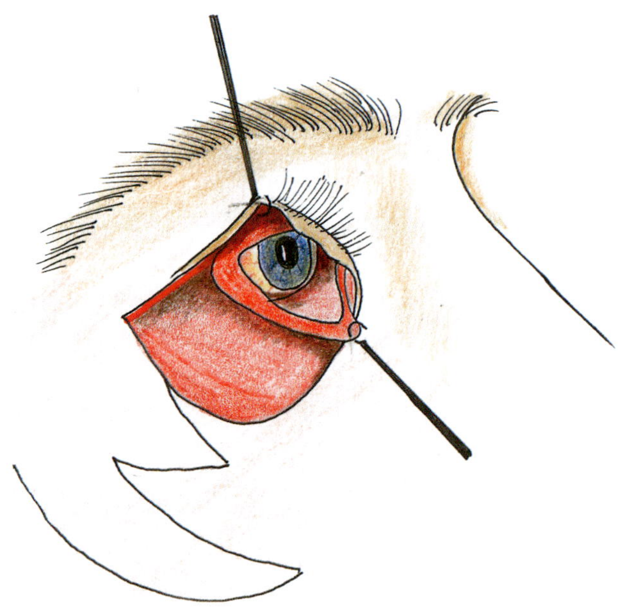

Figure 3.86c A transposition flap is planned for defect coverage. The remaining conjunctiva was mobilized completely in order to form the inner lining. A cranial pedicled skin flap is formed laterally to the lateral canthus in such a way that two flap tips are formed (one smaller for the upper eyelid and one larger for the lower eyelid). This represents a modification of Fricke's method.

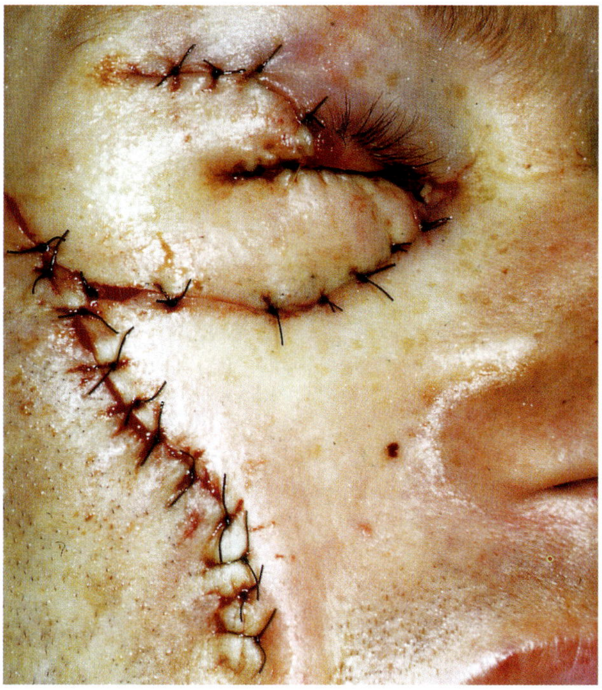

Figure 3.86d Appearance at the end of the operation: The secondary defect is closed primarily. The flap was thinned out at a later date.

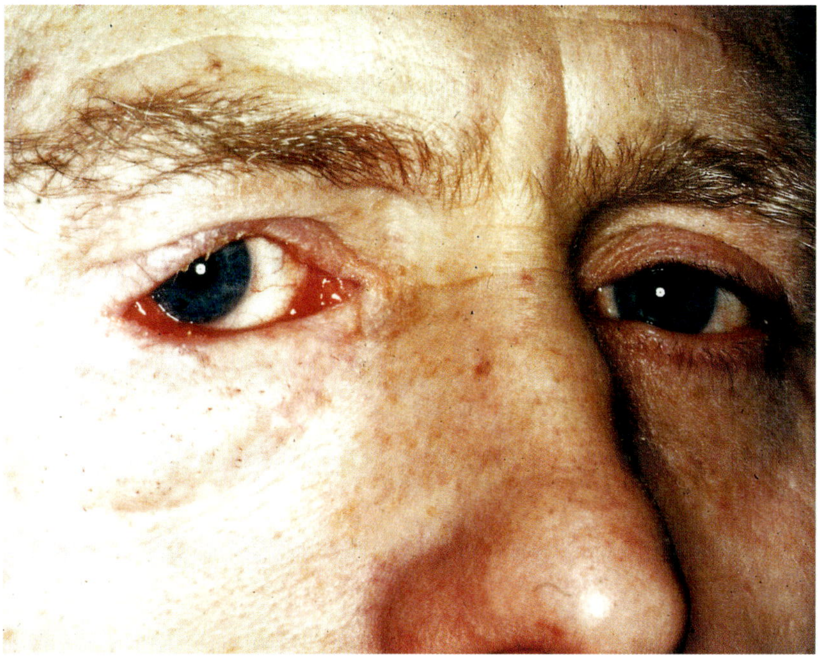

Figure 3.86e Appearance two years after the operation

Blepharoplasty

Blepharoplasty is one of the most frequent operations in plastic surgery. Most interventions are carried out under local anesthesia. This operation gives the patient a good aesthetic result provided the technique is correct.

One can not describe blepharoplasty as an easy operation. The learning curve is not short and aesthetic problems (usually temporary) resulting from poor technique are annoying both for the patient and the surgeon.
Amongst the most frequent causes of error are:

a) Inadequately sized incision and inadequate resection of the upper eyelid.
b) Excessive skin resection in the lower eyelid.
c) The prolapsed intraorbital fat, particularly in the medial part, is not resected or repositioned in the orbit.
d) The incisions in the upper and lower eyelid laterally should be 8 to 10 mm apart, otherwise a vertical scar might arise that produces "button eyes".
e) Too much intraorbital fat is removed.

Most blepharoplasties are carried out for aesthetic reasons. A smaller number (approx. 10 %) are indicated arising from medical conditions e.g. due to restrictions of field of sight.

The blepharoplasty is usually carried out under local anesthesia. It should be injected slowly to avoid pain during the injection. Hemostasis must be carried out by bipolar cauterization until absolute dryness is achieved at the end of the operation.

Incision in Blepharoplasty

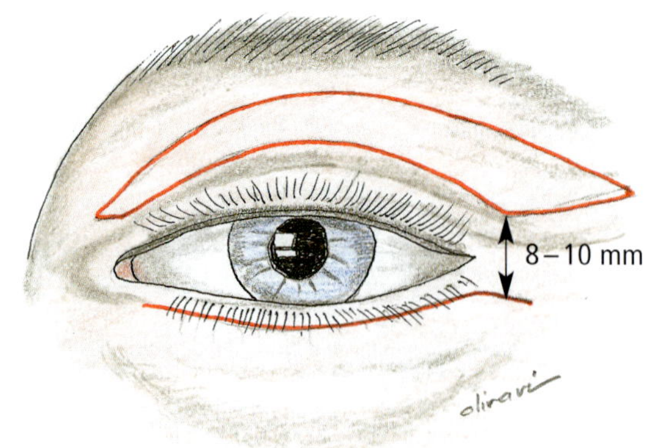

Figure 3.87 Incision for a blepharoplasty

In the upper eyelid the course of the lower arched incision (with raised eyebrows) runs in the middle area 8 to 10 mm above the eyelid margin, and lifts at the lateral commissure somewhat laterocranially to where it meets the upper incision.

The upper incision is determined by the surplus skin quantity to be excised. It should, however, be no higher than 15 mm from the raised eyebrow.

The incision in the lower eyelid runs 2 to 3 mm below the eyelid margin and is shorter than the incision in the upper eyelid.

In two thirds of blepharoplasty cases, it is necessary to remove the prolapsed fat in the medial and lateral area of the upper eyelid. It is even more important to remove the isolated medial fat cushion.

In the lower eyelid the fat is divided by two septa into thirds; all three parts should be removed. *Note:* Do not remove too much fat, but only the part that is spontaneously prolapsed. Otherwise there is a risk that a "hollow eye" might be produced. In older patients it is recommended that eyelid bags are treated as a hernia. Proptosis of fat can be repositioned by suturing of orbital septum and not by resection of fat.

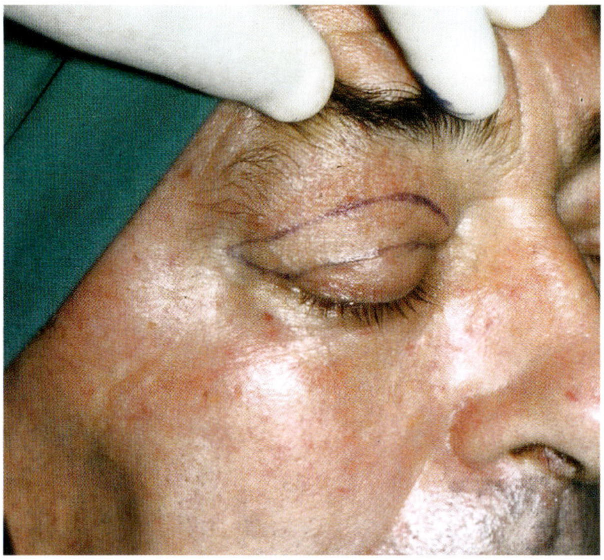

Figure 3.88a Incision line in the upper eyelid. The lower incision lies in the middle of the eyelid 8 to 10 mm away from the eyelid margin. The incision should proceed laterally. The upper incision is 15 mm away from the eyebrow.

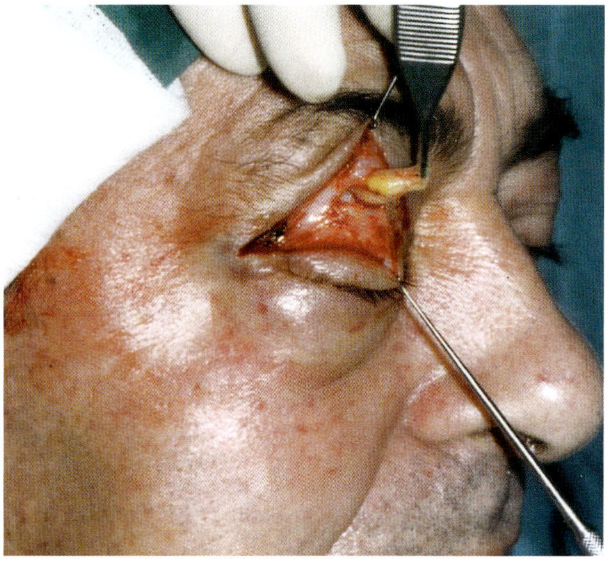

Figure 3.88b After resection of the skin, the fat in the middle part, but also very importantly that in the medial part, is removed. For this purpose the orbital septum must be incised transversely. The orbicularis oculi muscle can be resected in stripes (depending on the local situation).

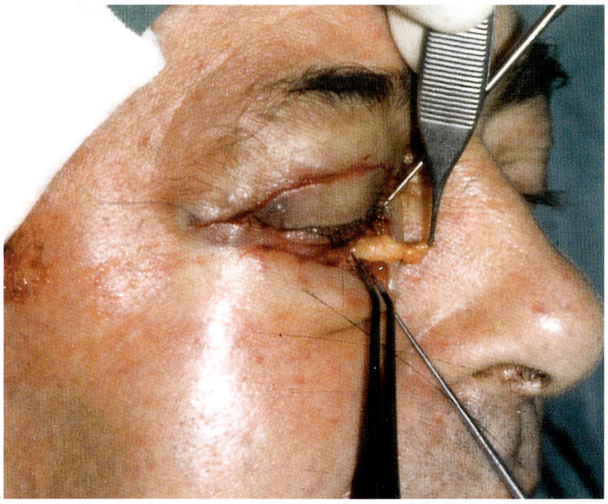

Figure 3.88c Fat removal in the lower eyelid proceeds medially and laterally. The incision in the lower eyelid is considerably shorter than that in the upper eyelid. The fat should never be grasped with a clamp. For fat removal coagulation is carried out before the incision!

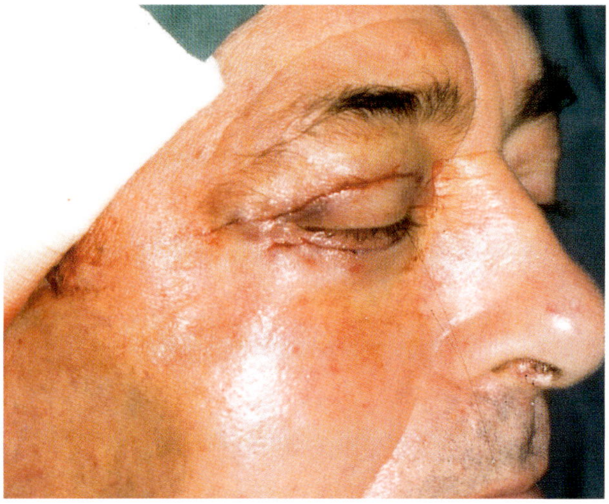

Figure 3.88d The skin excision in the lower eyelid is closed carefully without tension! There should be a distance of 8 to 10 mm between the upper lid and lower lid incisions. An inadequate gap can result in vertical scarring (button eyes). Intracutaneous suturing with 6×0 nylon. No interrupted sutures should be used because of the pain that may occur during suture removal.

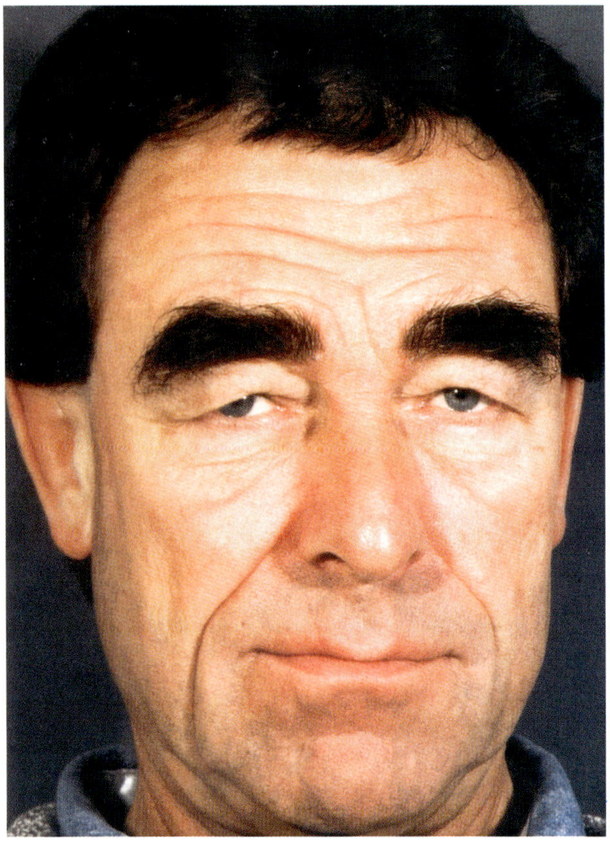

Figure 3.89a Blepharochalasis with restriction of field of view above and laterally. Clear medical indication.

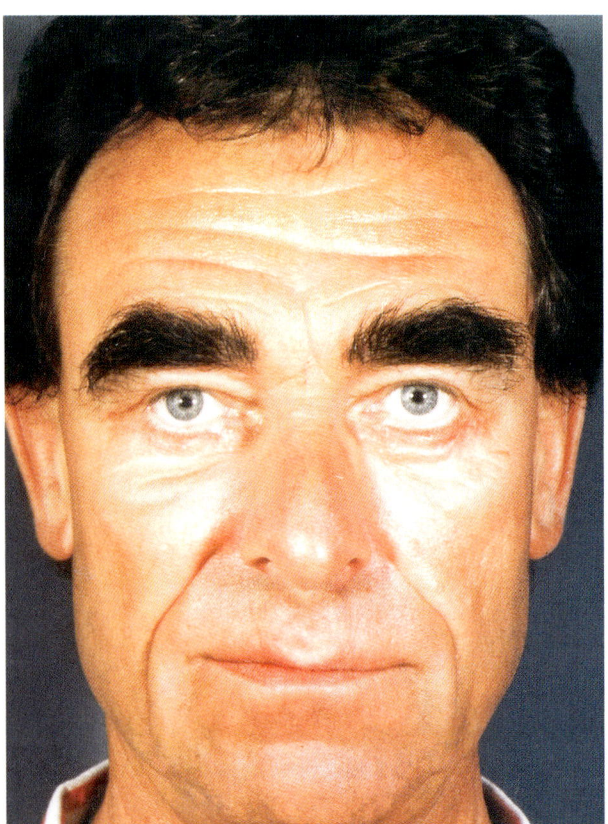

Figure 3.89b Appearance after blepharoplasty. Only the upper eyelids were corrected. A small amount of fat was removed.

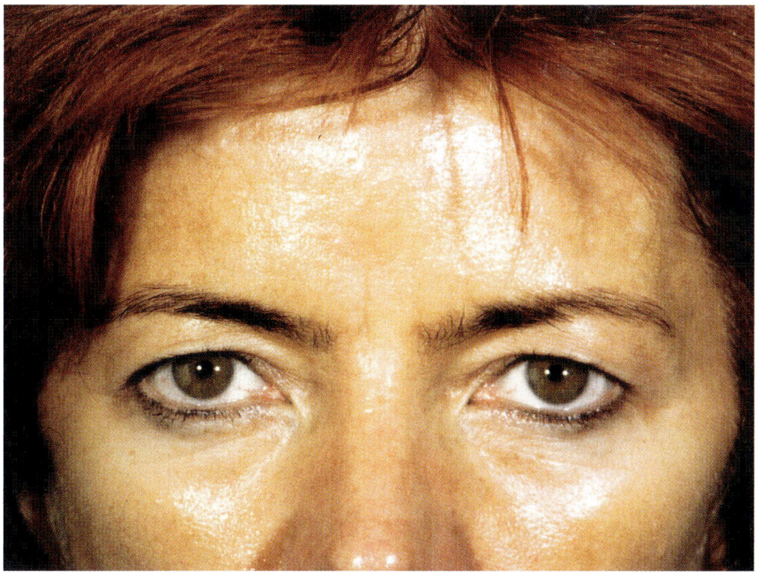

Figure 3.90a Moderate blepharochalasis (genetically caused). Aesthetic indication.

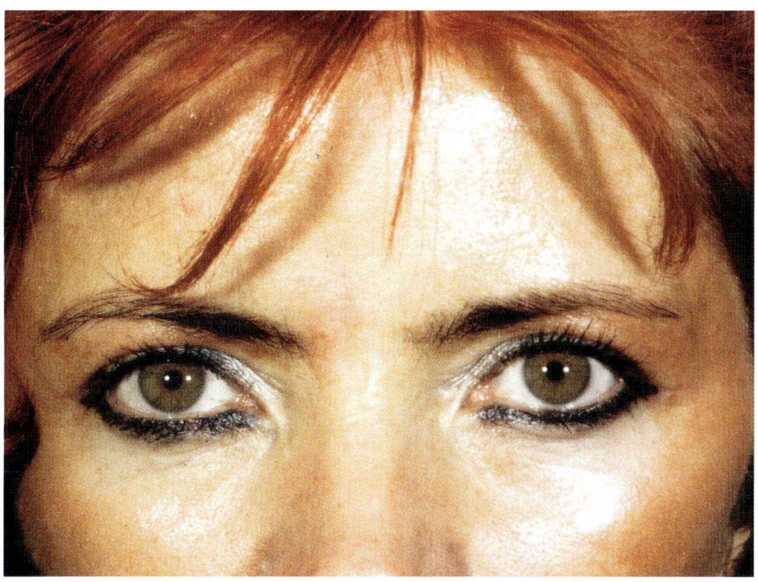

Figure 3.90b Appearance six months postoperatively. Only the upper eyelids were corrected. A small amount of fat was removed.

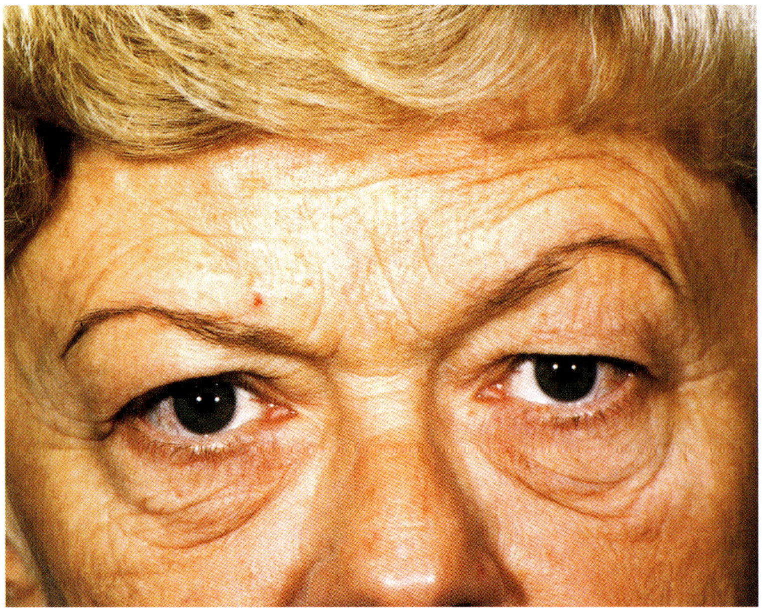

Figure 3.91a Asymmetric blepharochalasis (dermochalasis), slack lower eyelid skin. To the left there is a restriction in the visual field above and laterally. The patient has to lift his left eyebrow in order to see better.

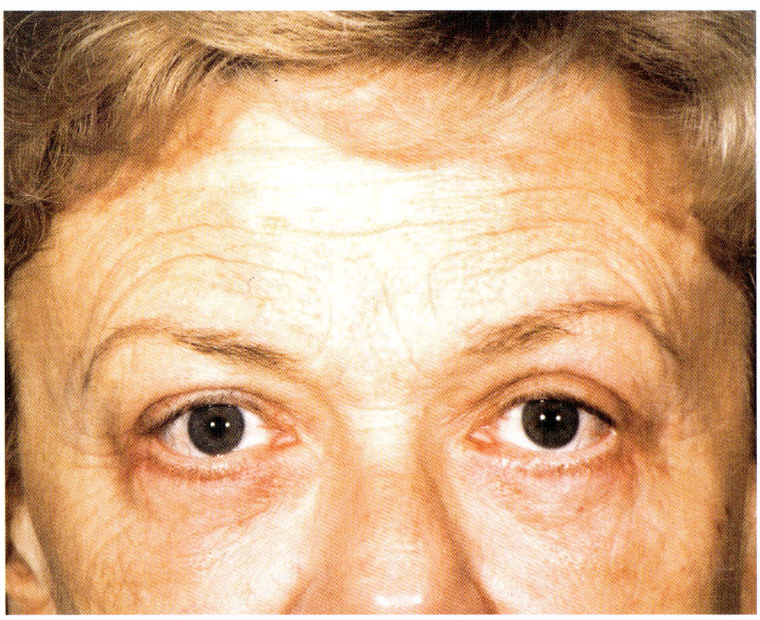

Figure 3.91b Appearance six months postoperatively. Generous excision of the upper eyelid skin as well as the lower eyelid skin. Minimal fat removal.

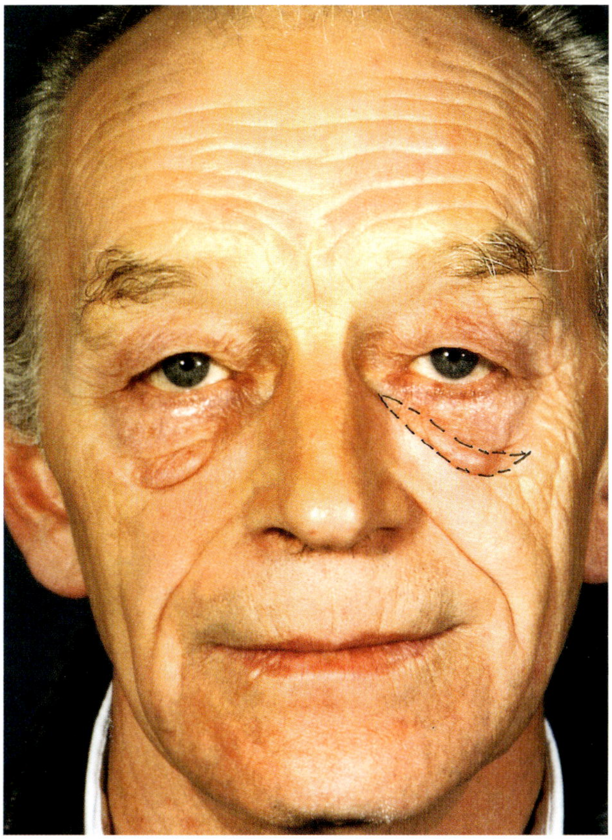

Figure 3.92a Slack skin in the upper eyelid as well as at the lower edge of the orbit. The upper eyelid is corrected in standard fashion. In the lower eyelid the surplus skin is excised after careful measurement. The resection is marked with a dashed line.

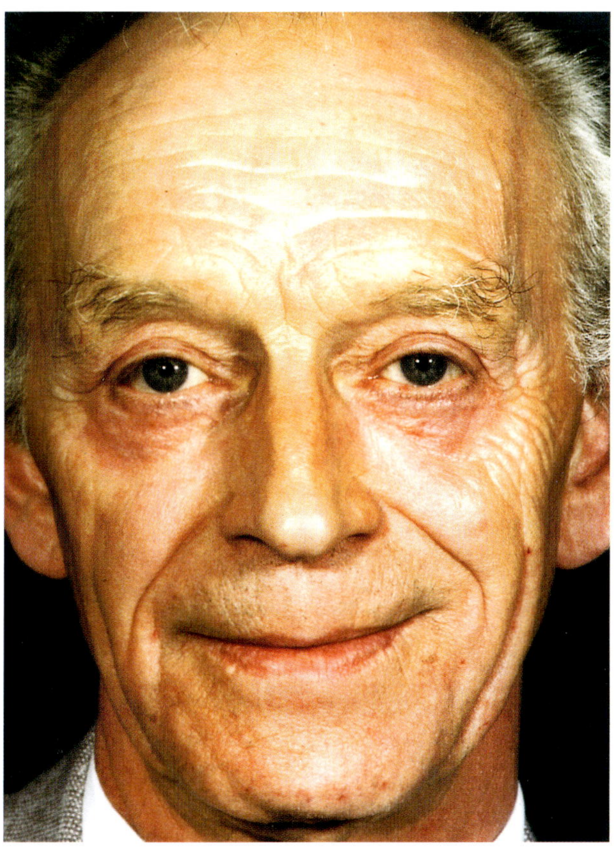

Figure 3.92b Appearance one year postoperatively. No fat tissue removal. Such a local excision can be carried out with older patients. The scars are barely visible after three months.

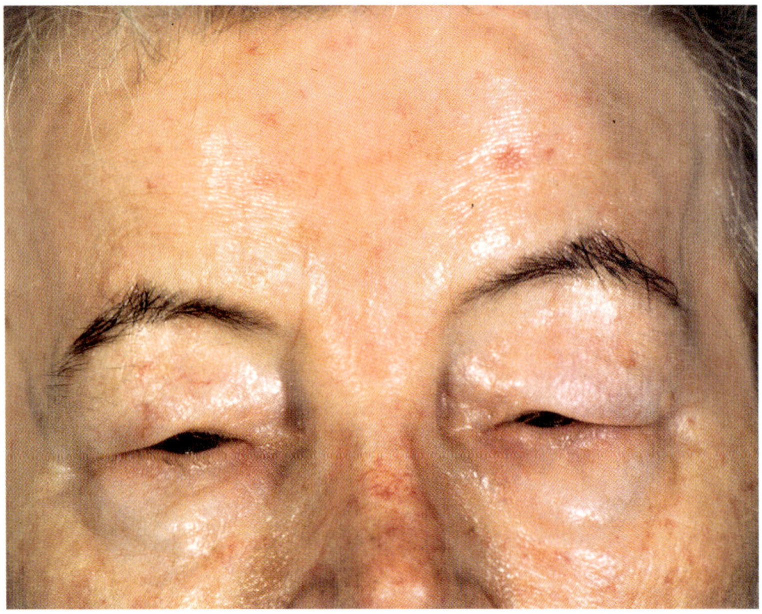

Figure 3.93a Blepharophimosis caused by excessive skin, but particularly by fat hernias above and below, that have arisen because of the lax orbital septum. Considerable restriction of field of sight. The operation was indicated for medical reasons.

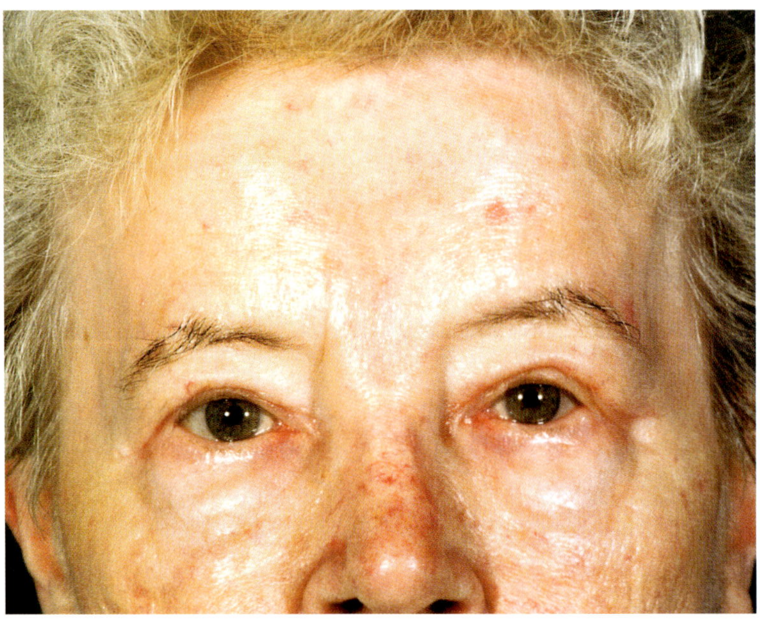

Figure 3.93b Appearance three months postoperatively. A lot of skin was excised in the upper eyelid area and prolapsed fat was removed. In the lower eyelid area a lot of fat was removed and only a minimal skin resection was carried out.

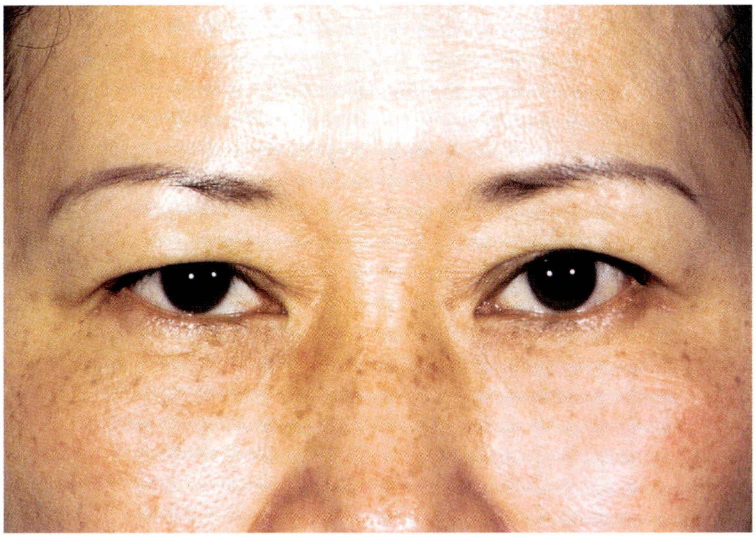

Figure 3.94a Asiatic eyes. In fact a normal, ethnically conditioned appearance.

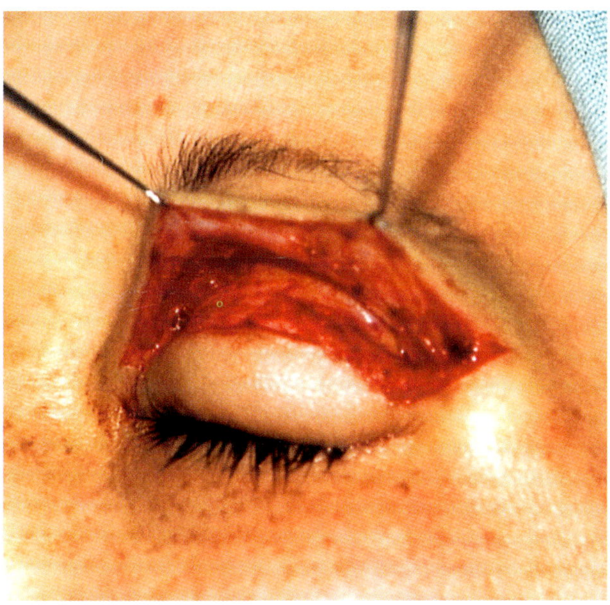

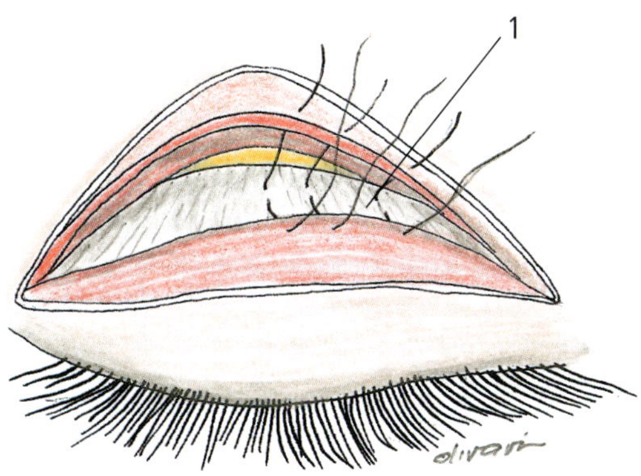

Figure 3.94b,c After moderate excision of the upper eyelid skin the orbicularis oculi muscle is transversely divided. In the area of the future fold the orbicularis oculi muscle is fixed to the levator aponeurosis (1) and an eyelid fold is shaped.

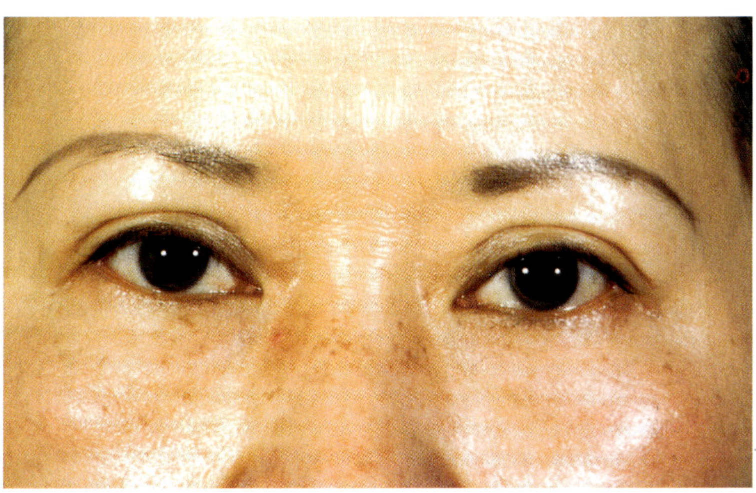

Figure 3.94d Appearance two years post-operatively

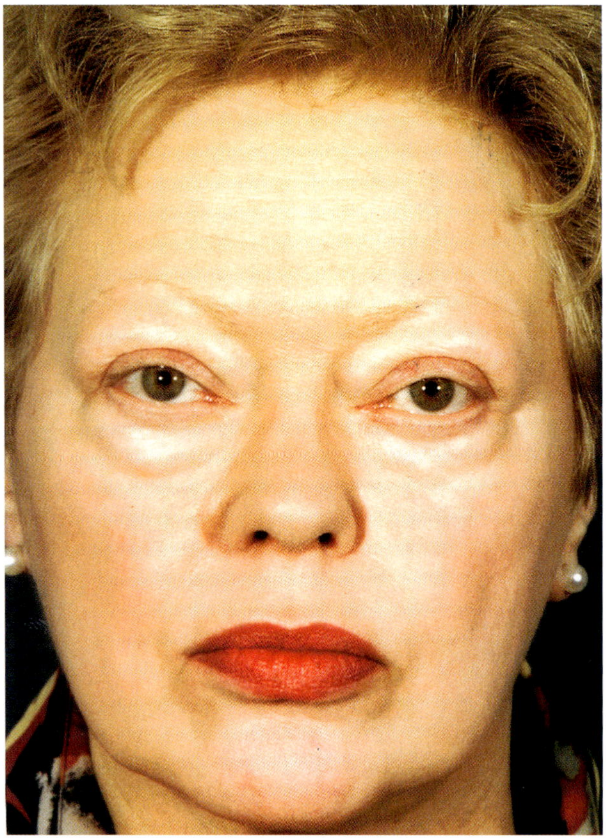

Figure 3.95a Severe fat herniation in the upper and lower eyelid with a weak orbital septum. Hardly any skin surplus exists.

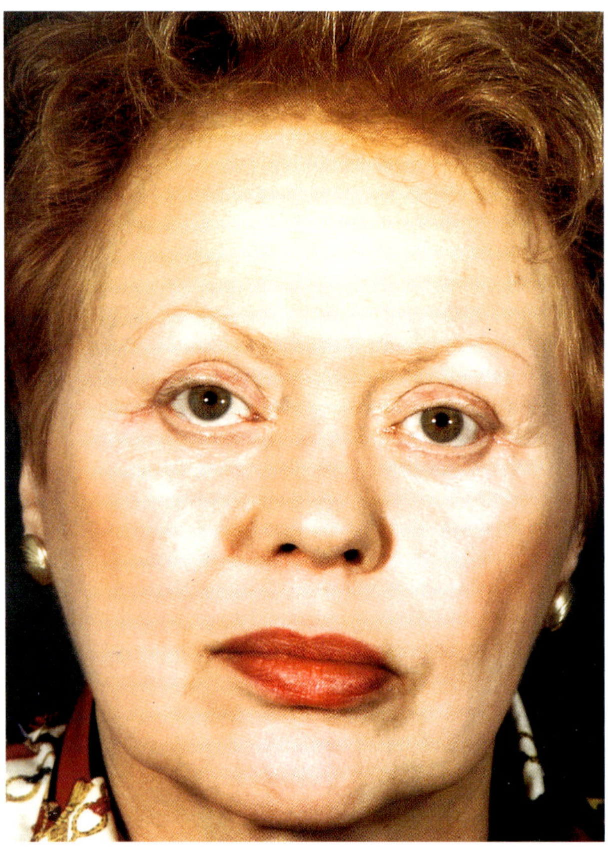

Figure 3.95b Appearance 16 months postoperatively. Small skin excision in the upper eyelid. Only fat is removed transconjunctivally in the lower eyelid medially and laterally.

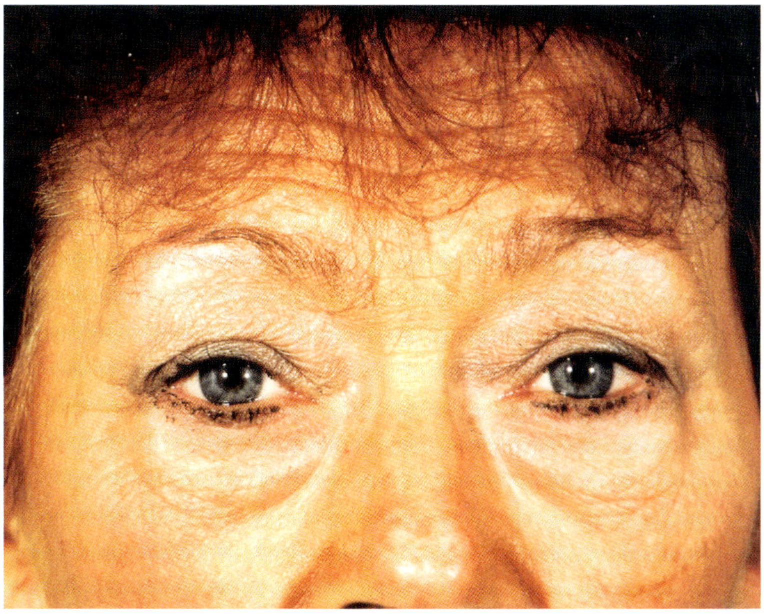

Figure 3.96a Slack eyelids and bulging orbital fat in the upper and lower eyelids with "eye bag". No disturbance of vision. Purely cosmetic indication.

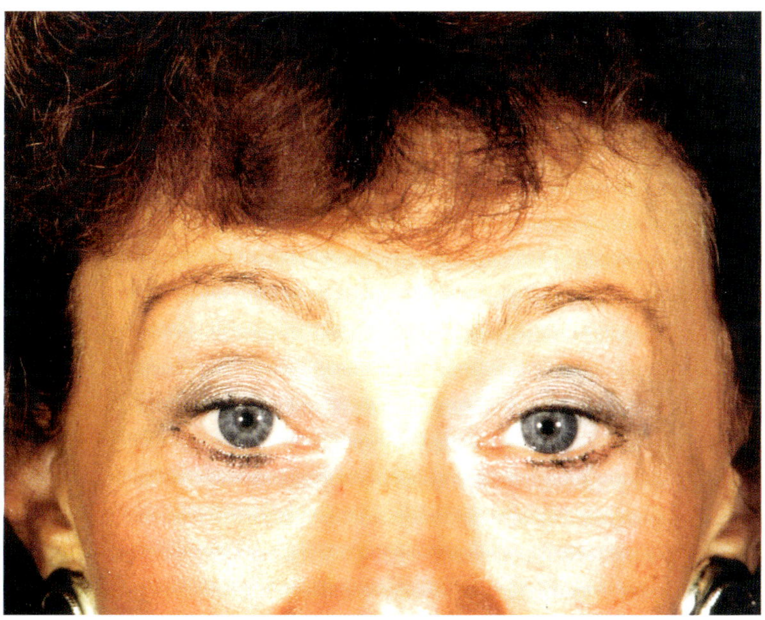

Figure 3.96b Appearance one year postoperatively. In the upper eyelid much skin was excised and fat was removed in the medial part. In the lower eyelid little skin but more fat was removed medially and laterally.

Transconjunctival Periorbital Fat Removal in the Lower Eyelid

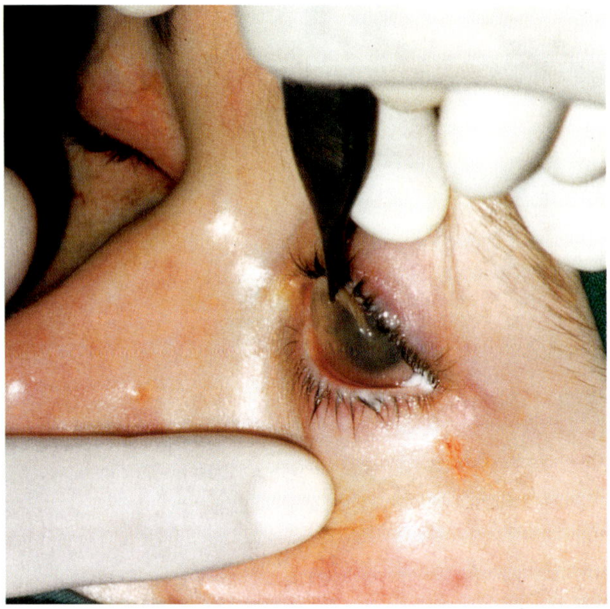

Figure 3.97a A silicon plate is introduced to protect the cornea.

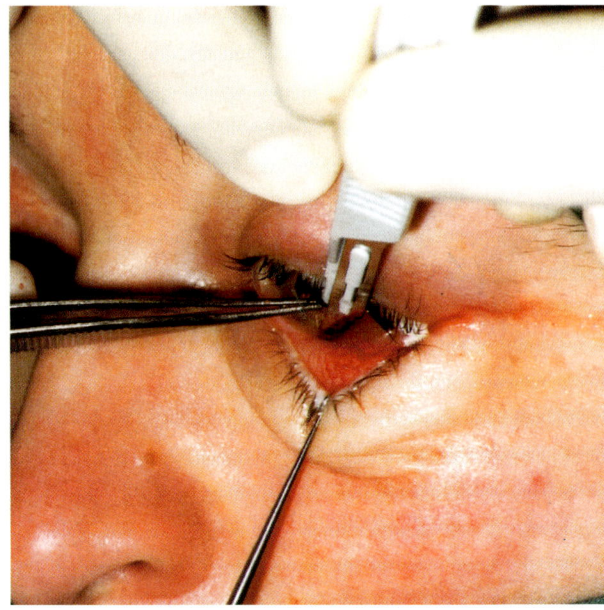

Figure 3.97b Under local anesthesia a transverse incision in the conjunctiva between the tarsus and fornix is carried out. The 1 cm incision runs transversely.

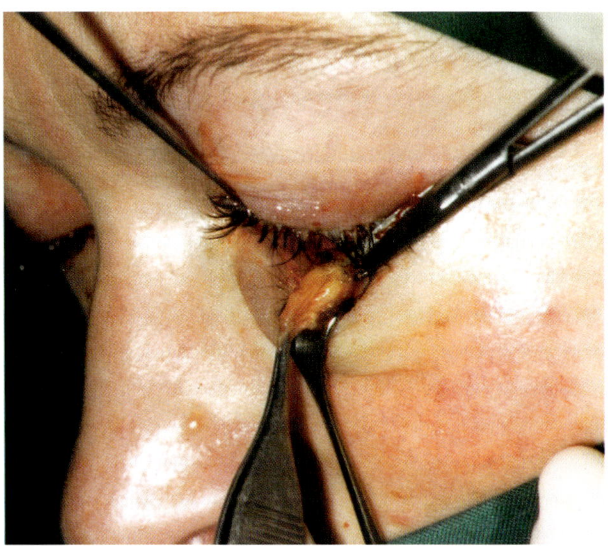

Figure 3.97c The fat is removed from the medial, middle and lateral part of the lower eyelid. By spreading with the scissors all three fat compartments can be easily reached.

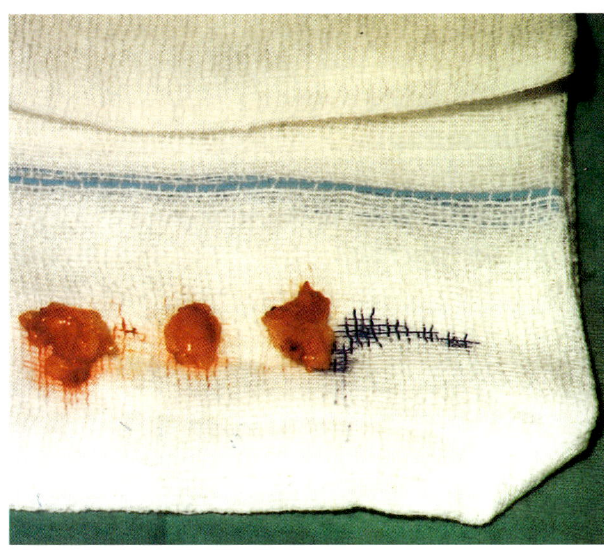

Figure 3.97d Fat cushion from the medial, middle and lateral part

Overview:

Transconjunctival fat removal in the lower eyelid has the following advantages:

1) The scar is invisible. Thus the method is indicated particularly for younger patients without excess skin.
2) Small wrinkles may be reduced after the operation.
3) The orbicularis oculi muscle remains unaffected.

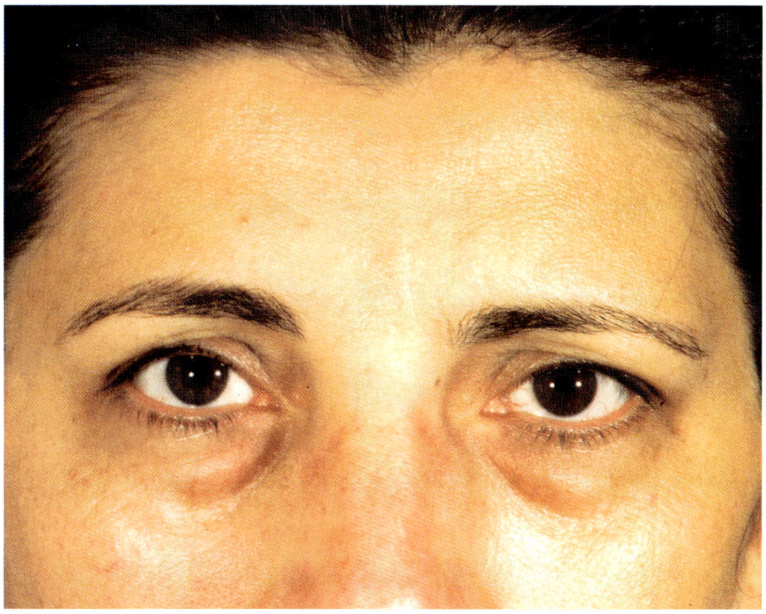

Figure 3.98a Local fat prolapse in the lower eyelid bilaterally

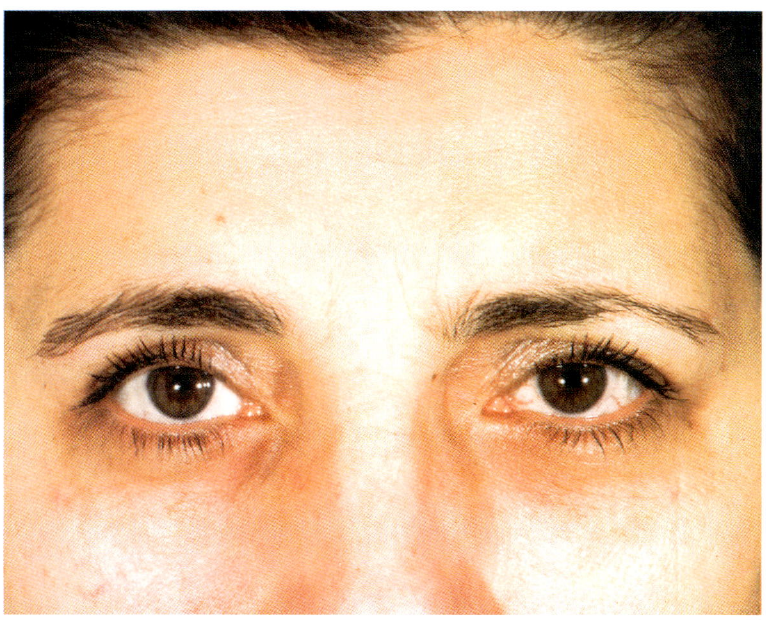

Figure 3.98b Appearance after transconjunctival fat removal

Table 3.1 Complications in aesthetic blepharoplasty (n=1470 patients from 1983–1995)

Complications	Number of Patients	Percentage
Lower eyelid ectropion	11	0.75
Hematoma – secondary hemorrhage	4	0.27
Local infection	2	0.13
Visual impairment due to hematoma	1	0.07

Eyelid Ptosis

Etiology of Ptosis

Eyelid ptosis arises because of:

- In most cases a congenital levator palpebrae dystrophy
- Paresis of the superficial branch of the oculomotor nerve (3rd cranial nerve). (Usually the superior rectus muscle is also affected.)
- More rarely due to myasthenia gravis.

Ptosis can occur unilaterally or bilaterally.

Ptosis Operation

The levator function (lifting of upper lid) is regarded as the most important parameter (normally 12 to 17 mm). With less than 10 mm a tightening of Mueller's muscle or better still the levator aponeurosis is the method of choice. With a levator function of less than 5 mm a resection and shortening of the levator is indicated.

The second parameter is the extent of the ptosis. If the upper eyelid is hanging down more than 2 mm over the upper limbus, the margin of the eyelid can not be raised sufficiently. A severe ptosis exists if the upper eyelid hangs by more than 4 mm over the upper limbus.

Beard has developed a scale indicating the quantity that must be resected from the levator aponeurosis.

Table 3.2 Beard-scale for levator resection

Ptosis [mm]	Levator function	Resection length of the levator fascia over upper limbus
Up to 2 mm	> 10 mm	approx. 10 mm
3–4 mm	> 8 mm	approx. 14–17 mm
> 4 mm	< 5 mm	approx. 20 mm

The better the levator function and the less the ptosis, the less is resected and vice versa.

Most errors are caused by an inadequate shortening of the levator, and rarely from an overcorrection. An overcorrection is frequently visible in the first 7 to 14 days. The final result is assessed after six weeks.

The goal of the operation is to achieve an eyelid margin position 1 to 2 mm below the upper limbus. The operation should not be carried out before the 5th year of life. An exception is if a very severe ptosis exists with a severe impairment of vision.

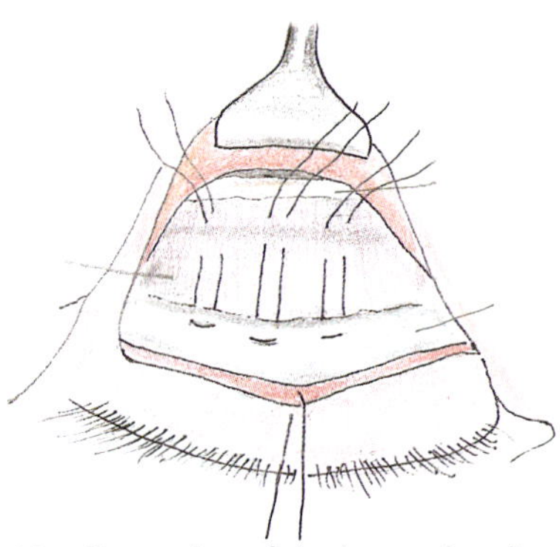

Figure 3.99a Shortening of the levator by plication

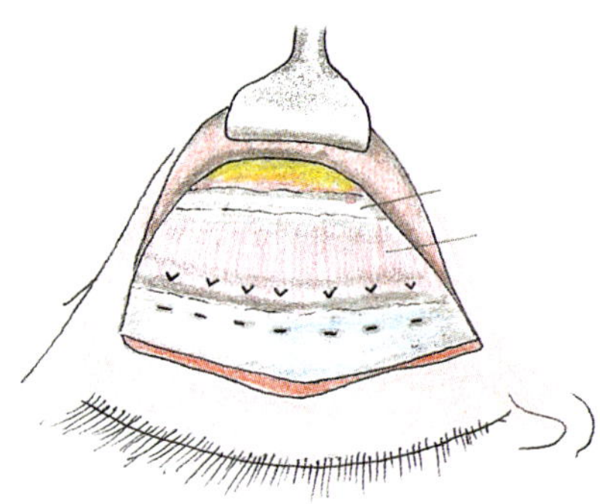

Figure 3.99b Appearance after plication of the levator fascia

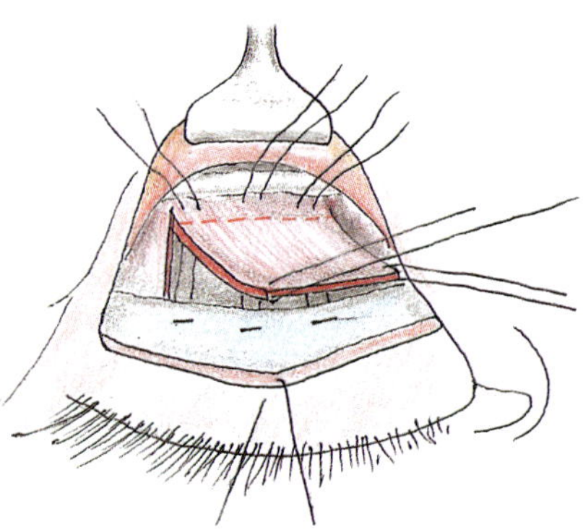

Figure 3.99c With severe ptosis the levator fascia is resected and fixed at the tarsus.

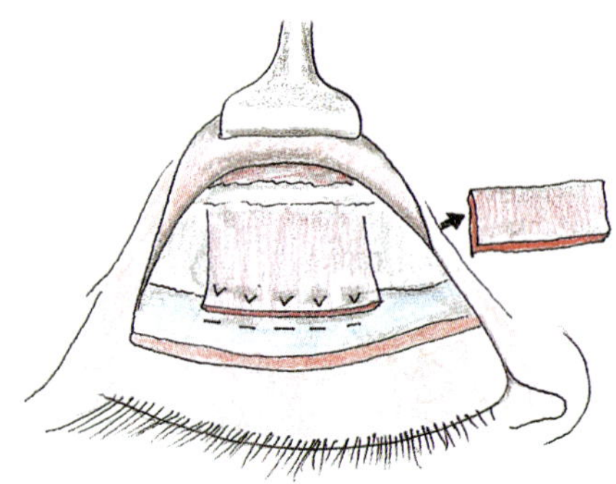

Figure 3.99d Fixation of the shortened levator fascia at the tarsus

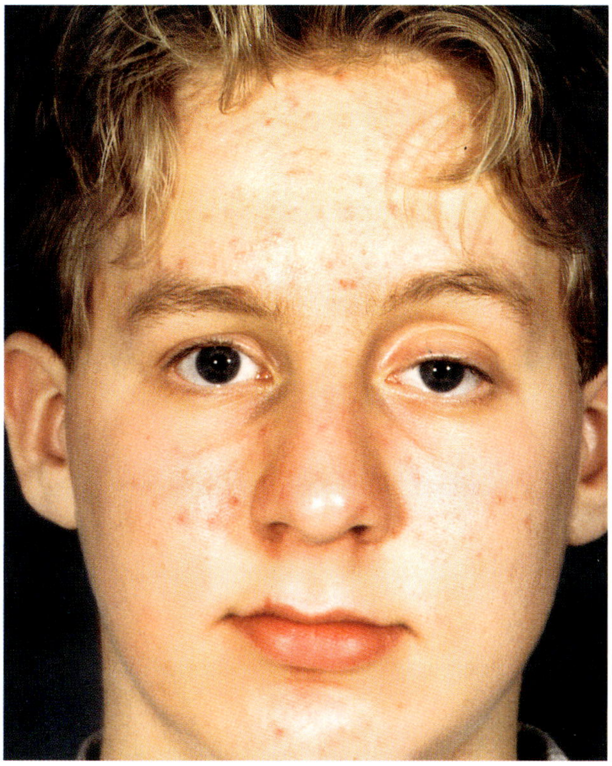

Figure 3.100a Congenital ptosis of the left upper eyelid of around 2 mm below the upper limbus

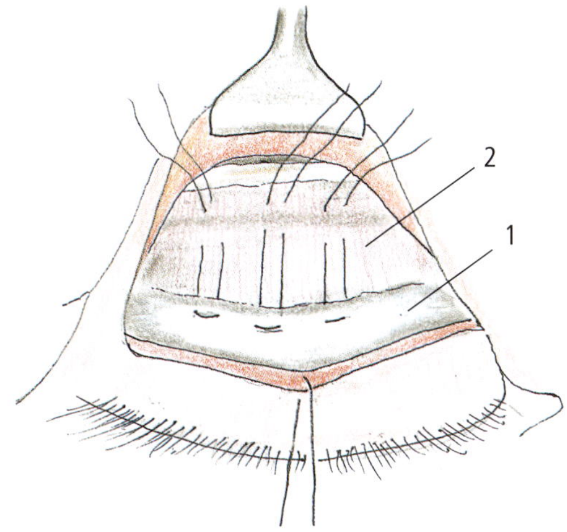

Figure 3.100b For minor to moderate ptosis, correction can be achieved by doubling (wrinkling) of the levator. In case of a 2 mm ptosis a shortening of the levator fascia should be 10 mm. Tarsus (1), levator aponeurosis (2).

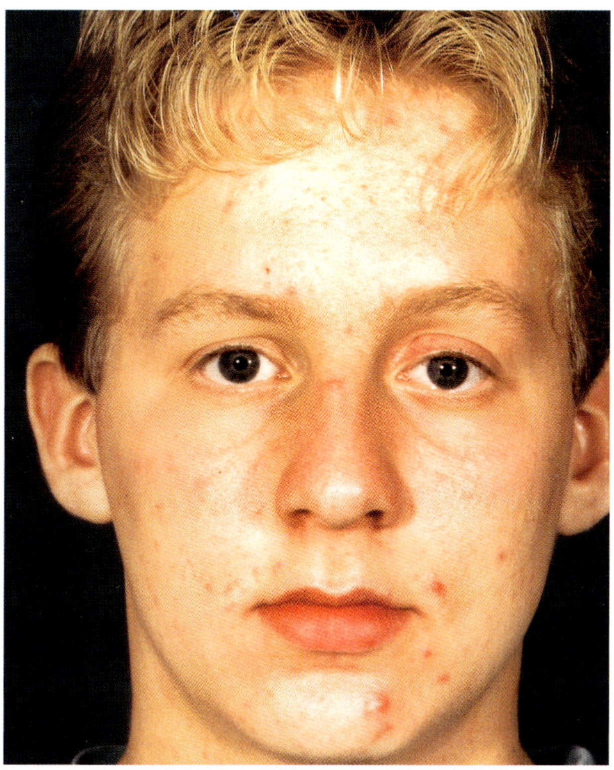

Figure 3.100c Appearance six months after the operation

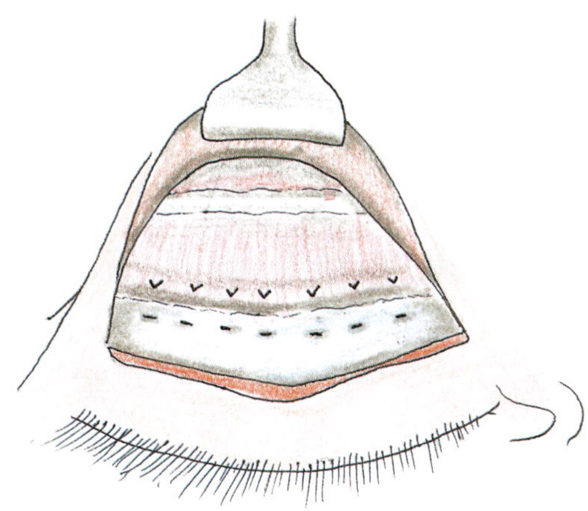

Figure 3.100d Plication of the levator which is fixed at the tarsus. This method suffices for a minor ptosis.

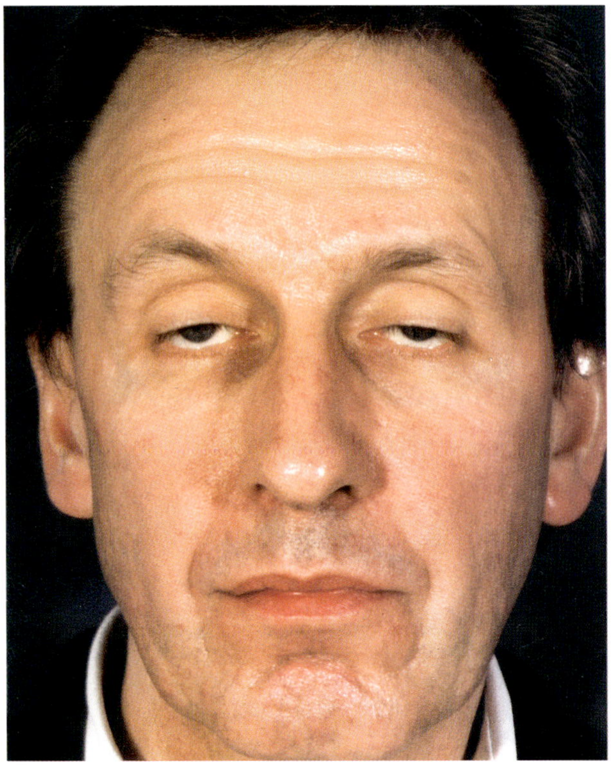

Figure 3.101a Bilateral ptosis of approx. 4 mm below the upper limbus

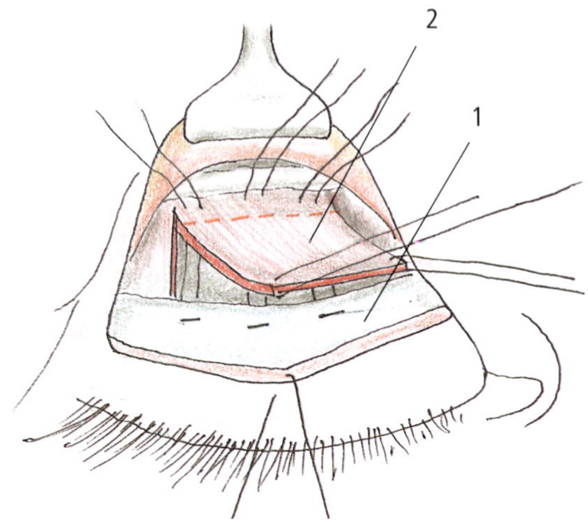

Figure 3.101b The levator is divided transversely just above the tarsus and mobilized widely. For this purpose lateral incisions are also necessary. Tarsus (1), levator aponeurosis (2).

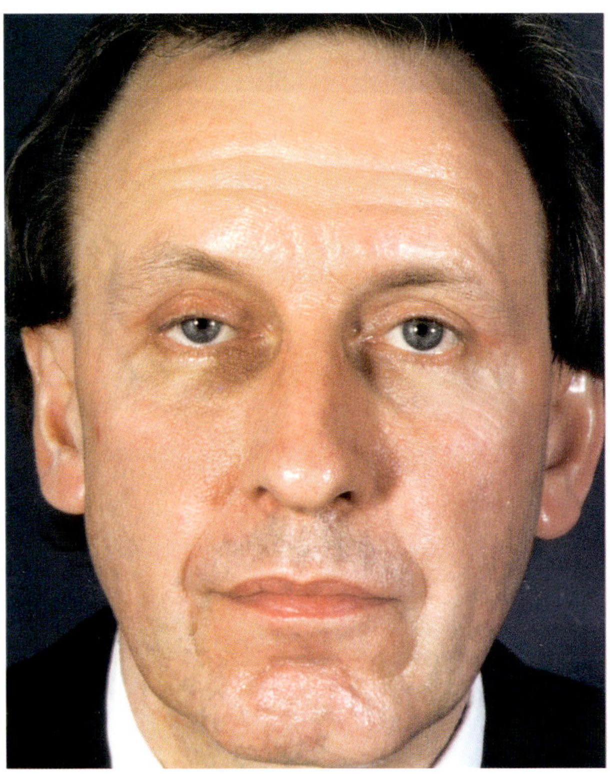

Figure 3.101c Appearance six months postoperatively after the resection of 20 mm of the levator

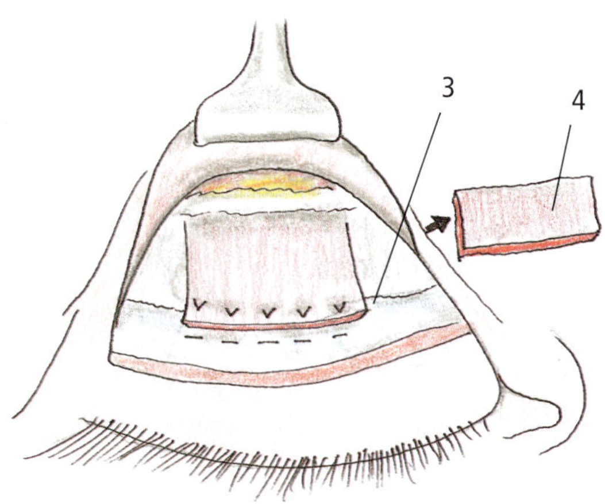

Figure 3.101d In order to correct a 4 mm ptosis, approximately 20 mm of the levator is resected (4) and the shortened muscle is fixed at the tarsus (3).

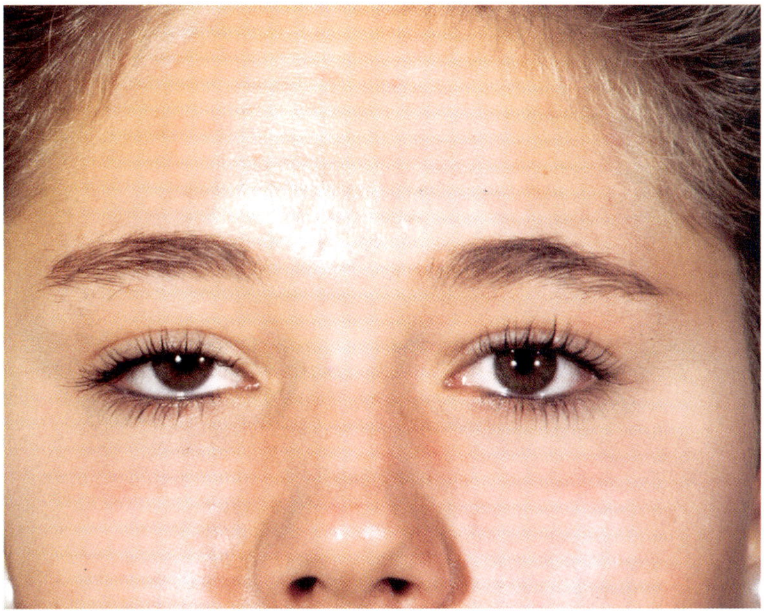

Figure 3.102a Congenital ptosis of the right upper eyelid approximately 2 mm

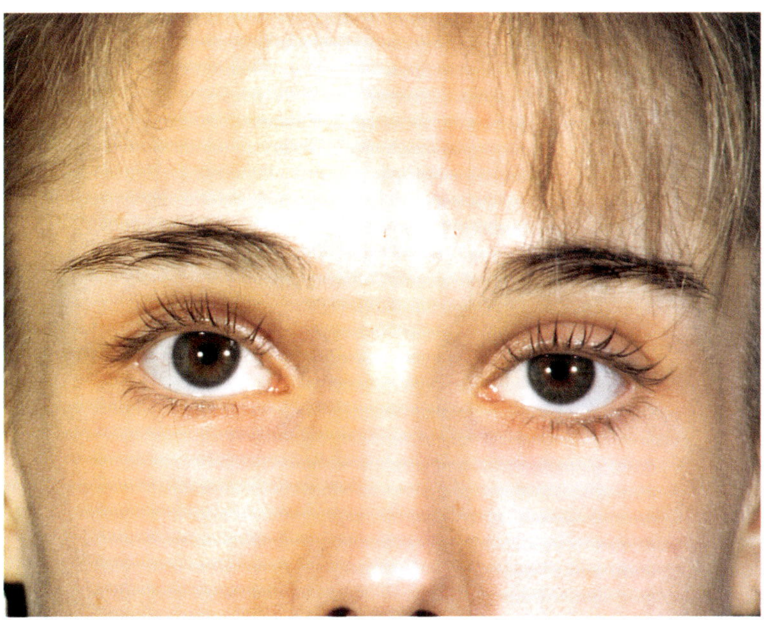

Figure 3.102b Status after shortening of the right levator approximately 9 mm two weeks after the operation. A slight overcorrection is still evident.

Facelifting

Skin slackening and increased wrinkling of the face can cause substantial problems in advanced age. The affected individuals often lose their self-confidence and also their capabilities when they can not deal with and compensate for these normal changes. Apart from advanced age, genetic factors also determine the extent of skin slackening.

More and more affected women and men seek help from plastic surgeons. This trend will certainly continue as more and more 50 to 70 year olds strive to keep themselves fit. Only the exposed face shows their true age. It seems unjust that the face skin ages considerably faster and more than e.g. the upper arm skin.

During counseling of patients even greater care should be exercised than is the case with eyelid or nose corrections. The patient needs to be informed fully about the normal postoperative course and any possible complications both verbally and in writing. In particular, unreasonable expectations should be warned against. The face may be lifted, but the human being as a whole is not rejuvenated. The written information using well-proven, legally tested explanatory forms should be presented to the patient during the first meeting so that they have sufficient time to become informed.

Caution must be exercised where major discrepancies exist between suffering and expected benefit. In cases of repeated face lifting, where, in the opinion of the patient, other doctor's had "bungled" their operations, it is sometimes wise to advise the patient not to have any further operations. Caution should also be exercised with patients who want to save their professional or personal lives by undergoing an operation.

Exceptions include actors and TV personalities for whom a facelifting is often very helpful in their profession.

Discussions regarding facelifting have proved very lively at medical congresses. New methods and variations are continuously being introduced, sometimes without any notable improvements. For decades, facelifting, as described by Lexer and Joseph, was only carried out in the form of a simple mobilization of the skin of the face. At the end of the 1970s the recommendation for the SMAS surgery arrived and it was almost impossible to admit that good facelifts could also be achieved without a SMAS elevation.

At the beginning of the 1980s bicoronal mask-lifting was introduced at the behest of the so-called French school (mainly craniofacial surgeons). This procedure was enthusiastically accepted and applied by us all. Afterwards, however, patients complained of loss of sensitivity on the head and sometimes also a temporary diplopia.

After many years, and hundreds of operations, I now ask myself, what is in fact really important for facelifting? The method? – The incision line? – Subperiostal mid-facelifting?: *These are all completely secondary aspects.*

The real question is: What procedure does the patient feel good and satisfied about, and which procedure has a short and relatively complication-free postoperative course? Then, secondarily, the result should last for a long time.

Some authors described that the skin (and SMAS) should be pulled cranially and dorsally, but, God forbid if tension should arise anywhere! Absolute nonsense! Tension must be present! Of course no tension should be so severe that it causes necrosis, but a facelifting without tension shows a poor long-term result.

So what now? Achieving a good result with the least trauma? The choice of procedure is of no interest to the patients. They just want to be satisfied and look good. The least invasive operation should be used, depending on local conditions, in order to achieve a good result.

This of course excludes surgeons who choose a 5 cm preauricular incision and who have the nerve to publicise this at congresses or on television as a "mini lifting".

This tiny incision with minimal undermining can only achieve a short lasting "smoothing" due to a temporary swelling of the face. Patients notice, at the latest two months after the operation, that they did not get the expected result. To operate in this way could be considered fraud committed on the patient.

Endoscopic facelifting promises the ideal of an operation without scarring. A lifting of the forehead can indeed be achieved with success. The durability of the results, however, appears to me to be debatable and in the cheek and throat area the applicability of this procedure is "restricted". In the forehead area this complicated – and thus expensive – method must also compete with botulinum toxin injection.

Mühlbauer remarked in Lemperle's book: "Of great importance is the choice of candidate. Younger people with good skin elasticity are preferred". The author wondered openly why young people with good skin elasticity would even want a lifting? Convincing results are still being waited upon.

A facelifting very frequently requires extensive mobilization of the skin, a quite long incision, an ample resection of the skin, an additional SMAS tightening and a mass-induced tension.

If problems arise in the eyelid area, a blepharoplasty should be carried out, if possible in the same session. This places great demands on the surgeon. If the eyebrows are lifted during the forehead lifting, the skin resection must be less broad in the upper eyelid than it would be in an isolated eyelid operation.

Therefore, if uncertainty exists, it is better to perform the eyelid correction and the facelifting as separate operations. This alternative entails more time and as such greater costs to the patient but could be better for both patient and surgeon overall.

In this chapter only two common routine procedures are described:

1. Standard lifting with modification, i.e. with considerably more mobilization in the forehead area. 90 % of the patients were operated on in this way.
2. Bicoronal incision line (mask lifting).

Very frequently the following interventions were carried out simultaneously:

- Blepharoplasty
- Dermabrasion of the perioral area or implantation of superficial temporal fascia into the lip
- Liposuction or lipectomy as well as platysmaplasty in the neck

Only very rarely is a nasal correction carried out simultaneously with a facelifting.

Anesthesia

90 % of our patients were operated on under general anesthesia (n = 635) and only 10 % under local anesthesia. For many surgeons this ratio is reversed. This depends primarily on the surgeon, while secondarily, experience has shown that the larger the clinic, then the more frequently is general anesthesia used.

The author is aware of the climbing trend in the percentage of operations done under local anesthesia.

The cost reduction to the patient is of course another important factor underlying this.

Also, patients that have surgery under general anesthesia receive a vasoconstrictor "cocktail" as follows:

Local anesthesia (also used as local infiltration with general anesthesia):

- One ampulla (2 ml = 2.5 IU) POR 8 (Ornipressin Sandoz)
- and 50 ml xylocaine 0.5 % with 1:200,000 adrenaline

Fifteen minutes should elapse between injection and operation. This pays dividends because hemorrhage is reduced considerably by such a measure. This "cocktail" proposed by Lemperle prolongs the local anesthesia time significantly while also reinforcing and prolonging the effect of the vasoconstriction.

Routinely we needed no more than 100 ccm for both facial sides (two ampullae POR 8 + xylocaine 0.5 % with 1:200,000 adrenaline). The same amount was given to patients having surgery under general anesthesia.

Because of two unexplained anesthetic incidents POR 8 is now under investigation, however, we have experienced no such incidents using this cocktail. Lemperle, who could boast a 25 year experience with this kind of vasoconstriction, also reported no complications.

Mottura recommends another mixture and has reported very good results:

- 7 ml lidocaine
- 7 ml bupivacaine in 150 ml saline
- 0.3 ml adrenaline
- 1 ml bicarbonate

Patients who were only operated on under local anesthesia also required sedation (usually with Midazolam). For various reasons the author prefers general anesthesia, but opinions vary and are open to debate.

On the second postoperative day the patient is discharged after the hair has been washed and any blood crusts have been removed. Patients are advised that they may be able to resume their normal activities after approximately three weeks.

a) Standard Facelifting

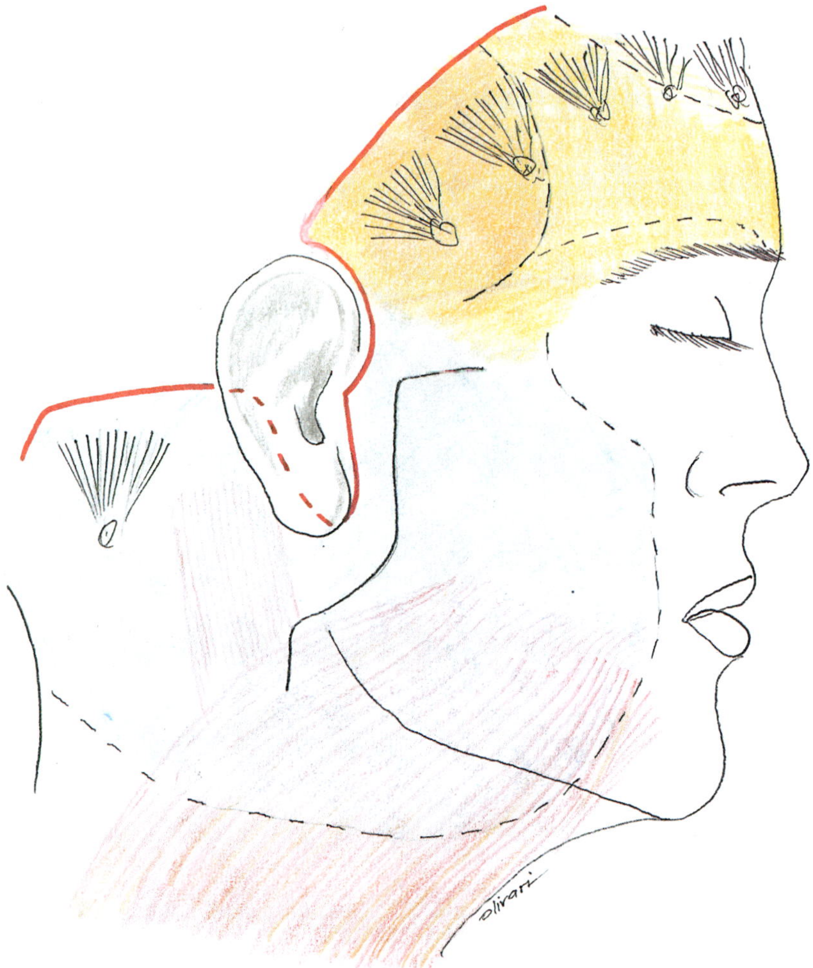

Figure 3.103 Standard facelifting – incision line (red).
The mobilization in the upper area runs initially below the superficial temporal fascia and then in the forehead area epiperiosteally up to the eyebrow. A subperiostal dissection is carried out 2 cm above the eyebrow (yellow) and in cases of hanging eyebrows over the orbital margin. In the cheek area dissection is carried out subcutaneously and extensively down in to the neck ventrally and caudally (blue). The incision course for the SMAS is marked with a black line.

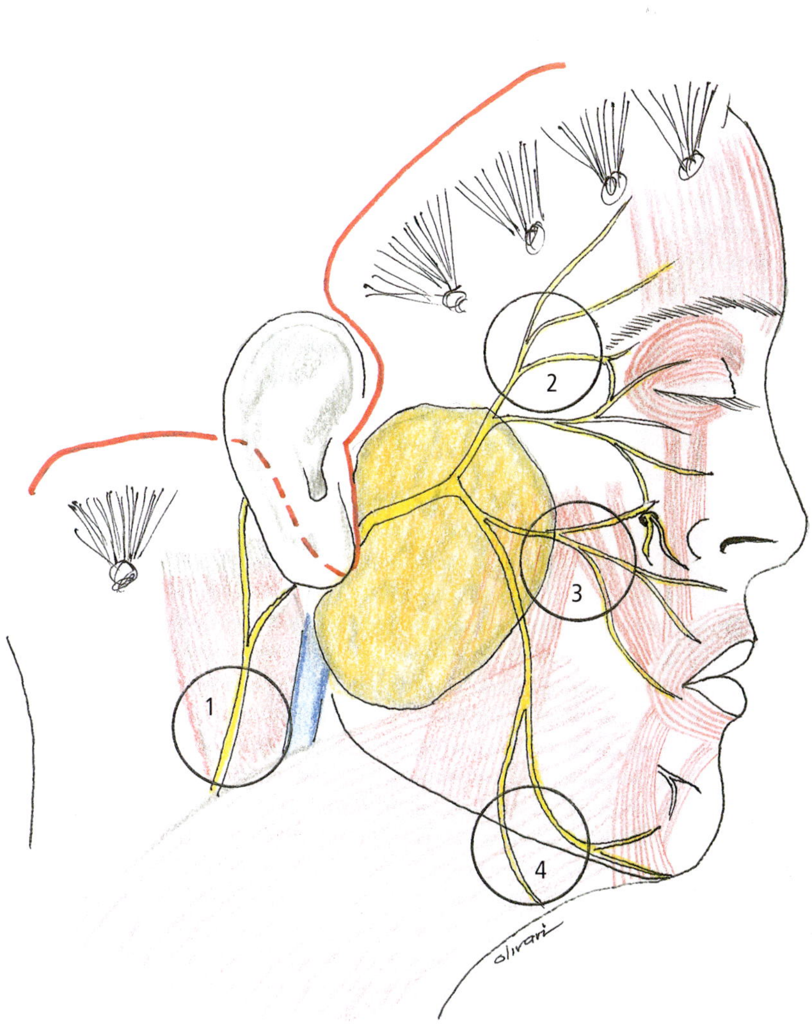

Figure 3.104 Risk of nerve injury during facelifting.

1) Injury to the greater auricular nerve is the most frequent. This nerve lies on the sternocleidomastoid muscle where the subcutaneous tissue is relatively thin. Dissection should therefore be carried out carefully. Injury will result in a loss in sensitivity of the lower two thirds of the ear concha as well as the skin of the surrounding cheek and the neck.
2) Damage to the frontal branch of the facial nerve.
This can be avoided if dissection is carried out precisely on the deep temporal fascia. Caution is called for especially when resecting above the zygomatic arch.
If injury occurs the frontal muscle can become paretic and the eyebrow can hang deeply.

3) Damage to the buccal branches of the facial nerves.
As a result of this a paresis of the upper lip can occur.
The buccal branches originate from the facial nerve through the parotid gland and lie on the masseter muscle.
4) Damage to the marginal branch of the facial nerve.
A paresis of the lower lip results. The marginal branch lies on the caudal part of the masseter, but under the platysma.
Injuries to the zygomatic branch or the infraorbital nerve are rare. With a bicoronal incision the supraorbital and supratrochlear nerves are endangered. Fortunately, permanent pareses of the above-mentioned nerves represent an exception. Re-innervation occurs almost always between week 8 and 12 postoperatively. One should never rely on this, however, and operations should always be carried out as precisely as possible.

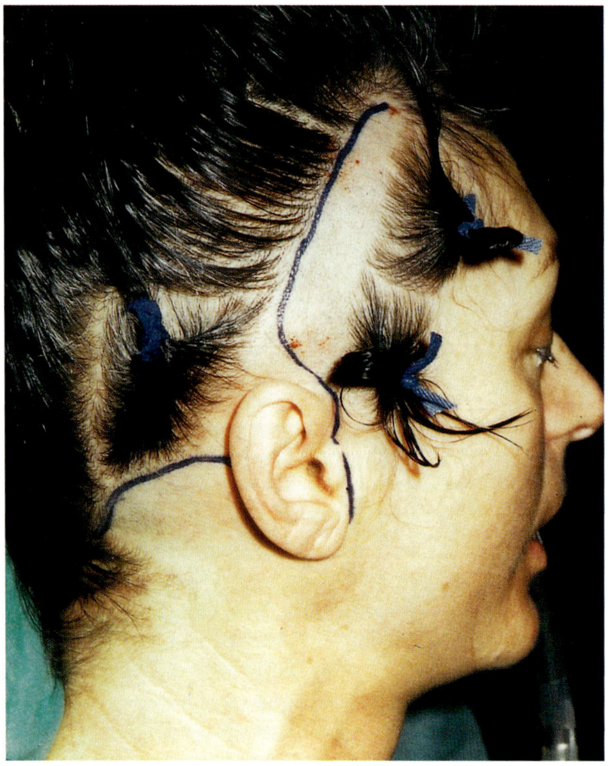

Figure 3.105a Modified standard incision by the author for facelifting. A relatively long incision in the upper part, diagonally in the ventral direction, allows an excellent mobilization of the forehead as well as the orbital margin under direct vision. In the postauricular direction the incision runs in the sulcus and then in a dorsal direction. At the end the incision should run slightly caudally. This prevents a "dog ear". The postauricular hairs are shaved.

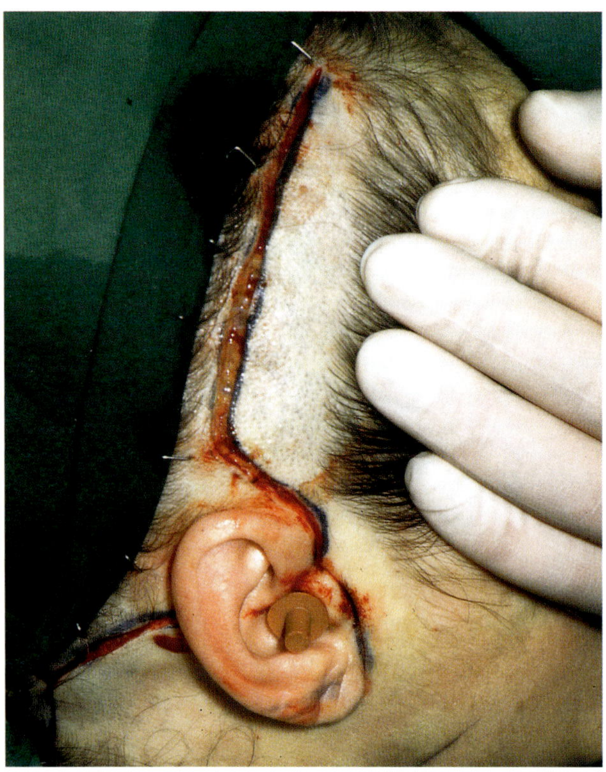

Figure 3.105b The preauricular incision proceeds immediately in front of the tragus. Incision behind the tragus is senseless. Often the tragus is displaced ventrally and it is possible to see right into the external auditory canal. The scar in the upper and lower preauricular area runs in the sulcus and the preauricular scars are barely visible if surgery has been carried out properly.

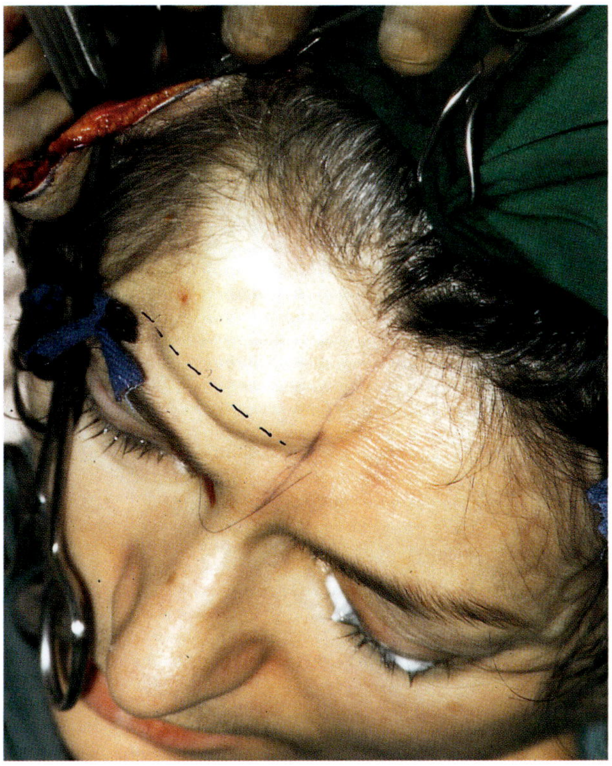

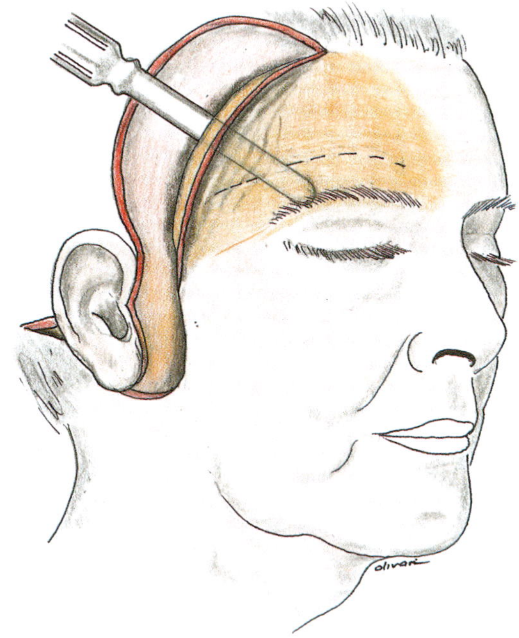

Figure 3.105c,d Mobilization in the forehead area with a "standard" incision. Dissection is carried out above the periosteum up to the broken line and caudally from there subperiosteally. The periosteum is raised under good direct vision (using a cold light retractor) from the orbital margin. At this point the eyebrow is mobilized and raised slightly by 5 to 7 mm. The mobilization occurs above the midline.

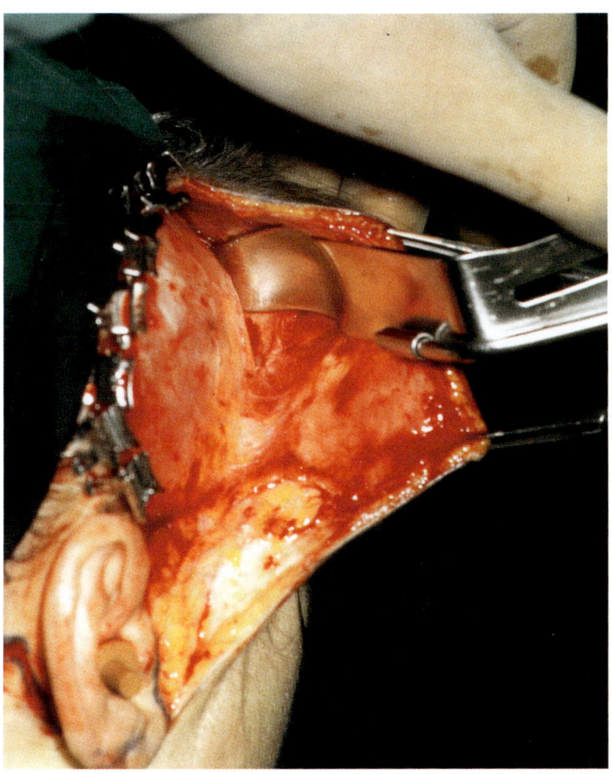

Figure 3.105e Using the cold light retractor one can dissect easily with good visibility up to the orbital margin, first above the deep temporal fascia and then above the periosteum. Dissection is carried out 2 cm above the eyebrow subperiosteally. Here the orbital margin is free and the eyebrow is mobilized. The effect of the eyebrow elevation is similar to that of a mask lifting.

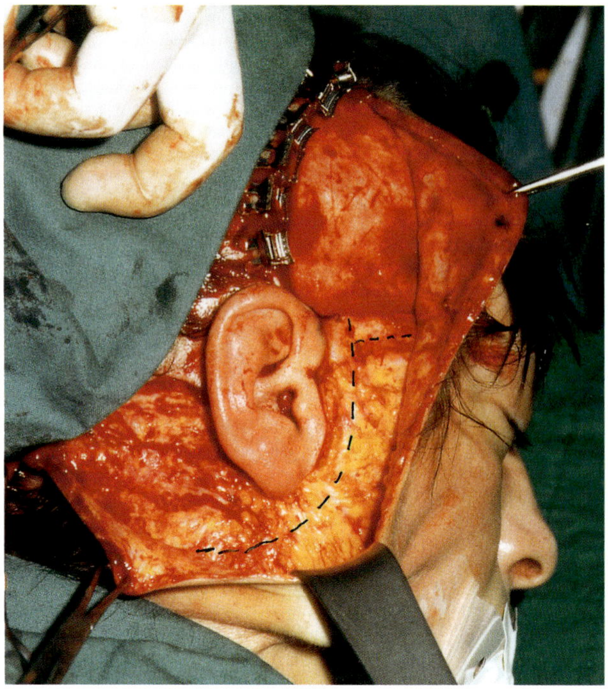

Figure 3.105f The broken line shows the location where the SMAS is incised. Dissection is carried out in the upper part laterally, above the deep temporal fascia, and medially, above the periosteum. In the cheek area and the neck the skin is mobilized extensively ventrally and caudally.

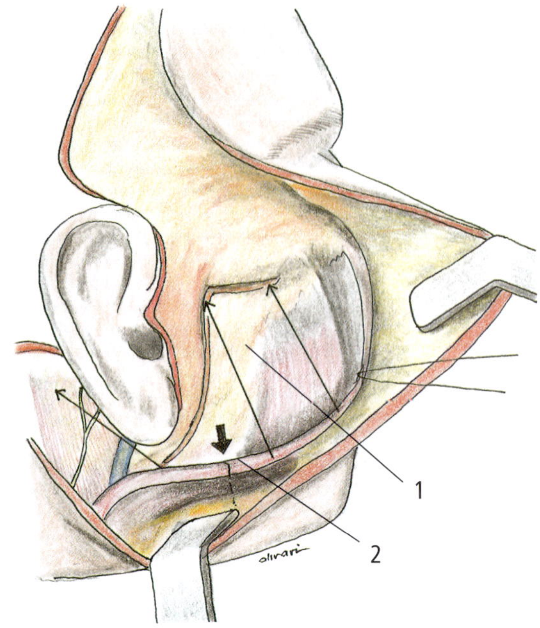

Figure 3.105g The main components of the SMAS are the parotid capsule (1) and the platysma (2). The arrow shows the site where the platysma is divided. The ventral part is pulled cranially and fixed in the area of the zygomatic arch. The dorsal part is fixed behind the greater auricular nerve retroauricularly.

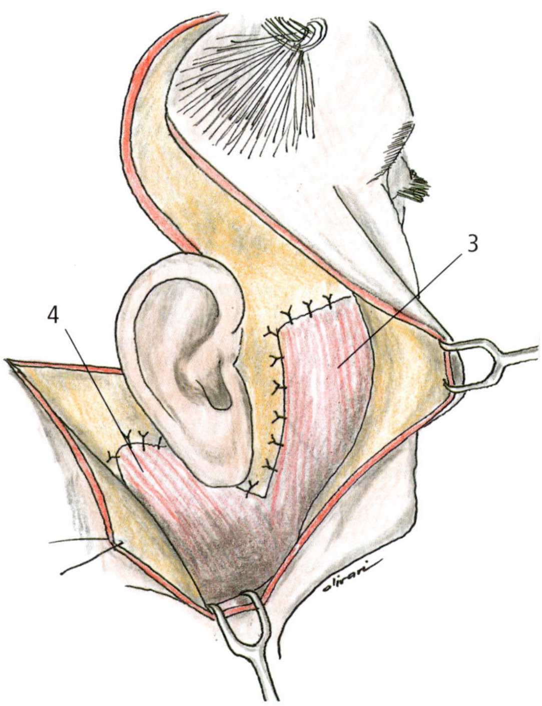

Figure 3.105h Appearance at the end of fixation of the SMAS that is divided into a ventral (3) and dorsal component (4)

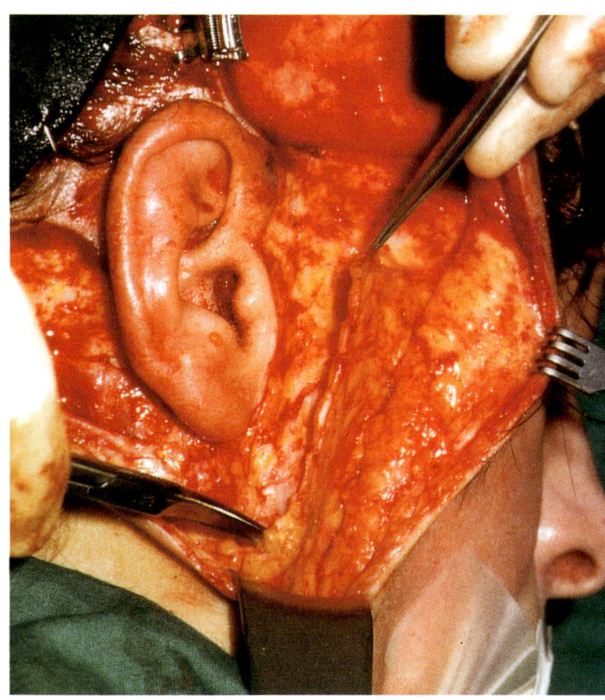

Figure 3.105i The cranial part of the SMAS is mobilized and fixed under tension

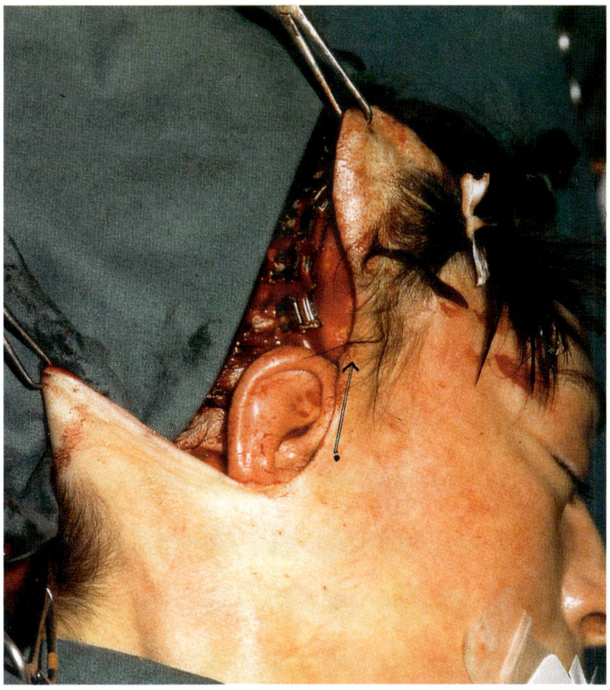

Figure 3.105j After mobilization in the forehead, cheek and neck areas, and after fixation of the SMAS, excision of surplus skin follows. In this case the pull is carried out more cranially than laterally. The arrow shows the point that was in front of the tragus and how far the skin has moved in the cranial direction.

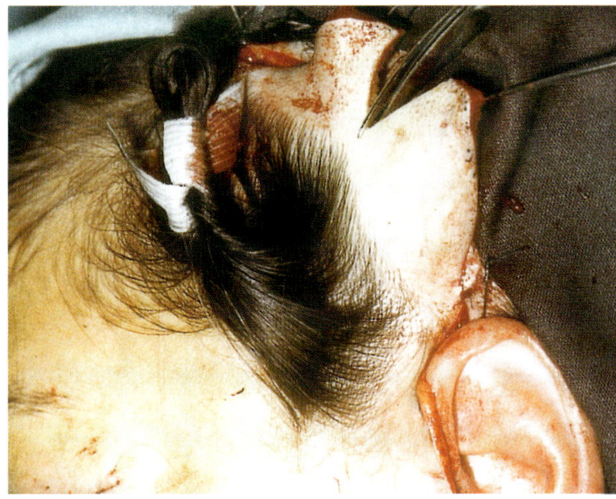

Figure 3.105k Above the ear, the hair bearing skin was resected by around 2 to 2.5 cm.

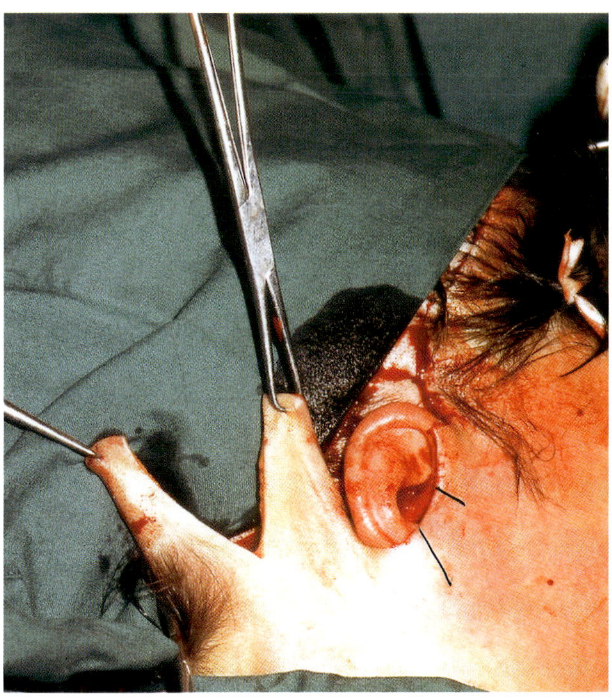

Figure 3.105l First two "key sutures" are placed supraauricularly and retroauricularly. Normally 2 to 2.5 cm of hairy skin is excised above the ear. The retroauricular resection amounts to 5 to 7 cm.

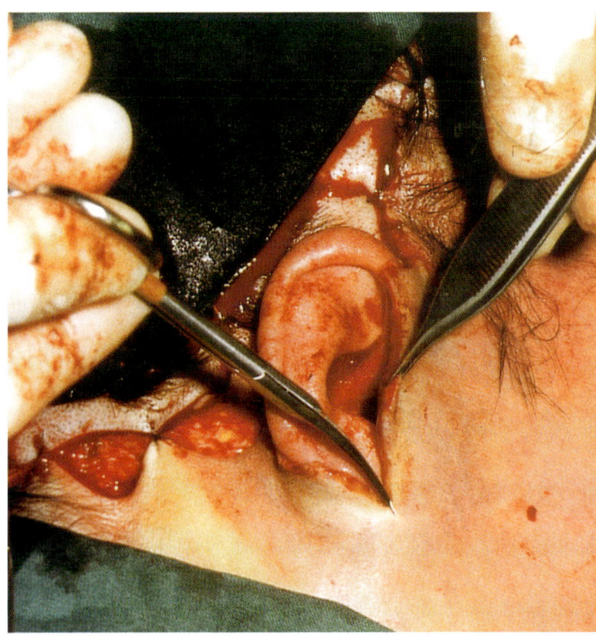

Figure 3.105m Careful incision in the region of the ear lobe! The incision must be as short as possible. Supraauricular (hairy skin): Interrupted sutures of 4 × 0 Trofilene, preauricular: intracutaneous suture of 6 x 0 Trofilene, retroauricular: Closure with 4 × 0 Vicryl and intracutaneous suture of 4 × 0 Trofilene.

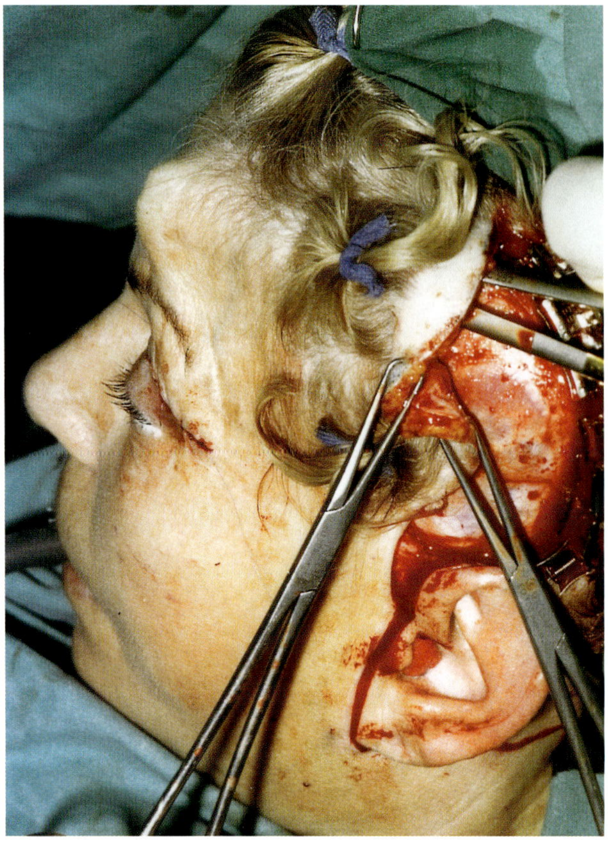

Figure 3.105n Epiperiosteal mobilization of the forehead skin in facelifting. Mobilization with the scissors up and over the midline.

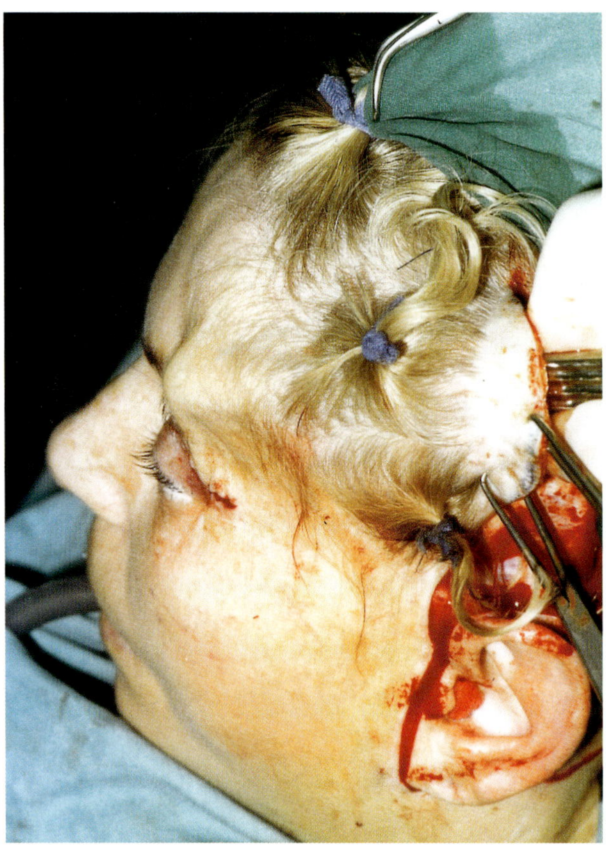

Figure 3.105o 2 cm above the eyebrow, subperiosteal mobilization is carried out using the raspatory. The mobilization can also be carried out above the periosteum. This patient had a blepharoplasty carried out at the same time.

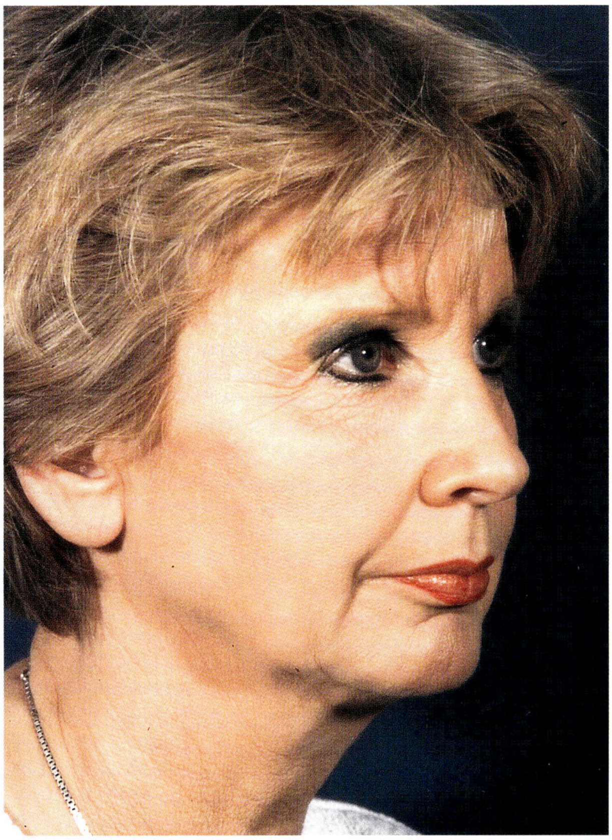

Figure 3.106a Slack facial as well as neck skin (formation of hanging cheeks), deep-lying eyebrows

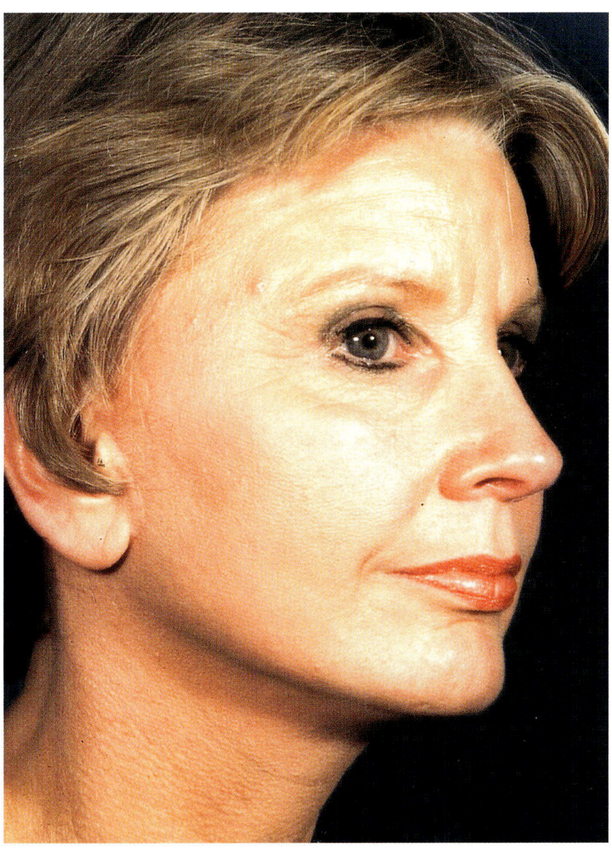

Figure 3.106b Appearance one year after the modified "standard" facelifting using SMAS, simultaneous lifting of the eyebrow and blepharoplasty

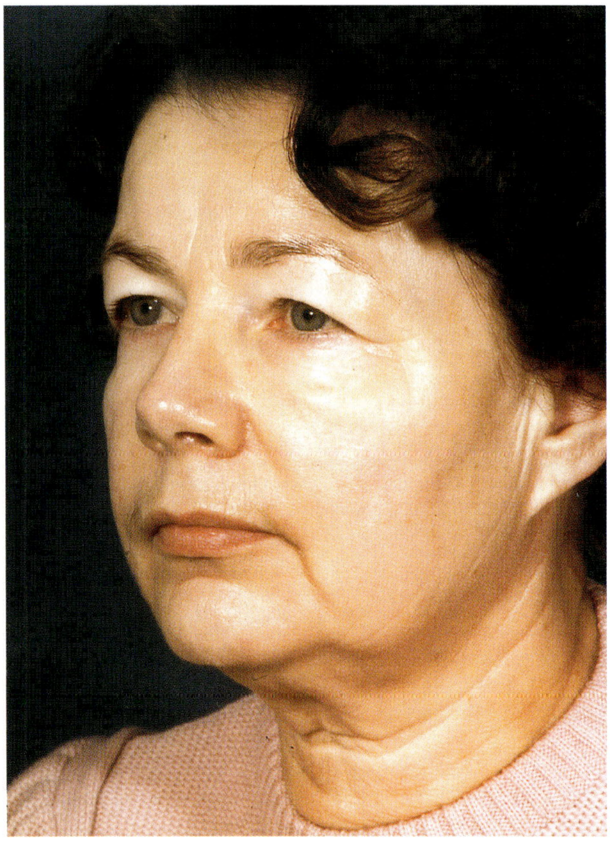

Figure 3.107a Blepharochalasis of the upper eyelids, sagging facial and neck skin, upper lip wrinkles

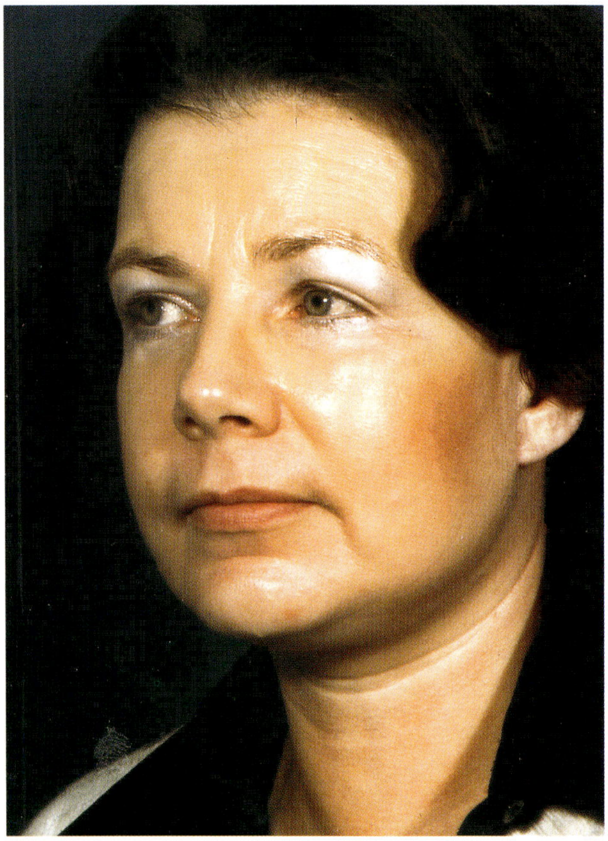

Figure 3.107b Appearance one year after modified facelifting with SMAS, eyebrow elevation as well as upper and lower lid correction. High-speed dermabrasion of the upper and lower lip.

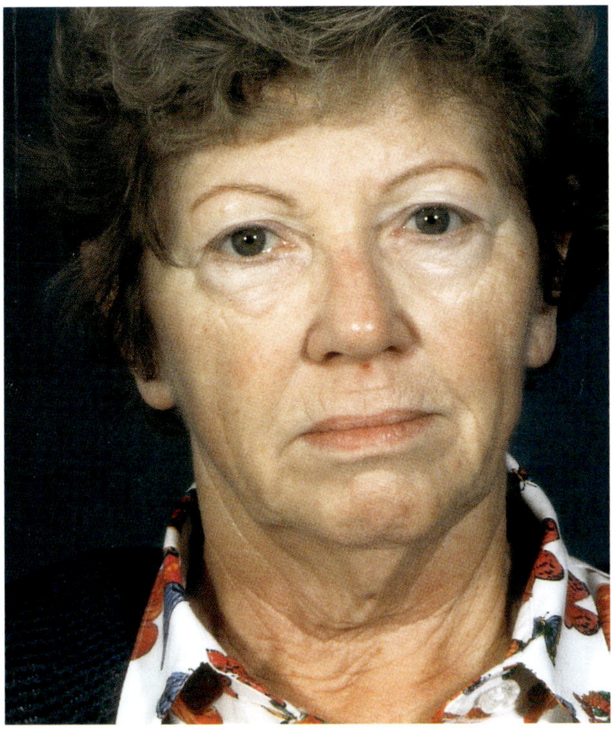

Figure 3.108a Blepharochalasis, "tear bags", severely sagging facial and neck skin

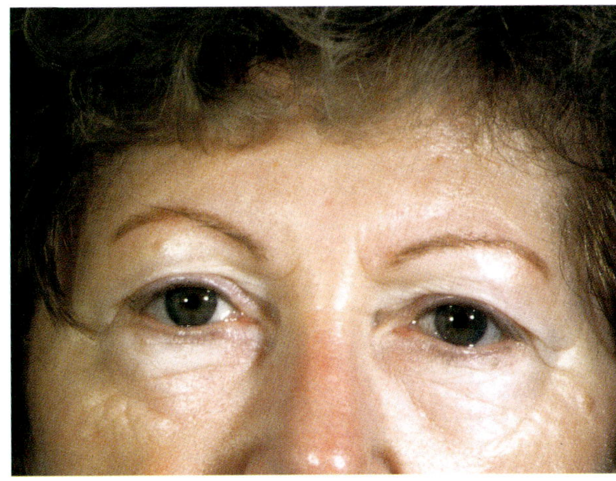

Figure 3.108b Detailed image of the eye area

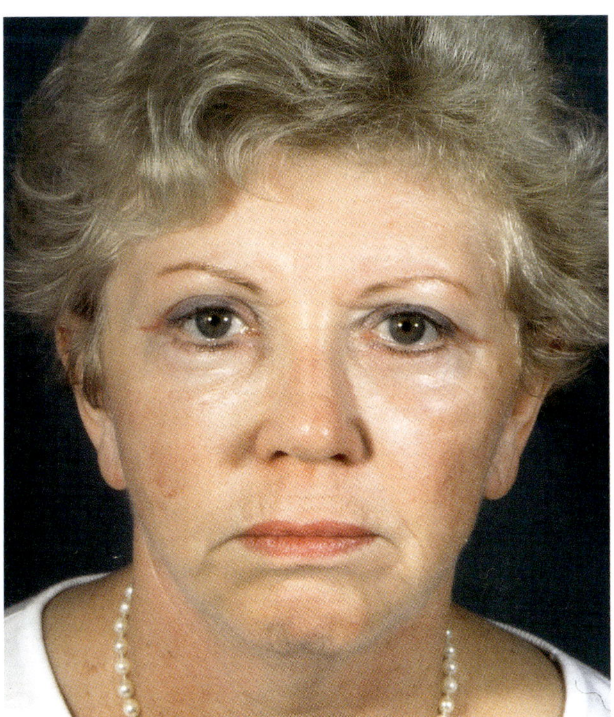

Figure 3.108c Picture after blepharoplasty and simultaneous modified standard facelifting with extensive neck skin lifting and SMAS. 8 cm of skin was excised retroauricularly.

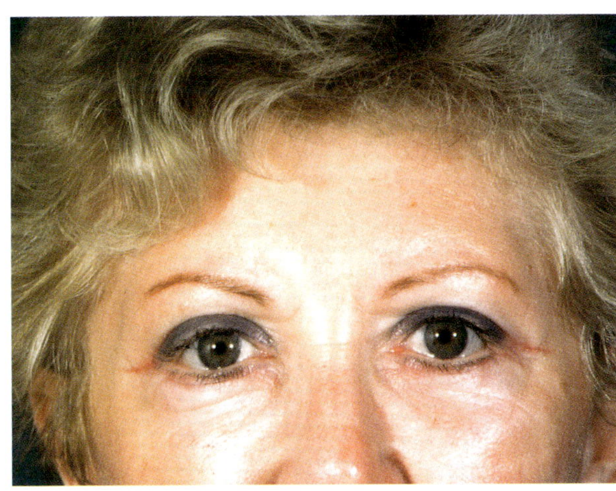

Figure 3.108d Considerable improvement after forehead elevation with modified standard facelifting as well as blepharoplasty. An extended supraauricular incision pays dividends for correcting the forehead area. The result hardly differs from the more extensive mask lifting.

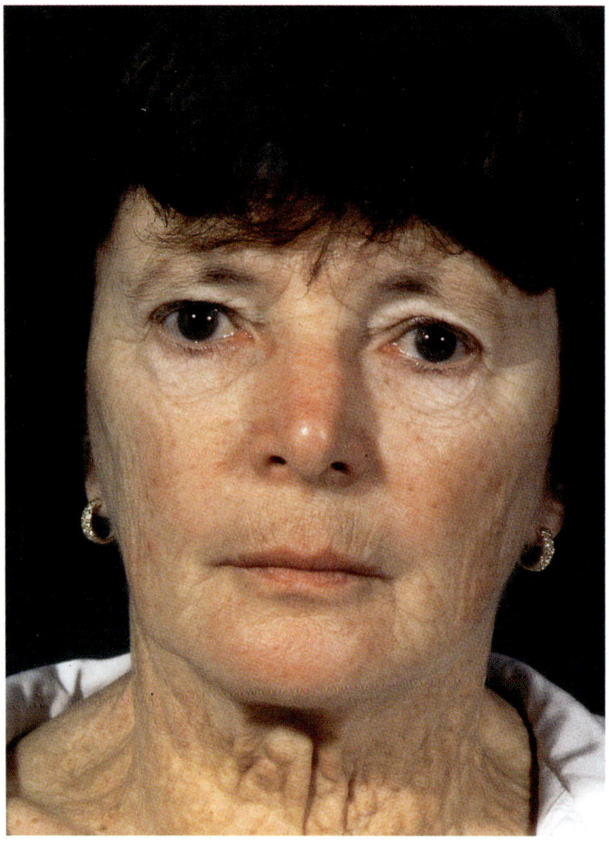

Figure 3.109a Blepharochalasis, sagging facial skin as well as extreme wrinkling of the neck

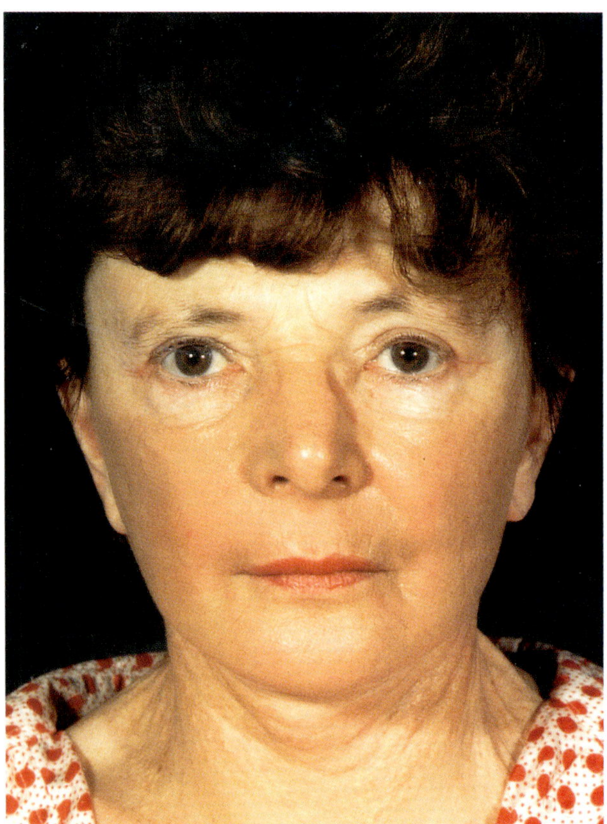

Figure 3.109b Appearance six months after blepharoplasty and modified standard facelifting with SMAS

b) Mask Lifting

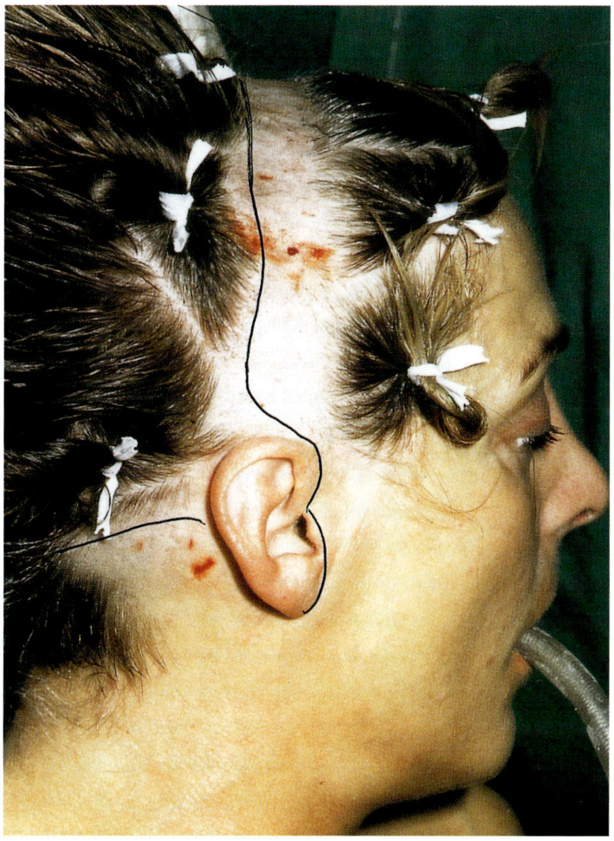

Figure 3.110a Bicoronal incision line in facelifting, so-called "Mask lifting".

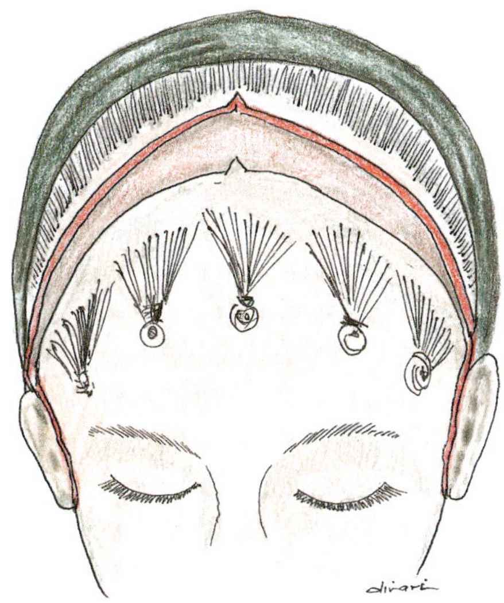

Figure 3.110b A small cusp was left in the middle for later orientation.

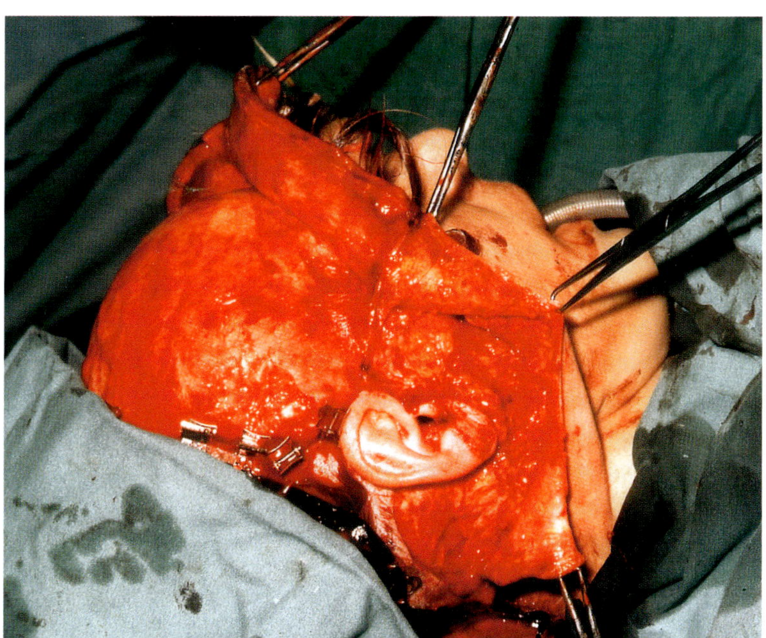

Figure 3.110c Mobilization of the skin of the head was carried out above the periosteum and into the temporal fossa up to the deep temporal fascia.

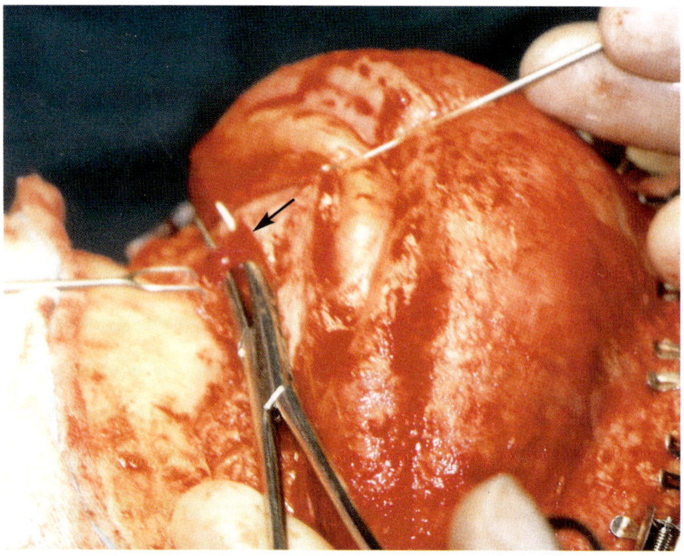

Figure 3.110d The corrugator muscle (arrow) is located cranio-laterally to the nasal root and medially to the supraorbital nerve (1).

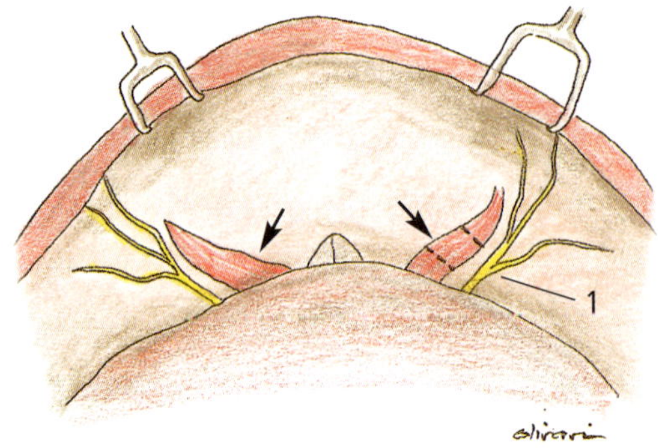

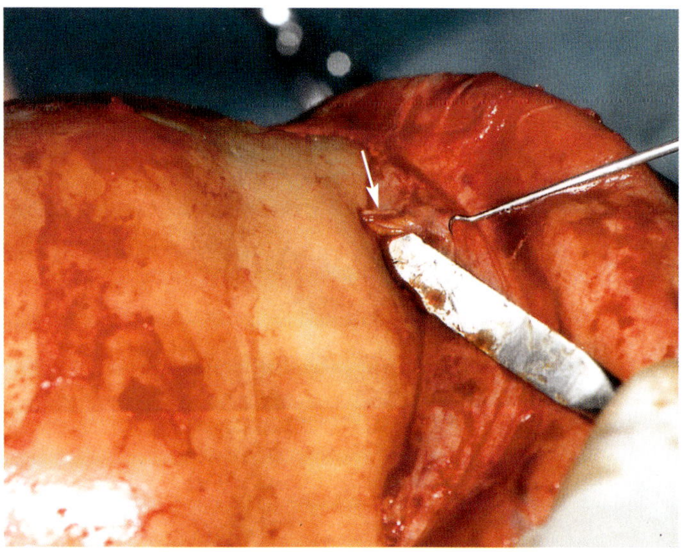

Figure 3.110e The corrugator muscle is not simply divided, but about 1 cm is resected.

Figure 3.110f Approximately 2 cm above the edge of the orbit a subperiosteal mobilization is carried out. The edge of the orbit is completely freed, as is the glabella and the lateral edge of the orbit up to the cheek bone. The supraorbital nerve (arrow) often runs in a foramen that is osteotomized to allow better mobilization.

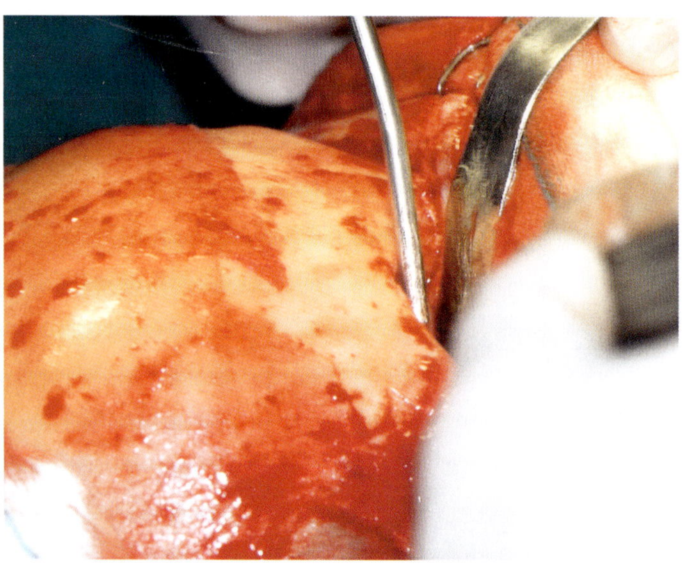

Figure 3.110g The edge of the orbit is completely free. Recently some authors have carried out corrections from an epiperiosteal approach. They maintain that a better mobilization of the eyebrow can be achieved.

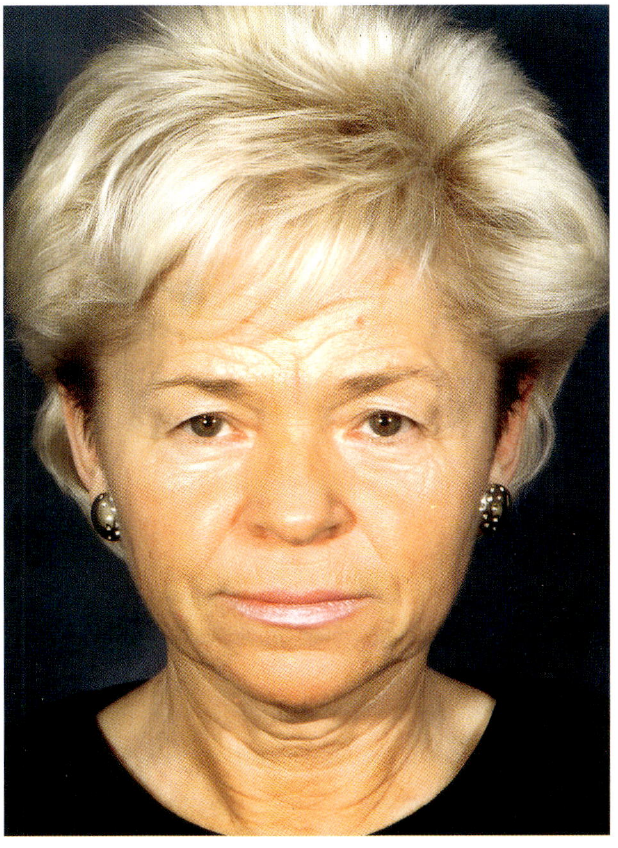

Figure 3.111a Forehead wrinkles, eyebrow ptosis of the upper eyelids, blepharochalasis, sagging facial and neck skin

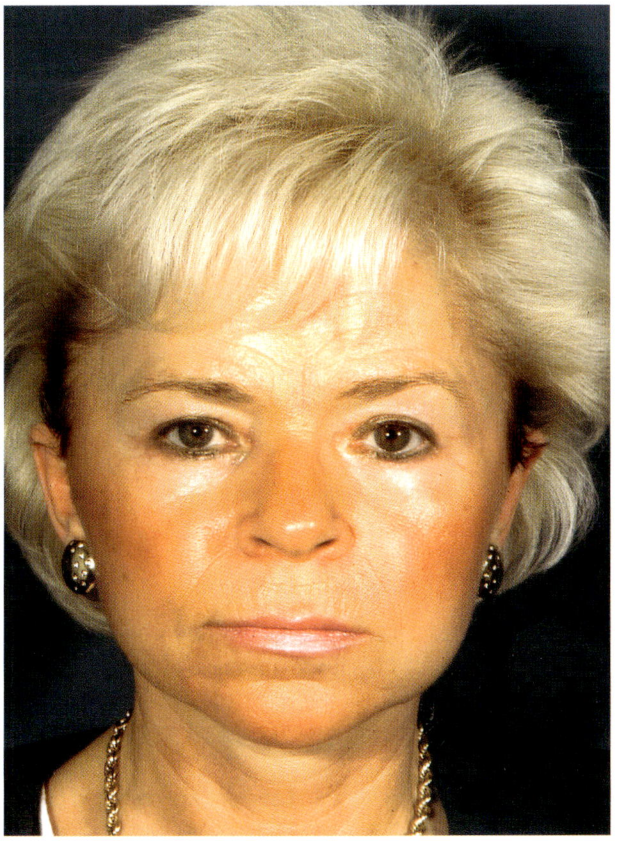

Figure 3.111b Appearance after bicoronal facelifting ("Mask lifting"), blepharoplasty and extensive neck skin lifting. It is an illusion to think that a neck skin lift can be achieved just by bicoronal incision in such cases. Here 7 cm of skin was resected postauricularly.

c) Upper Lip Wrinkle Abrasion

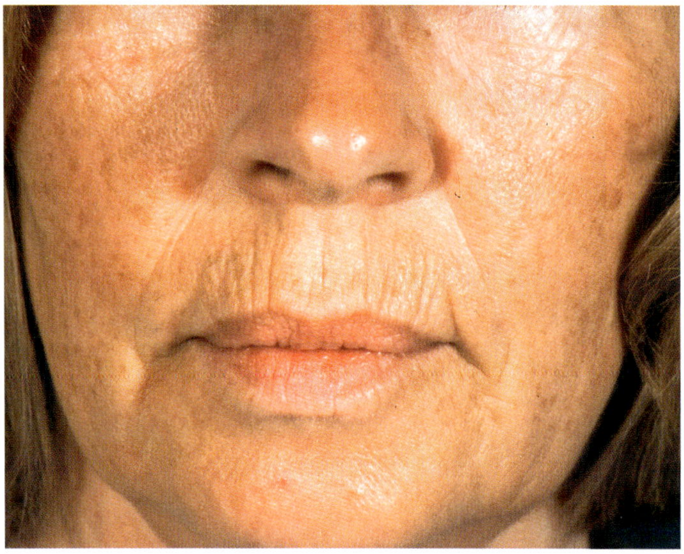

Figure 3.113a Upper lip wrinkles

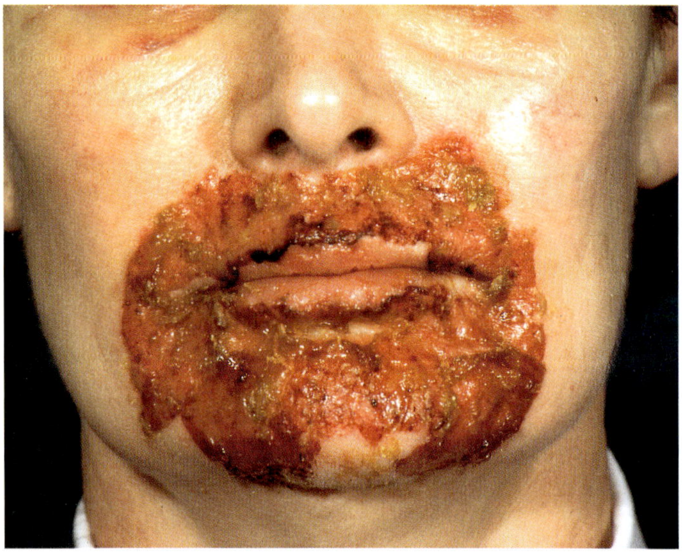

Figure 3.113b High-speed dermabrasion. Appearance two days after the deep dermal abrasion performed as an out-patient procedure under local anesthesia.

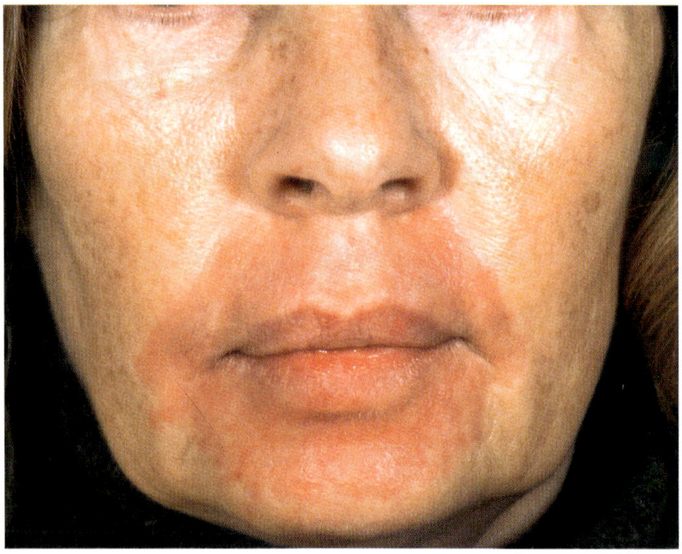

Figure 3.113c Appearance four weeks after the operation: One can still see a clear skin reddening. During the first six months the patient should keep away from the sun. The method is effective and economical (cheaper than laser and probably with less complications).

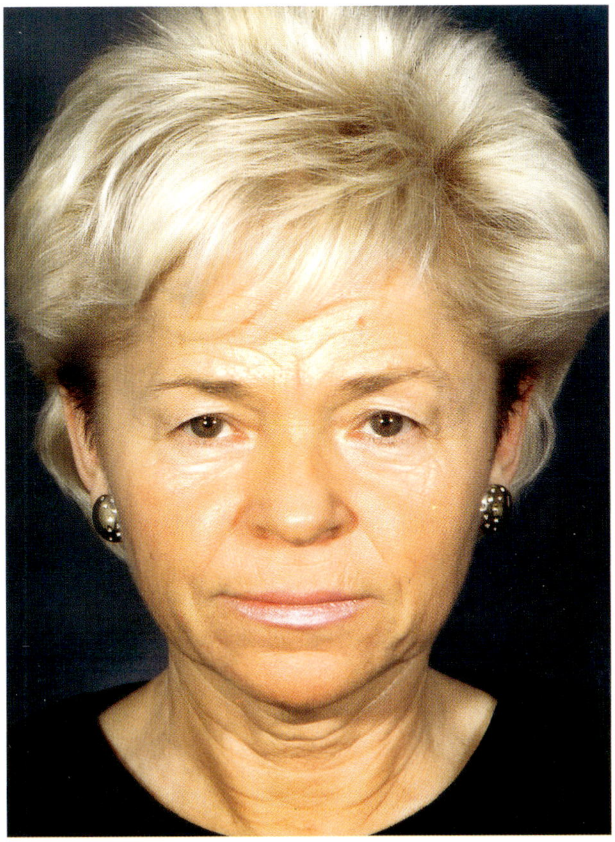

Figure 3.111a Forehead wrinkles, eyebrow ptosis of the upper eyelids, blepharochalasis, sagging facial and neck skin

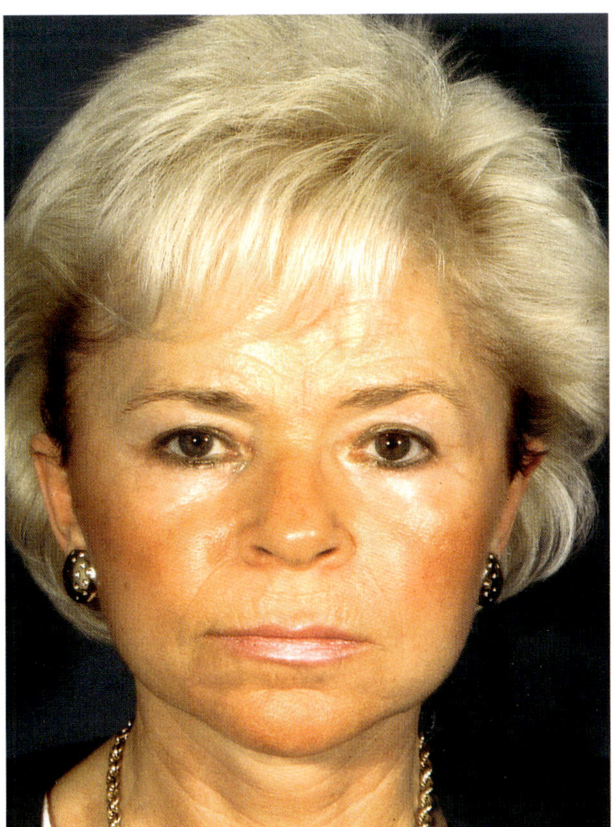

Figure 3.111b Appearance after bicoronal facelifting ("Mask lifting"), blepharoplasty and extensive neck skin lifting. It is an illusion to think that a neck skin lift can be achieved just by bicoronal incision in such cases. Here 7 cm of skin was resected postauricularly.

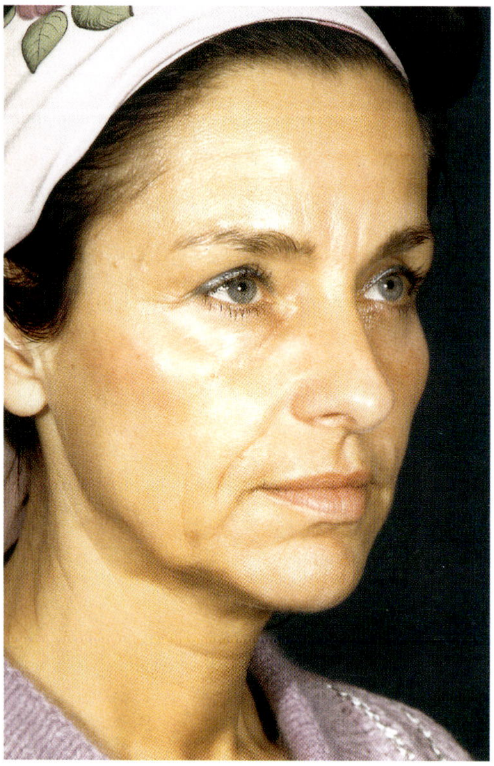

Figure 3.112a Sagging facial and neck skin, eyebrow ptosis

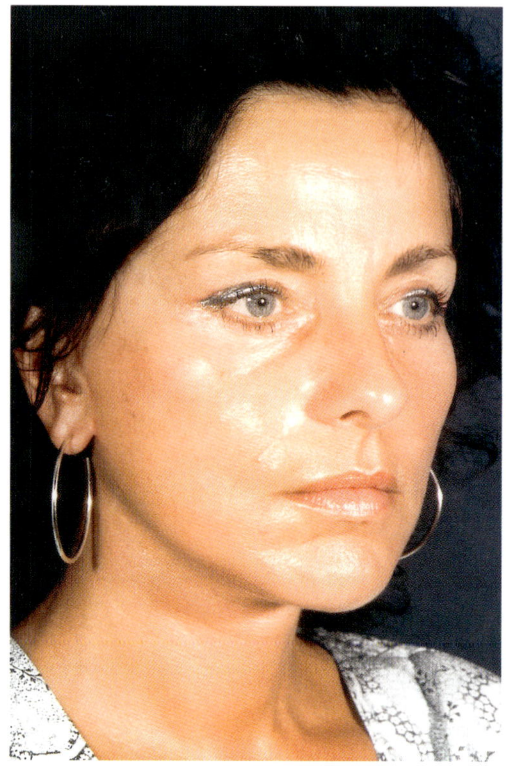

Figure 3.112b Appearance three years postoperatively after bicoronal mask lifting, neck skin lifting, and blepharoplasty.

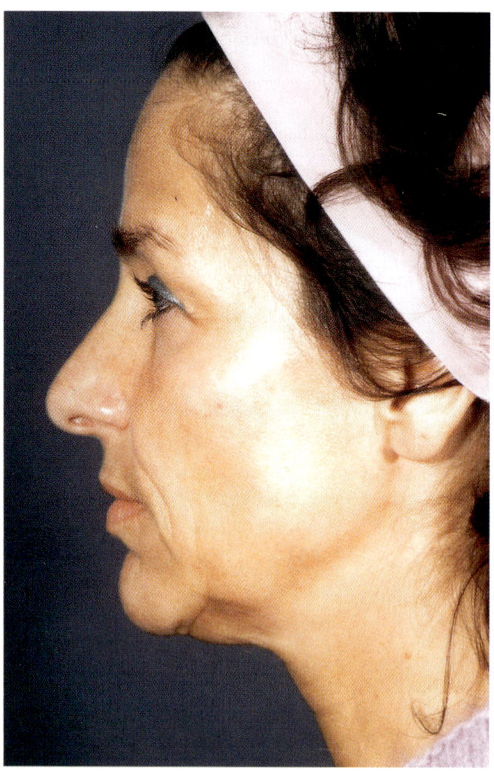

Figure 3.112c Preoperative profile

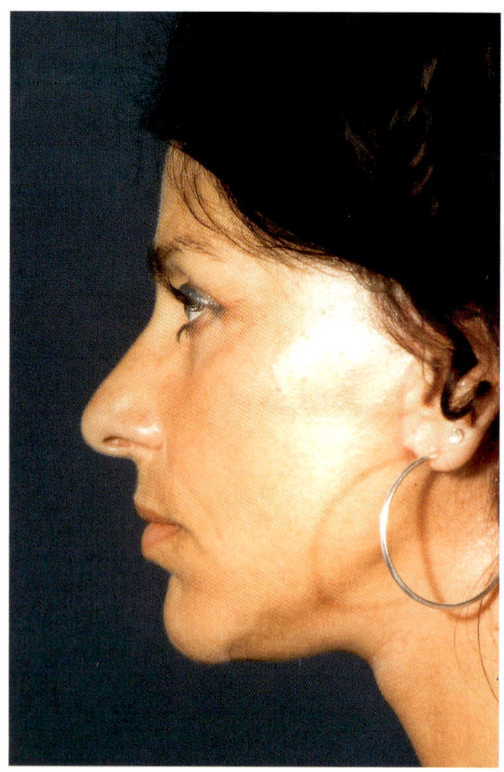

Figure 3.112d The forehead and midface are corrected by mask lifting. A neck lift was also carried out.

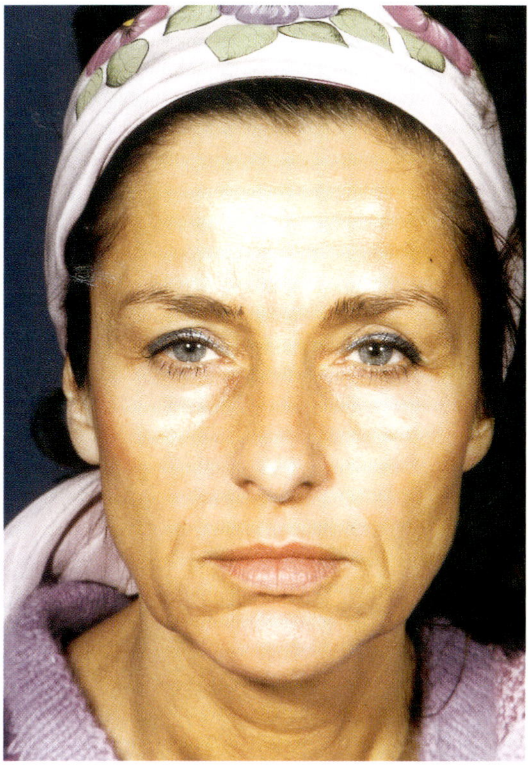

Figure3.112e The same patient before the first operation

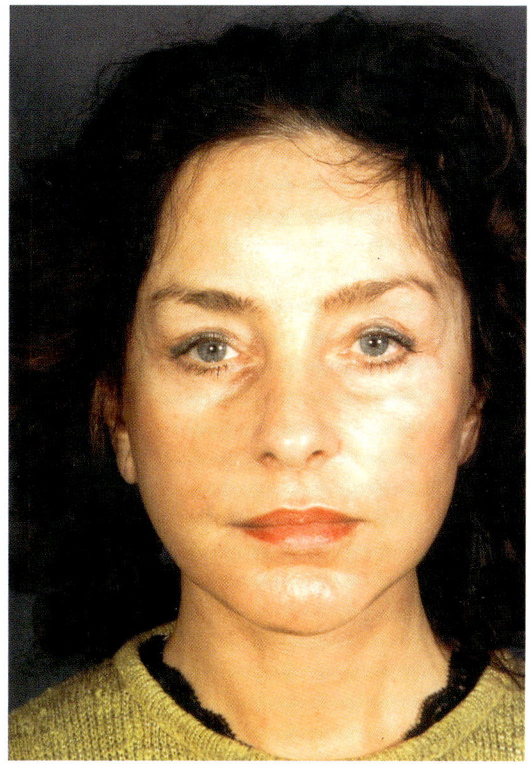

Figure 3.112f Appearance ten years after that and three years after the second minor lifting (only skin).

Second Facelifting:
Under no circumstances should a second facelifting be carried out earlier than three years after the first operation. At the second lifting one should only mobilize the skin and take a resection of approximately one to two centimeters. In most cases a second facelifting is a thankful and relatively simple operation (**no SMAS!**).

c) Upper Lip Wrinkle Abrasion

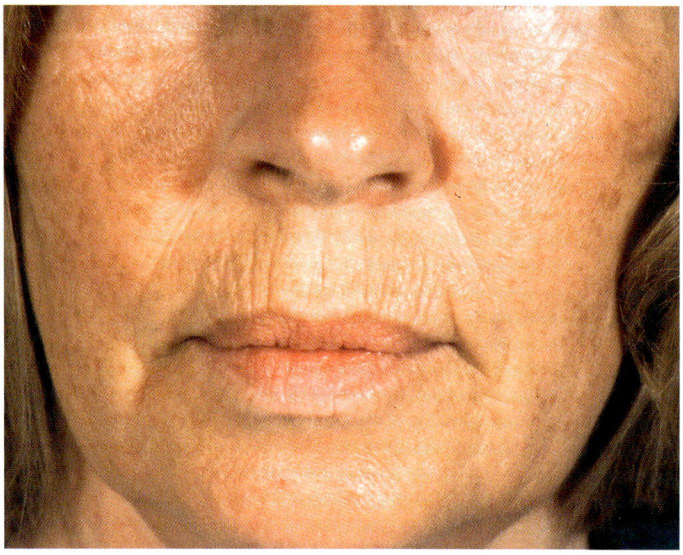

Figure 3.113a Upper lip wrinkles

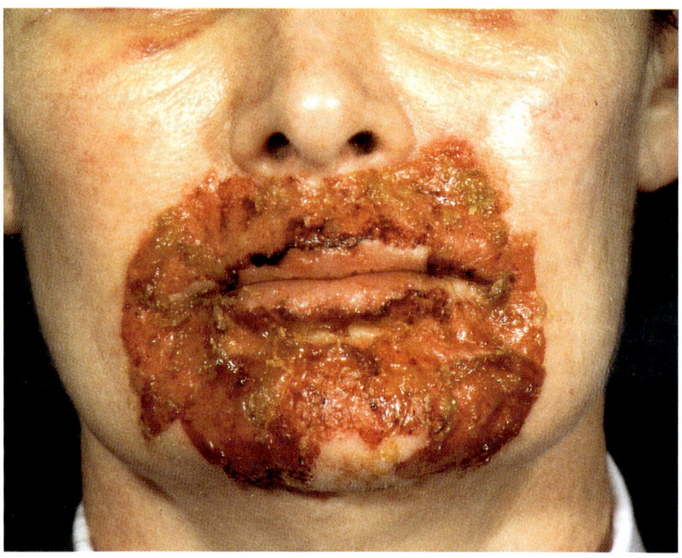

Figure 3.113b High-speed dermabrasion. Appearance two days after the deep dermal abrasion performed as an out-patient procedure under local anesthesia.

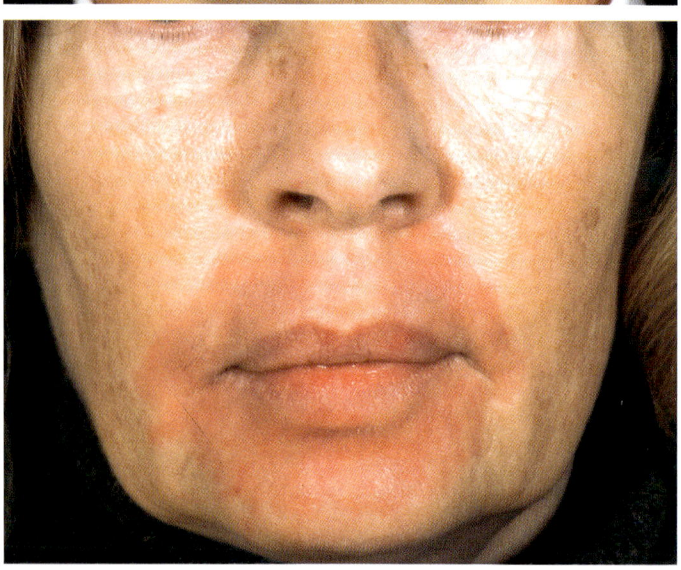

Figure 3.113c Appearance four weeks after the operation: One can still see a clear skin reddening. During the first six months the patient should keep away from the sun. The method is effective and economical (cheaper than laser and probably with less complications).

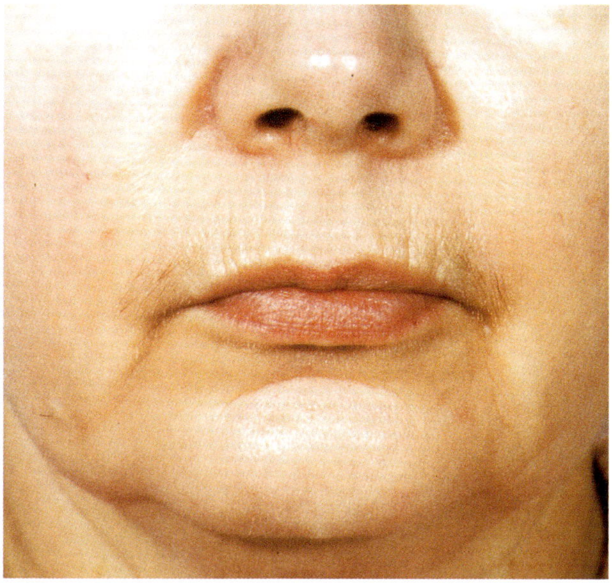

Figure 3.114a Upper lip wrinkle

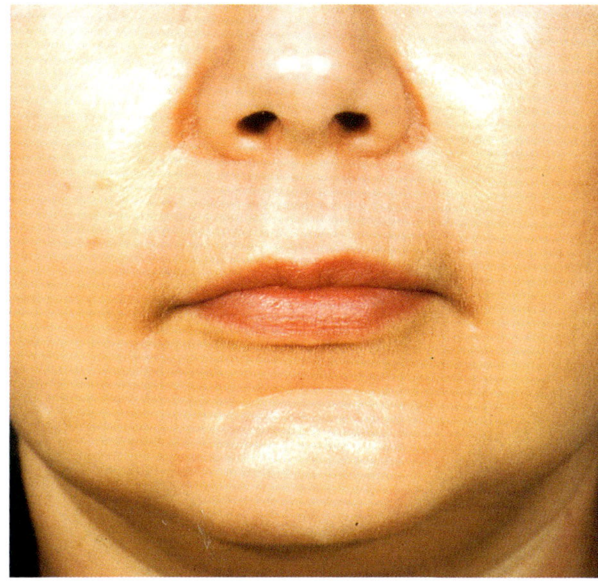

Figure 3.114b Appearance two years after the dermabrasion

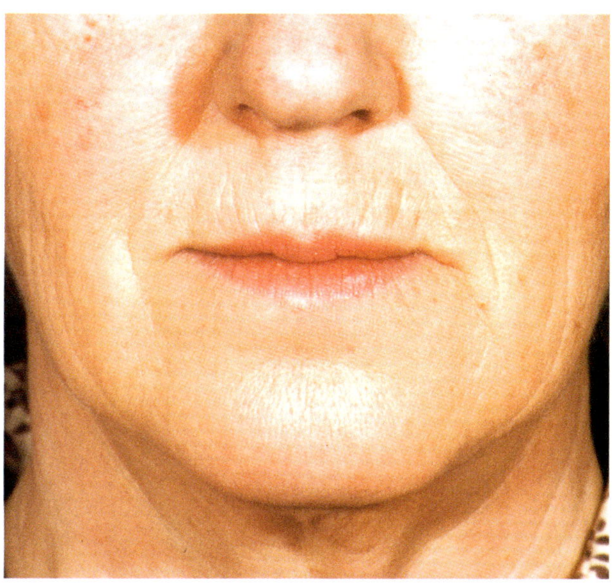

Figure 3.115a Upper lip wrinkle

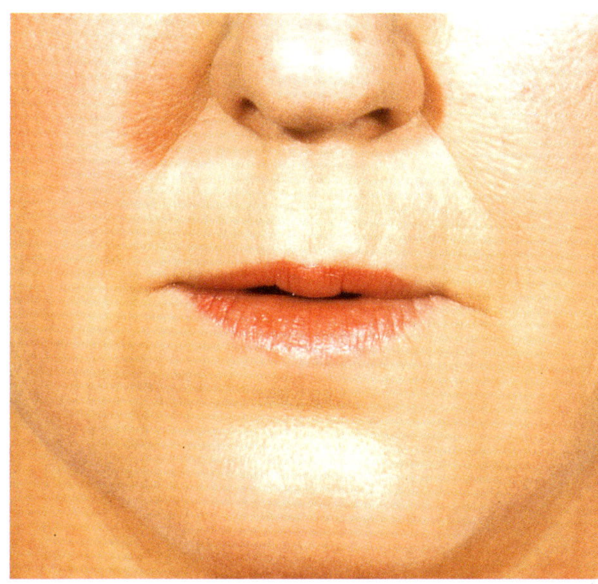

Figure 3.115b Appearance three years after the dermabrasion

d) Implantation of Superficial Temporal Fascia

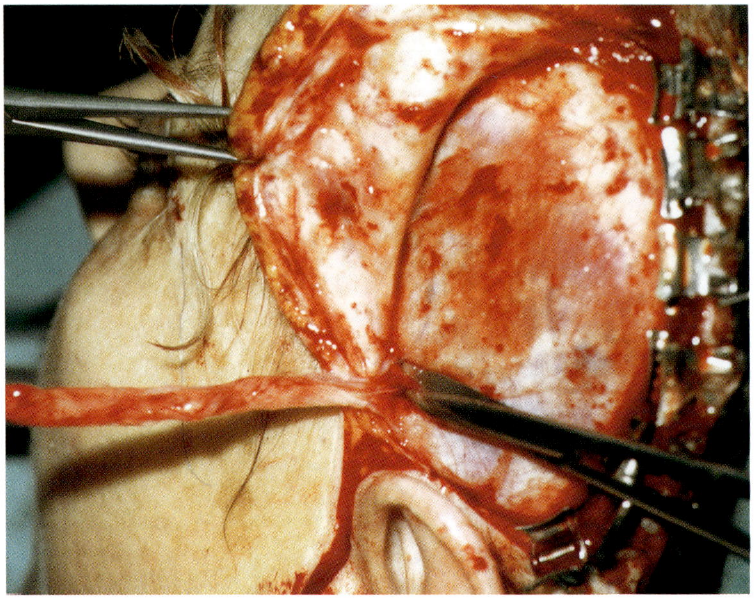

Figure 3.116a If during the facelifting a mildly wrinkled upper lip is apparent, a strip of superficial temporal fascia is removed bilaterally and used to fill the lip. This is of a very tender consistency. The healing rate of the fascia is approximately 90 %.

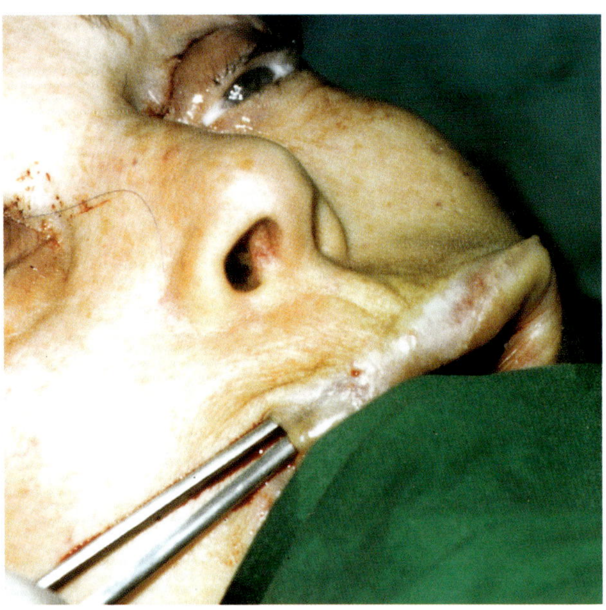

Figure 3.116b At the edge between the mucosa of the lip and the skin a tunnel is formed using some fine scissors (hand scissors). The incision is made in the area of the mucosa.

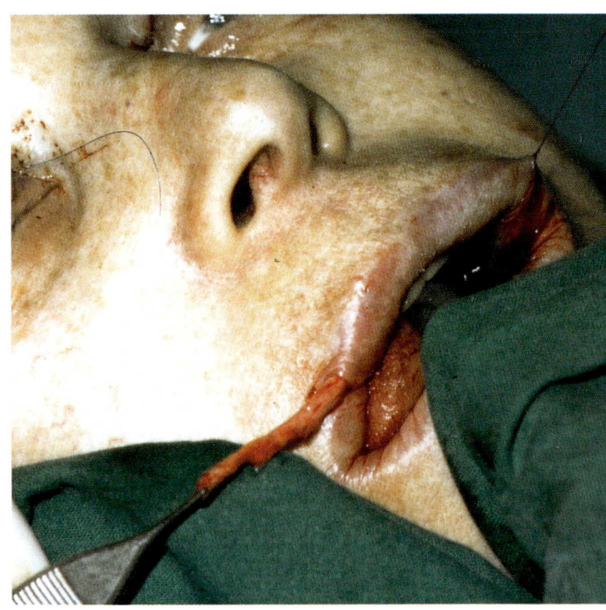

Figure 3.116c The superficial temporal fascia is implanted into the tunnel. The mucosa is sutured using 6×0 Vicryl suture. The scars are invisible and the result permanent. **This is a simple and economical method for correction of wrinkle of the lip if a facelifting is carried out at the same time.**

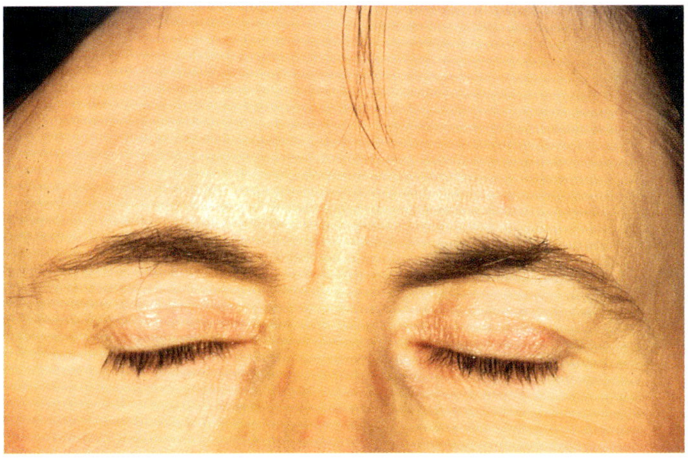

Figure 3.117a Vertical forehead wrinkle in the area of the glabella

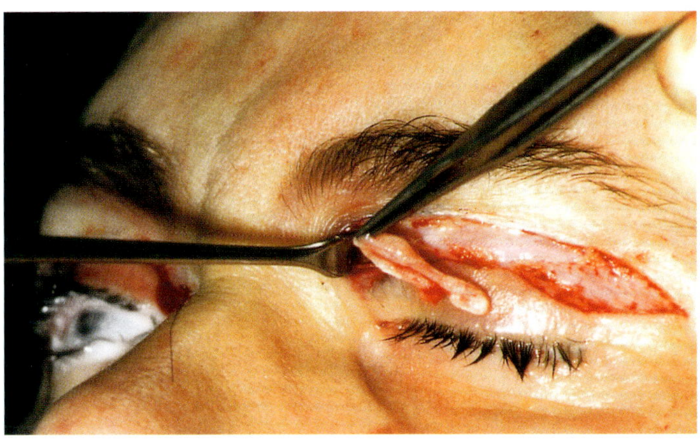

Figure 3.117b A strip of superficial temporal fascia is very suitable for correcting the vertical forehead wrinkle in the glabella area. The blepharoplasty incision allows the implant to be placed in the desired area. Through this incision it is easy to resect a part of corrugator muscle.

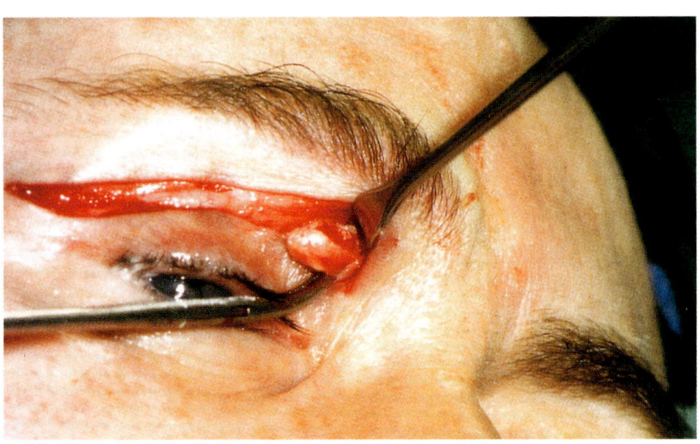

Figure 3.117c The fascia is pulled through into the prepared pocket. This problem is often dealt with nowadays by using botulinum toxin injections (every few months).

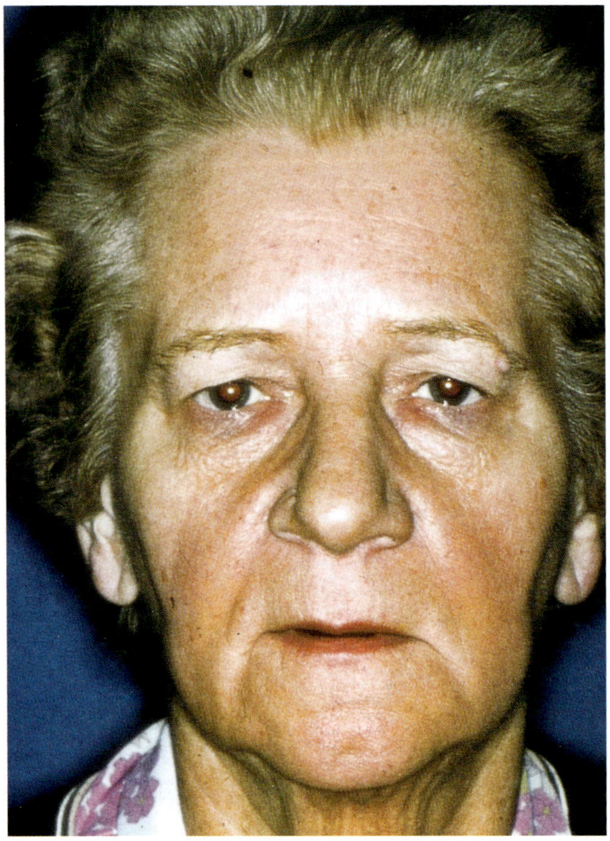

Figure 3.118a Blepharochalasis, ptosis of the eyebrows, sagging cheek and neck skin

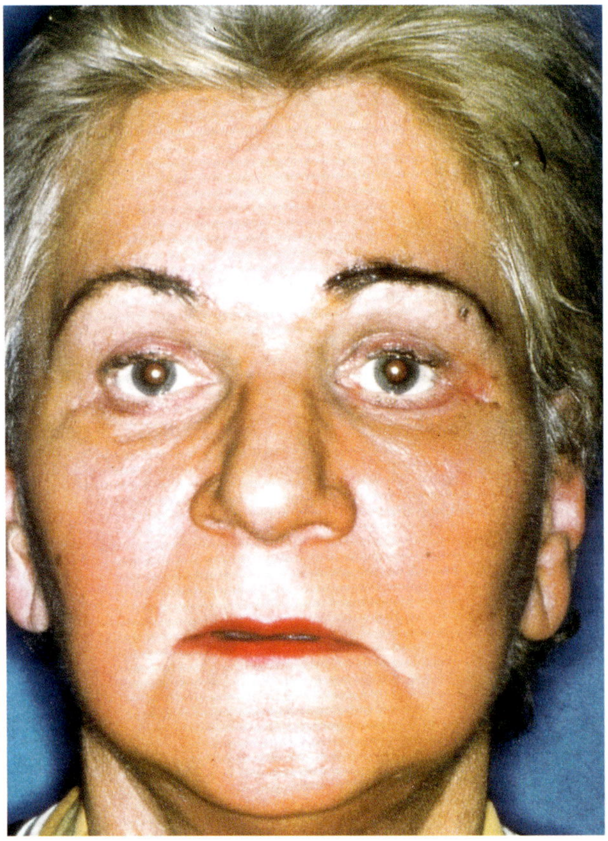

Figure 3.118b Appearance after forehead lifting as well as a face and neck skin lift. The blepharoplasty was carried out later.

e) Double Chin Correction

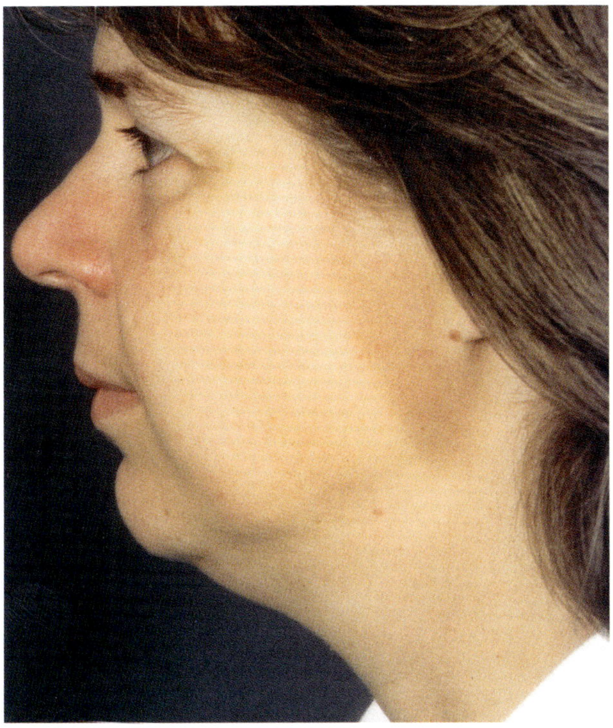

Figure 3.119a Double chin

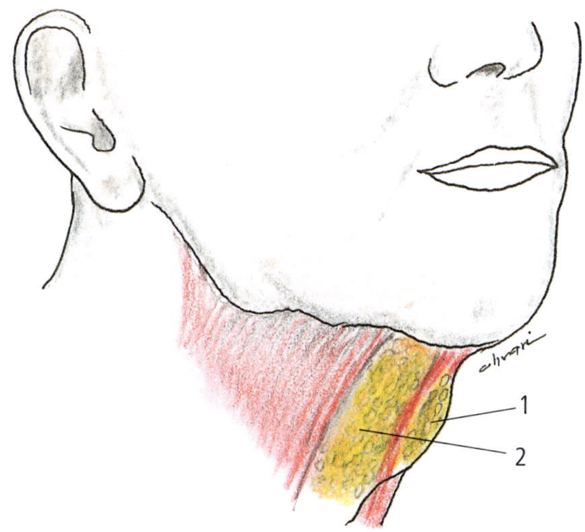

Figure 3.119b Distribution of the submental fat with a double chin. Only part of the fat is subcutaneous (1). The second part is localized behind the platysma diastasis (2).

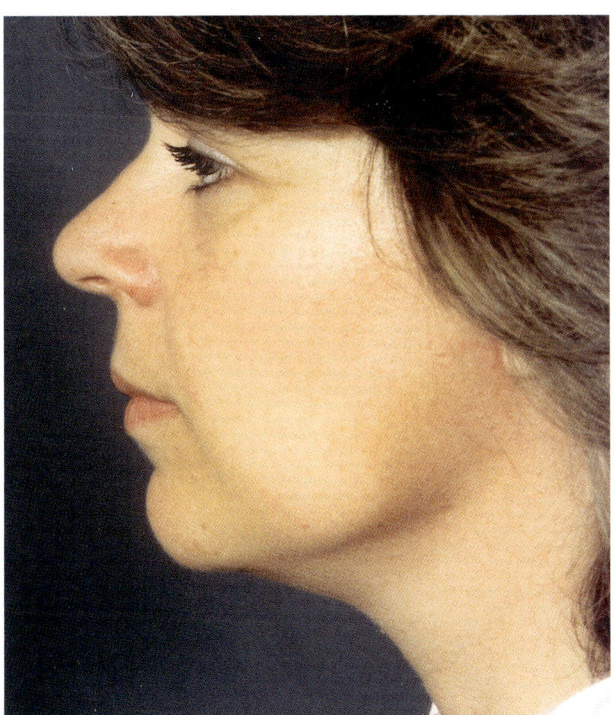

Figure 3.119c Appearance one year after the operation

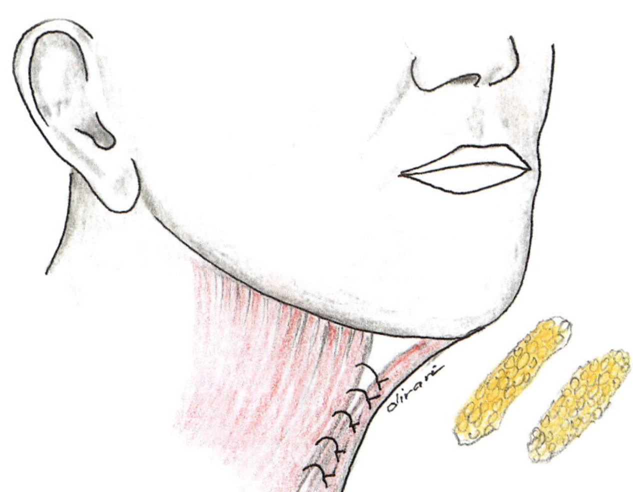

Figure 3.119d After removal of the subcutaneous fat and the fat behind the platysma a suture must always be made to reunite the dislocated platysma.

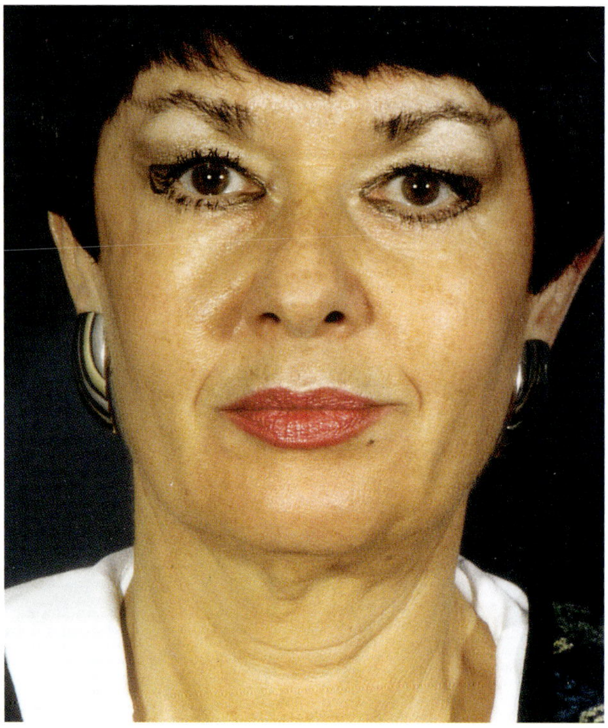

Figure 3.120a Problem zones: upper eyelids, nasolabial wrinkles, sagging lower part of the cheek as well as the neck

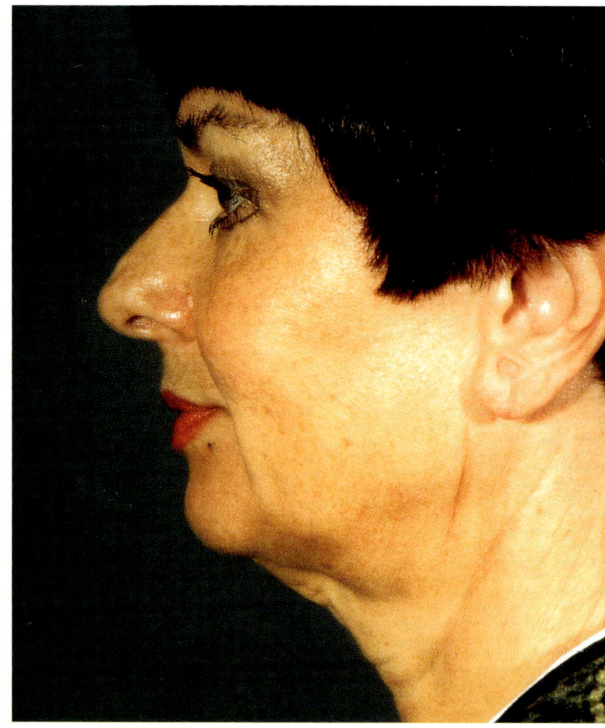

Figure 3.120b Sagging facial and neck skin as well as a somewhat excessively long humped nose

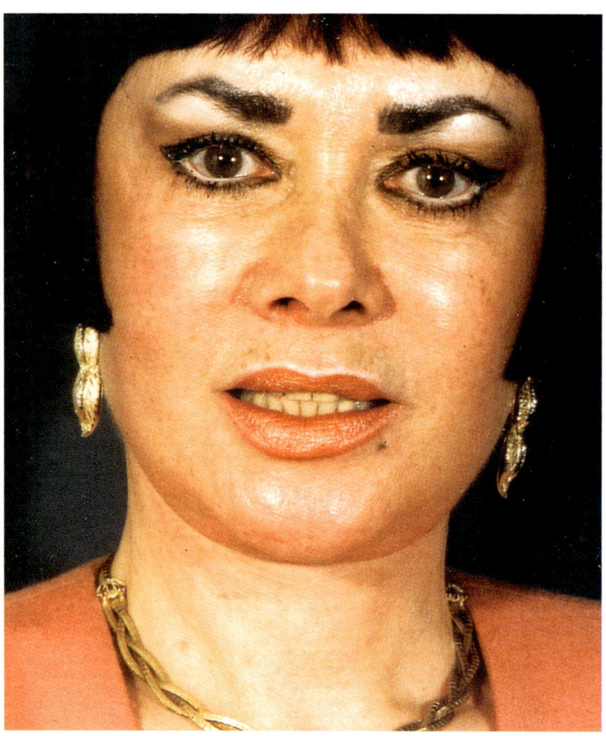

Figure 3.120c Appearance six years after the modified standard facelifting with SMAS, neck lift and blepharoplasty. Superficial temporal fascia was implanted into the upper and lower lips. Three months after the facelifting a nasal correction was carried out.

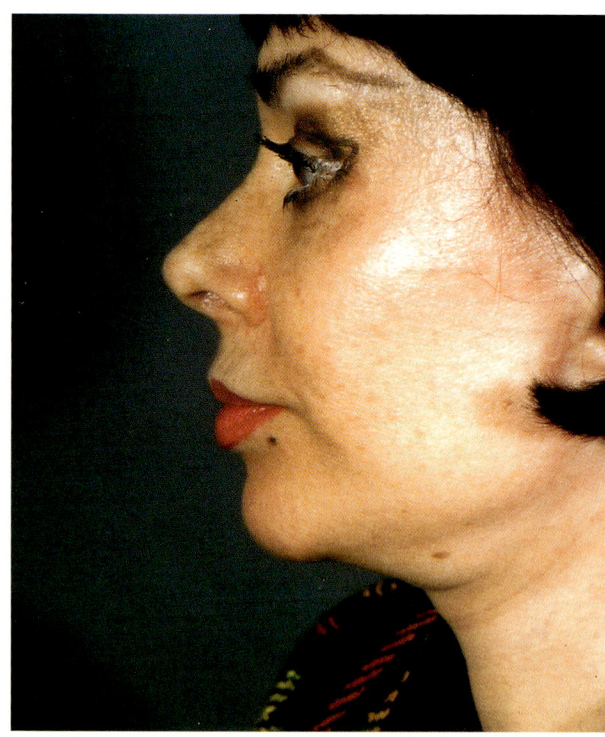

Figure 3.120d Appearance six years after the operation

f) Complications in Facelifting

From 1983 to 1997 we carried out 635 facelifting operations.

There are some surgeons, however, who never report complications, and such surgeons should never be believed!

1) Hematomas (3.1 %) usually occur during the first few hours after the operation. The revision should be carried out immediately. Any wait might be damaging and impair the outcome of the operation due to the significant extra stretching of the skin.
2) Partial nerve paresis (8 of 635 patients = 1.3 %) occurred more frequently with SMAS than it did without. Because, over the last decade, hardly any faceliftings have been carried out without SMAS, this statement is of little relevance. Of the injuries causing the eight pareses, four were of the frontal branch, three of the buccal branch and one was of the marginal branch
   All pareses were (fortunately) temporary and recovered spontaneously within six to 12 weeks. During this period the patients received intensive and friendly care. A reinnervation is almost always the rule particularly for the buccal branches that are multiple and anastomose with one another. With partial injuries or traction an amazing potential for reinnervation is also shown by the frontal branch, while this potential is considerably less for the marginal branch.
   Rule: If a nerve injury is found during an operation, nerve suturing should be carried out immediately. Statistics have shown that pareses of one of the above mentioned nerves (almost always temporary) occurs in 2.2 % of cases with SMAS and 1.0 % of cases without SMAS.
3) Skin necrosis arises due to excessive stretching and probably from nicotine abuse. Our 7 patients with skin necrosis were discharged very early on. We discovered, however, that our recommendation for patients to wash their hair on a daily basis was not followed. Where crusts became infected, these infections caused a marginal necrosis (Table 3.3).
   For this reason the hair must be washed 24 to, at latest, 36 hours after the operation.
4) Hair loss occurs due to marginal necrosis.

Table 3.3 Complications with facelifting (n = 635)

Complications	Number	Percent
Hematoma, secondary hemorrhage	20	3.1 %
Partial facial paresis (reversible)	8	1.3 %
Skin necrosis	7	1.1 %
Hair loss (partial)	6	0.9 %
In all		6.4 %

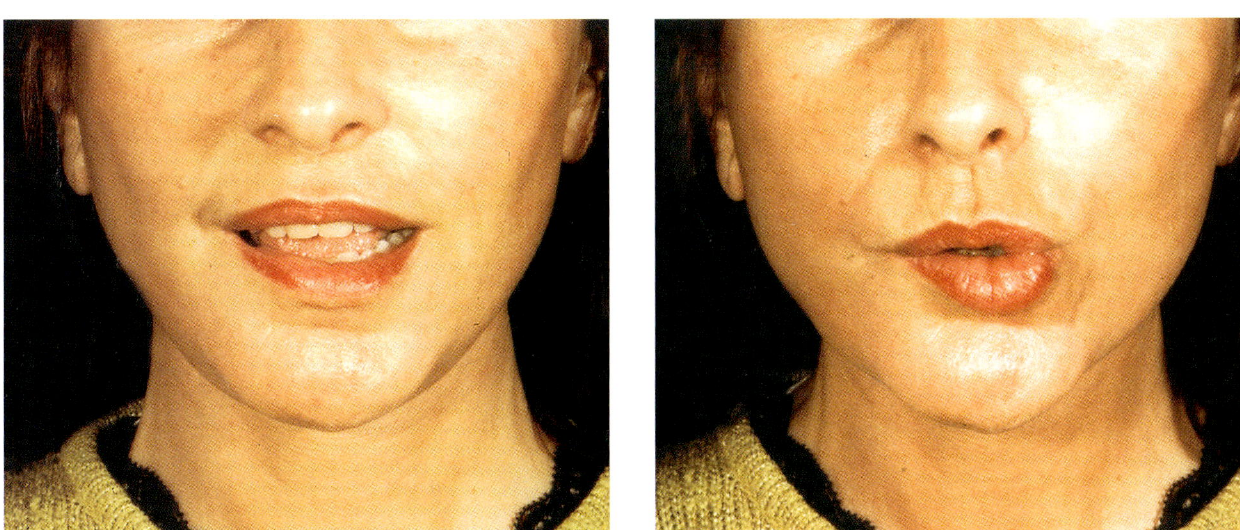

Figure 3.121a,b Typical damage of the marginal branch at three weeks postoperatively. After 12 weeks the innervation was fully intact again.

Laser Treatment

A laser consists of a source of light and a light amplifier, i.e. a generator and booster for coherent electromagnetic waves e.g. in the visible range, but also at infrared and ultra-violet frequencies that border on the visible range, and at other frequencies (maser, X-ray laser, free electron laser).

Laser types include CO_2, argon, krypton and others. A laser coagulates or vapourizes the tissue surface that consists of 80 to 90 % water. In simplified terms, laser therapy brings about a superficial burn.

The laser treatment of facial wrinkles is growing in acceptance. The results in the lip area are comparable with those of dermal abrasion.

In the eyelid area dermal abrasion is impossible. Laser treatment at the neck (see Figure 3.122) conveys no advantages, and pigmentation disorders can also arise.

Laser treatment is not surgery, so there is no reason to be extensively discussed in this book.

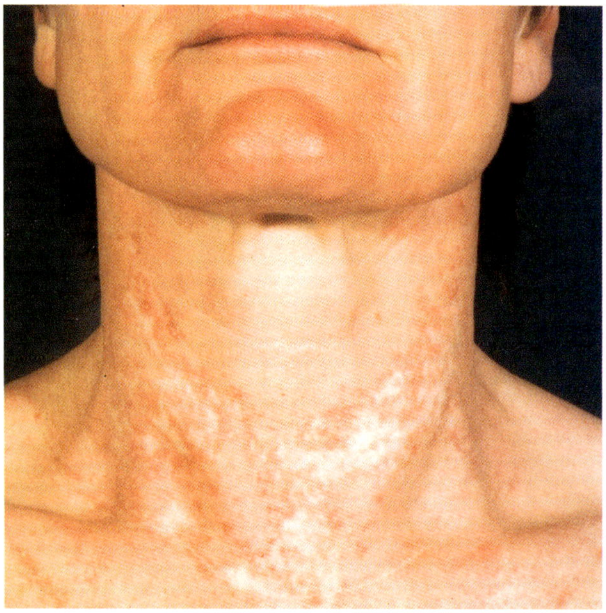

Figure 3.122a Appearance after an attempt to eliminate neck wrinkles using a CO_2 laser. Typical burn scars.

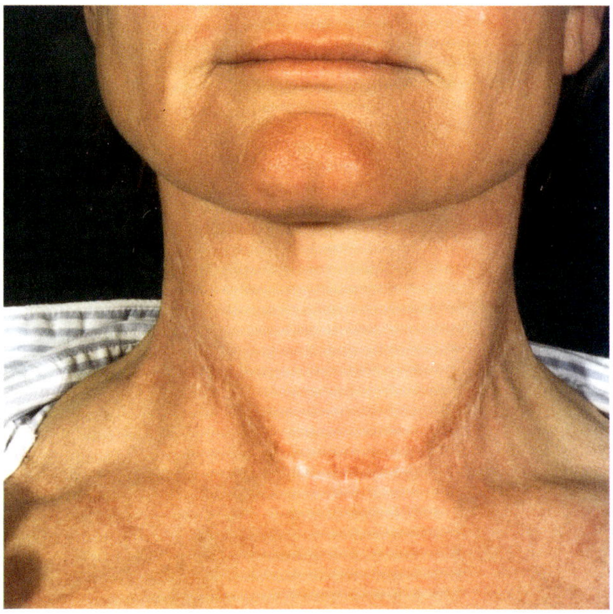

Figure 3.122b Appearance after excision of the burned area

Endocrine Ophthalmopathy – Surgical Therapy

Transpalpebral Decompression Through Removal of Intraorbital Fat

a) Pathogenesis

Endocrine ophthalmopathy (EO) is an autoimmune disease just as immunohyperthyreosis is, according to current knowledge. It still remains to be determined whether it is an independent clinical picture or whether EO is a manifestation of immunohyperthyreosis. In 90 % of individuals EO appears with an immunogenically-conditioned hyperthyreosis. It therefore appears logical to think that a common noxin (antigen) must exist, but this still remains to be verified. Because of the increasing volume of muscles and fat, combined with the venous and lymphatic congestion, the intraorbital pressure increases and the eyeball is displaced ventrally by around 5–10 mm (exophthalmos).

In Germany more than 100,000 patients suffer from this disease.

Probably 20,000 need operative treatment. This statistic is not exactly proofed.

b) Diagnosis

A careful medical history, clinical examination and precise determination of thyroid gland function all represent components for the initial diagnosis. All patients who came into our care had already been examined and treated, often many times, by endocrinologists, ophthalmologists and nuclear medicine specialists. Apart from two patients (see Figure 3.125), all others were euthyroid.

Table 3.4 Werner scale classification

Grade	Symptoms
Grade I	Upper lid retraction (Dalrymple's phenomenon), retraction of the upper eyelid when looking down (Graefe), convergence deficit
Grade II	With involvement of connective tissue (eyelid swelling, chemosis, tear dribbling, photophobia)
Grade III	With protrusion of the eyeball (pathological Hertel values, with and without eyelid swelling)
Grade IV	With eye muscle paresis (blurred and/or double vision)
Grade V	With corneal injury (mostly lagophthalmos with turbidity, ulcerations)
Grade VI	With losses in vision extending to blindness (involvement of the optic nerve)

c) Therapy

Primarily all patients should be treated by endocrinologist and ophthalmologist. The muscle and fat volume in the orbit must be defined by CT or MRI.

1) Conservative Therapy

Oral Glucocorticoid Therapy
Treatment of an EO in the acute phase using corticosteroids is reasonable. The corticosteroids also exert immunosuppressive, anti-inflammatory, and inhibitory effects on the synthesis of GAG fibroblasts.

Orbital Irradiation
The pathophysiological concept assumes that the lymphocytes infiltrating into the retrobulbar space become damaged by localized irradiation so that an anti-inflammatory effect can be achieved locally. In addition, the radiation effect should act antiproliferatively towards the fibroblasts and induce the production of glycosaminoglycans. Short-term results are apparently good during the acute phase, but long-term results are less convincing. Good results regarding protrusion, diplopia and vision are questionable. No long-term findings regarding possible irradiation injuries have been reported.

2) Surgical Therapy – Osseous Decompression (Enlargement of the Orbit)

Medial Wall Decompression
Medial decompression only corrects the proptosis by about 2 to 3 mm, but often causes diplopia or convergent squint. It does however represent a good procedure for decompression where the optic nerve is under pressure (1–2 % of patients)

In all osseous decompression periorbita (periost) is divided, so orbita content heriate into sinus maxillaries or ethmoid sinus.

Parts of this chapter are taken from the book by Neven Olivari (2001) "Endocrine Ophthalmopathy – Surgical Treatment". Kaden Verlag, Heidelberg

Two-Wall Decompression

The most frequently used method of bony decompression is two-wall decompression (75 % of bony decompression in the USA) Good results can be achieved in correcting proptosis as well as threatened loss of vision. Complication rate is relatively high. Diplopia is more common after surgery than before. Walsh and Ogura (1957) made this method popular. They performed medial and caudal osteotomy and allowed adequate room for displacement of the orbital content into the ethmoid sinus and the maxillary sinus, leaving the nasal function intact.

Three-Wall Decompression

Three-wall decompression is not used as often (20.5 % of all osseous decompressions in the USA). Using this procedure one can achieve a good correction of vision and the proptosis. However, because three orbital walls are resected, the complication rate is relatively high. An increasing number of diplopias have been described by most authors after the operation. The indication is restricted to patients who are threatened with loss of sight.

In all osseous decompressions the following complications are described: Oro-antral fistula, hematoma, perforation of dura, CSF leak, blindness etc.

3) Decompression Through Fat Removal – Method According to Olivari (Since 1985)

Decompression of the orbit through fat removal is designed to reduce pressure by lowering orbital content rather than enlarging the orbital volume. The globe remains in its central position. This is the only method in which the diplopia rate is drastically decreased. The complication rate is tolerable, the operation is complicated, and the learning curve is long.

Technique of the Operation

The operation is carried out under general anesthesia. As a rule only one orbit is operated on in one session, and seldom are both orbits operated on simultaneously. The operation is done using surgical magnifying glasses (loupes with 2.5 fold magnification).

In the evening before the operation, 250 mg dexamethasone is given intramuscularly, and just before the operation the same amount is given again.

The upper and lower eyelid skin is infiltrated with 0.5 % Scandicain and 1/200,000 adrenaline subcutaneously. No infiltration into the orbit. The eyelids are temporarily closed using a non-absorbable 5 × 0 suture.

The incision line in the upper eyelid is similar to that employed for a blepharoplasty, i.e. in the middle approximately 8 to 9 mm from the eyelid edge. In older patients with considerable amounts of excess skin a corresponding amount of surplus skin is also resected as for a blepharoplasty.

The orbicularis oculi muscle is divided transversely. Usually the orbital septum bulges like a hernia. The septum is divided transversely.

During division of the orbital septum, intraorbital fat appears ventrally upon application of pressure. The fat mass is mobilized dorsally between the orbital roof and the conus and removed medially and laterally en bloc. The tissue is ressected deeply to the apex.

In the lower eyelid the incision is carried out 4 to 5 mm below the eyelid margin. The orbicularis oculi muscle is transversely divided in the same way as the orbital septum.

The intraorbital fat is incised and removed first medially between the floor of the orbit and the conus, and then laterally up to the apex.

In the upper eyelid the superior oblique muscle, the supraorbital nerve, the supratrochlear nerve and the lacrimal gland must be identified and preserved.

In the lower eyelid the inferior oblique muscle as well as the inferior rectus muscle, the medial rectus muscle and the lateral rectus muscle are displayed.

The conus is divided up in the caudal part between the inferior rectus muscle and the medial rectus muscle. As a result of this the intraconal pressure reduces. The fat from the conus must not be removed. It now prolapses into the large new retrobulbar space. We never incise periorbit (periost) even in seldom cases of osteotomy (less than 1 %) to avoid diplopia.

At the end of the operation 3 to 5 mg dexamethasone is injected into each of all four rectus muscles. This apparently prevents any further muscular hypertrophy. The retrobulbar space is washed with a diluted solution including neomycin and dexamethasone.

If any upper eyelid retraction exists, an appropriate levator extension is carried out with or without interposition in the same session. The levator aponeurosis is divided completely up to the medial quarter, and the Mueller's muscle is also completely divided.

In the case of lower lid retraction, retractors should be transversely divided and if necessary ear cartilage is grafted in for lower lid support.

Postoperative Treatment

The operated eye is kept closed for four to five days with an eyelid suture. Mycinopred eye drops (Prednisolone, polymixin and Neomycin eye drops) are applied several times daily. On the first postoperative day 250 mg Solu Decortin (Prednisolone) is given intramuscularly.

The eyes are not bandaged!

The patients may get up the next day and move freely about since only one eye is usually operated on at a time. Usually the patients do not have postoperative pain.

Postoperative pain is always a cause for alarm (hematoma!) as it is unusual. In this case **immediately** operative revision is indicated (no tamponade!) On the 4th or 5th postoperative day the eyelid closure suture is removed.

For patients with simultaneous levator lengthening an overcorrection arises, i.e. there is a moderate ptosis of the upper eyelid. This normally settles spontaneously in two to six weeks. The other orbit may be operated on in the same way four to six days after the first operation. Exceptionally both orbits are operated at same time.

The suture closure of both eyelids for the first five days is designed to achieve two objectives:

- Fewer conjunctival reactions (chemosis) In the case of chemosis a small amount of Prednisolone should be injected into conjunctiva.
- The orbicularis oculi muscle exerts mild pressure on the globe in a dorsal direction where adequate space is now available.

Indications for Operation and Classification (N = 1000 orbits)

- Only 11 (1.1 %) orbits were operated on for severe lid retraction without clinically marked protrusion.
- 126 (12.6 %) orbits were operated on for severe protrusion. Many patients also had a concurrent lid retraction.
- 736 (73.6 %) orbits, i.e. the majority, simultaneously showed protrusion, a disturbance of motility (diplopia) and lid retraction.
- 73 (7.3 %) patients presented with corneal damage (keratitis, corneal ulceration) as well as protrusion and disturbance of motility.
- 54 (5.4 %) orbits presented with considerable loss of vision in addition to protrusion and disturbance of motility.
- 75 % of all patients were operated on because of lid retraction.

Patient Information

Ensuring the patient has full information requires a lot of time. Two, three or even more counselling sessions before the operation should be given if the patients are still unsure. A comprehensive patient information leaflet was developed on our part for this purpose.

The patient must undergo a comprehensive ophthalmological examination and must also be in a suitable endocrinological state (They should be euthyroid). A CT or MRI scan of the orbit is also regarded as a pre-requisite.

Fat Removal Through the Upper Eyelid

After incision of the orbital septum the fat is first bluntly separated from the orbit wall (We never touch periorbit). After that the globe is protected with a retractor (Martin 15-093-18). The fat between the orbit wall on the one hand and the conus on the other is deeply divided up to the apex. If possible, it is advantageous to remove the fat en bloc from each quadrant.

During the excision, coagulation is always carried out first, using bipolar forceps, before resection is performed using scissors. In this way hemorrhage is avoided. The lacrimal glands, the supraorbital nerve as well as the superior oblique muscle must all be protected and preserved. The fat must not be retracted or severed using a clamp, and instead one should carefully pursue, coagulate and resect up to the apex under full vision.

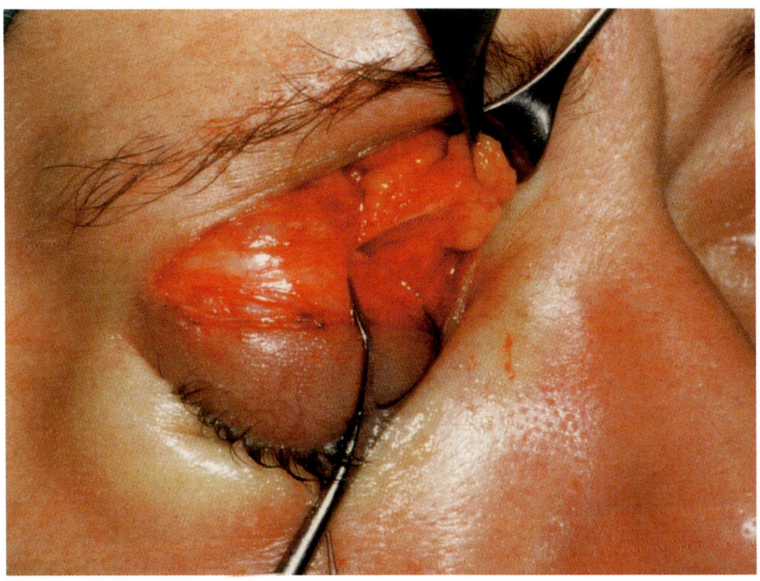

Figure 3.123a The globe is protected using the Martin retractor and the intraorbital fat is carefully resected.

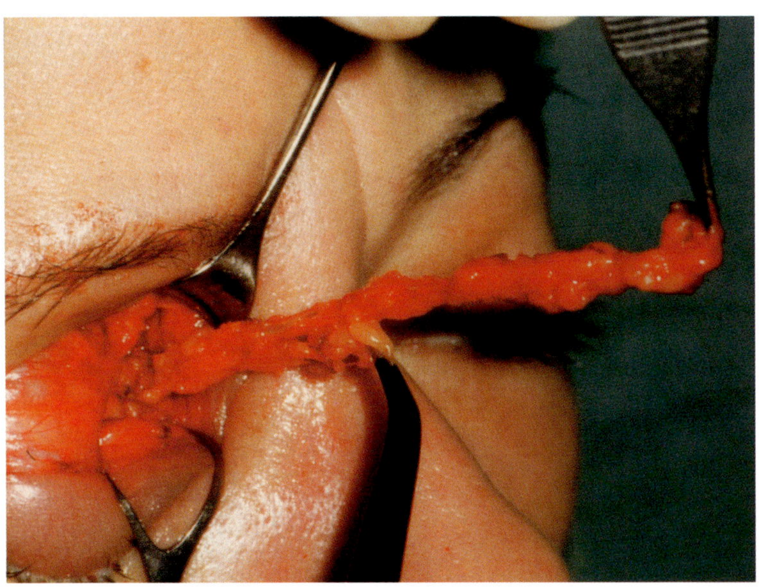

Figure 3.123b The fat mass is followed gradually downwards and is dissected from the important anatomical structures (muscles, nerves, vessels) using magnifying loupes. The fat quantity is greater in the medial upper part than it is in the lateral part.

Fat Removal Through the Lower Eyelid

The incision is made 4 mm below the lower lid margin. After division of the orbital septum the intraorbital fat is mobilized first from the orbital wall and after that from the conus in stages downwards. The largest fat quantity is found caudo-laterally.

After the fat between the orbital wall and the conus has been removed, a small longitudinal incision on caudally part of the conus (not cranially) while spreading the scissors. Here only the fat that spontaneously protrudes out of the conus under pressure come into new space. This decreases pressure on the conus.

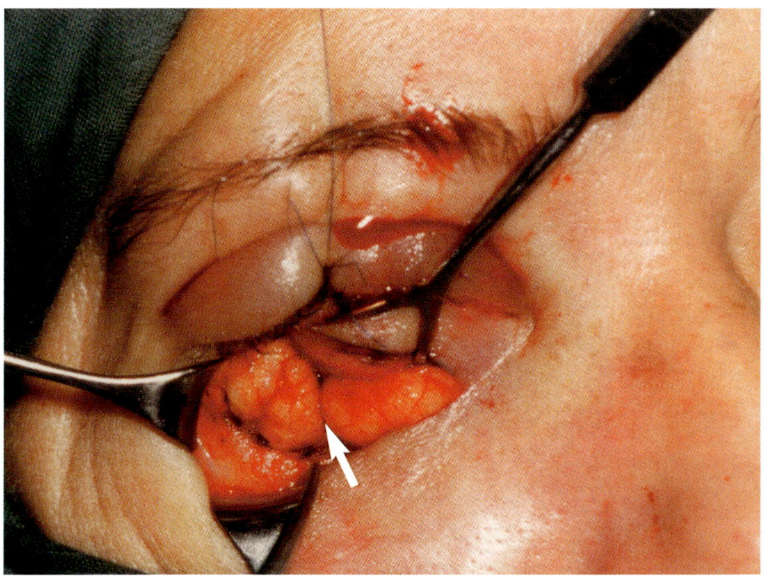

Figure 3.124a The largest amount of fat is found in the latero-caudal part of the orbit. One can clearly see the septum between the middle and lateral part of the fat (see arrow).

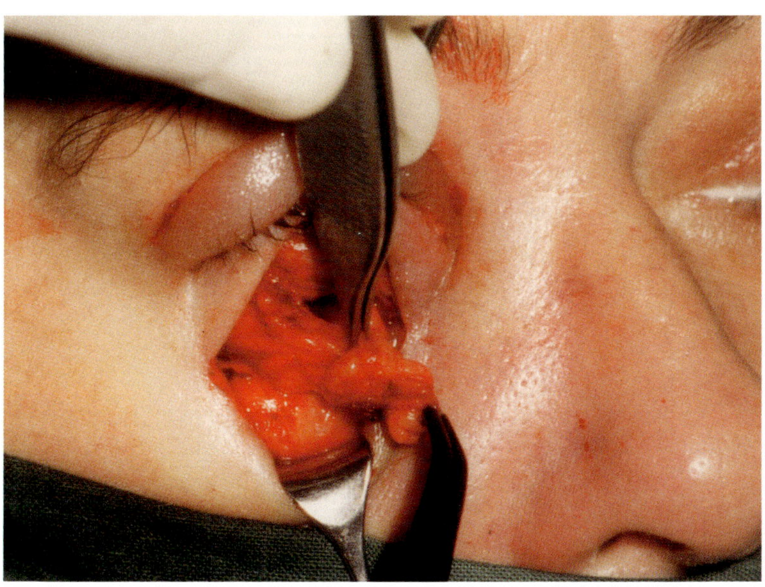

Figure 3.124b Also in the lower eyelid the intraorbital fat is first bluntly mobilized from the orbital wall on the periosteum up to the apex.

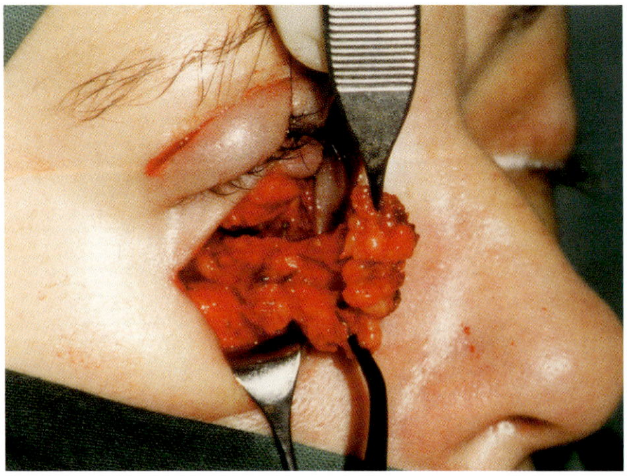

Figure 3.124c The fat mass is dissected free from the conus, the inferior rectus muscle and the lateral rectus muscle up to the apex.

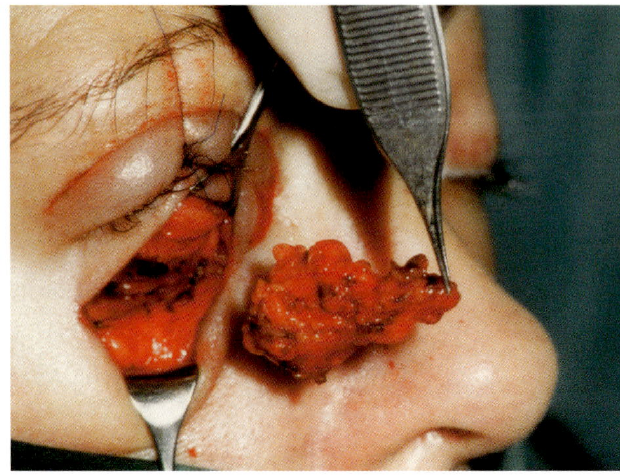

Figure 3.124d The fat mass is removed "en bloc". One should not attempt to remove the intraorbital fat in small pieces. This will complicate the operation considerably.

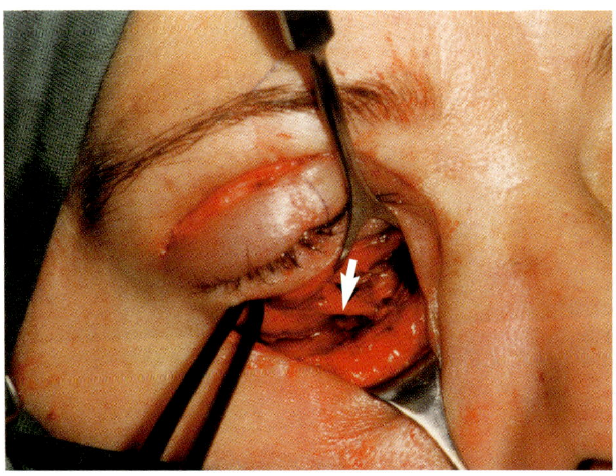

Figure 3.124e At the end of the operation one can see the inferior oblique muscle (see arrow).

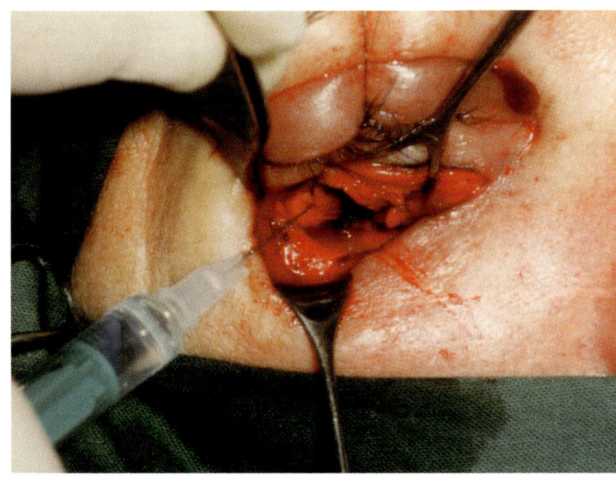

Figure 3.124f 5 mg of dexamethasone is injected into the lateral rectus muscle. The same amount is injected into all four rectus muscles. If there is severe upper lid retraction dexamethasone is also injected into the levator palpebrae muscle.

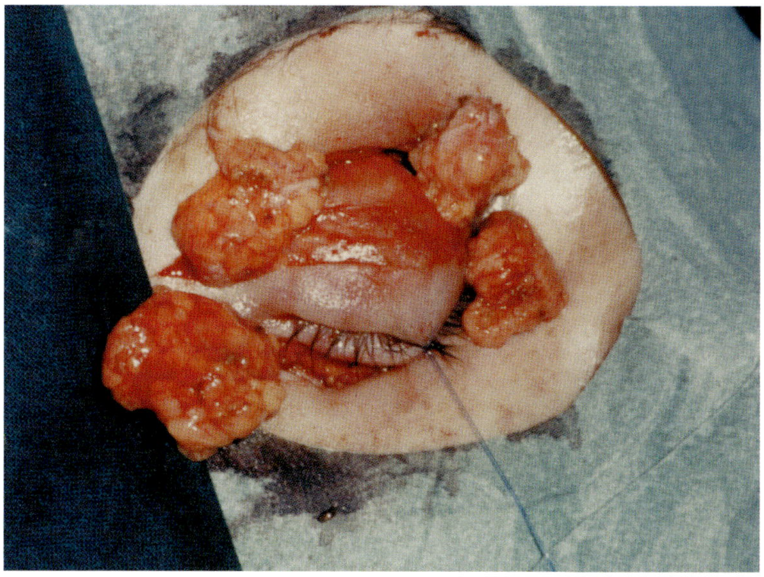

Figure 3.124g At the end of the operation one can see that the largest fat mass was removed latero-caudally. In all, 7.2 ccm of fat was removed. Experience shows that the removal of less than 4 ccm of fat produces an inferior outcome.

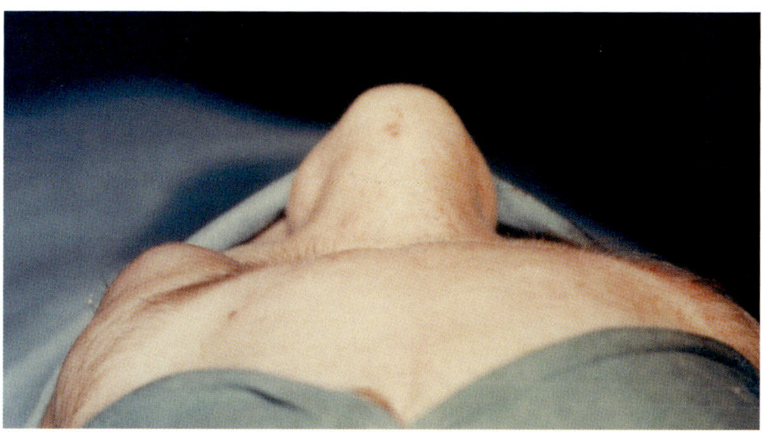

Figure 3.124h At the end of the operation the right globe has moved dorsally by about 8 mm. The left side has not yet been operated on.

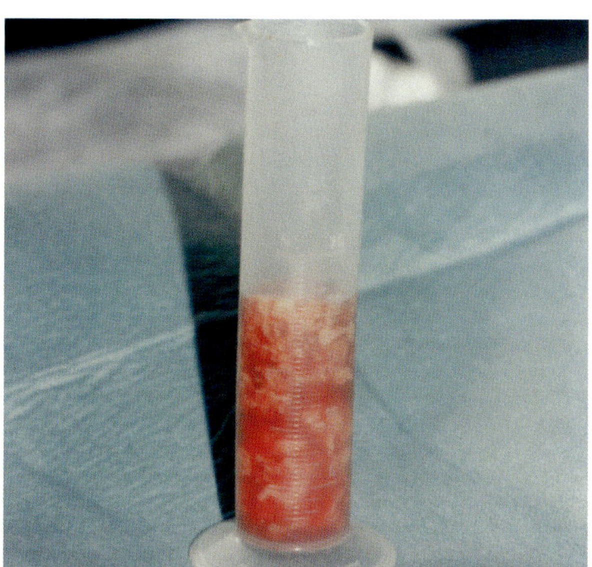

Figure 3.124i End of the decompression on the right side. 7.2 ccm of fat was removed. The measurement of the fat mass is carried out in a small measuring cylinder. The volume of the removed fat is important, not the weight. The Right globe has moved back about 8 mm at the end of the operation. Over the next few days the protrusion may increase again because of surgical edema. Approximately three months have to pass, and sometimes even longer, before the desired result is achieved. As a rule the other orbit is operated on four to six days later, and only rarely are both sides operated on at the same operation.

Exophthalmos and Its Consequences

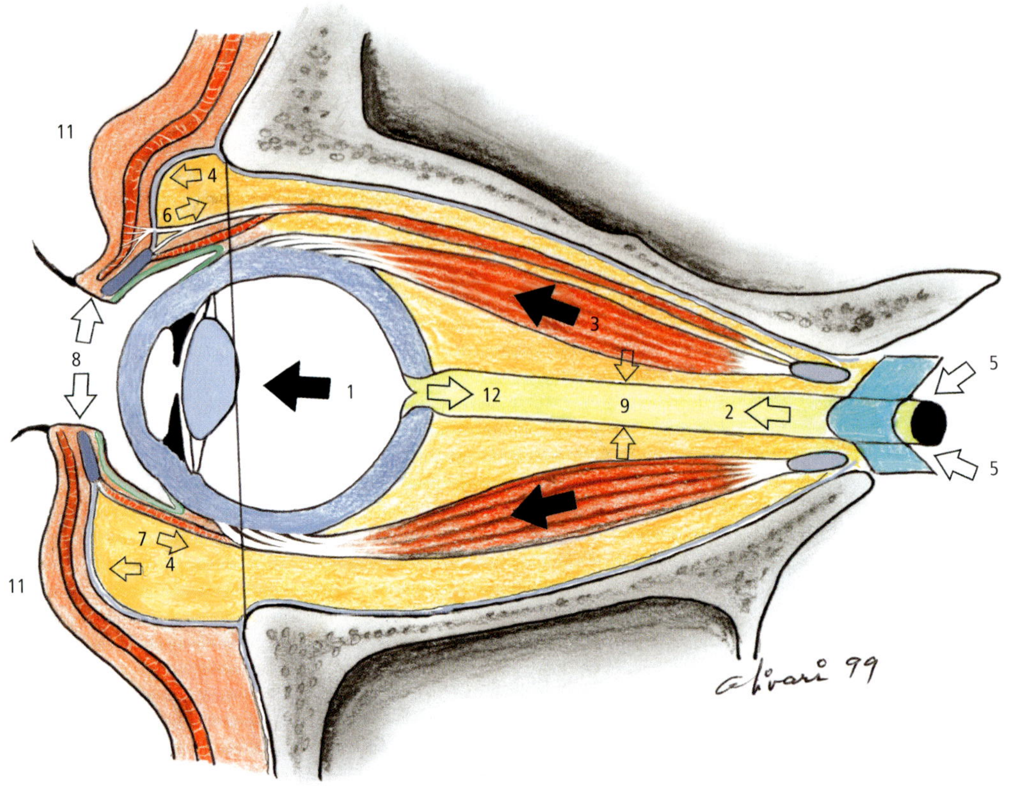

Figure 3.125

1) Because of the increased volume of muscles and fat, as well as the venous and lymphatic congestion, the intraorbital pressure increases and the globe is displaced ventrally by about 5 to 10 mm. (Globe has never pathological changes).

2) The optic nerve is stretched from the globe in a ventral direction. The nerve has almost no elasticity and is therefore already under tension in its primary position with EO. Upon movement of the globe, the tension on the optic nerve increases even more. The optic nerve exerts traction on the optic disc. The central retinal artery can be affected in this way leading to reduced blood supply.

3) The hypertrophic and fibrotic extraocular muscles have already lost their elasticity. With further stretching (of 5 to 10 mm) due to exophthalmos their mobility is restricted even further. This results in an indirect shortening of the muscles by about 5 to 10 mm; the results are eye motility disturbance (diplopia, strabism).

4) The intraorbital fat moves, due to intraorbital pressure, in a ventral (anterior) direction. The orbital septum bulges forward in the upper and lower eyelid. As a result a slight decompression occurs in the orbit. With a hard, inelastic orbital septum this possibility of spontaneous decompression is less likely and intraorbital pressure is even more extensive.

5) The optic nerve in dorsal part is covered by the dura mater and within its second part the dura mater is bonded to the periosteum in the optic foramen. A severe traction on the dura mater occurs via the optic nerve. This in turn induces retrobulbar pressure or burning and headache.

6) The hypertrophic and fibrotic levator palpebrae muscle pulls the upper eyelid cranially via its aponeurosis. The sympathetically innervated Mueller's muscle is also hypertrophic and is more contracted which produce lid retraction. The proptosis also aggravates the lid retraction.

7) The retractors of the lower eyelid become fibrotic and shortened. Through the additional tension of the inferior rectus muscle to which the retractors are fixed, a lower lid ptosis results which is aggravated by the proptosis.

8) Due to retraction of the upper and lower eyelids, an increase in the eyelid gap results which, can often lead to a lagophthalmos. If it becomes impossible to close the eyelid, particularly at night, conjunctivitis, chemosis, keratitis and scleral ulcerations can result.

9) A direct pressure on the optic nerve may result from muscle thickening (very rare.)

10) Frequently there is a raised internal ocular pressure (glaucoma).

11) A severe swelling of the upper and lower eyelids results from the fat prolapse.

12) The optic nerve exerts traction on optic disc.

Status After Decompression Fat Resection

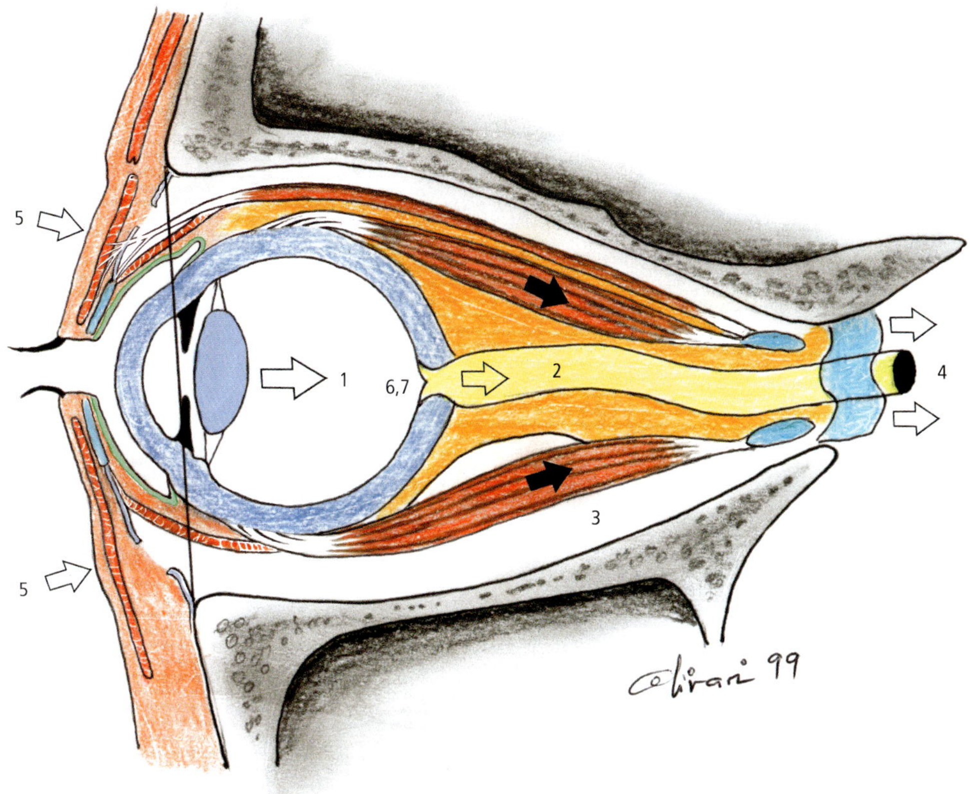

Figure 3.126 Appearance after fat resection from all four quadrants and a small part from the caudal part of the conus:

1. Following exstirpation of fat from all four quadrants and a small portion from the caudal part of the cone.
2. The optic nerve takes up a relaxed position. It can follow movements of the bulb easily.
3. All muscles are relieved of tension, thus improving eye motility.
4. The traction exerted by the optic nerve on the dura is eliminated, so that the retrobulbar pressure and the 'burning', as well as the headache, vanish rapidly following surgery.
5. The swelling of the upper and lower lids is eliminated following removal of the fat.
6. The pressure within the globe returns to normal or is reduced.
7. The globe is moved backwards
8. The tension on the optic disc is eliminated or reduced.

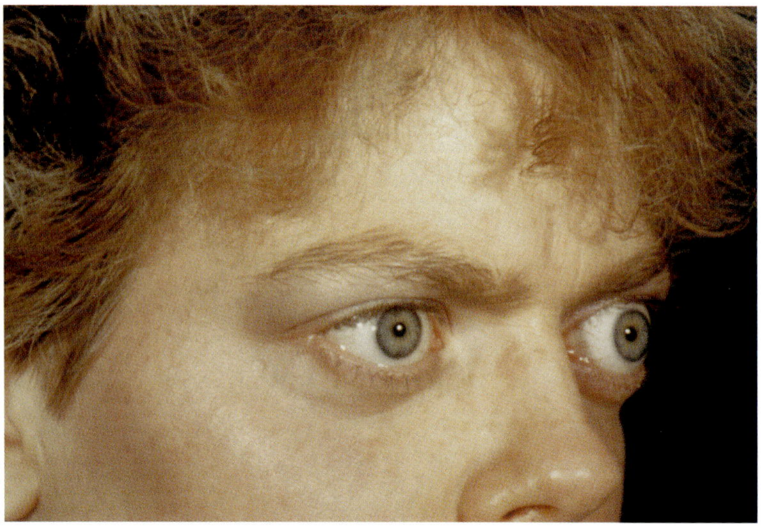

Figure 3.127a Anamnesis: Two years. Conservative treatment without success (orbital irradiation + corticosteroids). Symptoms: Protrusion, Hertel values 28 right, 30 left, diplopia, headaches, retrobulbar burn, chronic conjunctivitis, incomplete eyelid closure at night, severe psychological problems.
1st operation on 5/12/1989:
Decompression 5.4 cc fat right
2nd operation on 8/12/1989:
Decompression 6.3 ccm fat left.
3rd operation on 24/9/1990:
Bilateral levator aponeurosis elongation, division of Mueller's muscle bilaterally, bilateral retractor division in lower lid.

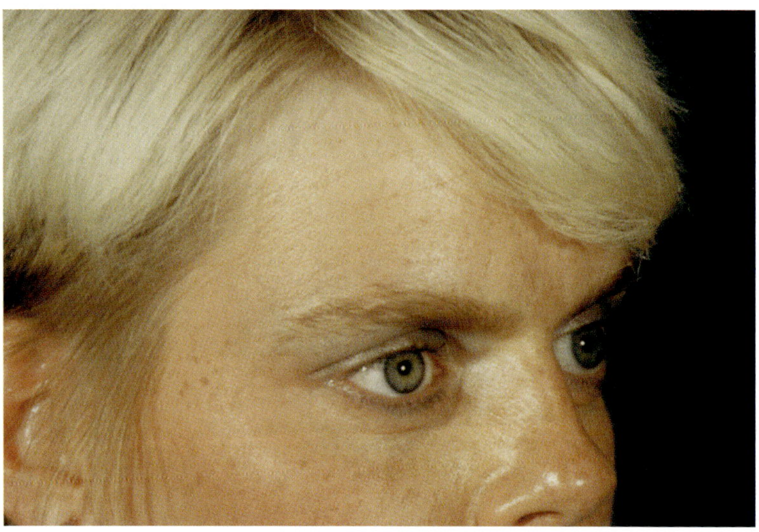

Figure 3.127b Appearance two years postoperatively (19/9/1991), Hertel values 18 right, 21 left, no double vision, complete eyelid closure, no headache, no retrobulbar pressure, no conjunctivitis, psychologically fully rehabilitated.

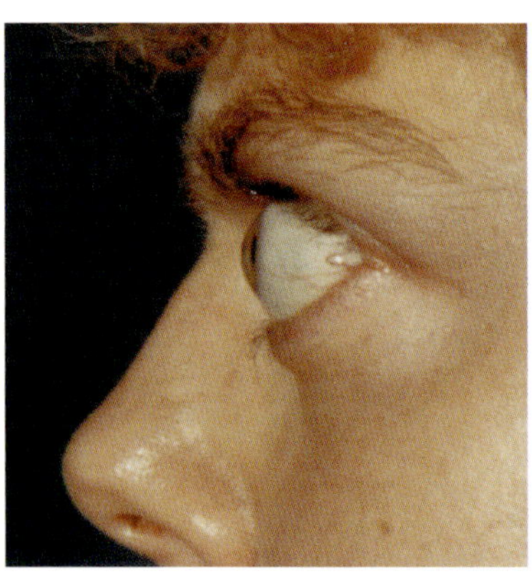

Figure 3.127c Preoperative profile (4/12/1989)

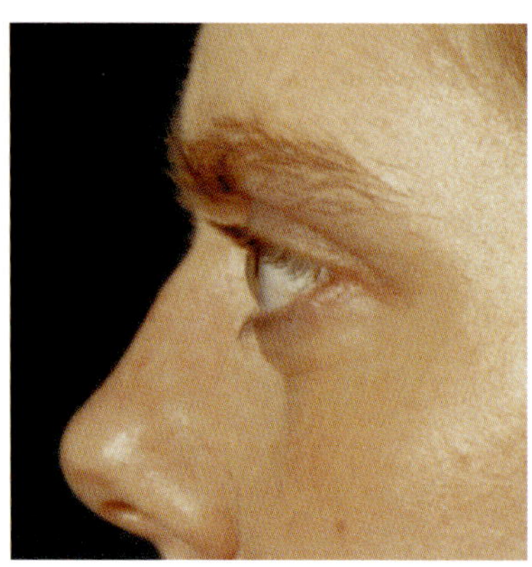

Figure 3.127d Two years after operation (19/9/1991)

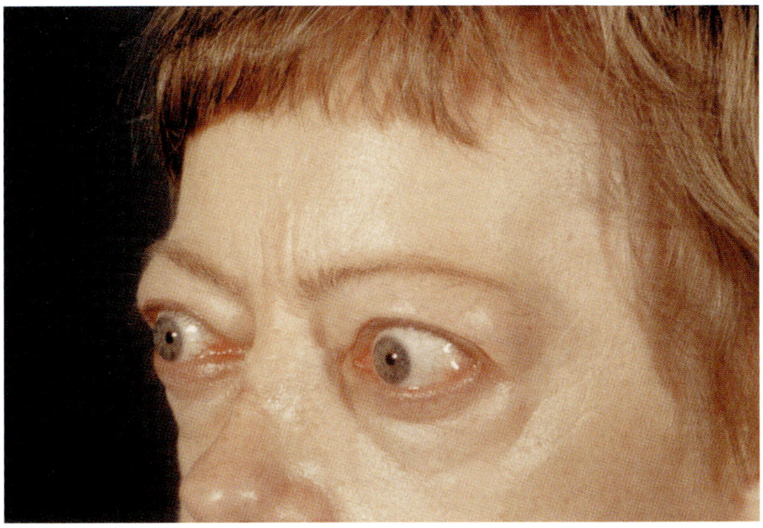

Figure 3.128a Anamnesis: 2.6 years. Conservative therapy (orbital irradiation + corticosteroids over four months).
Symptoms: Protrusion, Hertel values 29 right, 29 left, conjunctivitis, retrobulbar burn, headaches, bilateral lid retraction, lagophthalmos, aesthetic problems.
1st operation on 11/11/1993:
Decompression 8.4 ccm fat left
2nd operation on 18/11/1993:
Decompression 8.7 ccm fat right
3rd operation on 24/11/1993:
Lengthtening of the levator aponeurosis bilaterally and division of Mueller's muscle.

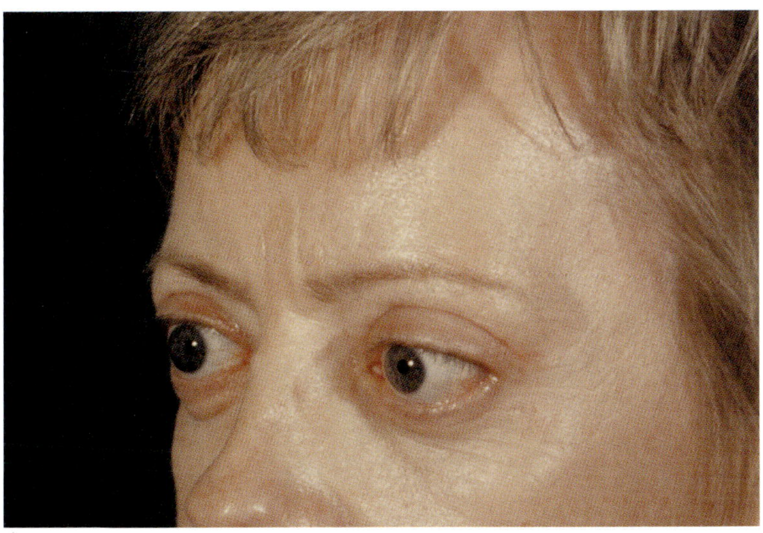

Figure 3.128b Appearance six months postoperatively. Hertel values 21 right, 22 left, slight upper lid retraction bilaterally, no conjunctivitis, no retrobulbar pressure, no headaches, no aesthetic problems.

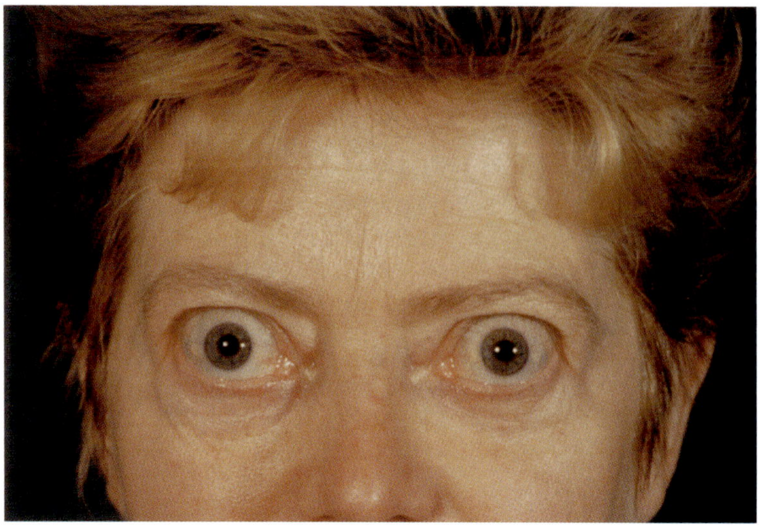

Figure 3.129a Anamnesis: 21 years
1989 Thyroidectomy, corticosteroid therapy (3 ×) without success, orbital irradiation without success, cardiac pacemaker for cardiac arrhythmias.
Symptoms: Protrusion, Hertel values 23 right, 24 left, retrobulbar burn, conjunctivitis, headaches, often keratitis, incomplete eyelid closure, internal ocular pressure bilaterally 29 mmHg (glaucoma), levator retraction
1st operation on 15/11/1994:
Decompression 6.8 ccm fat left, levator division, fascia lata interposition, division of Mueller's muscle.
2nd operation on 22/11/1994:
Decompression 7.2 ccm fat right, otherwise as with the left orbit

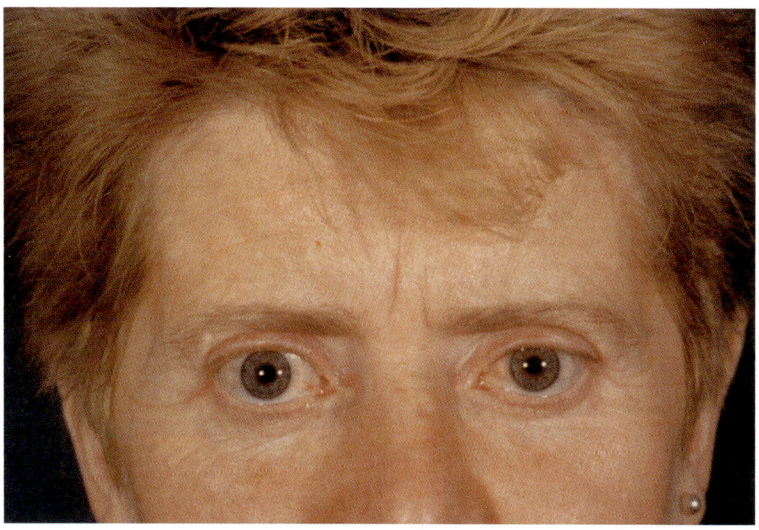

Figure 3.129b Appearance one year after the operation. Hertel values 17 right, 17 left, internal ocular pressure bilaterally 17 mmHg, no subjective complaints, no protrusion, no retrobulbar burn, complete eyelid closure, no glaucoma.

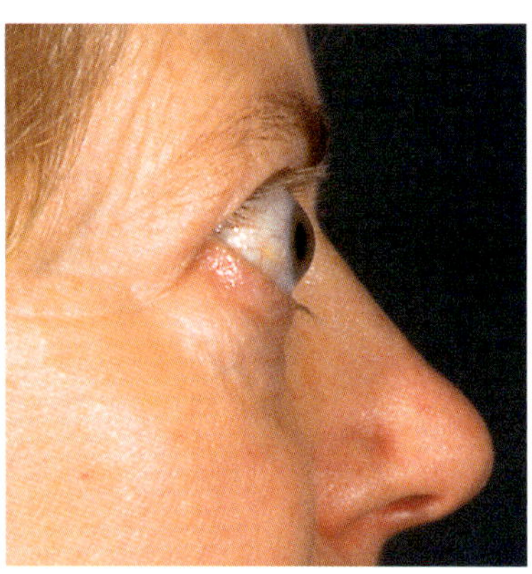

Figure 3.129c Preoperative profile

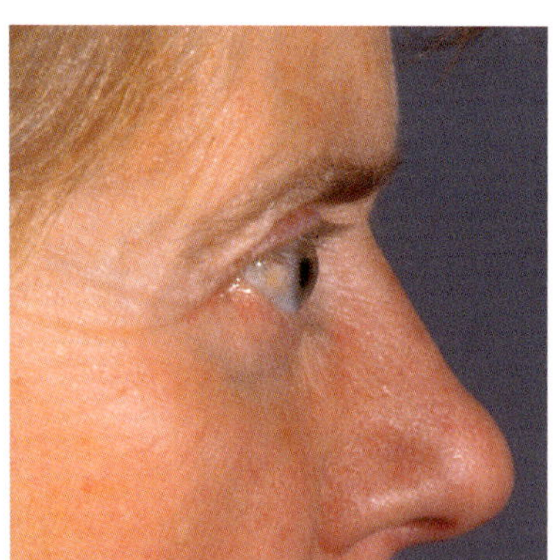

Figure 3.129c Profile one year postoperatively

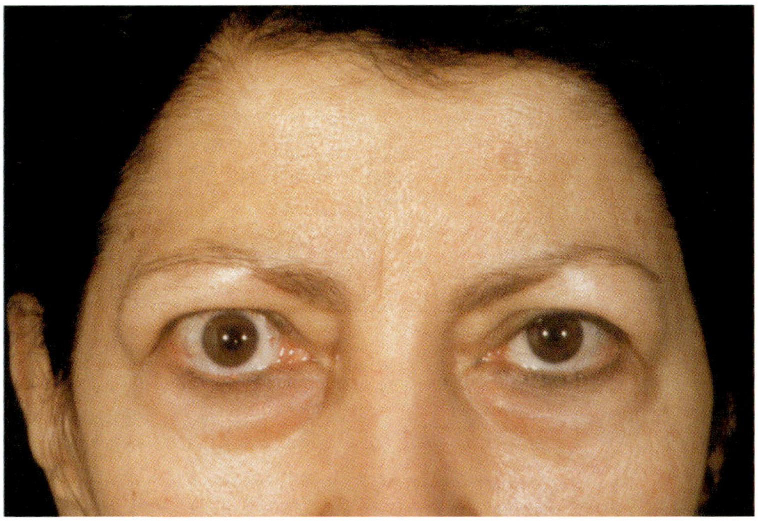

Figure 3.130a Anamnesis: One year. Conservative treatment (orbital irradiation + corticosteroids).
Symptoms: Diplopia, conjunctivitis on the right, sensitivity to light, incomplete eyelid closure on the right, lagophthalmos, protrusion, Hertel values 24 right, 20 left.
1st operation on 27/2/1996:
Decompression 7.4 ccm fat right, decompression 4.3 ccm fat left.
2nd operation on 30/5/1996:
Division of the levator aponeurosis bilaterally up to the medial segment. Division of Mueller's muscle bilaterally, retractor division in the lower eyelid bilaterally.

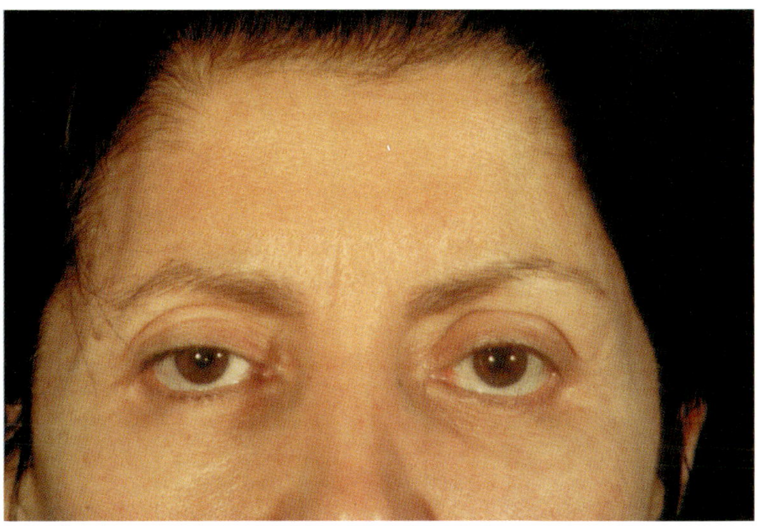

Figure 3.130b Appearance two years after the operation. Hertel values 18 right, 17 left, no diplopia, no conjunctivitis, complete eyelid closure bilaterally.

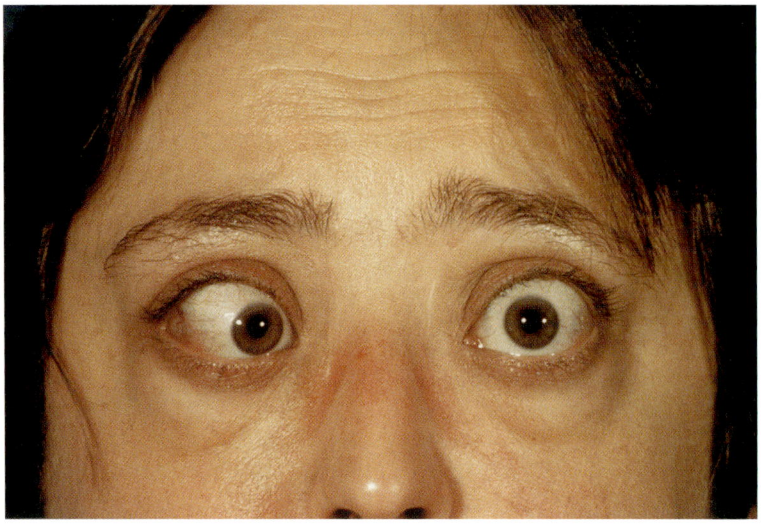

Figure 3.131a Endocrine orbitopathy. History: Six years. Osseous decompression of the medial orbital wall, after that deterioration (no strabismus before the osteotomy). Symptoms: Asymmetric exophthalmos, Hertel values 24 right, 26 left, convergant squint, extreme diplopia.
1st operation on 9/7/1992: Decompression 5.5 ccm fat right, levator extension with a interposition, division of Mueller's muscle.
2nd operation on 16/7/1992: Decompression 6.0 ccm fat left, otherwise as for the right.
3rd operation on 15/2/1994: Retractor division and cartilage grafting in the lower eyelid bilaterally.

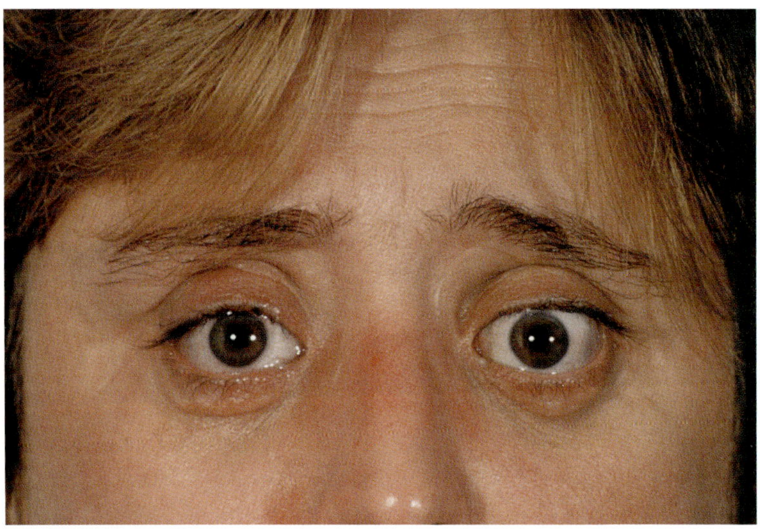

Figure 3.131b Appearance four years after the operation. Hertel values 17 right, 17 left, no diplopia, no strabismus (strabismus only corrected by fat removal and without any additional muscle operation).

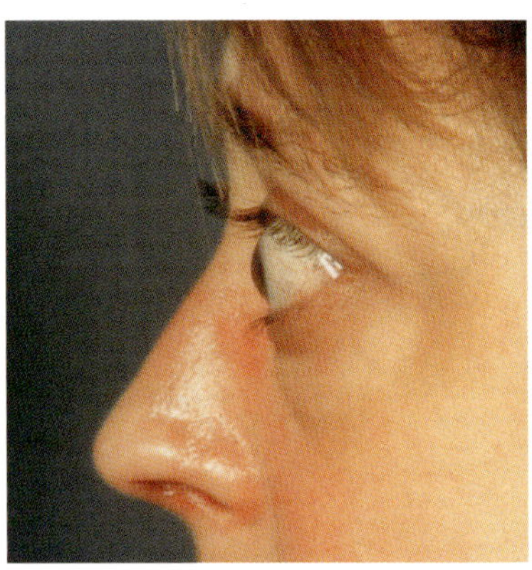

Figure 3.131c Preoperative profile (8/7/1992)

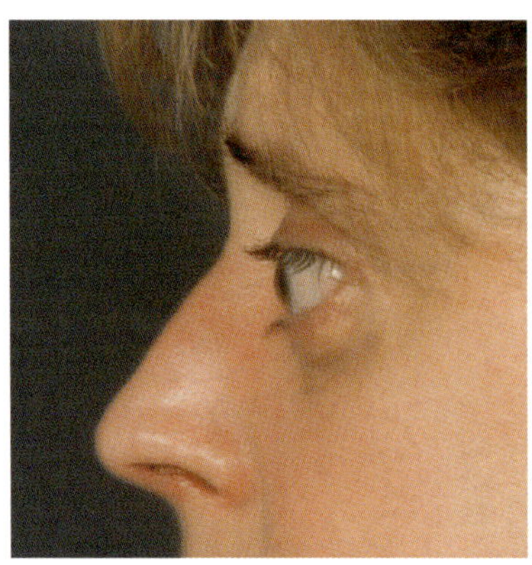

Figure 3.131d Profile four years postoperatively (11/11/1996)

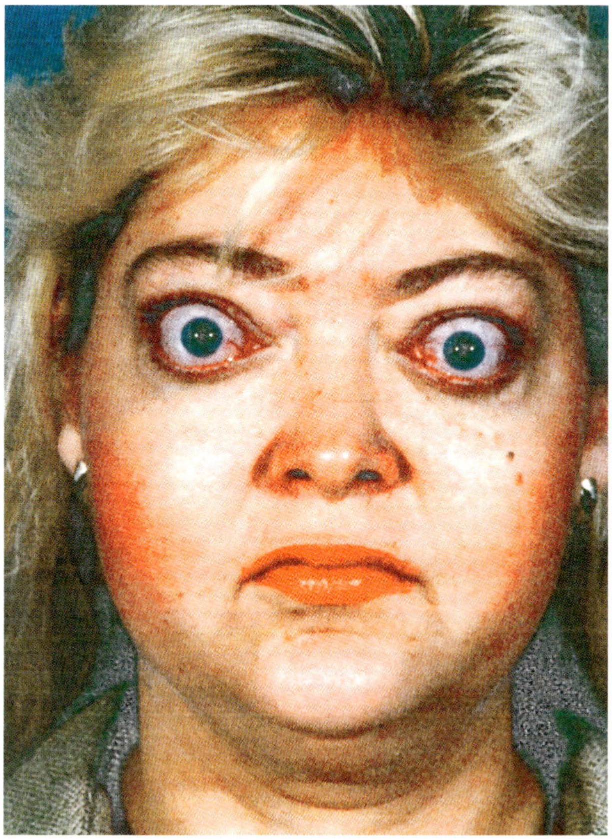

Figure 3.132a Symptoms: Protrusion, Hertel values 32 right, 31 left, diplopia, upper lid retraction, conjunctivitis, lagophthalmos, keratitis, severe headaches, severe depression. Operation: Decompression 7.8 ccm fat on the right, decompression 8.1 ccm fat on the left.
Upper eyelid: division of the levator aponeurosis to the medial part. Division of Mueller's muscle. Lower eyelid: Retractor division. Instillation of 5 mg dexamethasone directly into all four rectus muscles.

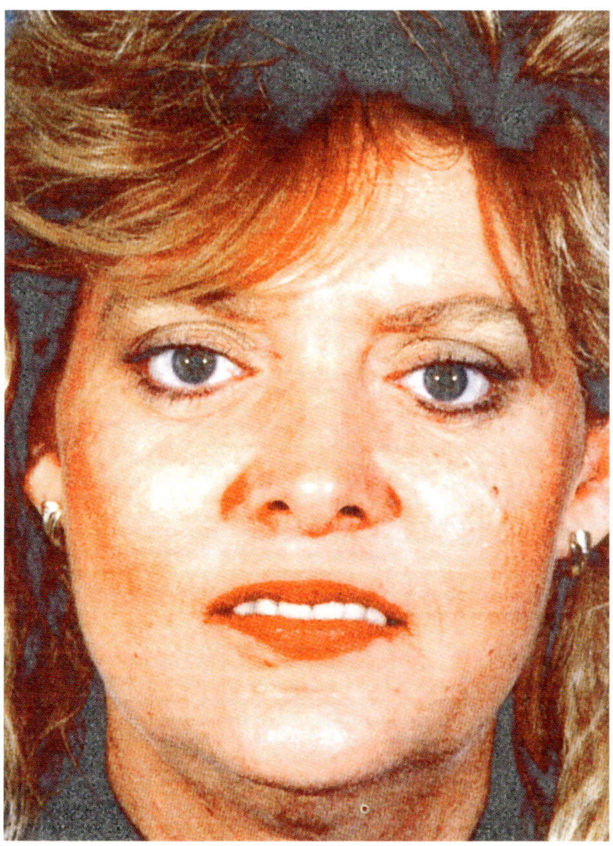

Figure 3.132b Appearance one year after the operation. No diplopia, no conjunctivitis, normal eyelid closure, Hertel values 19 right, 18 left, no headaches. Considerable psychological rehabilitation. This picture show that with this operation one can change personality.

Complications
(N = 1000 orbits with 511 patients).
Complications such as dura perforation, sinusitis, oroantral fistulae, paresis of the infraorbital nerve, meningitis and CSF leakage that are all common following osteotomy procedures, did not occur with transpalpebral fat decompression. There was never any loss of sight.

Three hematomas were revised immediately (not tamponaded!). Paresis of the supraorbital nerve occurred on 16 occasions during the first 150 operations, but not after that. This represents a clear complication of the operation learning curve. Two infections were successfully treated.

Twenty postoperative diplopias (4 % of the interventions) were of course a problem. However, there was a considerable improvement in the overall diplopia rate (368 patients preoperatively = 72 %, 90 patients postoperatively = 17.6 %).

Table 3.5 Complications in 1000 orbits (511 patients)

Complications	Number	%
Hematoma	3	0.6 %
Paresis of the supraorbital nerve	16	3.1 %
New diplopia	20	4.0 %
Infection	2	0.4 %
Total	41	8.1%

Summary
1067 patients with 2052 orbits were operated on because of an endocrine ophthalmopathy (exophthalmos) from 1985 to 2000 in the Department of Plastic Surgery, Dreifaltigkeits-Hospital, Wesseling. In order to bring about an intraorbital decompression, intraorbital fat was removed via a transpalpebral approach in the upper and lower eyelid.

An exact follow-up of 511 patients (1000 orbits) is available as a precise statistic. Only patients with a postoperative course of at least 6 months were included in this evaluation.

On average 6.2 ccm of fat was removed per orbit and an improvement in the Hertel values of around 6 mm was achieved.

Diplopia drastically decreased from a preoperative value of 72 % to 17.6 %.

An impairment of vision (<0.3) was experienced by 10.7 % of the patients preoperatively, whereas this figure was only 1.7 % postoperatively.

Conjunctivitis, retrobulbar pressure, lid swelling, photophobia as well as headaches were reduced by 80 to 93 %.

The complication rate was acceptable, particularly in comparison with osteotomy methods.

The operation can therefore be indicated on a more generous scale.

By applying the procedure of transpalpebral fat removal it became possible for the first time to remove great part of the sick tissue.

If a common antigen of thyroid gland and orbital tissue or an antigen acting specifically on orbital tissue exists, a large proportion of this antigen is removed by this procedure. In any case, T-cells, B-cells, macrophages, lymphocyte infiltration, glycosaminoglycans, HLA-DR and various adhesion molecules are considerably reduced in quantity, as are dendritic cells, cytokines and inflammatory mediators.

Through the routinely direct injection of dexamethasone into all four rectus muscles we were able to achieve a situation where no relapse of a muscle hypertrophy could be recorded due to the underlying disease over the last five years.

Preliminary examinations four years after the operation and injection of dexamethasone have revealed reductions in muscular volume, but further long-term studies still need to be carried out.

Although most patients are now corrected using this procedure, osteotomy remains an indication in certain exceptional cases (less than 1 % of patients).

Defect Coverage in the Lip Area

Cleft Lip, Jaw and Palate

Cleft lip, jaw and palate numbers amongst the most frequent deformities in man. Although a genetic predisposition definitely exists, external factors have also been implicated. Cleft lip, jaw and palate occurs with differing degrees of severity; from a simple one-sided isolated cleft lip to a bilateral, continuous cleft lip, jaw and palate. Prophylaxis has been attempted using various methods and a certain reduction in incidence amongst endangered pregnant mothers has been achieved through the application of vitamin B complex as well as vitamin B1. Cleft lip, jaw and palate becomes manifest in the fifth to the sixth week of gestation, i.e. prophylaxis must be applied at a time when most women are not even aware of their pregnancy.

Epidemiology

Cleft lip, jaw and palate occurs:

- In light skinned individuals at a frequency of 1 in 600 to 700 births
- In dark skinned individuals at a frequency of 1 in 1,500 to 3,000 births
- In Asians at a frequency of 1 in 450 to 800 births

Over the last 50 years the incidence has increased by around 30 %. This fact is ascribed to the increasing influence of chemicals and the environment. Another factor is that the now excellent surgical results have often lead to affected patients becoming married more often than they did 50 years ago.

In such cases a genetic factor also comes into effect. The probability that a child with cleft lip, jaw and palate shall come to the world is:

Table 3.6 Heredity and frequency of cleft lip, jaw and palate

	With cleft lip, jaw and palate	With cleft lip
1 sibling	4.5 %	2.5 %
1 parent	3.2 %	6.8 %
1 parent + 1 sibling	15.8 %	15.0 %
Both parents	23.0 %	50.0 %

Male children are affected more (60 %) than female children (40 %).

The distribution of the different cleft types (Fogh Anderson) is as follows:

- Only lips 25 %
- Only palate 50 %
- Cleft lip, jaw and palate 25 %

Table 3.7 Classification of cleft lip, jaw and palate

Group 1	Clefts of the front embryonic palate Lip: right and/or left Jaw: right and/or left
Group 2	Clefts of the front and rear embryonic palate Lip: right and/or left Jaw: right and/or left Hard palate: right and/or left Soft palate: medial
Group 3	Clefts of the rear embryonic palate Hard palate: right and/or left Soft palate: medial

It is unclear why left-sided clefts occur twice as often as right-sided clefts. Unilateral clefts are also more common than bilateral clefts.

Prenatal Diagnostics

Ultrasound diagnostics allow a cleft jaw or hard palate to be diagnosed in the 9th –12th weeks of gestation, whereas a cleft lip is first diagnosed in the 20th –24th weeks.

Cleft Lip, Jaw and Palate and Intelligence

About 60 years ago cleft lip, jaw and palate patients were still regarded as being retarded. This was due to operations that produced bad aesthetic results, speaking difficulties and social exclusion (open rhinolalia, or hypernasality).

Well operated and followed-up children do not differ from normal children with respect to their intelligence. As a rule an aesthetically good outcome can be expected these days. The scars are hardly visible and in most cases changes in speech are unnoticeable.

With severe cleft lip, jaw and palate it is often necessary to carry out a nasal correction at an age of 12 to 14 years. With open rhinolalia or "hypernasality" a pharyngoplasty may be indicated.

Treatment

Treatment depends on the severity of cleft formation. An isolated cleft lip without jaw involvement only requires a precise operation as a final treatment.

With severe forms involving the jaw and palate an interdisciplinary treatment concept is necessary, and indeed from birth to adulthood. Several subsequent treatments are necessary.

The key to a good outcome lies without a doubt in the surgical treatment. Orthodontists, speech therapists and ENT physicians are selectively consulted for this purpose.

Surgical Treatment

With cleft jaw and palates provision of a jaw plate is recommended before the operation. The gradual reforming of the cleft jaw results from the separation of the oral and nasal cavities.

The goal in this case is not to reduce the cleft, but rather to prevent a collapse of the bony cleft and restore the dental arches.

Most of our patients were operated on without this preparatory treatment. A precondition is an osteoplasty in the jaw cleft area that prevents the collapse of both jaw stumps and stabilizes the dental arch.

Lip Closure and Jaw Occlusion

This operation is carried out at the age of three to six months. A bilateral cleft lip is also operated on usually in a single surgical session. Exceptions are extreme bilateral clefts with a strongly protruding premaxilla. Here the broader cleft is operated on first. After a few weeks the second side is then operated on. A precise planning of the operation is absolutely necessary (see Figure 3.135). A planning that is off by just one millimeter can entail a bad outcome that is very difficult later on to correct.

Nomenclature and Severity

Table 3.8 Thallwitzer nomenclature for categorizing cleft forms

Clefts of the primary palate			
1) L = Lip	L1	Microform	left
	L2	Subtotal	bilateral
	L3	Total	right
2) K = Jaw	K1	Microform	left
	K2	Subtotal	bilateral
	K3	Total	right
Clefts of the secondary palate			
3) G = Cleft palate	G1	Microform	left
	G2	Subtotal	bilateral
	G3	Total	right
4) S = Soft palate	S1	Microform	
	S2	Subtotal	
	S3	Total	

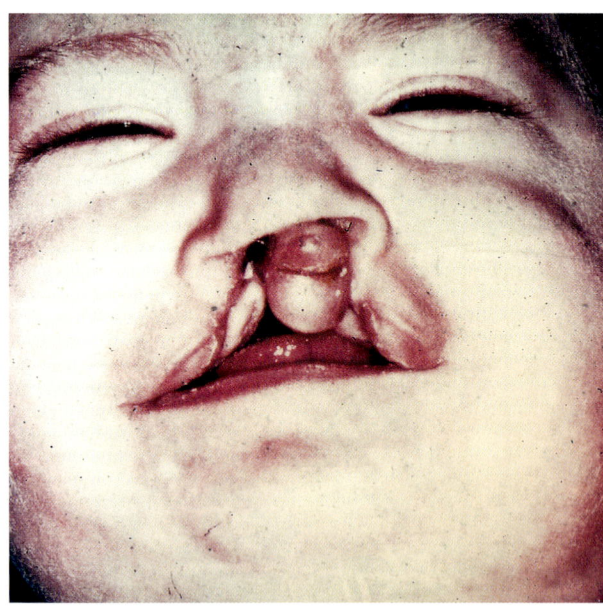

Figure 3.133 Example with a continuous bilateral cleft lip, jaw and palate: L3 K3 G3 S3 bilateral

Anatomy in the Mouth Area

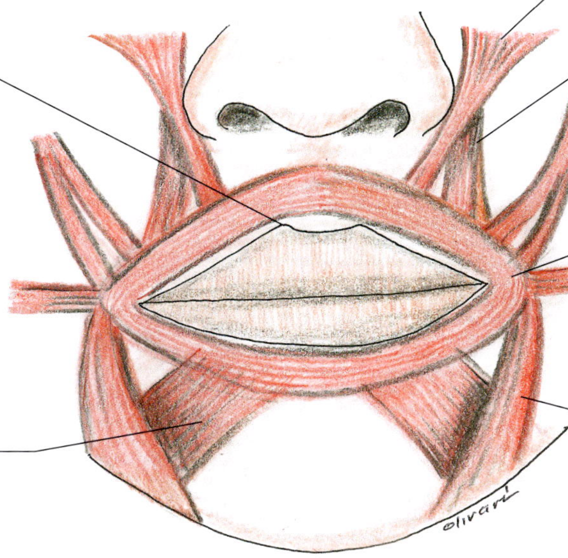

Figure 3.134a The musculature in the mouth area

Lip Closure and the Orbicularis Oris Muscle

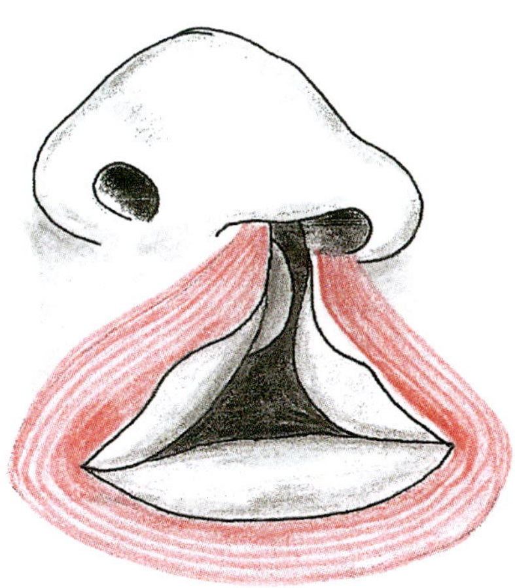

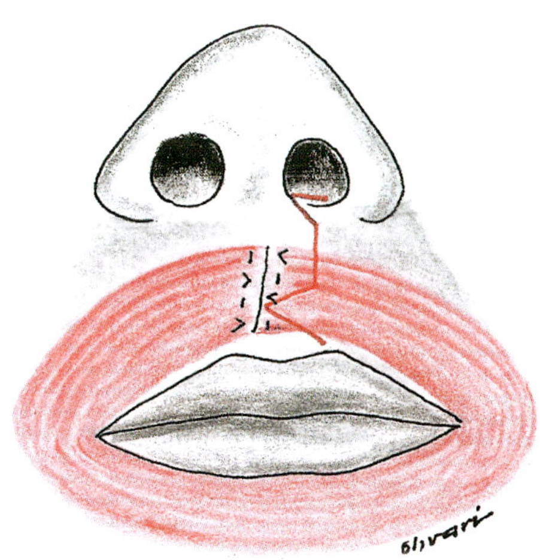

Figure 3.134b With cleft lip jaw the orbicularis oris muscle is severed and fixed bilaterally at the jaw stumps. Because of this it is no longer able to perform its function. A lip closure without muscle correction produces a poor aesthetic and functional result.

Figure 3.134c The orbicularis oris muscle must be released bilaterally and fixed in the middle after mobilization. In this way the function of the orbicularis oris muscle is restored.

Methods of Lip Closure

Procedure According to Tennison

The procedure according to Tennison with two triangular flaps originates initially from Hagedorn and was later modified by Le Mesurier. Tennison turned the procedure into a standard.

Precise Planning. The Tennison procedure is geometrically precise, functionally good and in our hands produces very good late results. It is easy to learn. For all these reasons the author of this work clearly favors the Tennison procedure. Of course other authors have produced equally good results using the Millard technique or others.

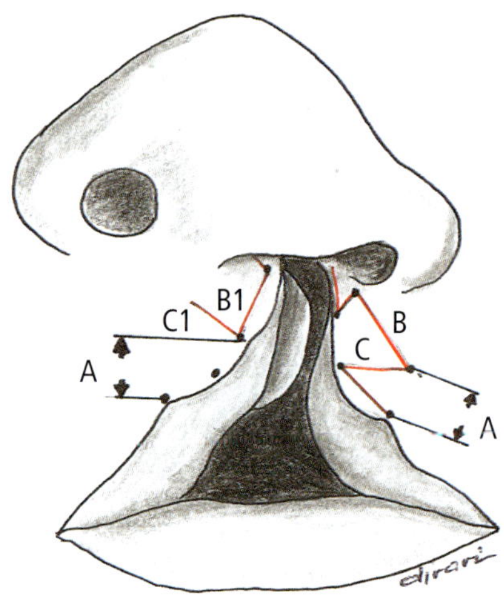

Figure 3.135a Lip closure according to Tennison. In order to bring the medial part of the vermillion on the right to the same level as it is on the left, the difference in height (A) is corrected using a triangular flap from the cleft side of the lip. The base of the triangular flap of the cleft side has the same width (A). The length of the triangular flap (C) is the same as the incision in the medial lip side (C1). Cut B is the same on both sides. The small triangular flap laterally and cranially serves for better shaping of the nostril.

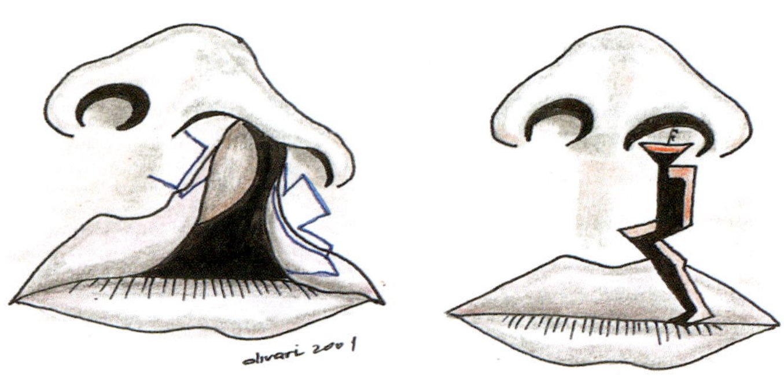

Figure 3.135b Incision line with a unilateral cleft lip, jaw and palate procedure according to Tennison. The nostril swellings are shaped by applying a triangular flap in the nostril area. The incision line in the red of the lip is carried out using a double Z-plasty, whereby in the upper part a triangular flap is formed from medial and in the vestibulum from lateral parts. As a result of this the prelabium gains some mucosal substance.

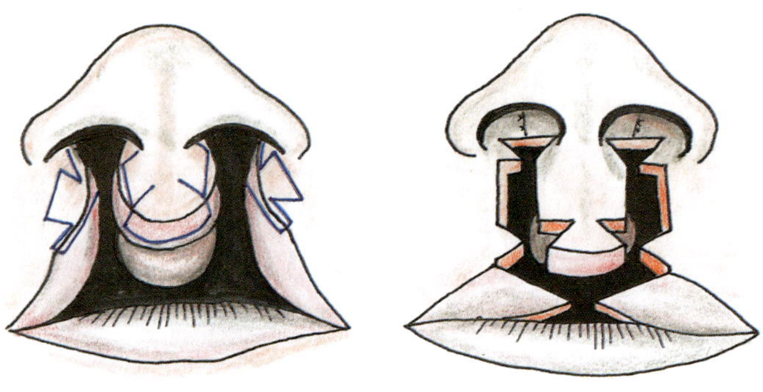

Figure 3.135c Incision line with bilateral cleft lip, jaw and palate. The Incision line does not differ in the white lip area from the incision line with a unilateral cleft lip, jaw and palate. In the mucosa of the lip area, however, a triangular flap is formed in the front area bilaterally from the lateral sides in order to form sufficient material in the medial part of the mucosa of the lip. Depending on the size of the prelabium the operation is carried out in one or two sessions. With a small prelabium the operation is carried out in two sessions. From: N Olivari, W Niermann (1980): The dependence of the lip form on the incision line in cleft-lip, jaw, and palate. Plastic Surgery Vol. 4: 3–10

Procedure According to Millard

Millard also uses a triangular flap in order to achieve a lip extension, but in the cranial part of the lip.

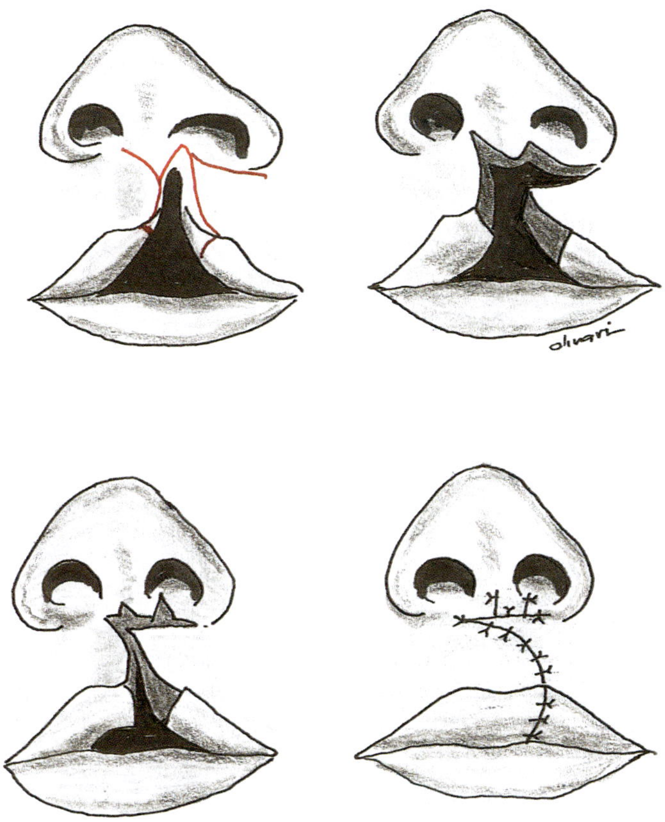

Figure 3.136 Procedure according to Millard. The triangular flap in the cranial part is used for the lip extension. The smaller scar in the lower lip area represents one advantage of this procedure. The disadvantage is that the length of the lip can not be determined as precisely as is the case with the Tennison procedure. This is of course personal opinion.

Osteoplasty and Cleft Surgery

The closure of the lip was largely perfected during the sixties; however, the problematic, mobile, unstable upper jaw still persisted as a problem. It was therefore attempted to stabilize the dental arch by applying an osteoplasty.

In 1956 Schmid and Nordin carried secondary osteoplasties in individual cases, i.e. some months after lip closure as well as after the palatoplasty.

The first systematic primary osteoplasty was developed by Schrudde. After a while the procedure proved to be highly effective for stabilizing cleft jaws.

A comprehensive study by Niermann (1985) unambiguously showed the following benefits:

1) The dental arch is stabilized by a primary osteoplasty.
2) The occlusion improves postoperatively in a manner depending on the time after the operation:

Same group of children	Year	Normal maxilla development
	1972	50 %
	1976	64 %
	1981	93.3 %

3) The good result depended on the healing of the bone graft material:

Same group of children	Year	Well healed bone graft
	1972	60 %
	1976	83.6 %
	1981	93.3 %

In the starting phase a few grafts were lost due to infection. This was due to the fact that the technique had not yet been perfected. The bone graft was sometimes not sufficiently covered with mucosa.

Overall a primary osteoplasty carried out synchronously with a lip closure is recommended if the correct technique is applied.

A secondary osteoplasty is possible later if the primary osteoplasty fails, although the results are less convincing.

a) Closure Techniques

Lip-Jaw Closure With Primary Osteoplasty (Schrudde)

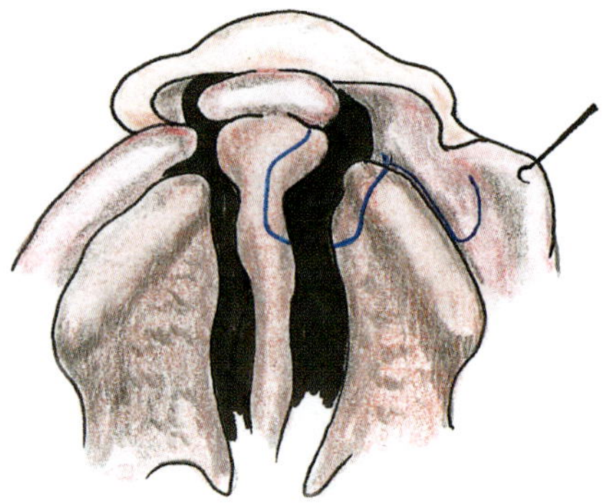

Figure 3.137a With an incision line according to Tennison in the lip area, the jaw area is operated on in the same session. The incision occurs at the lateral jaw stump and at the premaxilla.

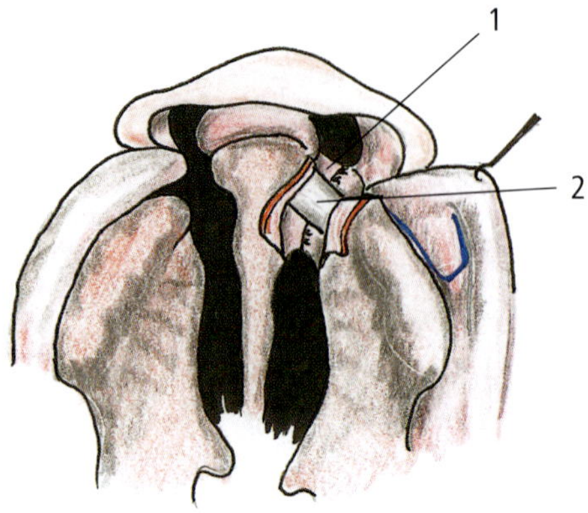

Figure 3.137b The mucosa along with the periostium are mobilized using the raspatory and sutured in the middle (1). Here a previously withdrawn piece of rib is implanted with compression between the lateral jaw stump and the premaxilla (2).

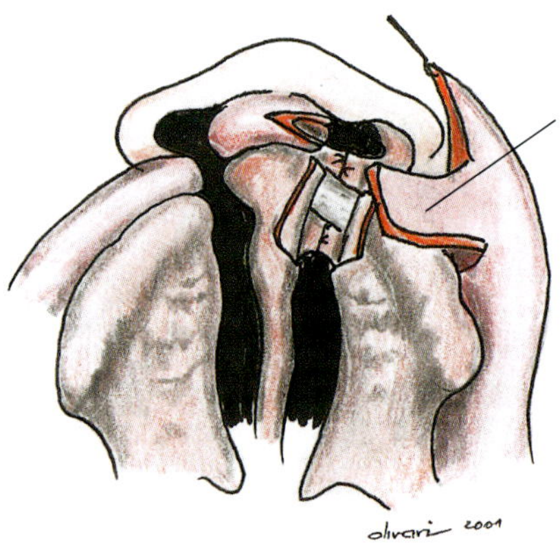

Figure 3.137c The bone graft is therefore covered from the nasal side. A mucosal flap (3) is formed from the vestibulum and using this the rib graft is sealed from the oral side.

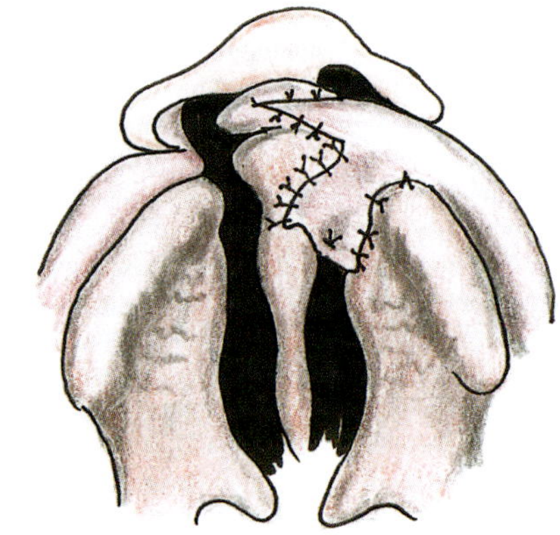

Figure 3.137d Status at the end of the lip jaw closure with a primary osteoplasty

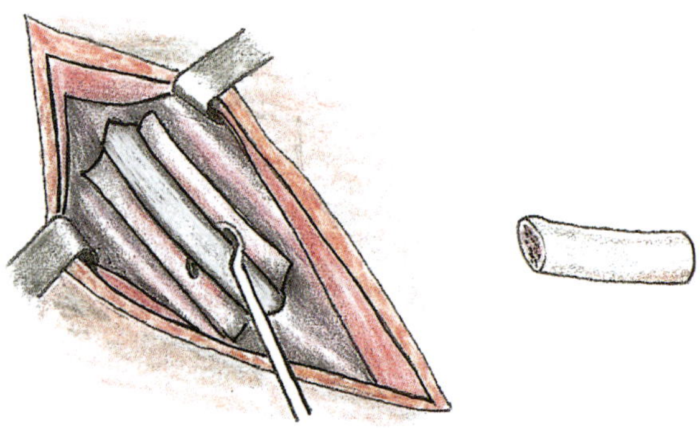

Figure 3.137e Bone withdrawal from the rib. The rib piece is removed subperiostally. The periostium is fixed with 5 × 0 Vicryl in its starting position. A new rib forms in the periostium in children within six weeks, and in adults within three to four months.

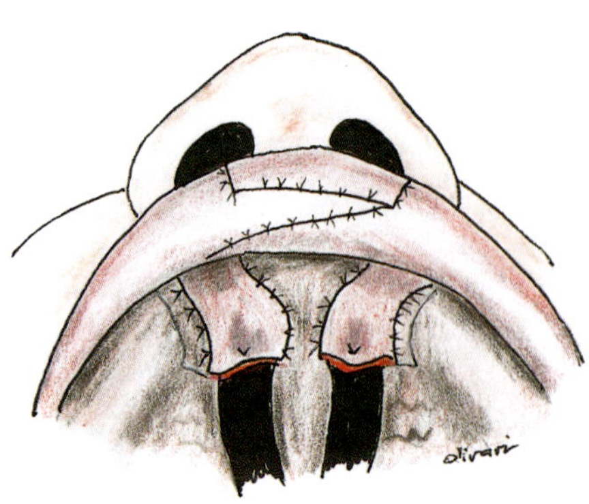

Figure 3.137f Status after bilateral lip jaw closure with primary osteoplasty. Note the precise covering of the oral side of the jaw cleft with a mucosal flap from the vestibulum. One can see the double Z-plasty in the lip area with which a sufficiently long lip was formed.

Bilateral Palatal Closure According to Langenbeck

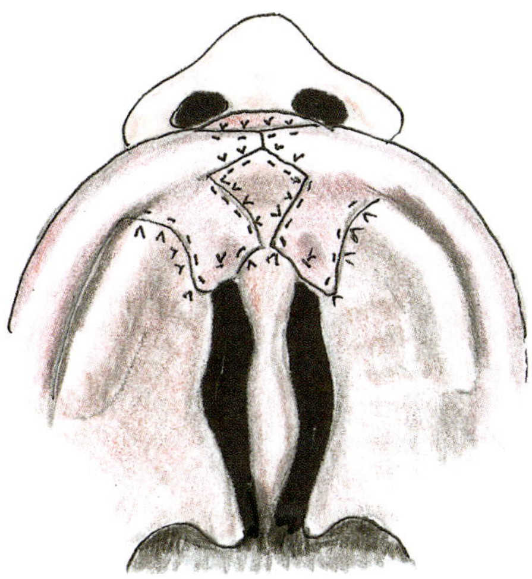

Figure 3.138a Between the 3rd and 6th month the lip and the jaw are closed; if possible with a primary osteoplasty.

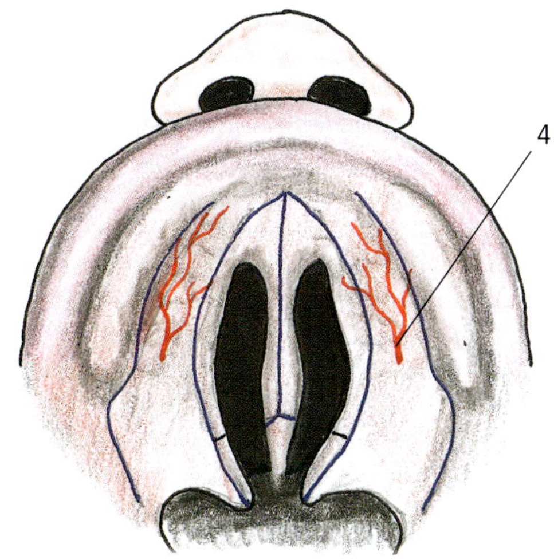

Figure 3.138b At 12 to 16 months the palate is closed (before the child starts speaking). The incision line occurs at the vomer, the palatal cleft margin as well as laterally. Note the position of the palatine artery (4) that must be protected from any damage.

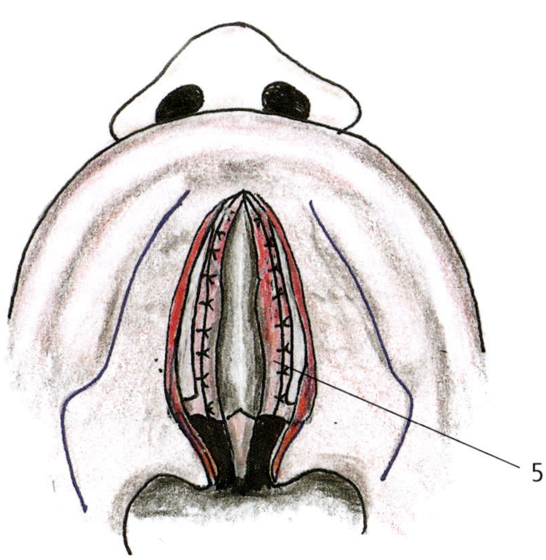

Figure 3.138c The mucosal periostium layer is closed (5) and in this way the nasal cavity is severed from the oral cavity. The incision line proceeds on up to the uvula.

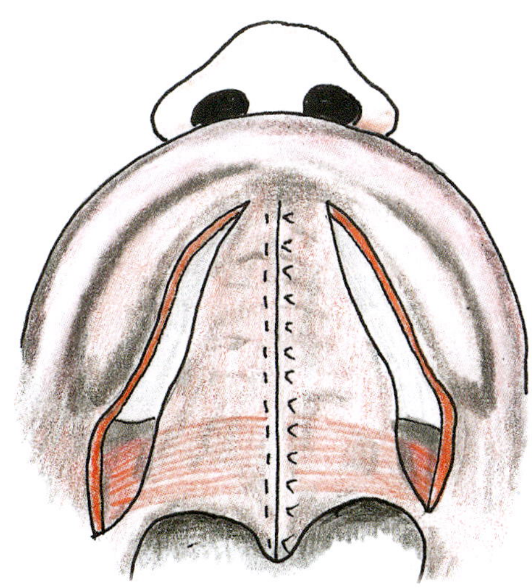

Figure 3.138d Two bridge flaps are formed by lateral incisions whereby these are completely mobilized from the hard palate. The palatine artery remains preserved. The tensor veli palatini muscle and the levator veli palatini muscle are severed from the edge of the hard palate and sutured together in the middle. The open wounds on both sides are tamponated using Sofratuell. They epithelialize after two to three weeks.

Cleft of the Hard and Soft Palate on the Left Side (Langenbeck)

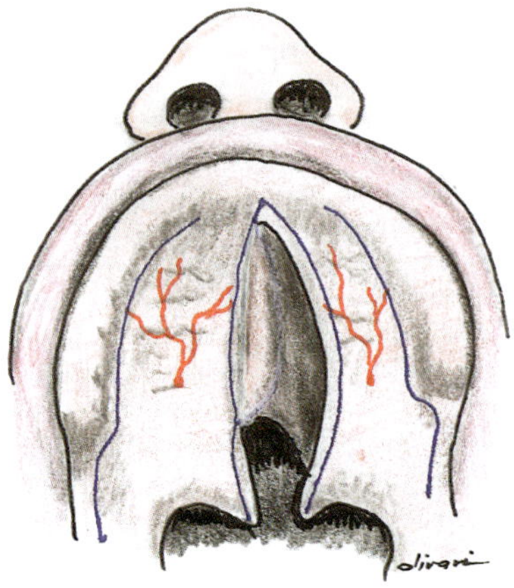

Figure 3.139a With a unilateral cleft palate (here to the left) the vomer along with the hard palate is arched to the right. Incision line (blue) with strict protection of the palatine artery.

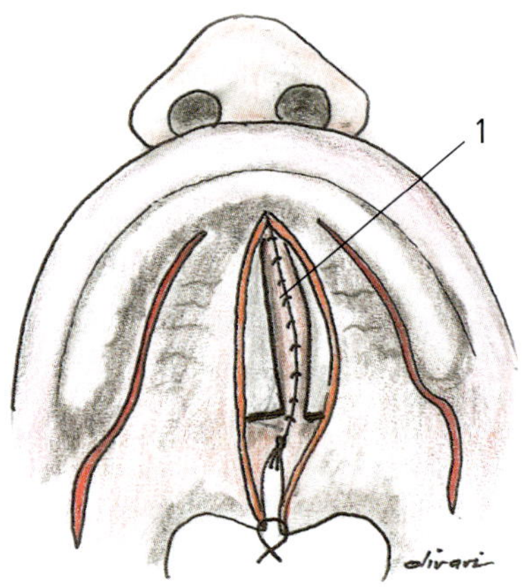

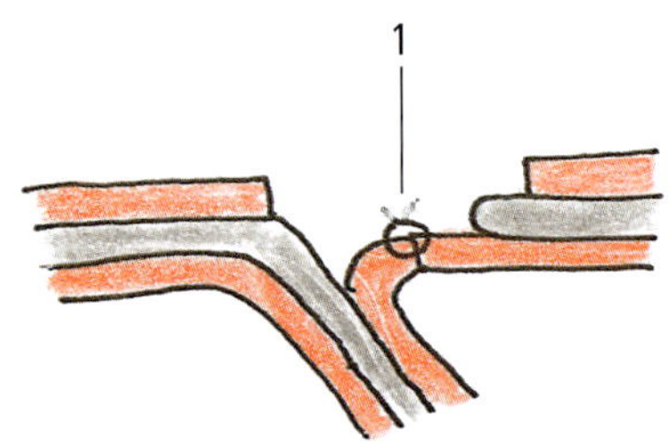

Schematic representation of the nasal layer

Figure 3.139b The nasal layer is formed by mobilization of the mucosa from the vomer (right) and the mucosa of the hard palate (left) (1).

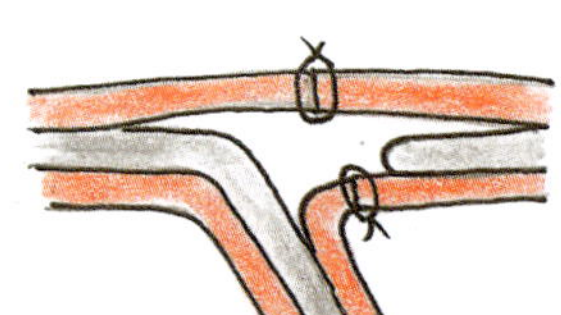

Schematic representation of the closure of the nasal and oral layers

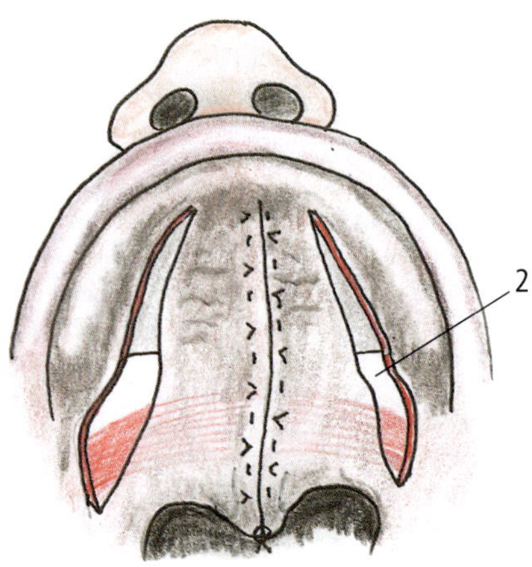

Figure 3.139c Two mucoperiostal bridge flaps from the hard palate are mobilized by lateral incisions. Both flaps must be sutured without any stretching. The lateral open wounds on both sides (2) are tamponated using Sofratuell (for four days) and become epithelialized within two weeks.

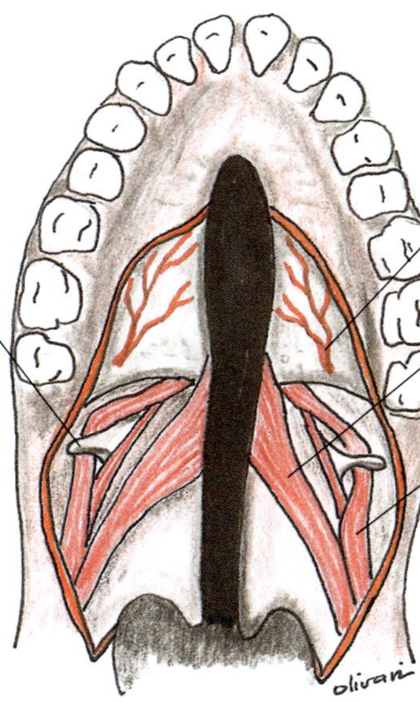

Figure 3.140a Distribution of the musculature with most cleft palates. The levator veli palatini muscle and the tensor veli palatini muscle are oriented longitudinally and fixed at the palatine bone. In this way they can not perform their normal function (pulling of the soft palate in a dorsal direction – a sphincter function).
1. levator veli palatini muscle
2. tensor veli palatini muscle
3. pterygoid hamulus
4. palatine artery

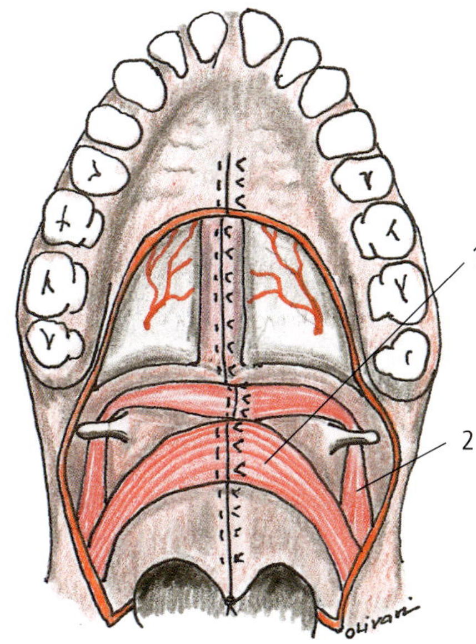

Figure 3.140b With the palatoplasty it is of essential importance to sever the tensor veli palatini muscle and the levator veli palatini muscle from the hard palate and to reconstruct it as a ring.

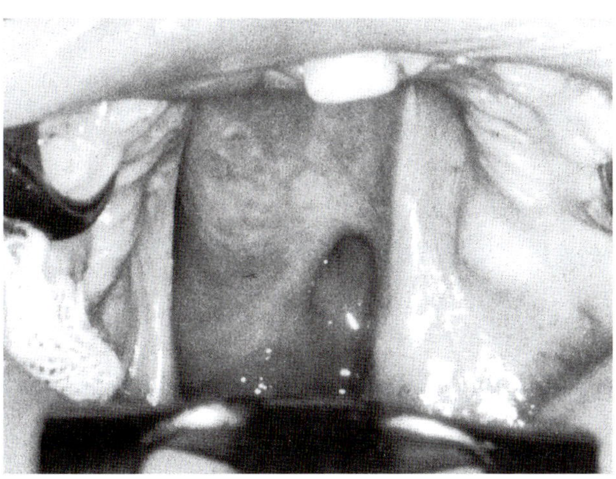

Figure 3.140c Right-sided cleft palate (L3 K3 G3 S3 right)

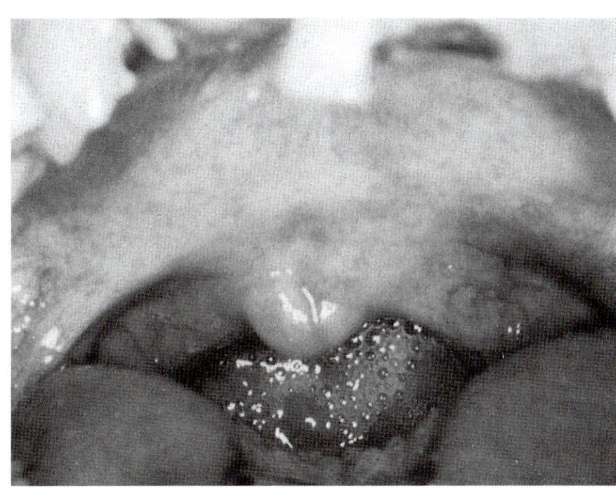

Figure 3.140d Status one year after palate closure (Langenbeck technique)

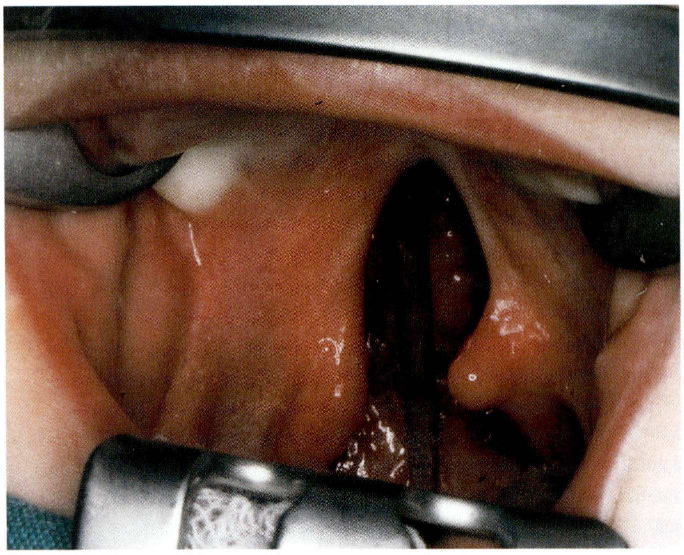

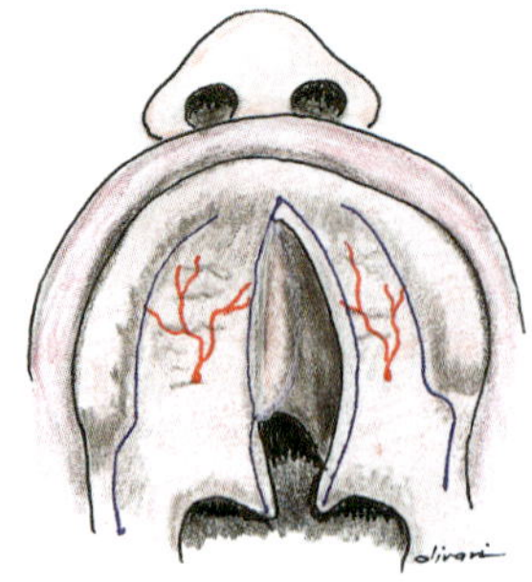

Figure 3.141a,b Left-sided cleft palate. The vomer along with the hard palate is arched to the right. Incision line (blue) with strict protection of the palatine artery.

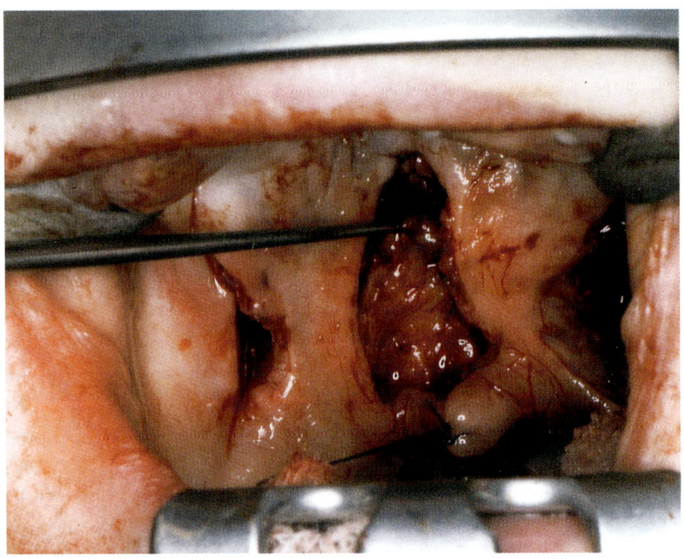

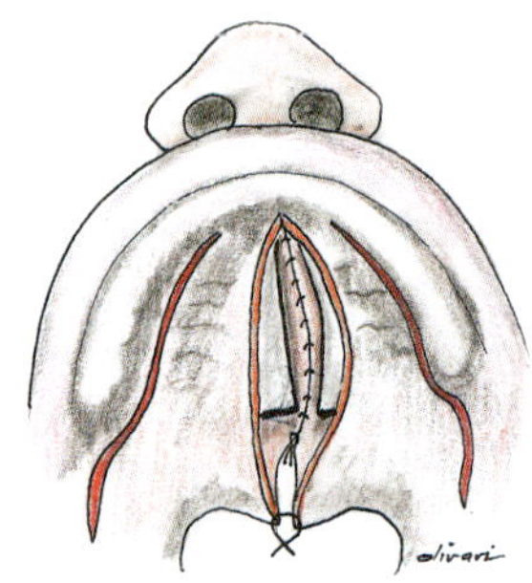

Figure 3.141c,d The nasal layer is joined in the middle by mobilization of the mucosa from the vomer to the right and from the palate on the left. In this way the nasal layer is closed.

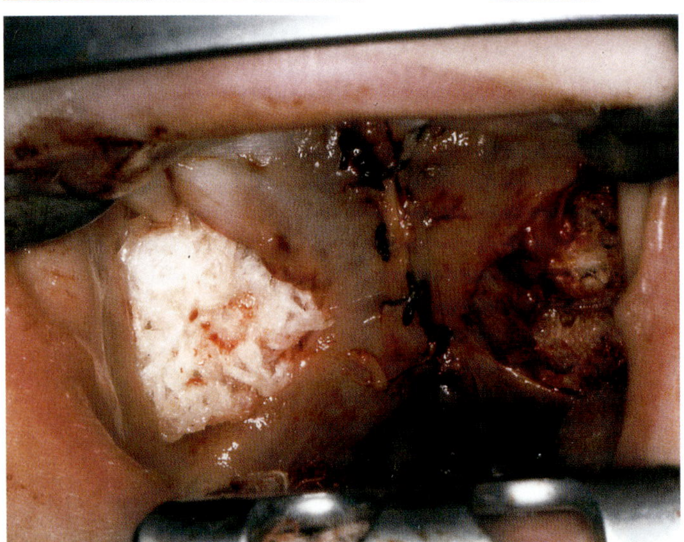

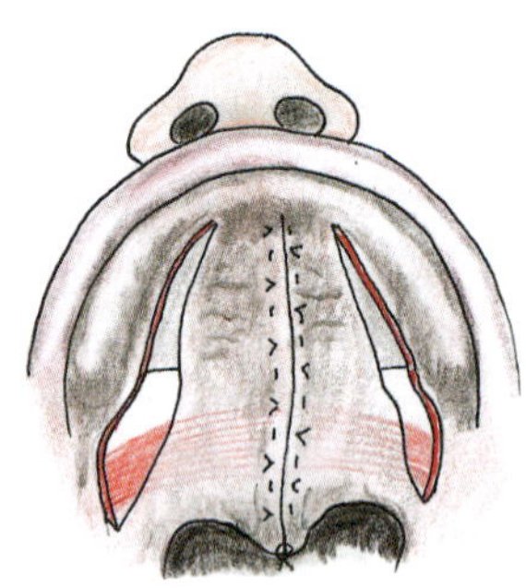

Figure 3.141e,f With the help of two lateral incisions two bridge flaps are mobilized completely medially and sutured without stretching. The open wounds are tamponated bilaterally with Sofratuell. After three weeks they become epithelialized.

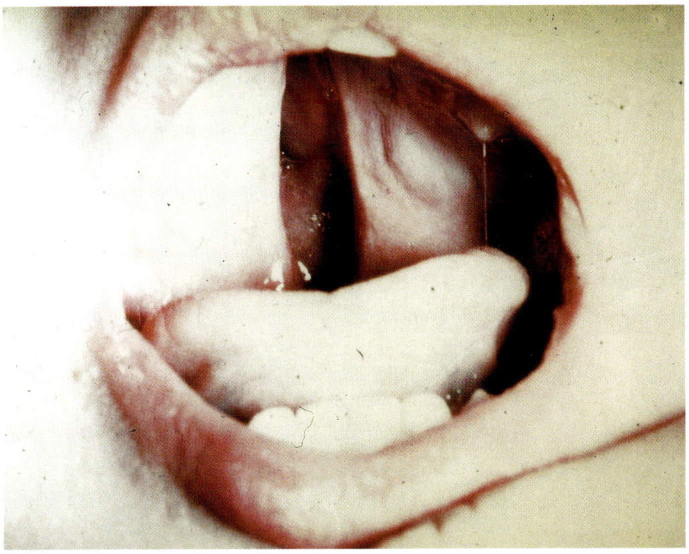

Figure 3.142a Status after left lip-jaw closure to the left at an age of six months. Status immediately before the palate closure at the age of 14 months.

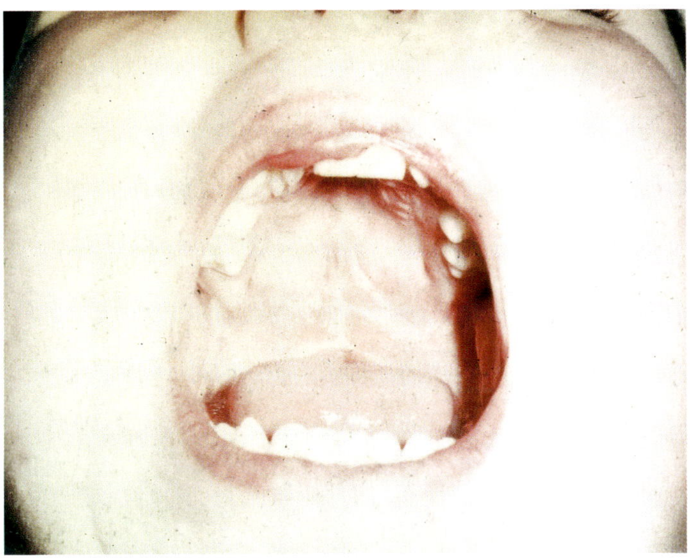

Figure 3.142b Status one year after palate closure (Langenbeck technique)

Primary Osteoplasty According to Schrudde

Healing of the Rib Graft in the Jaw Area

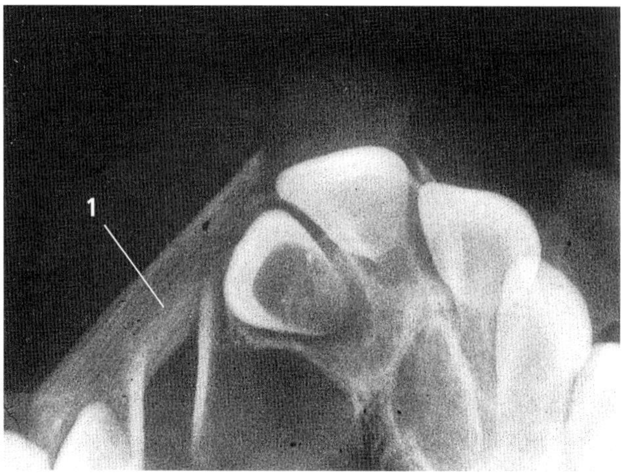

Figure 3.143a Incorporation of a bone graft in the jaw cleft area. Status immediately after the lip jaw closure with primary osteoplasty (see rib graft) (1).

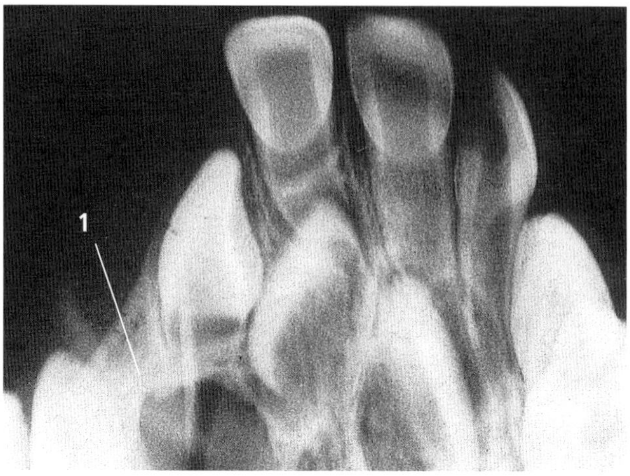

Figure 3.143b Status one year postoperatively. The rib graft was inserted by the reconstruction processes at the level of the dental arch (1).

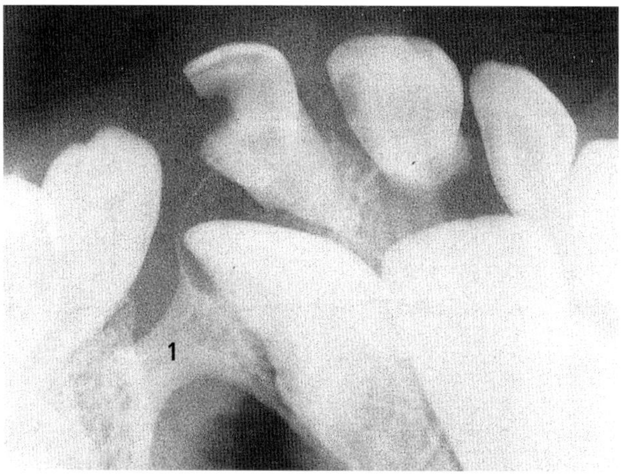

Figure 3.144 Status three years after the osteoplasty. The rib graft has become incorporated into the right side in the bone structure of the jaw. The collapse of the jaw stumps is prevented by the stable bone bridge.

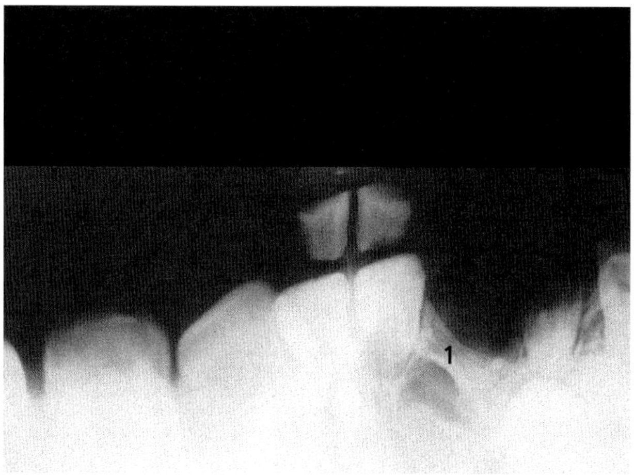

Figure 3.145 Same status as Figure 3.144, but here on the left side. The successful primary osteoplasty prevents pseudoprogenia.

b) Incomplete Cleft Lip

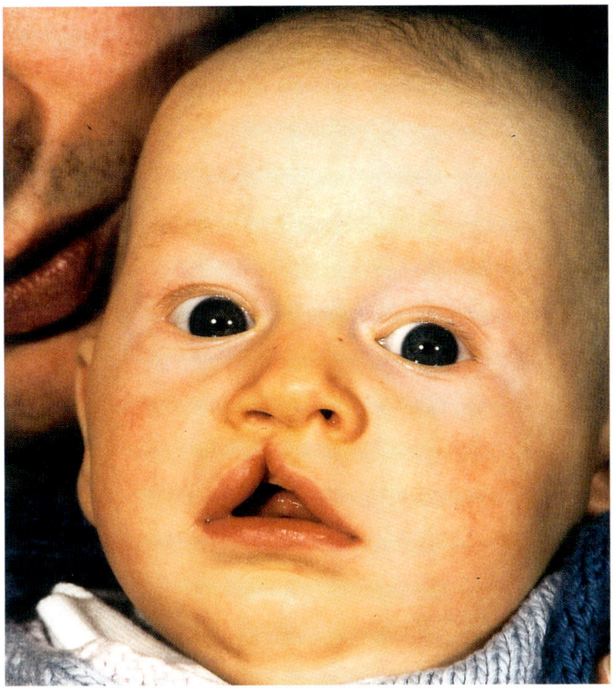

Figure 3.146a Incomplete cleft lip on the right. The notch in the jaw is functionally of no importance.

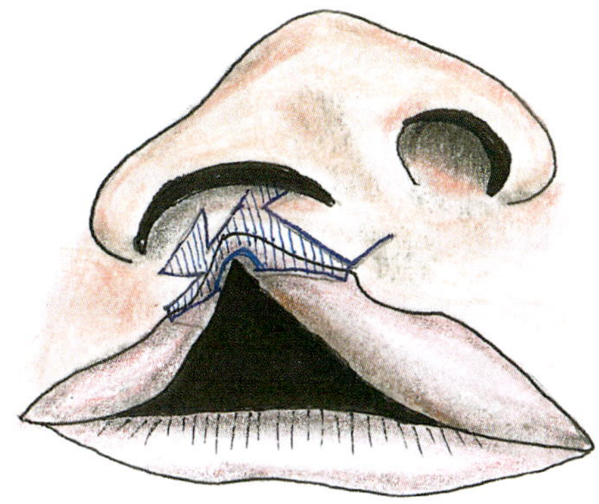

Figure 3.146b Incision line with an incomplete cleft lip. The shaded area is excised. Although the nostril is not affected, the incision goes into the nostril. Only in this way can the orbicularis oris muscle be reconstructed and the nasal wing be rotated medially.

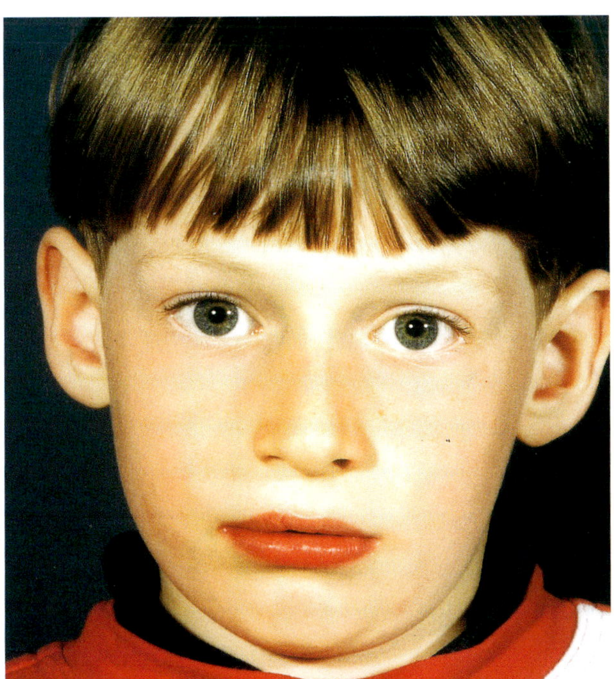

Figure 3.146c Status six years after the operation. Clear symmetry in the lip and nasal areas.

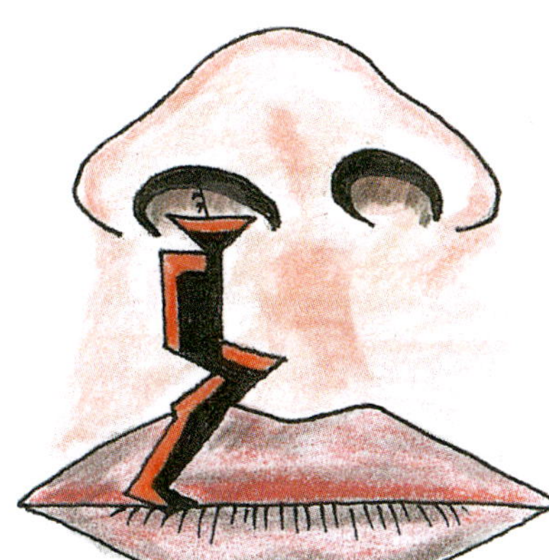

Figure 3.146d Status before the cleft lip closure (Tennison)

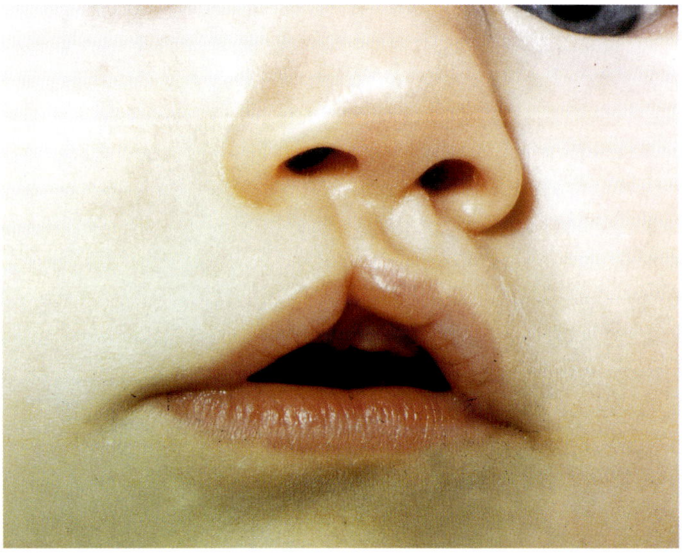

Figure 3.147a Incomplete cleft lip on the right and subcutaneous muscular cleft on the right. Here the orbicularis oris muscle is precisely fixed upon lip closure.

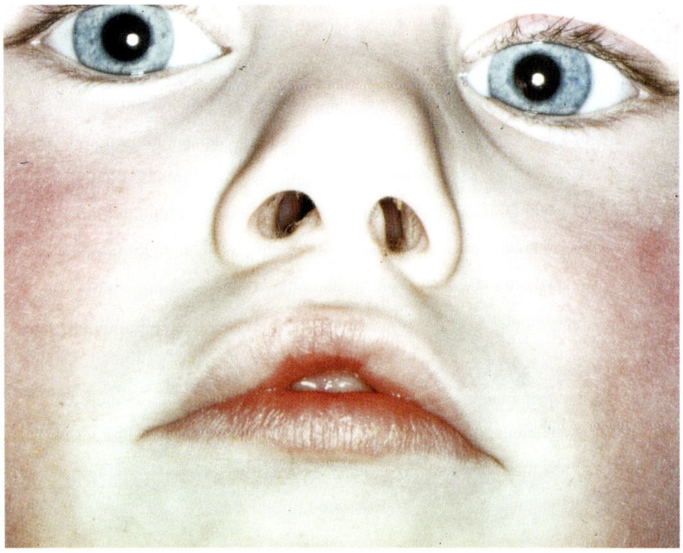

Figure 3.147b Status two years postoperatively

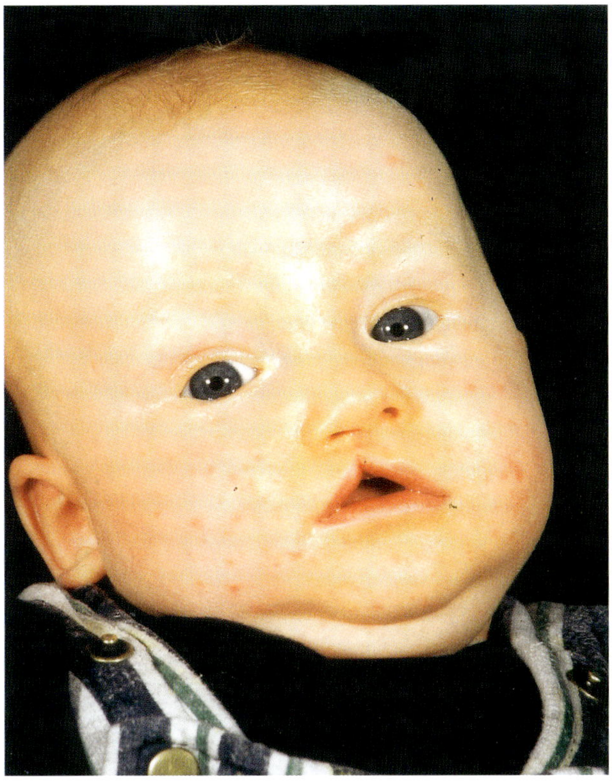

Figure 3.148a Incomplete cleft lip on the right. The jaw and palate are intact. Here a precise lip closure with a slight rotation of the right nasal wing medially is a good option. After surgery of an isolated cleft lip, later corrections are rarely necessary.

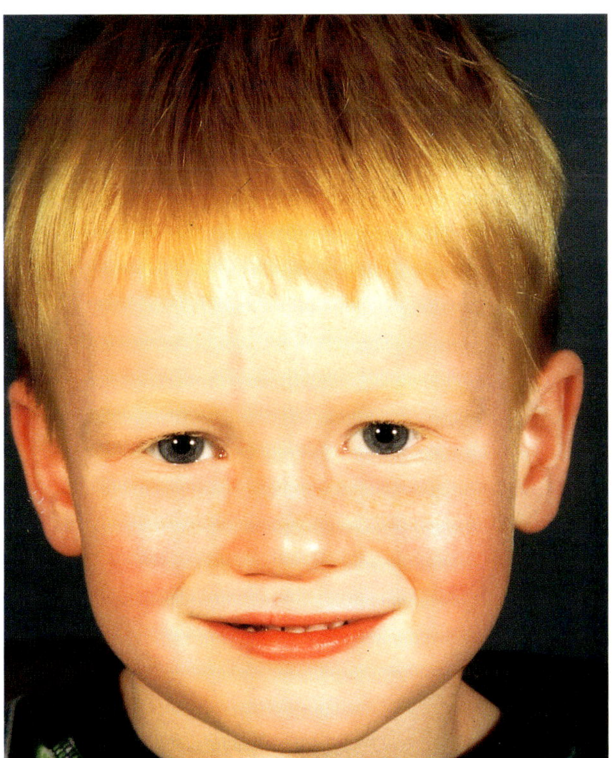

Figure 3.148b Status three years after the operation (Tennison)

c) Unilateral Cleft Lip, Jaw and Palate

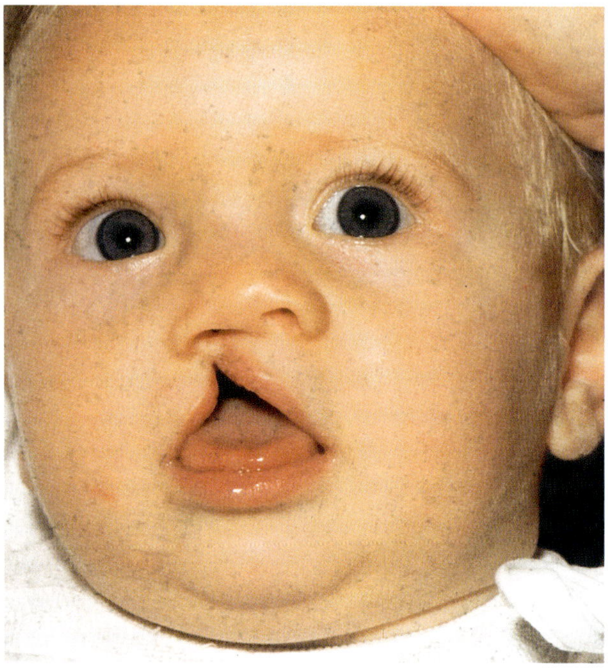

Figure 3.149a Incomplete right cleft lip as well as right cleft jaw and palate and a flat right nasal wing (L2 K3 G3 S3 right).

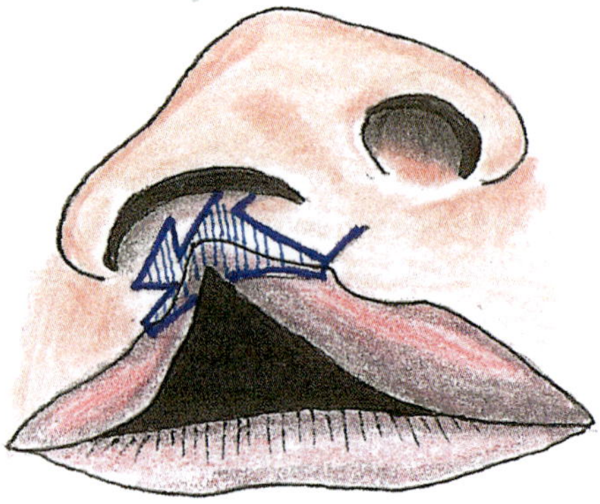

Figure 3.149b Incision line in the lip area according to Tennison. The shaded area is excised.

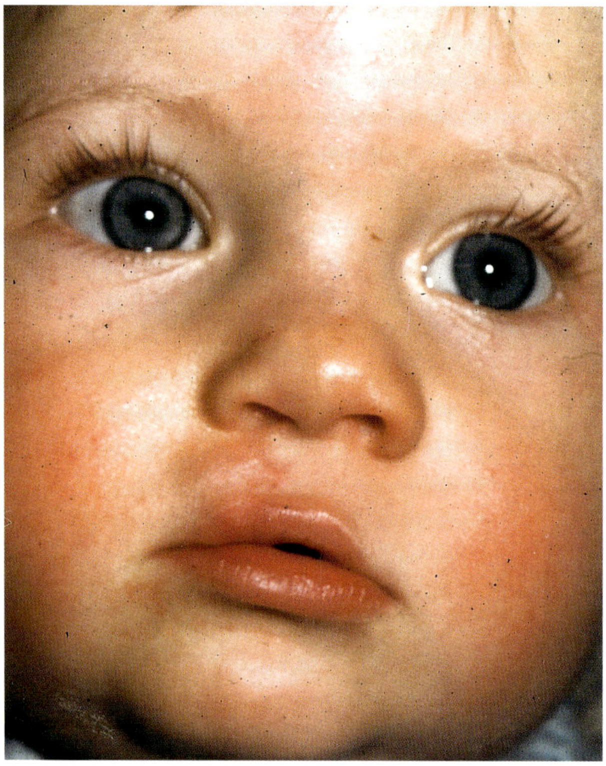

Figure 3.149c Status six months after the operation. Good lip form, the nose is symmetrical.

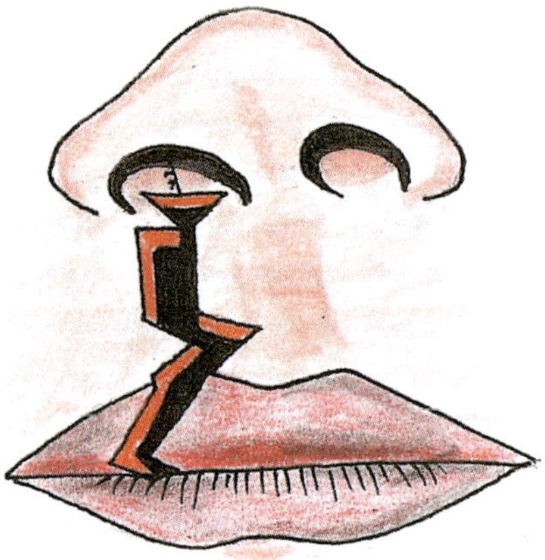

Figure 3.149d Lip closure according to Tennison

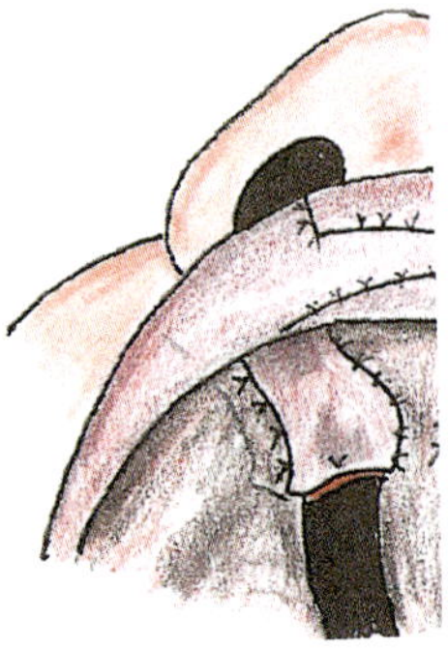

Figure 3.149e Jaw closure with osteoplasty

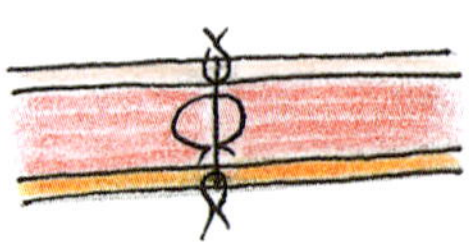

Figure 3.149f Lip closure:
Skin suture 6 × 0 Trofilene
Muscle suture 4 × 0 Vicryl
Mucosal suture 5 × 0 Vicryl

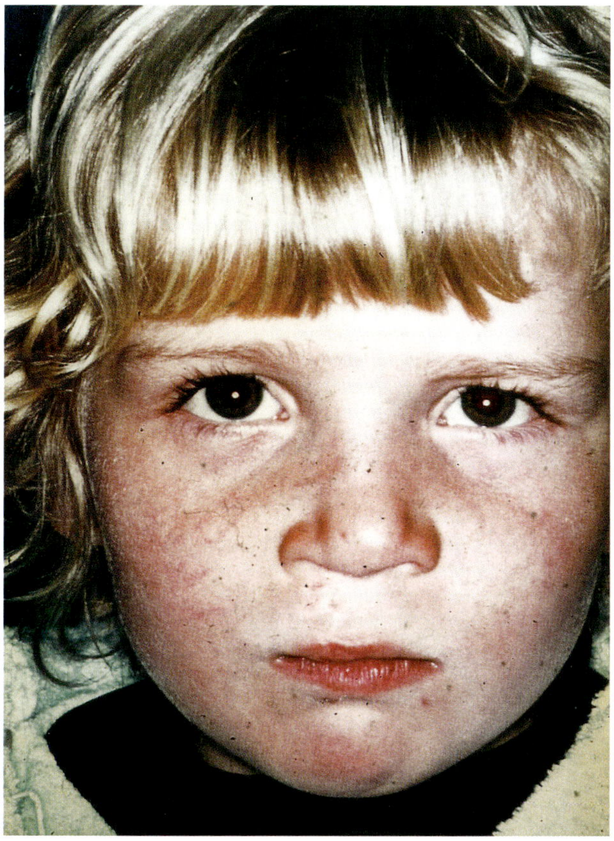

Figure 3.149g Status five years after the operation. The lip is symmetrical. The right nasal wing is flattened a little.

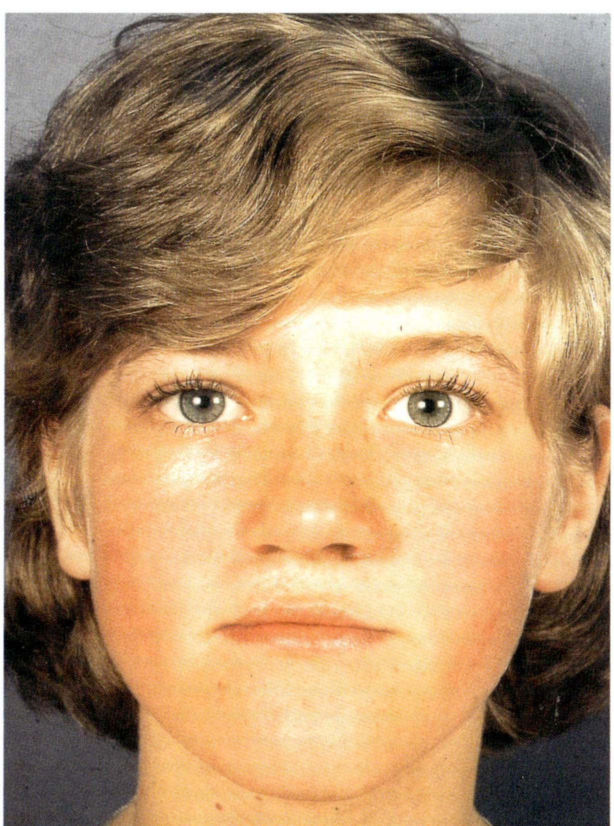

Figure 3.149h Status at 15 years. At 13 years a slight nasal correction was carried out.

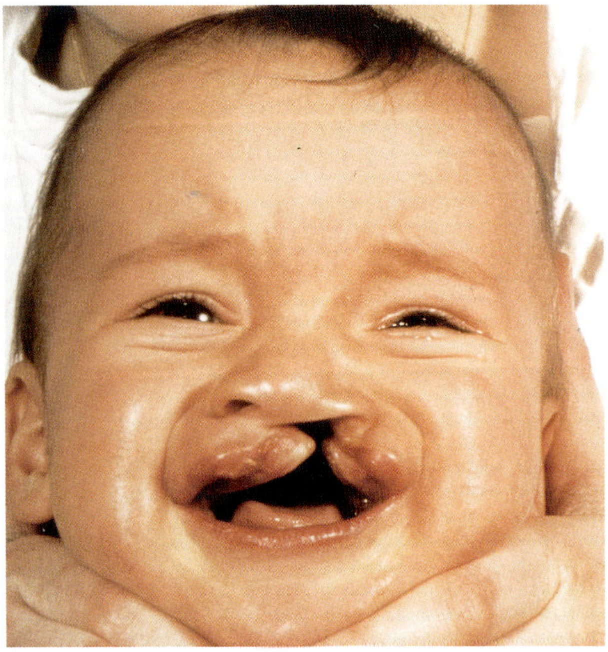

Figure 3.150a Cleft lip and jaw (L3 K3 G3 S3 to the left). Incision line in the lip area according to Tennison. The points on the Cupid's bow must be determined very precisely.

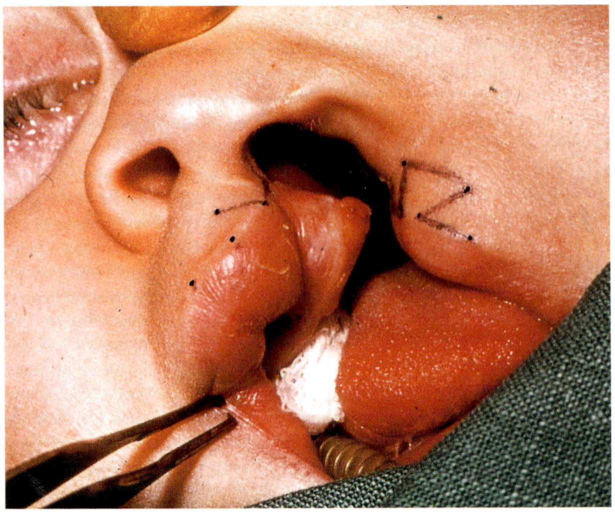

Figure 3.150b Precise preoperative measurement

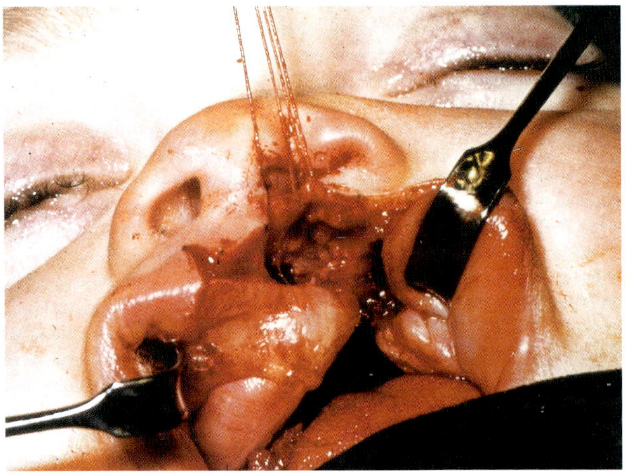

Figure 3.150c The severed orbicularis oris muscle is released from both jaw stumps and adapted after mobilization in the middle of the cleft. After that the floor of the nose is formed and the nasal side of the cleft jaw is closed.

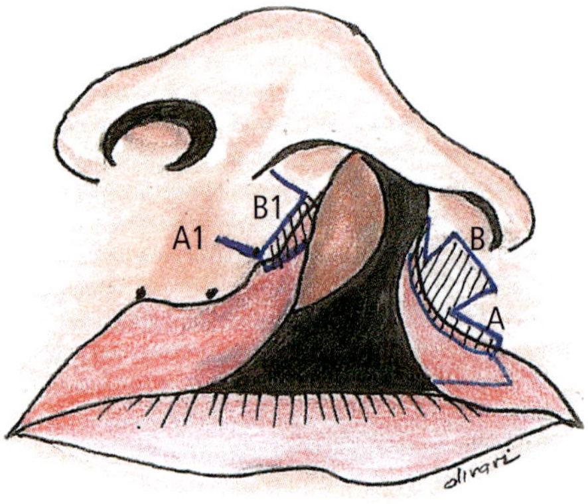

Figure 3.150d The shaded part is resected

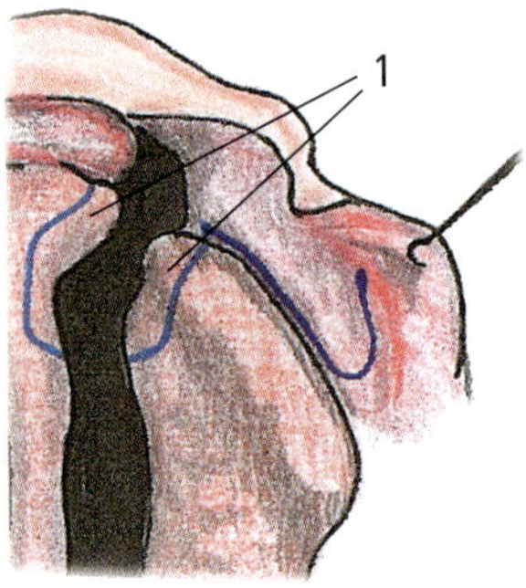

Figure 3.150e The closure of the cleft jaw occurs with formation of the nasal mucosa-periostium layer from both jaw stumps (1).

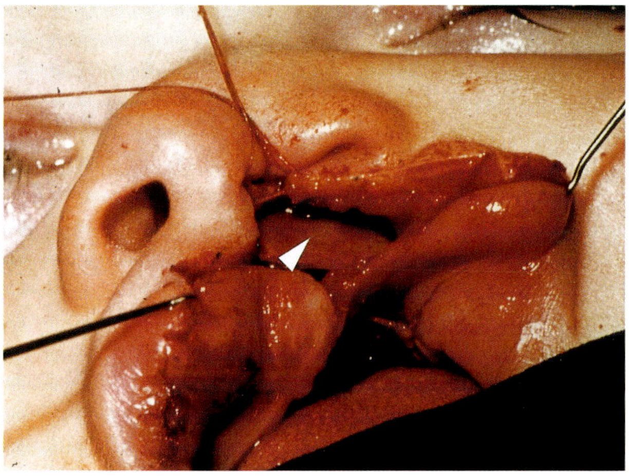

Figure 3.150f The nasal layer is formed. A piece of rib (see arrow) is implanted with moderate compression between the two jaw stumps. The rib ends are split in order to allow a better contact with the bone freed from the periostium. In order to close the oral side of the cleft jaw, a local mucous flap is used from the vestibulum. The hard and soft palates were closed at an age of 18 months.

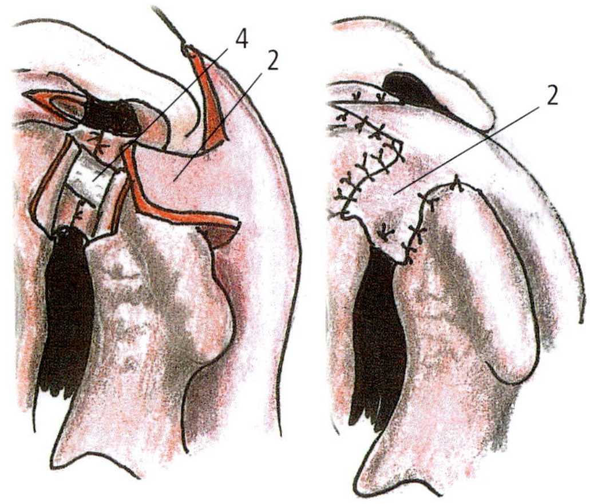

Figure 3.150g A piece of rib is implanted between both jaw stumps (4). The oral side of the cleft jaw is reconstructed using a local mucosal flap from the vestibulum (2).
The bone graft must be closed tightly.

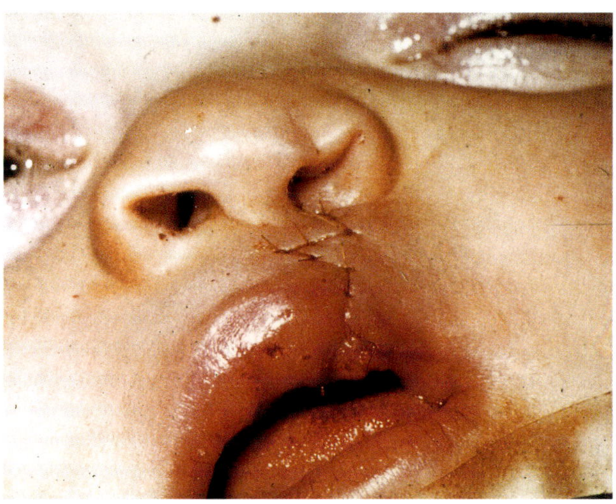

Figure 3.150h Status at the end of the operation. A symmetrical lip form is achieved. By rotating the nasal wing the nose has become symmetrical, but still with a denting in the area of the nasal wing cartilage. This usually corrects spontaneously within three to four months.

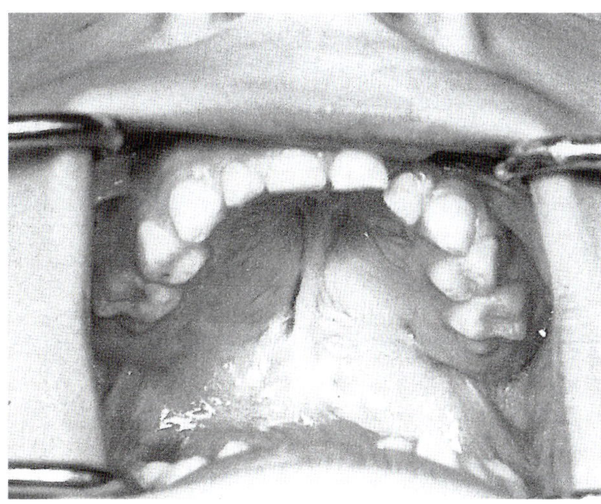

Figure 3.150i Status at the age of five years. Good upper jaw form after a primary osteoplasty. Normal dentition.

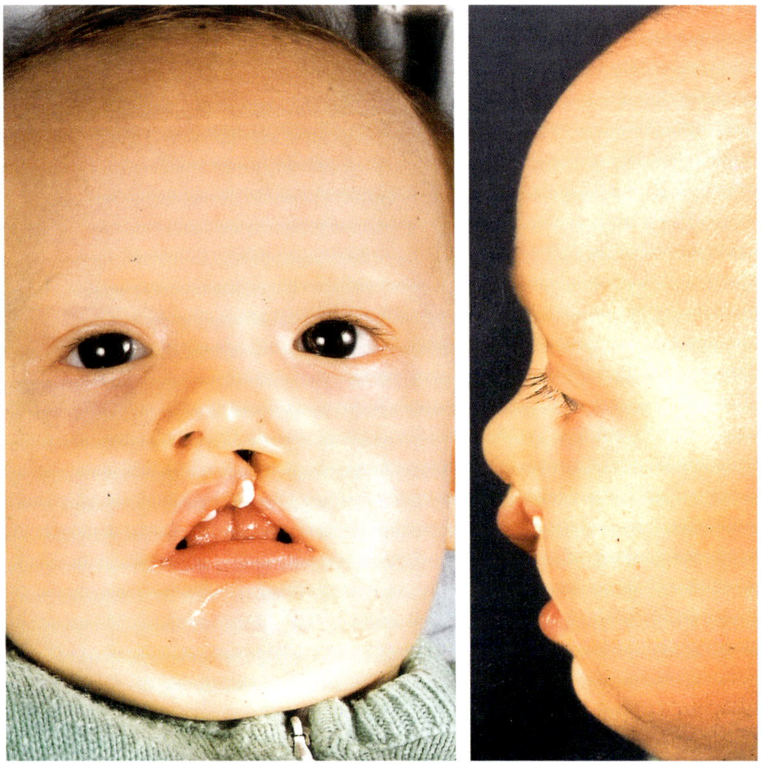

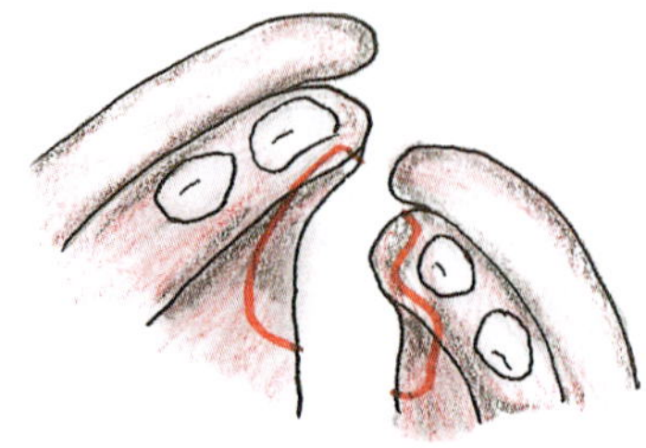

A

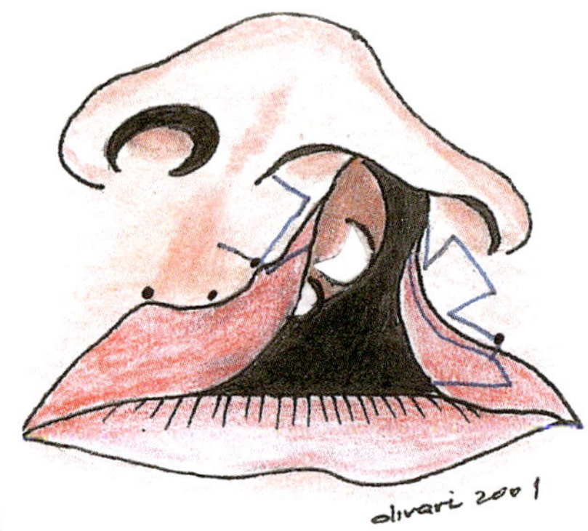

B

Figure 3.151a Left-sided cleft lip, jaw and palate with an unfavorable position of the jaw stumps (sketch A). The operation was carried out at an age of seven months (L3 K3 G3 S3 left).

Planning of the operation in the lip area

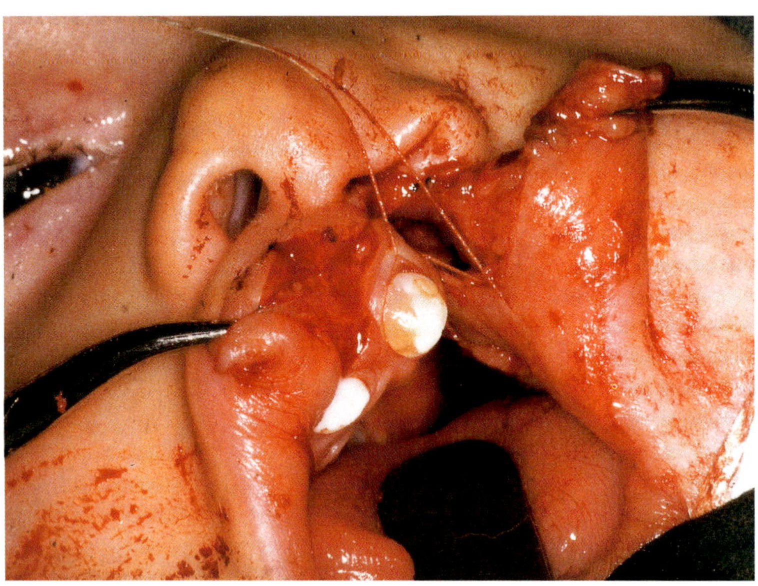

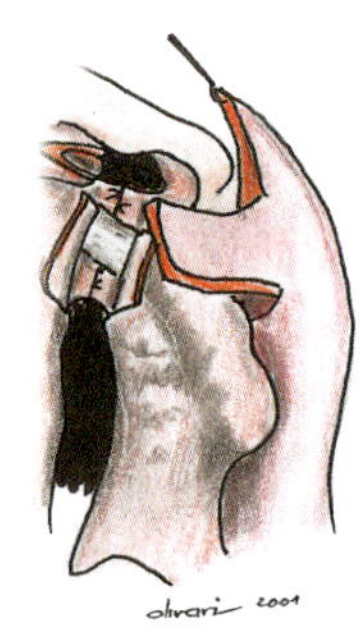

C

Rib graft

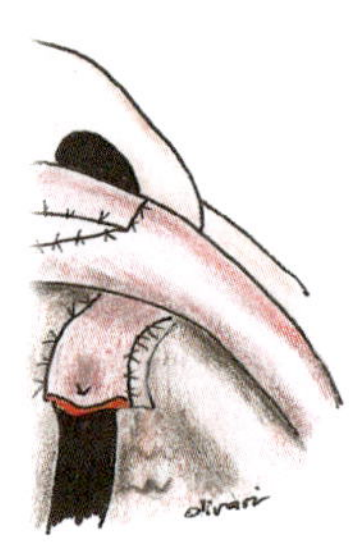

D

Figure 3.151b The floor of the nose in the jaw area is reconstructed and a rib is implanted. The bone graft is tightly closed from the oral side with a mucosal flap (sketch C). Age: Seven months.

Primary osteoplasty

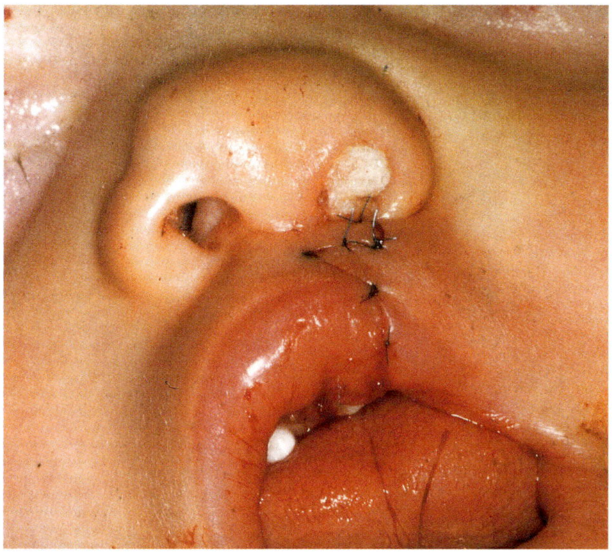

Figure 3.151c Status at the end of the operation. In the mucosa of the lip, triangular flaps are formed from both sides so that the prelabium and fornix can be reconstructed (see D).

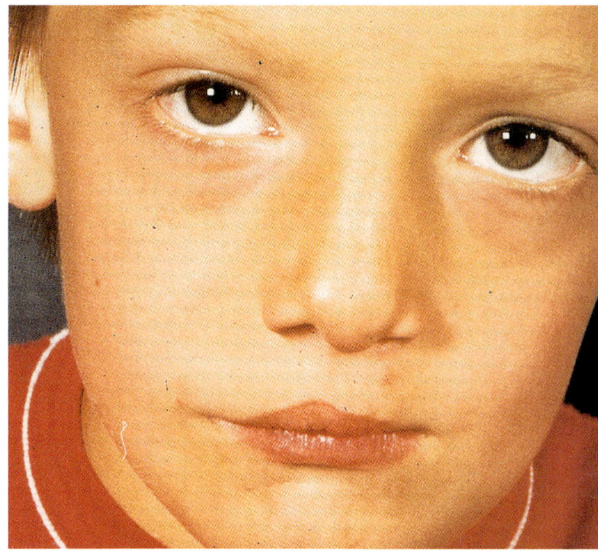

Figure 3.151d Status six years after the operation. A slight asymmetry of the red of the lip is corrected.

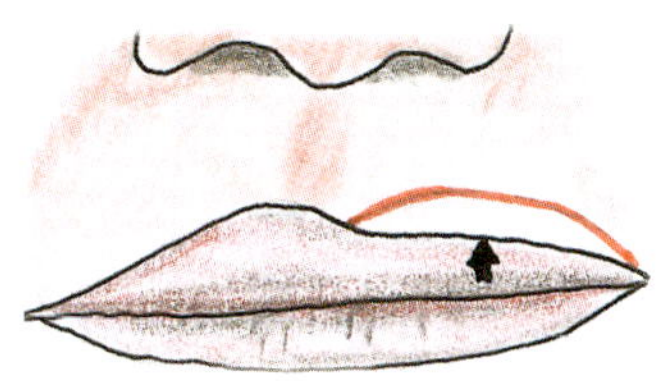

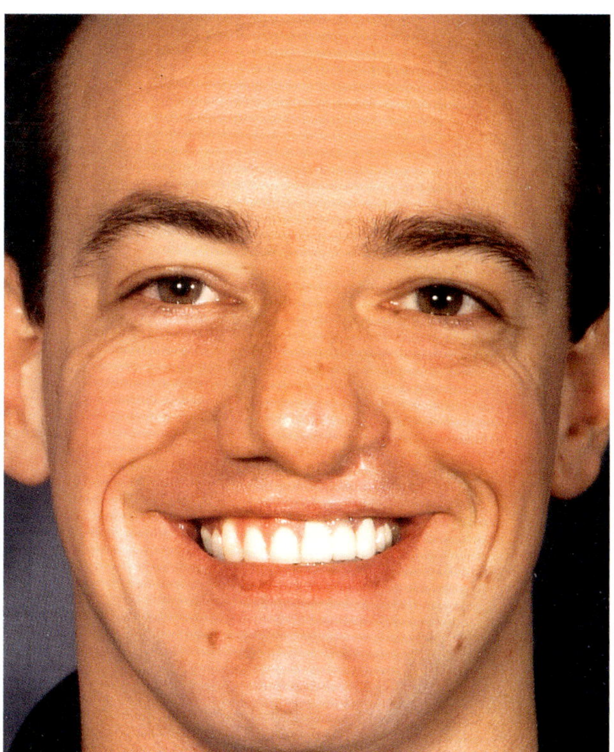

Figure 3.151e Status 26 years after the operation. The nose is symmetrical, the dental arch is well formed (no pseudo-progenia). The speech is unimpaired.

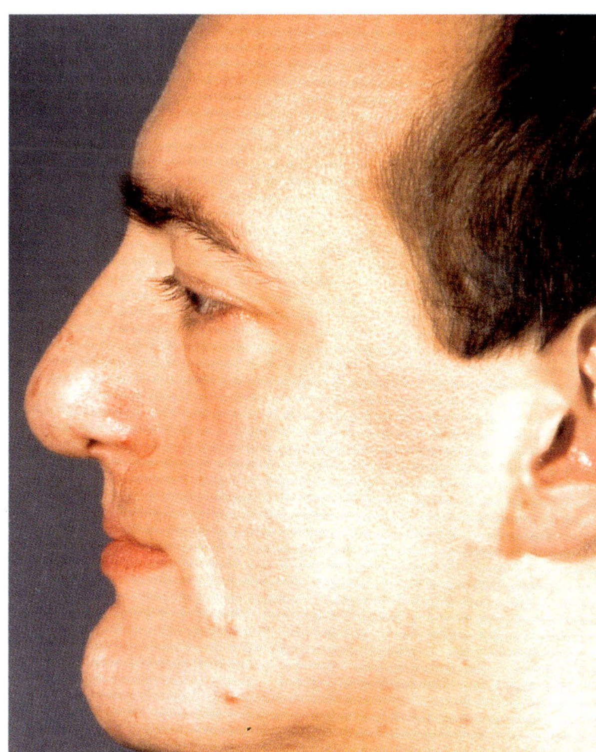

Figure 3.151f Status 26 years after the operation. Patient is now a lawyer.

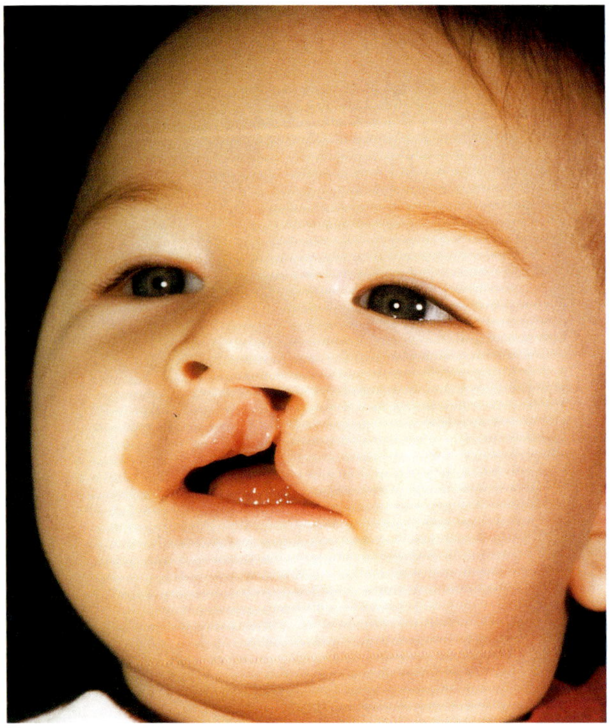

Figure 3.152a Left-sided cleft lip, jaw and palate. In the first session the lip closure as well as the jaw closure are carried out with a primary osteoplasty. The nasal wing is simultaneously rotated medially (L3 K3 G3 S3 left).

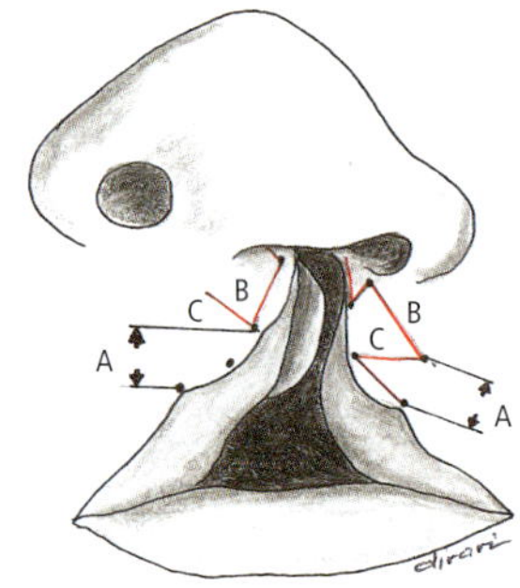

Figure 3.152b Operation planning

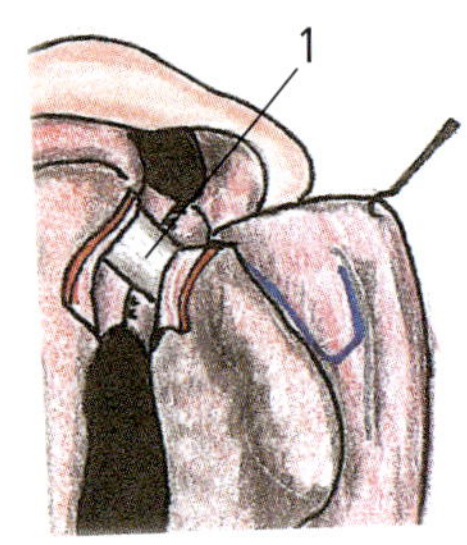

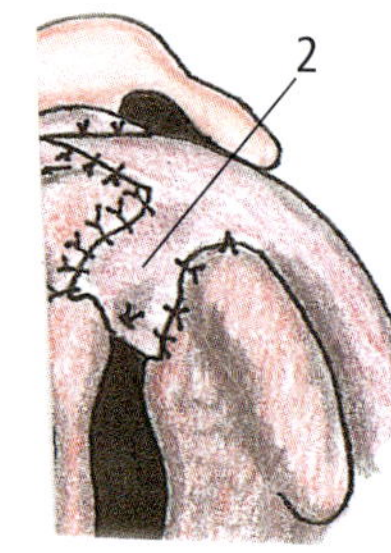

Figure 3.152c Closure of the nasal layer and osteoplasty (1)

Figure 3.152d Closure of the oral layer with a pedicular flap from the vestibulum (2)

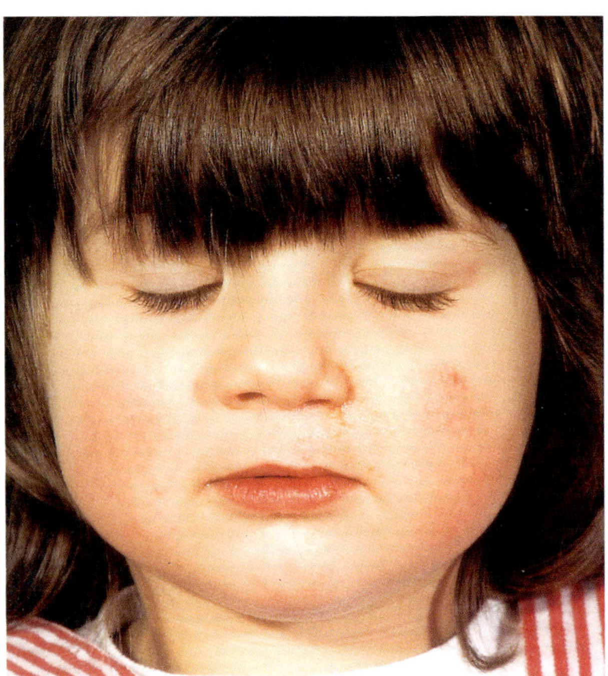

Figure 3.152e Status two years after the operation: Normal speech

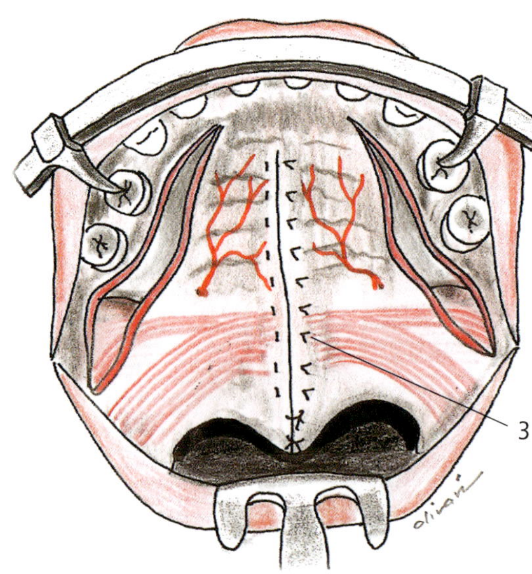

Figure 3.152f The palate closure occurred at the age of 14 months (before the child started speaking). **Note** the joining of the levator muscle and the tensor veli palatini muscle (3).

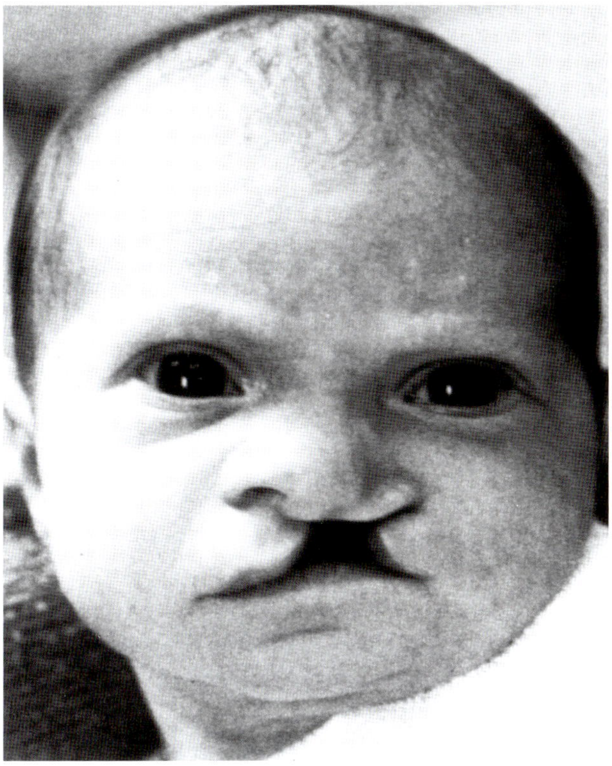

Figure 3.153a Total left cleft lip, jaw and palate with a very broad cleft in the jaw area. Lip and jaw closure occurred at five months, and palate closure at 14 months.

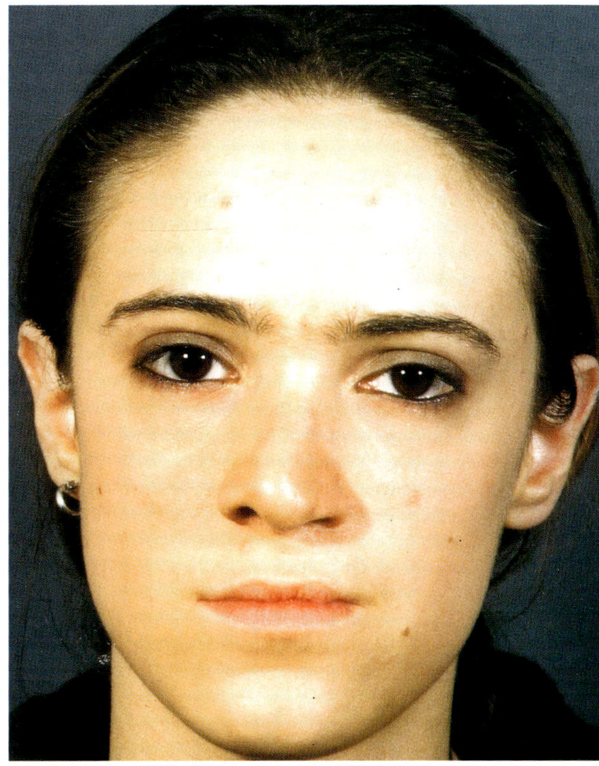

Figure 3.153b Status 16 years postoperatively. The lip form is aesthetically pleasing, the nose is symmetrical and the speech normal. The nasal correction was carried out at the age of 13 years.

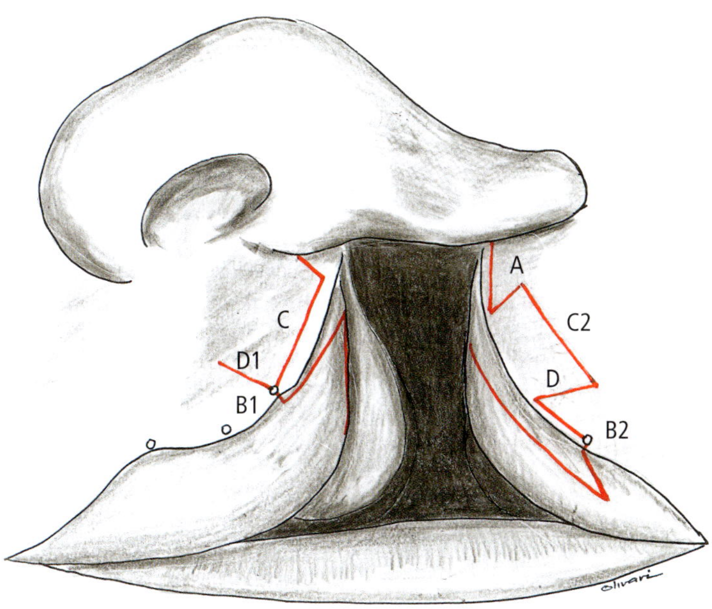

Figure 3.153c
B1: Philtrum point of the contralateral side

B2: Philtrum point of the cleft side

B1, B2: Philtrum points are brought together so that the philtrum can be shaped as a unit

A: Triangular flap at the nostril

C and C1 as well as D and D1 have in each case the same length

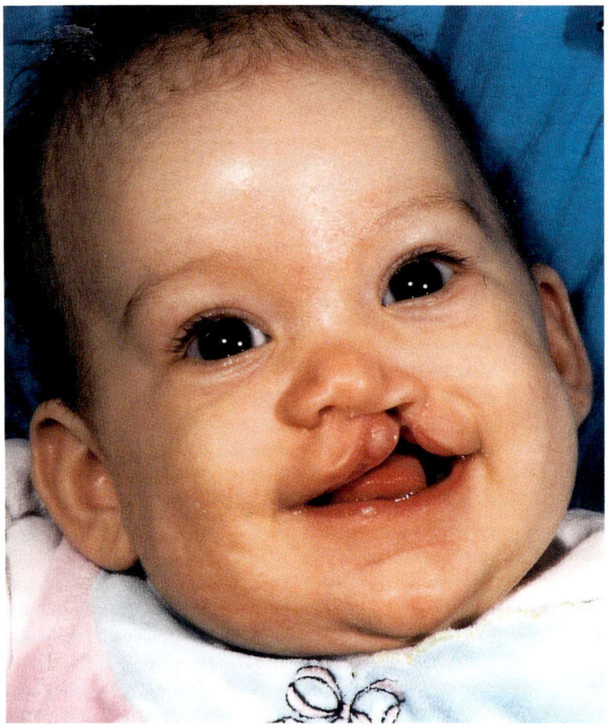

Figure 3.154a Left cleft lip, jaw and palate (L3 K3 G3 S3). The lip and jaw closure was carried out at the age of five months with a primary osteoplasty.

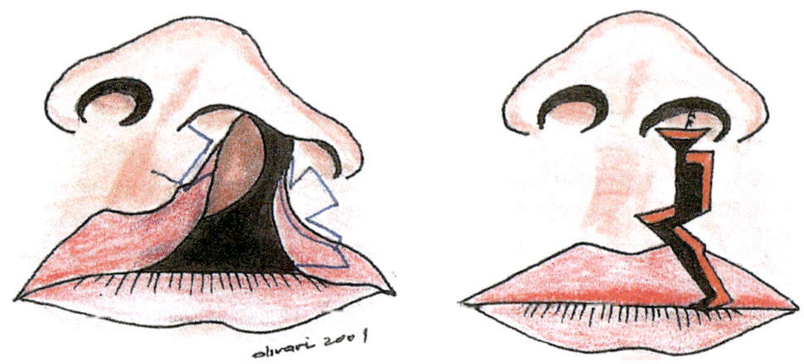

Figure 3.154b Incision line in the lip area with two triangular flaps (Tennison)

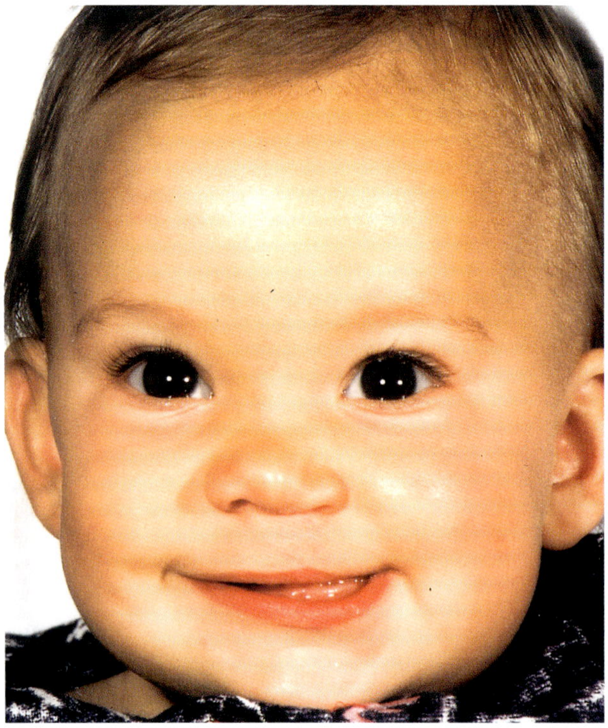

Figure 3.154c The cleft palate was closed at the age of 16 months (according to Langenbeck).

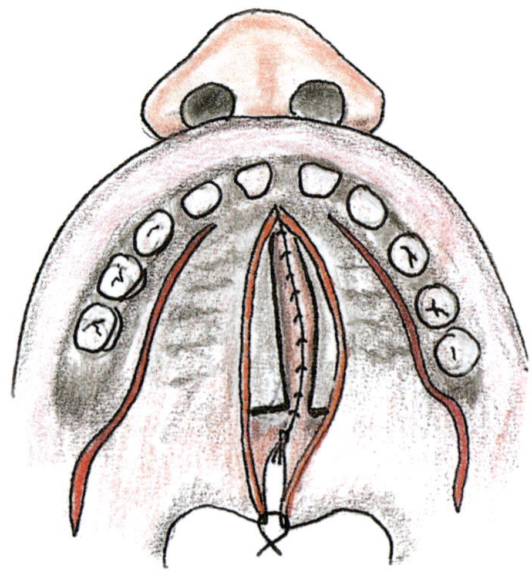

Figure 3.154d The nasal layer is closed. Closure of the oral layer follows.

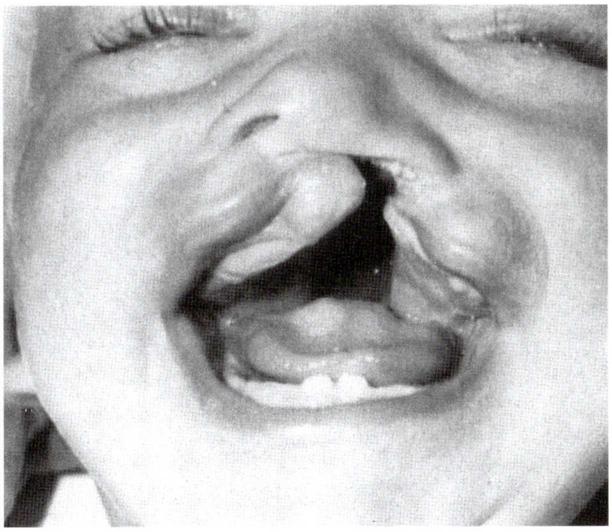

Figure 3.154e Status before the first operation

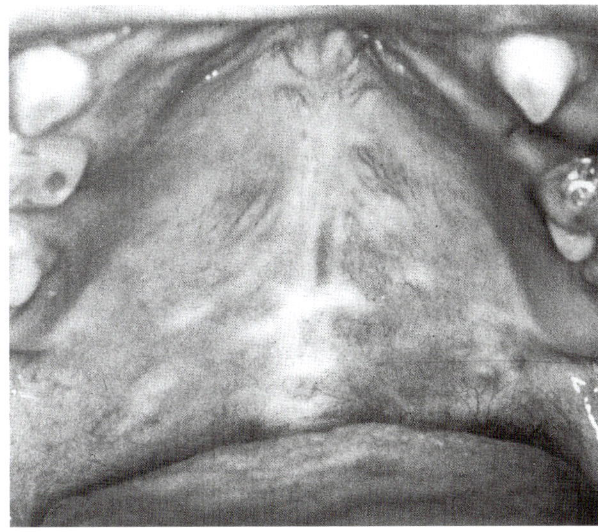

Figure 3.154f Status after the palate closure

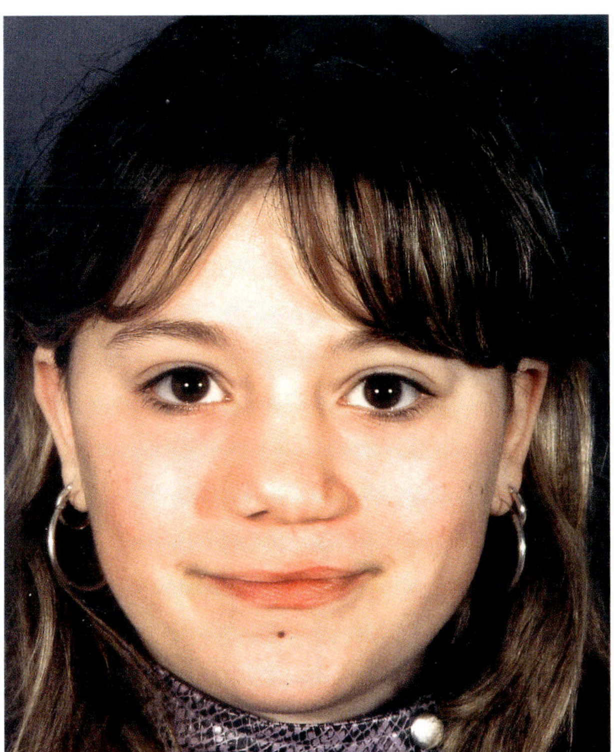

Figure 3.154g Status 12 years after the operation. Through an osteoplasty in the jaw area the collapse of the jaw stumps (i.e. a pseudoprogenia) is prevented. The speech is normal.

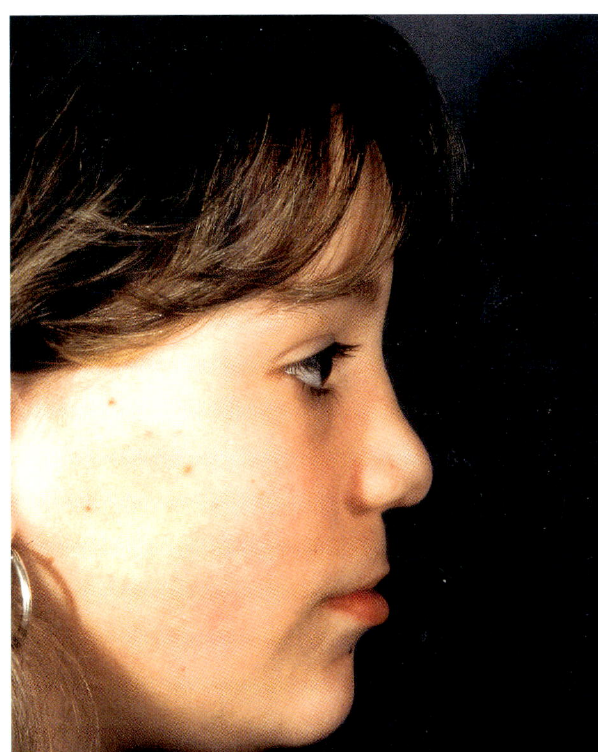

Figure 3.154h Status 12 years after the operation. No pseudoprogenia!

d) Bilateral Cleft Lip, Jaw and Palate

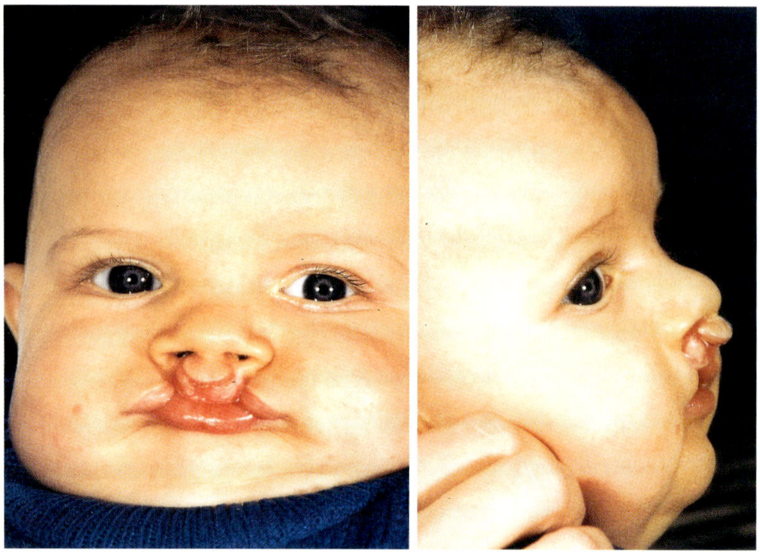

Figure 3.155a Bilateral cleft lip, jaw and palate with moderate dislocation of the premaxilla and an incomplete cleft lip (L2 K3 G3 S3)

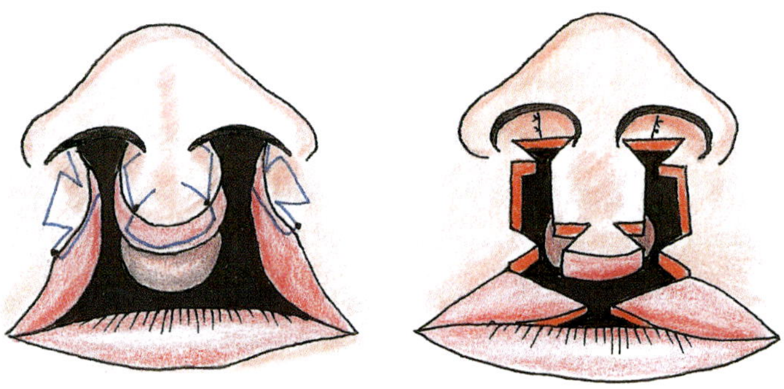

Figure 3.155b Incision line according to Tennison with a bilateral cleft lip, jaw and palate. The prelabium here plays an important role. Both incisions in the prelabium are carefully calculated.

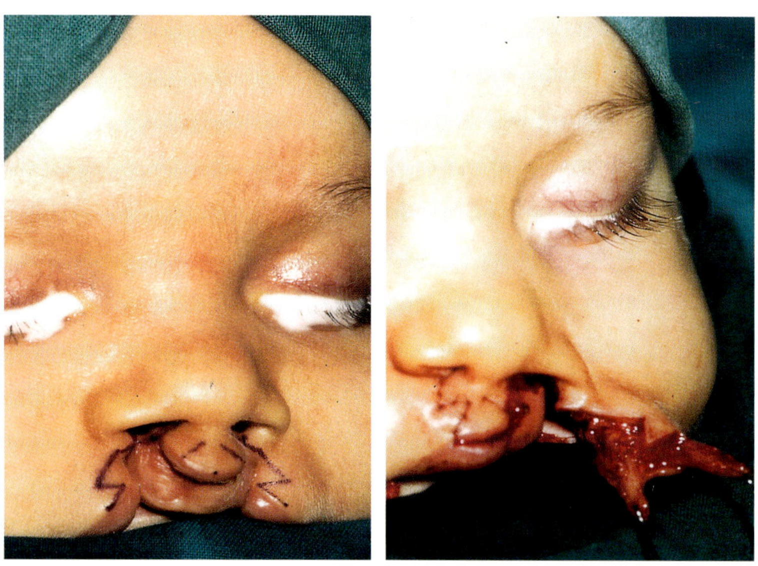

Figure 3.155c Precise incision line and lip jaw closure initially on the right. A rib implant is placed between the jaw stumps. The oral covering of the cleft jaw is carried out using a pedicular mucosal flap from the vestibulum. Both clefts are operated on simultaneously.

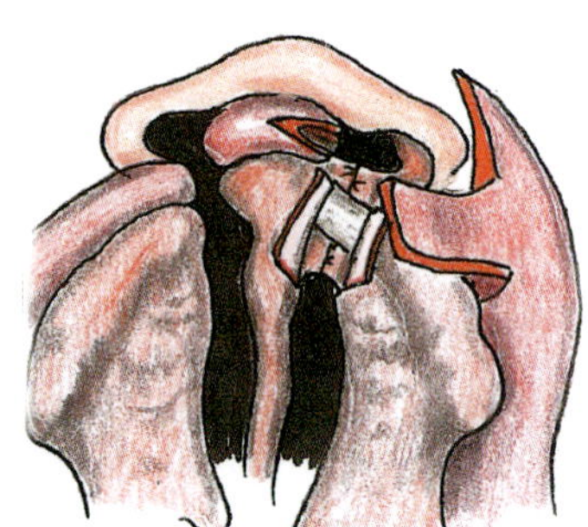

Figure 3.155d A rib implant is implanted between the jaw stumps.

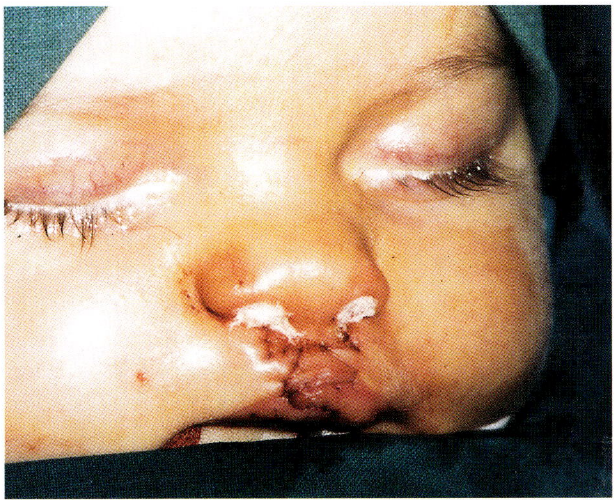

Figure 3.155e Status at the end of the operation. The Sofratuell tampon remains for approximately four to five days and is replaced on the second day.

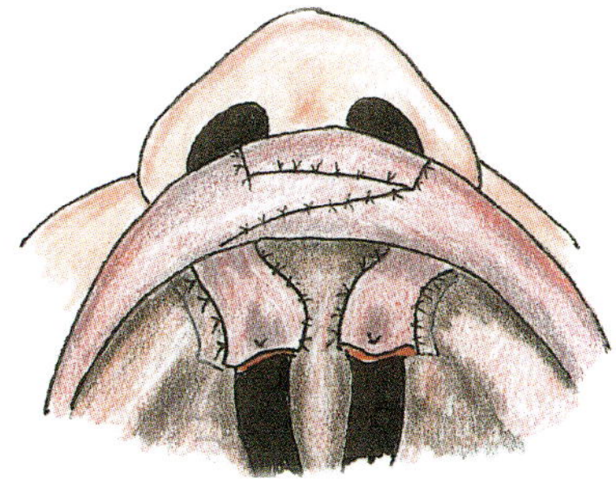

Figure 3.155f Lip jaw closure with osteoplasty on both sides

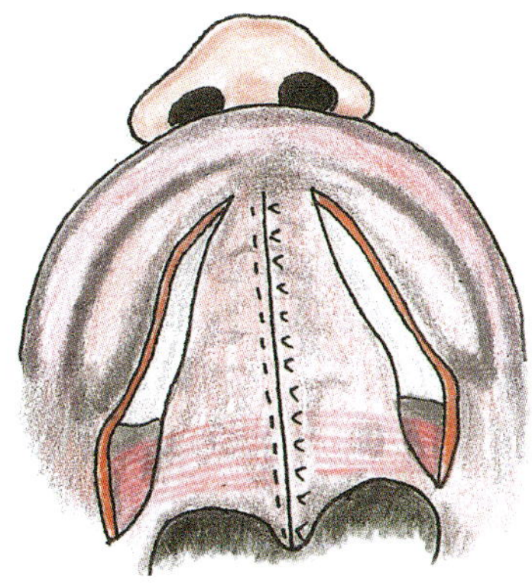

Figure 3.155g Palate closure with two bridge flaps at an age of 15 months

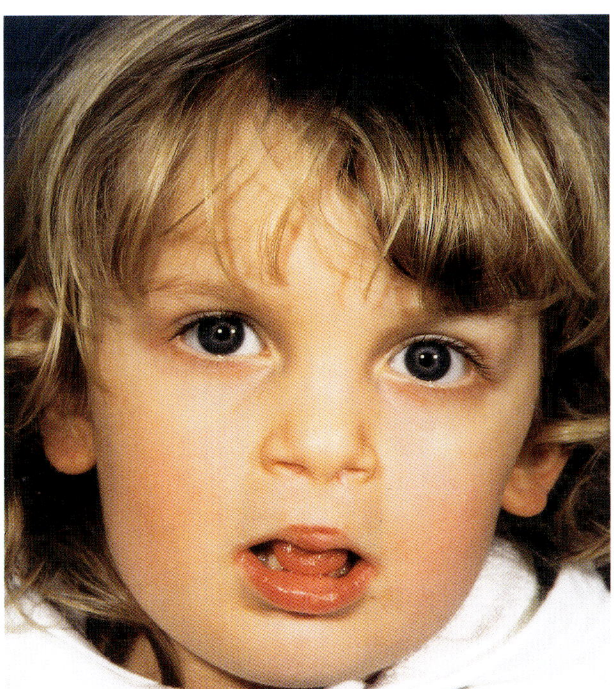

Figure 3.155h Status five years after the operation: The palate was closed at 15 months. The lip and nose are symmetrical. Slight speech problems at the start which improved after speech therapy.

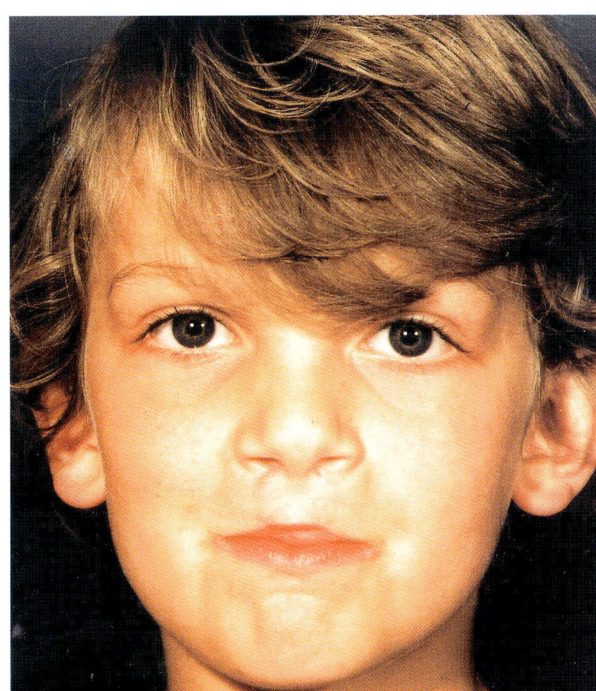

Figure 3.155i Status after ten years

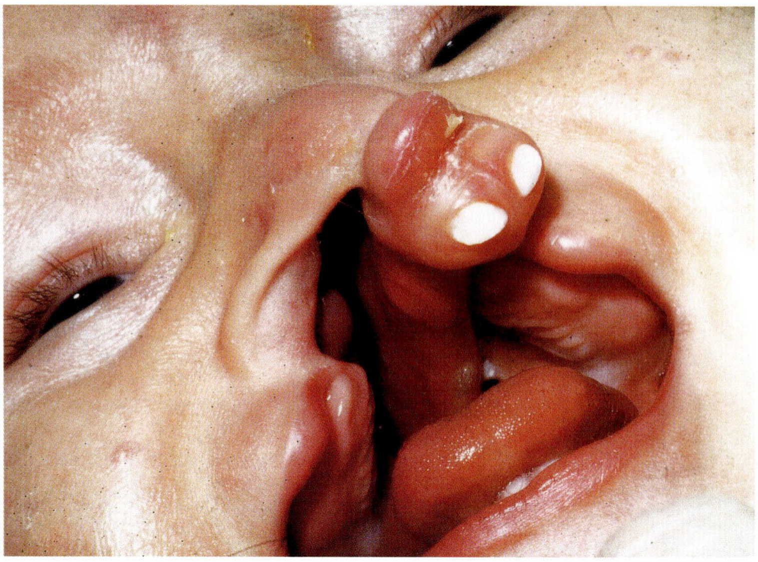

Figure 3.156a Bilateral cleft lip, jaw and palate with extreme dislocation of the premaxilla. Here the lip jaw closure is carried out first on the wider side, i.e. on the right. No partial resection of the vomer, as proposed by some authors. Although resection of the vomer seems reasonable in this state, this can cause an exacerbation of a pseudoprogenia later on.

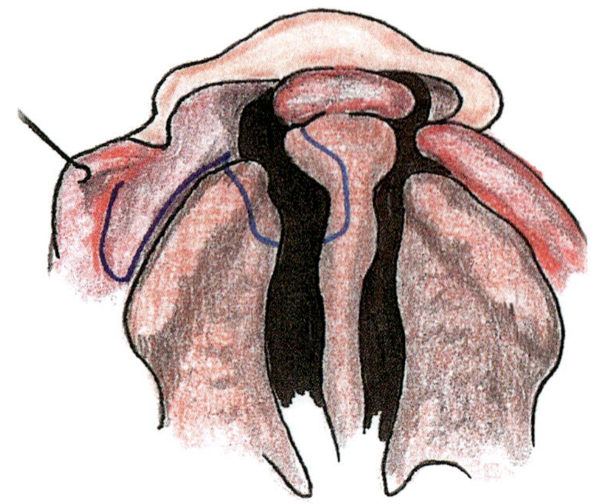

Figure 3.156b Planning of the demanding operation

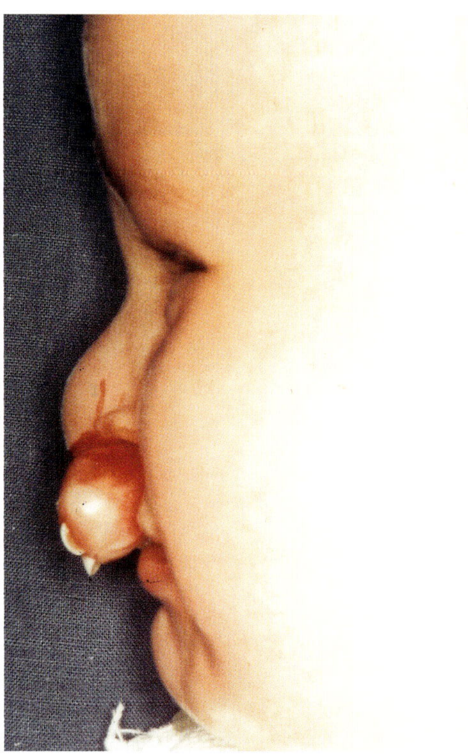

Figure 3.156c Dislocated premaxilla

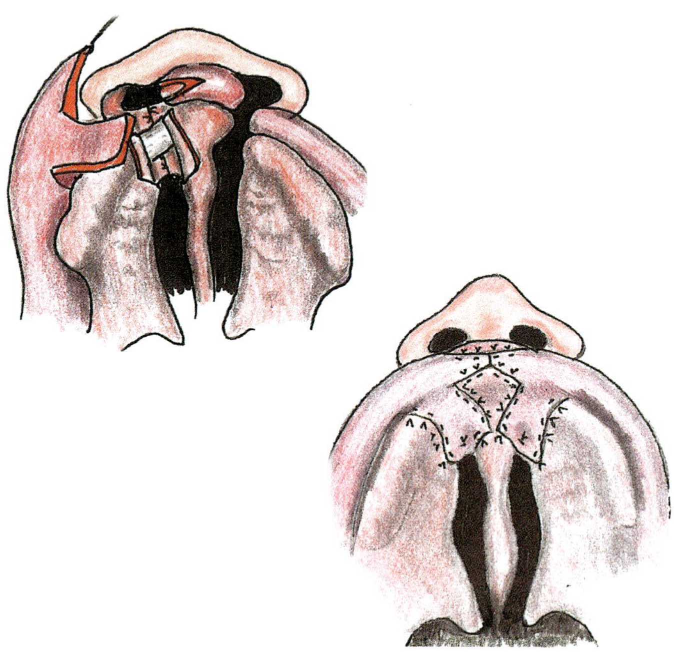

Figure 3.156d After lip closure the dislocated premaxilla is repositioned. The repositioned jaw stumps are also simultaneously displaced in the medial and dorsal direction. A previous orthodontic treatment is urgently recommended in such cases.

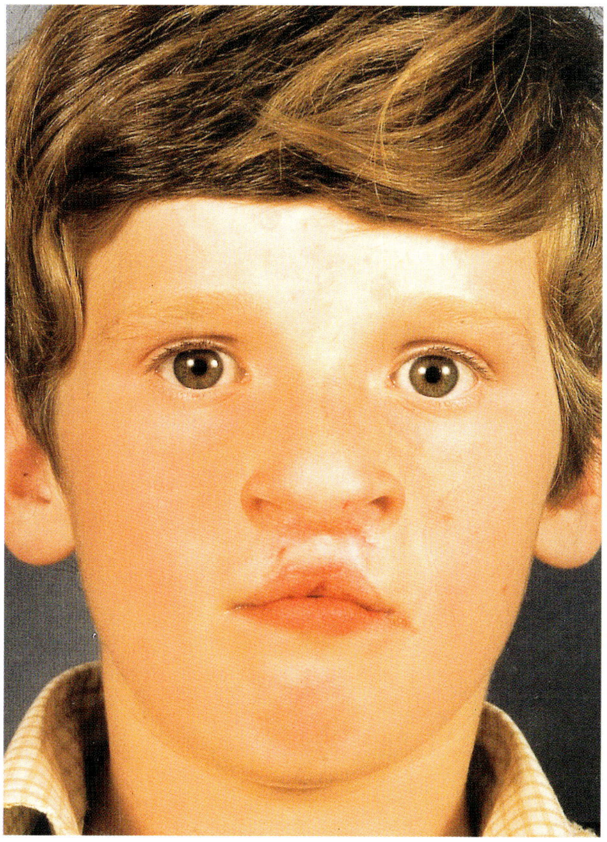

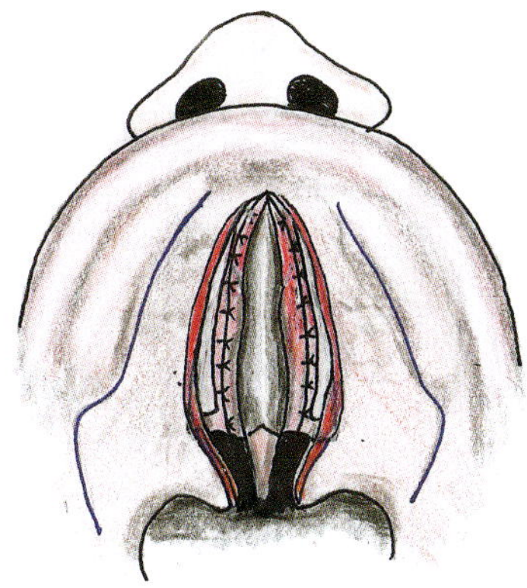

Figure 3.156e Acceptable result seven years after the operation with a very unfavorable starting state.

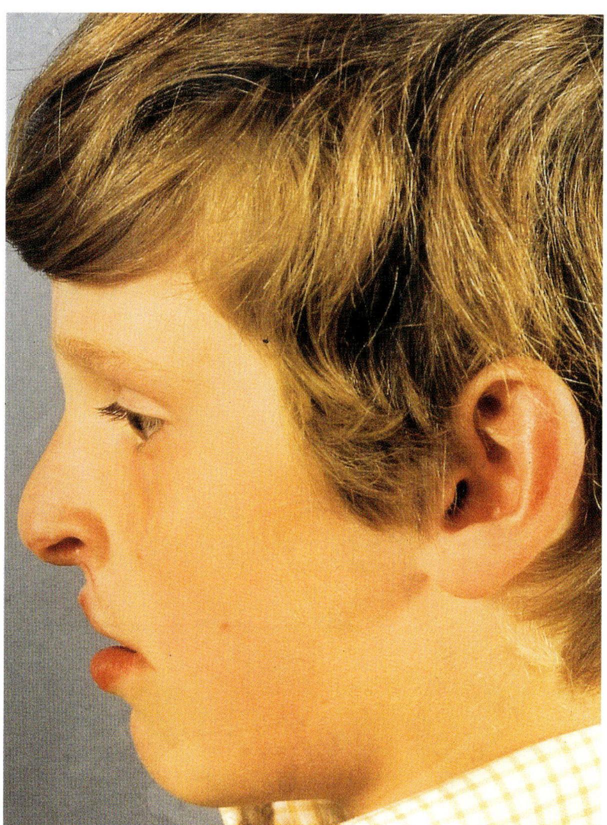

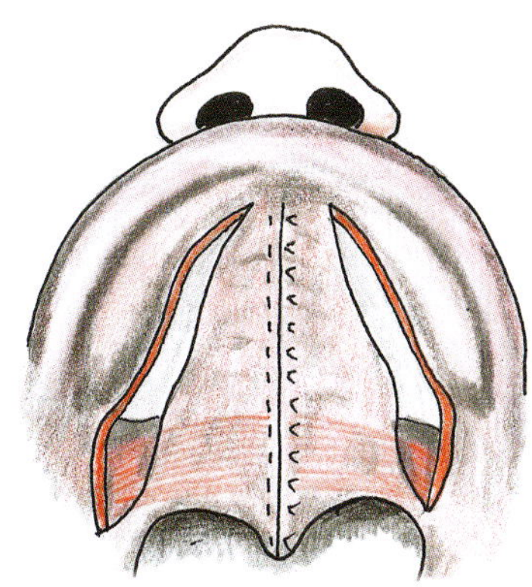

Figure 3.156f No pseudoprogenia arises, the upper lip is a little too short and the nasal form is in need of correction. These secondary interventions were carried out at the age of 14 years.

Abbe Plasty – Lip Correction – Nasal Correction

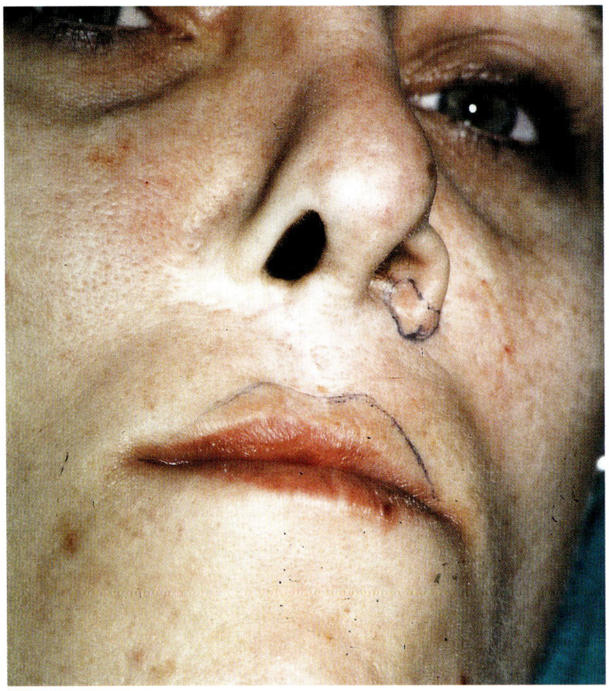

Figure 3.159a Status after cleft lip, jaw and palate. Planning: 1) Nostril correction, 2) Enlargement of the mucosa of the lip, 3) Abbe plasty.

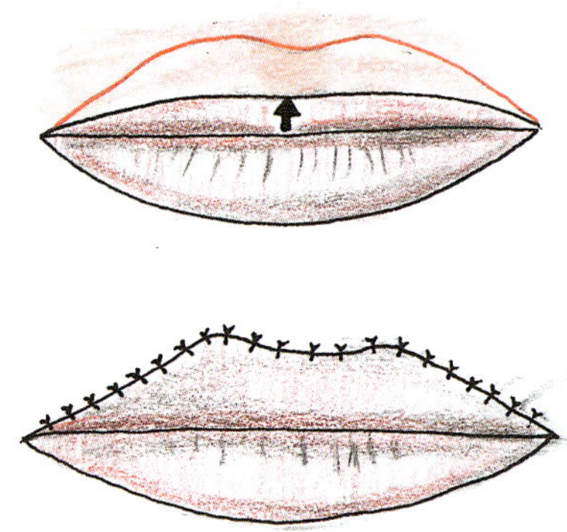

Figure 3.159b The very narrow upper lip is reconstructed by excision of the lip skin and mobilization and rotation of the mucosa of the lip cranially (not simultaneously with the Abbe plasty).

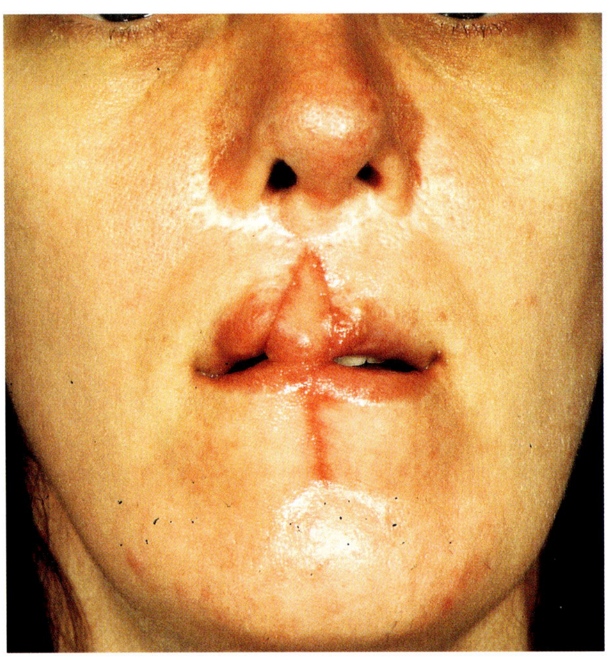

Figure 3.159c Two to three weeks after the operation the flap pedicle can be severed and the lip can be shaped. The inferior labial artery must be spared from damage. It can be easily palpated from the inner side of the lip, directly under the mucous membrane.

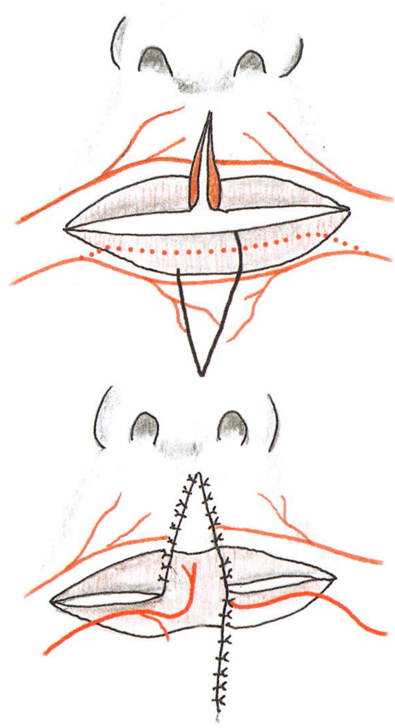

Figure 3.159d Abbe plasty for enlarging the upper lip. Consider the course of the inferior labial artery that must remain intact. When calculating the width of the Abbe plasty a simultaneous reduction in size of the lower lip should also be included in the calculations; i.e., smaller flaps than those initially planned.

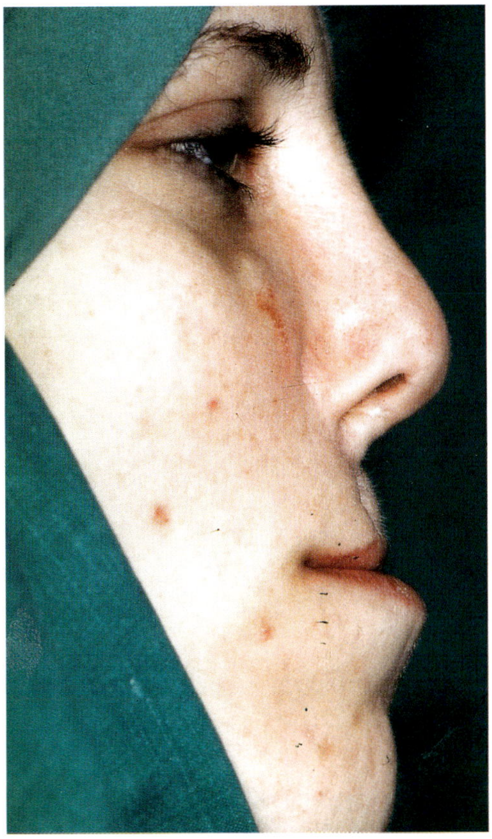

Figure 3.159e Pseudoprogenia after a LJP cleft. During the calculation of the Abbe flap it must be considered that the lower lip becomes reduced in size. As such one should not apply to large flaps.

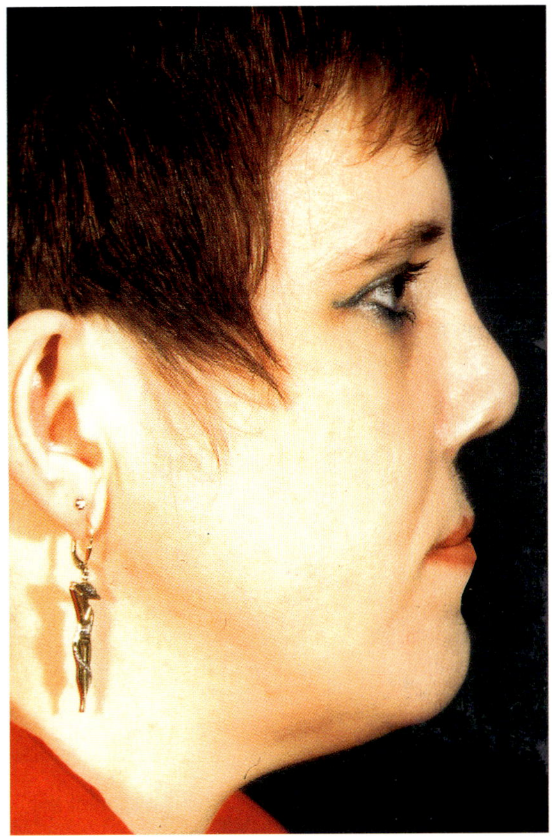

Figure 3.159f Three years after the Abbe operation, nasal correction and lip correction

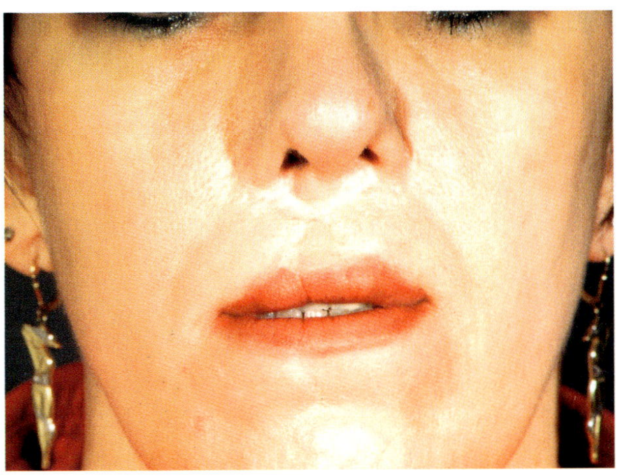

Figure 3.159g Status after Abbe flap and correction of the lip

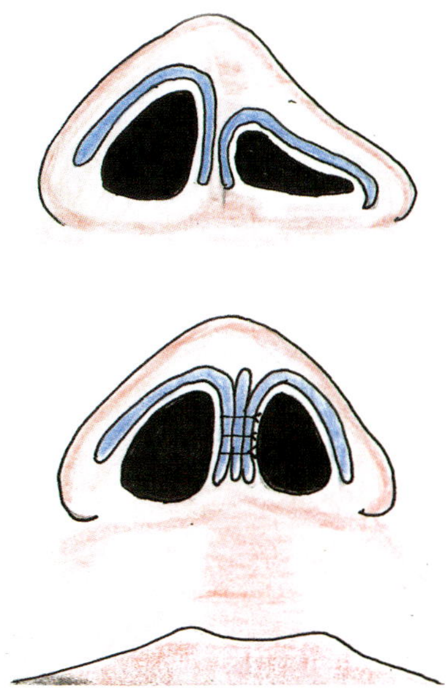

Figure 3.159h Rotation of the left nasal wing and cartilage implantation for improving the nasal form.

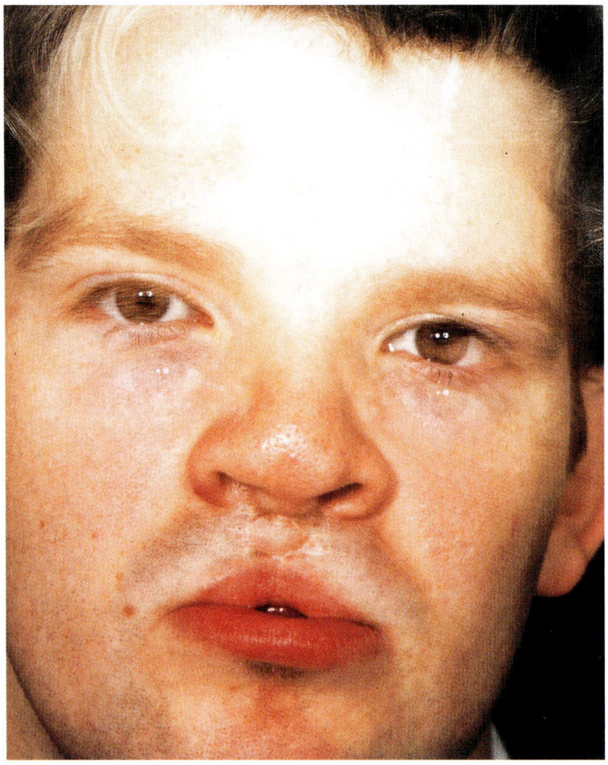

Figure 3.161a Abbe plasty: Status after bilateral cleft lip, jaw and palate. Pseudoprogenia.

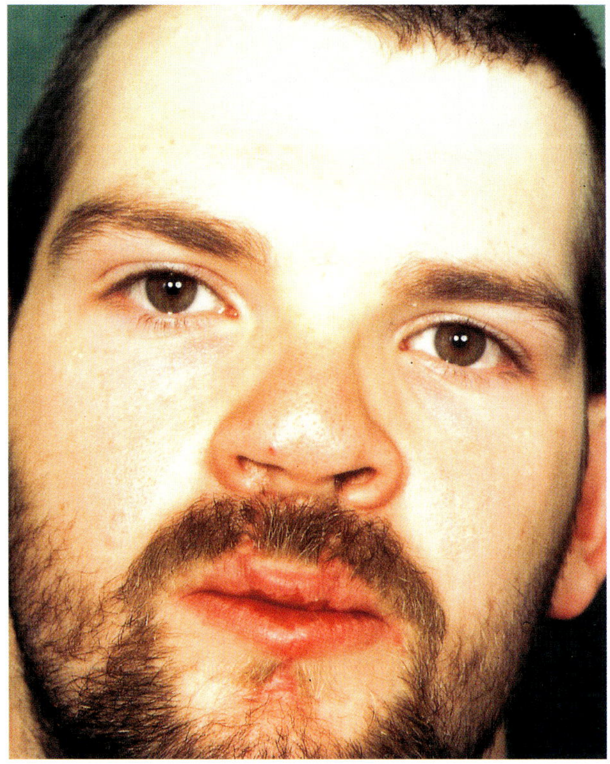

Figure 3.161b Status one year after the Abbe plasty: One can clearly see how severely (2 cm) the cupid's bow on the upper lip has been corrected.

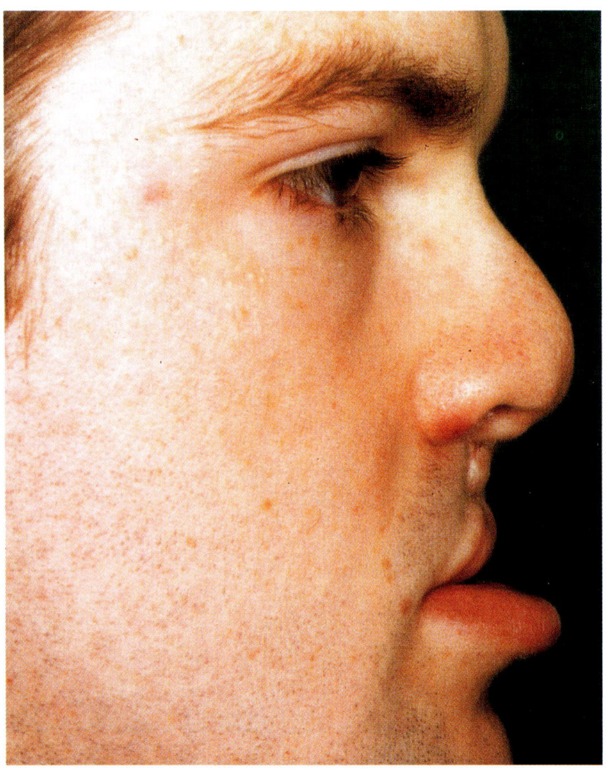

Figure 3.161c Status before the operation. An Abbe plasty with a W-shaped incision line was carried out.

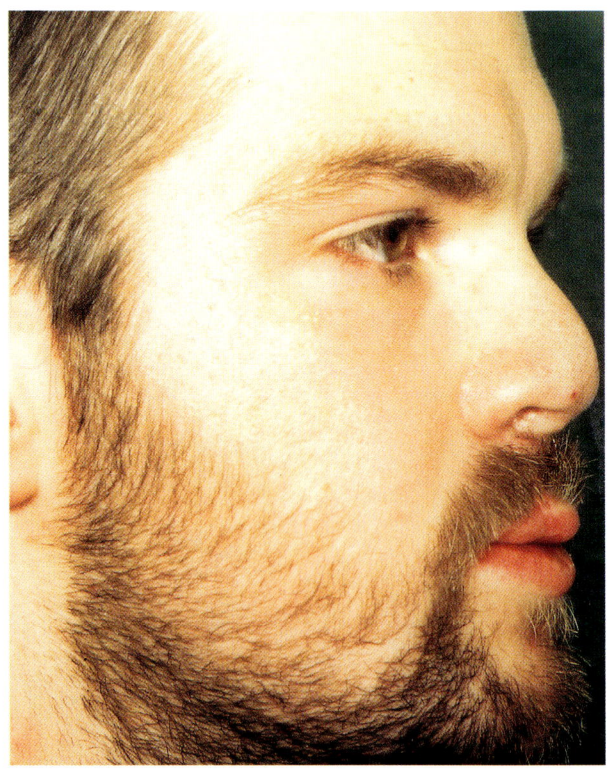

Figure 3.161d Status one year after the operation

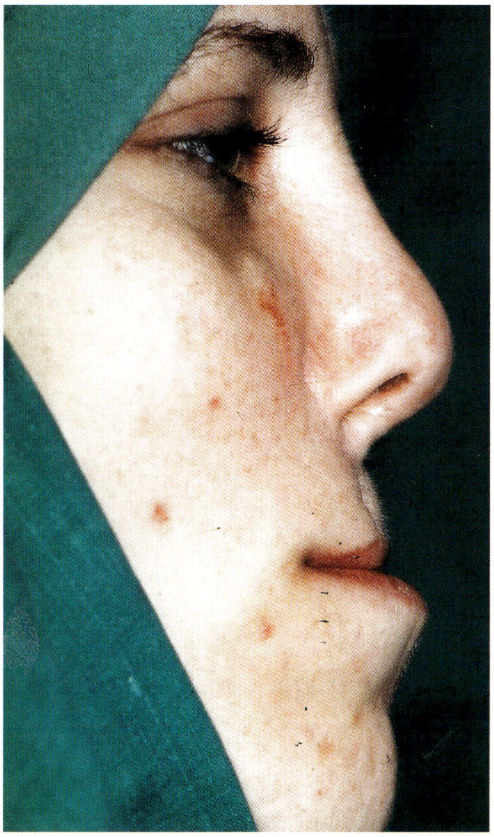

Figure 3.159e Pseudoprogenia after a LJP cleft. During the calculation of the Abbe flap it must be considered that the lower lip becomes reduced in size. As such one should not apply to large flaps.

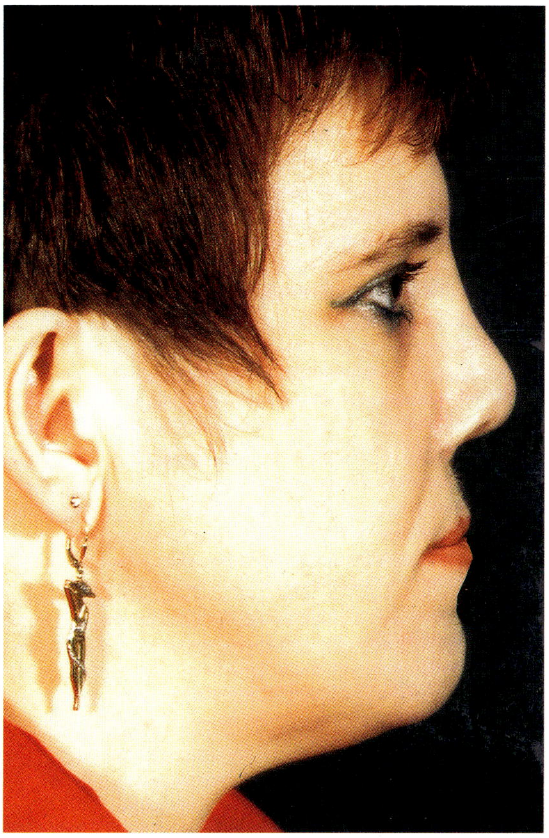

Figure 3.159f Three years after the Abbe operation, nasal correction and lip correction

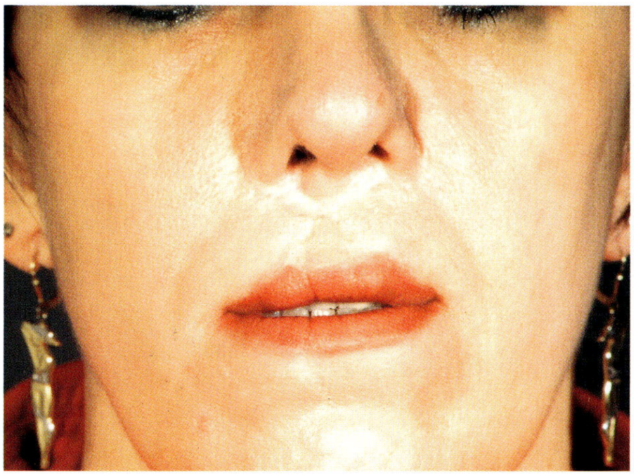

Figure 3.159g Status after Abbe flap and correction of the lip

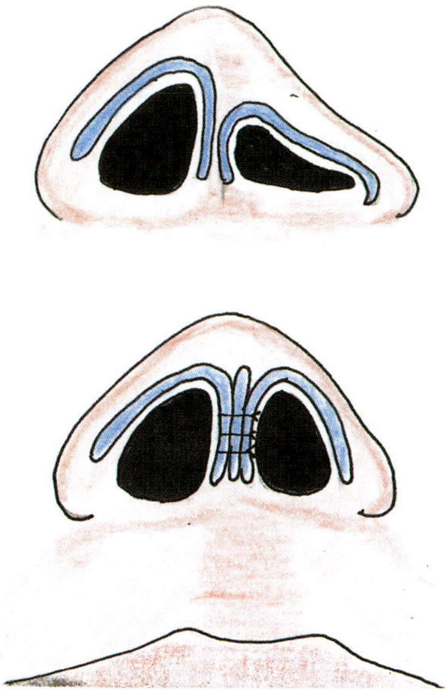

Figure 3.159h Rotation of the left nasal wing and cartilage implantation for improving the nasal form.

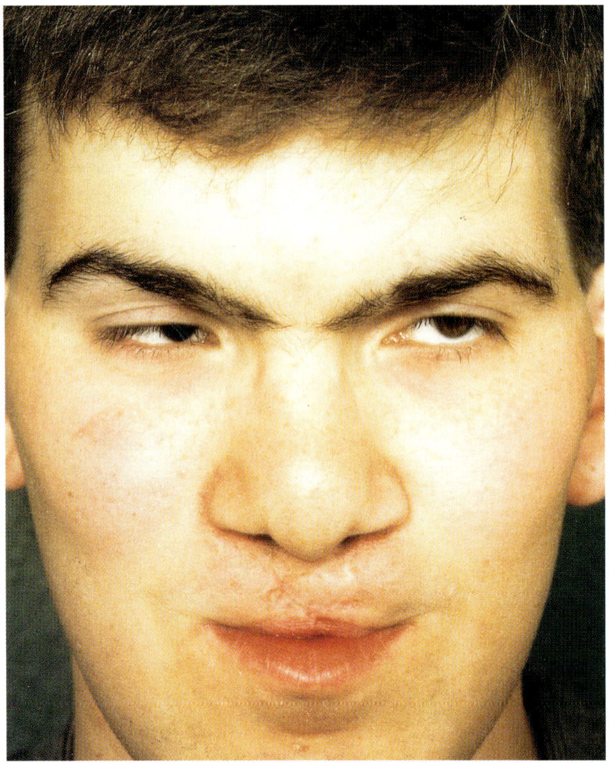

Figure 3.160a Severe pseudoprogenia after resection of the premaxilla after a LJP cleft.

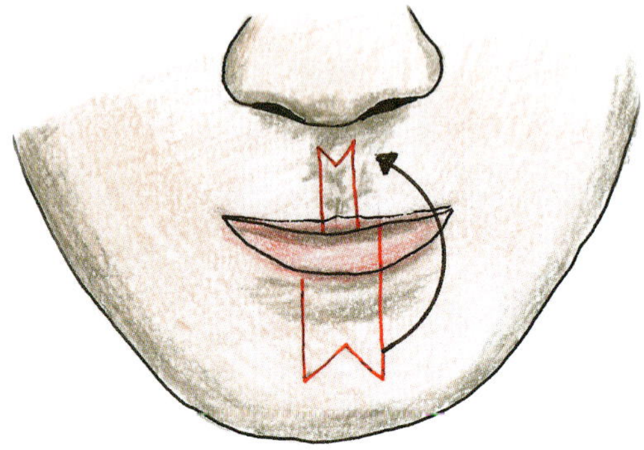

Figure 3.160b Planning of the Abbe plasty. A piece from the lower lip approximately 2 cm wide is mobilized by a W-incision and pediculated on the right lower lip artery.

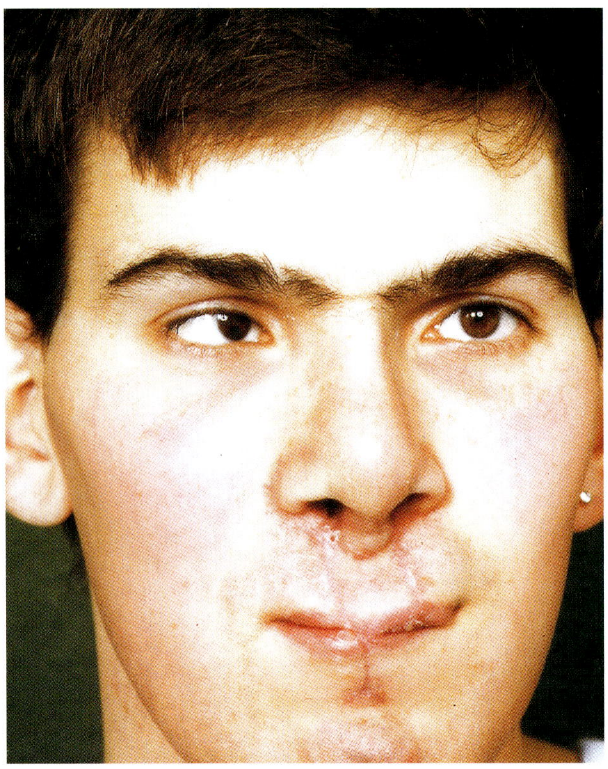

Figure 3.160c The arterial pedicle remains intact for two weeks. Then the lips are severed and modelled.

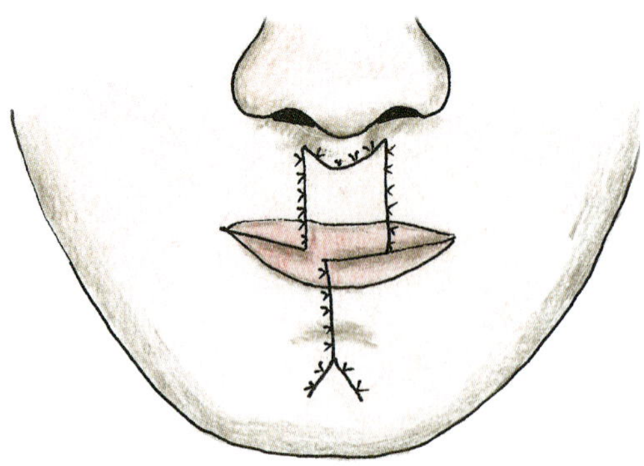

Figure 3.160d A part of the scarred tissue at the upper lip is resected and the Abbe plasty is carried out.

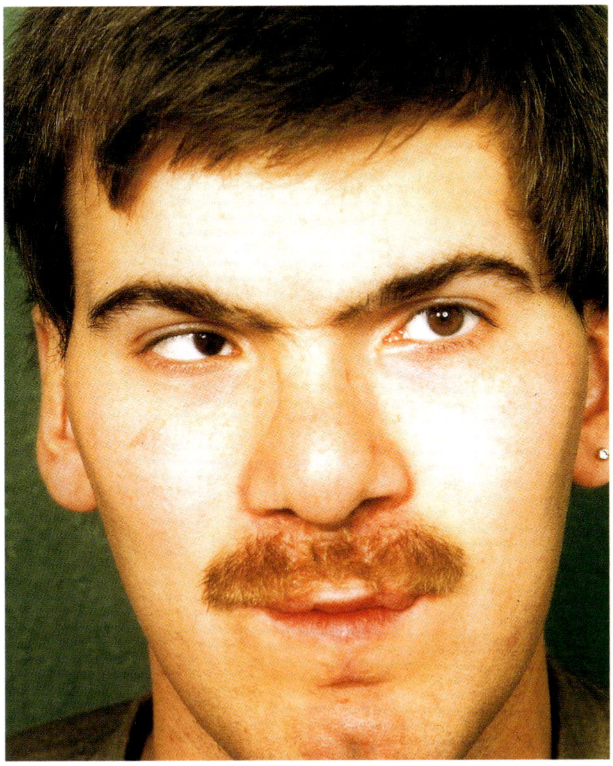

Figure 3.160e Status one year after the operation

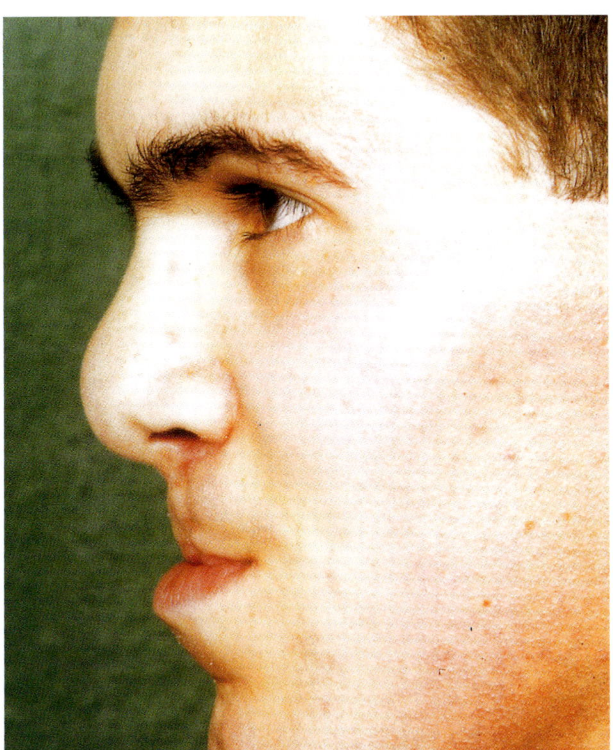

Figure 3.160f Profile before the operation

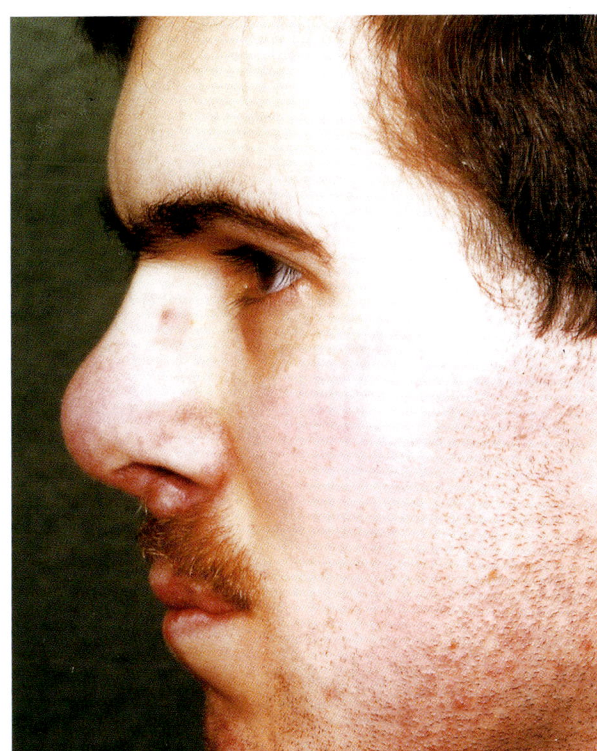

Figure 3.160g Profile after the operation. The nose was simultaneously corrected.

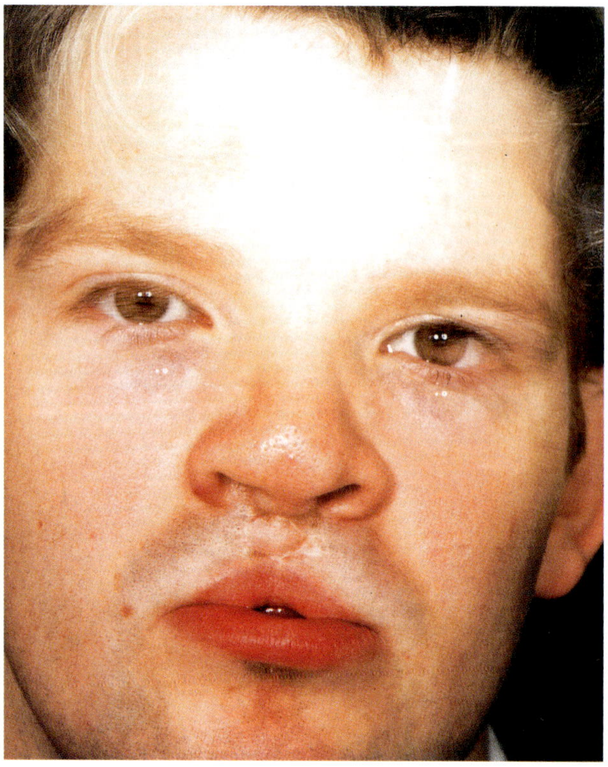

Figure 3.161a Abbe plasty: Status after bilateral cleft lip, jaw and palate. Pseudoprogenia.

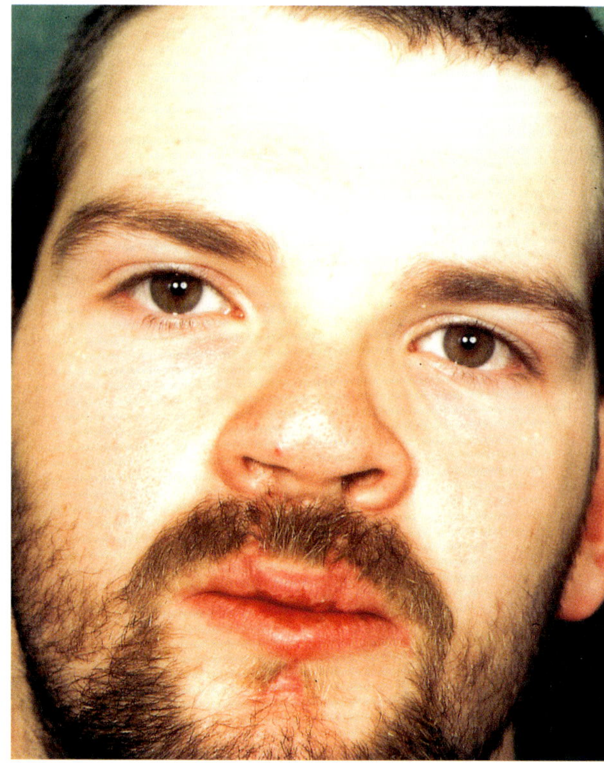

Figure 3.161b Status one year after the Abbe plasty: One can clearly see how severely (2 cm) the cupid's bow on the upper lip has been corrected.

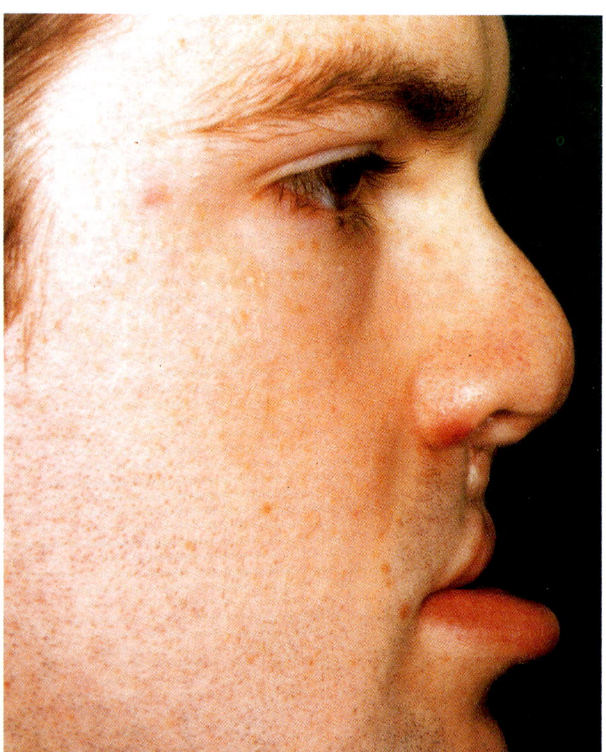

Figure 3.161c Status before the operation. An Abbe plasty with a W-shaped incision line was carried out.

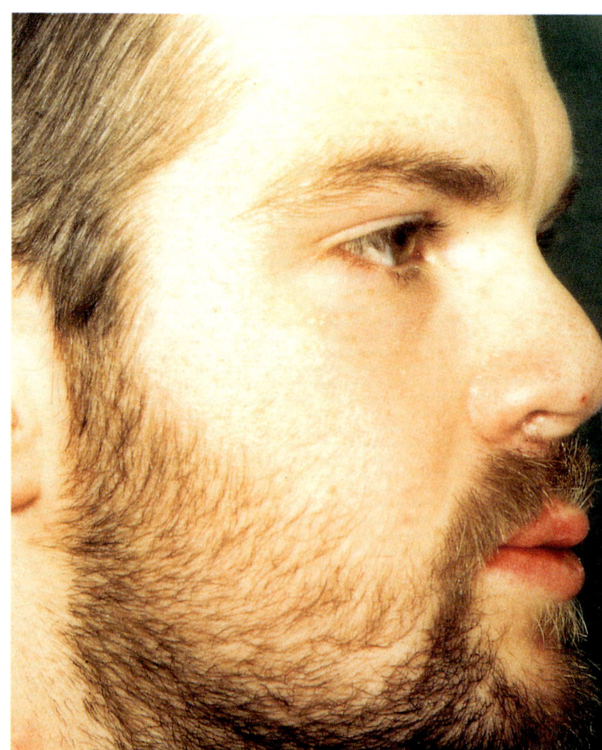

Figure 3.161d Status one year after the operation

Velopharyngeal Insufficiency

Speech problems arising from the inability to join the soft palate with the pharyngeal wall are designated as velopharyngeal insufficiency.

Velopharyngeal closure normally arises from the activity of the muscle loop of the levator veli palatini muscle that pulls the soft palate posterior-cranially in the direction of the pharyngeal wall.

In cleft patients the excessively short, and also scarred soft palate as well as the muscle dislocation are responsible for the insufficiency. Usually an imprecisely implemented operation in the palate area or a marked deformity are responsible for this. The levator and tensor veli palatini muscles are not completely separated from the hard palate and joined in the middle at the sphincter.

An open rhinolalia as well as nasal speech (hypernasality) were found in 31 % [Lindsay 1962] and 23 % [McEvitt 1971] of individuals.

One acquires the best speech results using a bridge flap when a proper joining of the levator veli palatini muscles is achieved [Koberg 1971].

Niermann in 1985 did not find a velopharyngeal insufficiency in any of the followed up cleft palate patients who were operated on with bridge flaps. The 5 % speech disorders amongst the patients were caused by articulation problems and not simply by a velopharyngeal insufficiency.

The best functional result after closure of the cleft palate is achieved if the levator veli palatini muscle is released from the hard palate and united to become an effective loop. Scarring should be decreased by an atraumatic technique in the velum area.

The surgical procedure with velopharygeal insufficiency:

1) Reoperation of the palate, release of the muscle periostium from the rear edge of the hard palate, precise joining of the musculature in the middle.
2) One can achieve here an extension of the palate by about 1 to 1.5 cm by employing a Z-plasty.
3) With an excessively short, scarred and immobile palate a pharyngoplasty should be applied for improving speech.
   The cranially pediculated velopharyngoplasty has clear benefits:
   a) The traction occurs in a dorso-cranial direction
   b) The flap can be selected to be very long

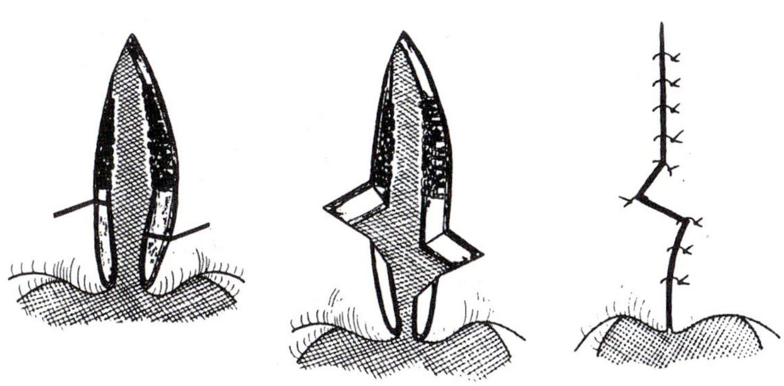

Figure 3.162a Palate extension by a Z-shaped incision

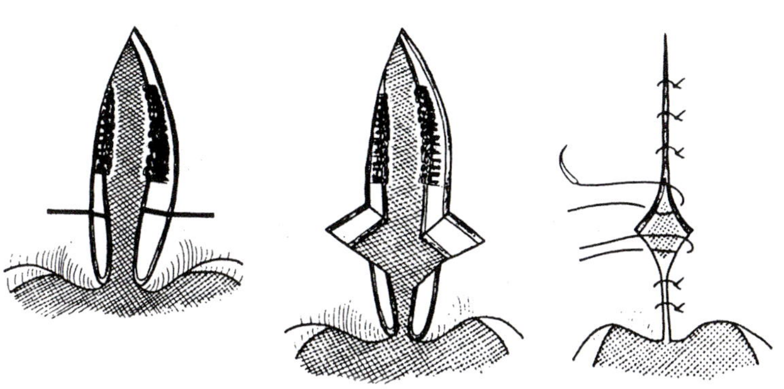

Figure 3.162b Palate extension by a transverse incision (Niermann 1985)

Pharyngoplasty

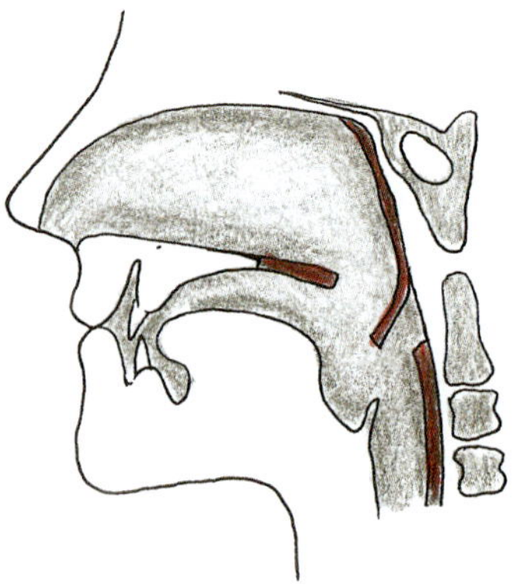

Figure 3.163a A velopharyngeal insufficiency arises with an excessively short soft palate.

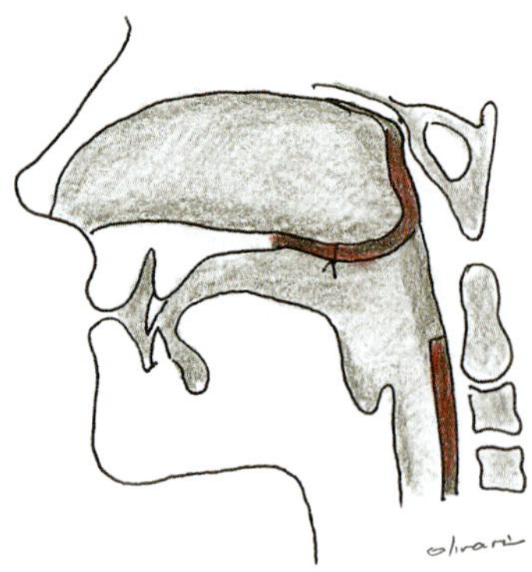

Figure 3.163b A velopharyngoplasty is formed with the cranially pediculated pharyngeal flap.

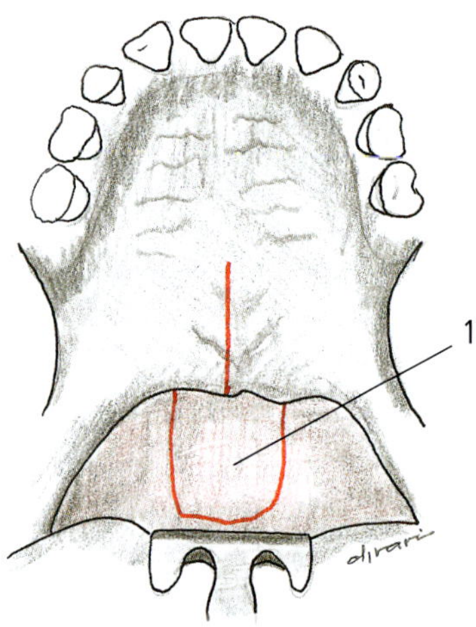

Figure 3.163c Planning of a cranially pediculated pharyngeal flap (1).

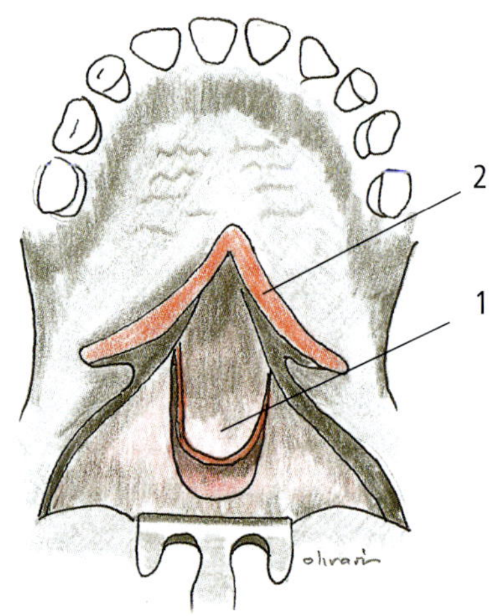

Figure 3.163d The pharyngeal flap is mobilized (1), the soft palate is split (2).

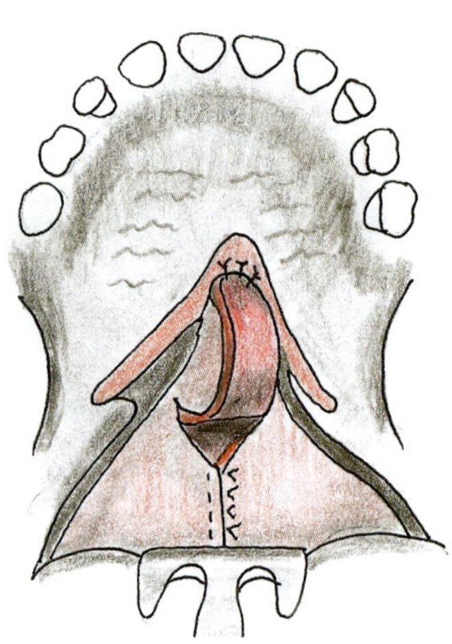

Figure 3.163e The pharyngeal flap is mobilized ventrally and sutured with the nasal layer of the soft palate (3). On both sides the airways remain preserved with a diameter of 1.2 to 1.8 cm.

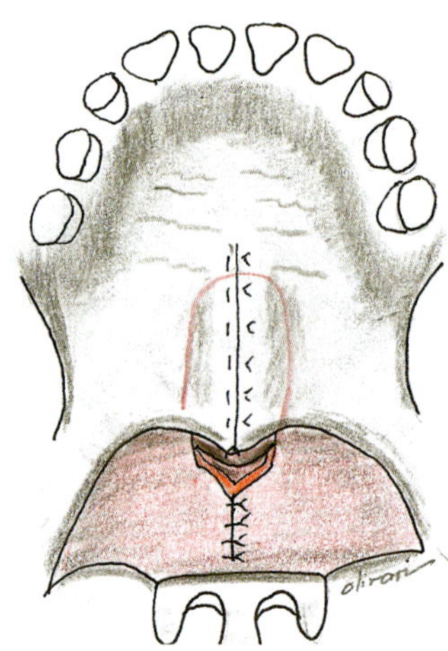

Figure 3.163f Status at the end of the operation

Defects of the Upper Lip

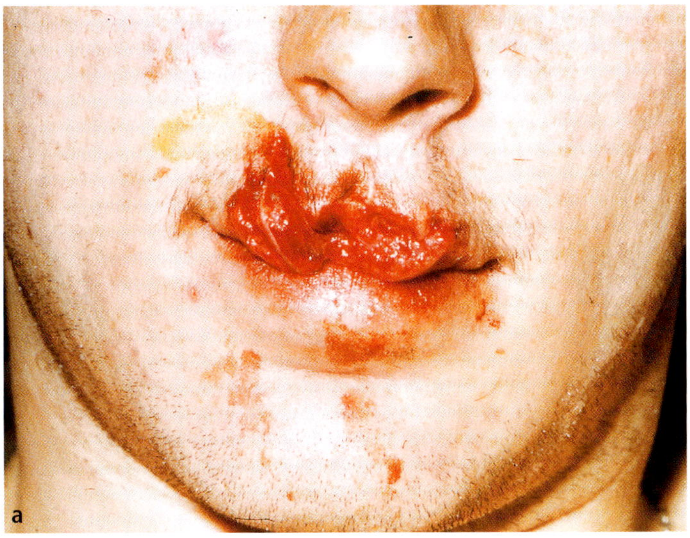

Figure 3.164a Defect at the upper lip after a dog bite. A part of the mucosa of the lip is missing as well. The skin shows several irregular small defects. Treatment: 1) Washing of the wound with medical soap, 2) disinfection with Betaisodona or other disinfectant, 3) local administration of antibiotics (e.g. Neomycin).
Every little piece of skin is used for reconstructing the upper lip. The old rule (in older textbooks), that dog bite wounds may not be closed primarily, is no longer applicable. Dog bite wounds should be primarily closed and no larger excisions should be carried out except devitalized tissue.

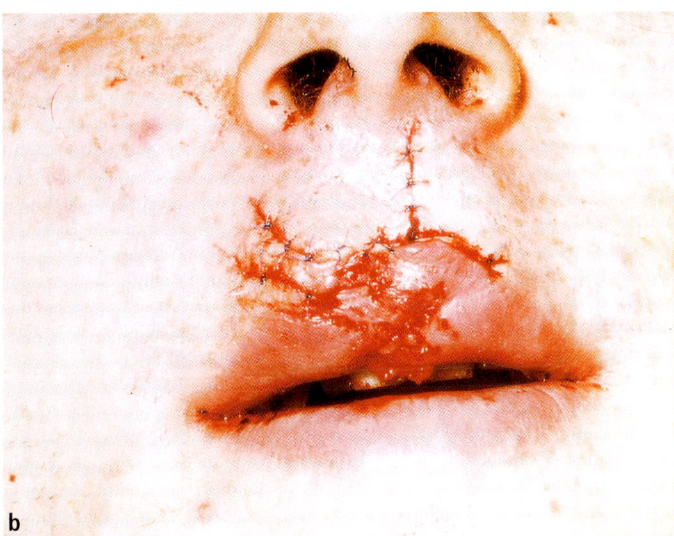

Figure 3.164b Adaptation of the skin of the upper lip with 6×0 nylon and defect of the mucosa of the lip is closed by a mucosa local flap from the oral cavity.

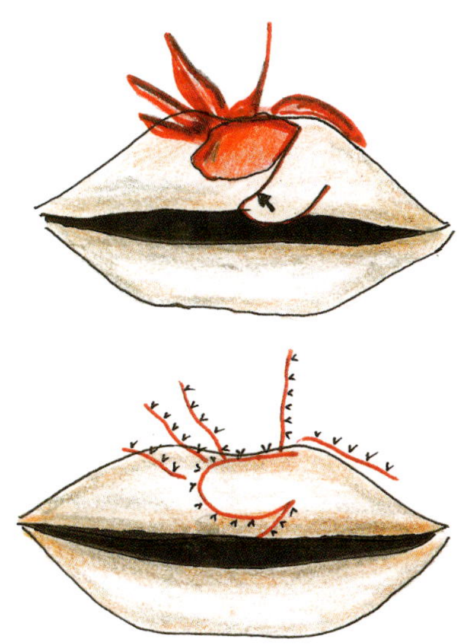

Figure 3.164c A local mucous flap is used to cover the defect.

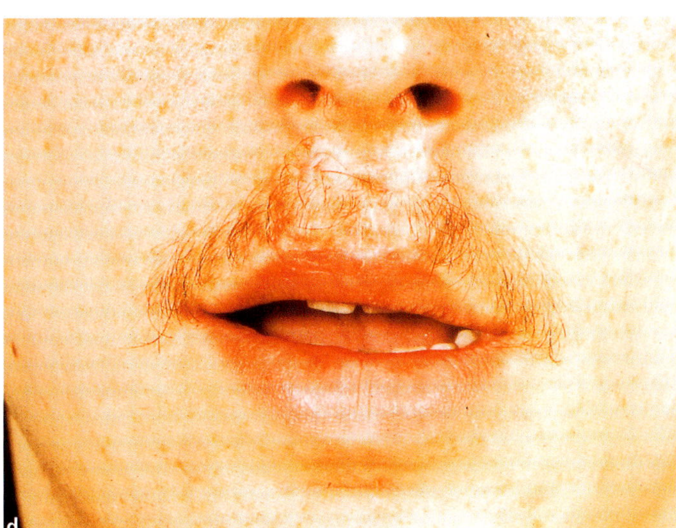

Figure 3.164d Status 20 months after the operation

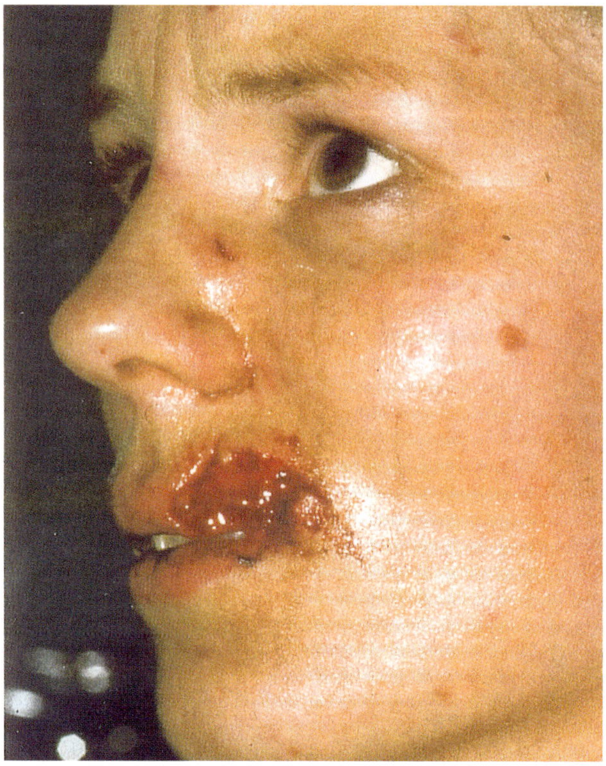

Figure 3.165a Defect at the upper lip on the left after a dog bite

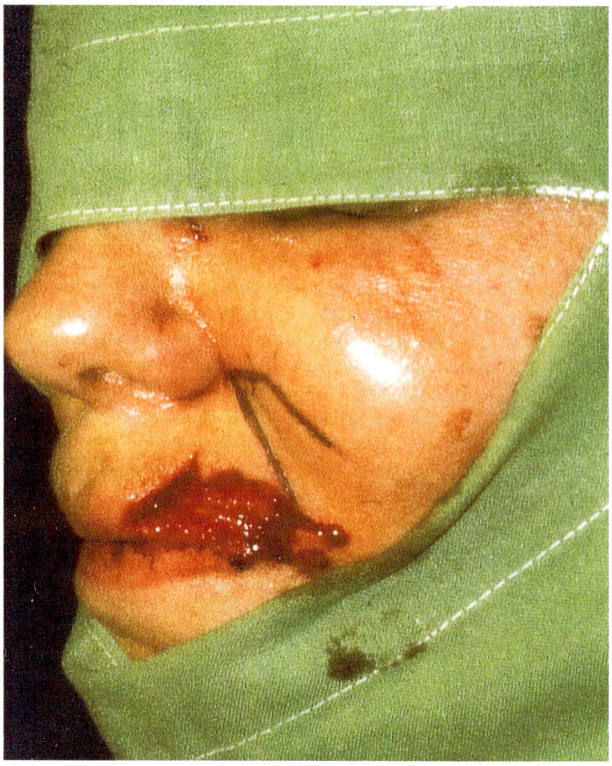

Figure 3.165b A caudal pedicle flap from the nasolabial fold is planned.

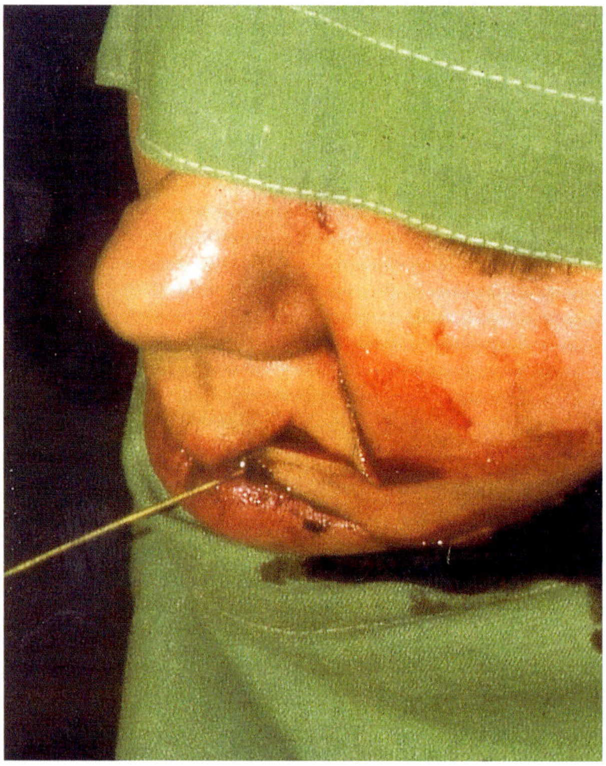

Figure 3.165c Mobilization of the flap and turning into the defect

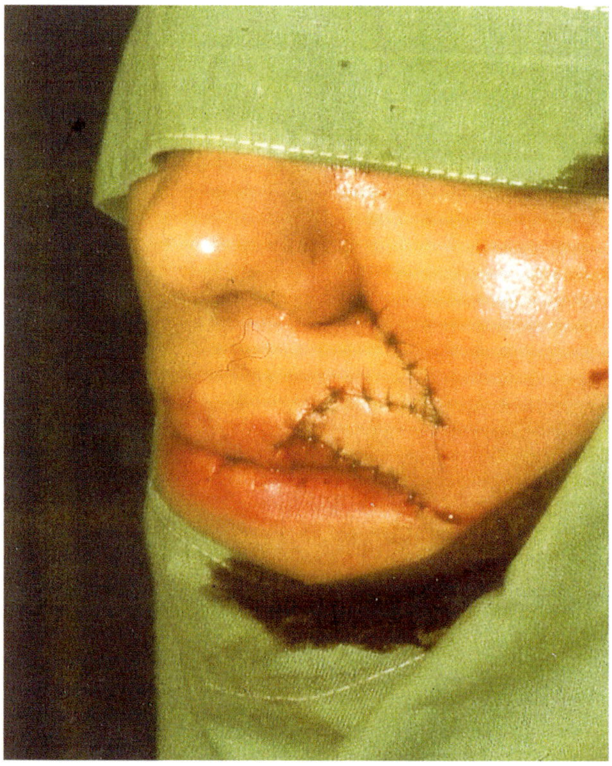

Figure 3.165d Situation at the end of the operation

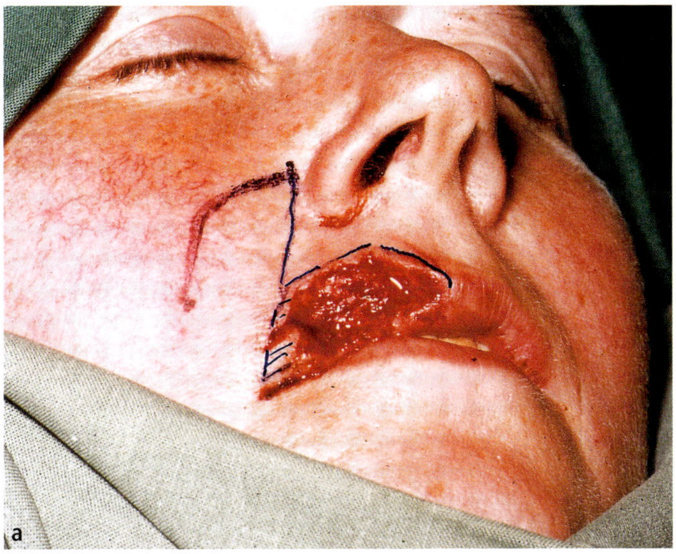

a

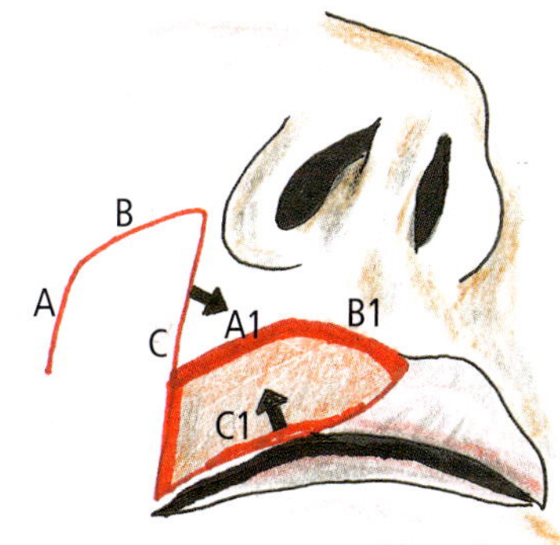

b

Figure 3.166a Defect at the upper lip after a dog bite. The skin as well as a part of the mucosa of the lip are missing. As always at dog bite the wound is washed first, disinfected (Betaisodona or similar) and treated locally with antibiotics (e.g. Neomycin). A minimal excision was carried out for regarding of the wound edges. At the same time the mucosa of the lip was mobilized from the mouth cavity and pulled cranially.

Figure 3.166b The flap for defect coverage is formed from the nasolabial fold and measured precisely: Length A must correspond exactly to length A1, length B exactly to length B1, and length C exactly to length C1.

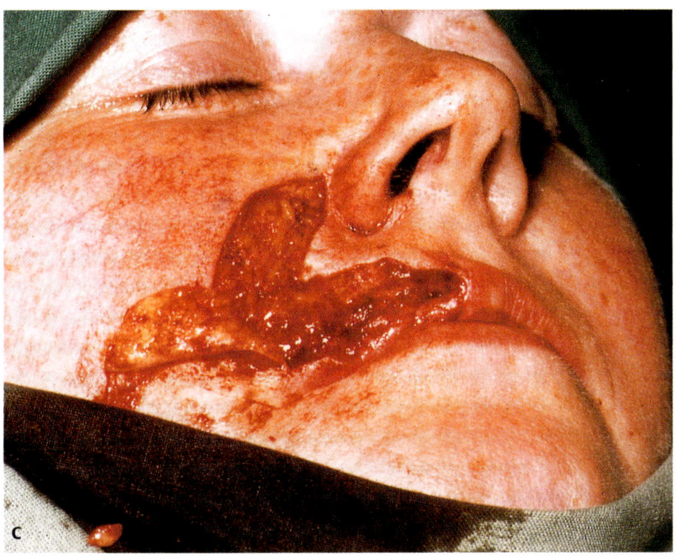

c

Figure 3.166c The flap is mobilized

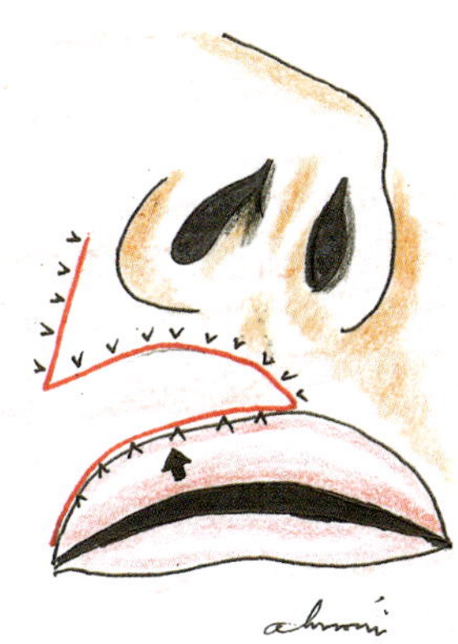

d

Figure 3.166d Secondary defect is closed primarily

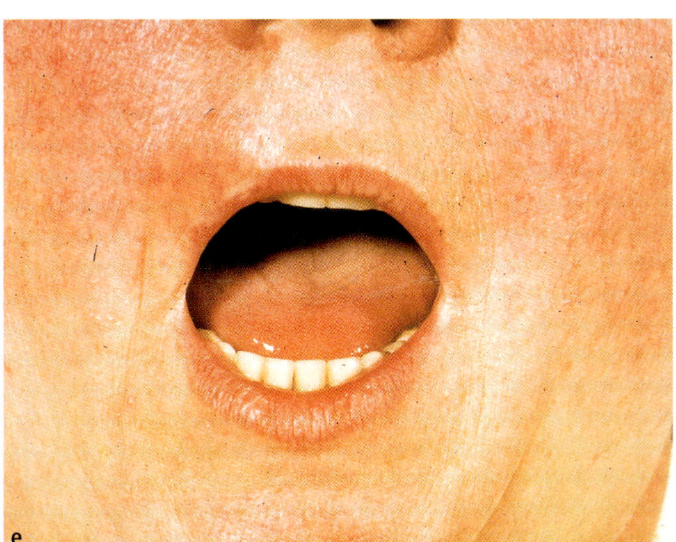

e

Figure 3.166e Functional result one year after the operation

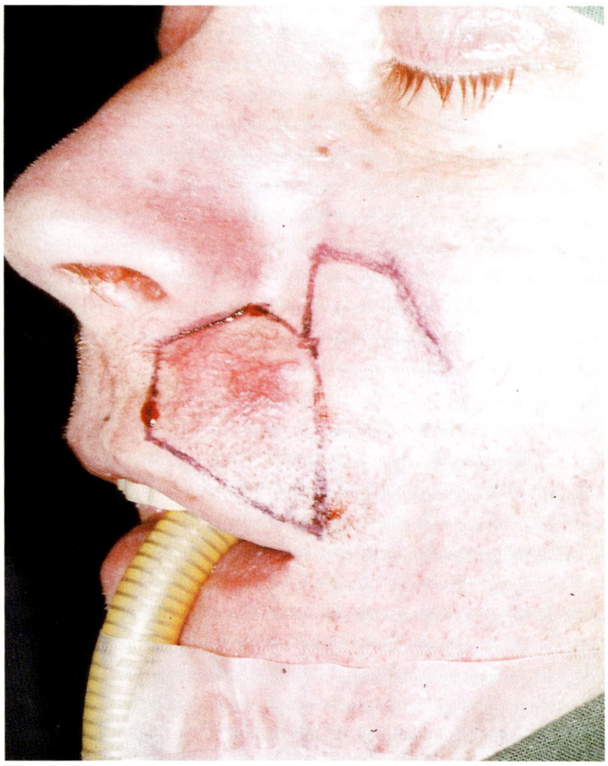

Figure 3.167a Tumor at the upper lip on the left side. Planning of the extirpation and the reconstruction.

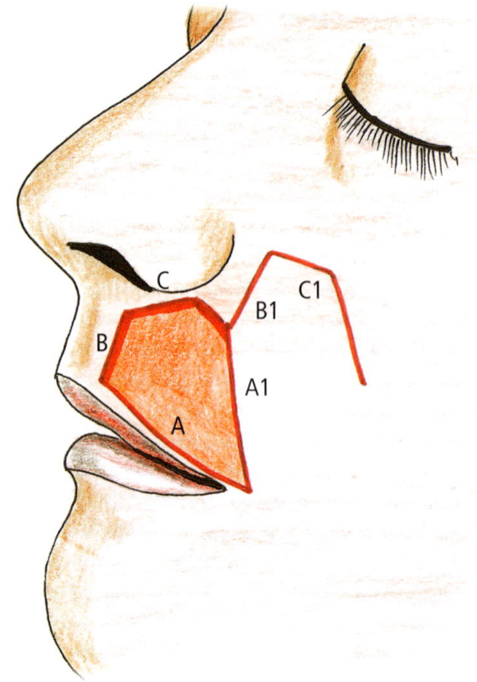

Figure 3.167b In order to cover the defect after an excision, a precisely calculated caudal pediceld flap is formed from the nasolabial fold. Length A must correspond exactly to length A1, length B exactly to length B1, and length C exactly to length C1. This is very important in order to avoid later deformations of the upper lip.

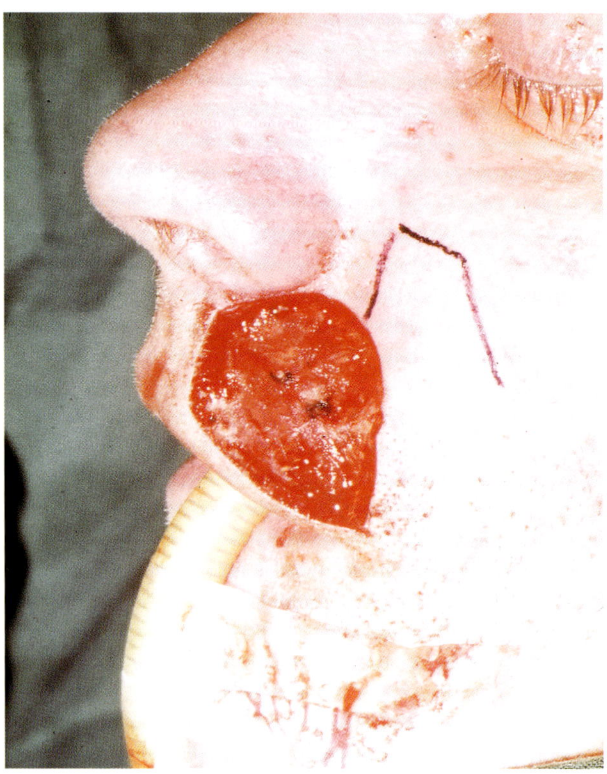

Figure 3.167c After the excision the defect enlarges due to skin elasticity. Thus the flap must be planned before the excision is done.

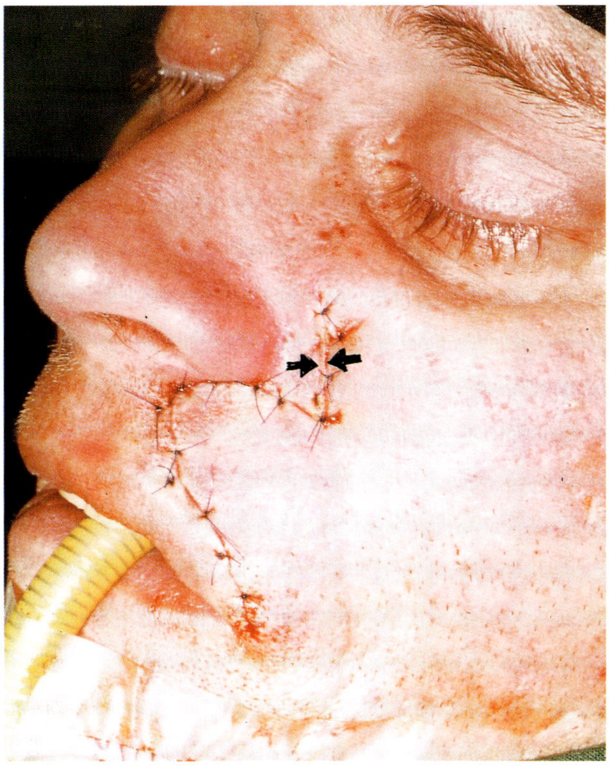

Figure 3.167d End of the operation

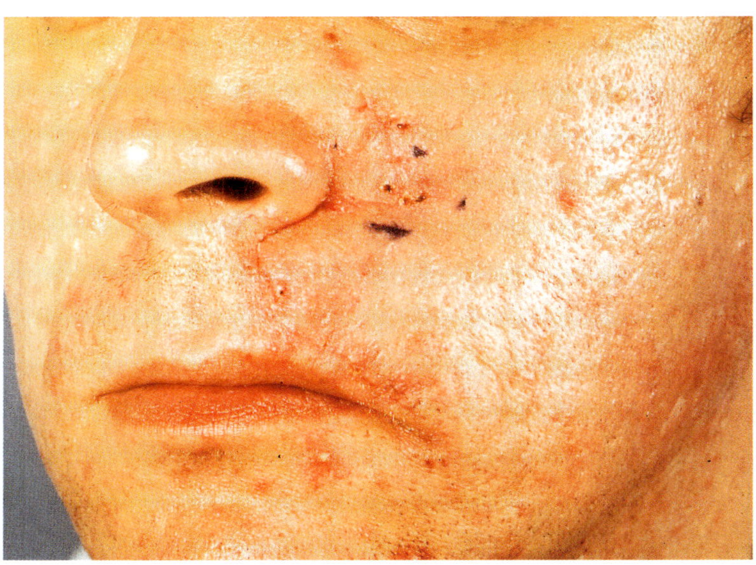

Figure 3.167e Aspect four weeks after the operation. No deformation of the upper lip.

Defect Coverage at the Lower Lip According to Burow

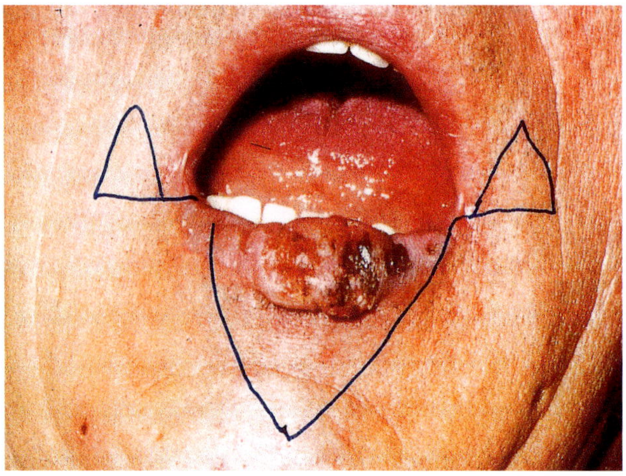

Figure 3.168a Squamous-cell carcinoma of the lower lip

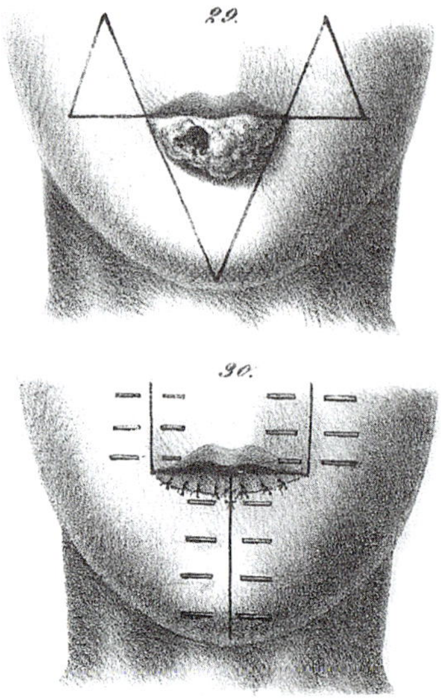

Figure 3.168d Burow's method. Originally illustration from the "Surgical atlas" of Victor Bruns (1857)

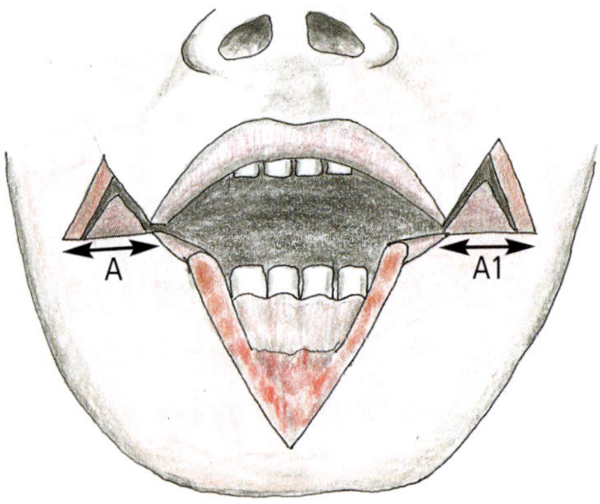

Figure 3.168b Scheme of the Burow's triangular excision.
The lower lip is extended by the length of A +A1.
Do not excise the mucosa!

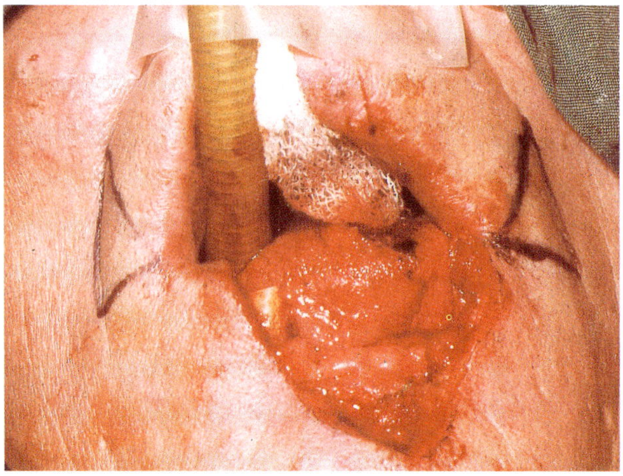

Figure 3.168c 80 % of the lower have been resected.
The excision is made in a V-shaped form. In order to close the very large defect, two Burow's triangles are excised laterally at the upper lip. The excision of the triangles occurs up to the mucous membrane. The mucosa is left as a caudally pedicular mucosa flap.

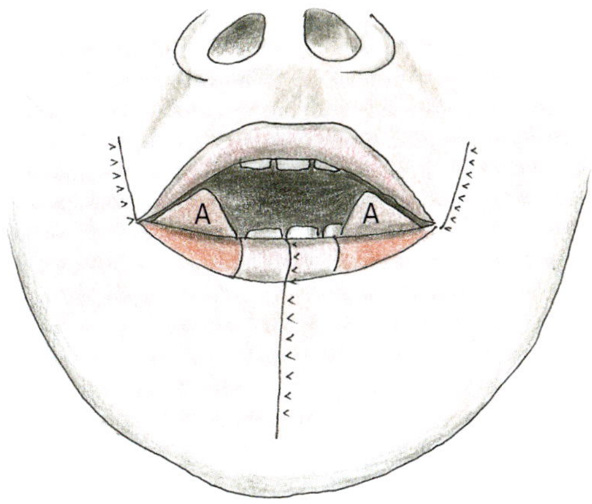

Figure 3.168e After excision of the Burow's triangle up to the mucosa, the lower lip is reconstructed. The remaining mucosal triangles are used for the reconstruction of mucosa of the lower lip (A).

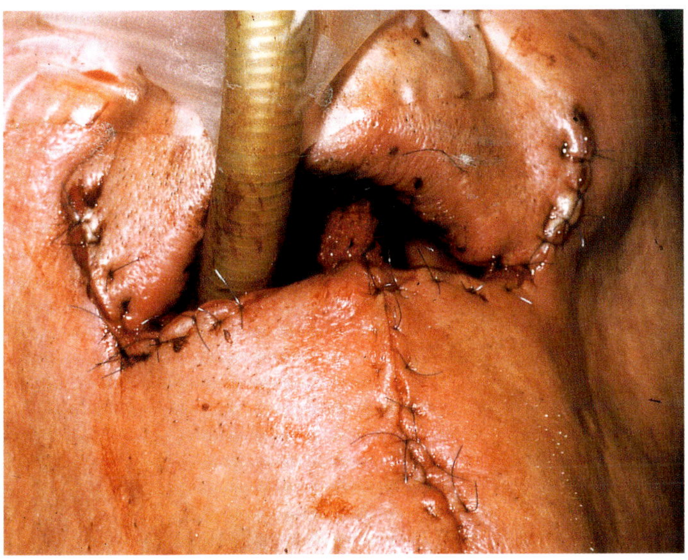

Figure 3.168f Situation at the end of the operation. The lower lip is reconstructed. In the lateral parts the mucosa from the Burow's triangle was used.

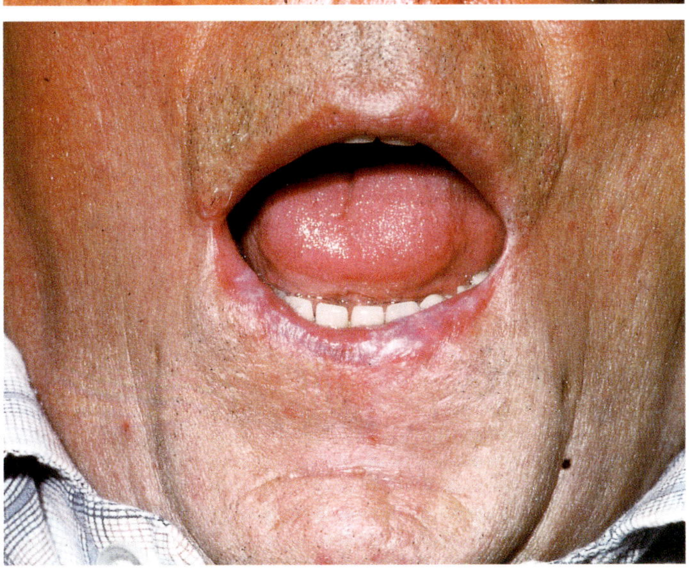

Figure 3.168g Status one year after the operation

Lower Lip Reconstruction According to Karapandzic

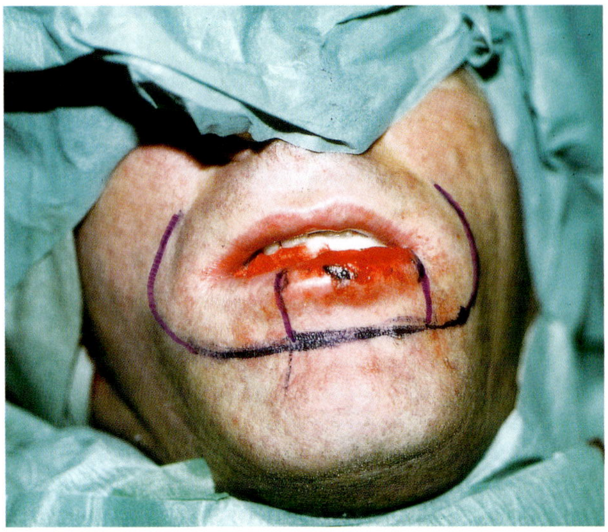

Figure 3.169a Carcinoma of the lower lip. Planning of the reconstruction with the Karapandzic method. This method is suitable for covering greater defects at the lower lip.

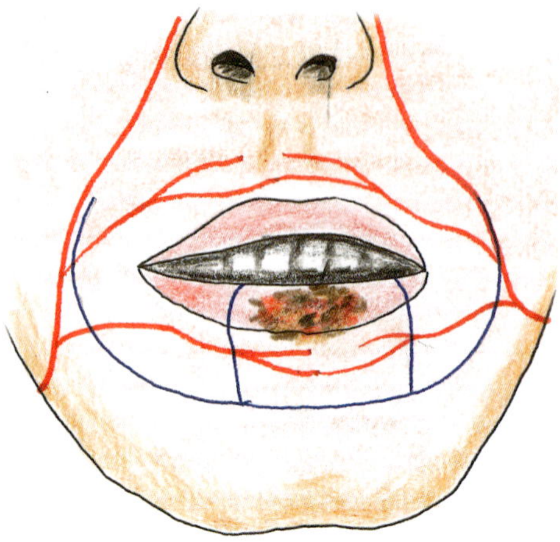

Figure 3.169b In reality these are two myocutaneous flaps, that are rotated mediocaudally. The vessel-nerve bundle is preserved.

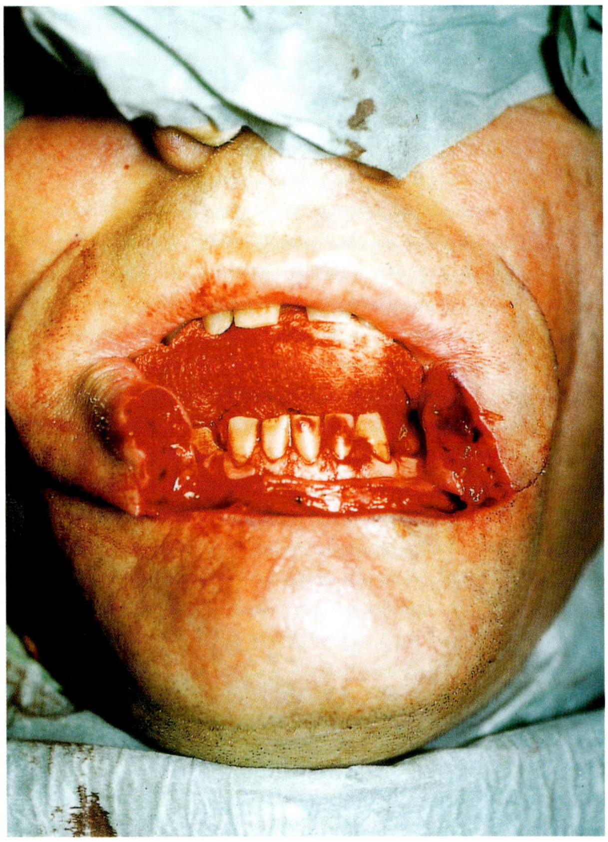

Figure 3.169c Situation after resection of tumor

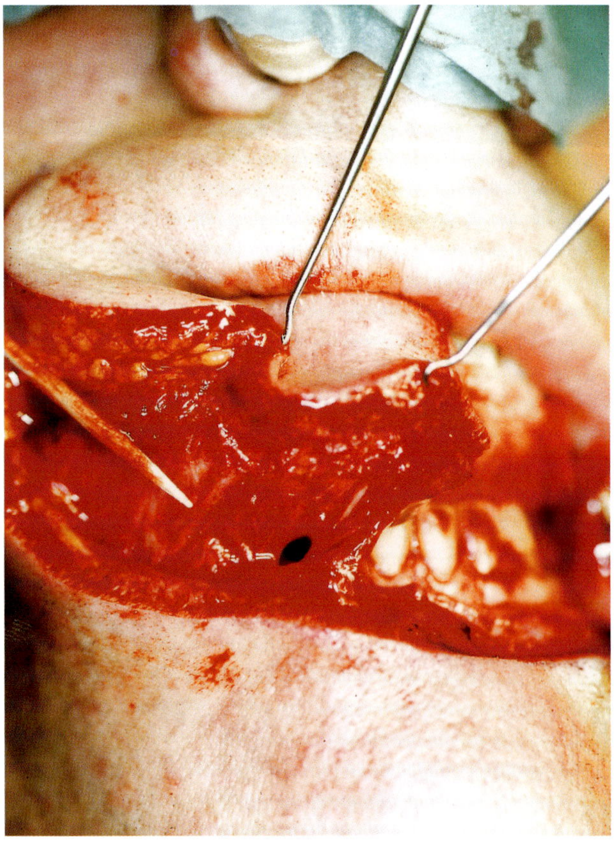

Figure 3.169d The vessel-nerve bundle is preserved. The inferior labial artery is identified.

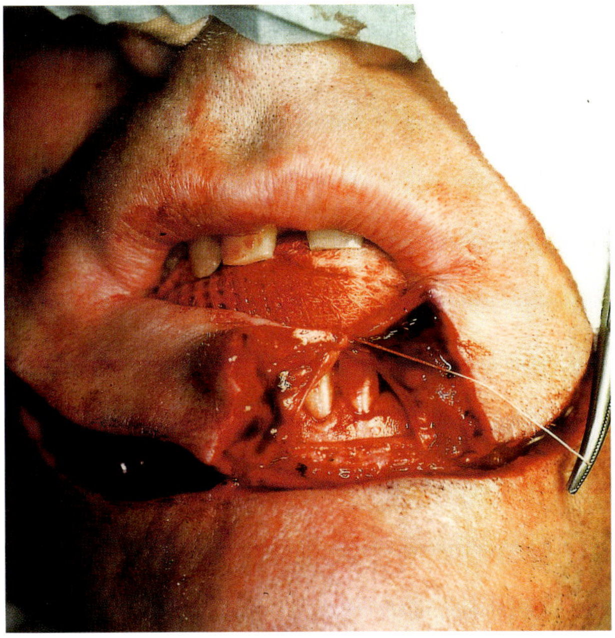

Figure 3.169e Rotation of the flaps

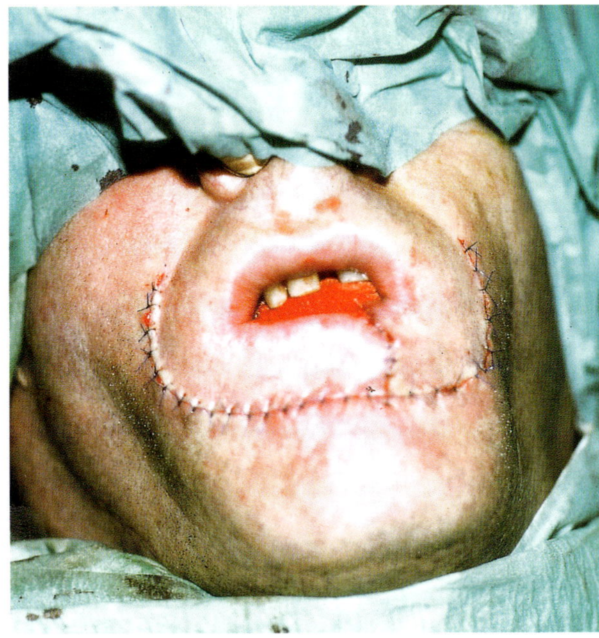

Figure 3.169f Picture at the end of the operation. The blood supply and the muscle function is preserved (sphincter). Sometimes a microstoma arises that should be corrected secondarily.

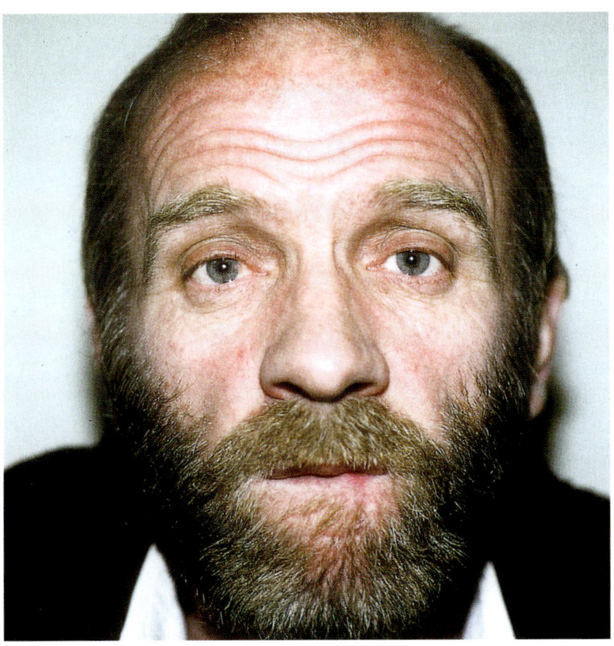

Figure 3.169g Picture one year after the operation

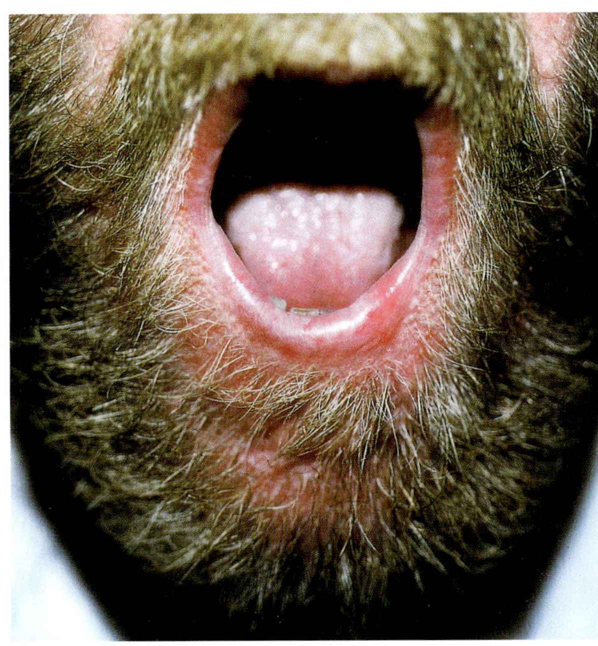

Figure 3.169h Functional result

Lower Lip Reconstruction According to Olivari

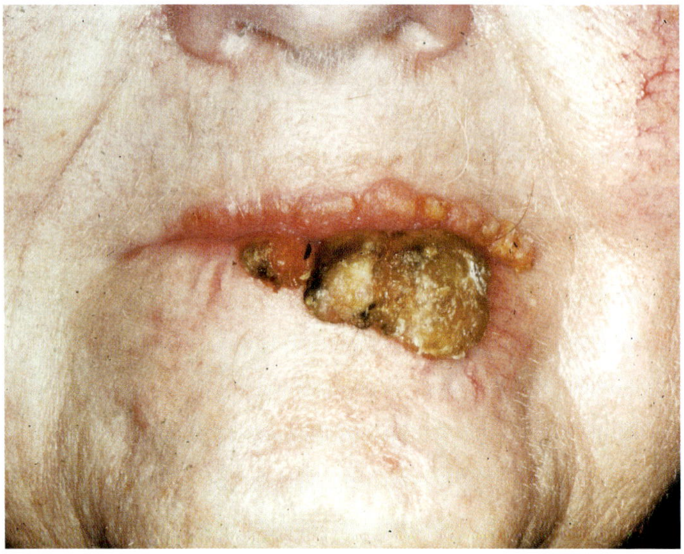

Figure 3.170a Lower lip carcinoma

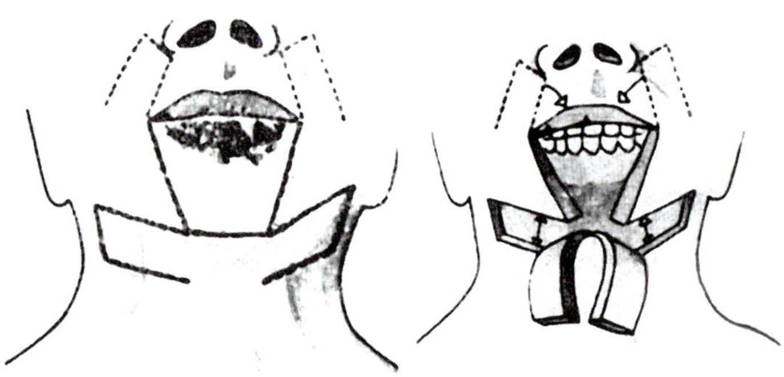

Figure 3.170b Planning of the operation: Tapered excision of the lower lip. Formation of two medial pedicular flaps from the neck. The dashed lines show where the mucosal flaps are formed for the inner lining. Synchronous regional lymphnode removal (histological negative).

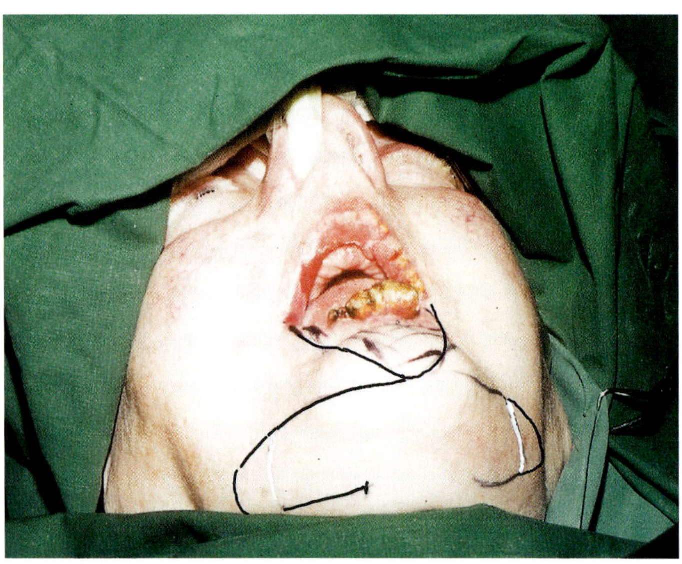

Figure 3.170c Intraoperative image. Two pedicular flaps from the submental area are used for skin reconstruction.

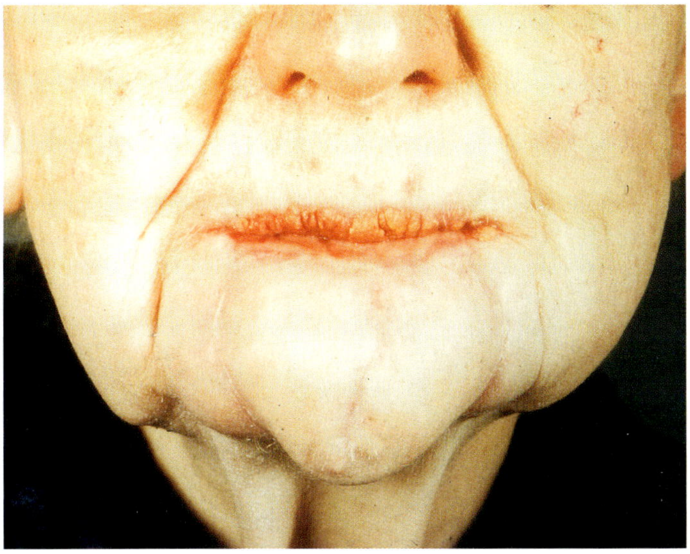

Figure 3.170d Status one year after the operation. The procedure functions only if mucosal flaps from the inner side of the nasolabial fold are used.

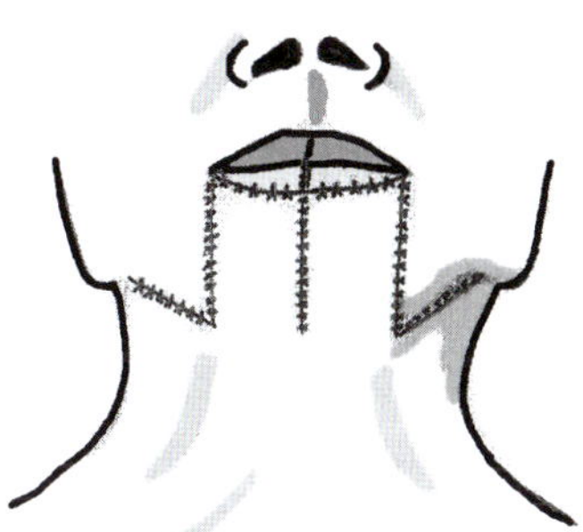

Figure 3.170e Secondary defect is closed primarily. Olivari, N. (1973) One stage reconstruction of the whole lower lip. Br J Plast Surg 26: 66

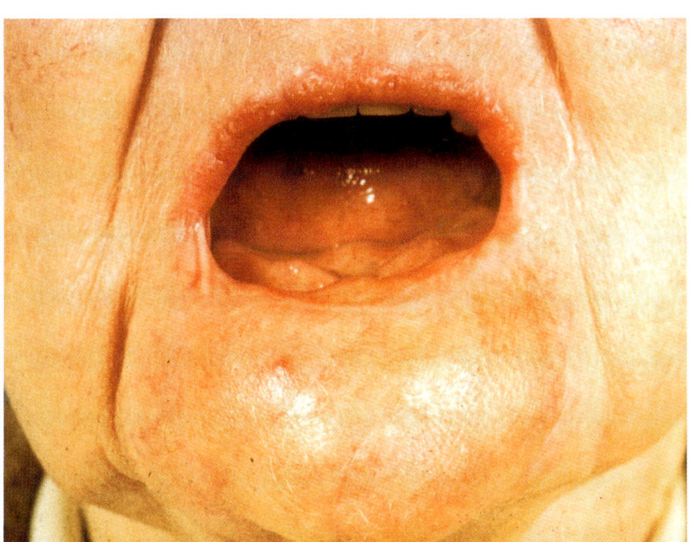

Figure 3.170f Functional result

Defect Coverage in the Face and Neck Area

Local Flaps – Blood Supply

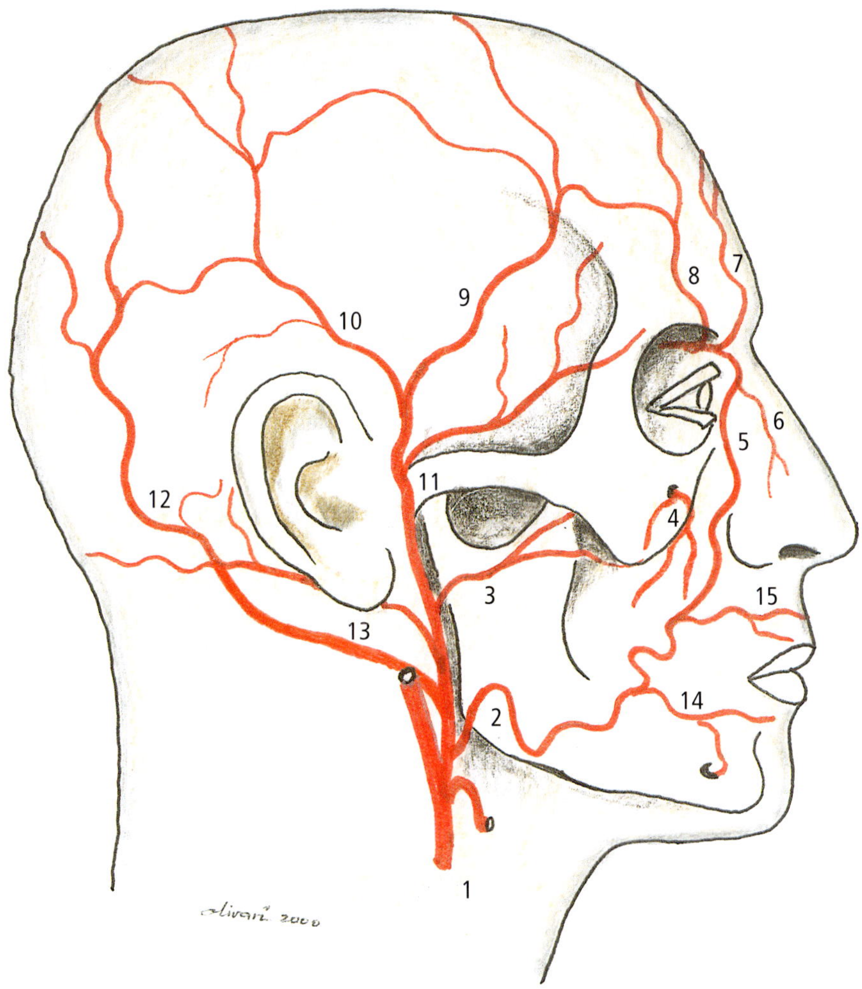

Figure 3.171 The superficial arteries
1. External carotid artery
2. Facial artery
3. Transverse facial artery (variable origin!)
4. Infraorbital artery
5. Angular artery
6. Dorsalis nasi artery
7. Supratrochlear artery
8. Supraorbital artery
9. Frontal branch of temporal superficial artery
10. Parietal branch of temporal superior artery
11. Superficial temporal artery
12. Occipital artery
13. Posterior auricular artery
14. Inferior labial artery
15. Superior labial artery

Rotation-Advancement Flap According to Schrudde

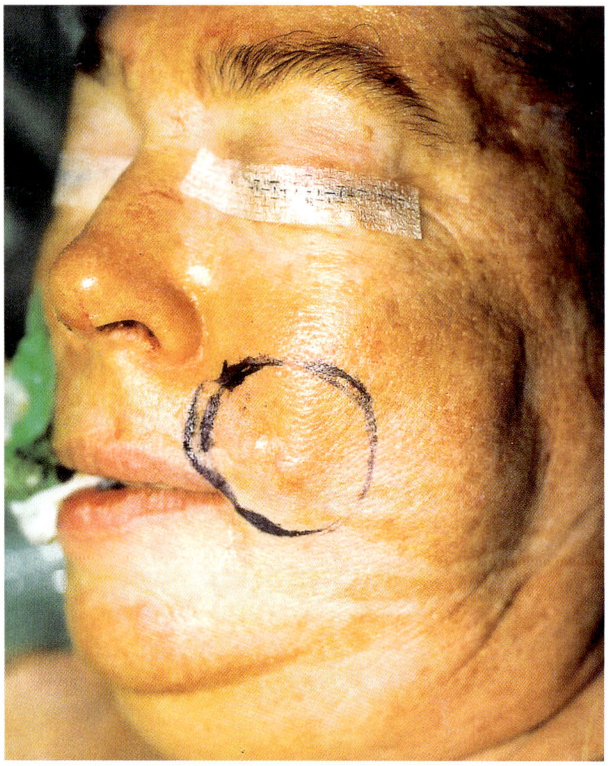

Figure 3.172a Metatypical basal cell carcinoma of the left cheek

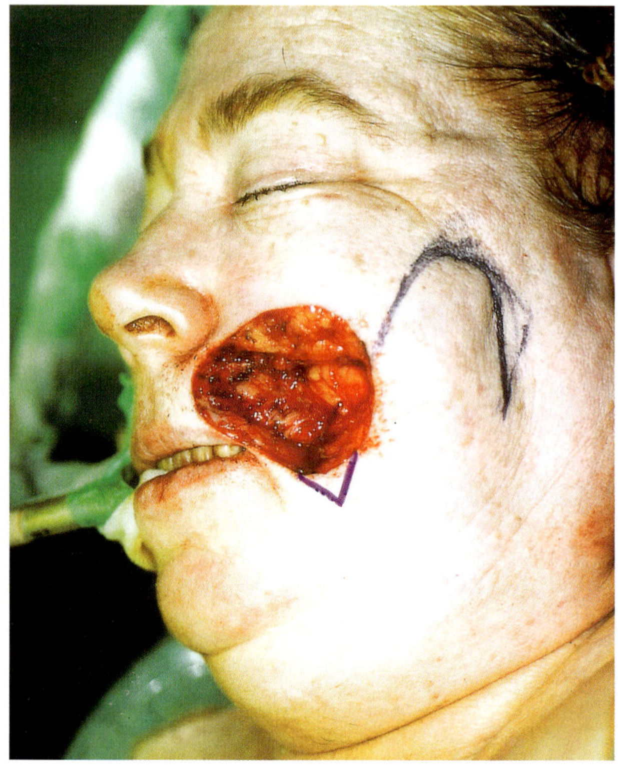

Figure 3.172b The tumor has infiltrated all layers. Planning of the local flap: The V-excision in caudal part (1). The flap is caudally pedicled and moved from the lateral part of the cheek. An additional excision of the caudal triangle prevents from a "dog ear".

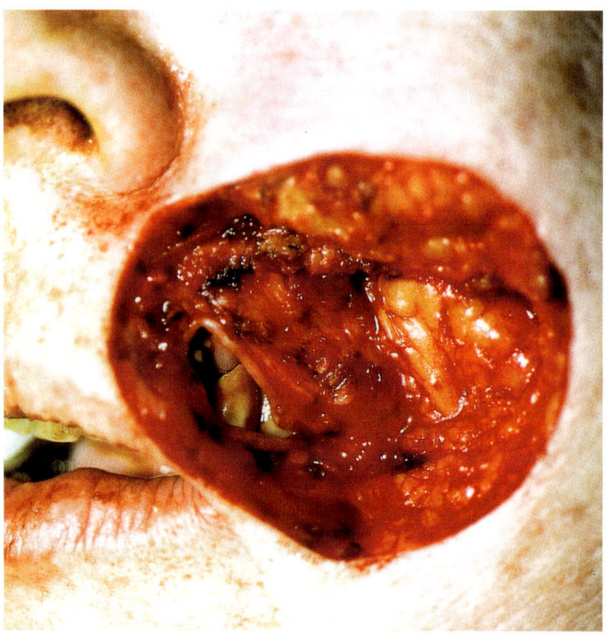

Figure 3.172c The tumor has infiltrated all layers. Also a part of the mucosa must be removed.

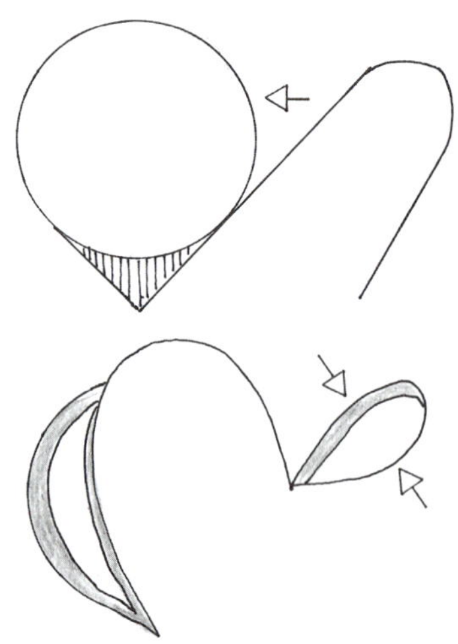

Figure 3.172d After the tumor excision the flap is fixed in the defect. Secondary defect closed primarily after mobilization. **Consider:** Only a transverse tension arises so that the lower eyelid remains in its normal position.

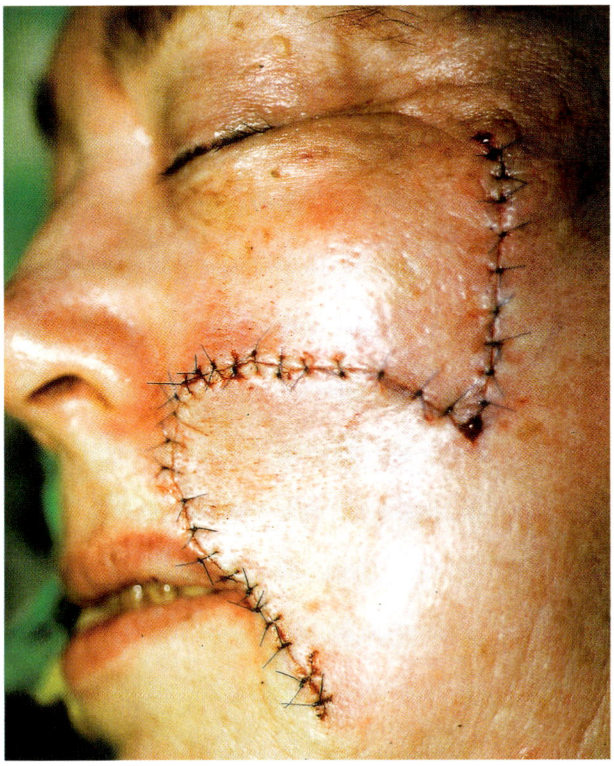

Figure 3.172e Picture taken at the end of the operation

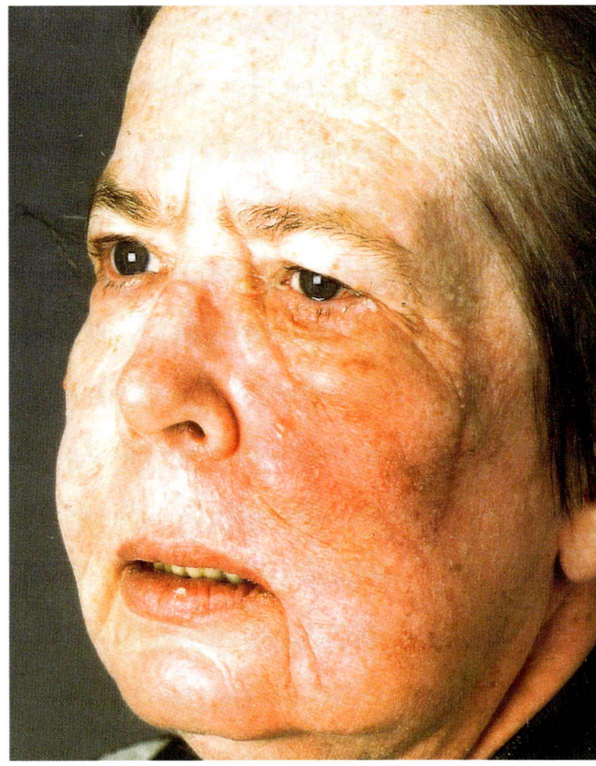

Figure 3.172f Aspect one year postoperatively

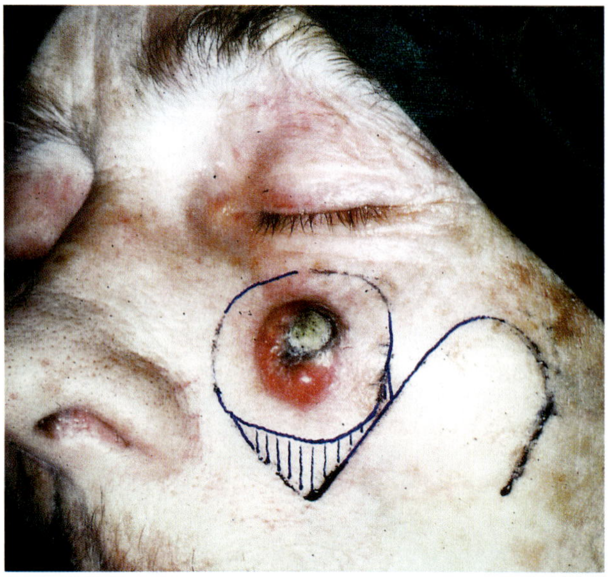

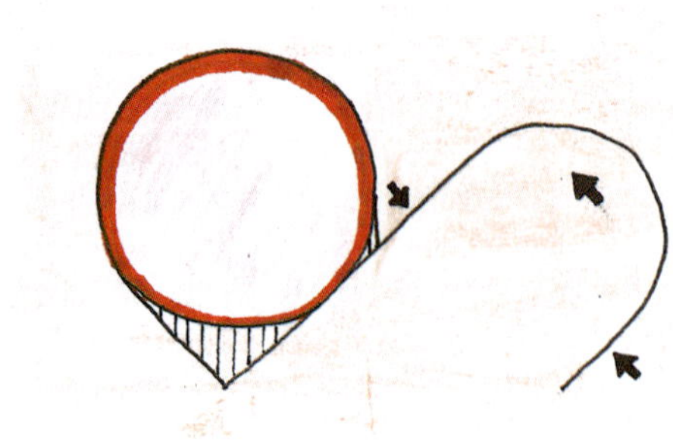

Figure 3.173a Basal cell carcinoma of the left cheek. Planning of the operation (cf. Figure 3.172b)

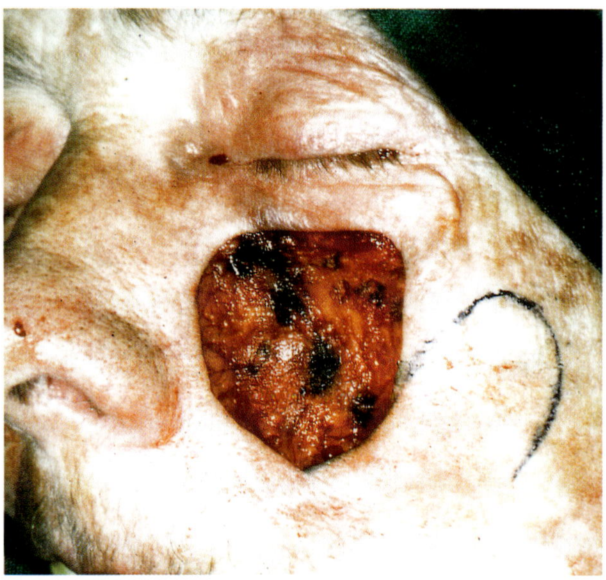

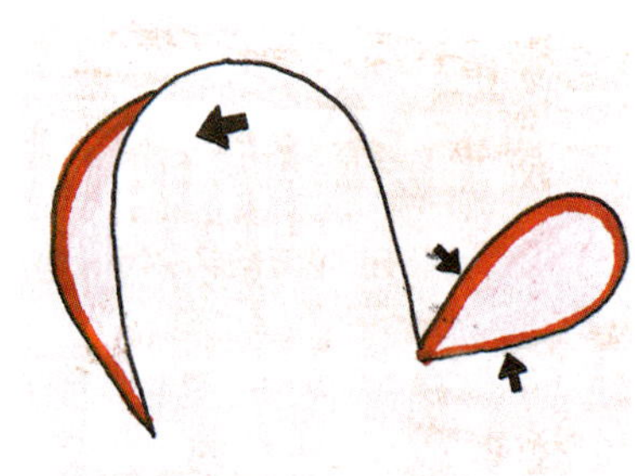

Figure 3.173b Situation after excision of the tumor with additional V-excision in the caudal part.

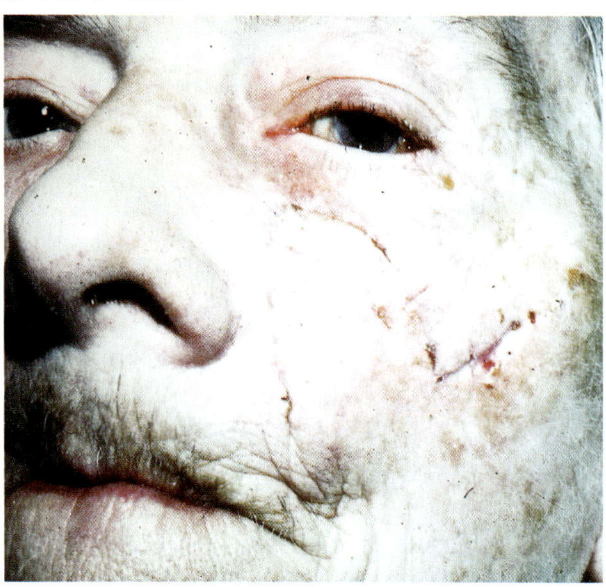

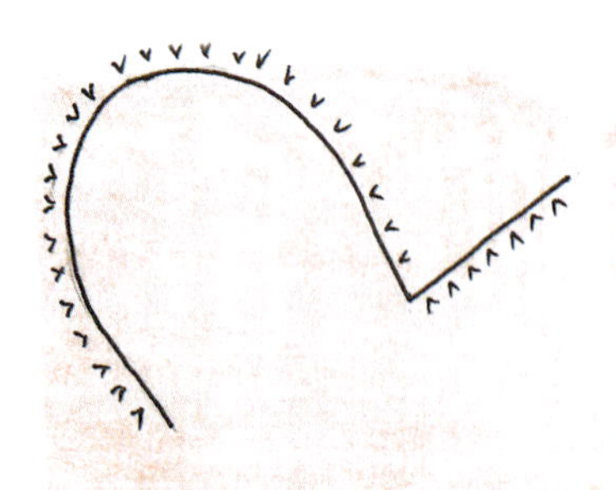

Figure 3.173c Secondary defect is closed primarily.

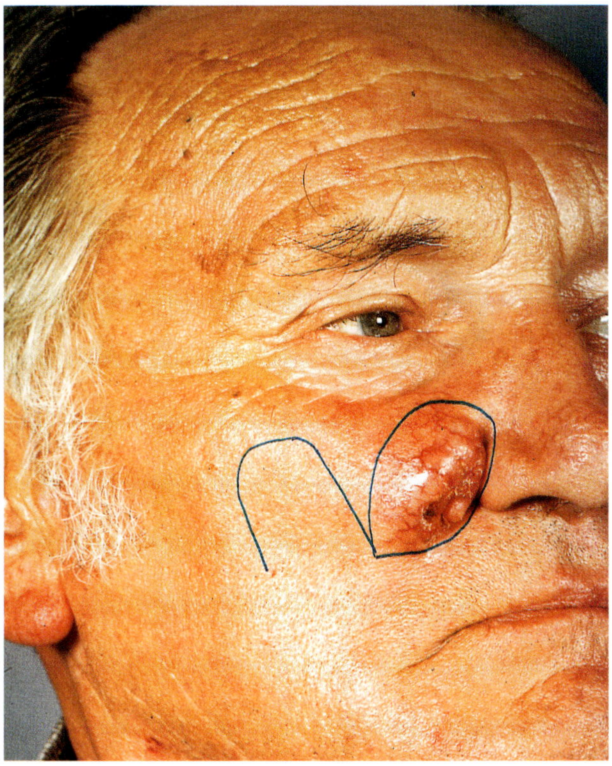

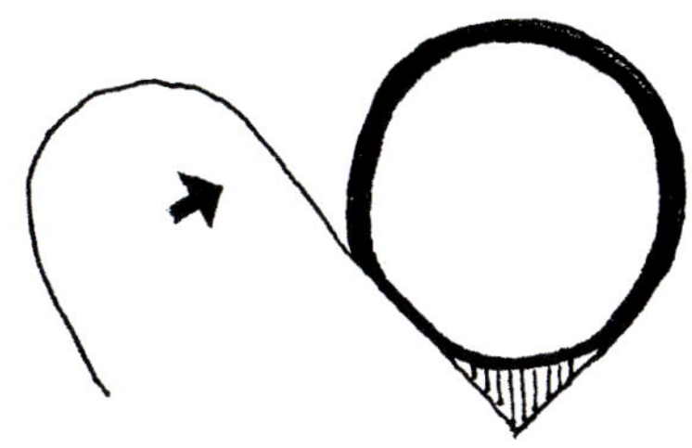

Figure 3.174a Chronically infected atheroma. In this case no incision is indicated, but excision.

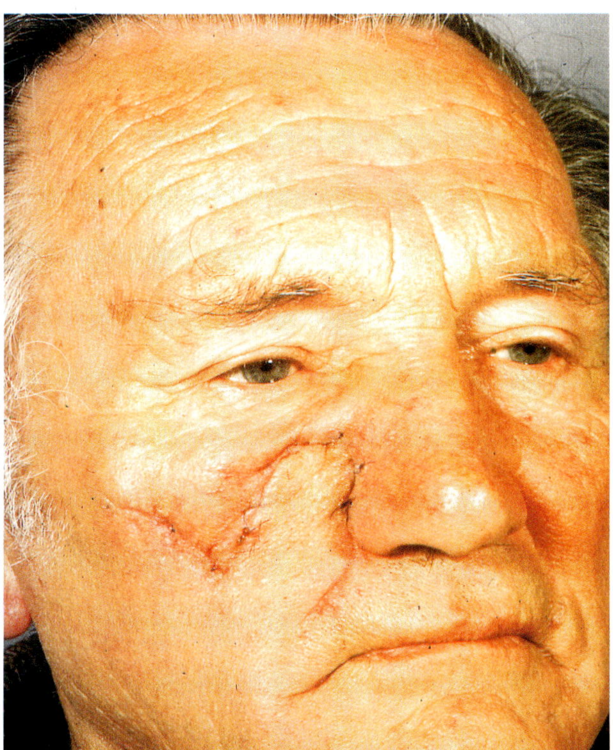

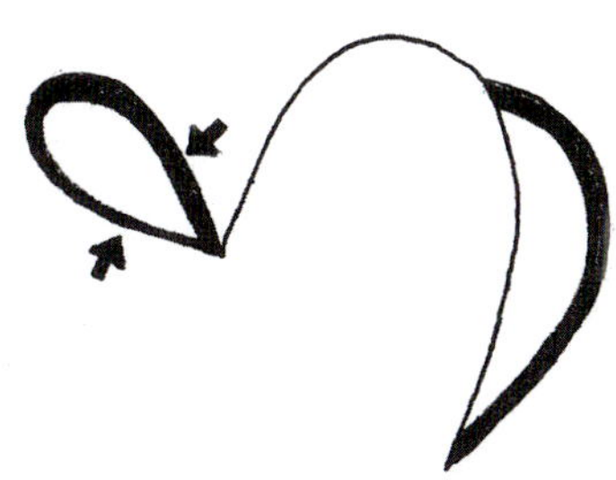

Figure 3.174b After excision coverage of the defect using a local flap

Transposition Flap

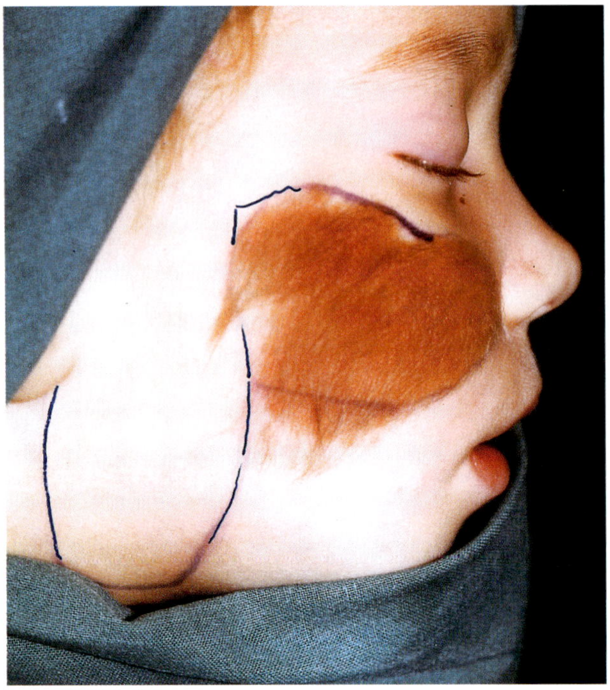

Figure 3.175a Giant nevus of the right cheek: Planning of the operation with the goal of defect coverage using tissues of the same color and quality. The flap was chosen in such a way that the tension after flap removal arises far from the lower eyelid and the corner of the mouth and runs transversally on the neck.

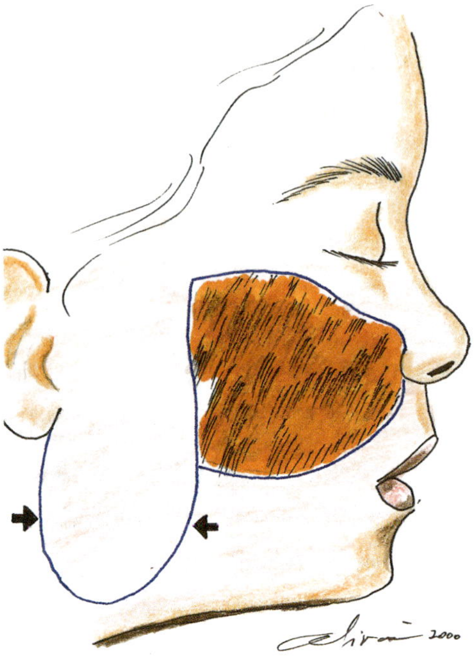

Figure 3.175b Schematic illustration: The flap is cranially pedicled and is formed from the preauricular area as well as the neck. It is a random pattern flap.

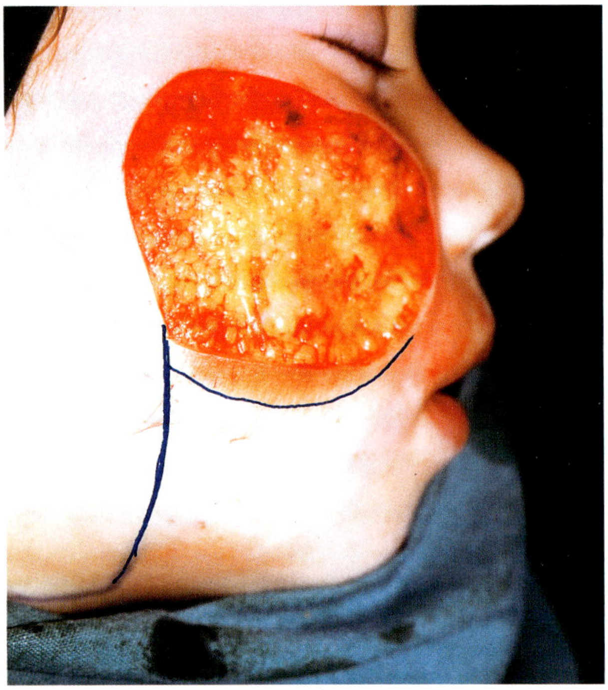

Figure 3.175c Situation after excision of the tumor

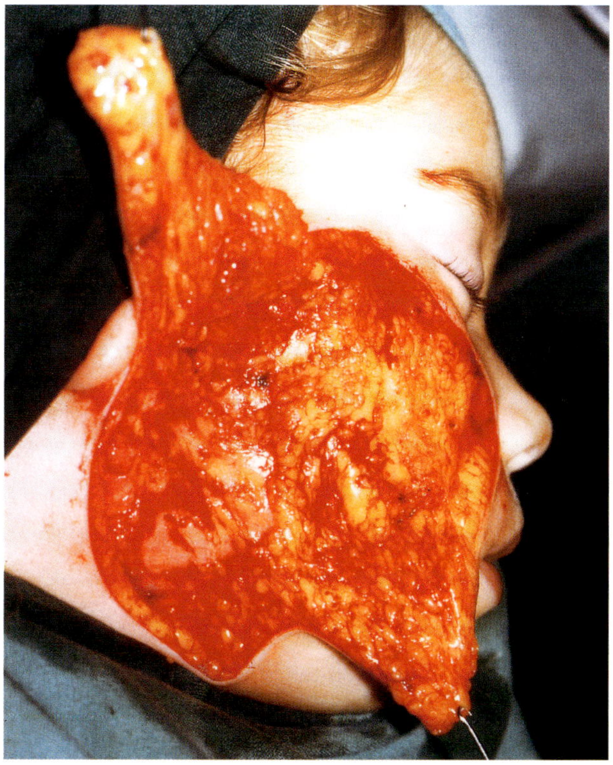

Figure 3.175d The picture shows how important the extensive mobilization of the flap and the edges of the donor site are

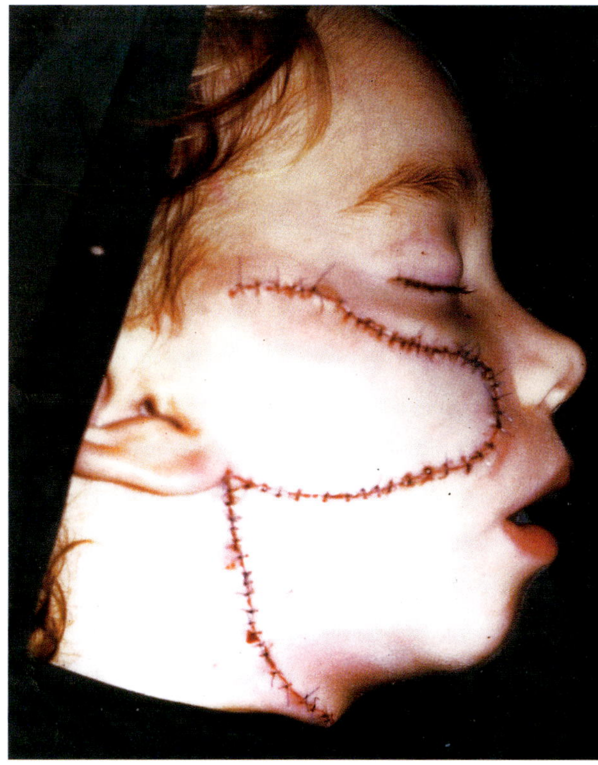

Figure 3.175e Fixation of the flap. The tension exist mainly in the neck transversally, where no problems are caused.

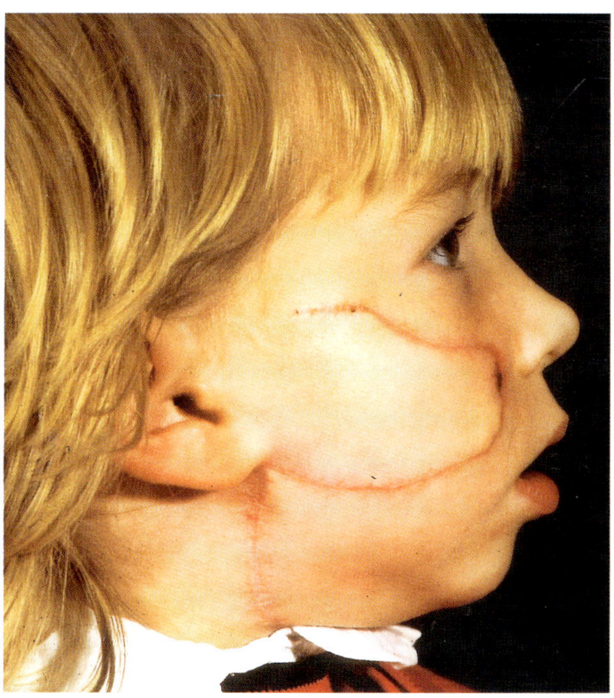

Figure 3.175f Picture taken three weeks postoperatively

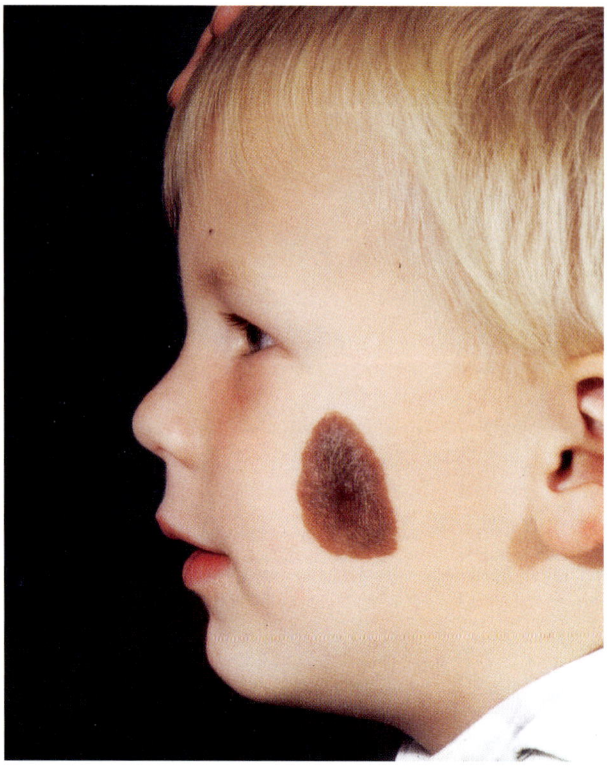

Figure 3.176a Giant nevus of the left cheek

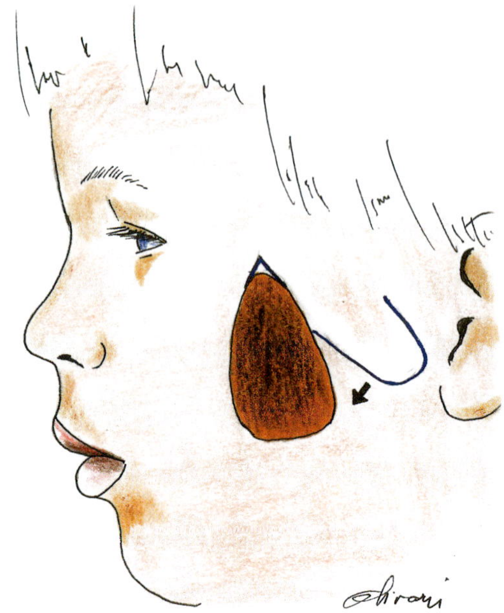

Figure 3.176b Planning of the operation. Because of the form of the tumor the flap is cranially pedicled.

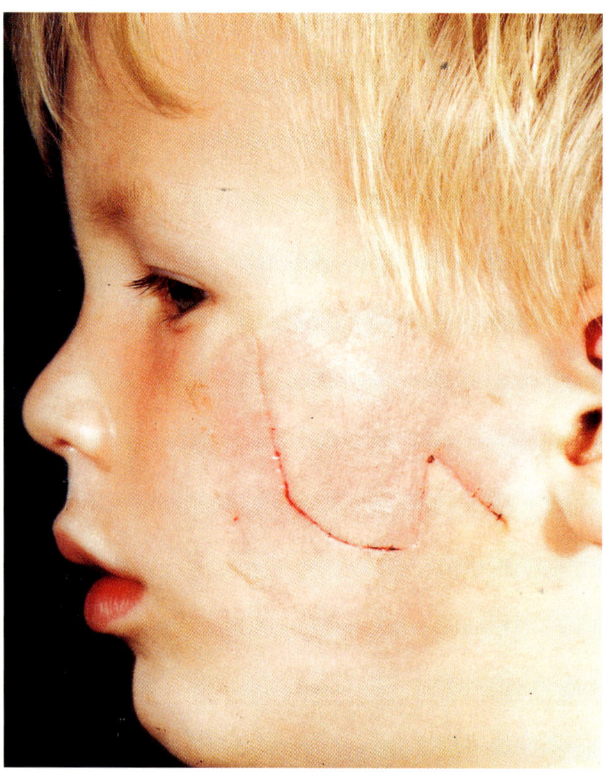

Figure 3.176c Aspect two weeks postoperatively

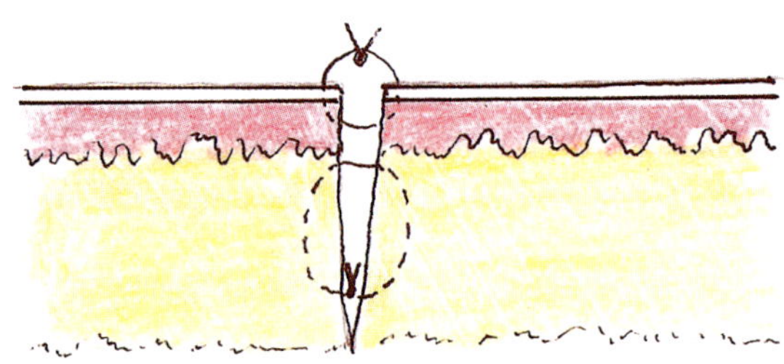

Figure 3.176d In the face the wound is closed as follows: First a subcutaneous suture with 5 × 0 Vicryl and sunken knots, then a skin suture with 6 × 0 nylon. The skin suture should be no further than 1 mm away from the wound margin. If there is no tension, intracutaneously suture with 6 × 0 is possible.

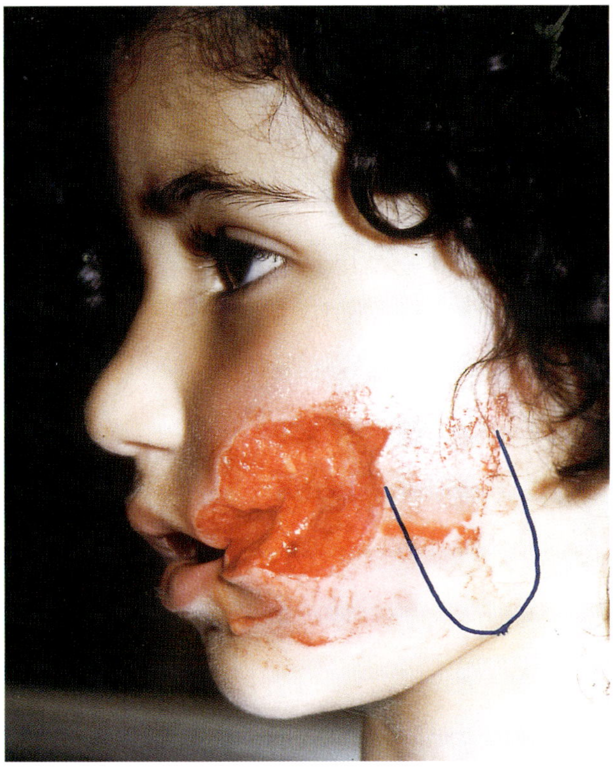

Figure 3.177a Dog bite injury of the left cheek with a 5 × 4 cm large defect. Treatment: Disinfection, local administration of antibiotics (Neomycin), sparing wound debridement.

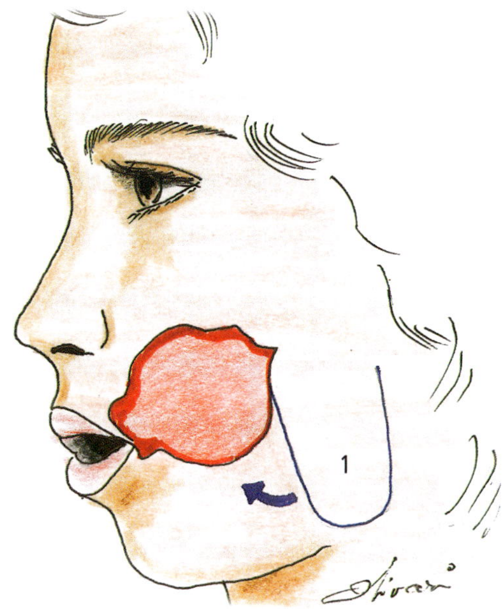

Figure 3.177b Formation of a cranially pedicled transposition flap of the preauricular region and the neck (1). The flap is sized so that it is large enough to avoid tension in the area of the left corner of the mouth.

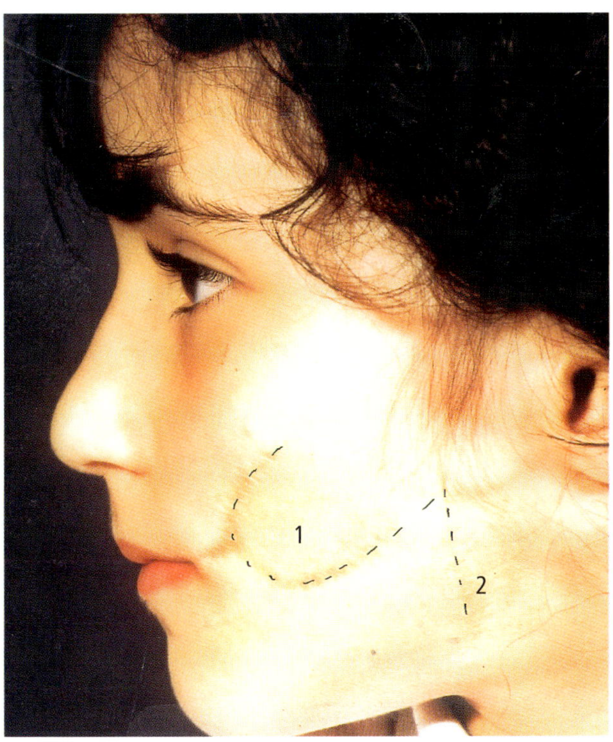

Figure 3.177c Picture one year after the operation: Positioning of the flap (1), secondary defect (2).

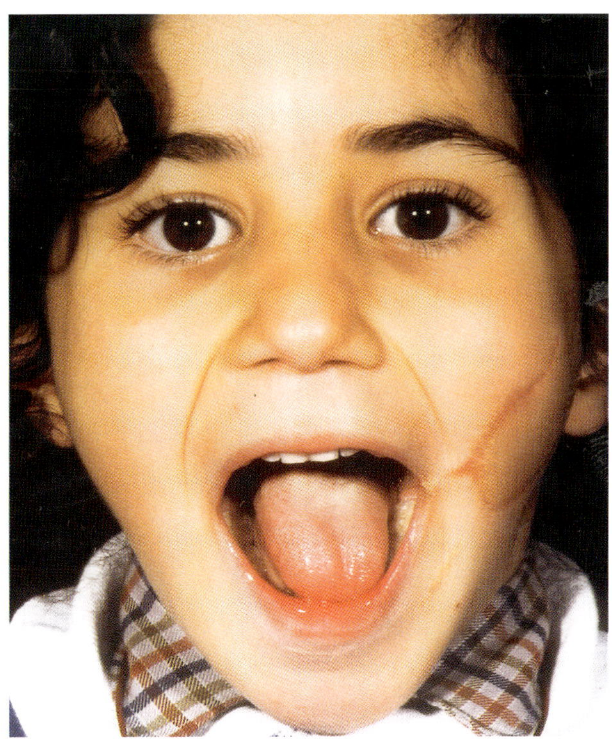

Figure 3.177d Functional result

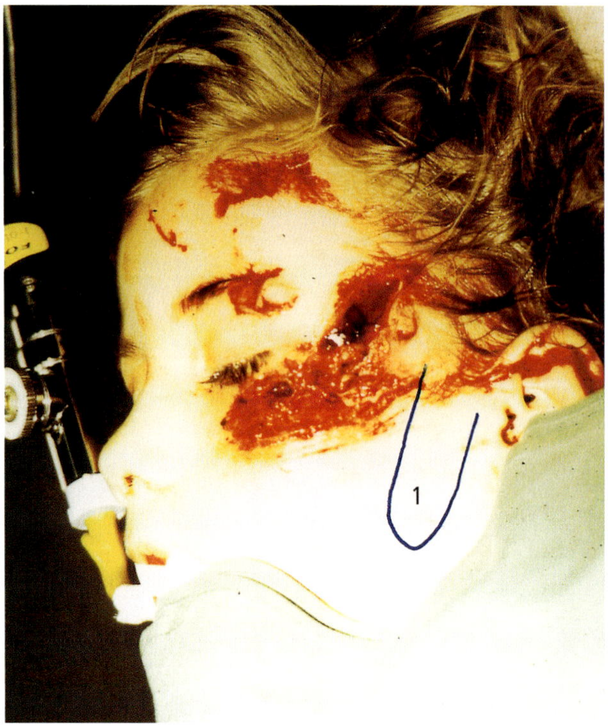

Figure 3.178a Status after a car accident.
Multiple lacerations and skin abrasions as well as a larger skin defect at the left lower eyelid and cheek. Lacerated skin should be fixed precisely in their initial position using 6 x 0 nylon. The larger defect below the left lower eyelid is closed with a transposition flap (1).

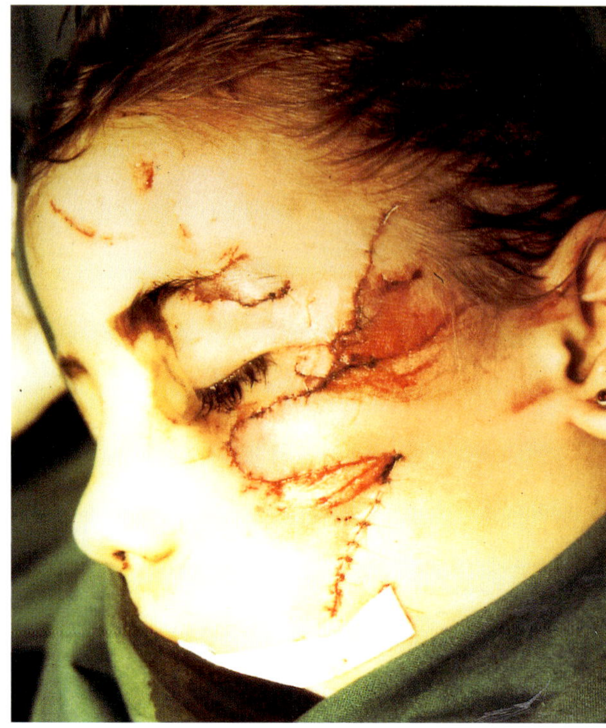

Figure 3.178b Primary multiple wound closure, precise adaptation of the transposition flap: The secondary defect is closed primarily.

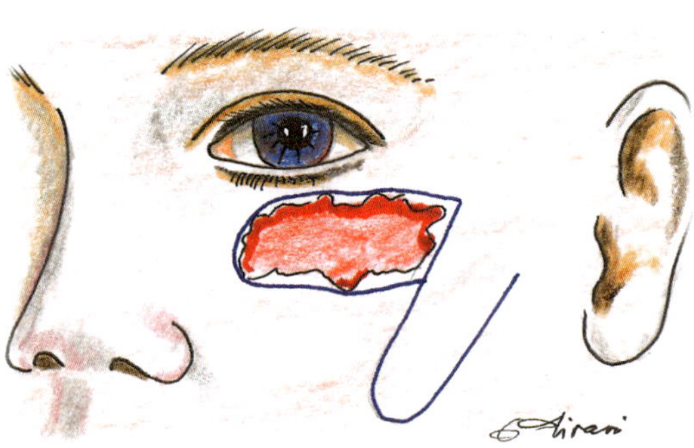

Figure 3.178c During the rising of the flap, as above, a transverse tension arises. The lower eyelid is not twisted downwards.

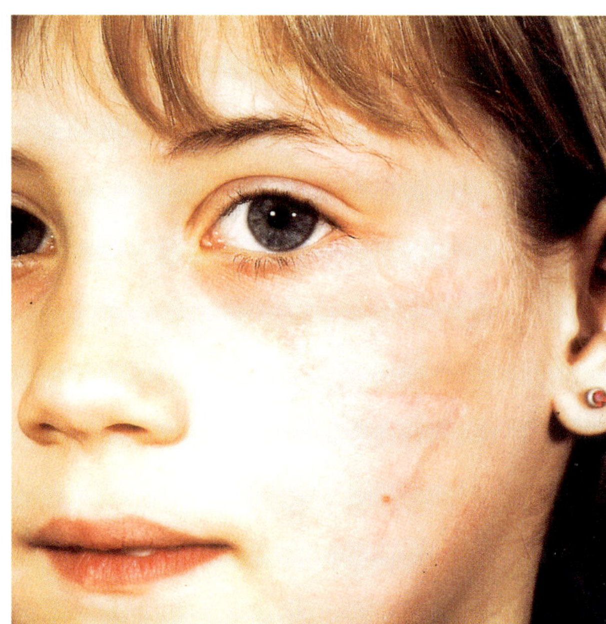

Figure 3.178d Aspect one year after the operation. The primary treatment strategy is of key importance.

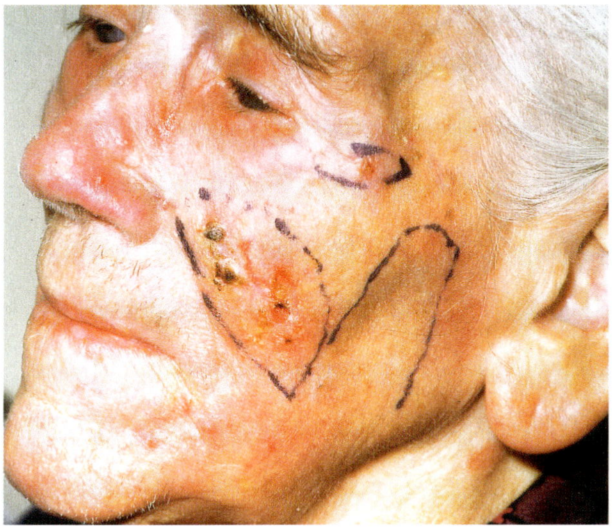

Figure 3.179a Multifocally growing basal cell carcinoma of the left cheek. Excision of the tumor in the region of the cheek and a smaller focus laterally to the left corner of the eye.

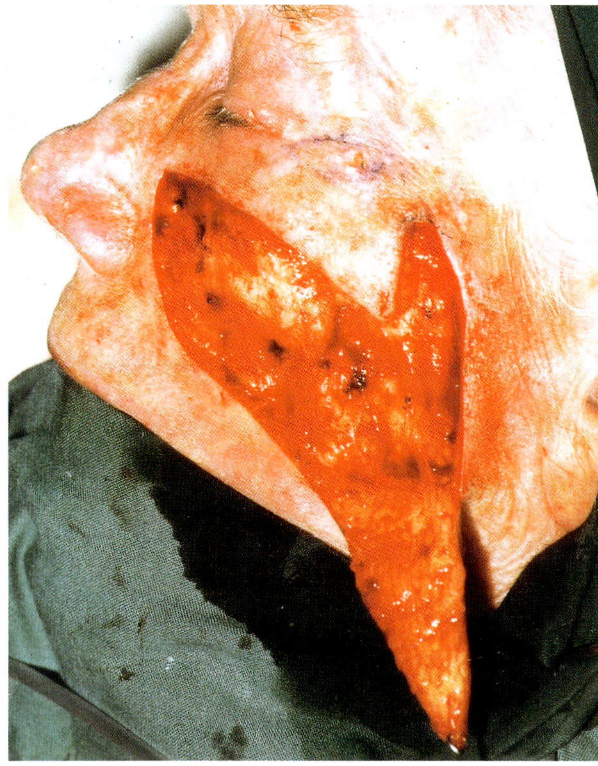

Figure 3.179b A caudally pedicled transposition flap is mobilized.

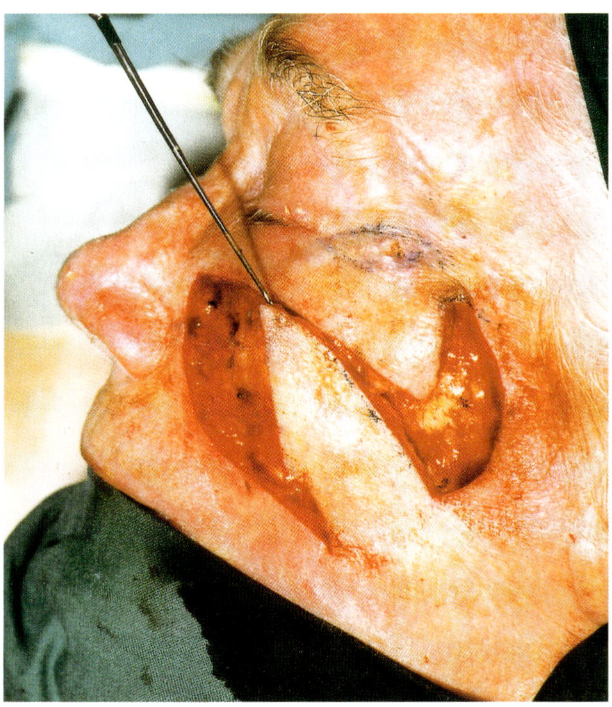

Figure 3.179c The flap is fixed into the defect, the secondary defect is closed primarily.

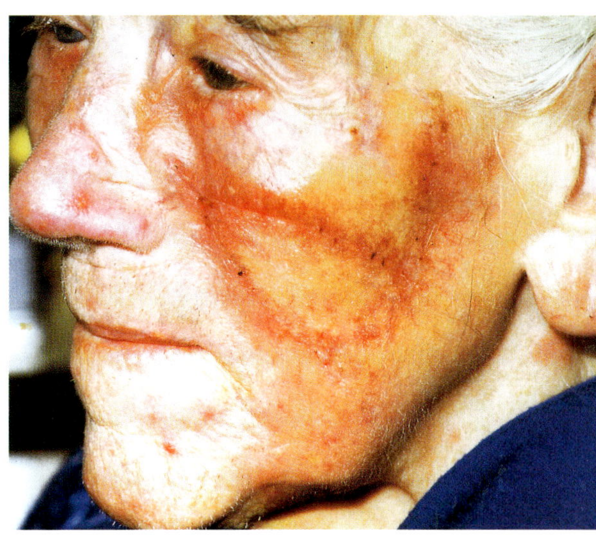

Figure 3.179d Picture three weeks postoperatively

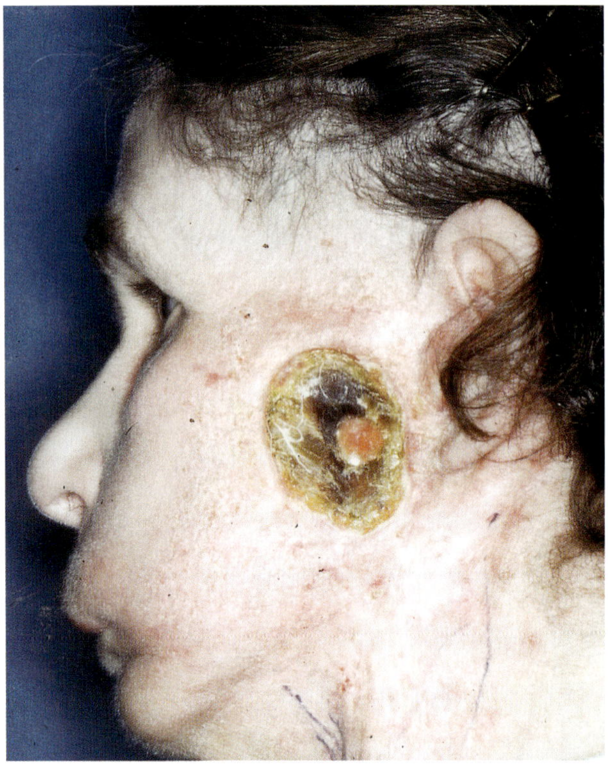

Figure 3.180a Situation ten years after irradiation of a basal cell carcinoma.
Three years after radiation, development of a radiation ulcer, facial palsy and restriction of mobility of the lower jaw due to joint stiffening.

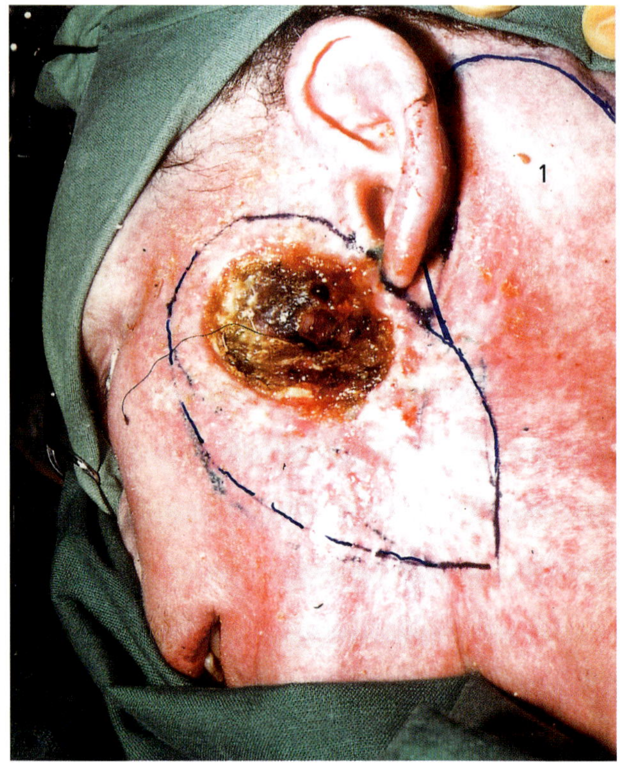

Figure 3.180b Planning of the operation. The defect should be closed with a transposition flap from the retroauricular area (1).

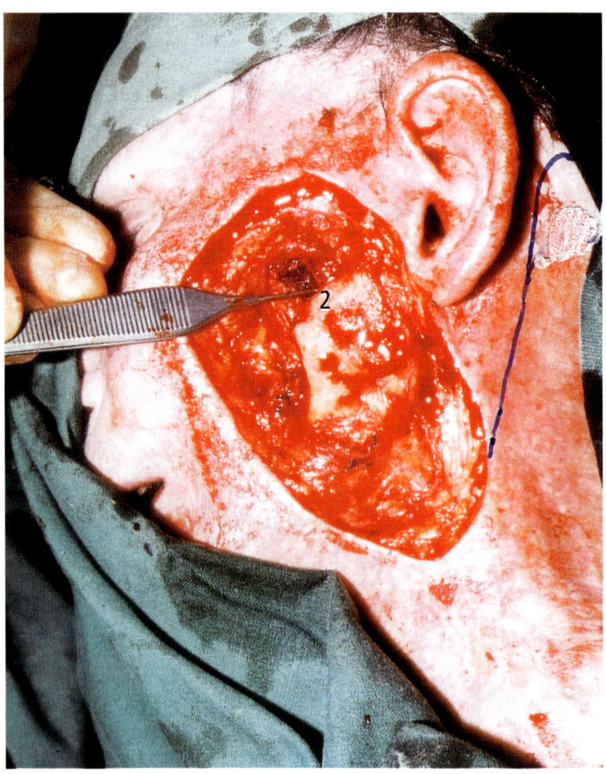

Figure 3.180c Situation after excision of the ulceration.
A part of the mandible (articular process) with radiogenic osteitis was resected (2). This allowed later on a easier mouth opening. Histological examination of the excised tissue did not show any signs of malignancy.

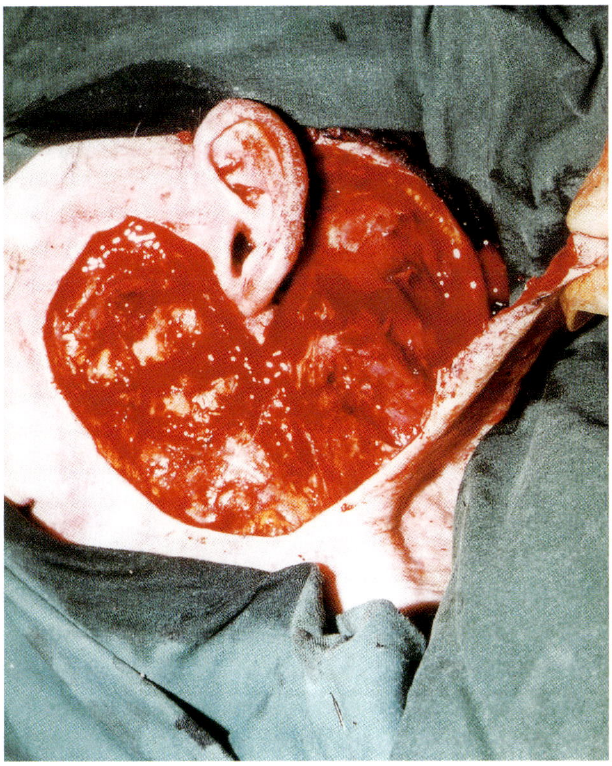

Figure 3.180d The transposition flap was mobilized.

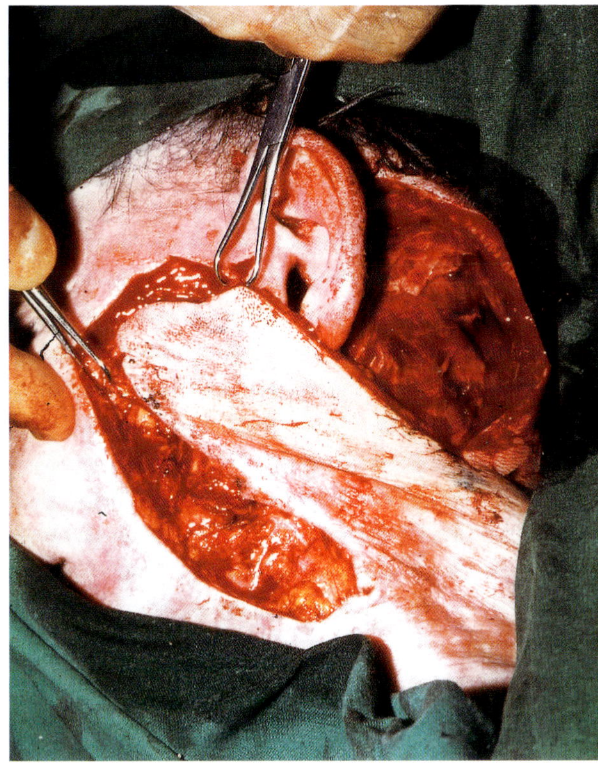

Figure 3.180e The long flap also contains hairy skin. After fixation in the defect, secondary defect is closed by a mesh graft (3).

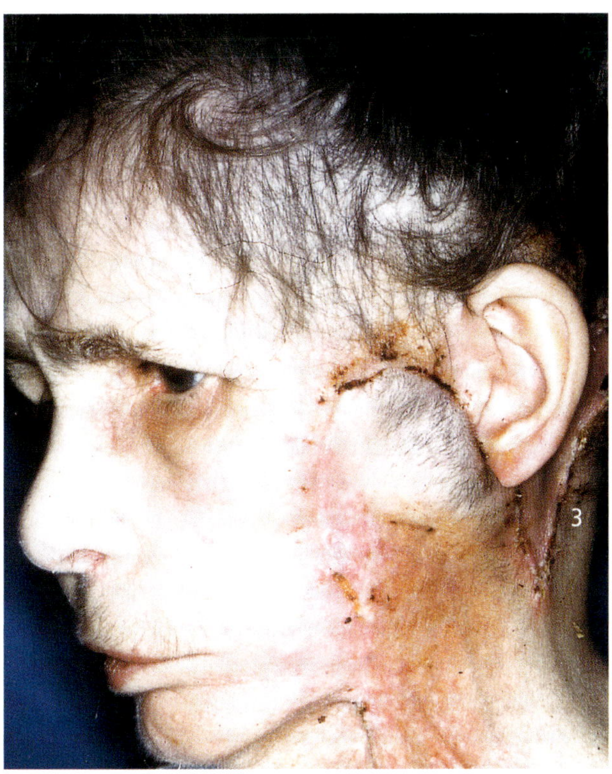

Figure 3.180f Situation three weeks postoperatively. Satisfactory result. The flap tip includes hairs. As an alternative a free radialis flap could be considered.

Supratrochlear Flap (Without Expanders)

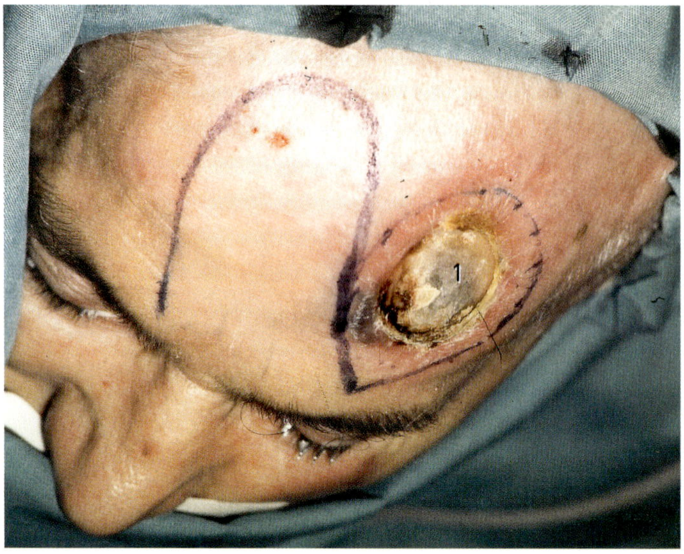

Figure 3.181a Defect in the left forehead area (irradiation of a basal cell carcinoma) in a 74-year old patient. The frontal bone is free; the external lamina is devitalized and infected (1).

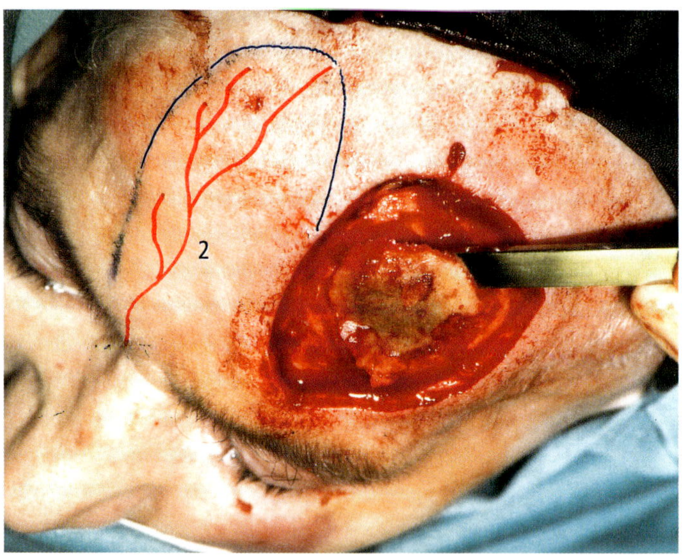

Figure 3.181b The defect should be closed by local (axial) flap. After the soft part debridement the necrotic part of the bone is removed with the chisel.
A supratrochlear flap is prepared (2). **Consider** the length of the flap. In the forehead and haired head area the flap must be planned longer because skin has poor elasticity.

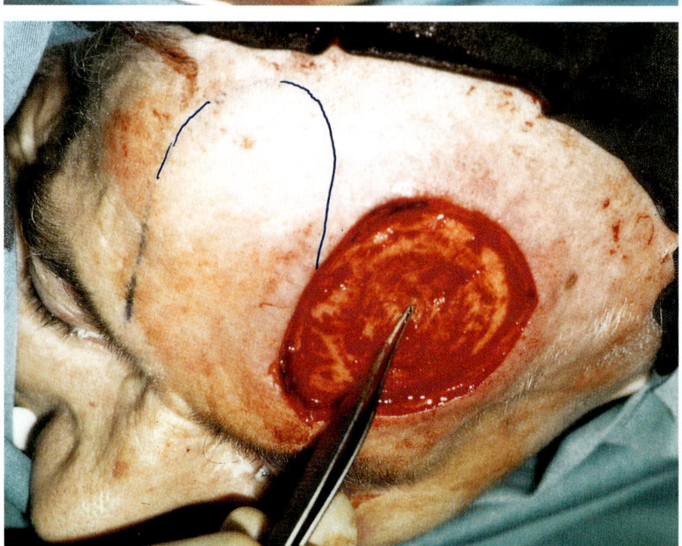

Figure 3.181c The internal lamina is well supplied by blood.

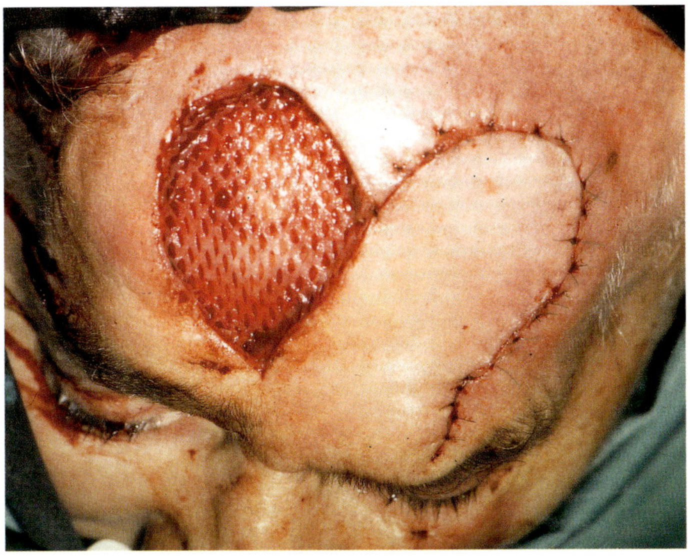

Figure 3.181d The defect is closed. Secondary defect is covered with a mesh graft.

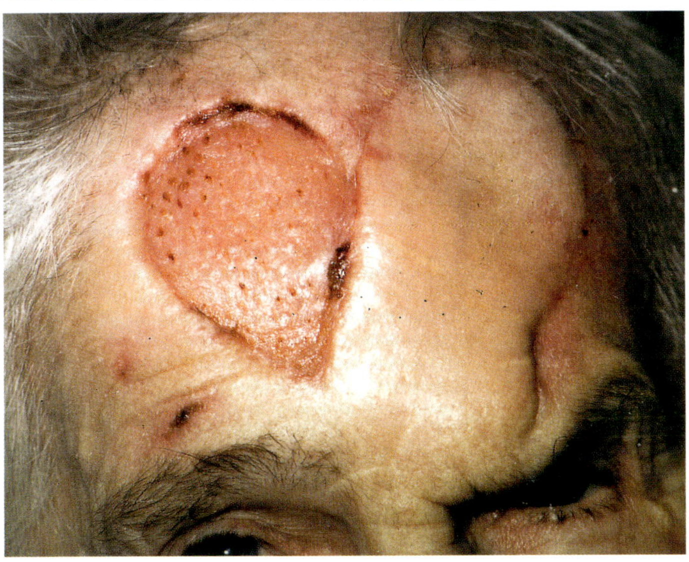

Figure 3.181e Status four weeks after the operation

Advancement Flap

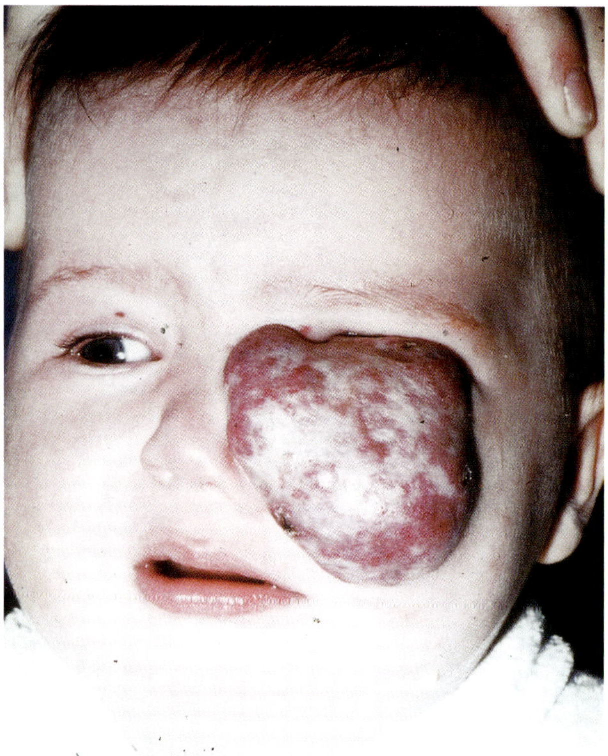

Figure 3.182a Tuberous hemangioma of the left cheek in a one-year old child. This kind of hemangioma frequently shows a spontaneous regeneration (more than 90 %).

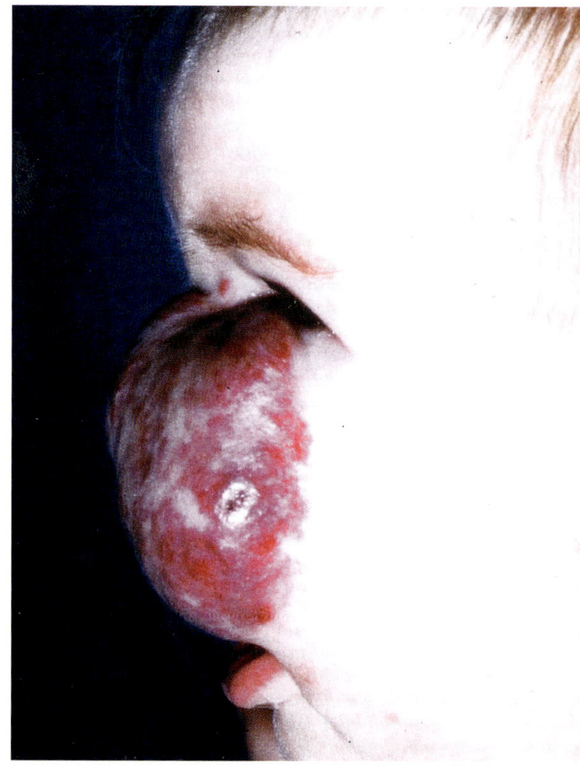

Figure 3.182b The operation was indicated urgently: The tumor conceals the left eye of the child. Since as a result of this no normal development of visual acuity so there was a danger of an amblyopia.

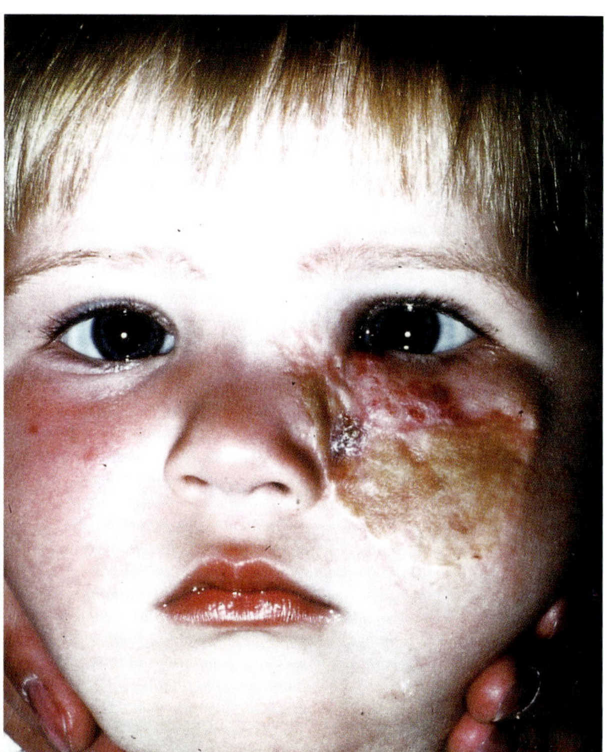

Figure 3.182c The hemangioma was excised. The area was covered temporarily with meshed skin graft.

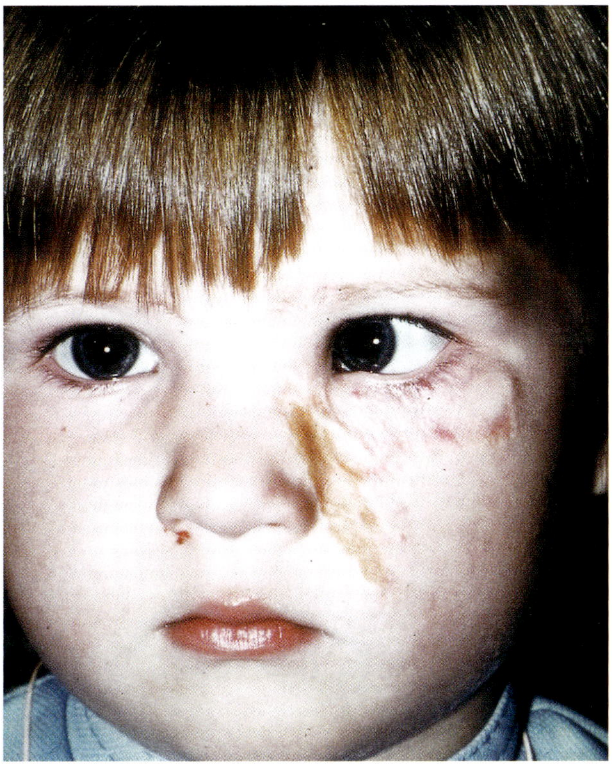

Figure 3.182d After healing, advanced flap from the cheek skin was mobilized from lateral three times within a year and the mesh graft was removed in stages.

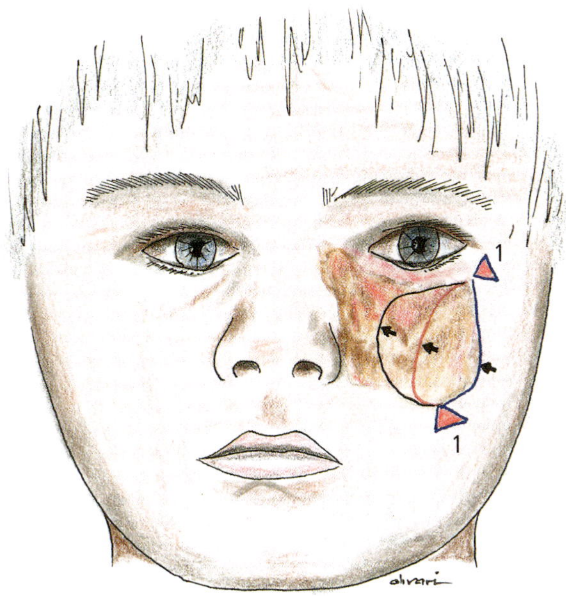

Figure 3.182e This was a multiply used advancement flap from the lateral with two Burow's triangle (1).

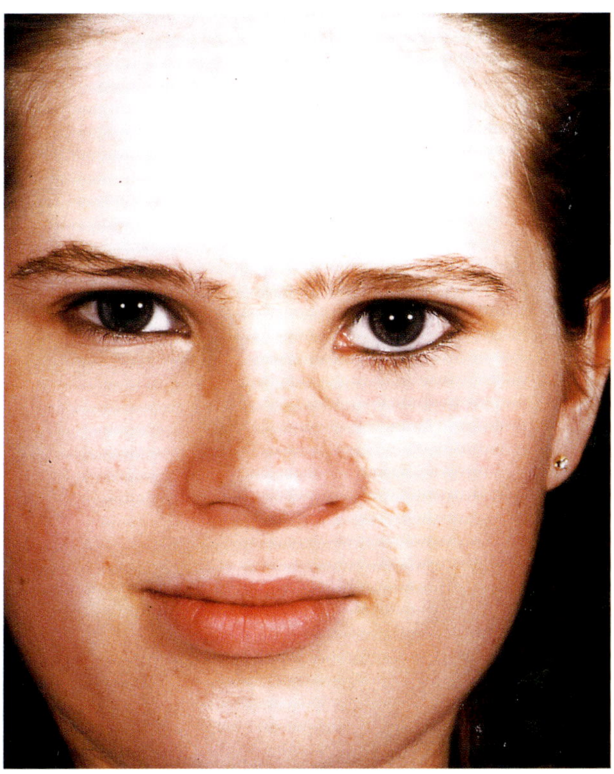

Figure 3.182f The patient at the age of 17 years. No further corrections were carried out at a later date. The patient shows a minimum "scleral show" on the left of no functional importance.

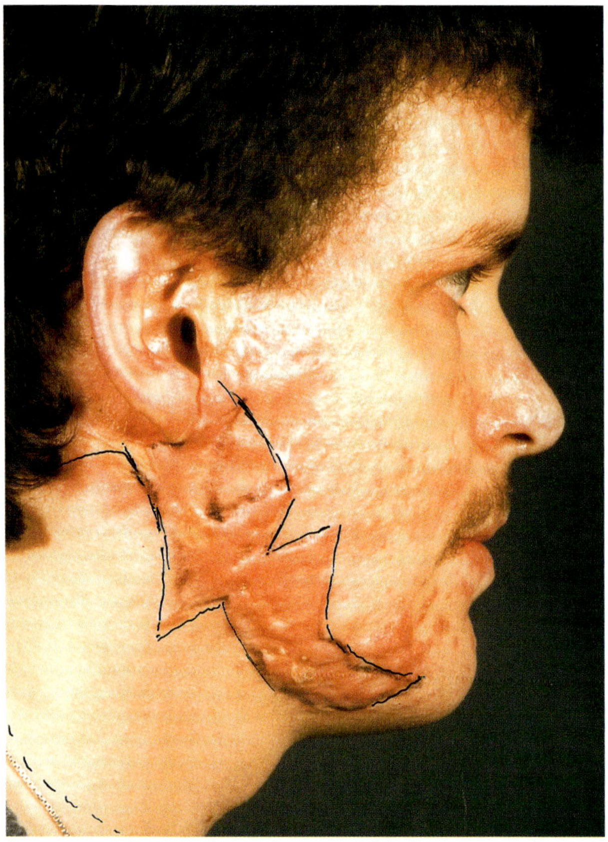

Figure 3.183a Burn scars of the right cheek that are partly keloid like. After excision of the scar an extensive mobilization of the neck skin down to clavicula was carried out. The facial skin must not be mobilized, otherwise lateral distortions can occur.

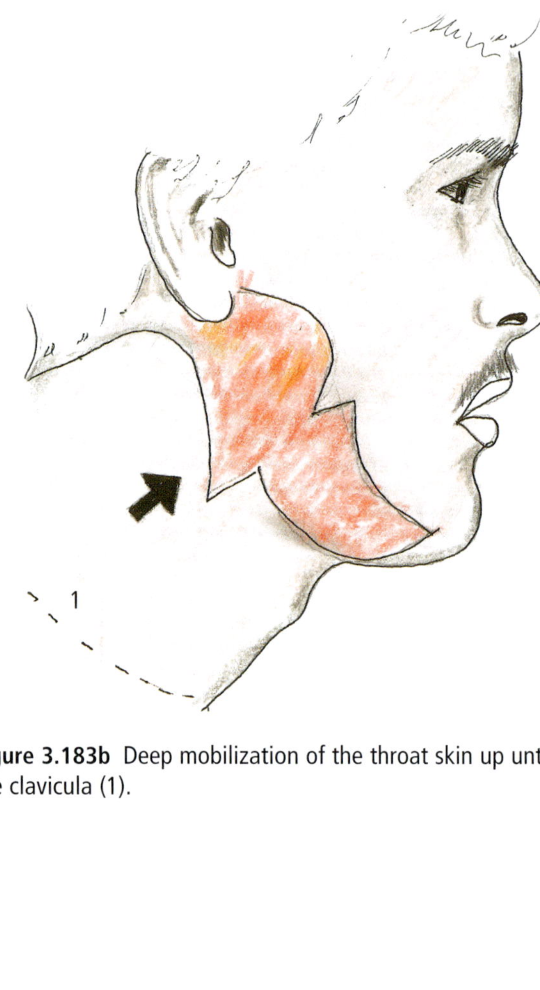

Figure 3.183b Deep mobilization of the throat skin up until the clavicula (1).

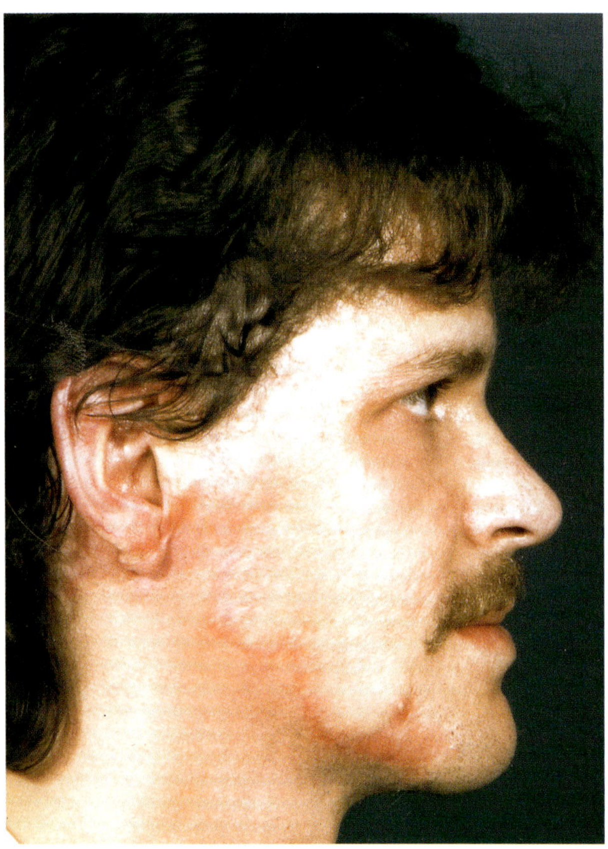

Figure 3.183c Status two years after the advancement flap

Multiple Z-Plasty + Dermabrasion

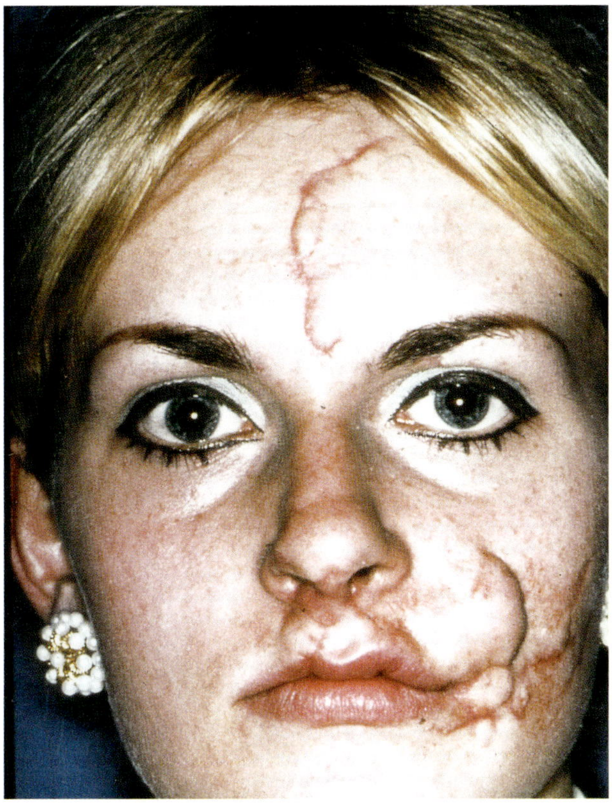

Figure 3.184a Post-traumatic scar formation (impacted windscreen) in the face. The scars are further deteriorated by the inadequate primary wound treatment. The treatment consists first of all of a six months wait. There are two reasons for this: 1) In the first weeks after the trauma the scars are in a proliferating phase. 2) After six months the tissue becomes softer and some scars disappear spontaneously.

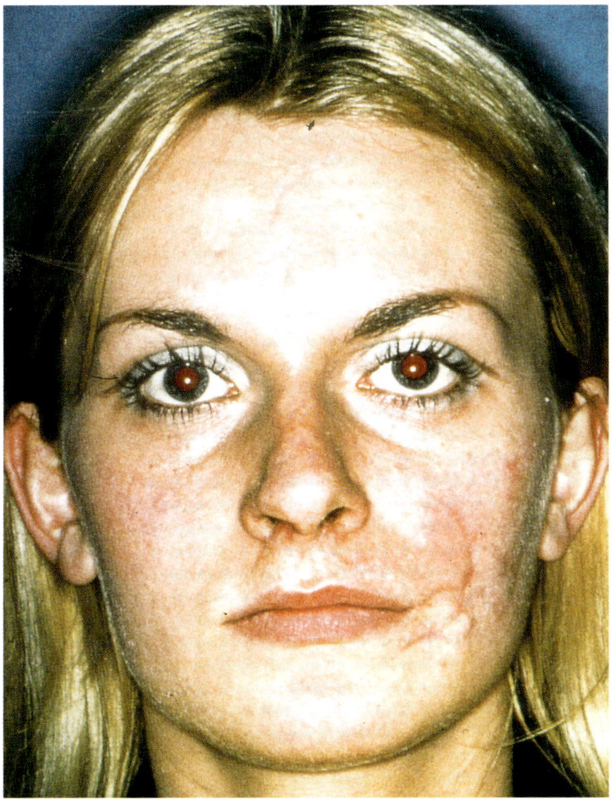

Figure 3.184b Situation one year after the treatment. Six months after the trauma the scar excision with Z-plasty occurred and a precise atraumatic wound margin adaptation occurred at the level of the skin. Three months later the scars were treated by dermabrasion.

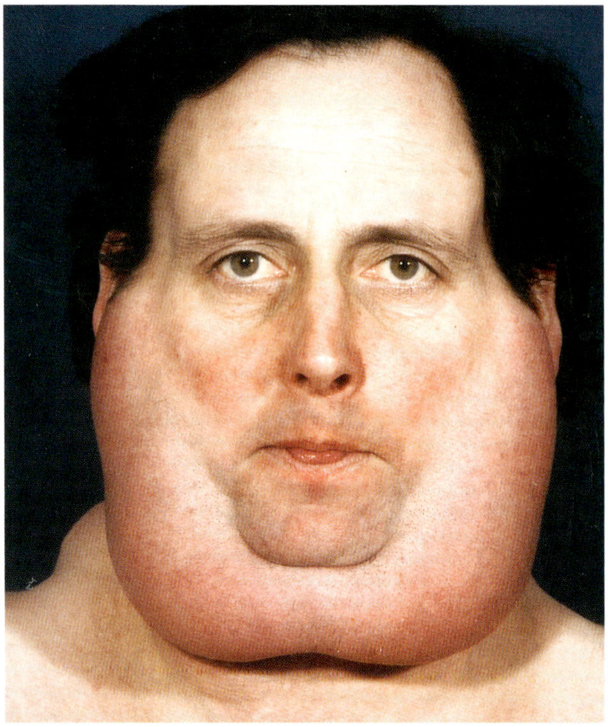

Figure 3.185a Cervical lipomatosis (Madelung's disease) or lipomatosis dolorosa. The disease is painful and greatly disfiguring. The tumor size caused considerable functional and psychological problems.

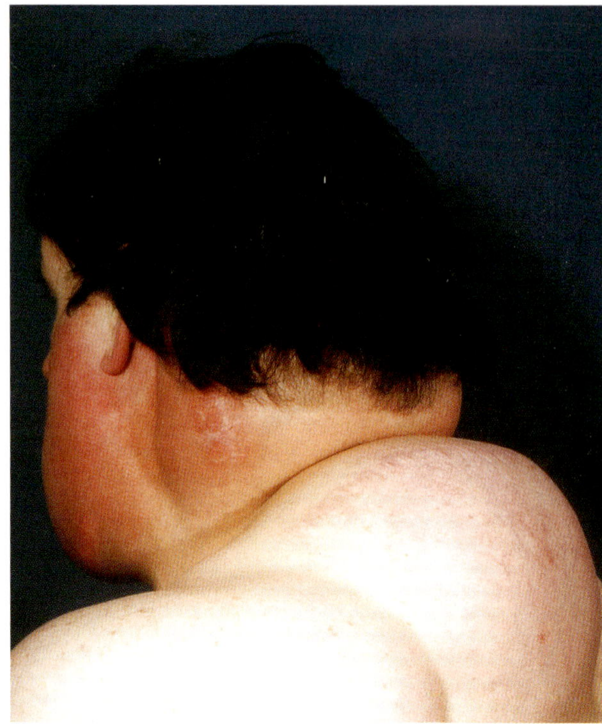

Figure 3.185b Because of the long duration of illness a fibrosis sets in parts.

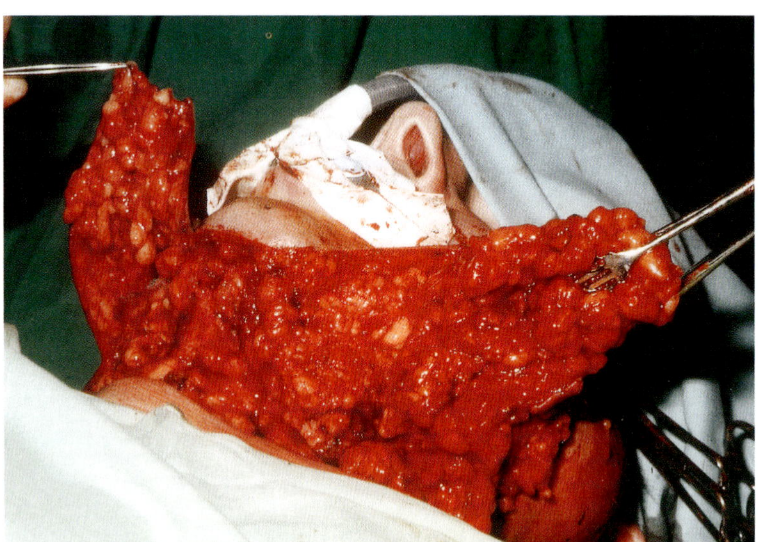

Figure 3.185c Since liposuction proved unsuccessful, an open operation was carried out. A very extensive and precise operation is necessary since the anatomical structures are partly dislocated. In dorsal part simple excision can be successful.

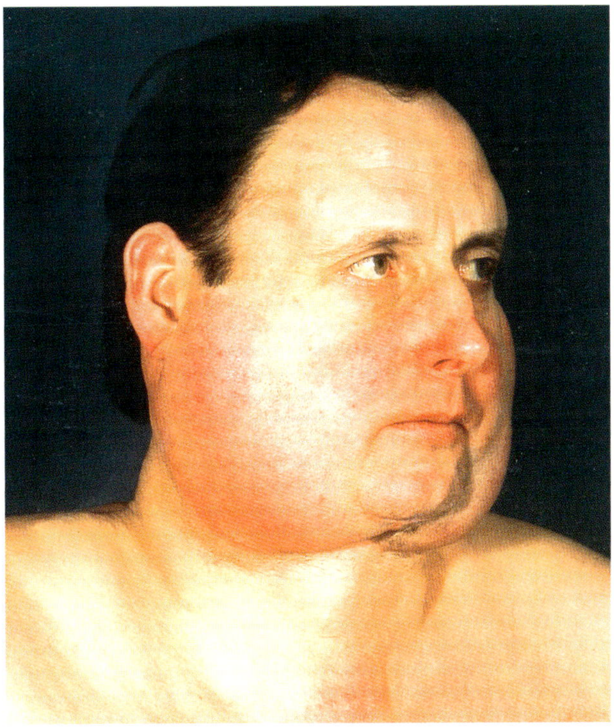

Figure 3.185d Status six months after the operation. A further surgical correction was intended in the cheek area, but was no longer desired by the patient.

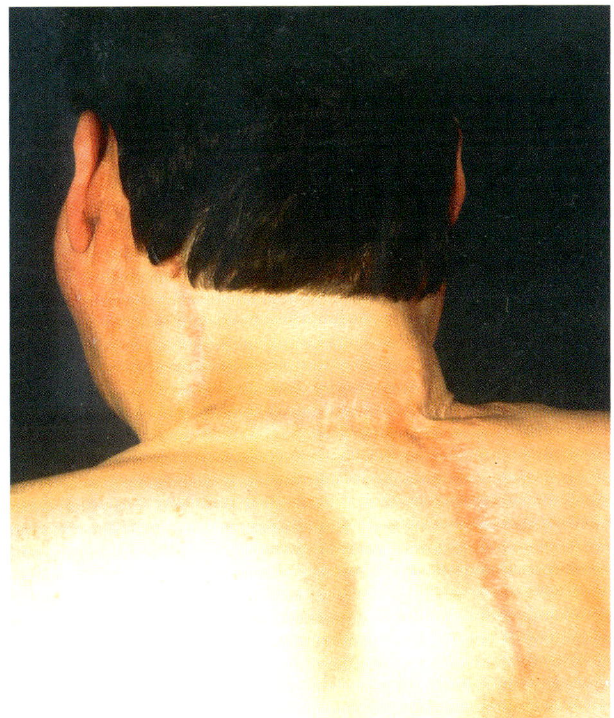

Figure 3.185e Therapy in the dorsal neck area: Partly liposuction, partly resection.

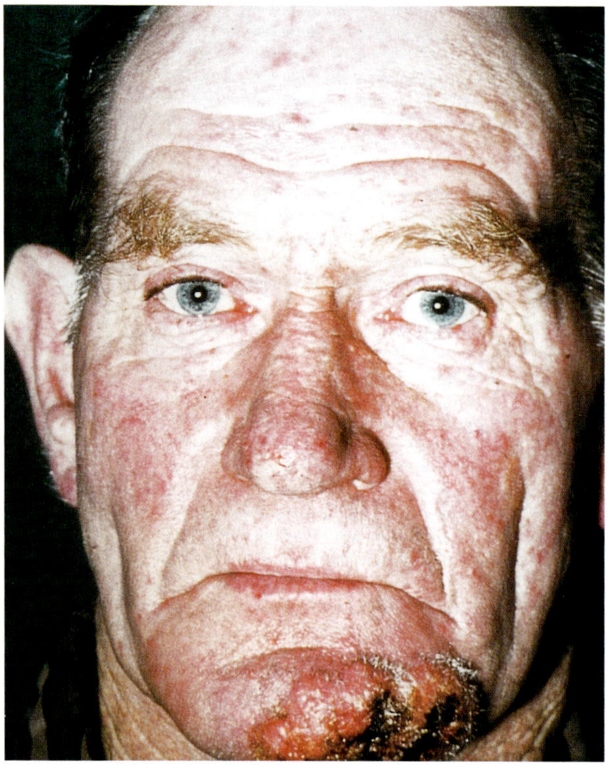

Figure 3.186a Four year-old infiltrative squamous-cell carcinoma on the chin

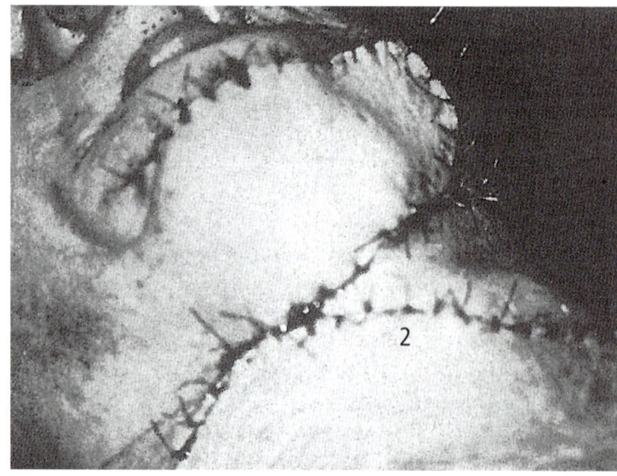

Figure 3.186c Coverage of the defect with a craniolateral pedicled flap from the neck area. The secondary defect is closed primarily (2).

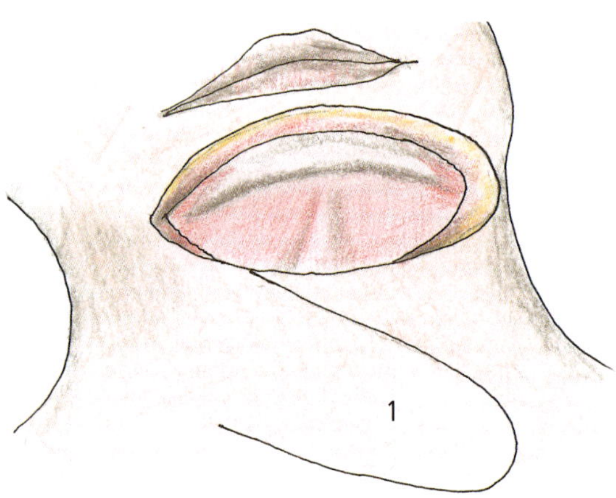

Figure 3.186b Resection in healthy tissue. A local lymph node removal follows on both sides. Histology: No regional metastasis. Transposition flap (1).

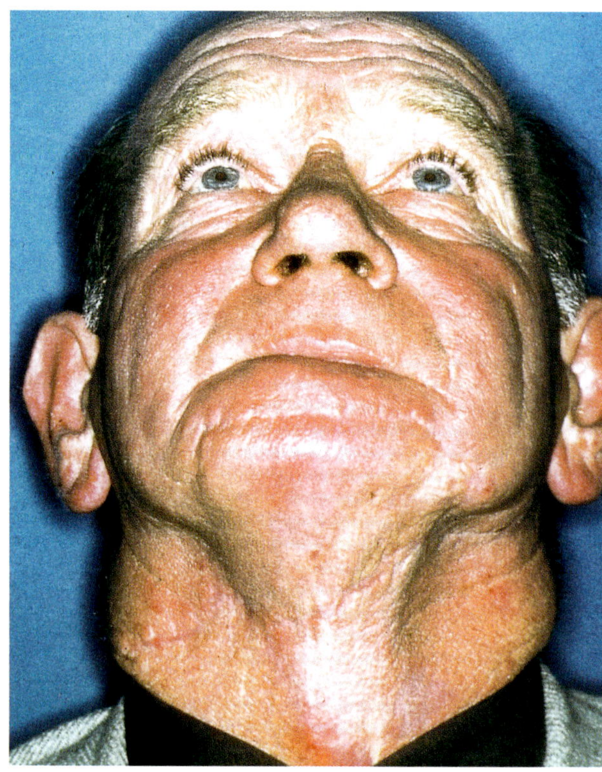

Figure 3.186d Status four years after the operation (This flap is described by Langenbeck in 1855; see page 17)

Double Triangle Flap (Olivari)

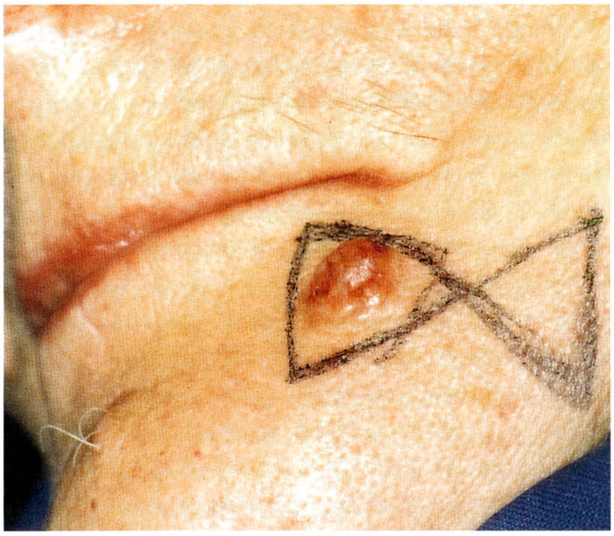

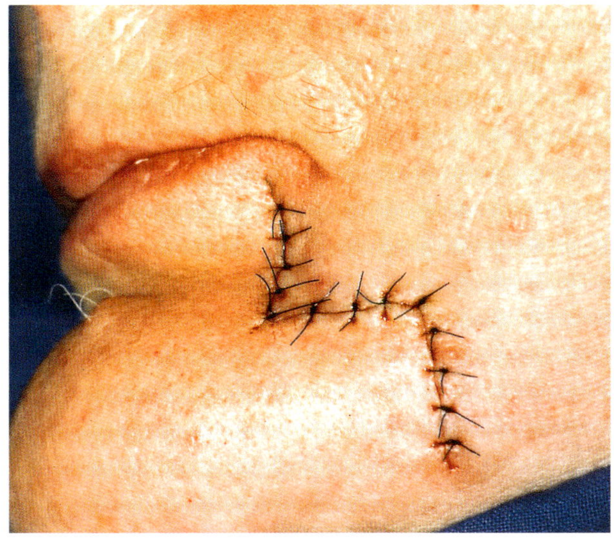

Figure 3.187a,b Double triangle flap

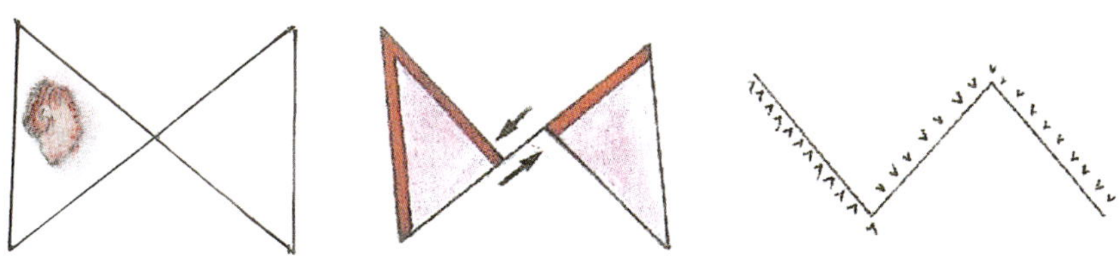

Figure 3.187c This is a double triangular flap. Its advantage is if one or two tumors of approximately the same size occur next to each other. The double triangular flap is an effective flap that is rarely used in medical practice. In such a delicate area this flap is feasible to perform without notable tension.

Rotation Flaps

Mustardé Type I

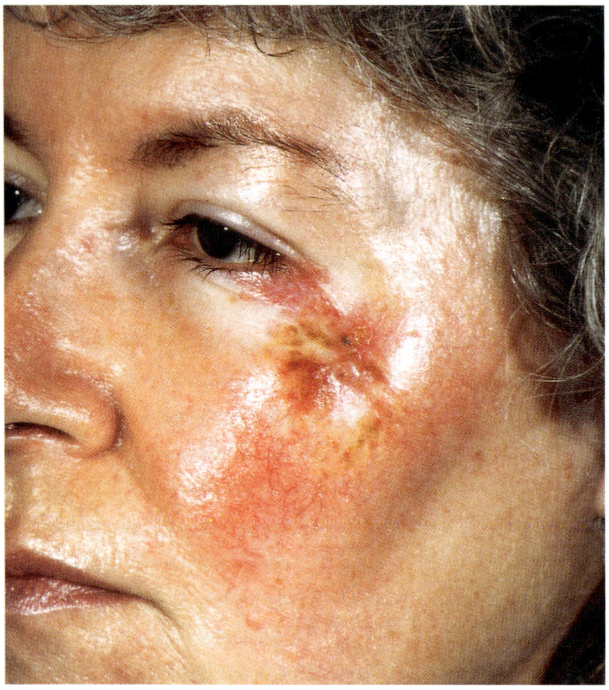

Figure 3.188a Recurrence of basal cell carcinoma in the lateral part of the left lower eyelid and the left cheek.

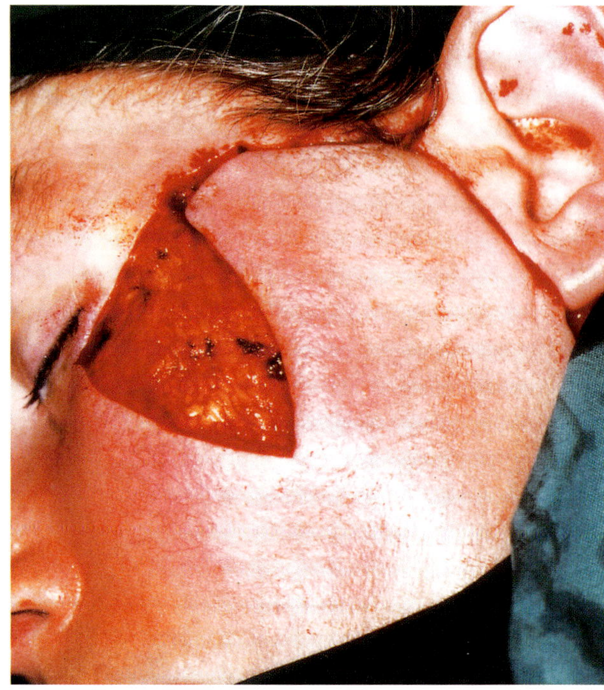

Figure 3.188b Histologically controlled excision. The cheek rotation flap (Mustardé type I) is formed up to the retroauricular area. It should be noted that the incision line runs laterally and above from the lateral cantus in order to avoid an ectropium.

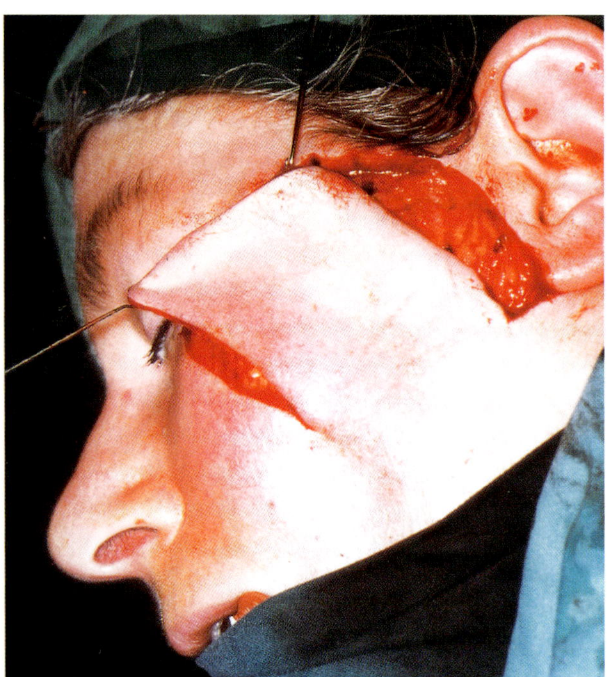

Figure 3.188c After rotation of the flap in the medial direction

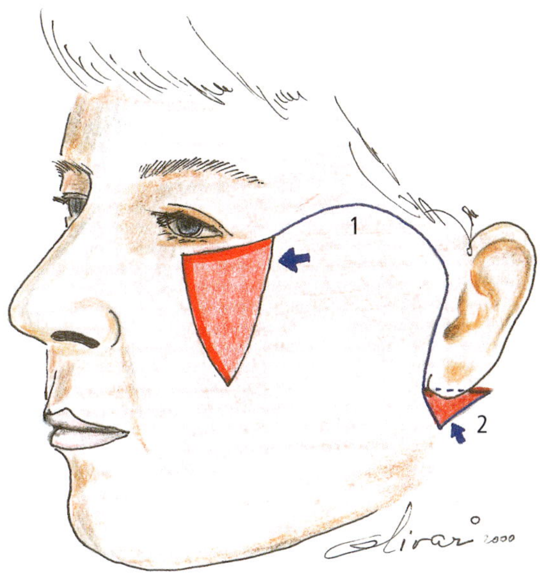

Figure 3.188d Mustardé type I – the incision line lateral to the defect must run in the latero-cranial direction (1), i.e. diagonally and upwards. A small triangle (2) below the ear lobe is excised in order to allow a better mobility of the flap.

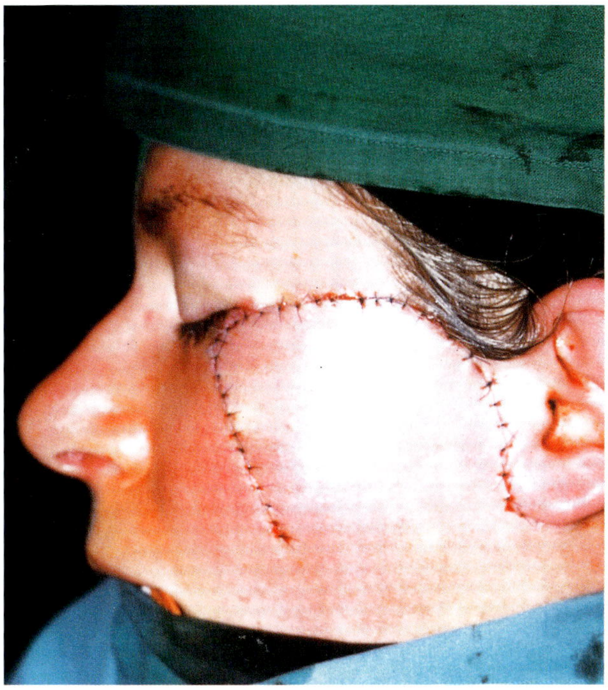

Figure 3.188e Picture taken at the end of the operation

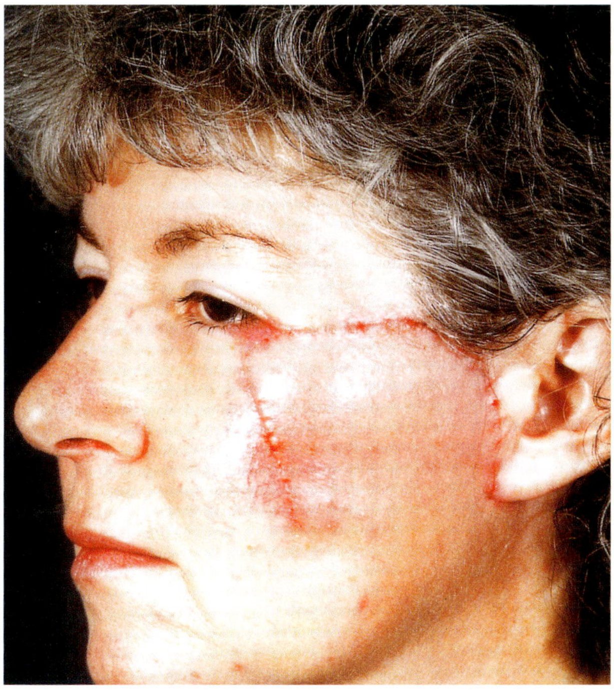

Figure 3.188f Picture taken 14 days after the operation

Mustardé Type II (Modification)

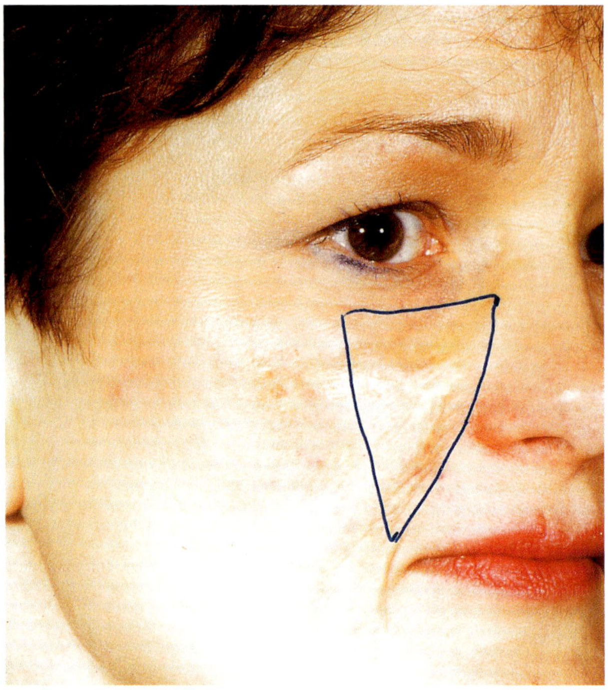

Figure 3.189a Basal cell carcinoma of the right cheek and the right nasolabial fold with a multifocal growth pattern that was operated on twice and irradiated.

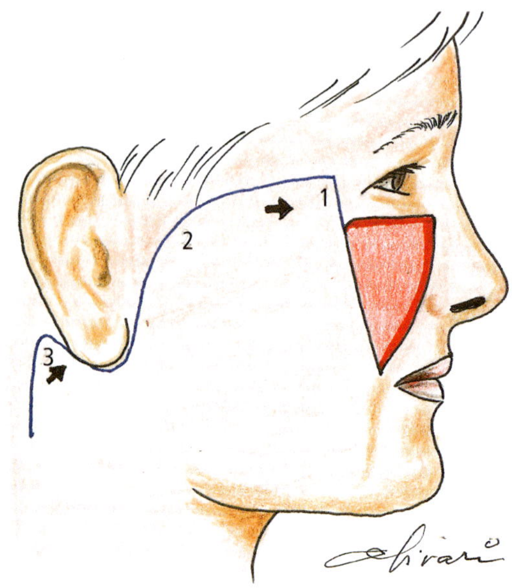

Figure 3.189b Incision line of the rotation flap from the right cheek (Mustardé type II). In order to achieve a large mobility medially, the incision does not end at the ear lobe, but extends retroauricularly a small flap in a V-form. It prolongs the rotation arch and allows a greater area to be covered. **Note:** The rotation flap begins higher up than the defect margin in order to prevent traction at the lower eyelid.

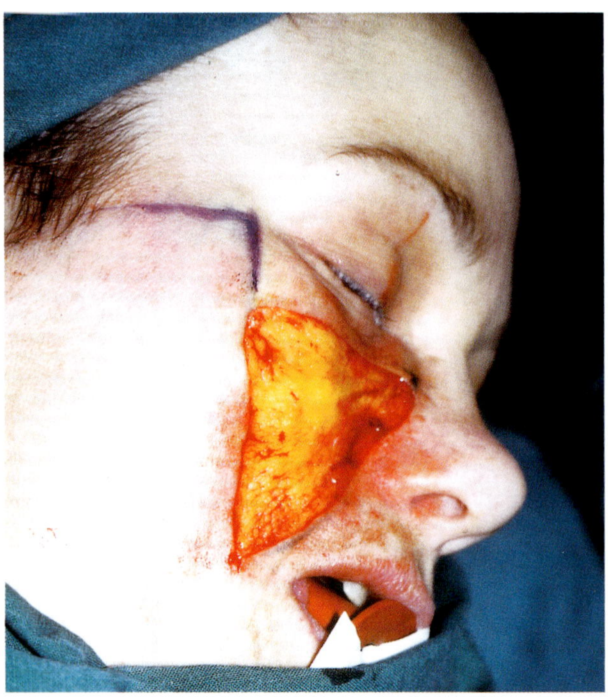

Figure 3.189c The excision is carried out

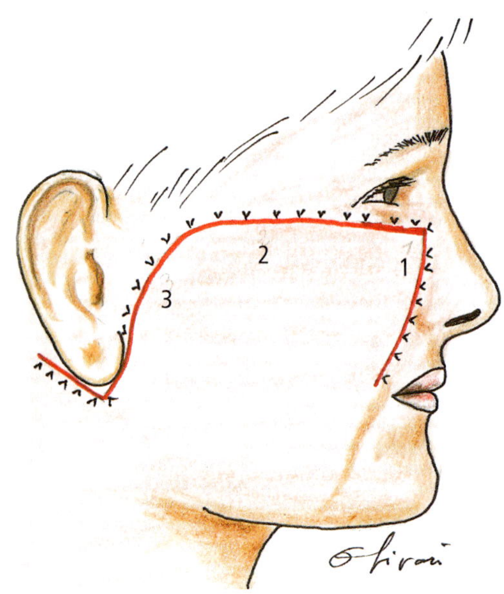

Figure 3.189d **Note** the displacement of points 1, 2 and 3

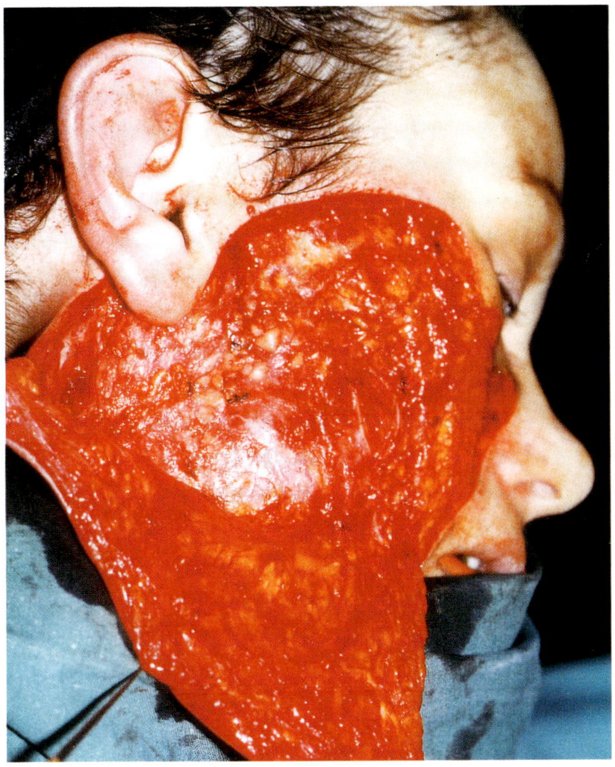

Figure 3.189e Considerable mobilization of the flap is extremely important.

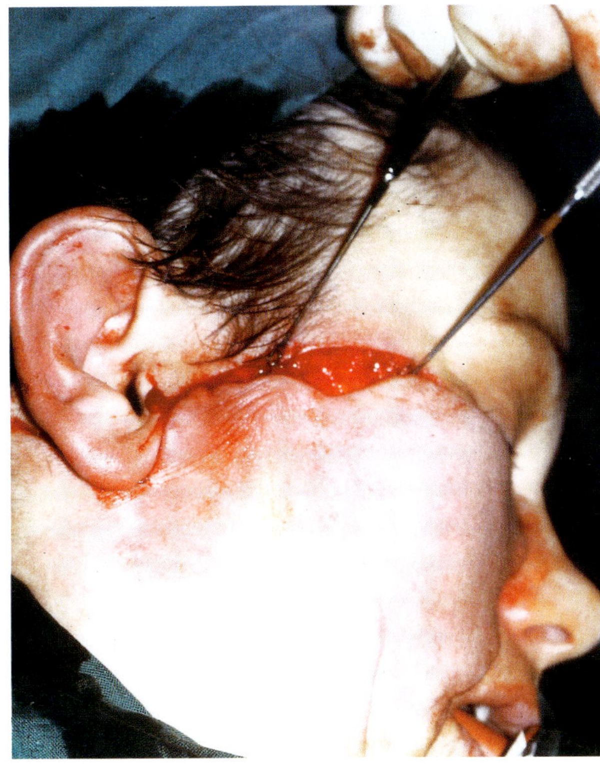

Figure 3.189f After extensive mobilization rotation can be carried out in the medial direction without tension. At the end of the operation the flap is sutured without tension at the lower eyelid.

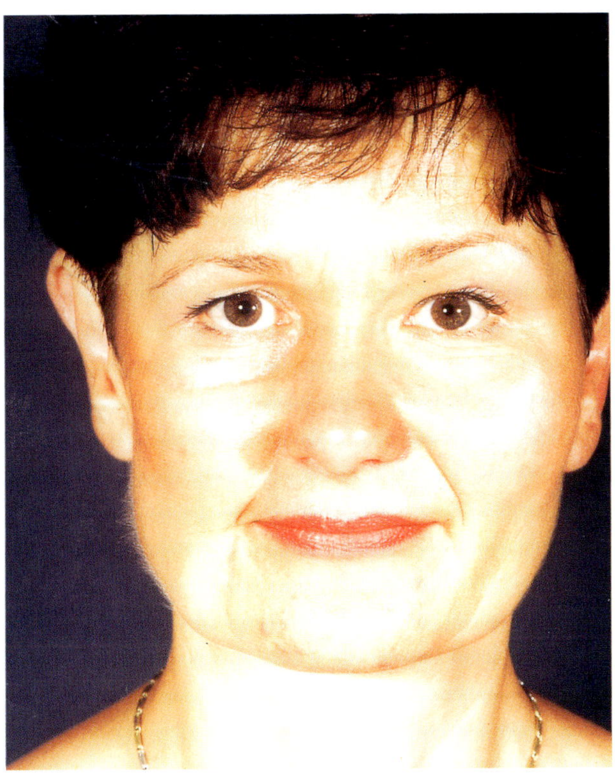

Figure 3.189g Picture taken 16 months after the operation. Note: The symmetry of the face is preserved.

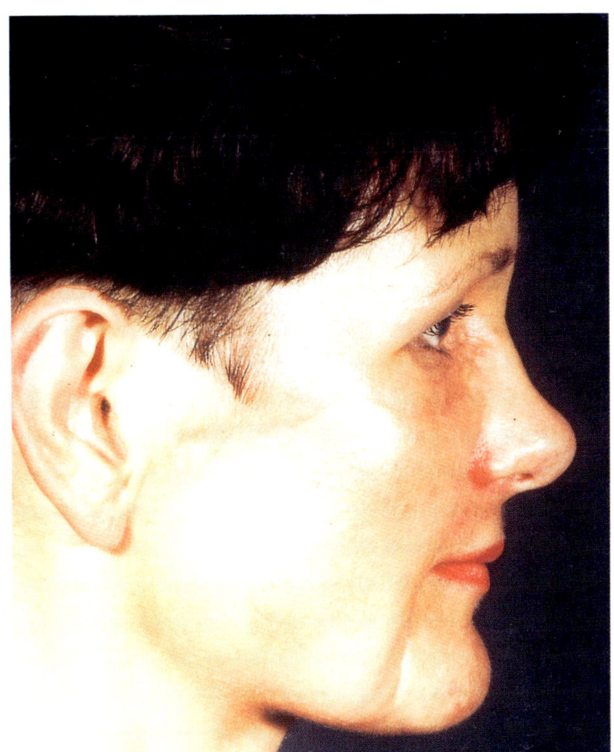

Figure 3.189h Profile

Mustardé Type II

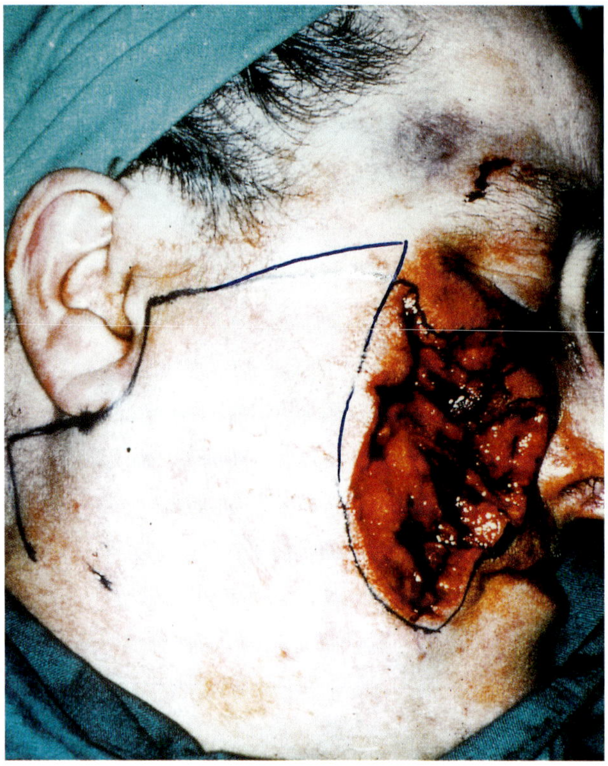

Figure 3.190a Defect of the right cheek after a dog bite. Treatment: Primary reconstruction:

1. Washing of the wound with medical soap
2. Disinfection with Betaisodona or another antiseptic
3. Local administration of antibiotics (for example Neomycin)
4. Only the minimal marginal excision in order to straighten the wound edges

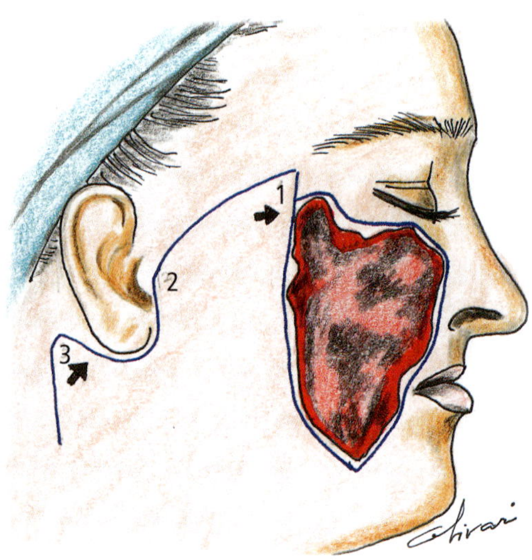

Figure 3.190b The rotation flap (Mustardé type II) from the right cheek must start higher laterally than the defect margin. The incision line is prolonged retroauricularly.

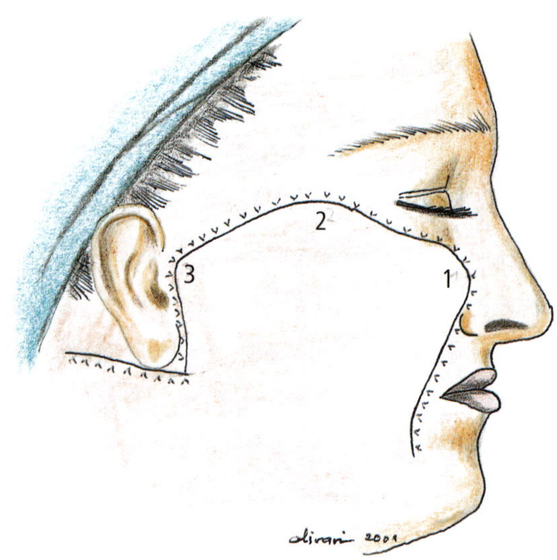

Figure 3.190c **Note:** Displacement of the flap as indicated by points 1, 2 and 3

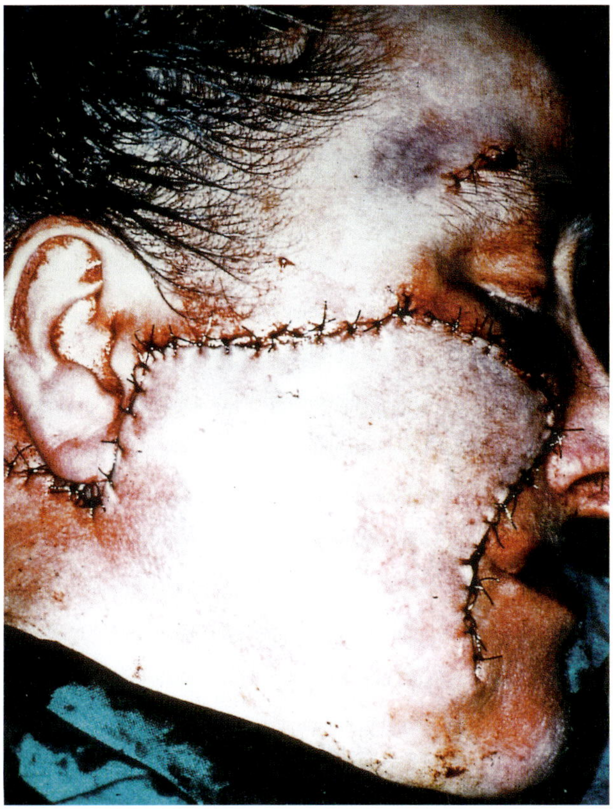

Figure 3.190d Situation at the end of the operation

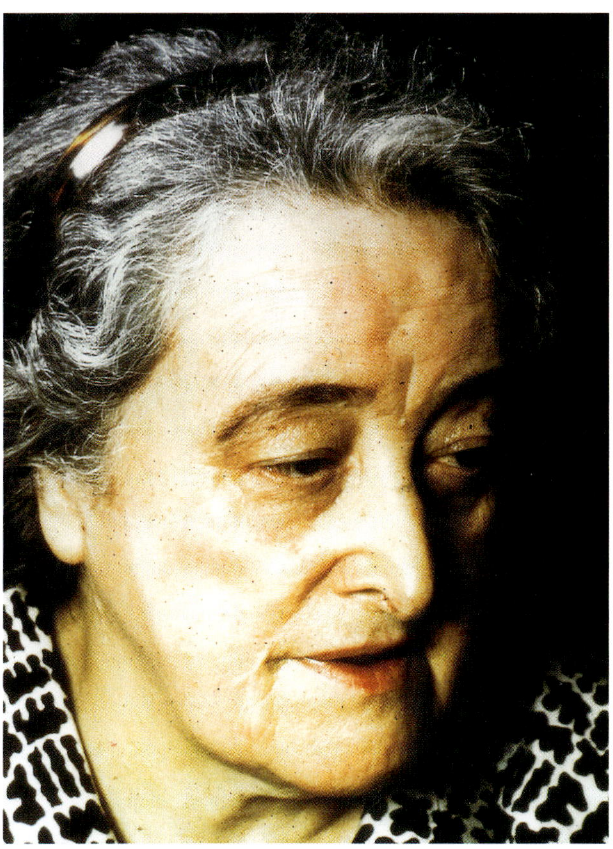

Figure 3.190e Aspect one year after the operation

Mustardé Type III

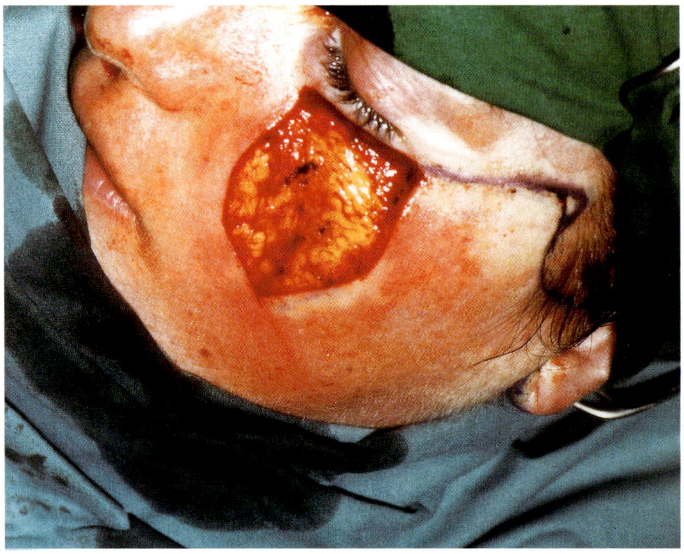

Figure 3.191a Situation after excision of a basal cell carcinoma of the left cheek and the left lower eyelid.

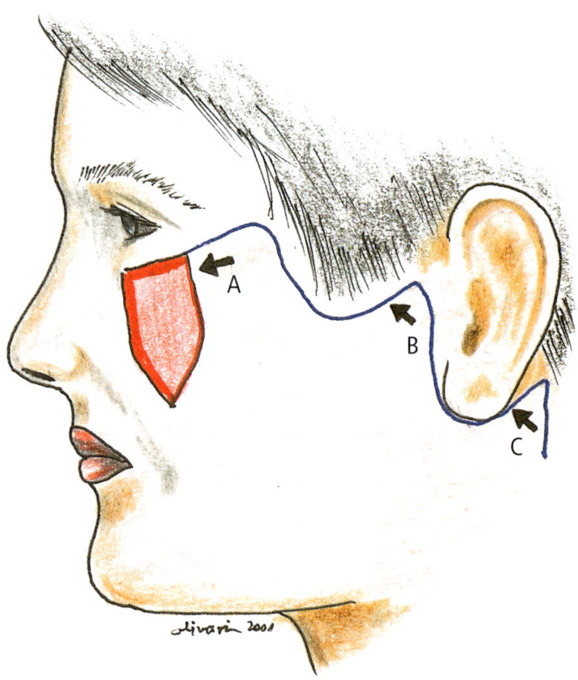

Figure 3.191b Planning of the operation (Mustardé type III). Because the patient has deep set preauricular hairs which with a normal rotation would come into the frontal part of the flap, the incision line is changes. The flap tip (A) is displaced medially in order to cover the defect. The preauricular part (B) is mobilized before the hairline and the retroauricular part (C) reaches the preauricular area.

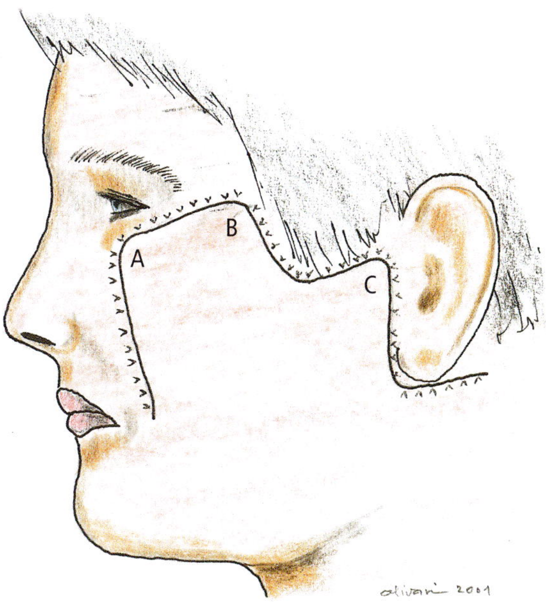

Figure 3.191c Consider: Rotation of points A, B and C. This rotation flap is indicated with severe preauricular hairiness.

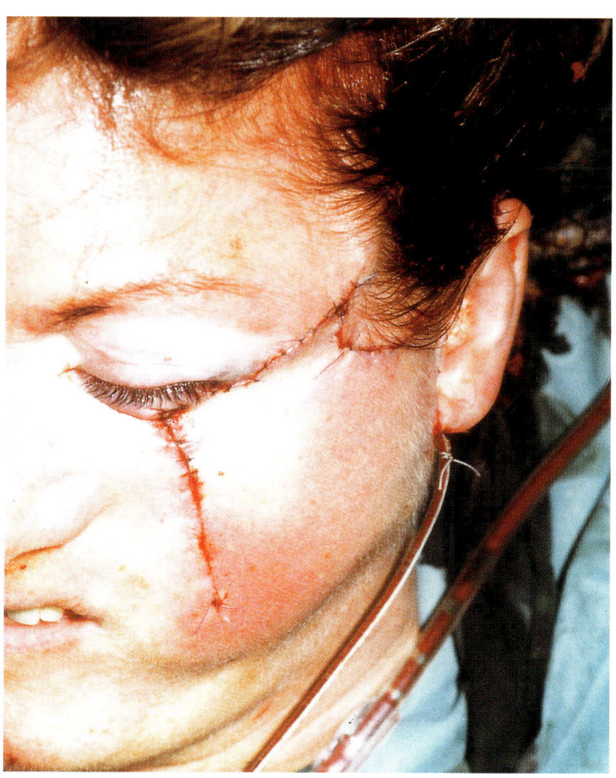

Figure 3.191d Picture at the end of the operation

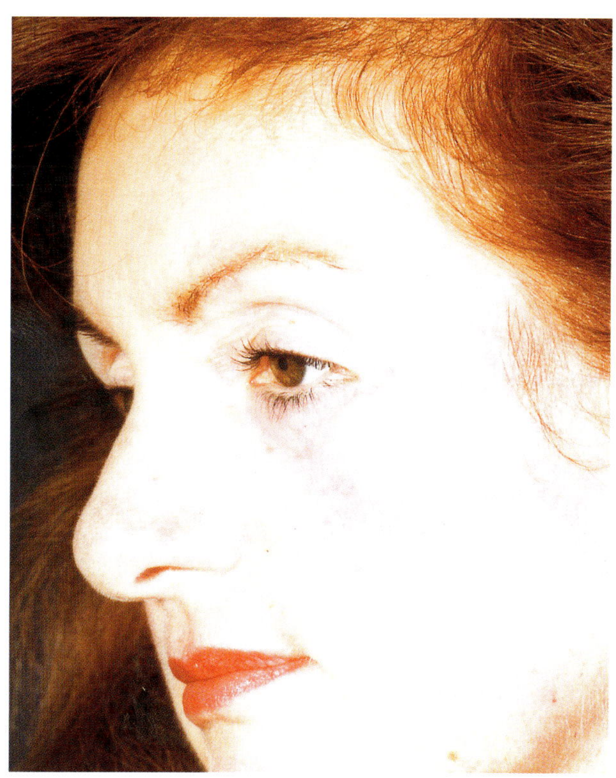

Figure 3.191e Aspect one year after the operation

Mustardé Type III Combined With a Full-Skin Graft

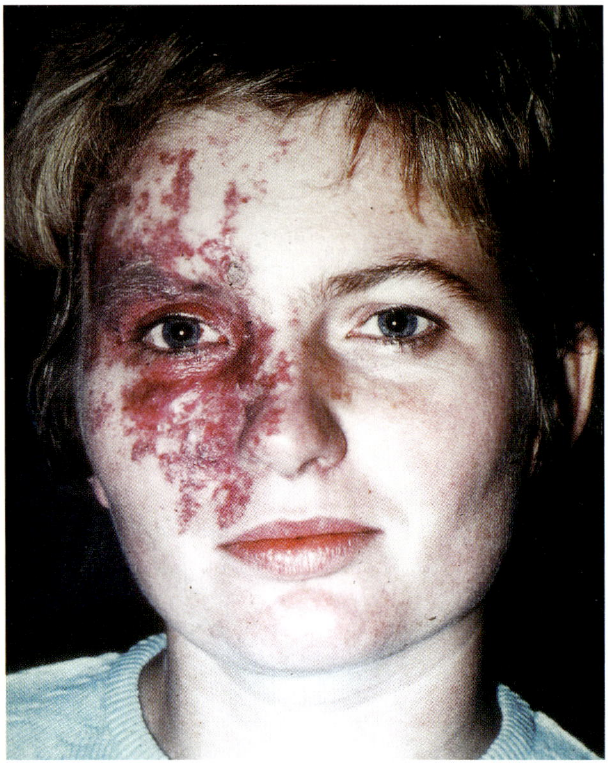

Figure 3.192a A so-called "Port-wine stain nevus" of the right cheek, nose, right side of the forehead as well as right upper and lower eyelid.

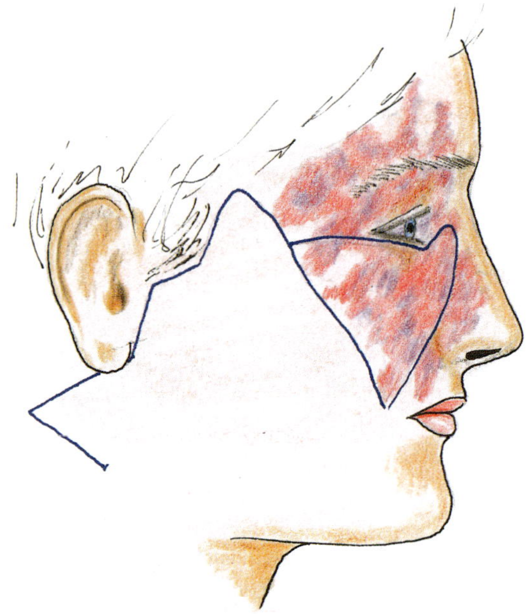

Figure 3.192b Planning of the first operation. By rotation flap from the right cheek a large part of the Port-wine stain nevus in the area of the right cheek, right nasal side as well as at the lower eyelid is treated.

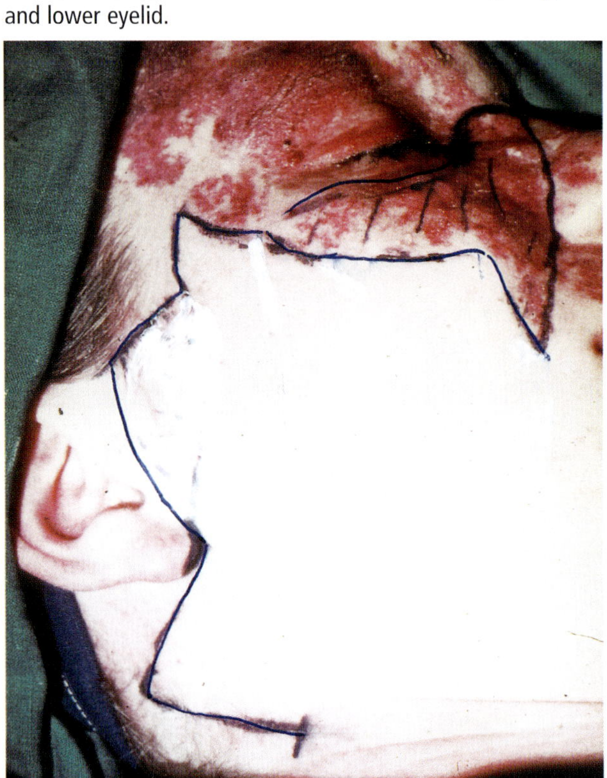

Figure 3.192c Planning of the flap

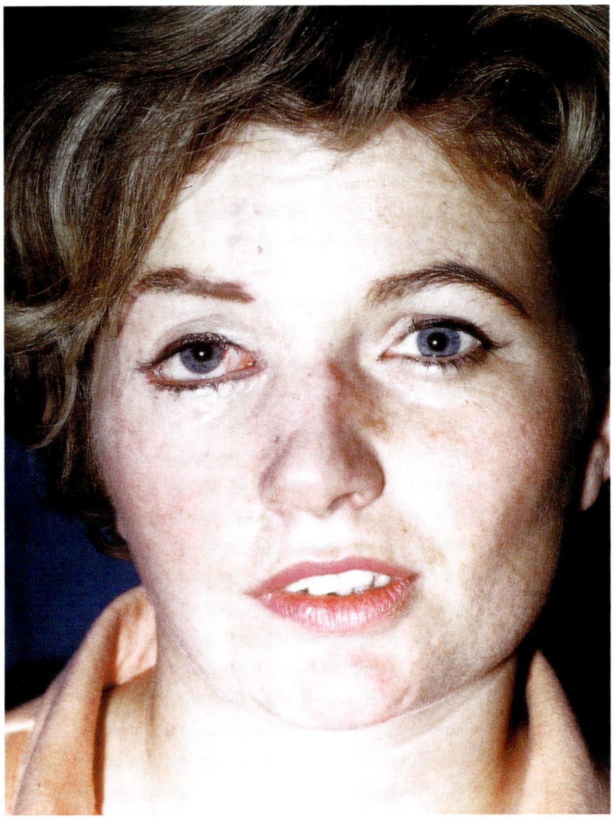

Figure 3.192d For a satisfactory result five operations are required within two years. Here the status two years after the last intervention.

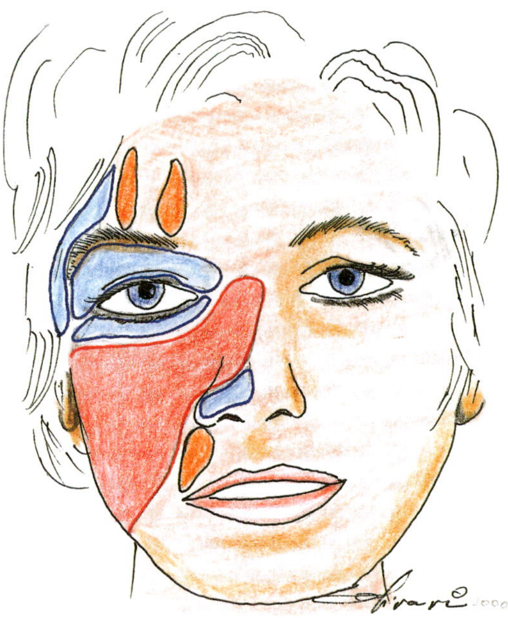

Figure 3.192e The following operations were carried out:
1. Rotation flap from the right cheek (red)
2. Excisions (orange)
3. Full thickness skin graft from the retroauricular area (blue)

Note: Laser therapy would of course be helpful these for small areas.

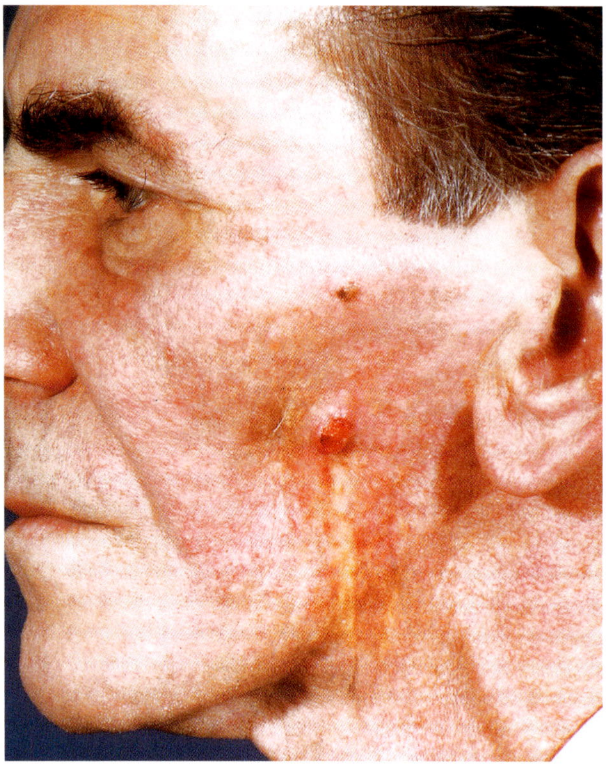

Figure 3.194a Relapse of a squamous cell carcinoma to the left preauricularly area – pre-irradiated

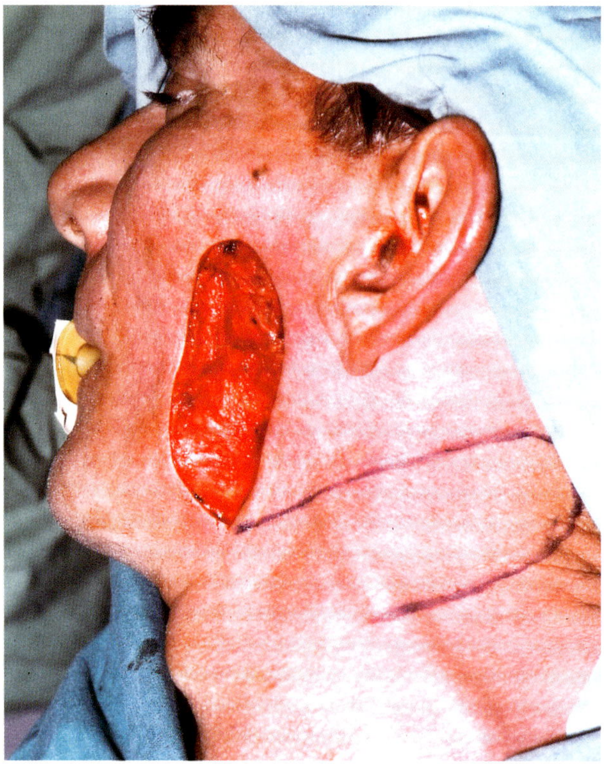

Figure 3.194b Excision of the tumor and planning of a medial pedicled platysma flap.

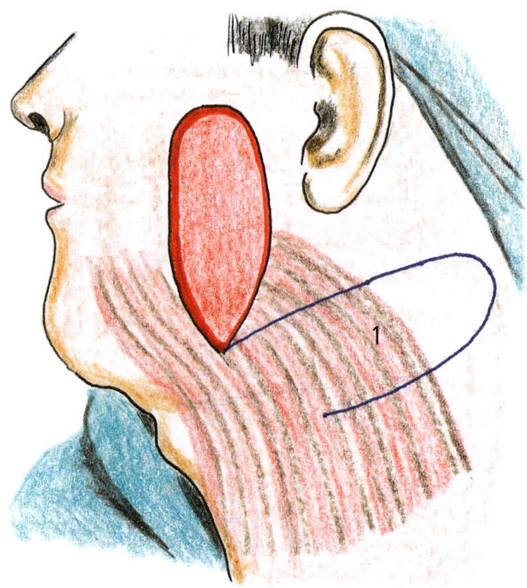

Figure 3.194c Cervico-retroauricular myocutaneous flap (1)

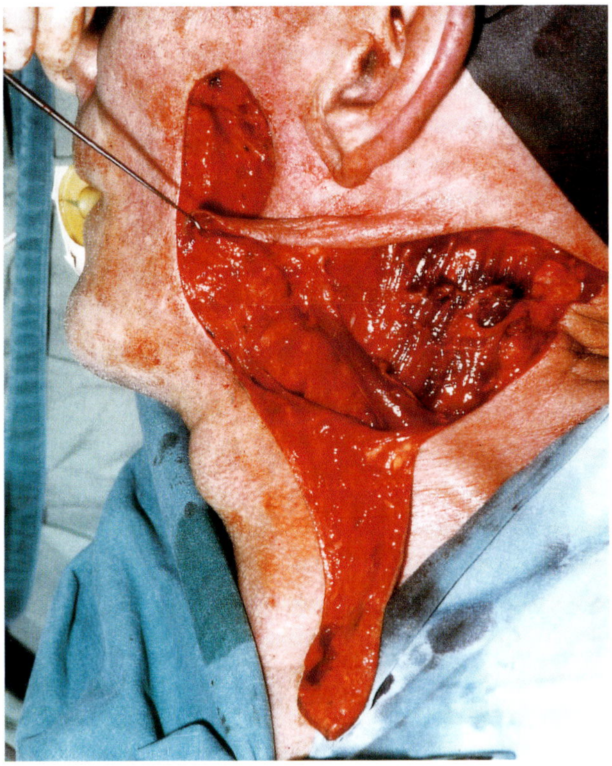

Figure 3.194d The flap is raised and a cervical lymphnode dissection is carried out. None of the 12 removed lymphnodes were afflicted.

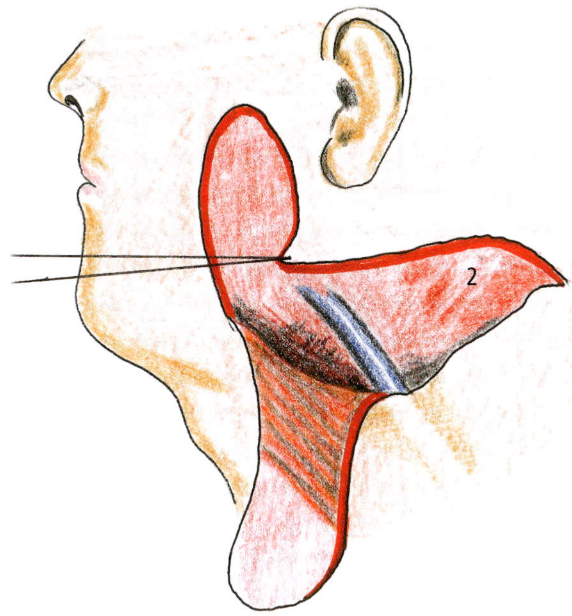

Figure 3.194e The secondary defect is closed primarily (2).

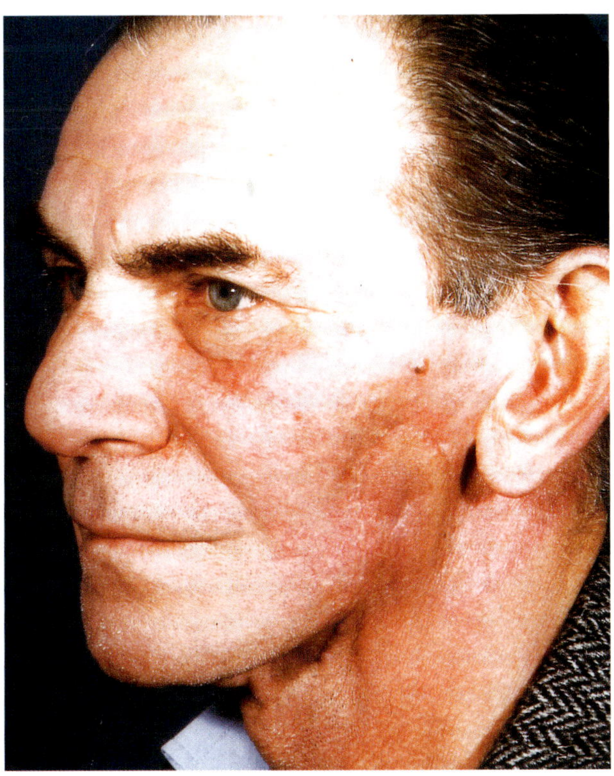

Figure 3.194f Aspect two years after the operation

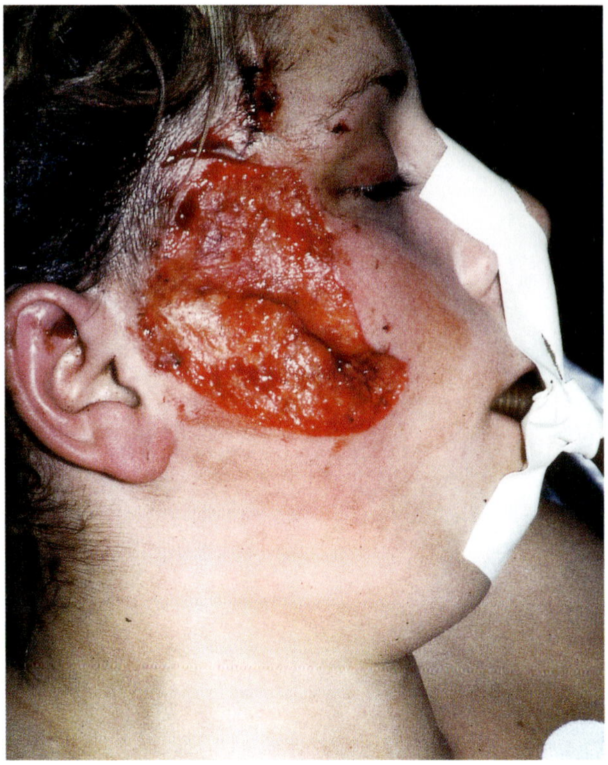

Figure 3.195a Defect of the right cheek, the preauricular area as well as the temporal region. A part of the hairy in temporal region is lost. The following therapies were discussed:
1. Mesh graft. Here however a well known dark pigmented coloring occurs as well as an irregular surface with unpleasant bad cosmetic results.
2. Free microsurgical flap (forearm flap). This procedure is technically favorable, since the superficial temporal artery is preserved; but there is almost always a severe thickening and varying color of the normal facial skin.
3. Local cervico-retroauricular flap

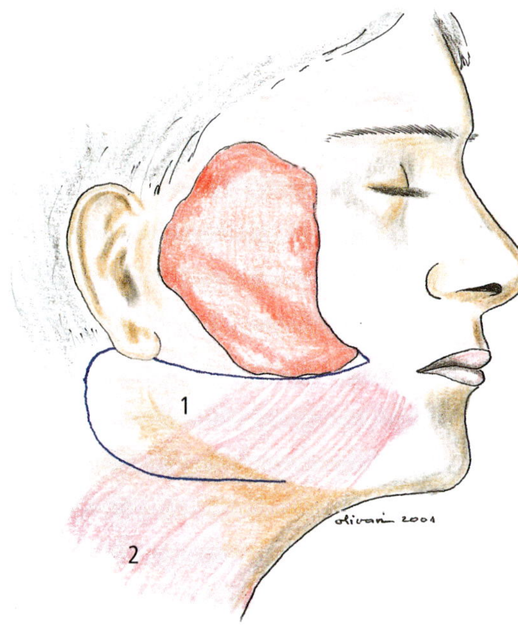

Figure 3.195b A cervico-retroauricular myocutaneous flap is planned (1) that is ventrally pedicled. In the frontal part of the flap the platysma is part of the flap. After flap removal the neck skin is mobilized far caudally (2) (as in a facelifting) so that a primary closure of donor site becomes possible and the scar is placed partly under the ear lobe and neck.

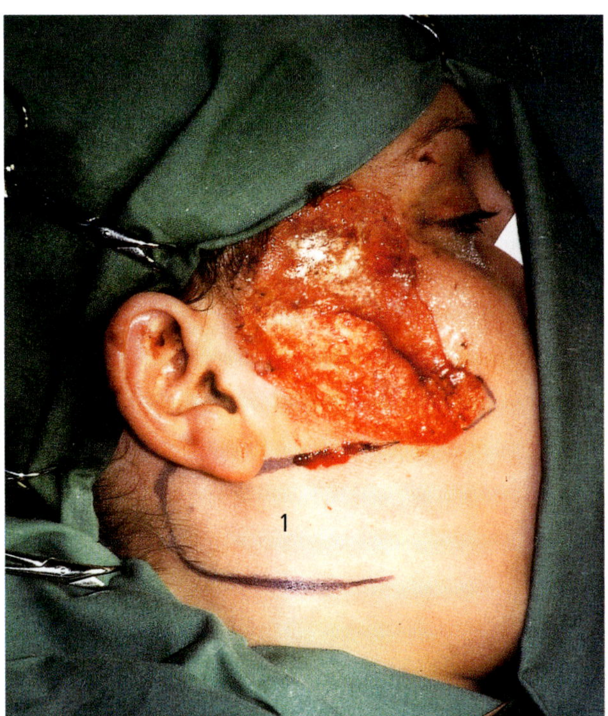

Figure 3.195c Planning of the cervico-retroauricular platysma flap. Tip of the flap includes retroauricular hairs.

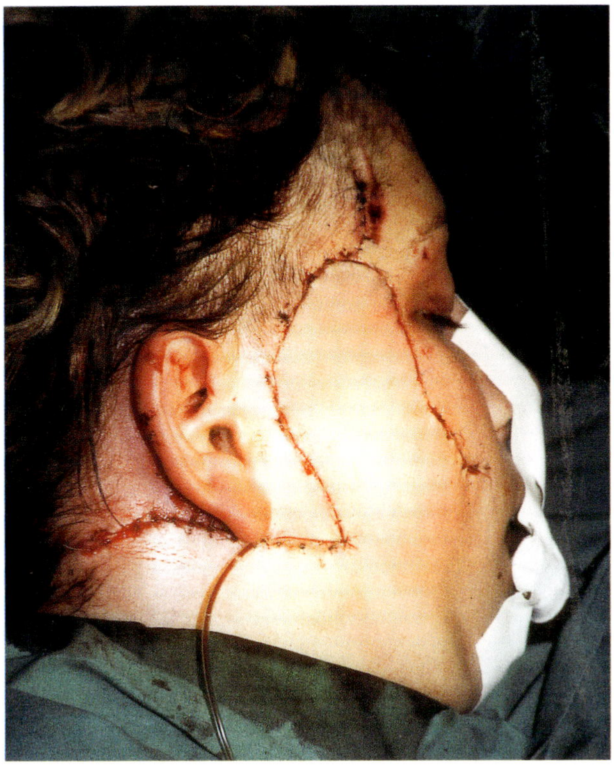

Figure 3.195d Picture at the end of the operation

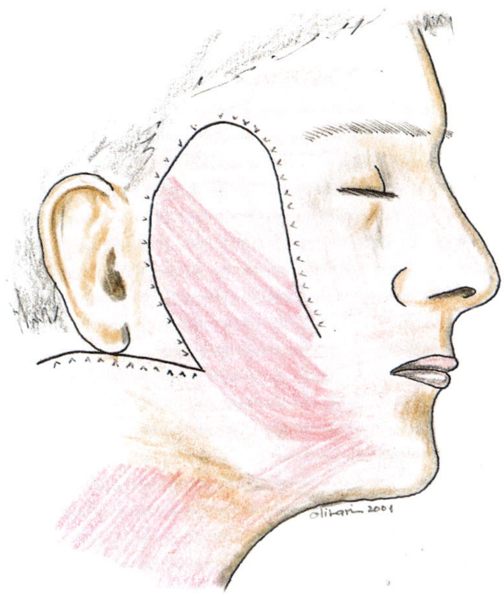

Figure 3.195e The schematic representation indicates how a part of the platysma remains incorporated in the flap.

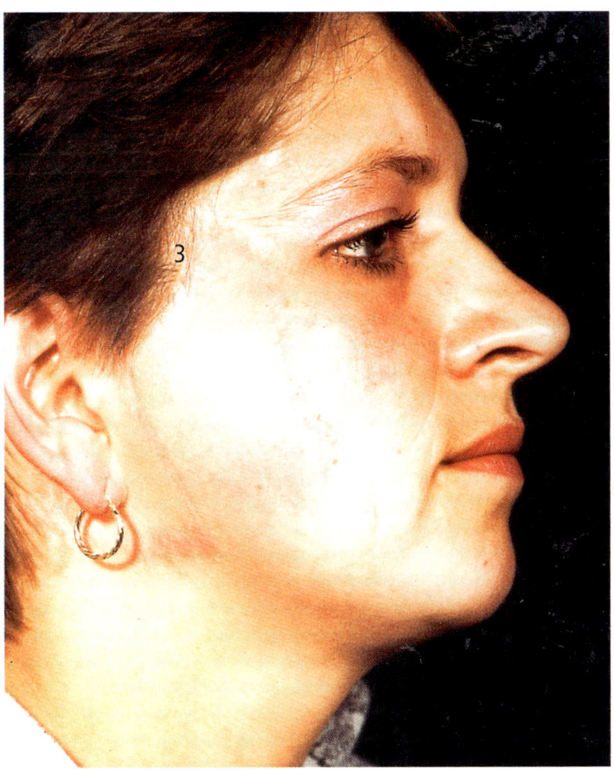

Figure 3.195f Aspect 14 months after the operation. Consider: The transposed retroauricular hairs grow out of the flap tip (3).

Result:
1) The defect is covered by a flap of the same color and quality.
2) Minimal scars.

b) Myocutaneous Pectoral Flap

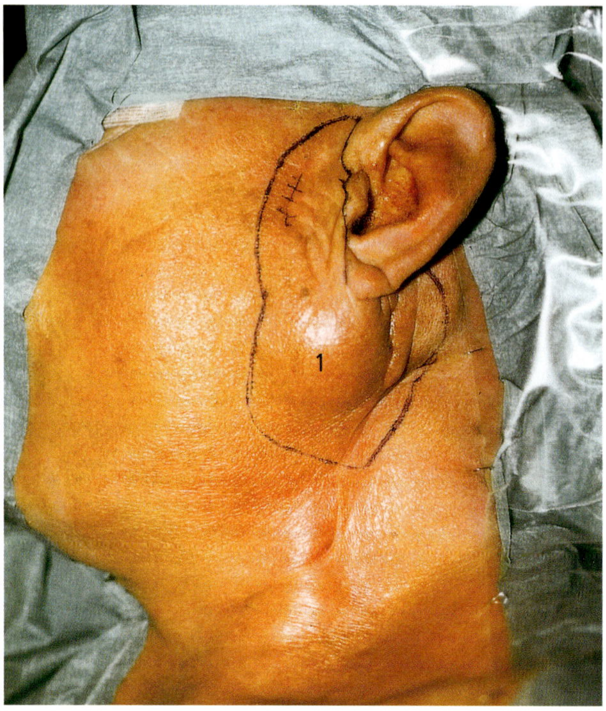

Figure 3.196a Preauricular basal cell carcinoma. The tumor grows in an infiltrating manner in the deeper layers with infiltration of the parotid gland (1).

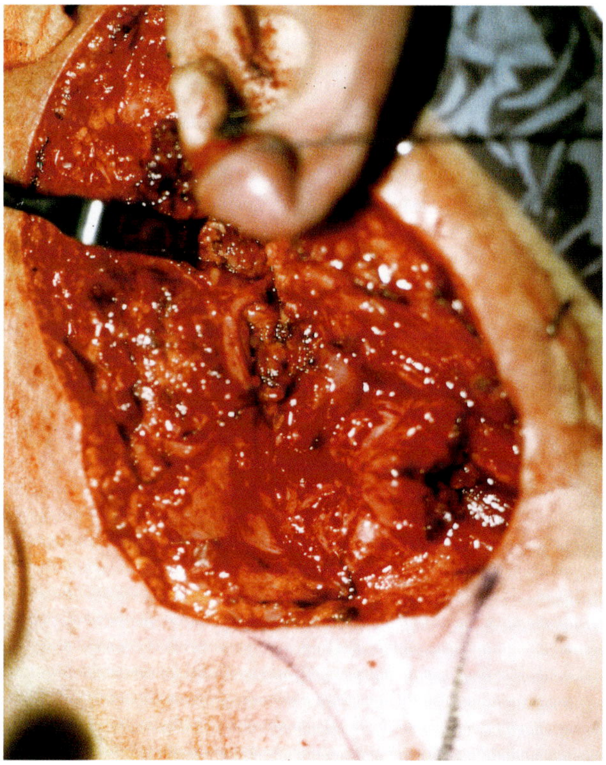

Figure 3.196b Situation after resection whereby the facial nerve is spared. The greater part of the parotid gland has been resected.

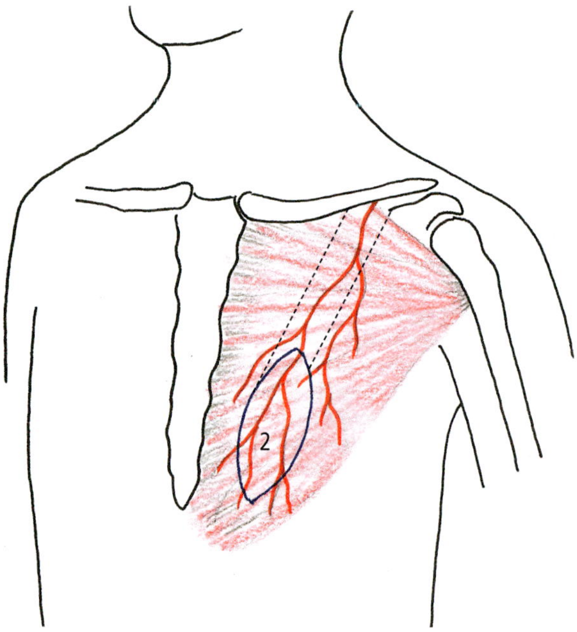

Figure 3.196c Preparation of a myocutaneous pectoral island flap (2), that is pedicled at the thoracoacromial artery. The vessels are long enough in order to reach the cheek.

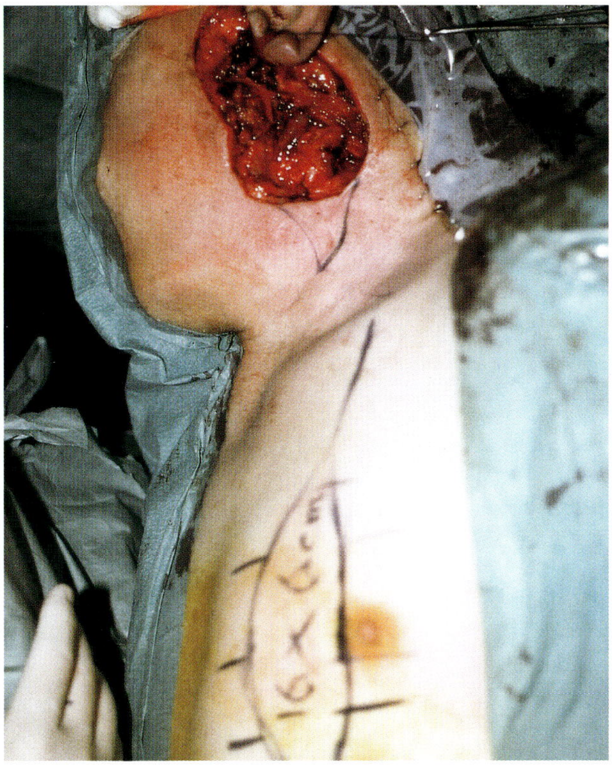

Figure 3.196d Formation of a myocutaneous pectoral flap (2) of 16 × 6 cm that is pulled into the defect area via a subcutaneous tunnel.

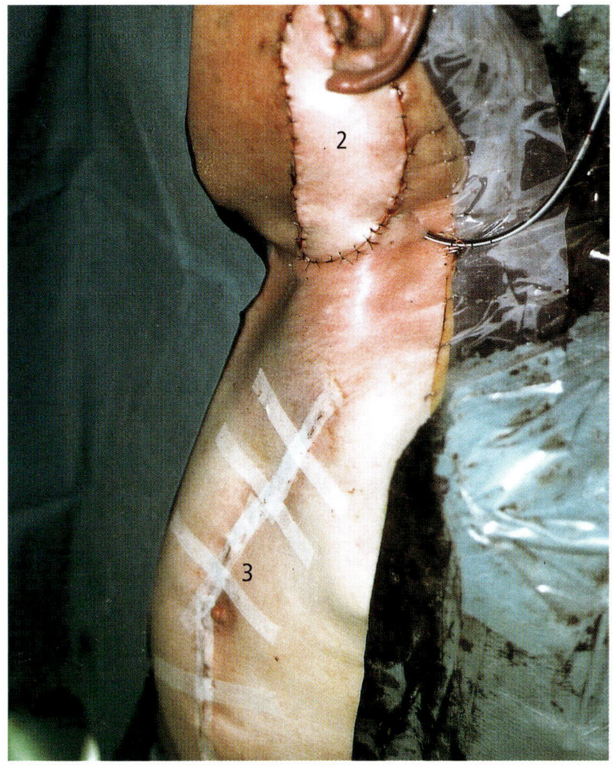

Figure 3.196e Status at the end of the operation. The secondary defect is closed primarily (3).

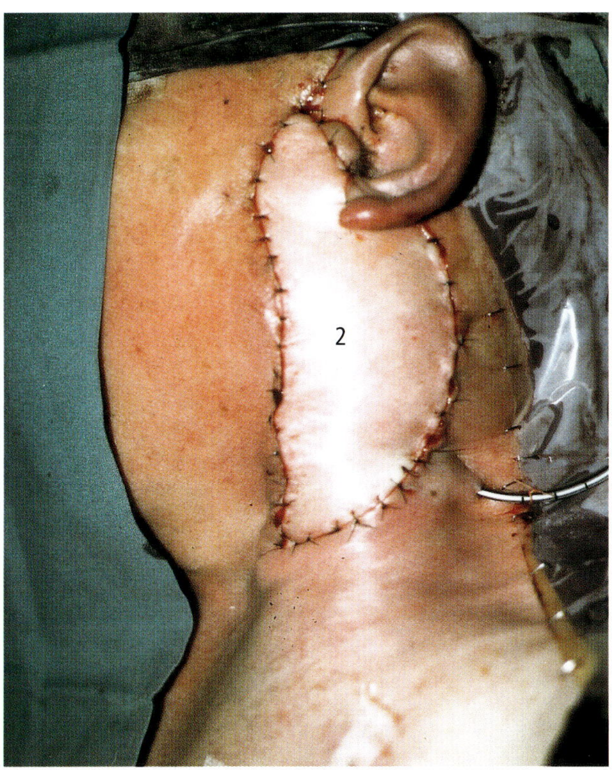

Figure 3.196f Excellent perfusion of the flap

Pectoral Island Flap

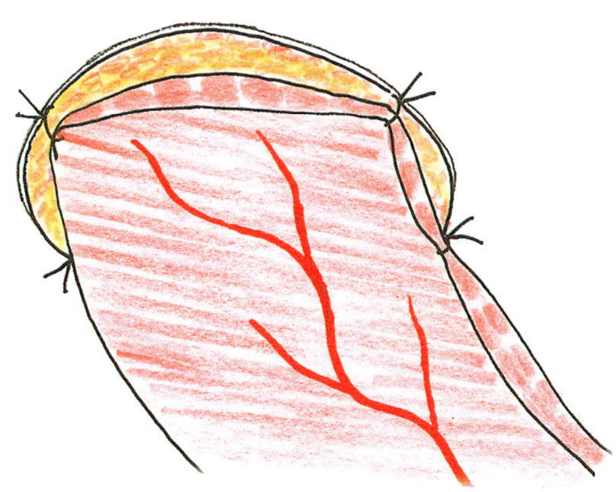

Figure 3.196g The island flap is fixed with a few sutures at the muscle to prevent damage of vessels during the manipulation.

Pectoral Island Flap

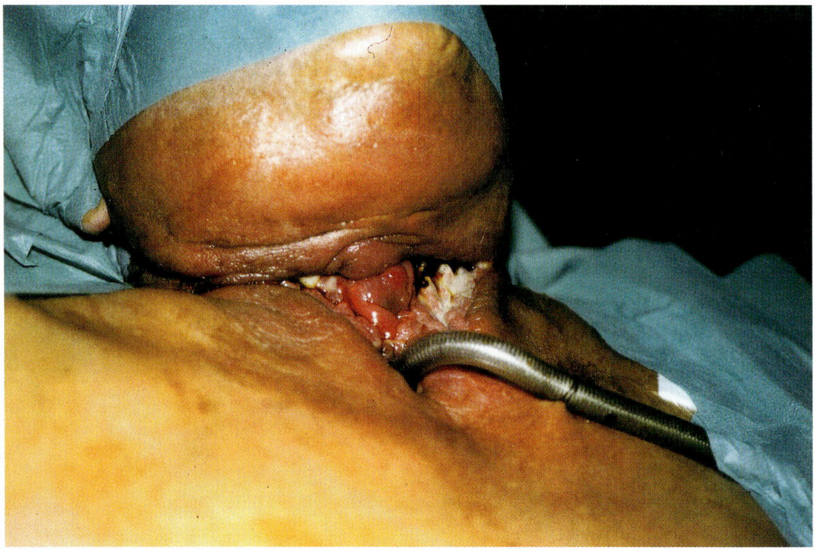

Figure 3.197a Defect at the neck two years after resection of a laryngeal carcinoma and following irradiation. Tracheostomy.

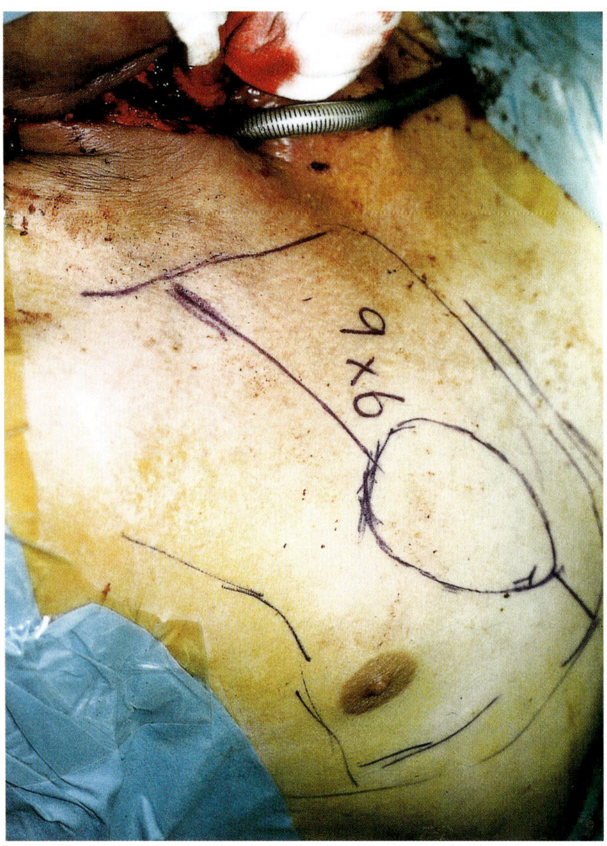

Figure 3.197b Planning of a pectoral island flap on the right side. The flap size is 9 × 6 cm.

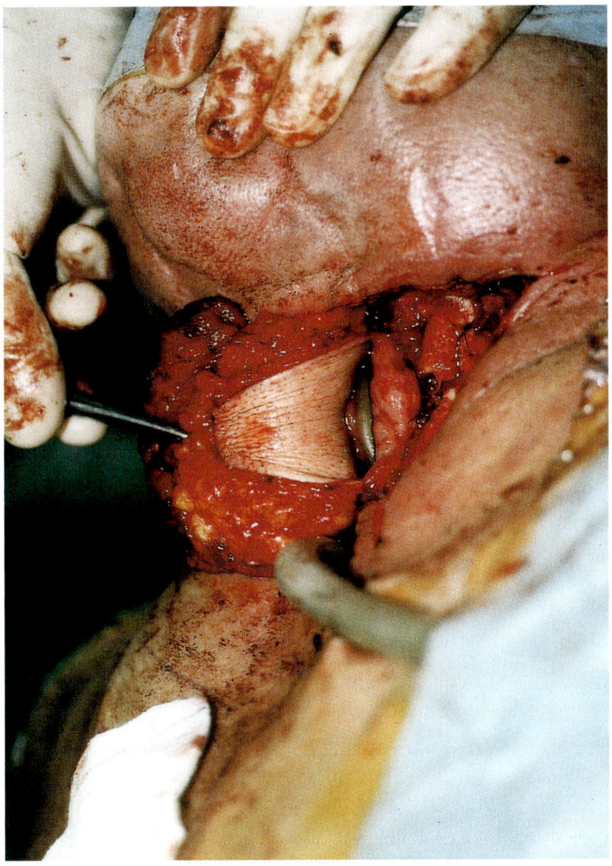

Figure 3.197c After debridement and a new tracheostomy, the pectoral island flap is pulled through a subcutaneous tunnel. The skin of the pectoral flap is used as an inner lining. The external part is covered with a mesh graft.

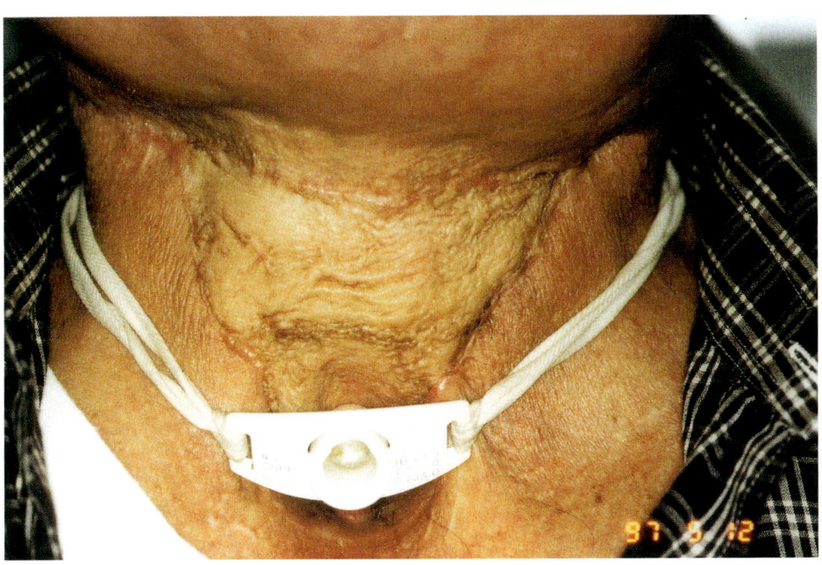

Figure 3.197d Status three years after the operation

Free Flaps

a) Free Parascapular Flap (Deepithelialized)

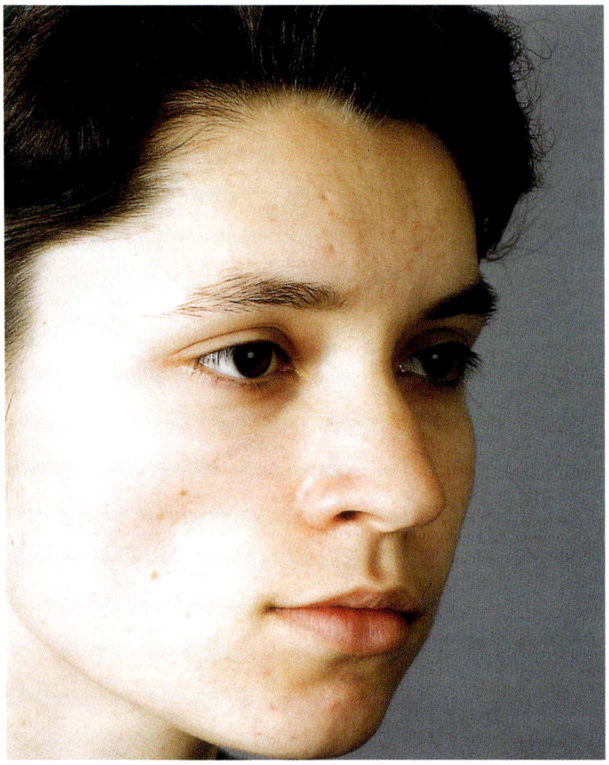

Figure 3.198a Romberg's disease (facial hemiatrophy) of the right cheek. Status after unsuccessful fat tissue implantation.

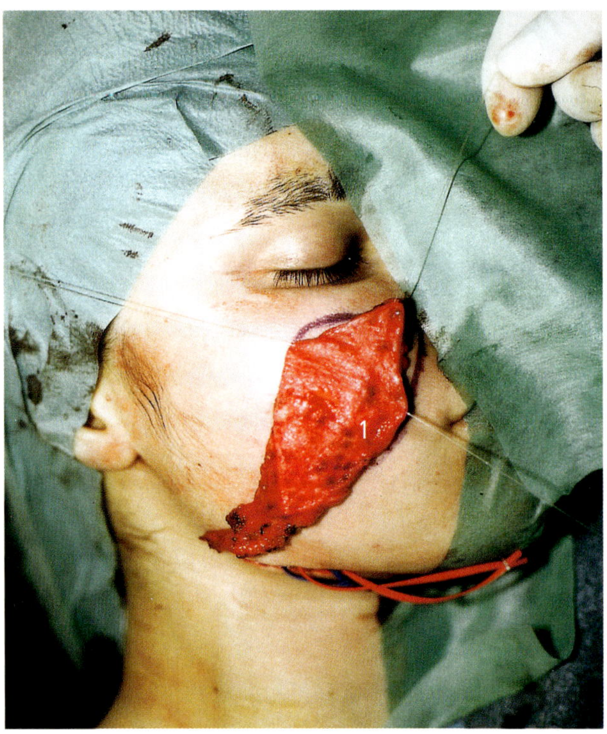

Figure 3.198b The deepithelialized parascapular flap (1) is used as a volume replacement into the cheek. The scapular circumflex artery is anastomosed with the facial artery. The flap is fixed through a subcutaneous tunnel into the affected cheek area without leaving a scar in the face. The incision is placed below the mandible.

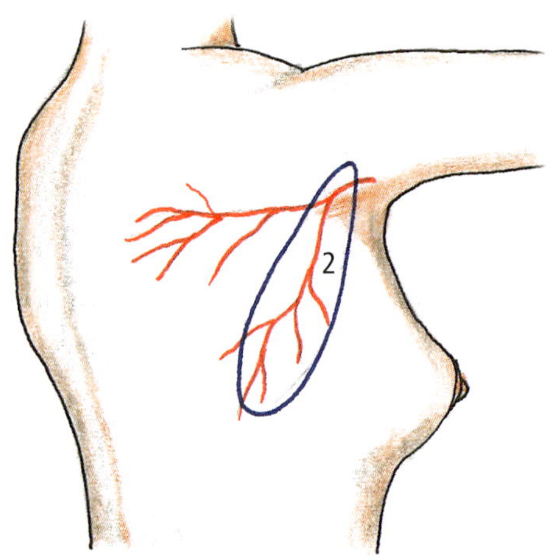

Figure 3.198c The deepithelialized parascapular flap is removed. **Note** the course of the inferior scapular circumflex artery in the flap (2).

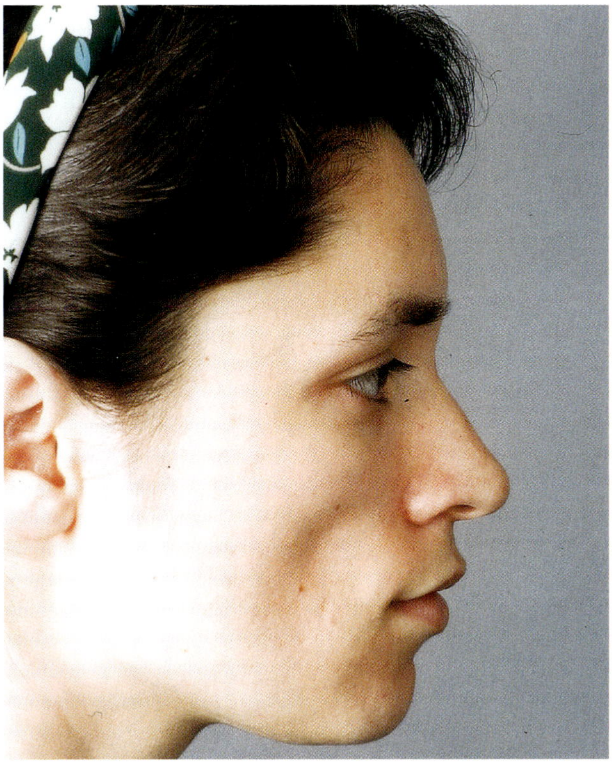

Figure 3.198d Situation before the operation

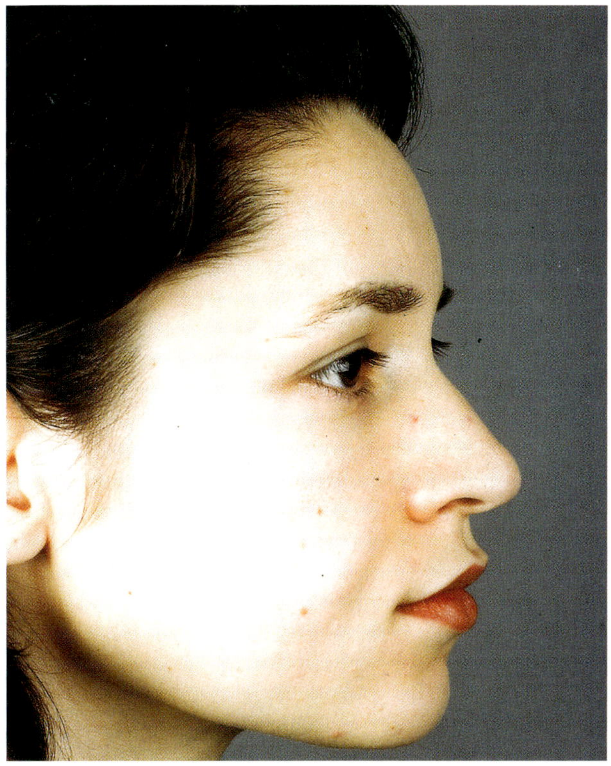

Figure 3.198e Picture taken two-and-a-half years after the operation. The face volume was adjusted. There are no signs of an atrophy of the graft.

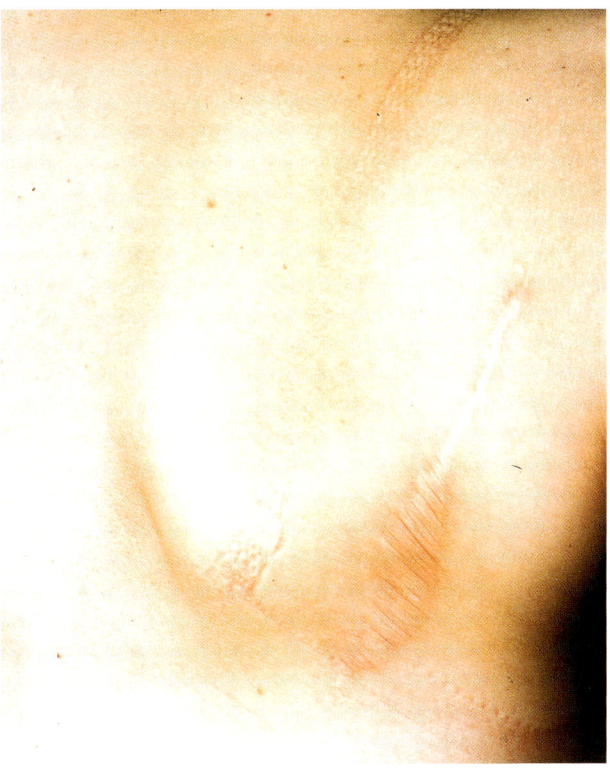

Figure 3.198f Secondary defect two-and-a-half years after the operation

b) Free Radial Flap

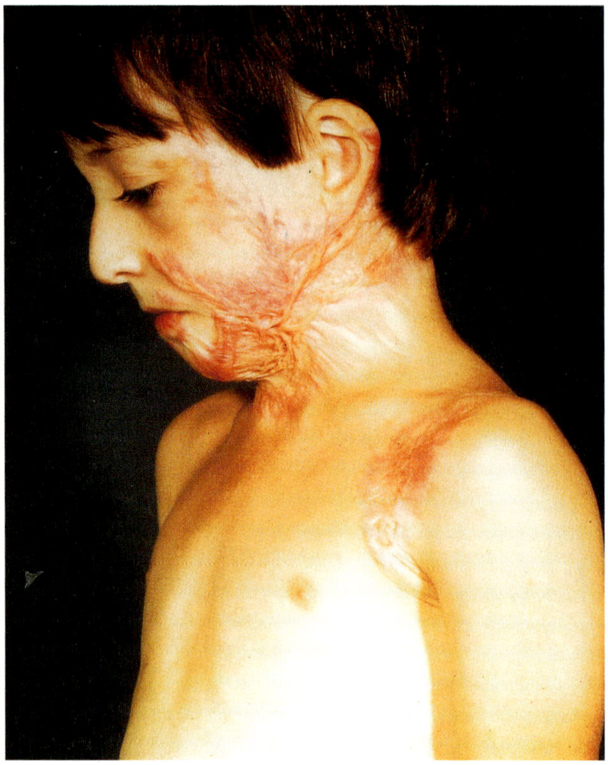

Figure 3.199a Contracting burn scars at the neck. Twice it was attempted to improve function using a skin graft.

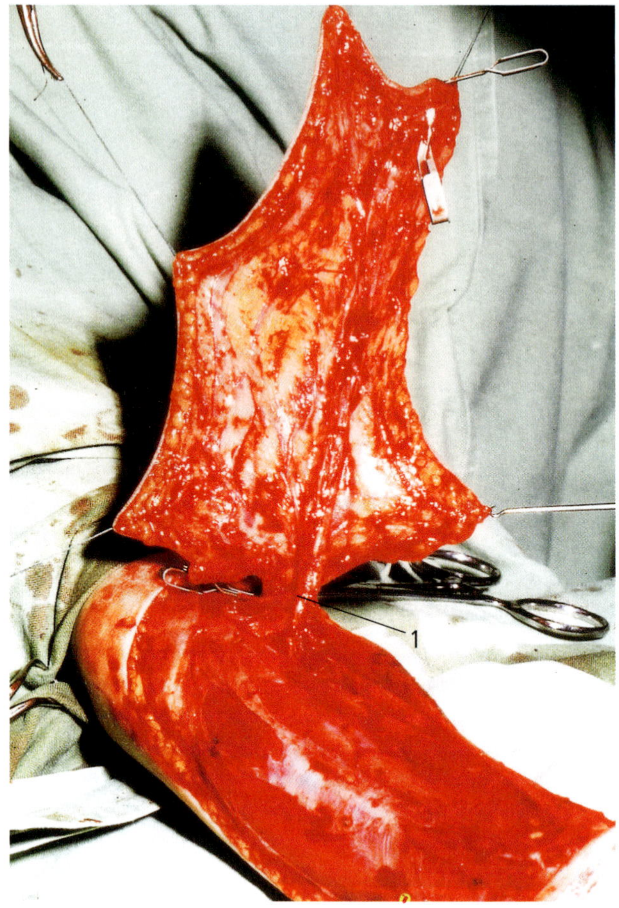

Figure 3.199b Preparation of a free radial flap, that on the illustration is only pediculated at the. radial artery and the comitant veins (1).

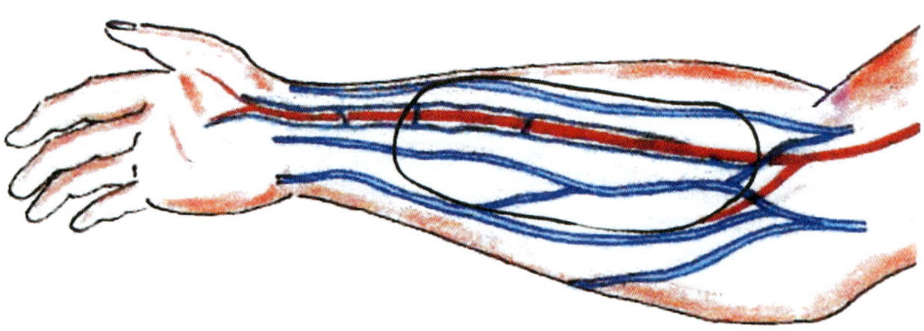

Figure 3.199c Before rising of the radial flap it must be tested whether the ulnar artery is intact and if the palmar arch is intact. In rare cases the ulnar artery does not suffice for a hand perfusion.

Test: Compress the radial artery tightly. If the hand after three minutes becomes white and pains occur, the radial flap can not be used. Or use Doppler.

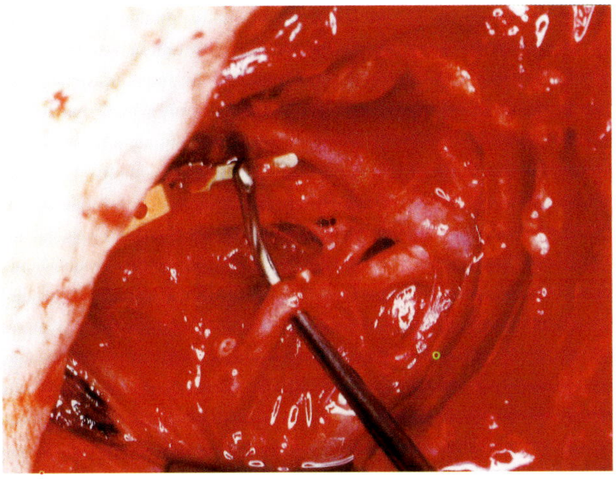

Figure 3.199d The superior thyroid artery is prepared for anastomosis. Radial flap is severed from its initial position and the radial artery is anastomosed with the superior thyroid artery, just as the accompanying veins are.

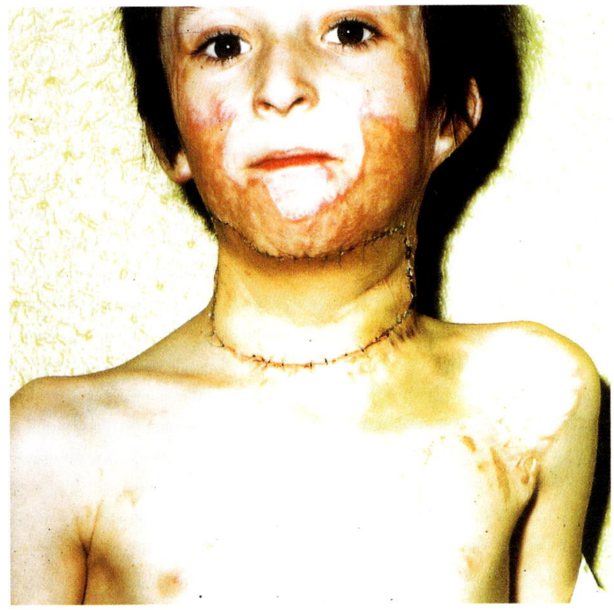

Figure 3.199e Situation ten days after the operation. Six months later two Z-flaps were carried out at both lateral sides of the flap in order to achieve a better aesthetic and functional result.

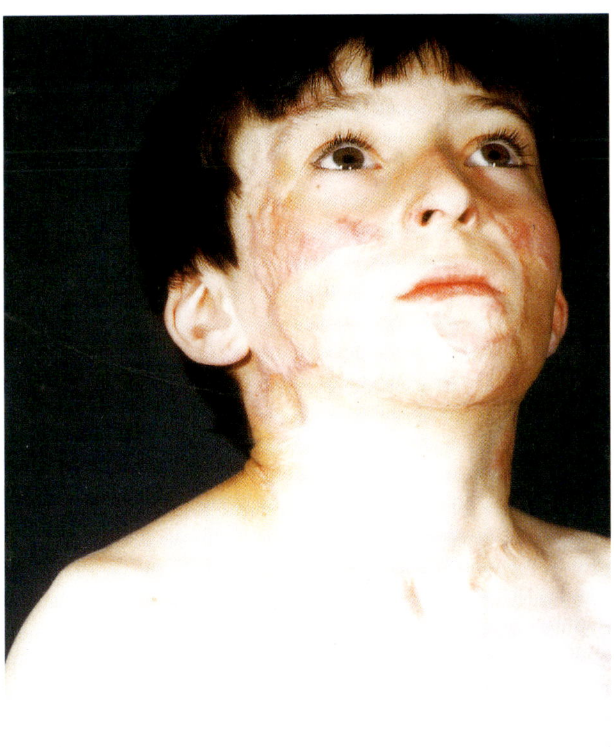

Figure 3.199f Picture taken two years after the operation. Functional and aesthetic result.

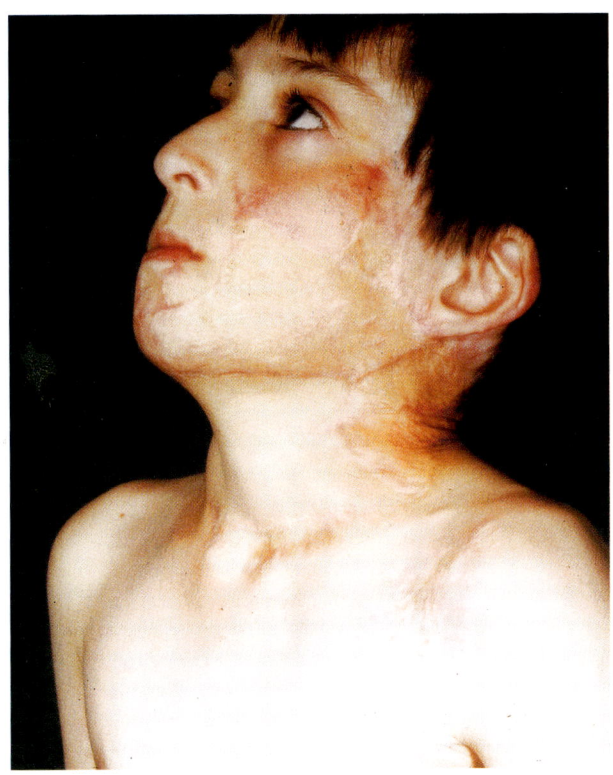

Figure 3.199g The radial flap is good indication for severe contractures in the neck area.

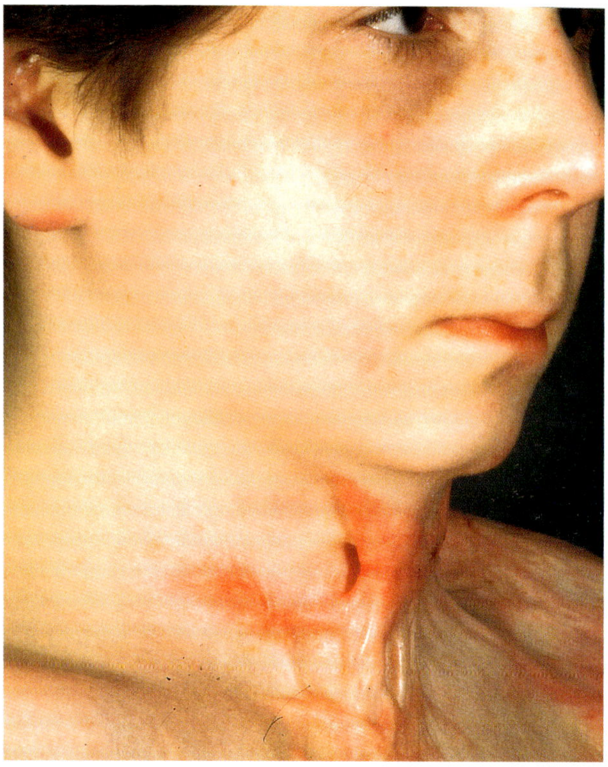

Figure 3.200a Neck contracture with keloids after burn injury

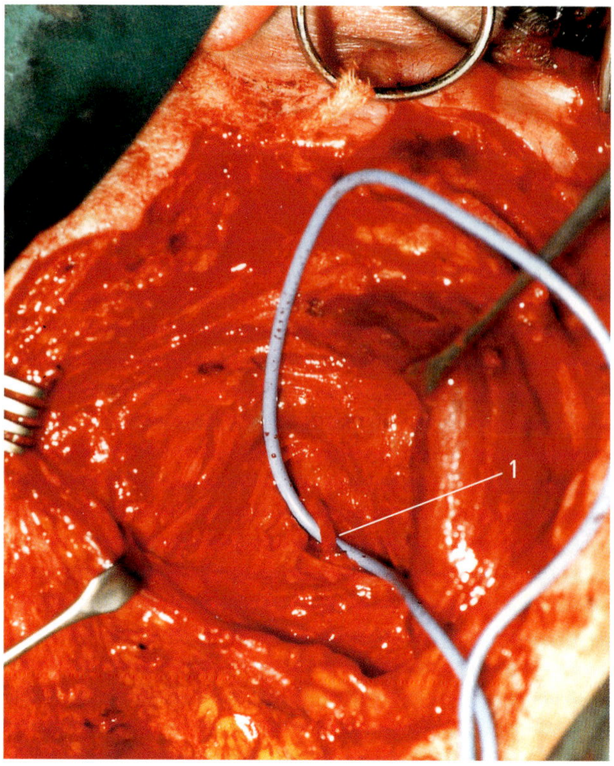

Figure 3.200b The scars are resected and at the same time the superior thyroid artery was prepared for the anastomosis (1).

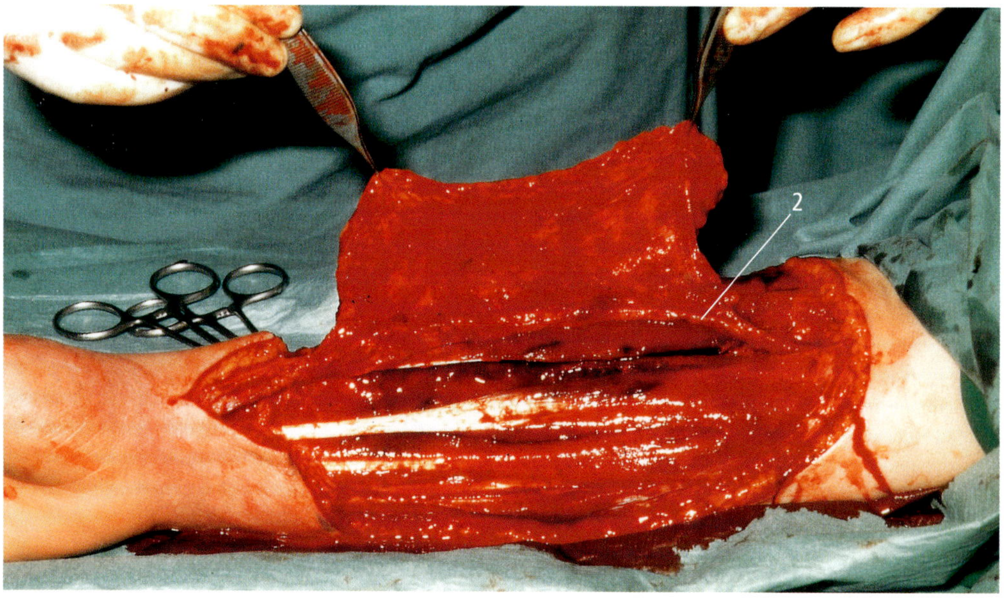

Figure 3.200c Preparation of a large radial flap.
The radial artery is visible with two accompanying veins (2).

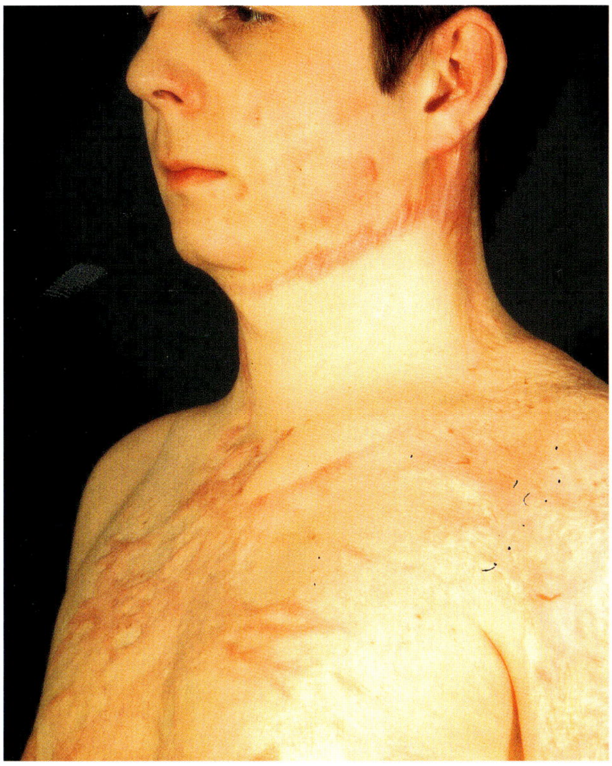

Figure 3.200d Aesthetic and functional result three years after the operation

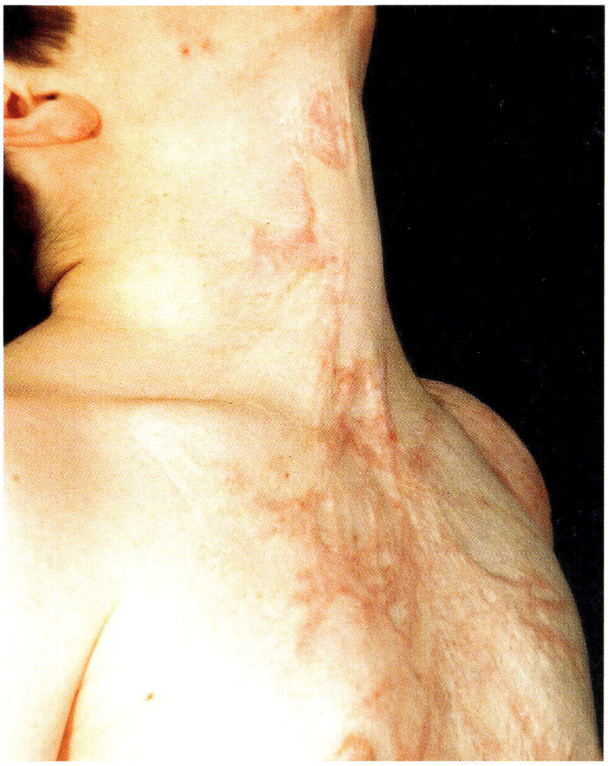

Figure 3.200e Aspect three years after the operation

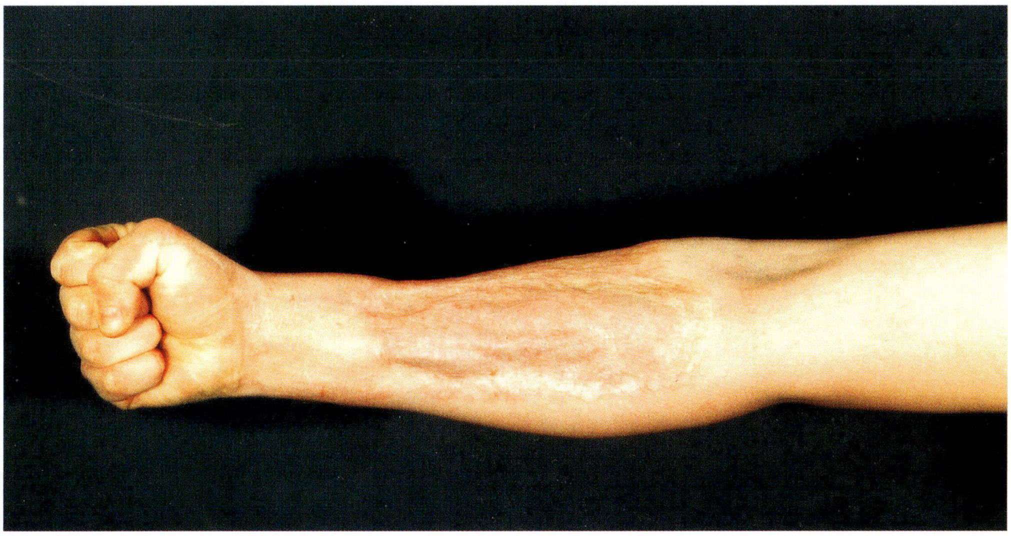

Figure 3.200f The secondary defect is tolerable

History of "Noma"

Classical authors such as Galen or Celsus already used the term "Noma", although still not specifically, for a rapidly spreading gangrenous inflammation of soft facial parts in children. In the 14th century the Flemish surgeon Jan Yperman in his "Chyrurgie" wrote about "water canker" in his chapter about diseases of the mouth. The first clinical description of this disease appeared in the "Handboeck der Chirurgyen" written by the Dutch doctor Carolus Battus in 1595. In Germany this disease that was endemic in Europe until the 19th century was described by Adolph Leopold Richter in his book "The water cancer of children" (Berlin 1828) – that up until then and for a further 173 years was the only work concerning itself with Noma. Due to the unknown cause the disease has received many synonymous names, such as cancrum oris, water cancer, mouth cancer, gangraena scorbutica, burning mouth ulcer, aphthae serpentes, Todtenwurm and many other names over the course of history. Because of its appearance, Noma is often falsely associated with cancer.

One of the First Surgical Attempts to Treat a Noma Defect Dated Back in 1781

Contrary to frequent assumptions, the term Noma that is often used today and that first emerged from the Dutch surgeon Cornelis van de Voorde in 1680 is not an acronym, but is much rather a term of Greek origin that meant "grass" or "meadowland", and is metaphoric for the rapid disappearance of soft facial parts due to the disease. The term "cancrum oris" that is still on occasion used today is a grammatical error which has strangely haunted the literature since 1649, whether it be due to tradition or pure ignorance, as was already noted by an American physician at the beginning of the 19th century. In 1765 the Swedish physician Gabriel Lund presented a series of 11 diseased children in the Proceedings of the Royal Academy of Sciences, and almost at the same time a British physician observed that measles frequently precedes a Noma infection. One of the first surgical treatments dated 1781 was carried out by the surgeon Leendert Stelwagen, who successfully closed a lip defect caused by a Noma using a surgical technique employed for the treatment of cleft lip, jaw and palate. Approximately 100 years later a number of surgeons, particularly in Germany, dealt intensively with the surgical therapy of Noma, including Johann Friedrich Dieffenbach, Victor von Bruns and Friedrich von Esmarch. With the gradual improvement in living conditions for the poorer classes since the end of the 19th century, Noma ultimately disappeared little by little from European and North American hospitals.

Noma: Necrotizing or gangrenous inflammation of the oral mucosa and cheeks. In its advanced stage jaw and facial bone defects also arise. The illness occurs exclusively amongst children after infections (measles, typhoid fever, scarlet fever), malnutrition and poor hygiene.
Pathogen: Borrelius and Fusobacteria.
Primary therapy: Antibiotics.

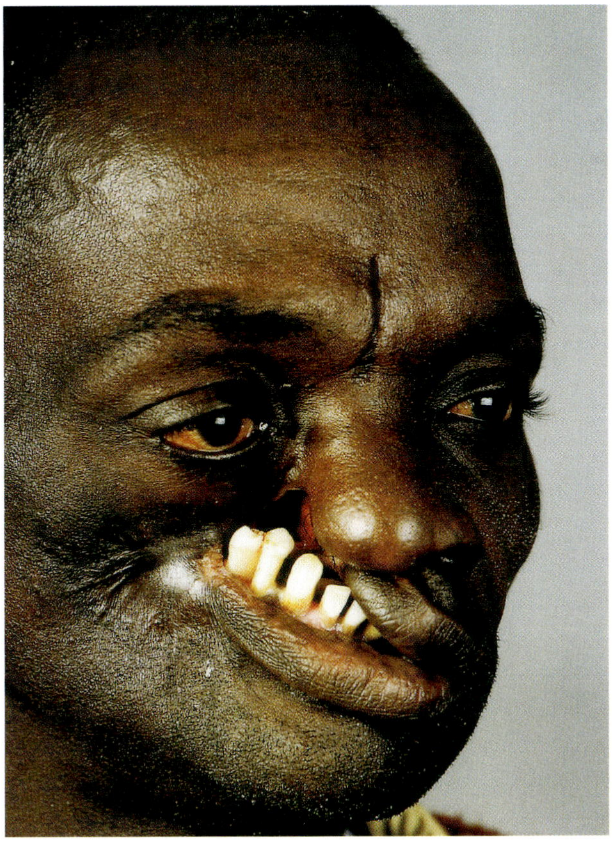

Figure 3.201a Noma of the right facial side. Anamnesis of approximately eight years. Lacking tissues: Upper lip, part of the right cheek, part of the upper jaw.

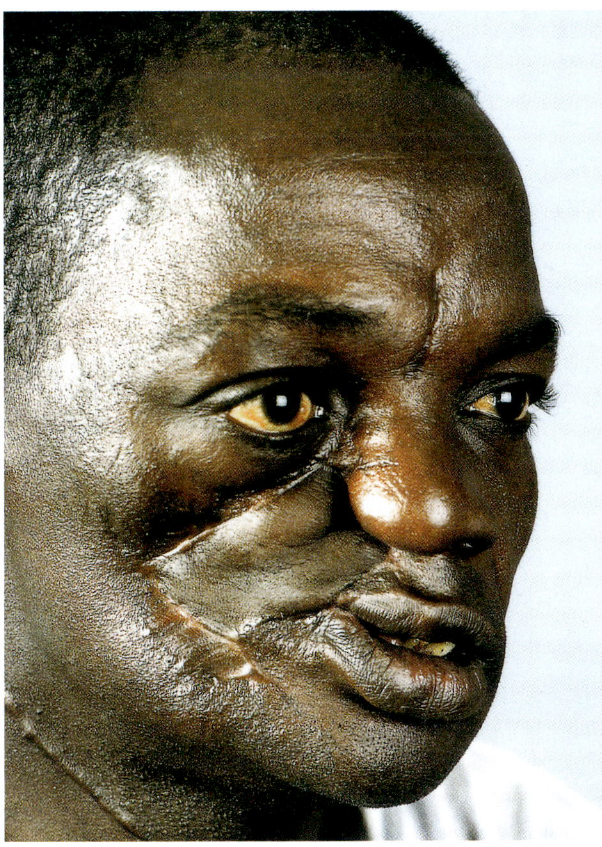

Figure 3.201b Status four months after the operation. The temporal fascia was applied for the inner lining and the free radial flap was used for the outer cover. Connection to facial vein and artery.

Expander and Defect Coverage

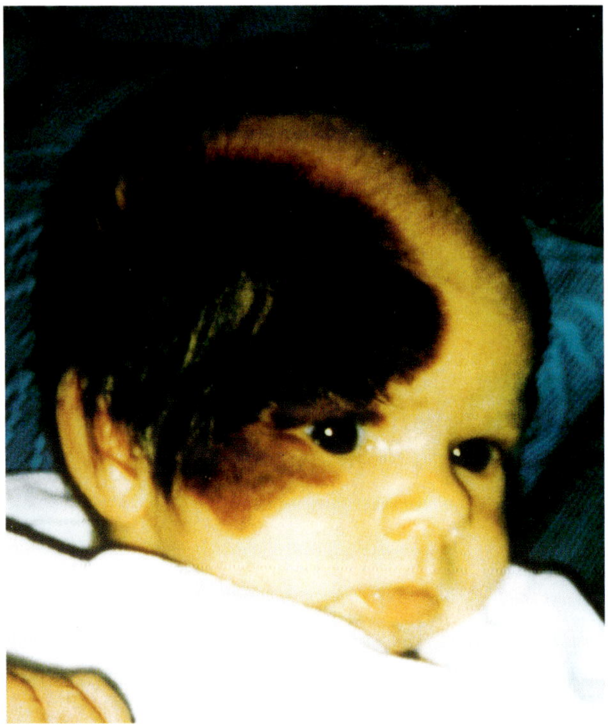

Figure 3.202a Giant nevus of the right cheek, right side of forehead, temporal region as well as the right upper and lower eyelids

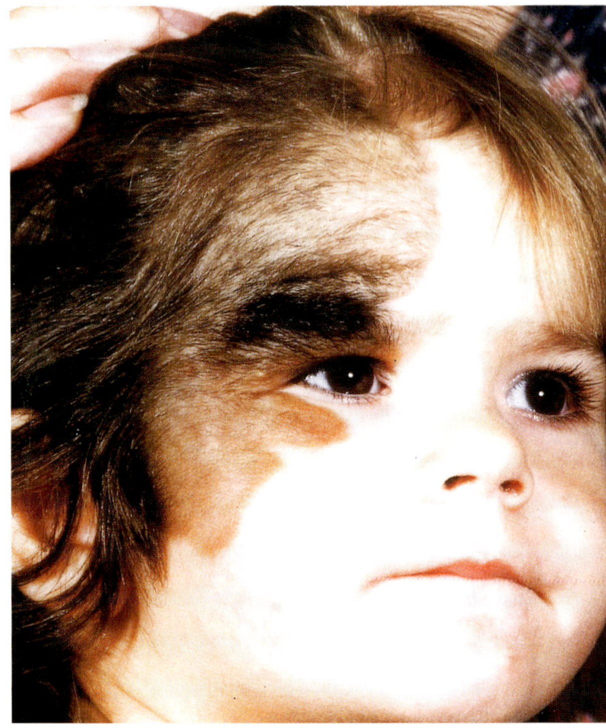

Figure 3.202b Different procedures such as grinding off and laser therapy were attempted without success. The nevus is only a little paler and the area has become smaller.

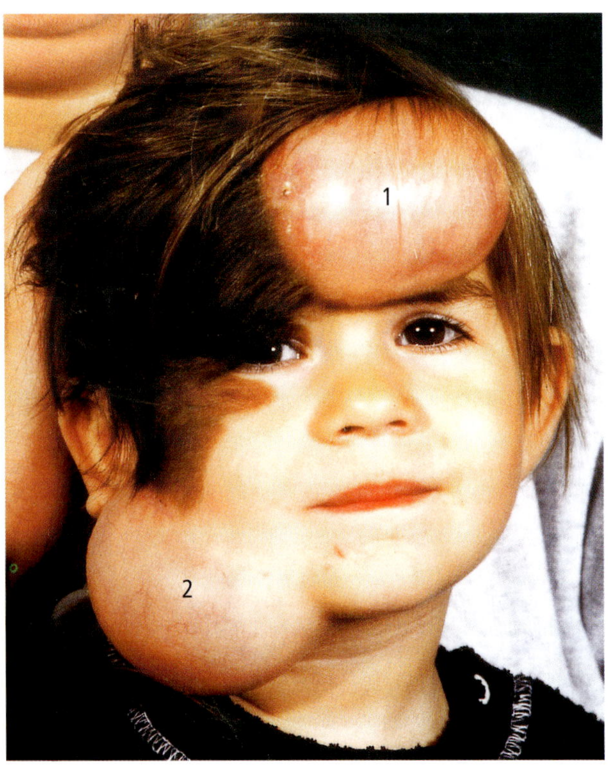

Figure 3.202c Two expanders were implanted:
– In the forehead area an rectangular expander of 180 ccm (1)
– On the neck area an oval expander of 220 ccm
During the course of four weeks the expander was filled in the forehead to 170 ccm and at the throat to 230 ccm (2). In this way a large area of healthy skin could be won.

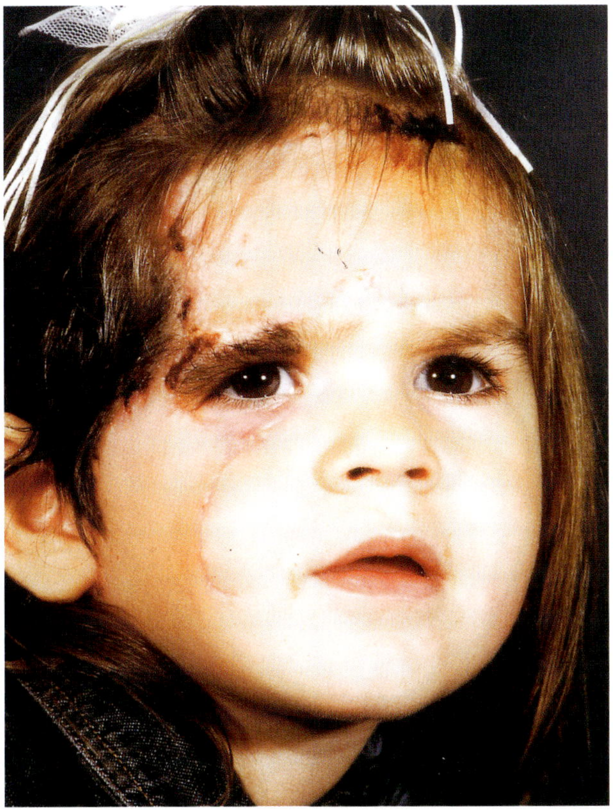

Figure 3.202d After removal of the two expanders the stretched healthy skin was expanded in the forehead area up to the temporal area. The stretched skin of the right cheek as well as the throat area was expanded so that the entire right cheek, the right preauricular area and the right lower eyelid could be covered. A residue still remained at the right upper eyelid and the right temporal area.

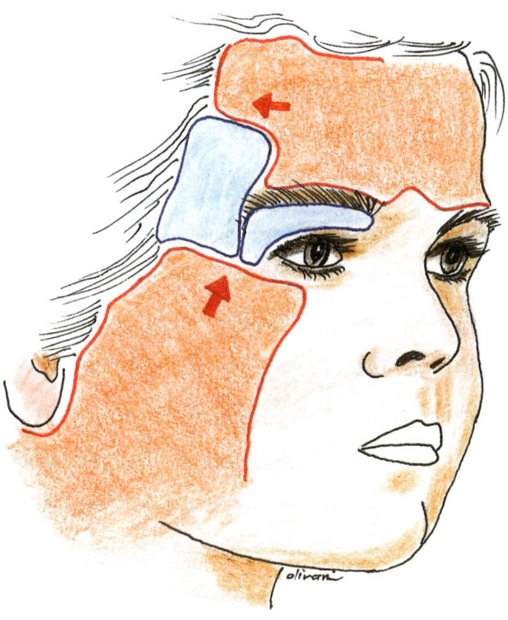

Figure 3.202e Red: Areas that could be covered by skin obtained through expansion. Blue: Full skin thickness graft from the retroauricular area.

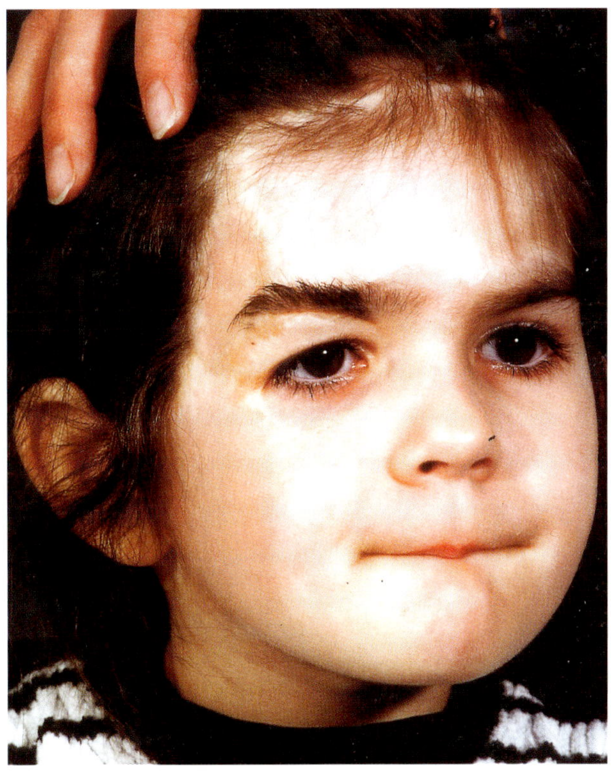

Figure 3.202f Status two years after the operation: Good aesthetic and functional results. The full skin grafts at the temporal area and the upper eyelid hardly showed any difference in color to the normal skin. In all only three operations within three months result was achieved

1. Expander implantation
2. Expander removal and forming
3. Full skin thickness graft

Coverage of Large-Area Defects Using Different Techniques

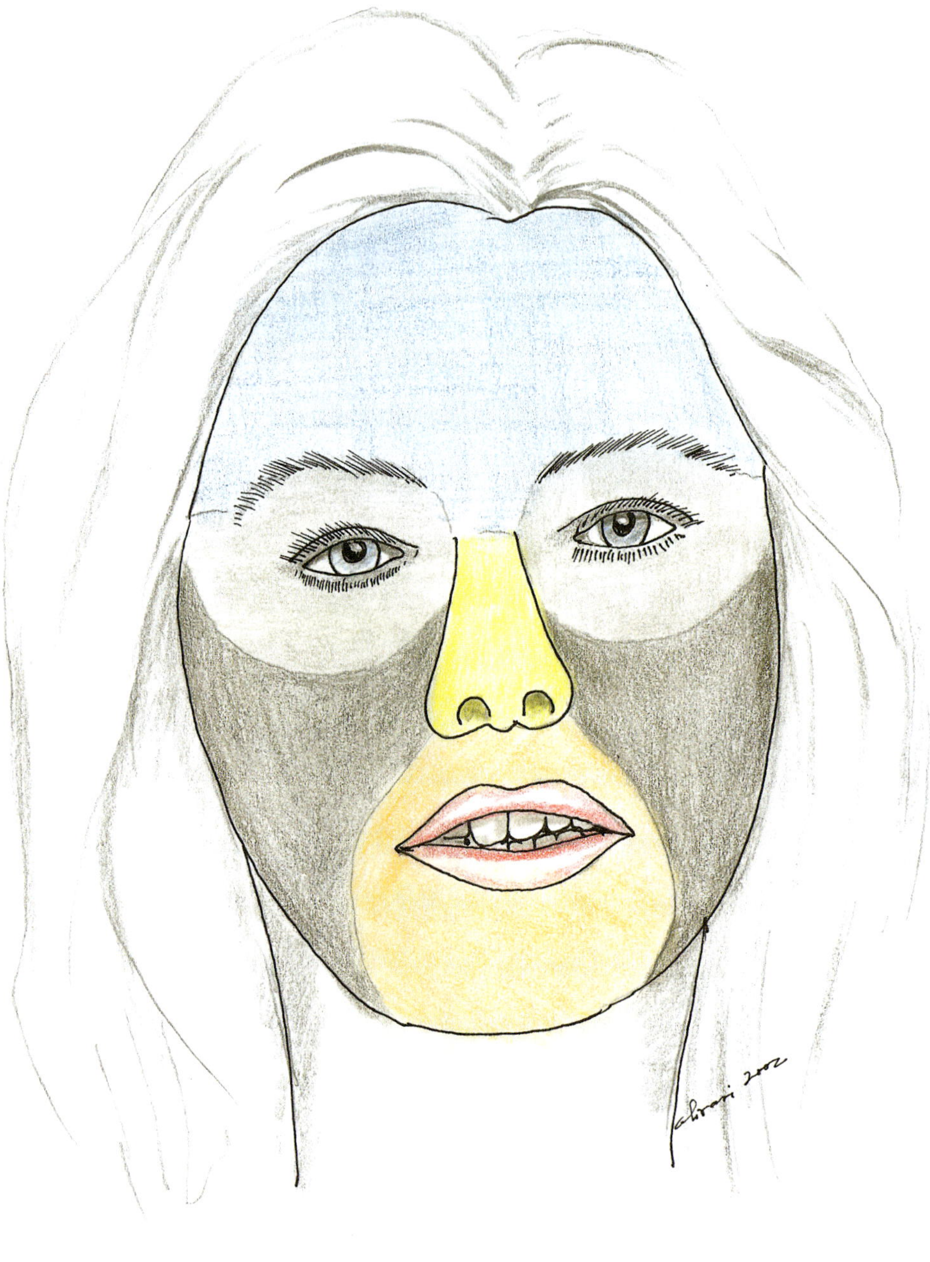

Figure 3.203 Aesthetic zones in the face: Upon coverage of larger areas in the face it is important to respect the aesthetic zones. In large burn scars in particular it is not useful to use graft that is smaller than the aesthetic zone.

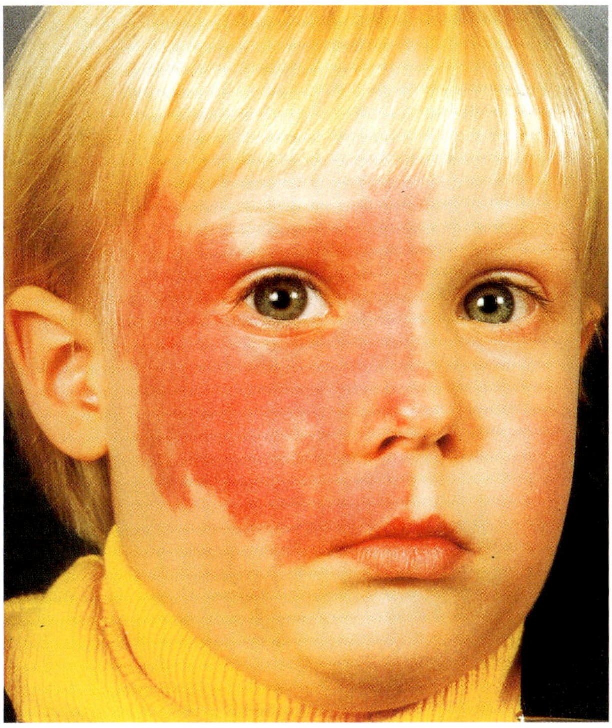

Figure 3.204a Port-wine stain nevus of the right cheek, upper lip and right nasal side

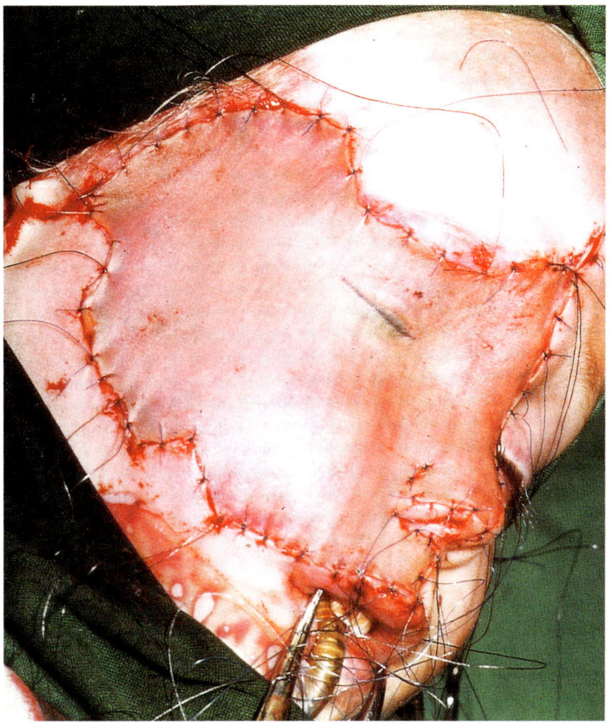

Figure 3.204b The Port-wine stain nevus is removed and a split skin graft is fixed in one piece to the defect. Above the right eyelid the graft is incised only horizontally. A full thickness skin graft that is better regarding coloring and quality is not available in this size!

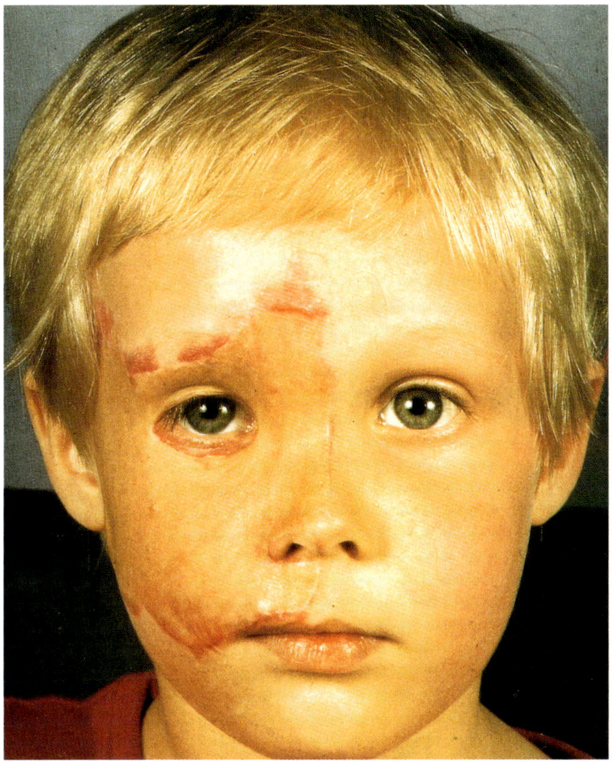

Figure 3.204c Situation six months after the first operation The graft has healed completely. Typically for the Port-wine stain nevus, at the edge of the graft a small relapse has arisen that should be eliminated by further surgical corrections or laser treatment.

Important: If a skin graft is used in the Port-wine stain nevus, this should only be carried out as a large graft. With several smaller grafts a relapse can be seen between each of the grafts. Laser therapy represents another good option.

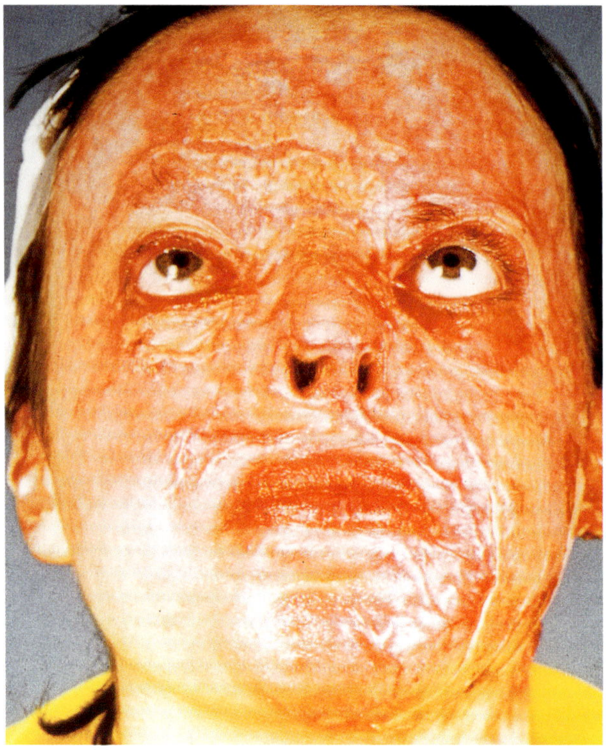

Figure 3.205a Burn multiple scars in the face with deformation of the nose, lid ectropion, absence of eyebrows and partial loss of the ear concha.

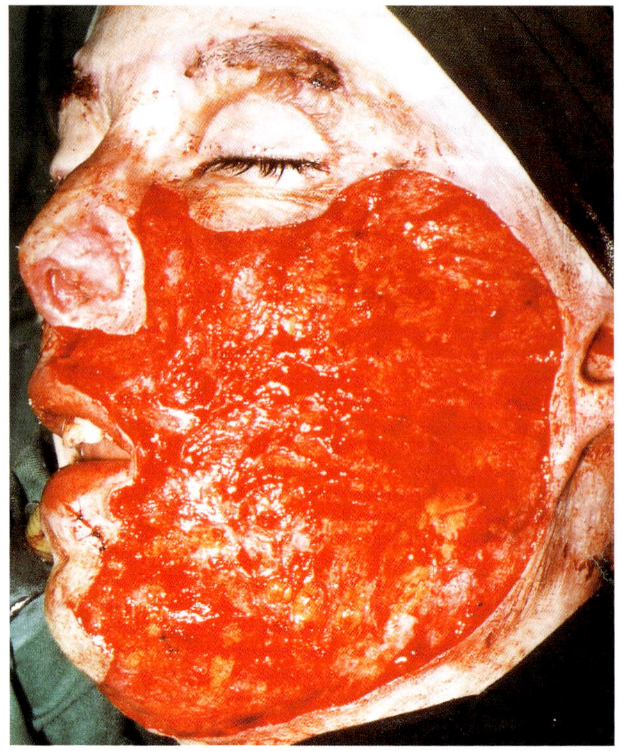

Figure 3.205b Large excision of the scar area with careful consideration of the aesthetic zones. At the same time a relatively thick split skin graft is removed and kept 24 hours at 4 °Celsius.

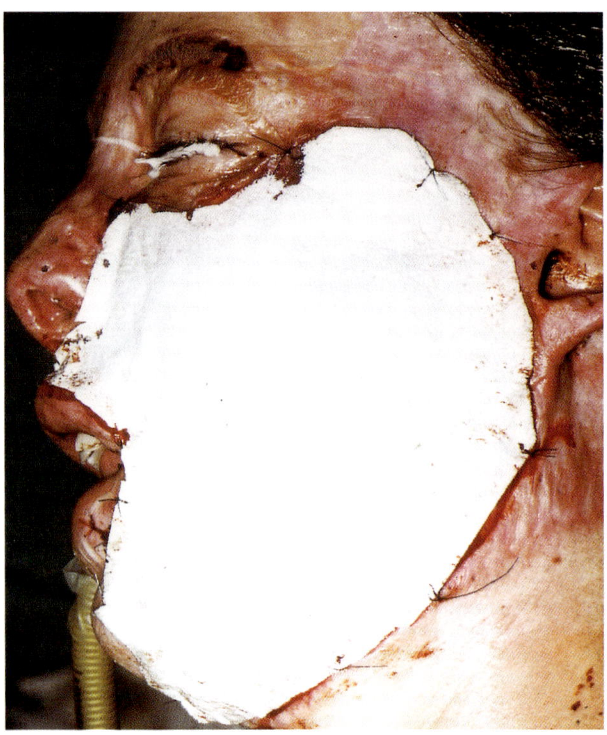

Figure 3.205c For 24 hours the excised area is covered with Epigard to avoid development of a hematoma.

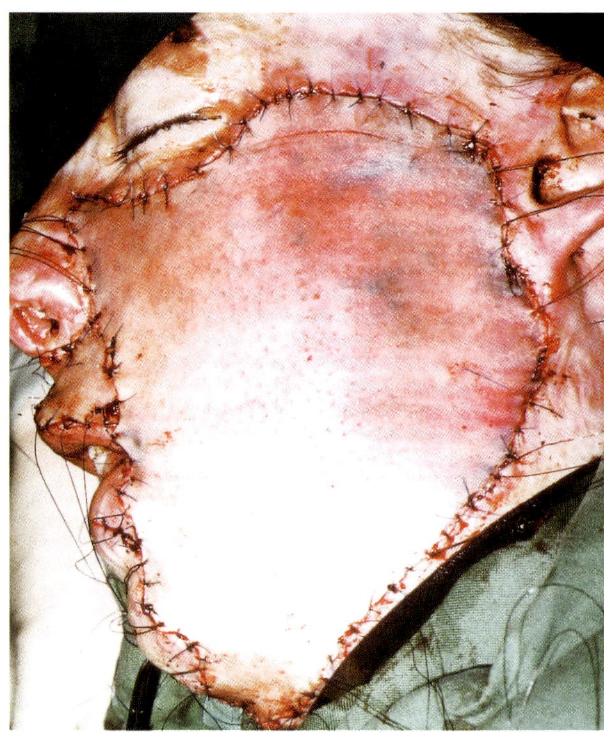

Figure 3.205d After removal of the epigard the split skin graft is fixed. Only large-area grafts are fitting for the aesthetic zones. Not mesh graft.

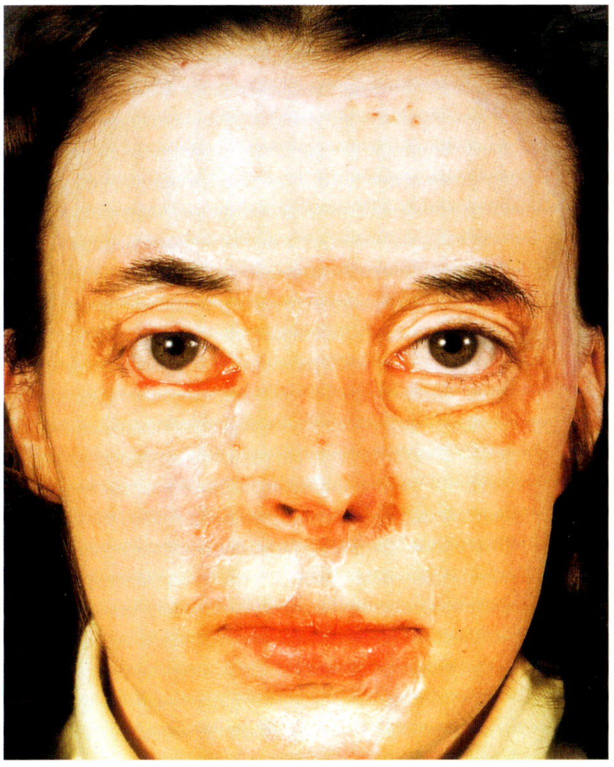

Figure 3.205e Status after two-and-a-half years and four operations.
1) The forehead was treated with a large split skin graft.
2) Both eyebrows were reconstructed with a pedicled temporal hairy island flap.
3) Both the upper and lower eyelids and the nose were covered with a full-thickness skin graft from the groin.
4) The left cheek and upper lip were covered with large split skin grafts.

The improvement in nasal form from the full-thickness skin graft is remarkable. The scarred contractures were completely removed down to the subcutaneous tissue.

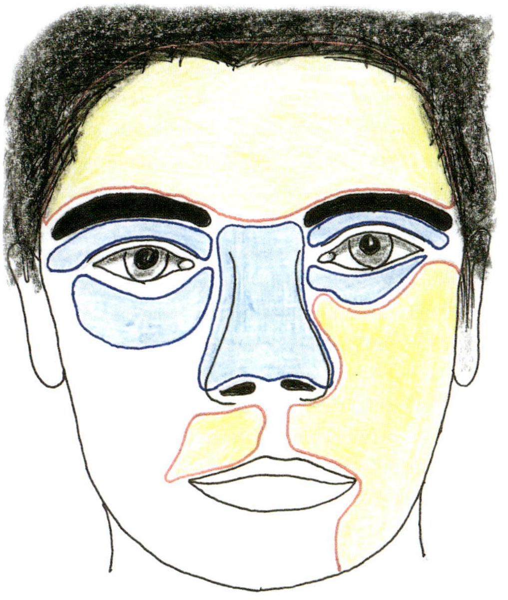

Figure 3.205f Yellow: Split skin graft. Blue: Full-thickness skin graft. Black: Pedicled island flap of hairy skin.

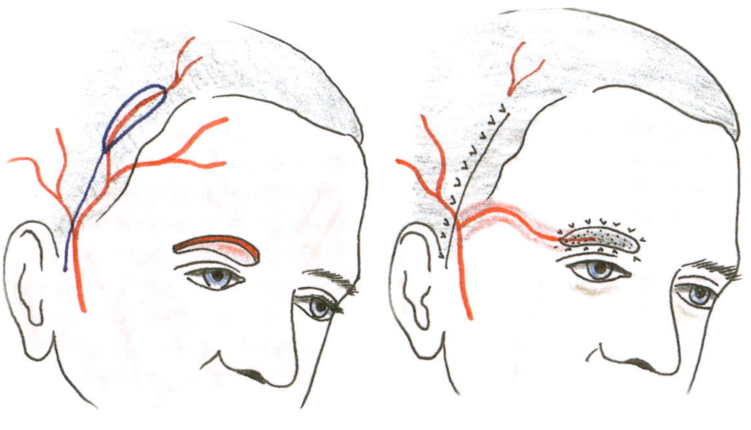

Figure 3.205g Reconstruction of the eyebrow with a hair bearing temporal island flap according to Monks (1950)

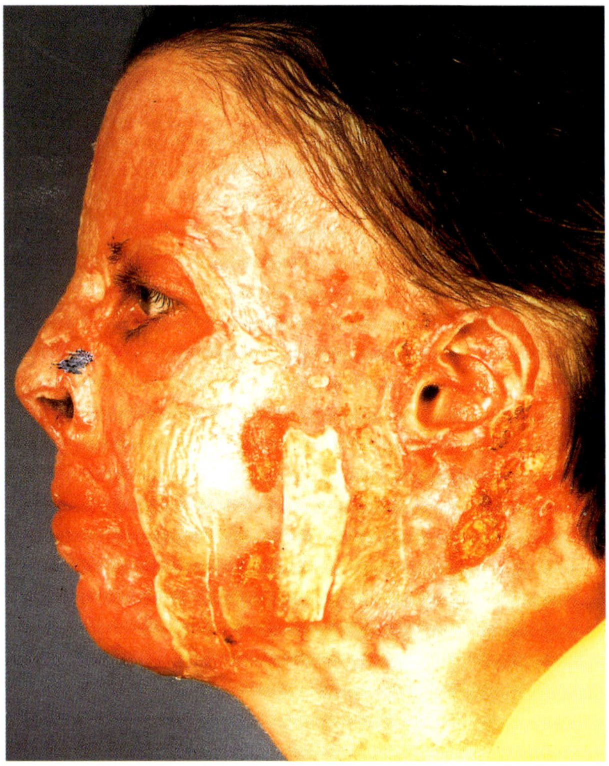

Figure 3.205h Preoperative state

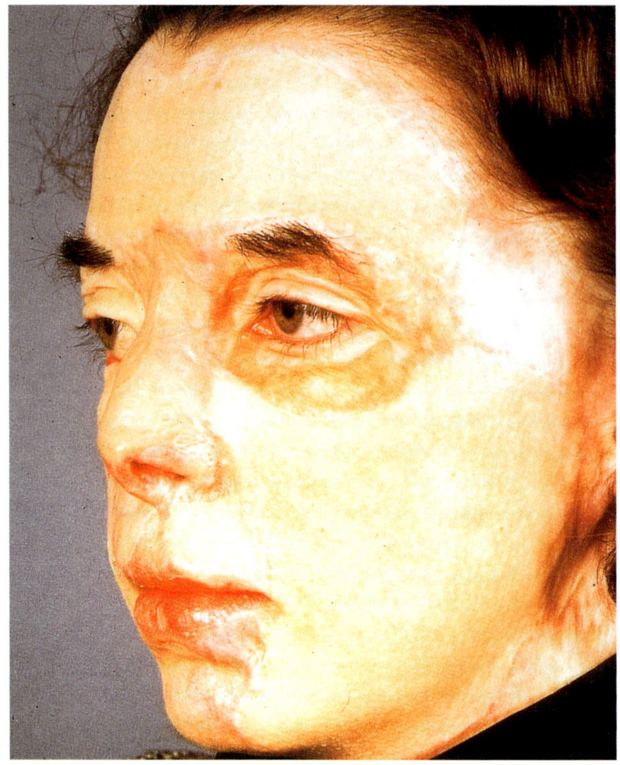

Figure 3.205i Status two-and-a-half years postoperatively

Combined Reconstruction in Complex Defects

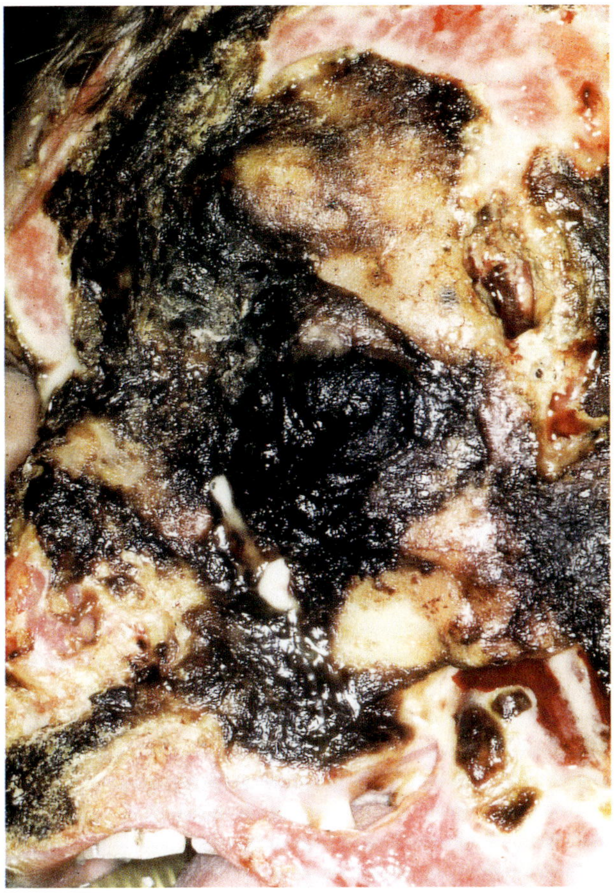

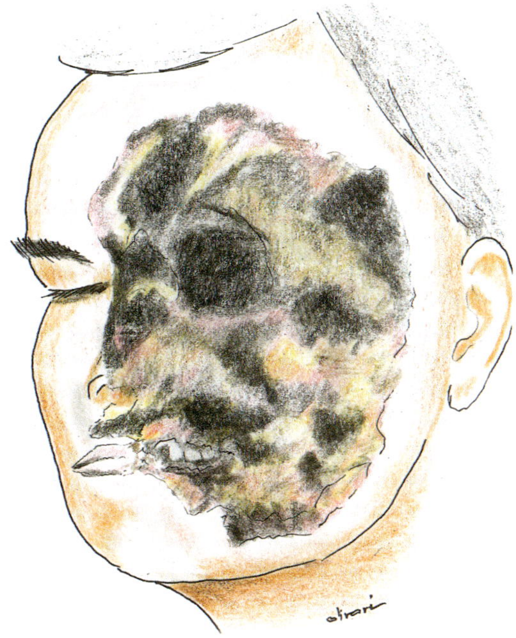

Figure 3.206a,b Third degree contact burns (coagulation) of the left cheek, nose, left eye and orbital region due to an exhaust muffler.
Complex facial defect with coagulation of the nasal frame (cartilage, bone). Parts of the frontal bone and the zygomatic bone was devitalized by the effects of the heat, just as the parotid gland. The content of the left orbit was also coagulated. Situation 14 days post burn trauma.

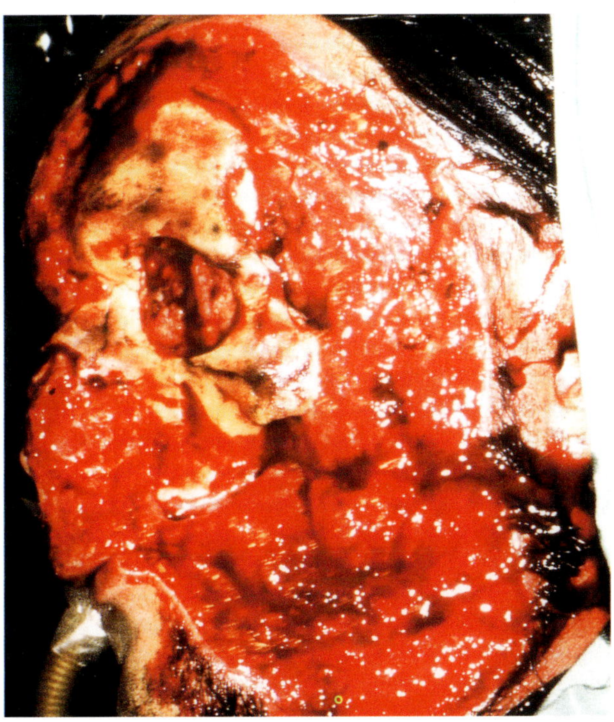

Figure 3.206c First operation: Debridement of necrotic tissue of the coagulated areas. Great part of the nose had to be removed, just as the nasal bone. The orbital exenteration occurred at the same time.

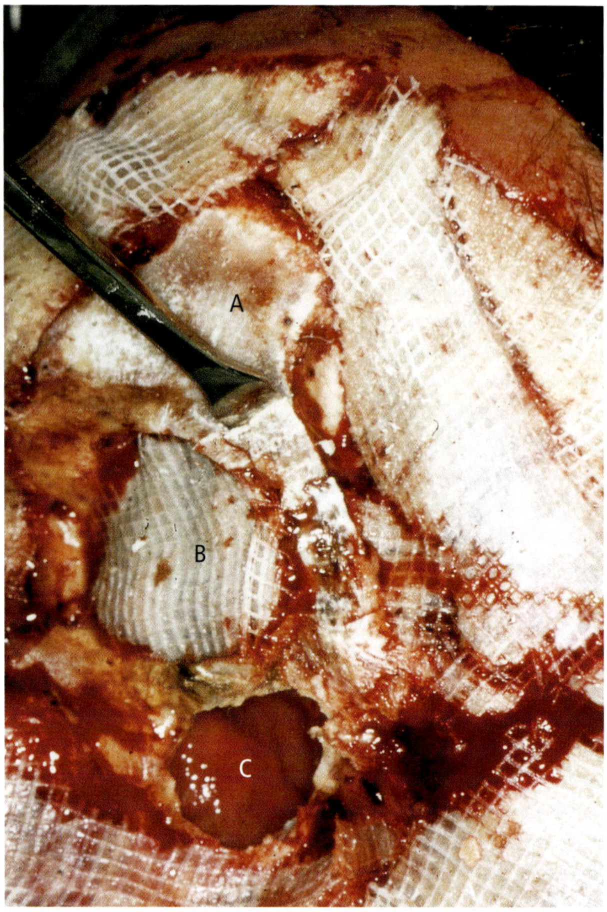

Figure 3.206d The heat denatured bones in the area of the frontal and zygomatic bones were removed (A). After enucleation the orbital tissue which was still well supplied with blood (B) was covered split skin graft. Maxillary sinus is open (C) due to maxilla necrosis.

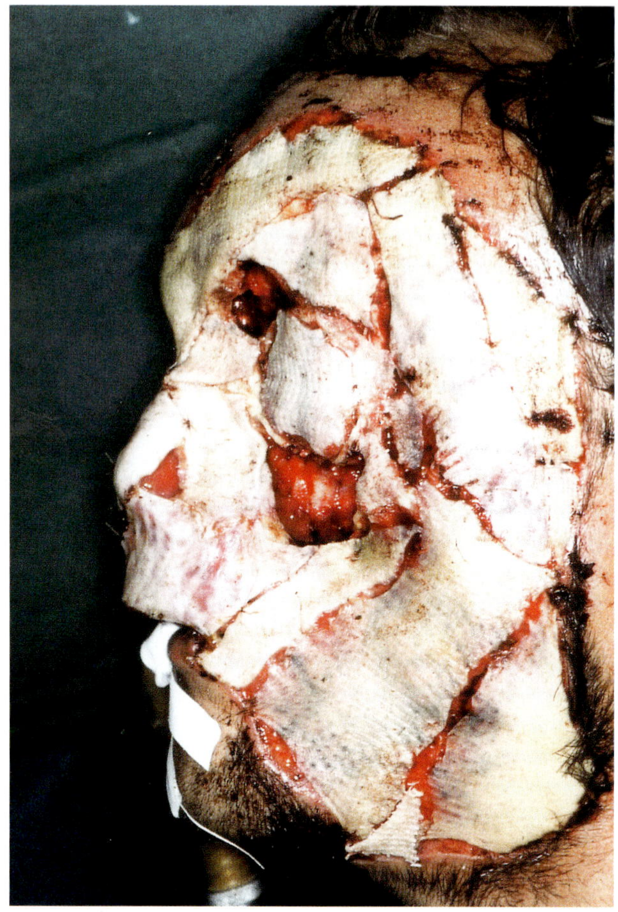

Figure 3.206e Status at the end of the first operation. After debridement of necrotic tissue, surfaces are covered with split skin graft. In the same way the bone was covered with mesh grafts after chiseling down to the layers well supplied with blood.

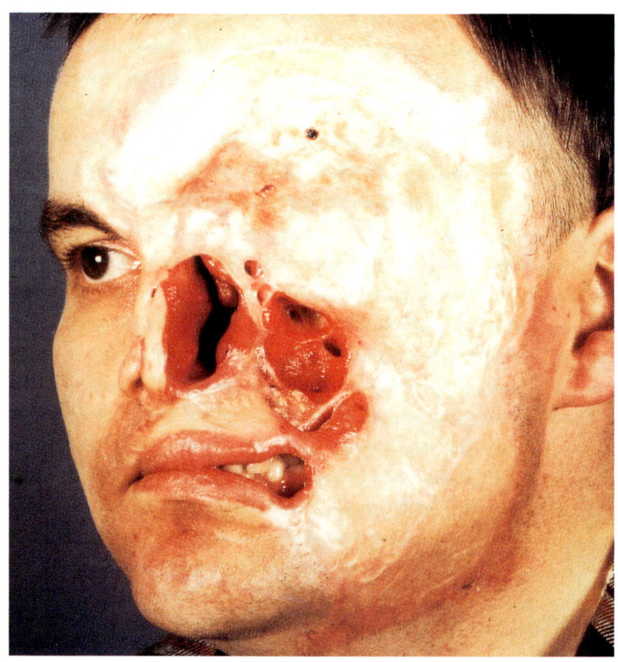

Figure 3.206f Status four months after the first operation. The patient had to be given an intensive psychological treatment.

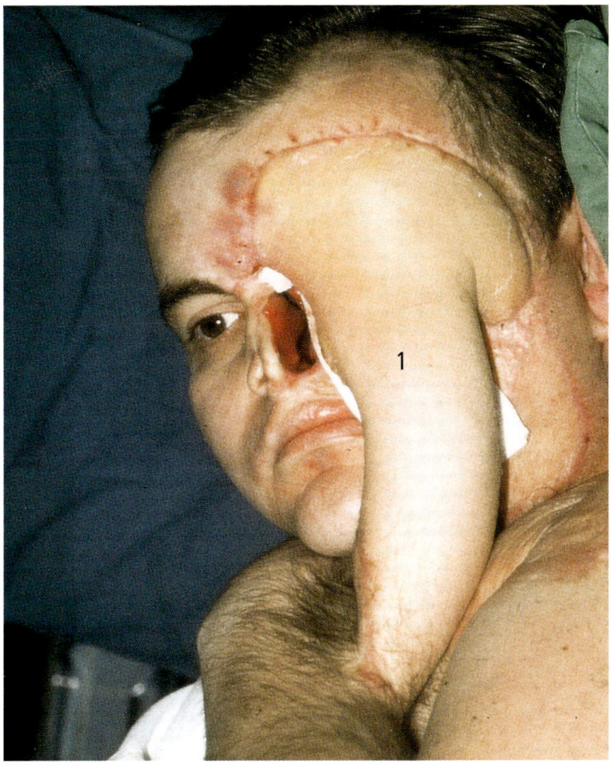

Figure 3.206g The soft-tissue defects on the left facial half were reconstructed using a pedicle tube flap from the left groin (1) as well as the abdomen. The flap was advanced over the left forearm.

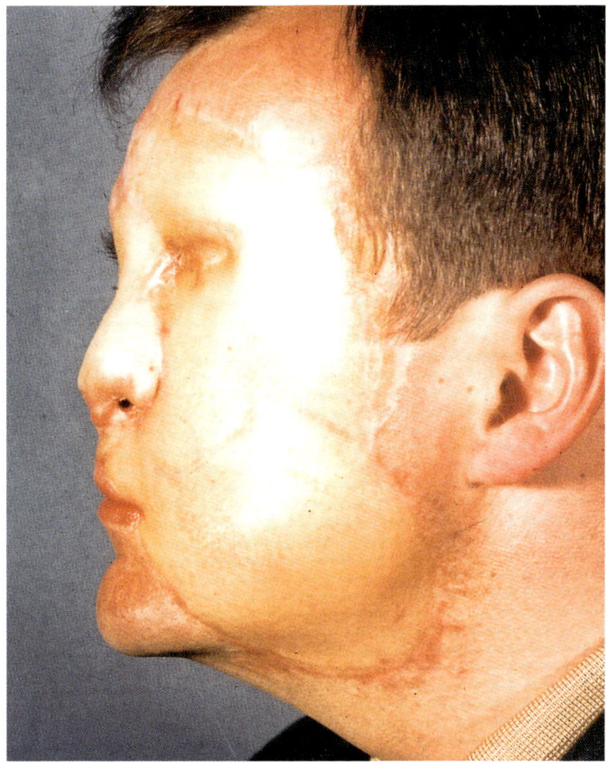

Figure 3.206h Status after reconstruction of the left facial side as well as a part of the nose.

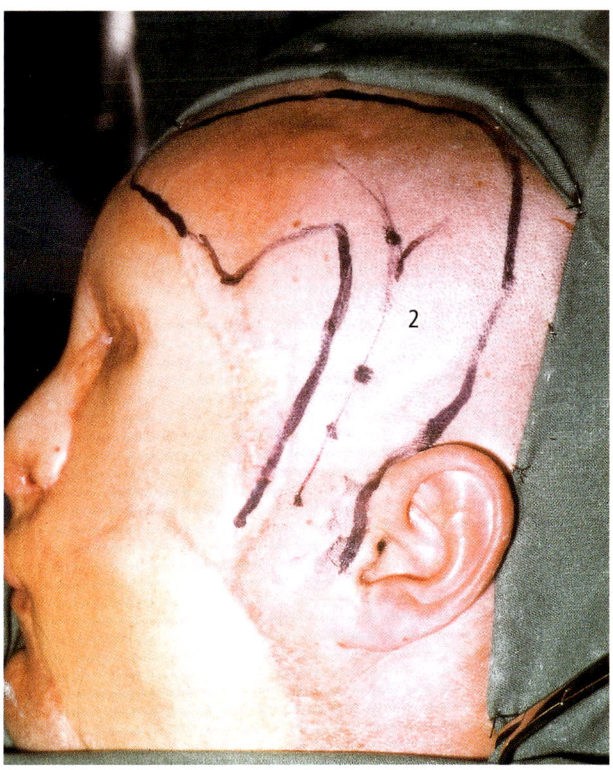

Figure 3.206i For reconstruction of the nose a forehead flap (supratrochlear flap) was refused by the patient. He did not want any scars in the middle of the forehead or on the right side of the forehead. So a decision was made to perform a temporo-frontal flap (New's sickle flap) (2). The superficial temporal artery was identified using the Doppler device.

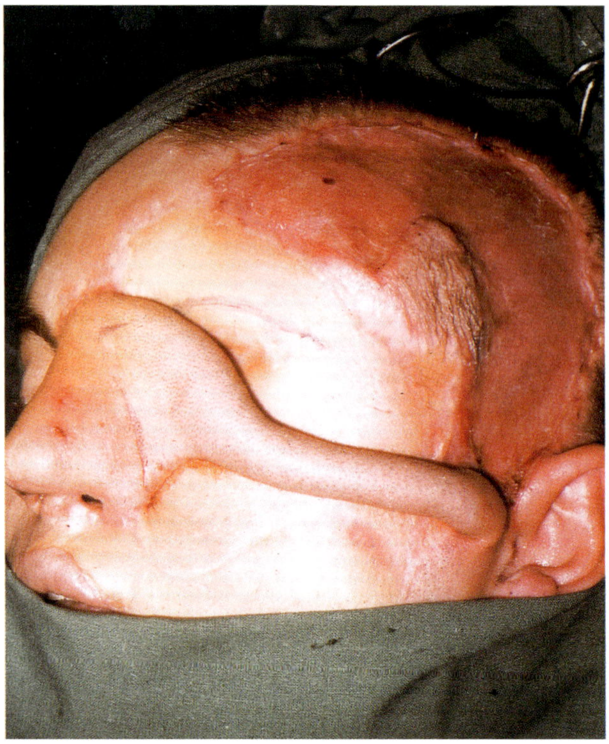

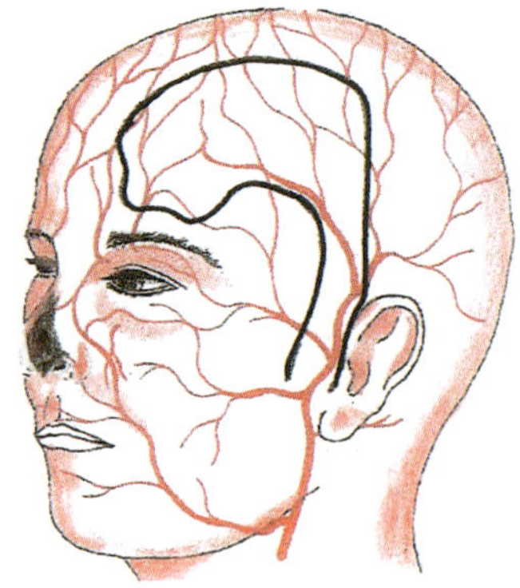

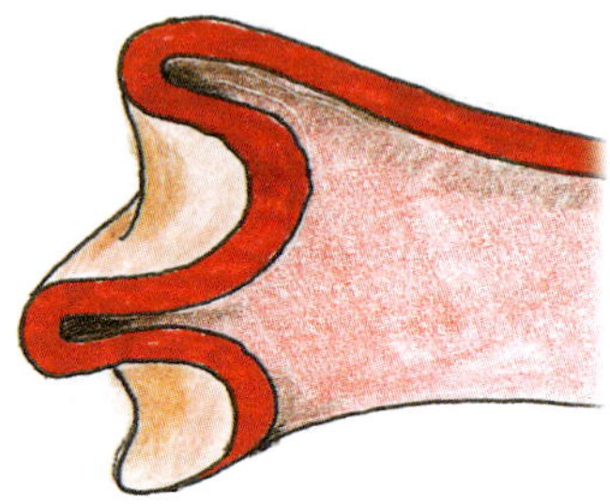

Figure 3.206j Mobilization of the temporo-frontal flap and forming of the nose. The remaining part of the flap was tubed in order to avoid a local infection. The secondary defect was temporarily covered with meshed graft.

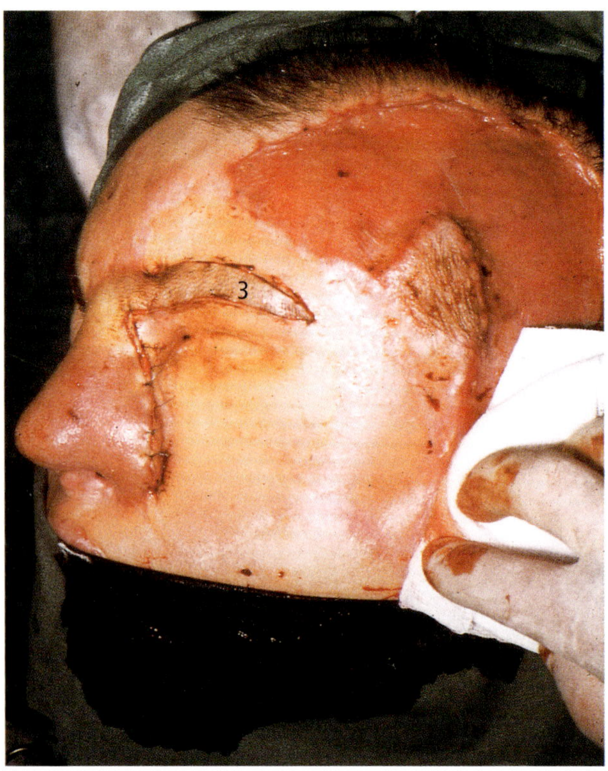

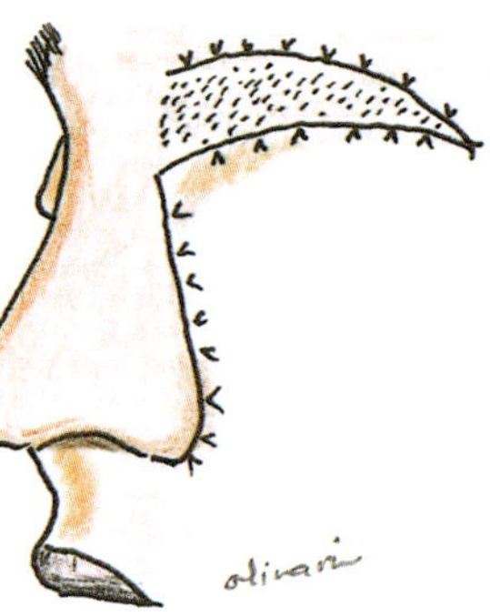

Figure 3.206k The temporofrontal flap (sickle flap) was severed after four weeks. The nose was formed and a part of the hair bearing flap was used for eyebrow reconstruction (3). The remaining part of the flap was rotated forwards so that the secondary defect appeared smaller than the material employed for the nose and eyebrow reconstruction.

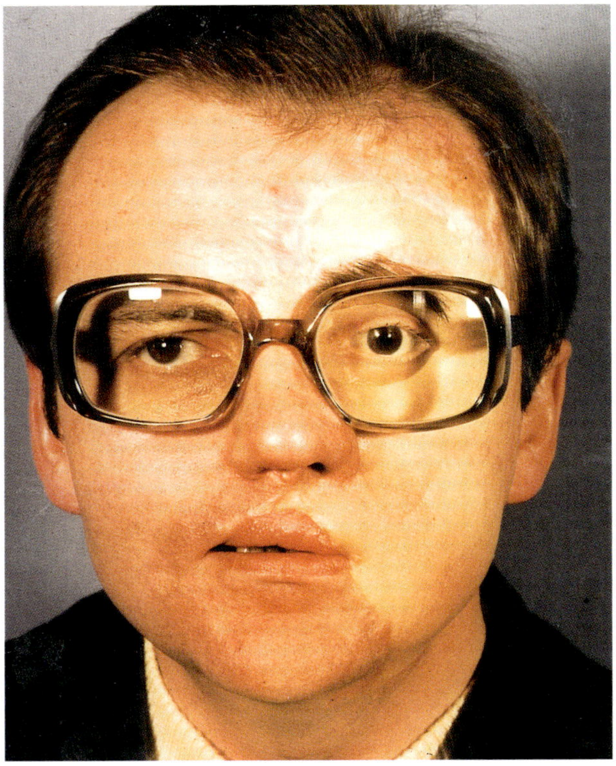

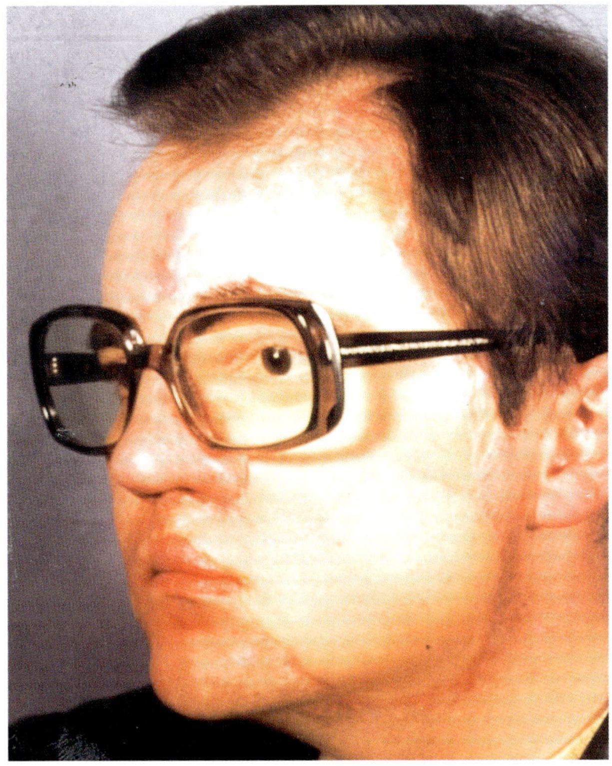

Figure 3.206l, m Situation after 19 months of treatment and seven operations. The patient bears an ocular epithesis. Few scars have occurred in the area of the flap donor site on the left side. The patient was rehabilitated as much by the operations and the psychological treatment that he could return successfully to his job as an engineer.

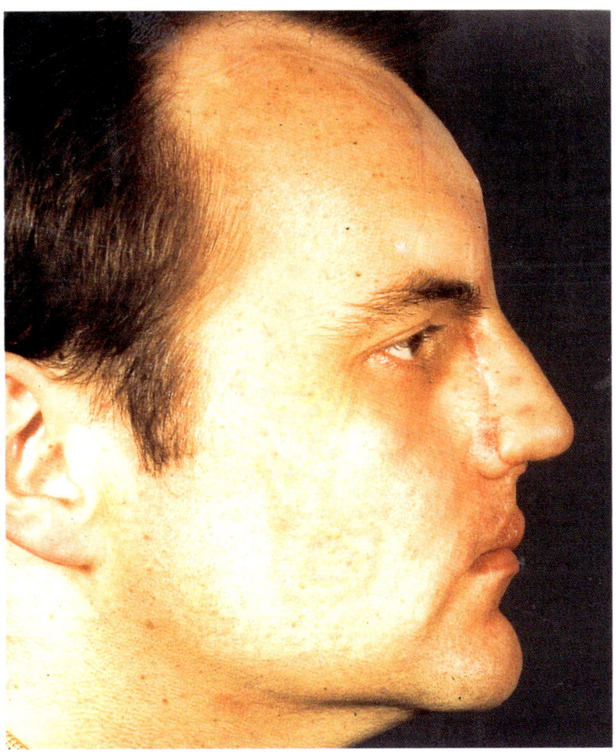

Figure 3.206n Good profile on the right side

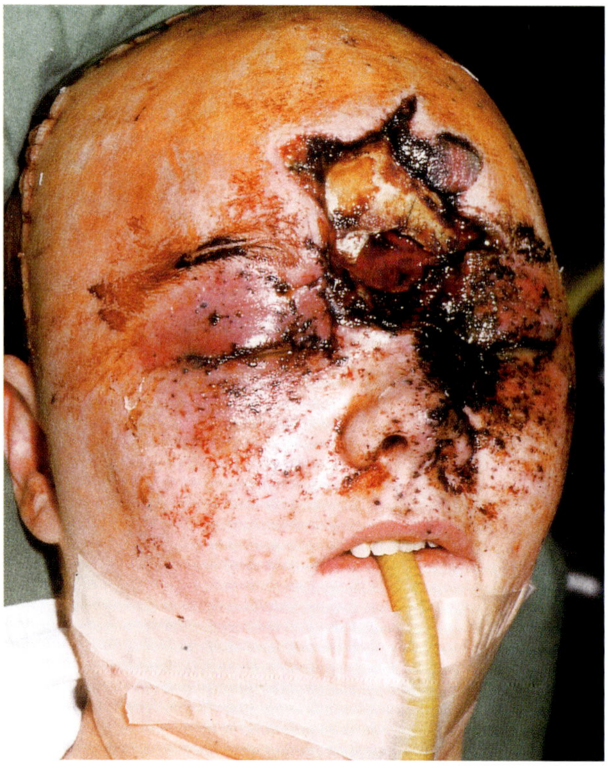

Figure 3.207a Ballistic injury (old fashioned shotgun) in the forehead and nasal area. Because of the intracranial injury in the area of the frontal lobe the patient was treated first by a neurosurgeon (see bicoronary incision).

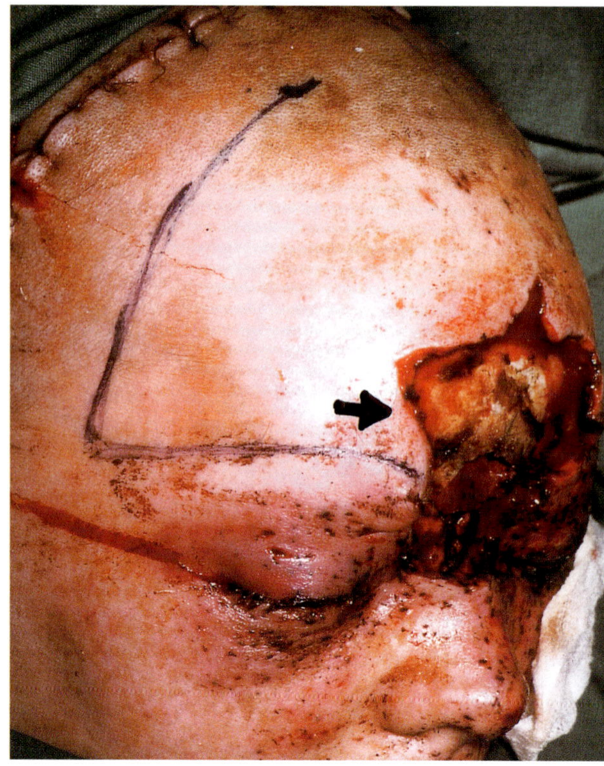

Figure 3.207b A defect at the frontal bone with opening of the frontal sinus and a liquor fistula were present. After debridement, forehead and head skin were mobilized from the right side in the medial direction to cover the defect. Meshgraft for residual defects.

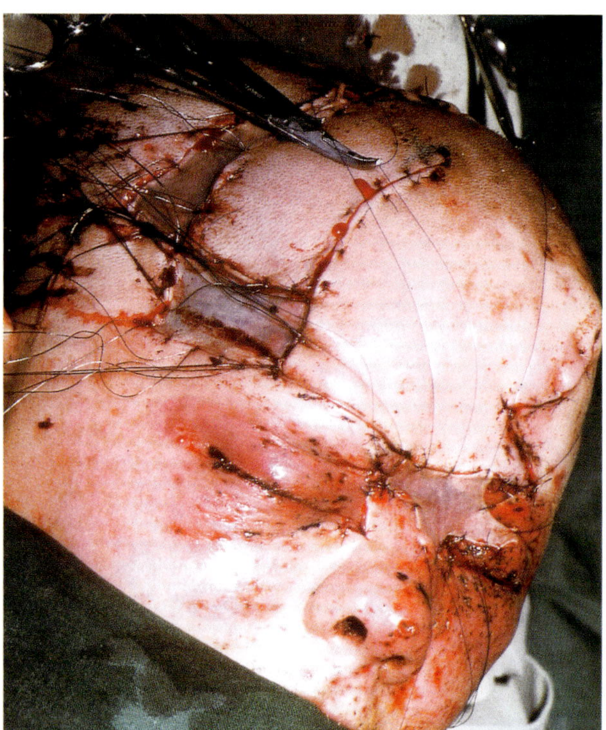

Figure 3.207c Situation at the end of the first operation. Particles of lead shot was removed by multiple single excisions and brushing out. A rotation flap was able to close the major part of the defect. In the glabella area mesh skin was applied temporarily.
Consider: If small lead shot particles are not removed immediately, they can remain permanently as "dirty pigmentation" in the skin.

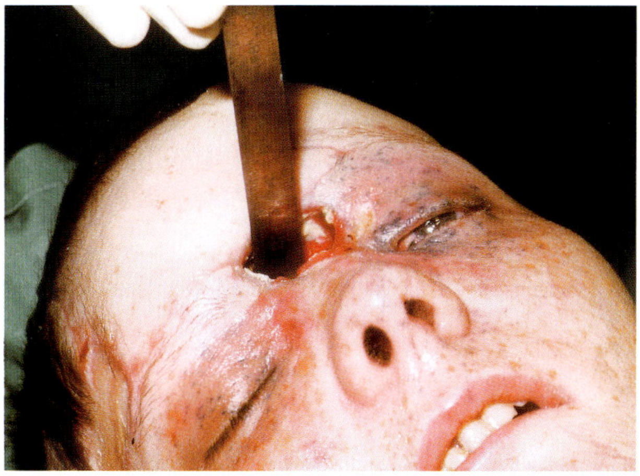

Figure 3.207d In the area of the glabella a defect with minor liquor fistula remains for four weeks after the operation.

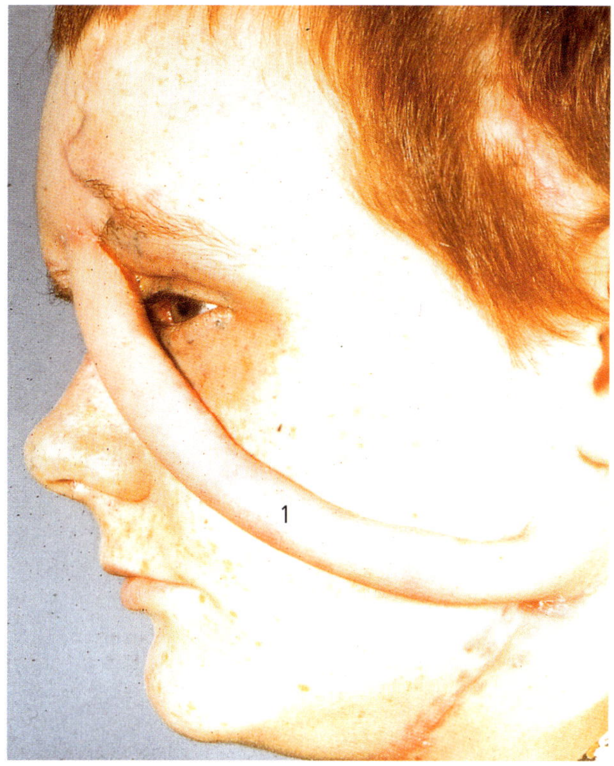

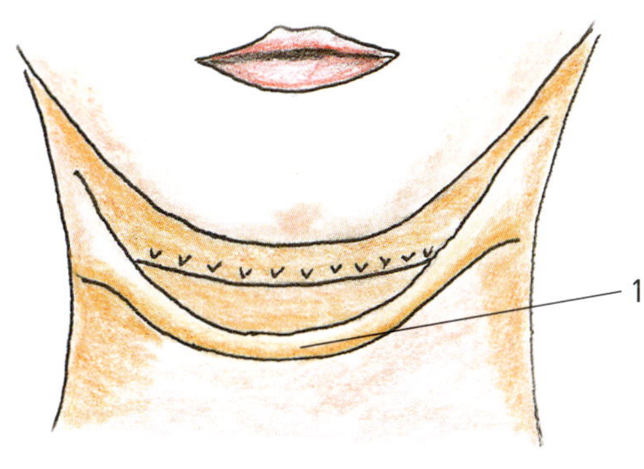

Figure 3.207e Because no local flap was available due to vessel destruction, we decided for this occasion to use exceptionally a pedicle tube flap from the neck (1).

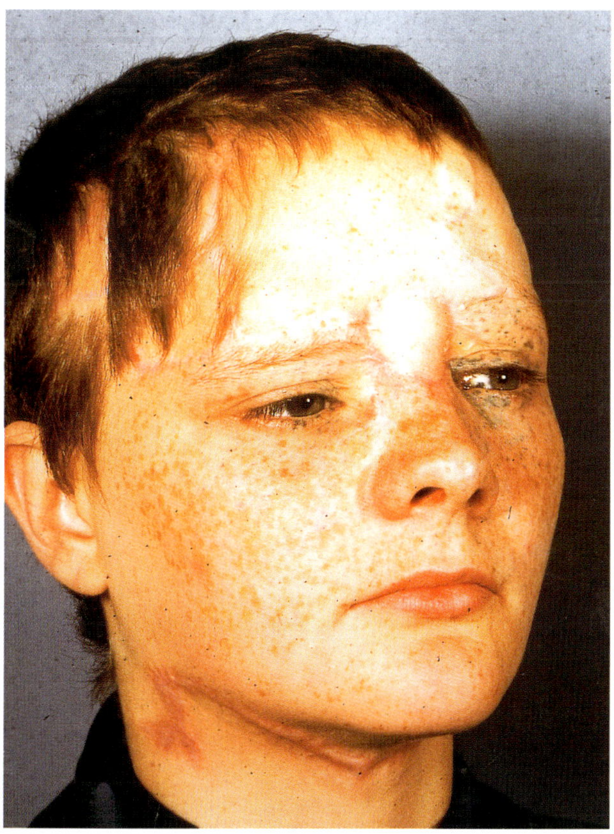

Figure 3.207f Status seven months after the accident. The patient is free of complaints. The scars at the neck are still clearly visible. At the left upper and lower eyelid, where not all the lead shot particles could be removed, a residue of "dirty pigmentation" remains.

Facial Nerve Paresis

Anatomy of the Facial Nerve

The facial nerve passes from the cerebello-pontine angle through the long facial nerve canal in the temporal bone, which runs in the wall of the middle ear and comes extracranially from the stylomastoid foramen.

Immediately after exit from the stylomastoid foramen the facial nerve sprouts three branches, namely the posterior auricular nerve, the stylohyoid branch and the digastric branch.

After that the facial nerve passes through the parotid gland in a ventral direction. Here it divides into four main branches (frontal branch, zygomatic branch, buccal branch, marginal branch) as well as numerous peripheral branches and in so doing innervates 24 mimic muscles.

Its long path through the temporal bone renders it sensitive; to infections in the middle ear. Here the nerve can be damaged by compression in the narrow canal where it is unable to swell. The result is that motor defects may develop.

Etiology

The anamnesis of a facial nerve paralysis is of prognostic significance regarding the cause, the type and duration of the paralysis. The following clinical pictures may be encountered.

1) Traumatic or iatrogenic paralysis of the facial nerve
2) Infection-induced paralysis of the facial nerve
   a) Herpes zoster
   b) Borrelliosis (Lyme disease)
   c) Meningitis
   d) Poliomyelitis
   e) Otitis media
3) As a result of an acustic neurinoma or glomus tumor
4) As a result of a surgical removal of a parotid tumor
5) Congenital unilateral or bilateral paralysis of the facial nerve
6) Idiopathic paralysis of the facial nerve (Bell's palsy)

Table 3.11 Causes of facial paralysis in our patient collective (N=65)

Cerebellar-pontine angle tumors	21
Idiopathic facial nerve paralysis	9
Otitis media	8
Traumatic damage	7
Congenital facial nerve paralysis	6
Parotid tumor	3
Acoustic neurinoma	4
Unknown origin	7
Total	65

The cause of peripheral facial nerve paralysis is of central importance to the treatment. Peripheral nerve damage is subdivided into five subcategories (Sunderland in [May 1986]).

Grade I

Neuropraxia: This is an injury to the nerve caused by external pressure or by an intraneural edema. This leads electrophysiologically to a block in transmission. Distal to the obstruction normal response to an electric stimulus is possible. A complete remission is usual provided that the external or intraneural pressure is relieved.

Grade II

Axonotmesis develop if the increased intraneural pressure is not overcome. The increased intraneural vascular permeability leads to a degeneration of axonal structures. The endoneurium in this stage is intact so that complete neural regeneration is still possible.

Grade III

Neurotmesis: Continuing external compression or an increase in intraneural pressure can lead to a degeneration of the endoneurium so that regenerating axons are misdirected on their way to the target organ. As a result neural healing is retarded and incomplete, and there is a risk of synkinesis in which axons connect with the wrong muscles.

Indication for Operation

The grade, localization as well as the duration and prognosis of the facial nerve paralysis determine the nature of the surgical treatment to be chosen.

1) Traumatic Severance of the Facial Nerve

A direct unstretched epineural nerve suturing is the therapy of choice during the acute phase. If the nerve suture can not be carried out in a stretch-free manner or larger defects exist, a bridging with a nerve graft is indicated. Here the sural nerve or the greater auricular nerve can be used. Is must be noted that the chances for recovering a normal, symmetrical function in the area supplied by the marginal branch and the frontal branch are worse than is the case with the branches supplying the midface.

2) Complete Facial Paralysis

One can reckon on a complete, spontaneous functional recovery in 56 to 70 % of the cases of idiopathic, complete facial paralysis up until the end of the third month [Anderson 1991, May et al. 1986, Rubin et al. 1986]. If no clinical signs of a re-innervation should become visible after the third month of the disease, an EMG and EneG examination is recommended in order to obtain important information about the remaining muscular and neural function [Burgess and Goode 1994].

The indication for a surgical treatment of a complete face paralysis must consider the age and possible accompanying-diseases of the affected patient, as well as the duration, extent and prognosis of the disease. It is especially important to determine the expectations of the patient regarding postoperative outcome. At the same time it is recommended during the ***patient information session to point out unambiguously that none of the available surgical, modern techniques are able to completely restore the symmetry of the face in its resting state or when carrying out mimic movements.***

Surgical Treatment

1) The Midface

Static Methods

The suspension of the paralyzed upper or lower lip, the corner of the mouth as well as the nasolabial fold using a strand of broad fascia from the thigh, or a GoreTex loop fixed to the temporal fascia or the zygomatic bone is considered to be a static procedure for the surgical treatment of a facial paralysis.

Static surgical procedures have the disadvantage that no voluntary or involuntary motor activity of the affected facial half can be expected. A satisfactory symmetry of the oral fissure at rest is the goal of the operation [Gillies 1934, Petroff et al. 1992].

An exclusive indication of static procedures is, however, seldom made. Such procedures are, however, justified with advanced tumor diseases of the face if extensive resection of the mimic musculature become necessary and no distal end-branches of the facial nerve are available any more.

Static procedures are often carried out in combination with microsurgical methods, in order to provide the patient some muscular tone in the midface, as well as to allow a better starting position of the corner of the mouth at rest during the period up until re-innervation occurs.

Dynamic Methods

Motor substitution plasty – the age and accompanying diseases of a patient with a complete irreversible facial paralysis determine the nature of the possible surgical reanimation of the paralyzed facial half. If the affected individual is in the age-group beyond the sixtieth year of life, a favorable result is rarely to be expected from microsurgical neural and muscular reconstructions for treating involuntary motor movements, so that a decreased quantitative growth of axonal potential to the target organs should be expected [Frey 1999].

This patient group is treated preferably using techniques designed to bring about a voluntary reanimation. To this end muscles innervated by the trigeminal nerve are used for the transfer (temporal muscle).

A voluntary smile, as well as an improved initial state of the corner of the mouth at rest can be achieved through a partial transfer of temporal muscle.

Facial Nerve Paresis

Anatomy of the Facial Nerve

The facial nerve passes from the cerebello-pontine angle through the long facial nerve canal in the temporal bone, which runs in the wall of the middle ear and comes extracranially from the stylomastoid foramen.

Immediately after exit from the stylomastoid foramen the facial nerve sprouts three branches, namely the posterior auricular nerve, the stylohyoid branch and the digastric branch.

After that the facial nerve passes through the parotid gland in a ventral direction. Here it divides into four main branches (frontal branch, zygomatic branch, buccal branch, marginal branch) as well as numerous peripheral branches and in so doing innervates 24 mimic muscles.

Its long path through the temporal bone renders it sensitive; to infections in the middle ear. Here the nerve can be damaged by compression in the narrow canal where it is unable to swell. The result is that motor defects may develop.

Etiology

The anamnesis of a facial nerve paralysis is of prognostic significance regarding the cause, the type and duration of the paralysis. The following clinical pictures may be encountered.

1) Traumatic or iatrogenic paralysis of the facial nerve
2) Infection-induced paralysis of the facial nerve
   a) Herpes zoster
   b) Borrelliosis (Lyme disease)
   c) Meningitis
   d) Poliomyelitis
   e) Otitis media
3) As a result of an acustic neurinoma or glomus tumor
4) As a result of a surgical removal of a parotid tumor
5) Congenital unilateral or bilateral paralysis of the facial nerve
6) Idiopathic paralysis of the facial nerve (Bell's palsy)

Table 3.11 Causes of facial paralysis in our patient collective (N=65)

Cerebellar-pontine angle tumors	21
Idiopathic facial nerve paralysis	9
Otitis media	8
Traumatic damage	7
Congenital facial nerve paralysis	6
Parotid tumor	3
Acoustic neurinoma	4
Unknown origin	7
Total	65

The cause of peripheral facial nerve paralysis is of central importance to the treatment. Peripheral nerve damage is subdivided into five subcategories (Sunderland in [May 1986]).

Grade I

Neuropraxia: This is an injury to the nerve caused by external pressure or by an intraneural edema. This leads electrophysiologically to a block in transmission. Distal to the obstruction normal response to an electric stimulus is possible. A complete remission is usual provided that the external or intraneural pressure is relieved.

Grade II

Axonotmesis develop if the increased intraneural pressure is not overcome. The increased intraneural vascular permeability leads to a degeneration of axonal structures. The endoneurium in this stage is intact so that complete neural regeneration is still possible.

Grade III

Neurotmesis: Continuing external compression or an increase in intraneural pressure can lead to a degeneration of the endoneurium so that regenerating axons are misdirected on their way to the target organ. As a result neural healing is retarded and incomplete, and there is a risk of synkinesis in which axons connect with the wrong muscles.

Grade IV

Partial nerve division severance results in malfunctions typical of those of untreated lesions.

Grade V

Complete nerve severance causes total functional loss without spontaneous recovery.

Symptomatology

Complete Facial Nerve Paralysis

1) Loss of the temporal branch results in an inability to raise the eyebrow. In the resting state and during mimic movements a clear asymmetry of the position of the eyebrows is evident. The paretic eyebrow flattened and there are no wrinkles on the forehead.
2) Loss of the zygomatic branch results in paralysis of orbicularis oculi muscle. The eyelids do not close and tearing is present, as the pump function of the orbicularis oculi muscle is absent. The loss of muscular tone in the lower eyelid results in ectropion in older individuals.
   The eyelid closure is incomplete (lagophthalmos) and rapid blinking of the upper and lower eyelid is absent. Patients suffer from dry eye, increased weeping, conjunctivitis and keratitis. Frequently a pressure sensation is described in the external orbit and temple area (Bell's phenomenon), as well as a subjective restriction in the visual field laterally (restricted lateral field of vision).
3) The loss of the buccal branch results in the cheek and the corner of the mouth hanging down slackly when at rest. A collapse of the affected nasal wing with concurrent nasal obstruction can often be observed. The nasolabial fold is raised. Everyday oral hygiene is complicated and older people in particular report that they often bite themselves in the paralyzed cheek, since the mouth on the healthy side feels displaced. Saliva can run from the corner of the mouth. Intake of food as well as speech can be disrupted so that not uncommonly such problems can lead to a psychosocial isolation of the affected individual.
4) The loss of the marginal branch entails that the depressor function of the lower lip is removed. This is expressed as a lowering of the lower lip upon mimic movements.

Partial Facial Nerve Paralysis

A partial facial paralysis can occur due to a traumatic injury to individual branches of the facial nerve, or can result as a final state of a complete paralysis.

Accordingly symptoms occur on many levels since the degree of partial damage can vary quite substantially. An age-dependent compensation of functional defects can be observed. Children and adolescents compensate a partial loss in the function of the facial nerve better than older people. Tiredness or stress allows facial paralytic symptoms or synkinesias to be expressed more vividly. Other functional defects can be perceived to varying extents by the patient. A discrete asymmetry of the corner of the mouth during smiling can entail a marked restriction of quality of life for a human being involved in public life. Every patient presents their own special situation so that precise information has to be obtained from the various facial areas to allow a customized, specific surgical treatment to be provided.

In conclusion it can be stated that the degree of impairment of a partial facial paralysis is experienced differently and individually by the patients.

Diagnostics

The concrete extent of a facial paralysis along with the functional, motor and aesthetic effects is difficult to describe clinically using a simple scheme.

The classification according to House and Brackman is a coarse classification of the possible symptoms, but does not provide any information about the complexity of the motor defects that occur during mimic movements [House 1985] (Table 3.12).

The diagnostics and treatment of facial paralysis is carried out by a team of specialists from various disciplines: i.e. otorhinolaryngology, ophthalmology, neurosurgery, electrophysiology, neurology and plastic surgery.

Here it should be pointed out that a patient with a complete traumatic peripheral facial paralysis should be referred as early as possible to a plastic surgery or ENT clinic so that a timely indication for a surgical revision can be made before an atrophy of the facial musculature sets in.

Duration of the Paralysis

One can distinguish between the acute state (0 to 3 months), the subacute state (3 to 12 months) and the chronic state (more than 12 months) after the occurrence of the paralysis.

If the motor innervation is removed, the muscular end organ suffers a trophic transformation that is reversible up to a certain point. If no re-innervation occurs within 12 months after the occurrence of the paralysis, an irreversible slack muscular atrophy can be expected. This means that 18 months to two years after the occurrence of a complete facial paralysis there is no longer any functional muscular motor activity.

Conservative Treatment

The conservative treatment of the eye of the paralyzed facial half must be given the highest priority. In order to protect the eye against the risk of a corneal ulceration, the upper and lower eyelid should be fixed at night using a small plaster strip. The repeated daily provision of artificial tear fluid or eye ointment helps to ameliorate the subjective symptoms. If the patient carries an eye chamber, this can preclude any draining of the eye. With longer lasting complaints the indication for an eyelid correcting intervention is given the utmost priority.

Table 3.12 The clinical grading of the facial nerve paralysis according to House and Brackman

Grade	Nerve paralysis	Characteristics
I	No	Normal function
II	Slight malfunction	Rest: Good symmetry and muscular tone Facial expression: Forehead: good; Eye: complete eyelid closure; Corner of the mouth: slight asymmetry
III	Moderate malfunction	Rest: Good symmetry and muscular tone, synkinesias, possibly hemifacial spasms Facial expression: Forehead: slight weakness; Eye: complete eyelid closure possible with effort; Corner of the mouth: Slight raising under maximal effort
IV	Moderate malfunction	Rest: Clear asymmetry Facial expression: Forehead: functionless; Eye: incomplete eyelid closure; Corner of the mouth: asymmetric under maximum effort
V	Severe malfunction	Rest: Asymmetry Facial expression: Forehead: functionless; Eye: incomplete eyelid closure; Corner of the mouth: discrete raising
VI	Complete functional loss	No function

Indication for Operation

The grade, localization as well as the duration and prognosis of the facial nerve paralysis determine the nature of the surgical treatment to be chosen.

1) Traumatic Severance of the Facial Nerve

A direct unstretched epineural nerve suturing is the therapy of choice during the acute phase. If the nerve suture can not be carried out in a stretch-free manner or larger defects exist, a bridging with a nerve graft is indicated. Here the sural nerve or the greater auricular nerve can be used. Is must be noted that the chances for recovering a normal, symmetrical function in the area supplied by the marginal branch and the frontal branch are worse than is the case with the branches supplying the midface.

2) Complete Facial Paralysis

One can reckon on a complete, spontaneous functional recovery in 56 to 70 % of the cases of idiopathic, complete facial paralysis up until the end of the third month [Anderson 1991, May et al. 1986, Rubin et al. 1986]. If no clinical signs of a re-innervation should become visible after the third month of the disease, an EMG and EneG examination is recommended in order to obtain important information about the remaining muscular and neural function [Burgess and Goode 1994].

The indication for a surgical treatment of a complete face paralysis must consider the age and possible accompanying-diseases of the affected patient, as well as the duration, extent and prognosis of the disease. It is especially important to determine the expectations of the patient regarding postoperative outcome. At the same time it is recommended during the ***patient information session to point out unambiguously that none of the available surgical, modern techniques are able to completely restore the symmetry of the face in its resting state or when carrying out mimic movements.***

Surgical Treatment

1) The Midface

Static Methods

The suspension of the paralyzed upper or lower lip, the corner of the mouth as well as the nasolabial fold using a strand of broad fascia from the thigh, or a GoreTex loop fixed to the temporal fascia or the zygomatic bone is considered to be a static procedure for the surgical treatment of a facial paralysis.

Static surgical procedures have the disadvantage that no voluntary or involuntary motor activity of the affected facial half can be expected. A satisfactory symmetry of the oral fissure at rest is the goal of the operation [Gillies 1934, Petroff et al. 1992].

An exclusive indication of static procedures is, however, seldom made. Such procedures are, however, justified with advanced tumor diseases of the face if extensive resection of the mimic musculature become necessary and no distal end-branches of the facial nerve are available any more.

Static procedures are often carried out in combination with microsurgical methods, in order to provide the patient some muscular tone in the midface, as well as to allow a better starting position of the corner of the mouth at rest during the period up until re-innervation occurs.

Dynamic Methods

Motor substitution plasty – the age and accompanying diseases of a patient with a complete irreversible facial paralysis determine the nature of the possible surgical reanimation of the paralyzed facial half. If the affected individual is in the age-group beyond the sixtieth year of life, a favorable result is rarely to be expected from microsurgical neural and muscular reconstructions for treating involuntary motor movements, so that a decreased quantitative growth of axonal potential to the target organs should be expected [Frey 1999].

This patient group is treated preferably using techniques designed to bring about a voluntary re-animation. To this end muscles innervated by the trigeminal nerve are used for the transfer (temporal muscle).

A voluntary smile, as well as an improved initial state of the corner of the mouth at rest can be achieved through a partial transfer of temporal muscle.

The transposition of temporal muscle can be conceived in two ways:

a) The temporal muscle can be released from the temporal fossa and fixed over the zygomatic bone via a subcutaneous tunnel at the corner of the mouth. Strips of fascia lata from the thigh serve to prolong the temporal muscle [Gillies 1934]. This technique entails the disadvantages of visible strand formation, swelling above the zygomatic bone as well as the formation of hollows in the temporal fossa. It should also be mentioned that the transposed temporal muscle has a tendency to stretch over time, so that an overcorrection is initially offered. A secondary surgical stretching of the transferred strips is often unavoidable with the passage of time. In order to circumvent this disadvantage, we used temporal fascia to extend the temporal muscle in our patients. The relatively coarse broad fascia of the thigh is not necessary (Figure 3.220 c-f)

b) Using the procedure of McLaughlin the connection of the temporal muscle to the coronoid process is released and fixed using a fascial loop with the corner of the mouth and the lip segments (Figures 3.208, 3.211, 3.221) [McLaughlin 1953]. The advantage of this procedure lies in the fact that the fascial strip can be placed in the depth of the fasciocutaneous layer (SMAS) of the cheek, so that a less visible cord formation occurs in the area of the cheek. The amplitude of the voluntary raising of the corner of the mouth is not very large. However, it is possible, through mimic training before a mirror, to create a satisfactory symmetric smile provided that the patient voluntarily learns to adapt the excursion of the healthy corner of the mouth on the reconstructed side. Lexer and Eden (1911) fixed the ventral part of the masseter muscle to the corner of the mouth and achieved some symmetry and mobility (Figure 3.211f). Lexer's idea was also to apply two strips of temporal muscle as a motor substitute for the orbicular ocular muscle and to transpose it to the upper and lower eyelid. This method is still today the method of choice for reconstructing a voluntary eyelid closure (Figures 3.210, 3.213).

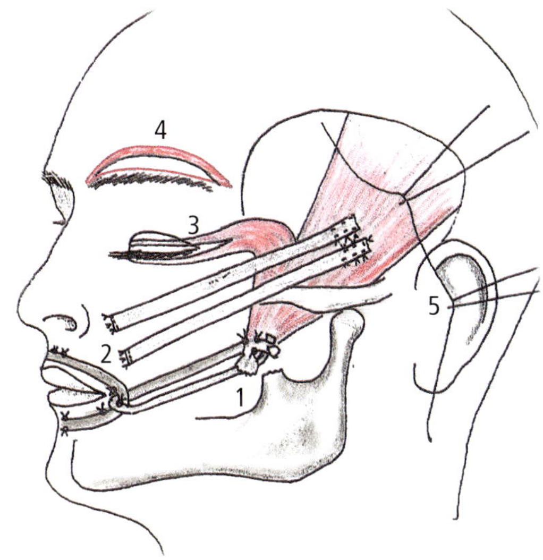

Figure 3.208 Combination of dynamic and static operation procedures favored by the author:
1. Dynamic suspension of the corner of the mouth according to McLaughlin
2. Static suspension of the nasolabial fold using two fascial strips
3. Correction in the eyelid area with two strips of temporal muscle (Lexer)
4. Frequent eyebrow elevation
5. Modified facelifting

The masseter transposition has the disadvantage that only a very small amplitude of mobility in the corner of the mouth is possible. The vector of the raising of the corner of the mouth is also directed laterally and does not correspond to the excursion of the corner of the mouth with a normal smile, entailing that this procedure is no longer applied as the only method for transposition.

In the following the procedures favored by the author are described. The dynamic suspension of the corner of the mouth is carried out according to McLaughlin (Figure 3.208). The nasolabial fold is fixed using two fascial strips onto the temporal fascia. The coronoid process is released from the mandible together with its temporal process. Through an arched incision lateral to the corner of the mouth a submuscular tunnel is formed under the orbicular oris muscle. Beyond the midline a broad fascia strip is fixed to the orbicular oris muscle at the upper and lower lip and fixed via a broad fascia loop to the process of the temporal muscle. The correction in the eyelid area is carried out using two strips of temporal muscle. The eyebrow is lifted with the help of a sickle-shaped skin excision, while a face lifting with SMAS completes the operation. The combination of the different procedures entails for the patient an immediate drastic improvement in the previously existing asymmetry of the midface and an eyelid closure directly after the operation. The patients can start exercises before a mirror for synchronizing their masticatory movements with eyelid closure and smiling on the first day after the operation. After a suitable training period this is satisfactorily mastered by most patients [Olivari 1979].

Correction of the Eye Contour.

Tarsorrhaphy is very frequently recommended. In practice, however, this brings barely any improvement in the eyelid ptosis and lagophthalmos, but does reduce kerato-conjunctivitis.

Magnet implantation was indeed a brilliant idea of Mühlbauer, but unfortunately all 22 magnets implanted by us perforated through the thin eyelid within six weeks to a year. After that temporal strips were applied.

Silastic loops have also been talked about for some time, but these are also not to be recommended.

The application of two temporal loops shows that the oldest procedure is still far superior to all the other procedures. With a good operation technique the results are not only functionally good, but also permanent (Figure 3.210a-e).

Gold implants in the eyelid area are also not to be recommended. In a standing position the ptotic eyelid becomes even more ptotic due to the weight of the gold implant. In the lying position the gold weight exerts force in a dorsal and cranial direction. At nighttime the eye is opened even more.

Microsurgical Reconstruction

1) Re-Innervation of the Affected Side Using a Nerve Graft

In the seventies the re-innervation of the paralyzed facial half using nerve grafts from the healthy side was described independently by Smith (1971), Anderl (1973) and Scaramella (1971). Using grafts of the sural nerve the branches of the facial nerve of the healthy side are bridged microsurgically with corresponding branches of the paralyzed side using 10 × 0 synthetic suture material (Cross-face). The number of grafts selected varies from author to author. The procedures were carried out either in one or two sessions (Figure 3.209a-d).

The idea was to reconstruct a spontaneous, involuntary function of the paralyzed facial half. Since only approx. 50 % of the nerve branches of the healthy side can be used for the microsurgical connection, the potential of the axons transferred to the paralyzed side is reduced to far less than 50 %. This entails that even with a successful sprouting of nerve tissue to the paralyzed side one can only reckon on a weaker, uncoordinated function compared to the healthy side. The time taken for nerve tissue to sprout from the healthy to the paralyzed facial half is about 12 to 16 months. After this time it is unlikely that sprouting axons will encounter still functional muscles because of the atrophy that ensues. This might at least partially explain the results reported up until now.

Conley's successes amongst ten patients treated using this technique were unsatisfactory and comparably worse than the results of a hypoglottal nerve – facial nerve plugging [Conley 1979]. Such poorly optimistic results were also confirmed by other authors. Gary-Bobo (1983) achieved only a poor function in 11 of 16 cases 18 months postoperatively and Fisch (1976) also reported disappointing results in seven cases. Cross-face nerve grafting has been largely abandoned today as a sole surgical procedure in favor of neuromuscular grafting.

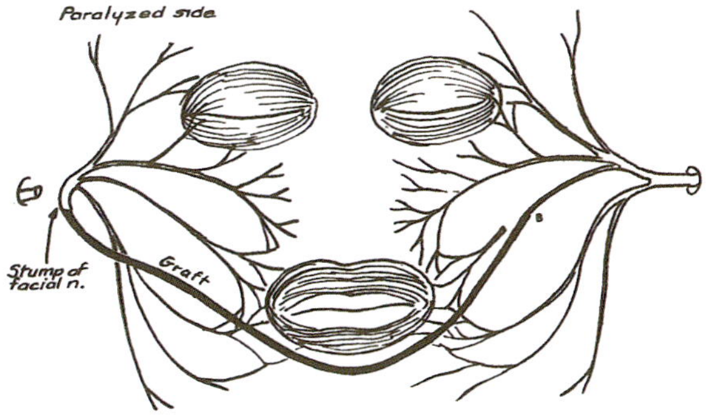

Figure 3.209a Scaramella (1971)

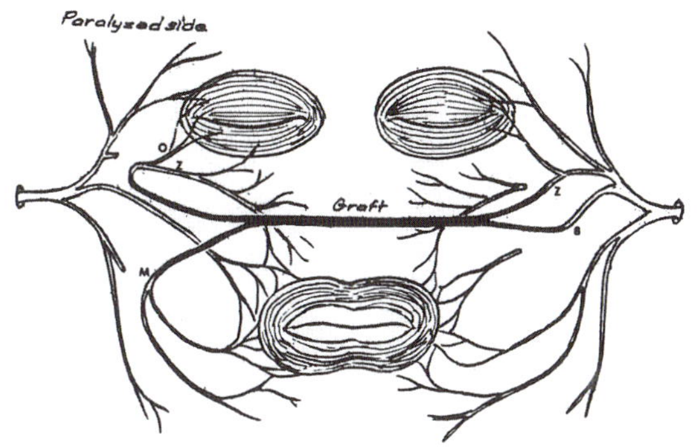

Figure 3.209b Fisch (1974)

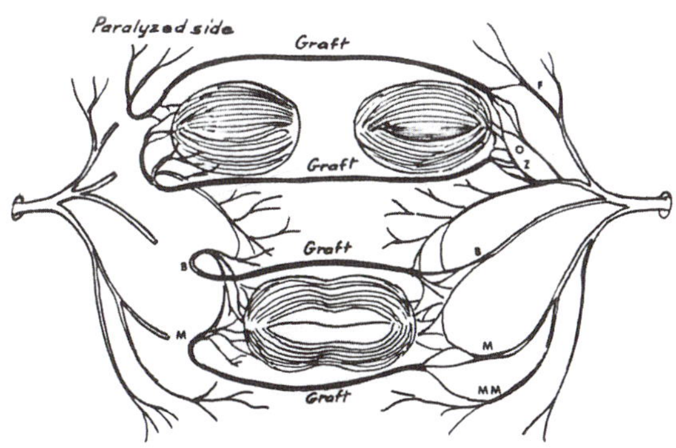

Figure 3.209c Anderl (1973)

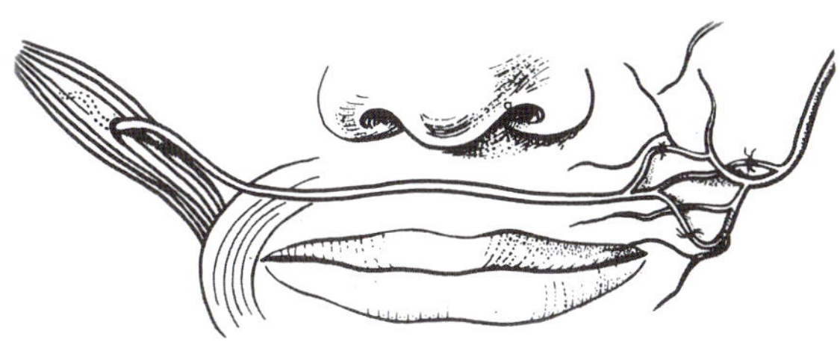

Figure 3.209d Freilinger (1975)

Figure 3.209a–d Different options for cross-face nerve grafts with facial paralysis

2) Neuromuscular Grafting

Restoration of a spontaneous, involuntary smile can be achieved using a neuromuscular graft, whose motor is the facial nerve of the healthy side. The first reports using a one-session procedure came from Thompson (1976) who employed the extensor digiti minimi muscle and the branch of the anterior tibial nerve. Vedung and Hakelius (1984) also reported on a two-session procedure. The results of this procedure remained at first unsatisfactory since no revascularization of the muscle graft had been carried out. It was shown, however, that even an improved muscular perfusion through creation of microvascular anastomoses did not produce any lasting improvement [Mayou 1981]. Further investigations in this field showed that the choice of the muscle to be transplanted was of key importance. The ideal muscle should be flat, show a long as possible neurovascular pedicle, and should possess parallel aligned muscle fibers. Muscles with these qualities include the gracilis, the pectoralis minor muscle, the latissimus dorsi muscle, the serratus anterior muscle and the rectus abdominis muscle.

Harii in 1976 described a two-session reconstruction using a sural nerve and a gracilis graft. A revascularization of the muscle was carried out via microsurgical connections to the temporal vessels or to the facial vessels [O'Brien 1990, Frey 1999, Harii 1976].

I. The Two-Session Procedure for Facial Reconstruction with Facial Nerve Paralysis. The sural nerve is removed in smaller, separate incisions over the entire length from the foot up until the proximal lower leg as a graft. The use of a nerve stripper is not recommended so that the nerve does not become damaged. The sural nerve can be lifted both unaided (freely) in smaller incisions, or with the aid of an endoscope. The endoscopic operation lasts longer than the free operation does, but does have the advantage that more extensive scars at the lower extremity can be avoided. The indication can be made for children from the fourth year of life since from this age the nerve graft is of sufficient length. The facial nerve of the healthy facial half serves as a donor nerve.

a) Nerve Grafting. The incision course is made in the same way as that for a facelifting. In the area of the throat the incision is made slightly arched in a forward direction in order to allow a clear exposure of the branches of the facial nerve. In the front of the parotid gland all emanating branches of the facial nerve are exposed and checked separately for function using a nerve stimulator at 25–50 Hz (Aaron Neuro-Pulse™, Ref 0003Y). For this it is important that the patient recieves no muscle relaxant medication during the anesthesia. Branches that induce a raising of the corner of the mouth as well as a narrowing of the lips, as might occur during whistling, should not be used. It is recommended to feel the muscular tone of the lips upon nerve stimulation so that only those branches which innervate the levator musculature are identified. Branches that cause a mass movement of the face should also not be considered as donor nerves. Nerve branches that raise the corner of the mouth for smiling and in so doing induce eyelid closure as minimally as possible, are preferentially chosen as donor nerves. The nerve graft is initially subcutaneously inserted through the upper lip until the paralyzed facial half via two small incisions parallel to the nasal wings. A preauricular incision course in the area of the paralyzed facial side facilitates the placement of the graft end up until the height of the tragus. The graft end is marked with a 5 × 0 suture so that it can be located more easily in the second session. In individual cases it may make sense to displace the nerve graft submentally or directly under the mucosa of the upper lip. The nerve suturing between two branches of the facial nerve and the sural nerve is carried out in a stretch free manner using the surgical microscope. Synthetic suture material with thicknesses of 9 × 0 or 10 × 0 are used as thread material. As a rule the diameter of the proximal end of the sural nerve is twice as large as that of the donor branches. The distal end of the sural nerve, which is frequently divided into two tender branches, has proven effective when adapted to the donor branches. For this purpose an epineural suture material is used and the suture site is safeguarded with a biological adhesive. It can not be considered as guaranteed that the retrograde positioning of the nerve graft, unlike the anterograde positioning, prevents a potential sprouting of axons through collateral branches [Mantkelow 1999]. In this surgical session the operation according to McLaughlin is also carried out with complete facial paralysis, as well as the temporal muscle transfer to the upper and lower eyelids. This allows a certain improvement in the patient's defects during the time it takes for the nerve tissue to sprout to the paralyzed side. After the coaptation of the sural nerve with the branches of the healthy facial half, approx. 8 to 10 months pass before the patient observes a feeling of a slight electric shock upon tapping of the nerve end in front of the tragus of the paralyzed facial half (Tinel test). During the course of the sprouting one can in this way determine exactly how far the re-innervation process has proceeded. The withdrawal of the sural nerve has the effect that the outer side of the back of the foot becomes numb. In addition visible scars remain at the lower leg after removal of the nerve.

b) Muscle Grafting. The characteristics of the smile are studied preoperatively, and before the operation the nasolabial fold is recorded symmetrically with the healthy side. The vectors characterizing the raising of the corner of the mouth and the upper lip during smiling are marked preoperatively on the paralyzed facial half. It is recommended that photos should be at hand during the operation which depict the face in a position of rest and during facial expression.

In the following the elevation of the gracilis as a neuromuscular graft shall be described. Regarding the elevation of the latissimus dorsi muscle [Harii 1998] and the pectoralis minor muscle [Terzis 1989 and 1997, Harrison 1985] appropriate literature is referred to.

The employment of two surgical teams considerably reduces the operating time. While one team prepares the recipient facial side, the other operation team extracts the gracilis from the same side. In this way the donor muscle can be positioned into the facial half in such a way that a neuromuscular pedicle is placed under the muscle. A potential later revision for the purposes of thinning the muscle endangers neither the neural or the vascular pedicle, since both are located under the muscle. During preparation of the paralyzed facial half it must be ensured that the re-innervated nerve graft is not damaged.

The facial flap is raised above the parotid fascia as well as above the levator musculature in order to avoid a fusion of the muscle graft with the skin. We expose the nerve graft up until the ala nasi and remove the distal neuroma. Then the facial vessels are exposed. In this way submuscular channels for introducing the gracilis strips are formed via two separate incisions at the upper and lower lip at the height of the midline. The orbicular muscle is exposed at the height of the commissure.

The gracilis is exposed with the help of a slightly arched incision at the inner side of the thigh. The obturator muscle should be cut away in its entire length of 10 to 12 cm. The vascular pedicle of the gracilis, approximately 6 to 9 cm below the pubic tuberculum, is cut free as long as possible. Its length is approx. 6 to 7 cm. The two accompanying veins have a diameter of 2 to 3 mm, the artery approx. 2 mm. For the reconstruction of the paralyzed facial half a muscle of approximately 9 cm length and 3 to 4 cm width is needed. The muscle volume is dependent on the degree of muscular atrophy present, or any possible muscle loss of the paralyzed facial half. If it should become necessary to thin out the gracilis, this muscular resection shall be carried out before the transfer to the face. In this way the perfusion of the muscle can be better assessed and a correct hemostasis can be carried out. The obturator nerve is shortened so far that the path of the regenerating axons to the transplanted muscle becomes as short as possible. The proximal part of the gracilis is adapted to the periosteum of the zygomatic bone using 4 × 0 non-resorbable suture material. The distal muscle end is adapted using 4 × 0 non-resorbable suture material at the orbicular oris muscle from the upper and lower lip as well as at the lip commissure. The muscle tension should correspond to that which was present in the thigh at its starting position. With complete paralysis, a muscle strip can also be fixed laterally at the nasal wing. The future nasolabial fold is thinned out up until the dermis and fixed to the surface of the gracilis using 4 × 0 non-resorbable suture material.

A checking of the perfusion of the muscle occurs during the first five days after the operation using a Laser-Doppler, where the probe is stitched to the muscle using the threads that pass out of the cheeks. The first signs of re-innervation of the transplanted muscle become clinically noticeable after four to six months in the form of a slight raising of the corner of the mouth. In all the entire process of reanimation of the paralyzed facial half with the two-session procedure lasts about two years before the patient can expect any functional recovery.

II. The One-Session Procedure for Facial Reconstruction With Facial Nerve Paralysis. The above-described two-session procedure is a standardized procedure with the disadvantage that two years must pass before a functional recovery occurs. For this reason ways have been sought to accelerate the pace of re-innervation. Various authors have chosen one-session procedures, whereby the long motor nerve of the transplanted muscle is coapted directly with the contralateral facial nerves. Guelinckx employed the gracilis (1986), Harii the latissimus muscle (1998), while Koshima used the rectus muscle (1994).

The length of the obturator nerve is approximately 12 cm and is therefore not always sufficient to reach facial branches of the healthy side without stretching. A nerve suture is only possible at the height of or medial to the nasolabial fold so that the axonal potential may not be sufficient to allow a strong contraction of the gracilis. The latissimus muscle appears better suited since the thoracodorsal nerve can be openly resected up to a length of 15 cm [Harii 1998, Dellon 1999, Wei 1999]. The re-innervation of the transplanted muscle with one-session procedures has proven itself not to be inferior to that seen with the two-session techniques. The fear of a muscular atrophy before the onset of re-innervation with a one-session procedure proved to be unjustified. The results are not inferior compared to those of the two-session reconstruction [Harii 1998].

The classification according to House did not prove itself to be satisfactory in practice for comparing postoperative results with one another since it only provides an incomplete picture about the details of mimic movements. In order to be able to illustrate the movement processes one needs video equipment. In 1999 Frey introduced a three-dimensional video analysis for allowing a better comparison of postoperative results with one another [Frey 1999, Deutinger 1995].

2) The Upper Facial Third

The improvement in asymmetry of the forehead at rest and during facial expression is the goal of treatment. In discreet cases of partial facial paralysis one finds with some patients a sunken eyebrow, synkinesia in the area of the upper and lower eyelid as well as an absence or weaker pronouncement of forehead wrinkles.

Synkinesias of the eyelids can be successfully treated using botulinus toxin (Botulinum toxin type A, Allergan).

Botulinus toxin can induce an allergic state of shock in some extremely rare cases.

The overall outcome of a microsurgical reanimation of the midface can be improved if the upper facial third is also modeled as harmoniously as possible. Improving the asymmetry of the forehead with an open or endoscopic forehead lift has proven to be effective over the last years. During the endoscopic operation it must be ensured that the paralyzed side is fixed permanently in a lifted position. A functional lifting in this case is not sufficient [Keller 1997].

The best outcome in the upper facial third is achieved by employing two temporal muscle strips and an eyebrow elevation with the help of a supraorbital skin excision. Here the oldest procedures are the best.

Conclusion

In an ideal situation, the reconstructive operations in the paralyzed face should restore a harmonious expression in a resting state and during facial expression. This expectation, however, is not realistic and as operating surgeons we must satisfy ourselves with much more modest results.

New procedures have raised hopes that a natural mobility of the paralyzed face may become possible. The results are, however, only modest. No procedure can restore the natural movement of the face. Many patients can imitate a kind of smile after the operation and achieve a certain degree of facial expression with hard training. All postoperative images, including our own, have demonstrated a kind of smiling. However, objective analyses using a video camera have made the results look more modest.

Despite that, operations intended to reanimate a paralyzed face are entirely justified. The patients enjoy a considerably better condition than they did before the operation:

- relatively good symmetry in a resting state
- often a certain degree of mobility in the corner of the mouth, that is often not spontaneous, but much rather trained
- improvement in speech, food intake and oral competence
- improved eyelid closure
- considerable psychological rehabilitation; no patient regrets having the operation.

With facial nerve paralysis two surgical options are available at this time:

a) Cross-face nerve implantation with free muscle transfer
It is barely possible to compare the success of the various procedures and it is not our intention to carry out such a comparison here. Theoretically the procedures of cross-face nerve grafting as well as of free muscle grafting are logical and as such physiological. For any result, however, one has to wait 1 1/2 to 2 years and the result is also not completely satisfactory. These procedures belong to the future.

b) Classical procedure of local muscle transfer of the masseter and static suspension
We have frequently employed this procedure.
- Dynamic suspension of the corners of the mouth according to McLaughlin
- Static suspension of the nasolabial fold using two fascial strips
- Correction in the eyelid area using two strips of the temporal muscle (Lexer)
- Eyebrow elevation
- Modified facelifting + SMAS

None of the above-mentioned classical operations on their own produce a satisfactory result. If all procedures are carried out in an operation process, however, a drastic improvement can be registered for the patients immediately after the operation.

Already from the first postoperative day the patients practice a synchronization of masticatory movements and smiling before the mirror. This is more or less mastered by most patients after practice.

Patients can of course only move the voluntarily reconstructed face (and eyelids).

A reconstruction in the eyelid area according to the old Lexer procedure still remains a procedure of choice.

Reconstruction of Eyelid Function (Lexer)

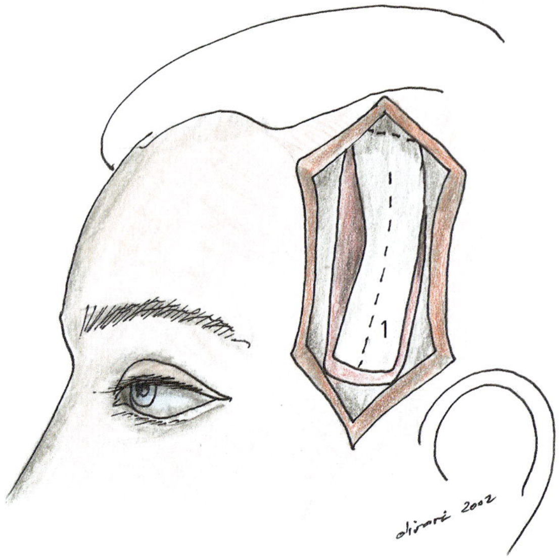

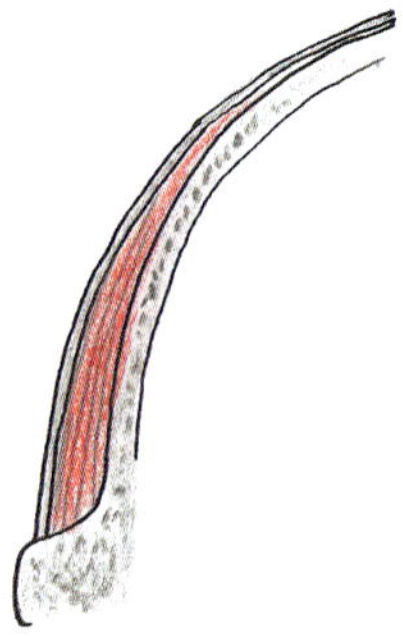

Figure 3.210c

Figure 3.210a Reconstruction in the eyelid area according to Lexer (modification):
Preparation of two temporal strips for treatment of the upper and lower eyelid. The superficial temporal fascia (1) is cut around caudally and folded up. The upper incision is carried out in the periostal area; in this way the fascial strips remain connected to the temporal muscle.

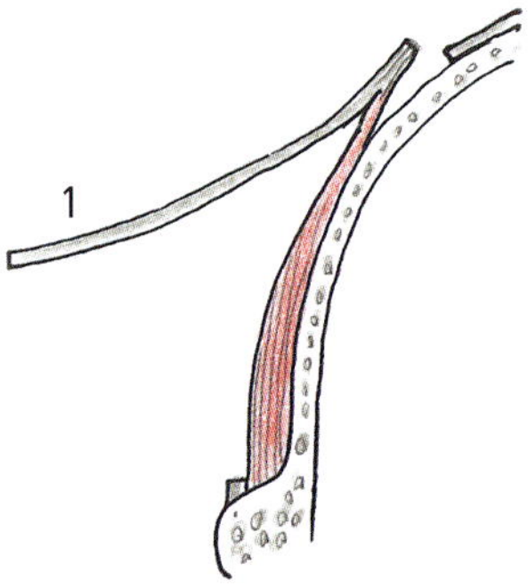

Figure 3.210d

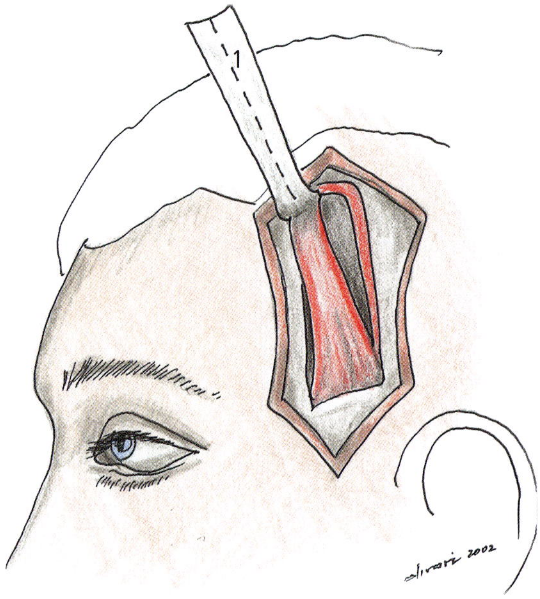

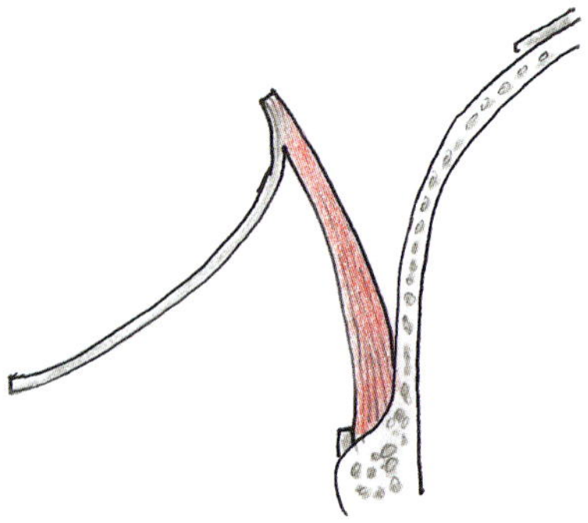

Figure 3.210e

Figure 3.210b With the extension of the temporal muscle using its own fascia, two loops of sufficient length arise that can be guided around the eye in a sufficient length. An additional fascial transplant is not necessary.

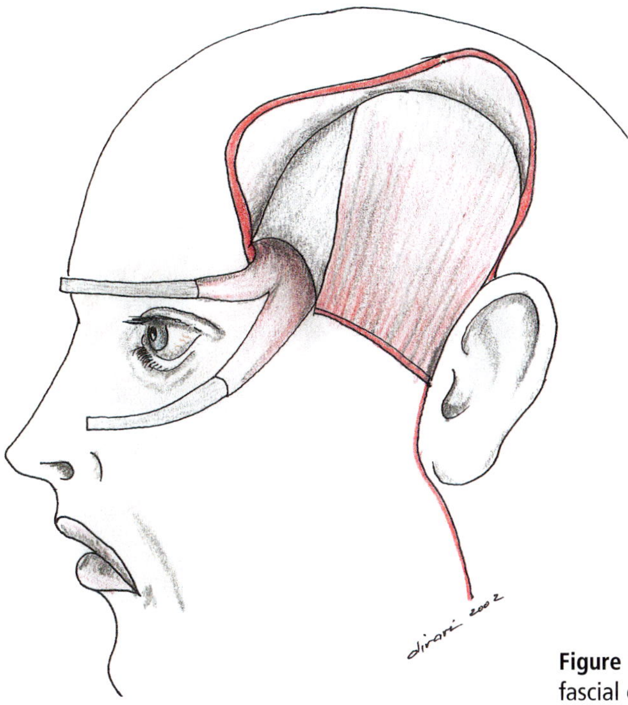

Figure 3.210f The divided temporal muscle strips with their fascial extensions reach the base of the nose.

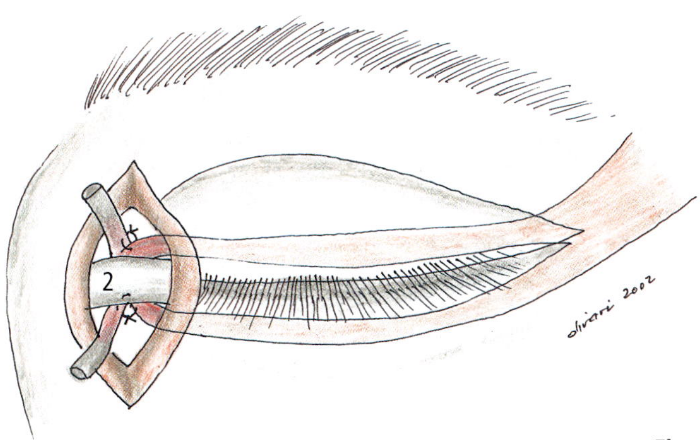

Figure 3.210g Both temporal muscle strips are led through the upper and lower eyelid before they are pulled and fixed under the medial ligament (2).

Dynamic-Static Operation

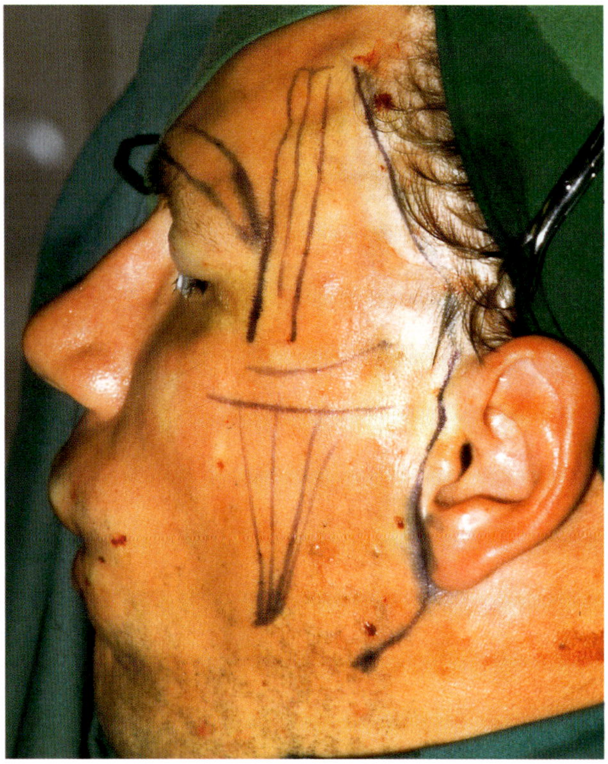

Figure 3.211a Planning of the operation with facial palsy

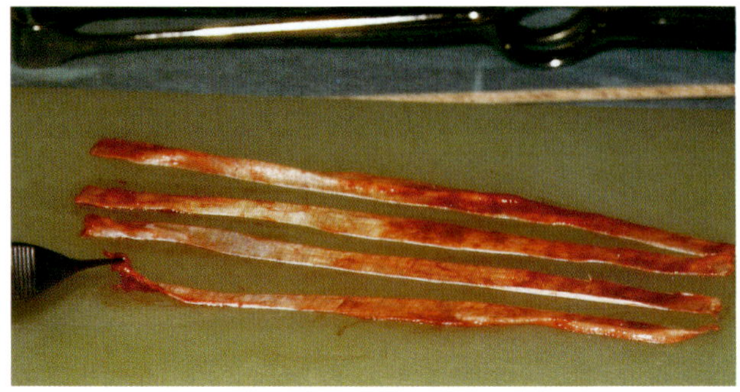

Figure 3.211b Four fascia lata strips are prepared:
1) Circular around the mouth
2) Connection of the temporal muscle with the corner of the mouth
3+4) For the static suspension of the nasolabial fold

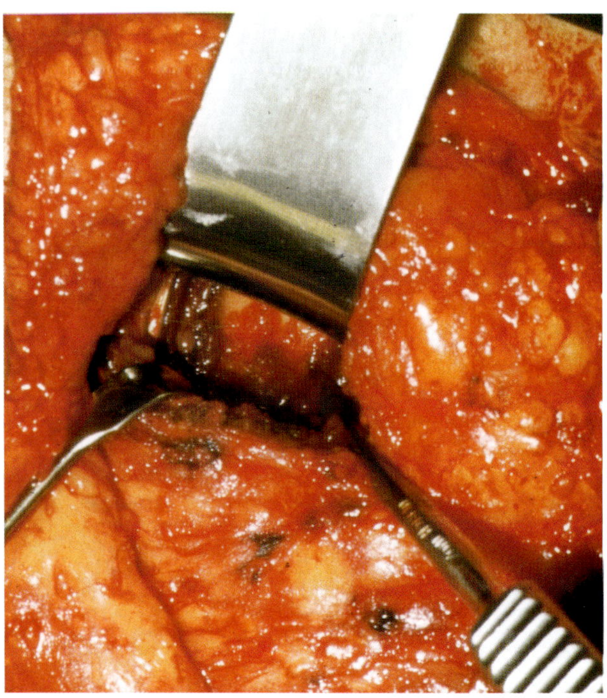

Figure 3.211c The masseter is transversely split below the zygomatic arch in its front part and the coronoid process is sought after.

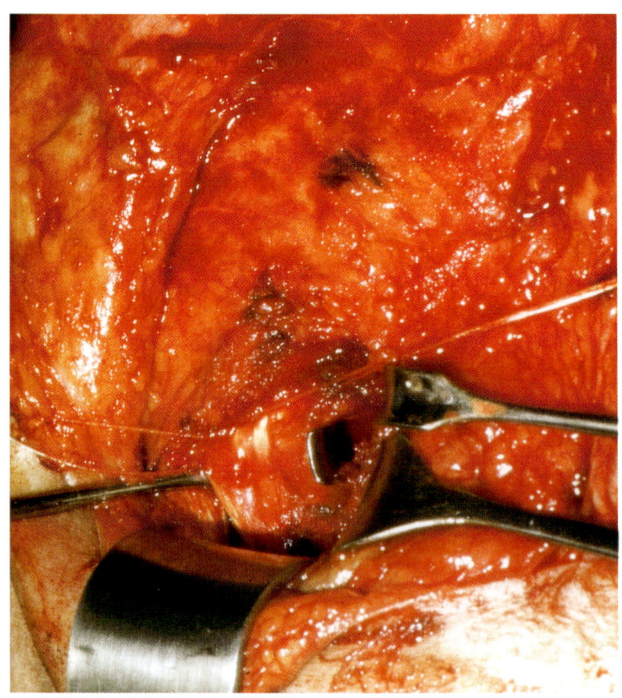

Figure 3.211d The coronoid process is severed along with the temporal muscle from the mandible.

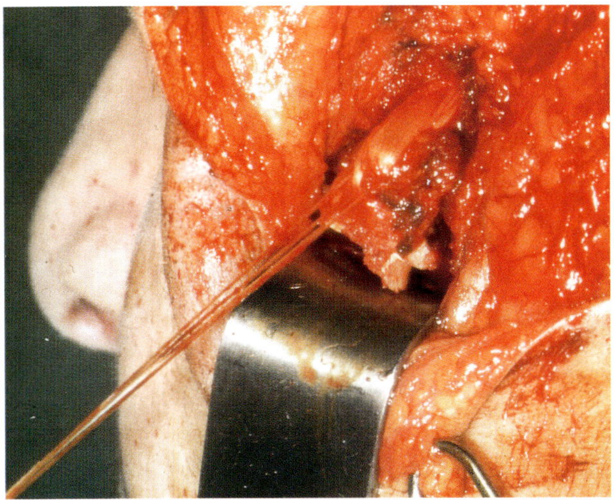

Figure 3.211e The coronoid process is mobilized

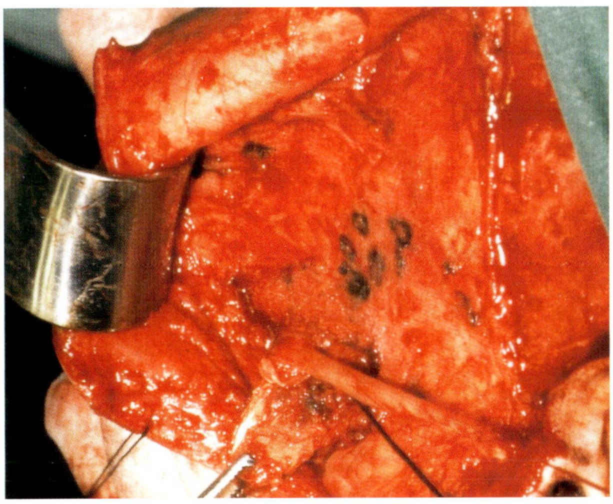

Figure 3.211g The coronoid process is fixed at the corner of the mouth using fascial strips.

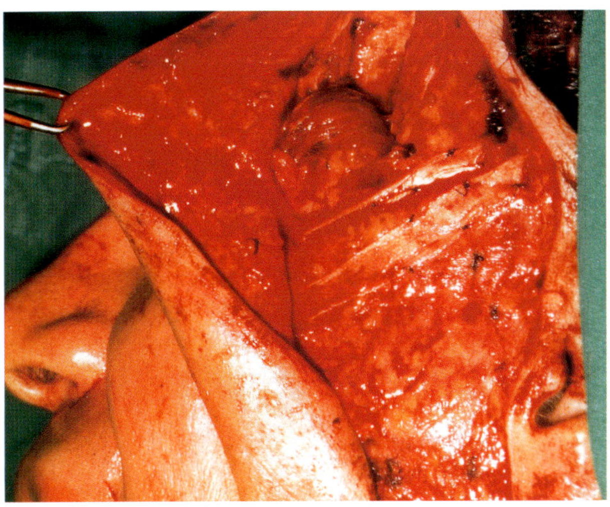

Figure 3.211i Two temporal muscle strips are pulled through the lower and upper eyelid.

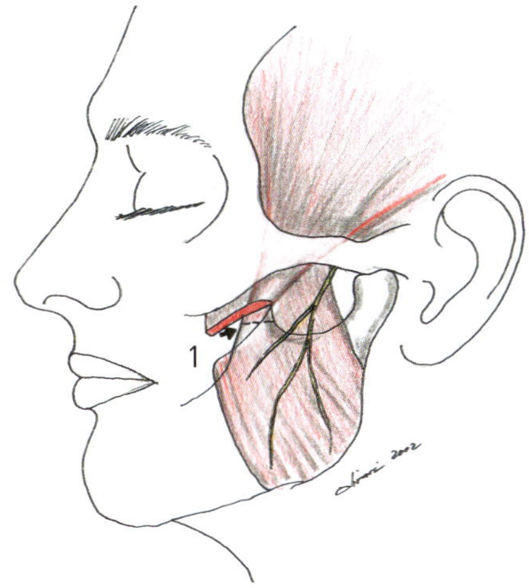

Figure 3.211f The masseter is only divided ventrally (1). The masseteric nerve is located dorsally.

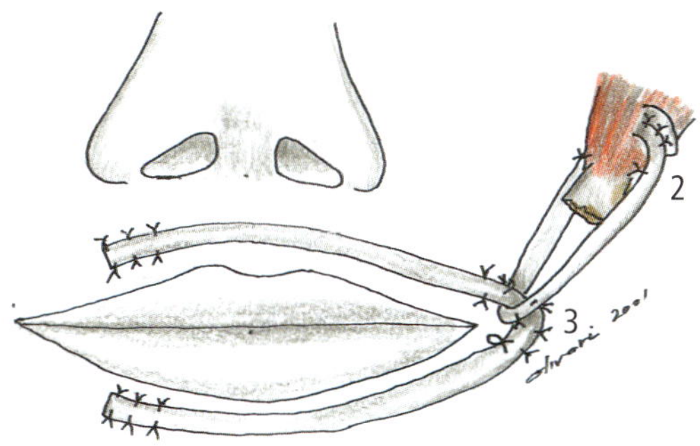

Figure 3.211h McLaughlin-procedure: A fascia lata strip is pulled between the temporal muscle and the sawn-off coronoid process (2) and fixed at the corner of the mouth using fascial strips (3).

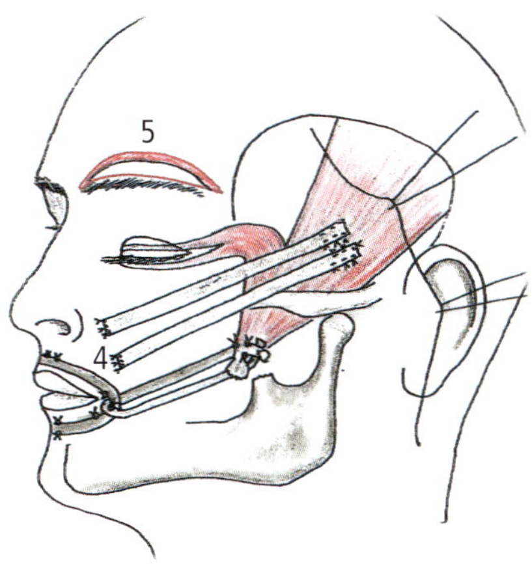

Figure 3.211j Two fascial strips are fixed at the nasolabial fold (4) and attached with extensive stretching to the temporal fascia. Two temporal muscle strips are pulled at the upper and lower eyelid. The eyebrow elevation occurs by skin excision (5).

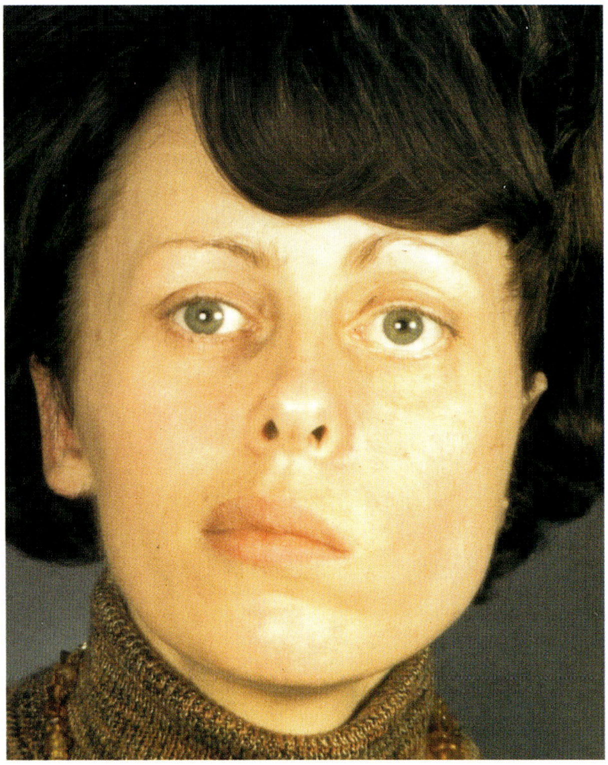

Figure 3.212a Since four year facial paralysis on the left side (acoustic neurinoma)

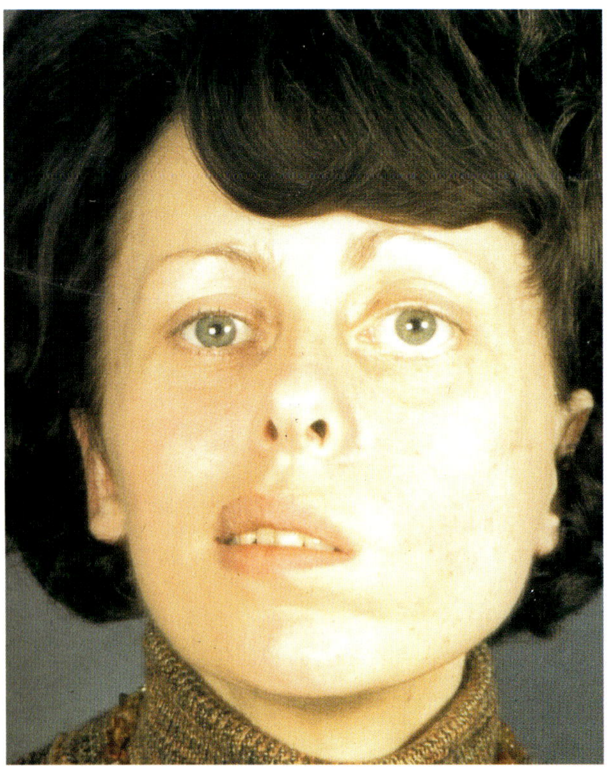

Figure 3.212b Severe asymmetry upon smiling "scleral show"

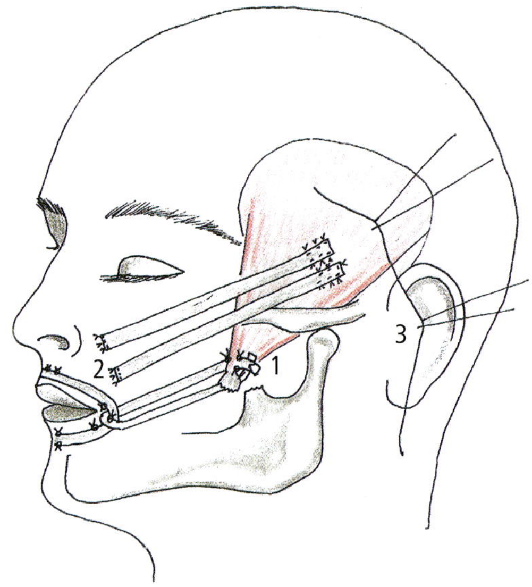

Figure 3.212c Planning of the operation:

1) The temporal muscle is severed with a part of the coronoid process and fixed with fascia lata strips under strain at the corner of the mouth (McLaughlin).
2) Two fascia lata strips are fixed under strain between the nasolabial fold and the temporal fascia (overcorrection).
3) Facelifting on the left side

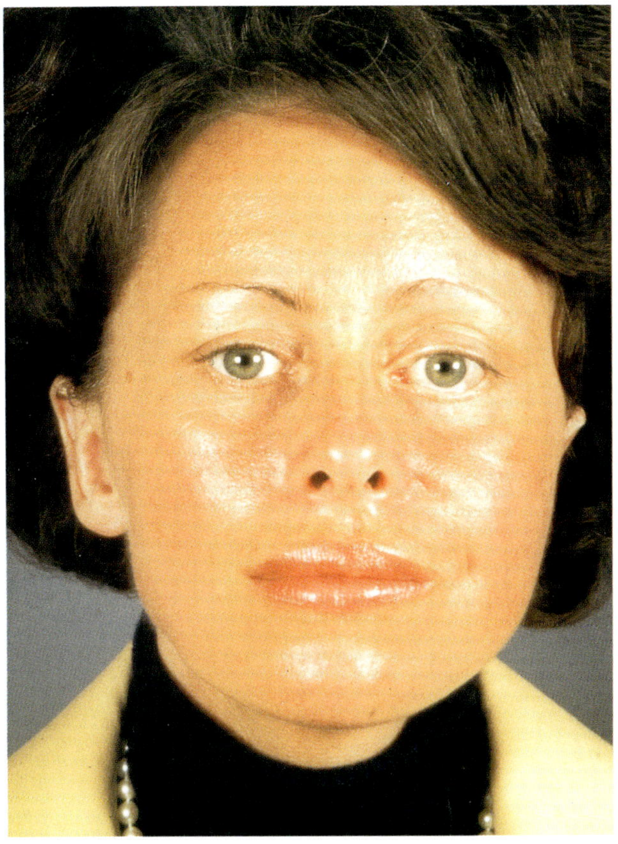

Figure 3.212d Situation 18 months after the operation

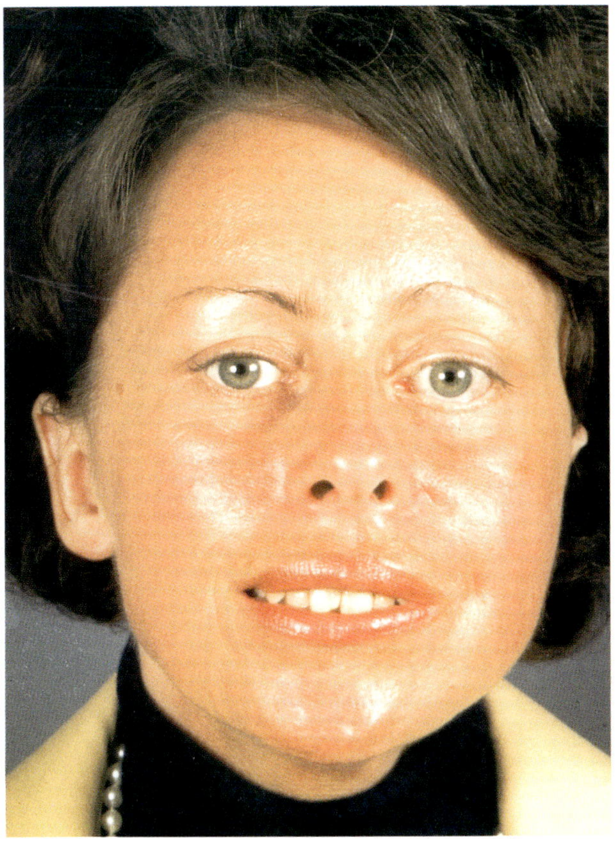

Figure 3.212e Satisfactory facial expression in a very intelligent patient who learned to synchronize her movements.

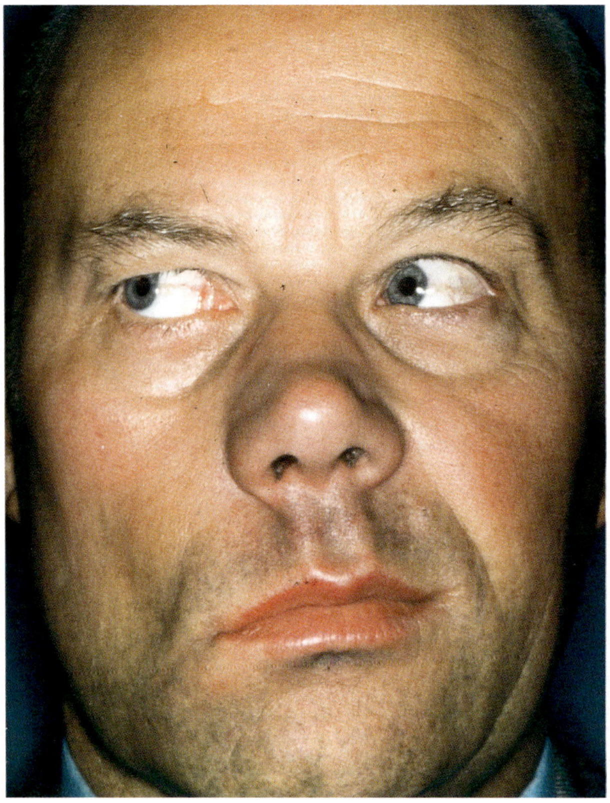

Figure 3.213a Complete facial nerve paralysis on the right

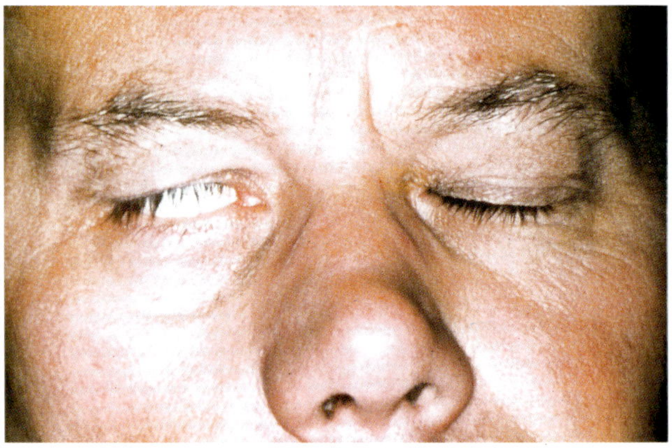

Figure 3.213b Incomplete eyelid closure on the right with Bell's phenomenon

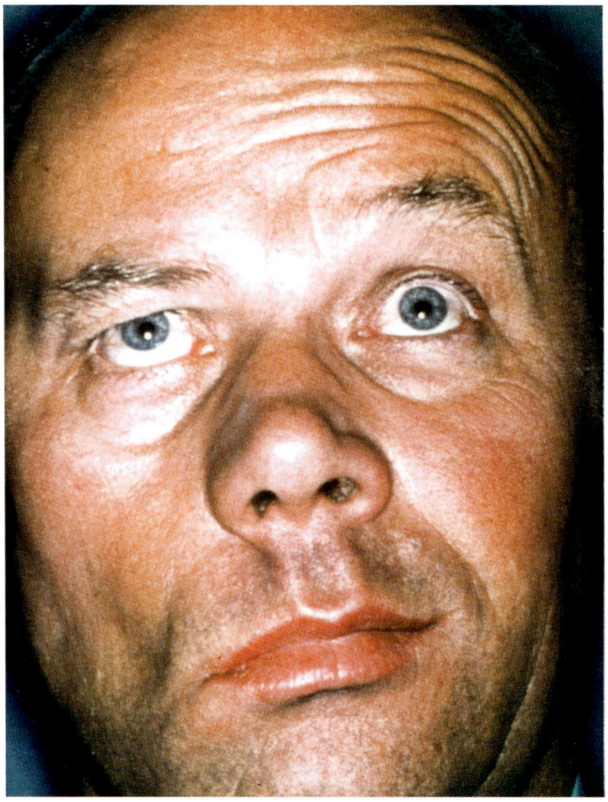

Figure 3.209c Defective facial expression

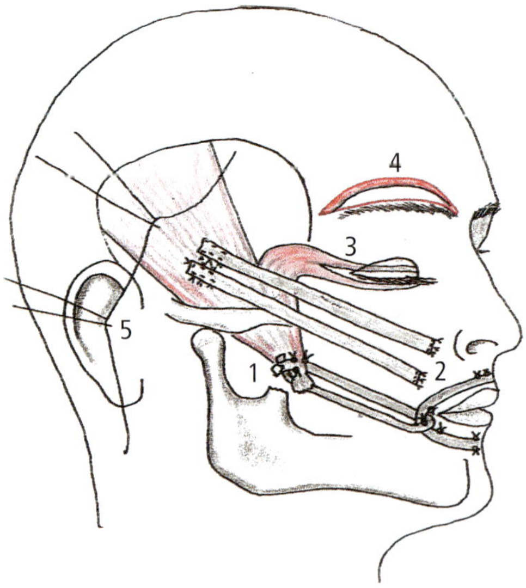

Figure 3.213d Operation technique:

1) Dynamic suspension of the corner of the mouth according to McLaughlin
2) Static suspension of the nasolabial fold using fascial strips
3) Drawing of temporal strips into the upper and lower eyelid
4) Spindle-shaped excision above the eyebrow (eyebrow elevation)
5) Facelifting

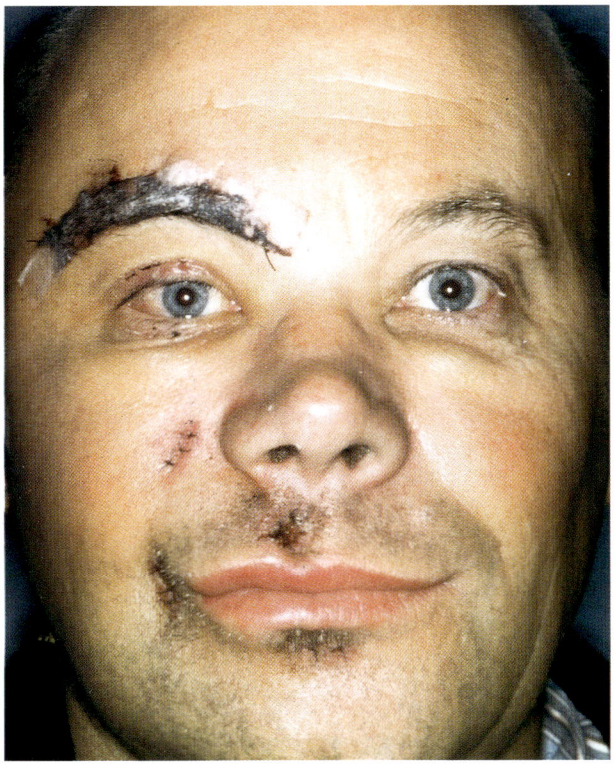

Figure 3.213e Status nine days after the operation. Training begins on the first day after the operation.

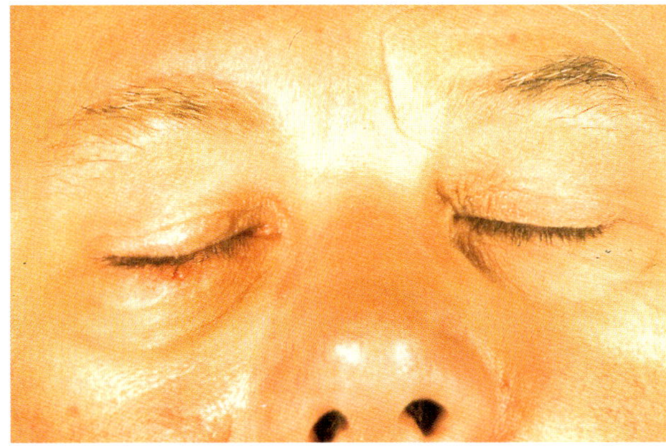

Figure 3.213f Complete eyelid closure one year postoperatively

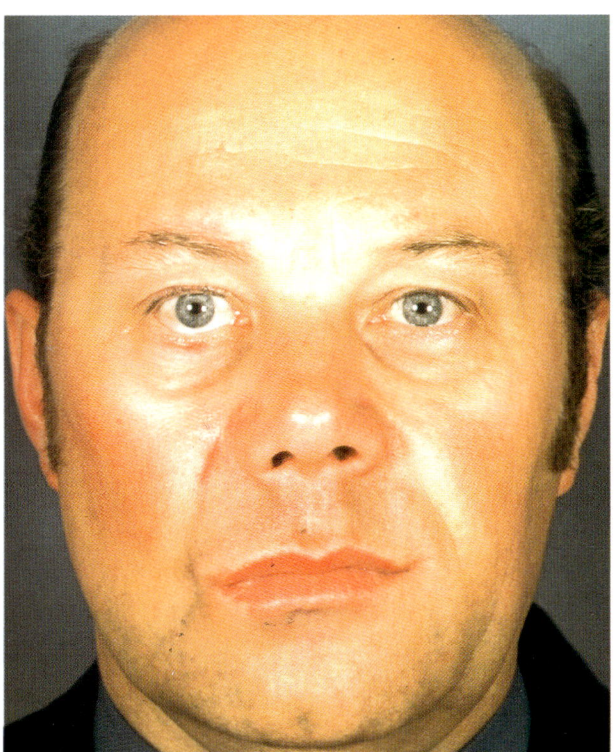

Figure 3.213g Status one year after the operation

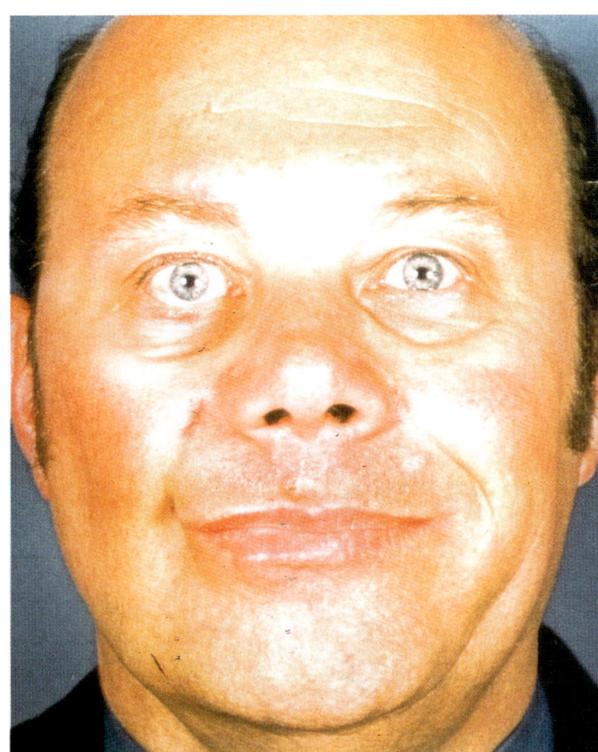

Figure 3.213h Sufficient facial expression

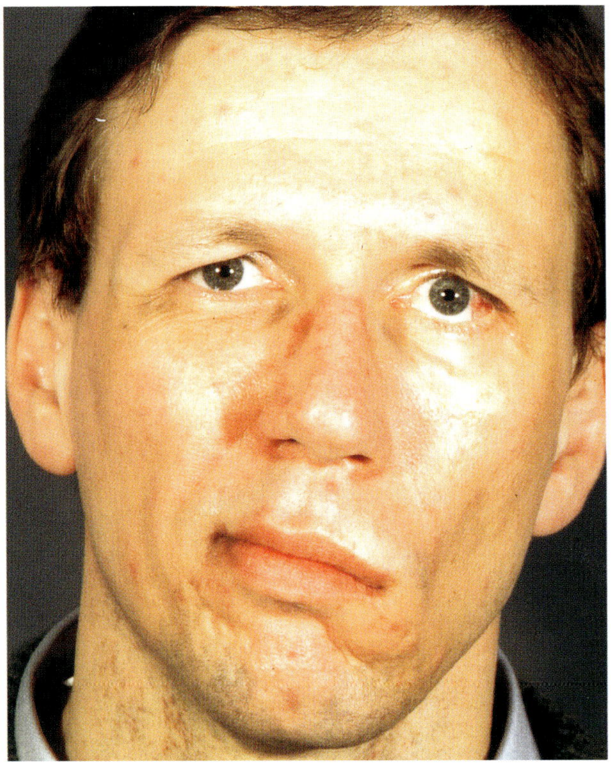

Figure 3.214a Facial nerve paralysis on the left side

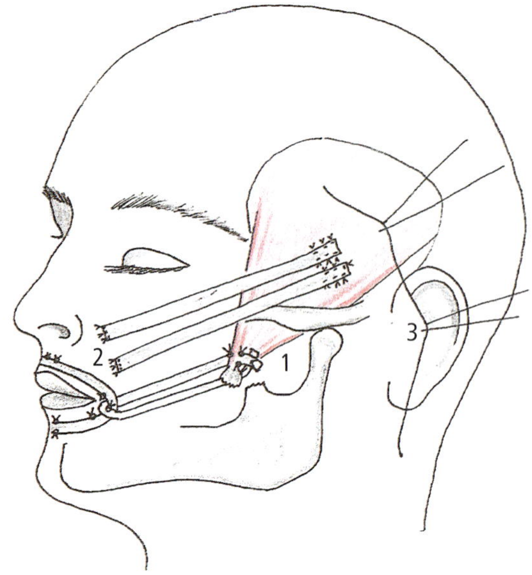

Figure 3.214b Operation:

1) Suspension of the corner of the mouth according to McLaughlin (dynamic)
2) Static suspension of the nasolabial fold with fascia lata strips
3) Facelifting

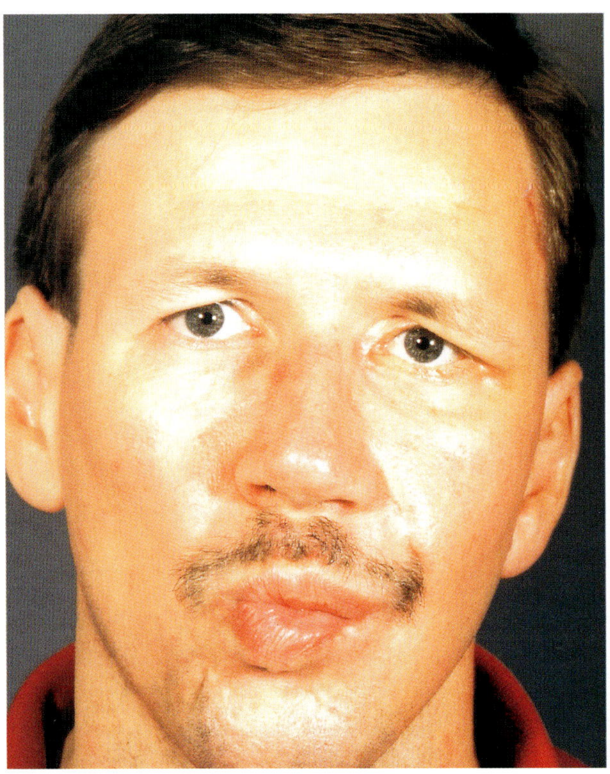

Figure 3.214c Status 18 months after the operation

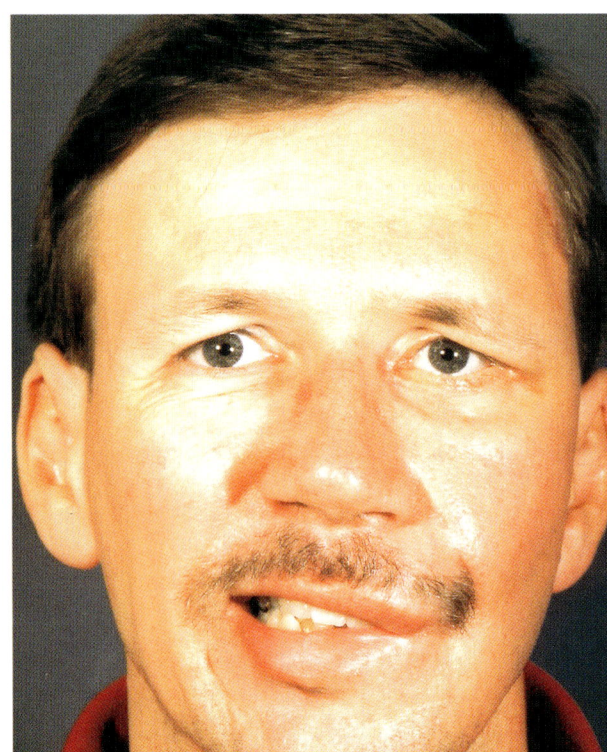

Figure 3.214d Satisfactory facial expression

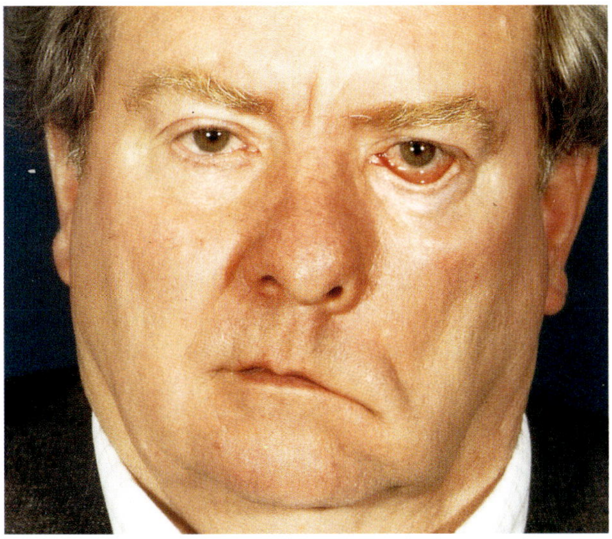

Figure 3.215a Facial nerve paralysis on the left side already lasting nine years

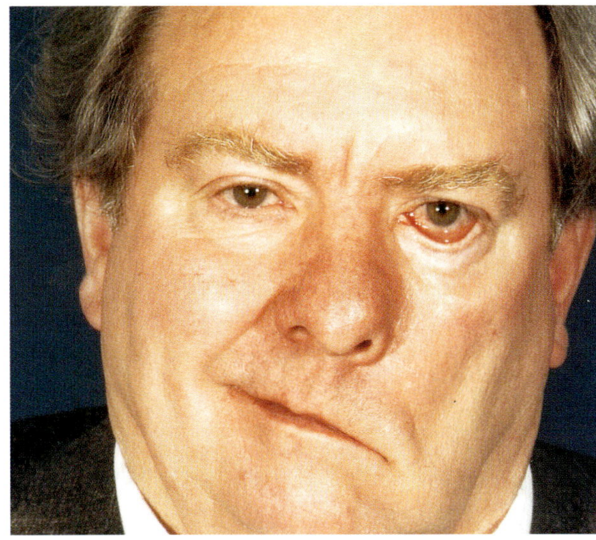

Figure 3.215b Severe eyelid ptosis, chronic conjunctivitis. Typical facial expression when attempting to smile.

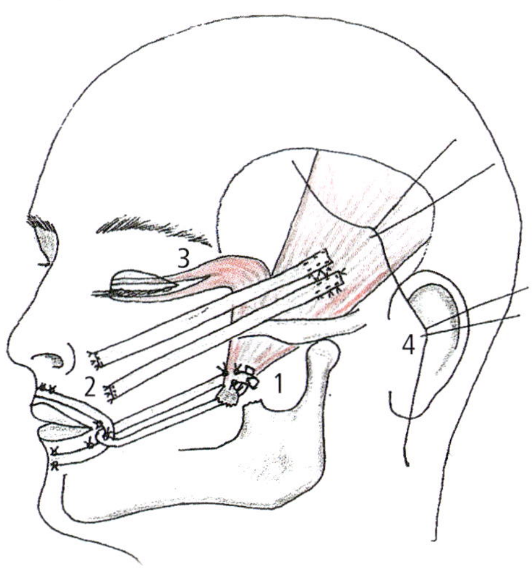

Figure 3.215c Operation:
1) Suspension of the corner of the mouth according to McLaughlin
2) Suspension of the nasolabial fold with fascial strips
3) Correction in the eyelid area using two temporal muscle strips
4) Facelifting

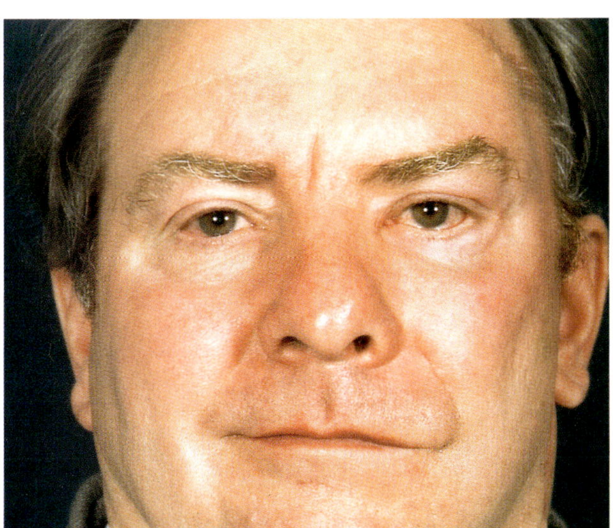

Figure 3.215d Status one year after the operation: Static symmetry.

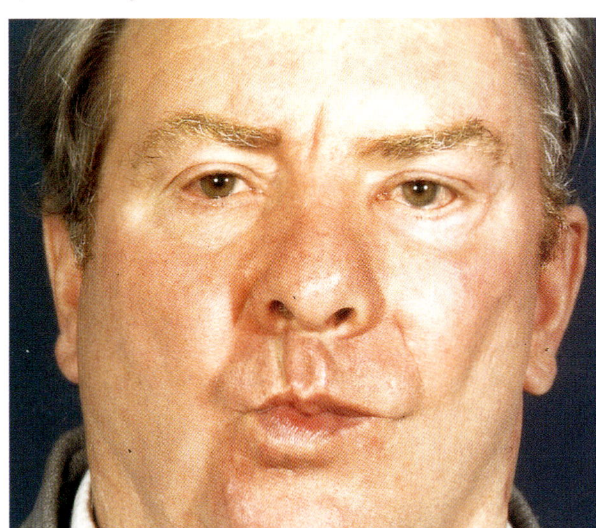

Figure3.215e Status one year after the operation

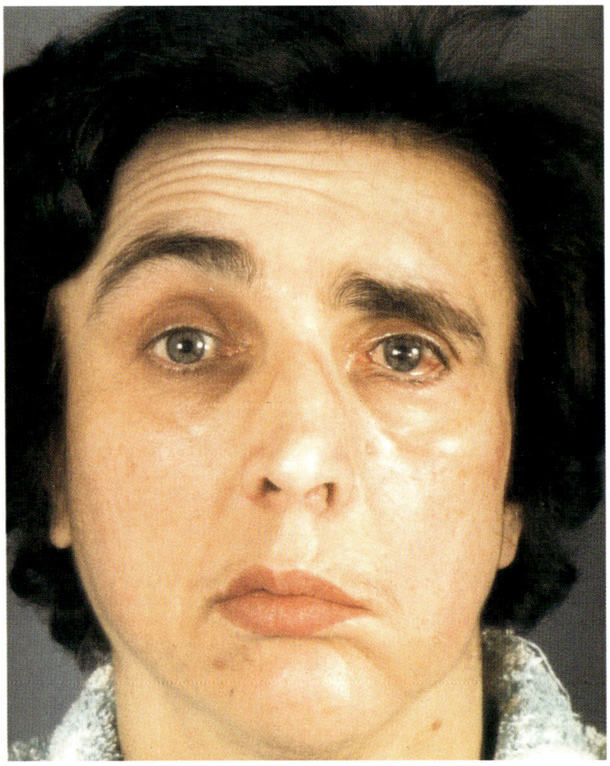

Figure 3.216a Facial nerve paralysis on the left side

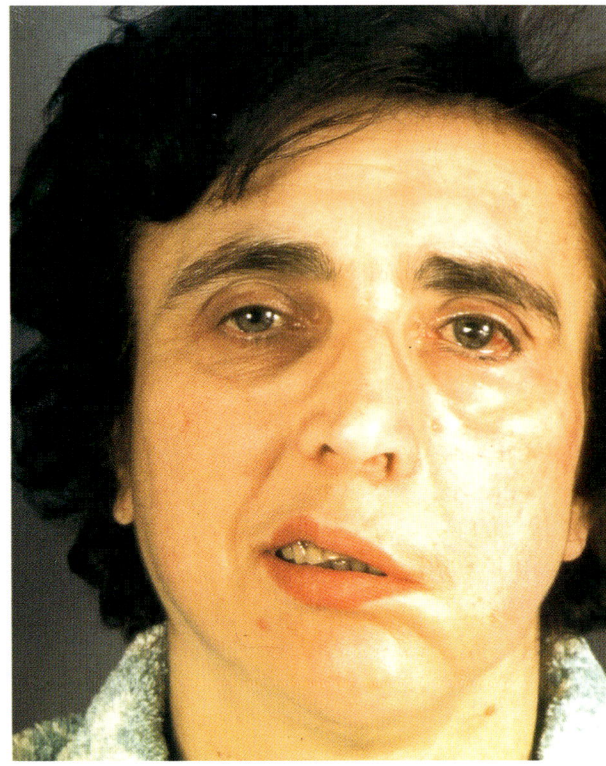

Figure 3.216b Anamnesis: Five years

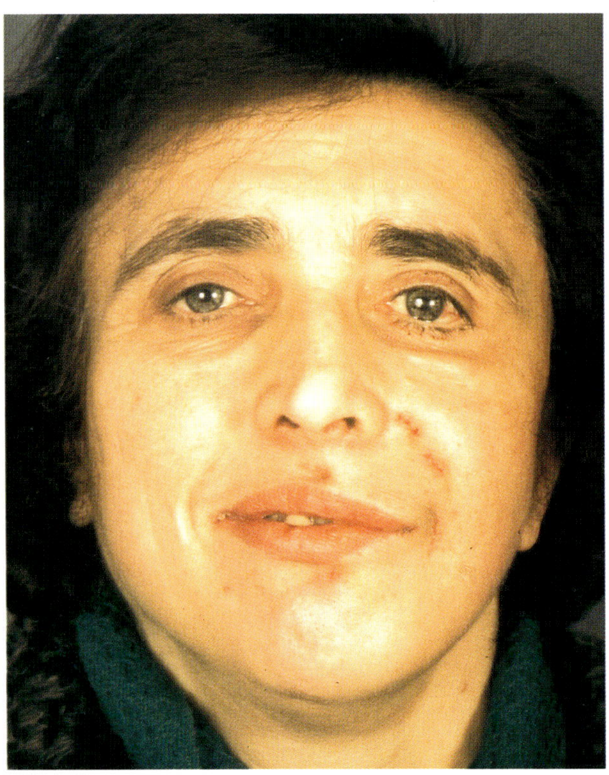

Figure 3.216c Important! Early practice already one day after the operation. Here the status ten days after operation.

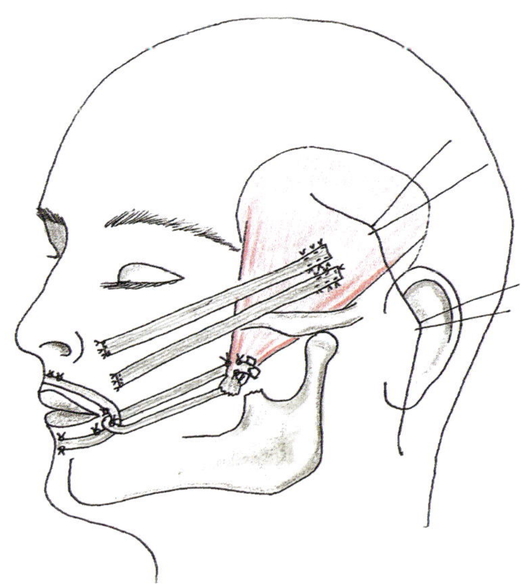

Figure 3.216d Operation:
1) Suspension of the corners of the mouth according to McLaughlin
2) Suspension of the nasolabial fold with two fascia lata strips
3) Modified facelifting

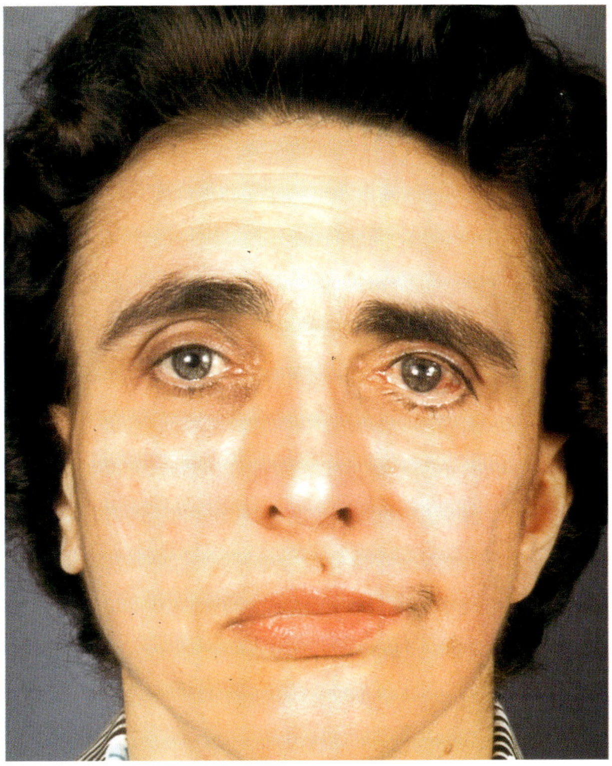

Figure 3.216e Status 16 months postoperatively. Modest symmetry at rest.

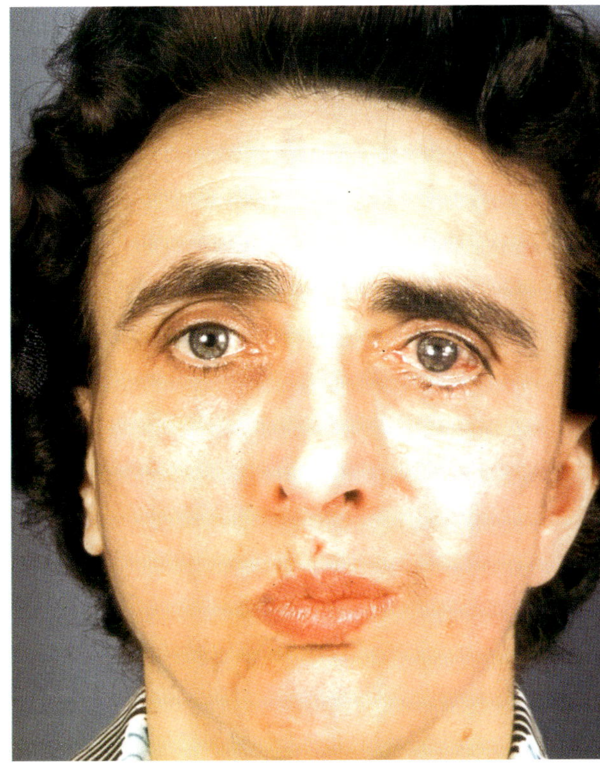

Figure 3.216f Sufficient facial expression accomplished after long practicing by the patient.

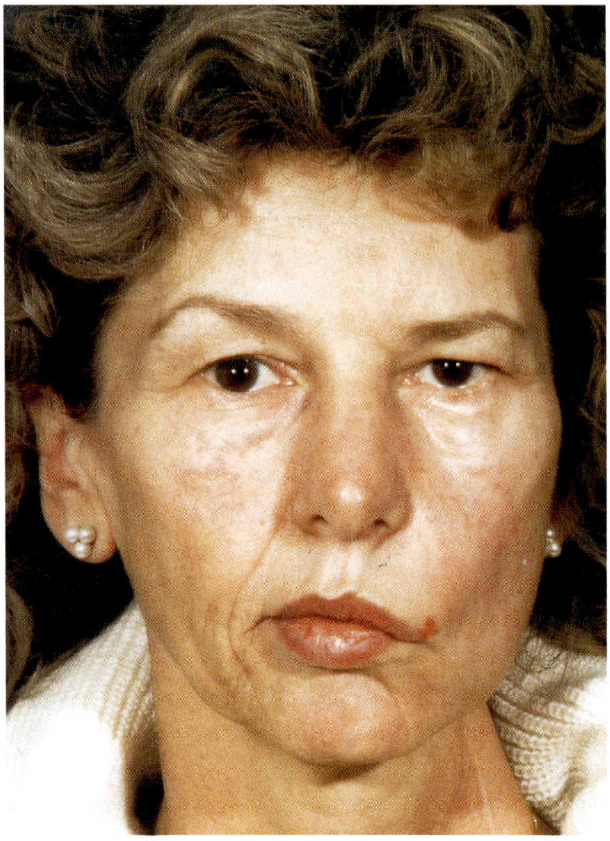

Figure 3.217a Complete irreversible facial palsy on the left side

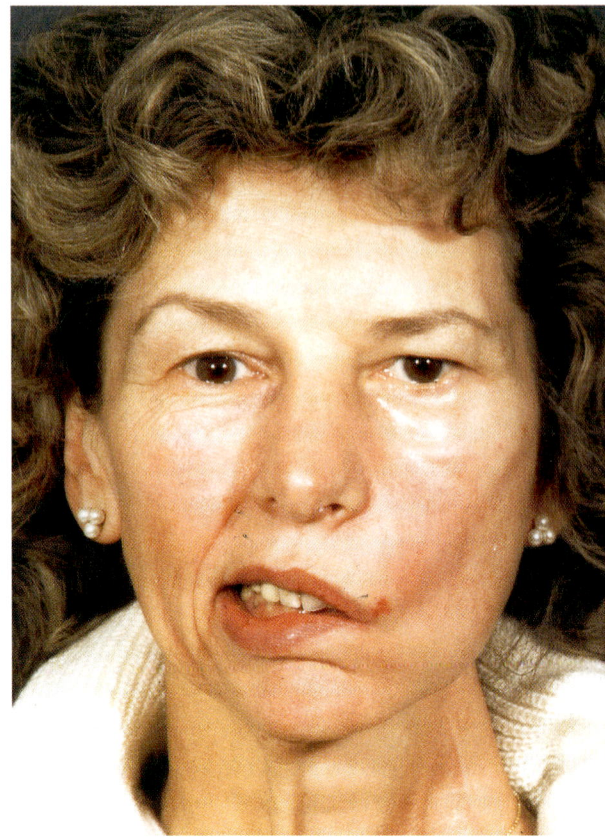

Figure 3.217b Striking, typical facial expression

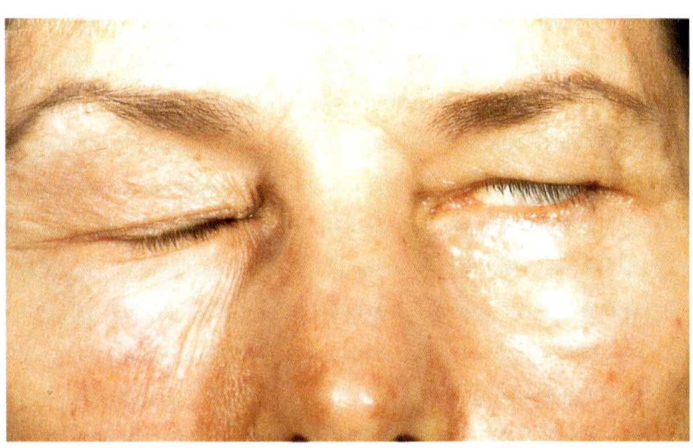

Figure 3.217c Eyelid closure on the left side is not possible

Operation:
1) McLaughlin
2) Suspension of the nasolabial fold with two fascial strips
3) Eyelid correction according to Lexer
4) Facelifting

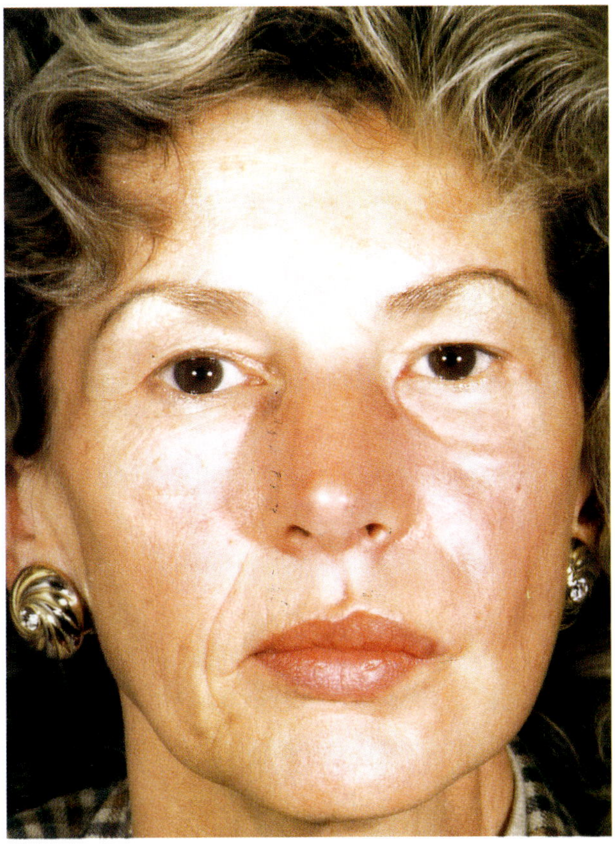

Figure 3.217d Status one year after the operation: Good symmetry at rest.

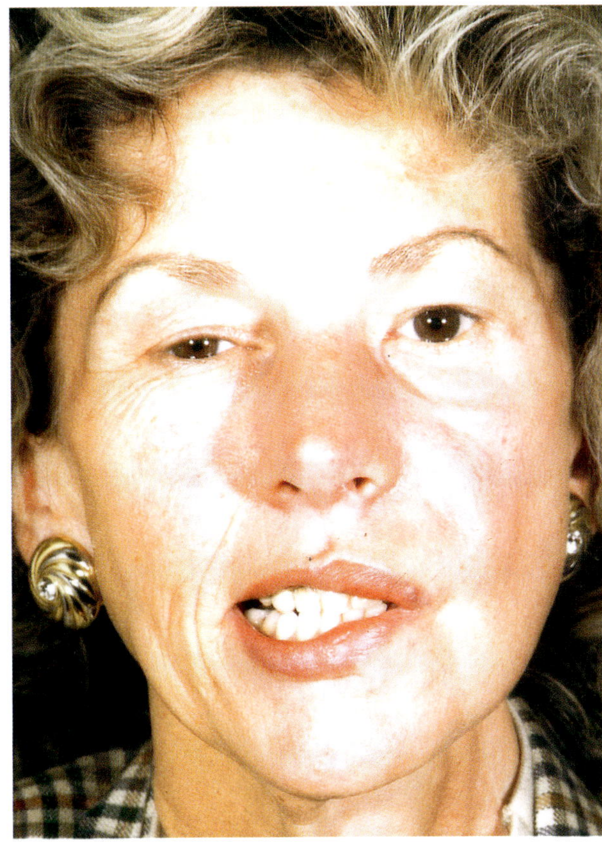

Figure 3.217e Acceptable symmetry when smiling

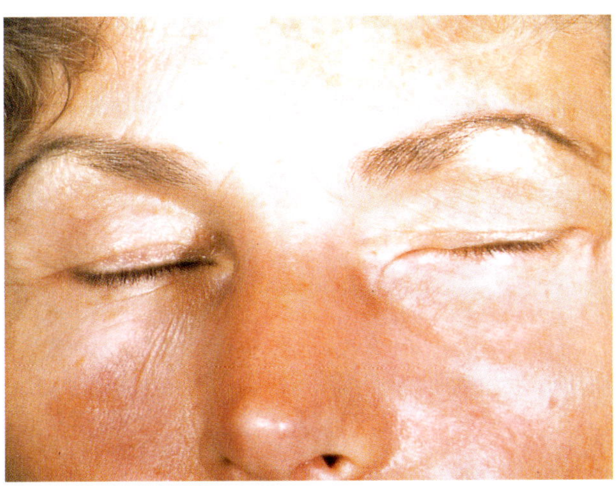

Figure 3.217f Eyelid closure is complete after two strips of the temporal muscle are transferred, but out of sync with the right side. A long training is absolutely necessary in order to achieve a good outcome.

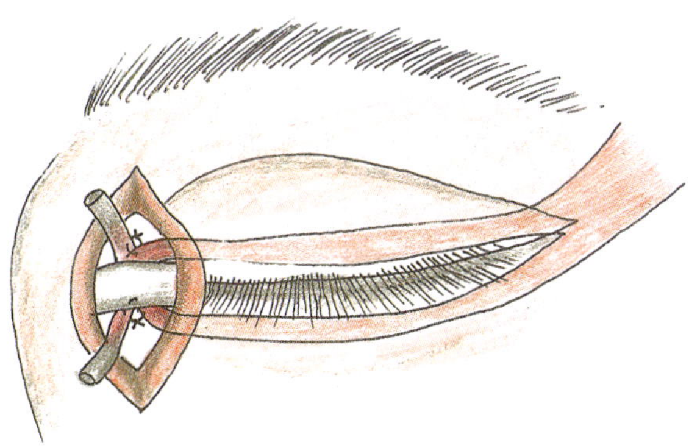

Figure 3.217g The temporal muscle strips are pulled through under the medial ligament and fixed under moderate strain.

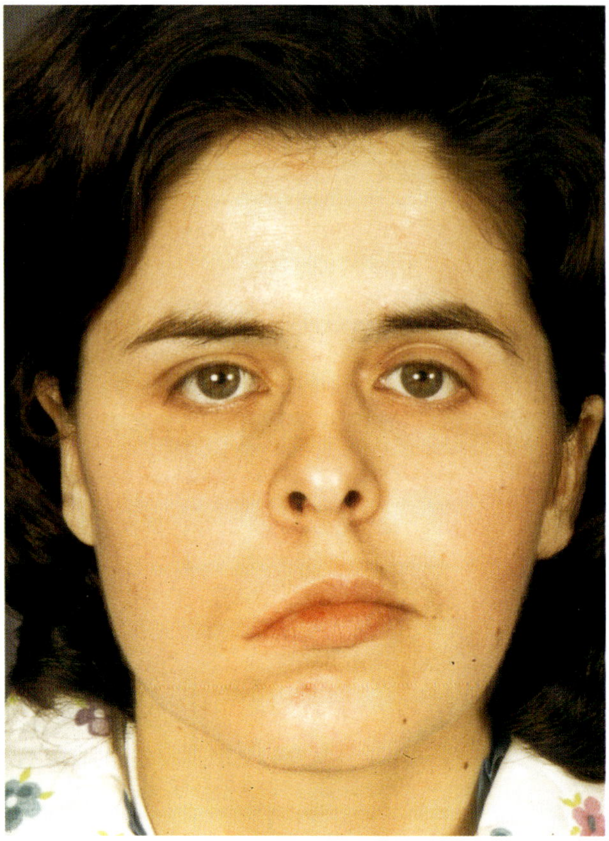

Figure 3.218a Completely facial palsy on the right side

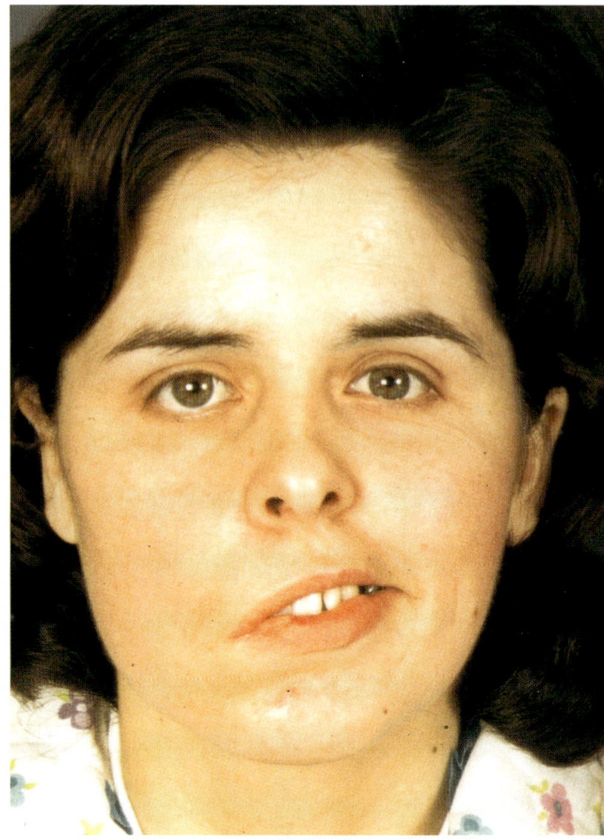

Figure 3.218b Anamnesis: Five years (status after acoustic neurinoma operation)

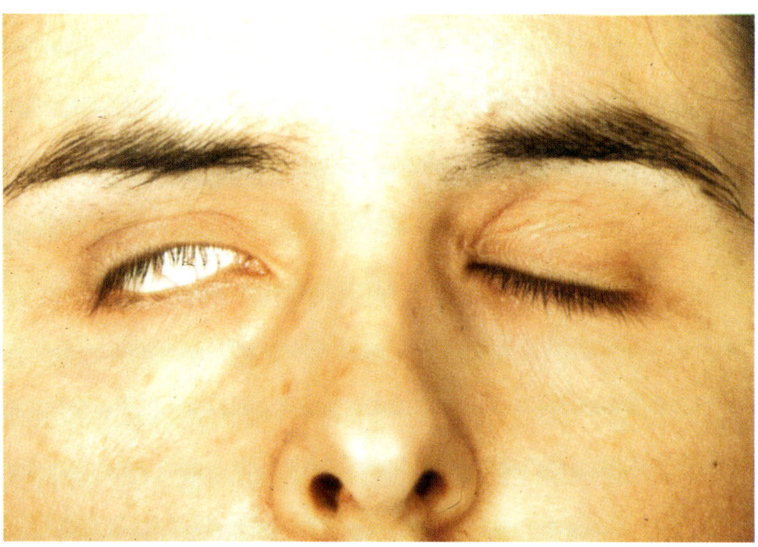

Figure 3.218c Incomplete eyelid closure preoperatively

Planned operation:

1) Modified McLaughlin operation
2) Static suspension of the nasolabial fold with fascia lata strips
3) Facelifting
4) Strips of temporal muscle in the eyelid area

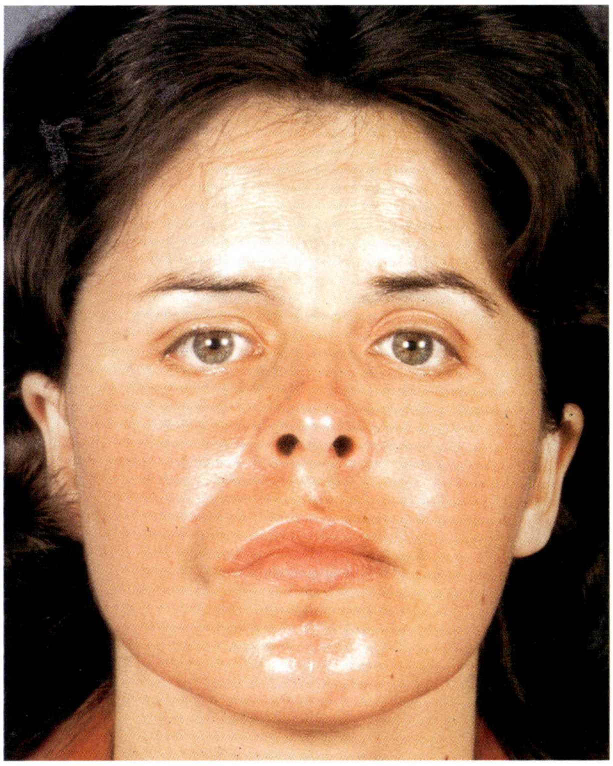

Figure 3.218d Status six months after the operation: Symmetry at rest.

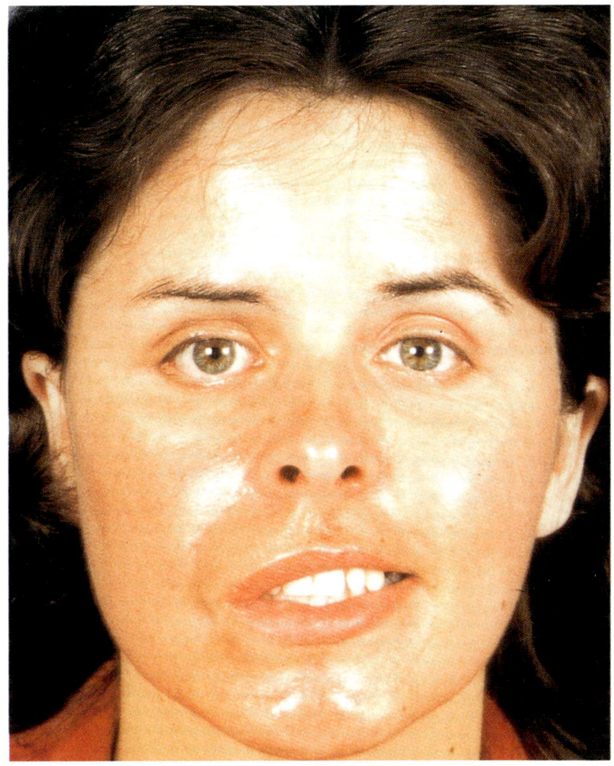

Figure 3.218e Acceptable facial expression

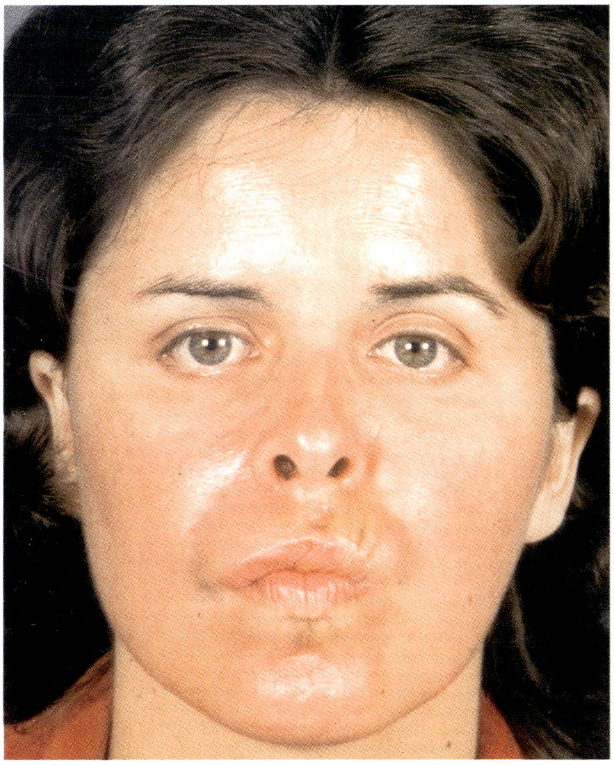

Figure 3.218f Status six months after the operation

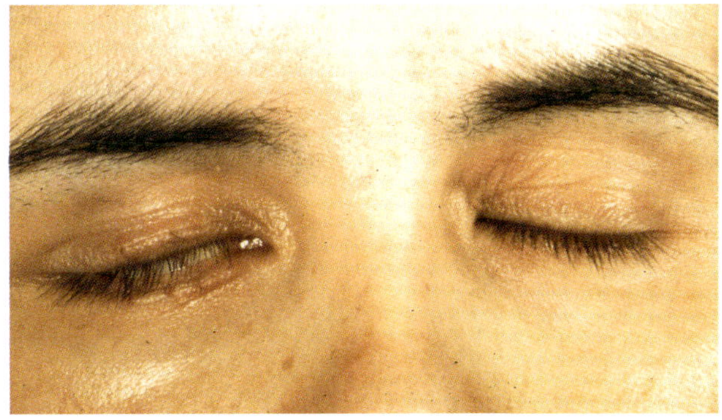

Figure 3.218g Improved but still incomplete eyelid closure

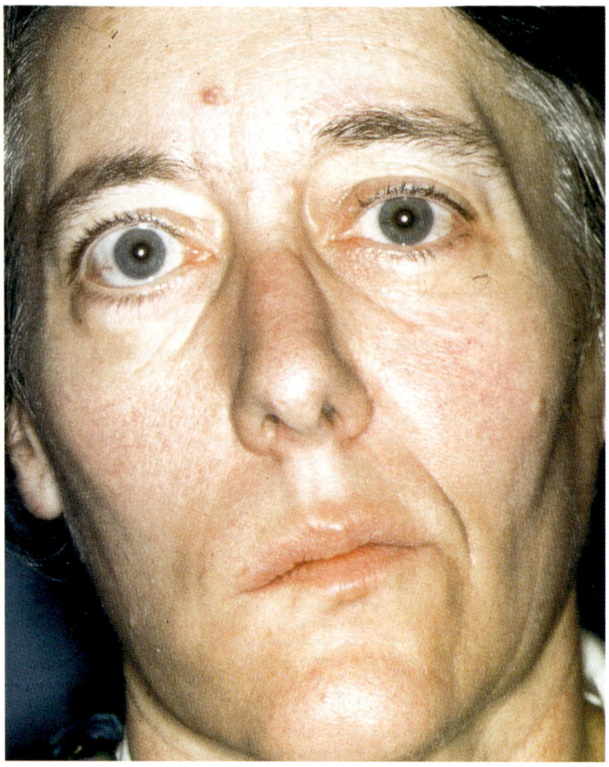

Figure 3.219a Complete facial nerve paralysis on the right side.
Anamnesis: Five years.
Planned operation:
1) Dynamic suspension of the corner of the mouth according to McLaughlin
2) Static suspension of the nasolabial fold with two fascia lata strips
3) Implantation of Mühlbauer magnets in the upper and lower eyelid
4) Facelifiting on the right side

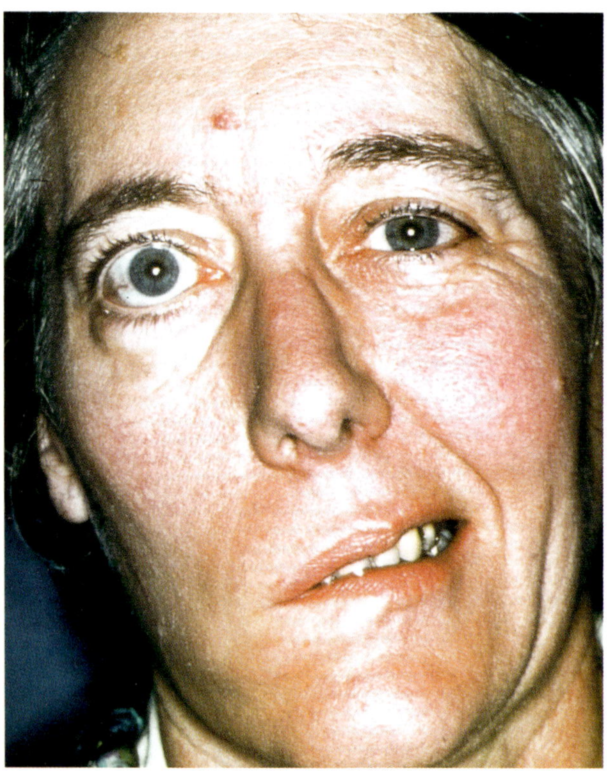

Figure 3.219b Preoperative facial expression

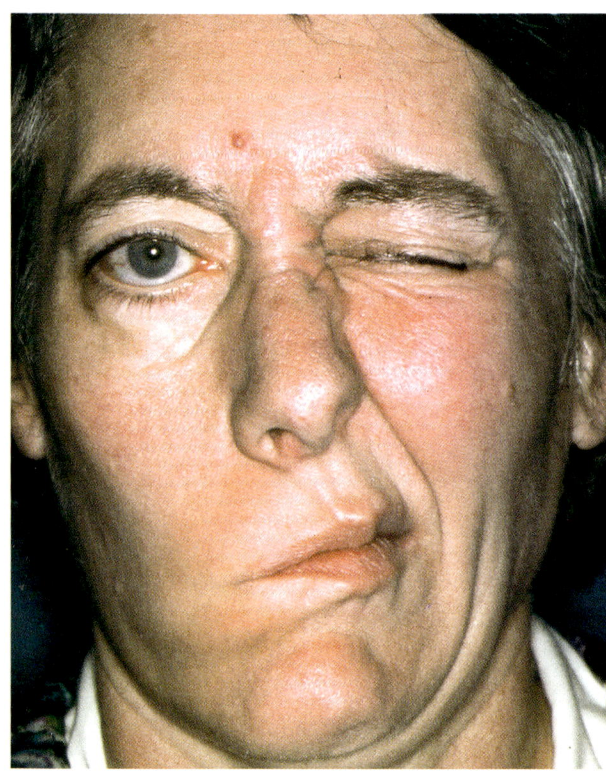

Figure 3.219c Incomplete eyelid closure

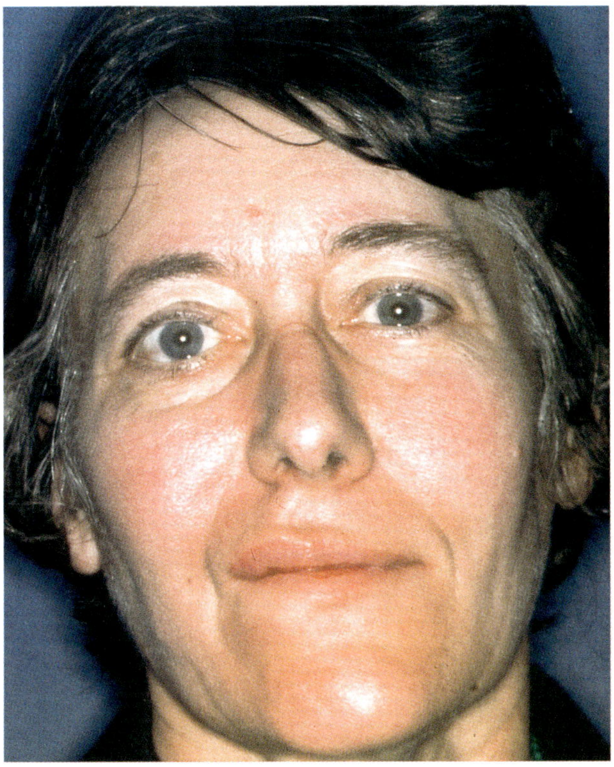

Figure 3.219d Status six months after the operation: Symmetry at rest.

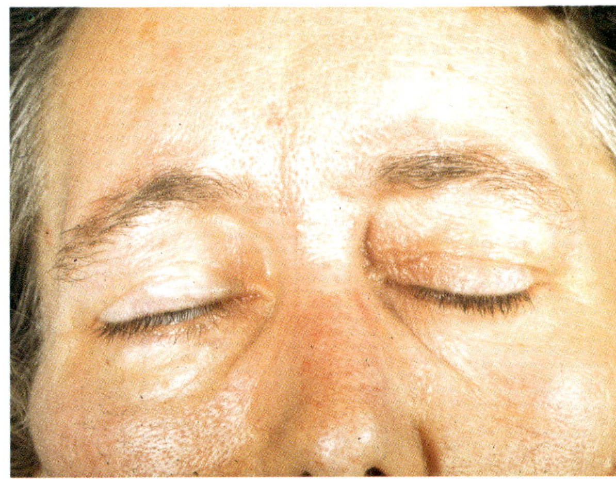

Figure 3.219e Good closure function with implanted magnets. After a further six months the magnets perforated and were removed. After that two temporal muscle strips were drawn into the upper and lower eyelid.

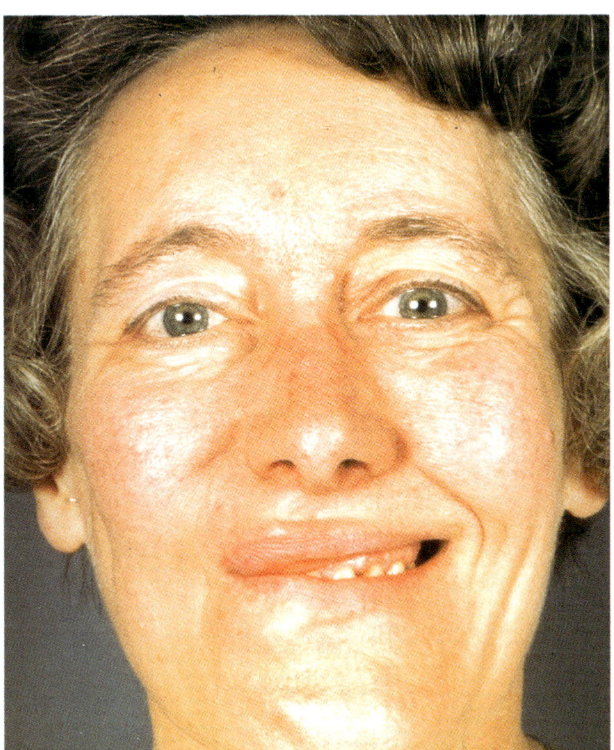

Figure 3.219f Status three years after the operation

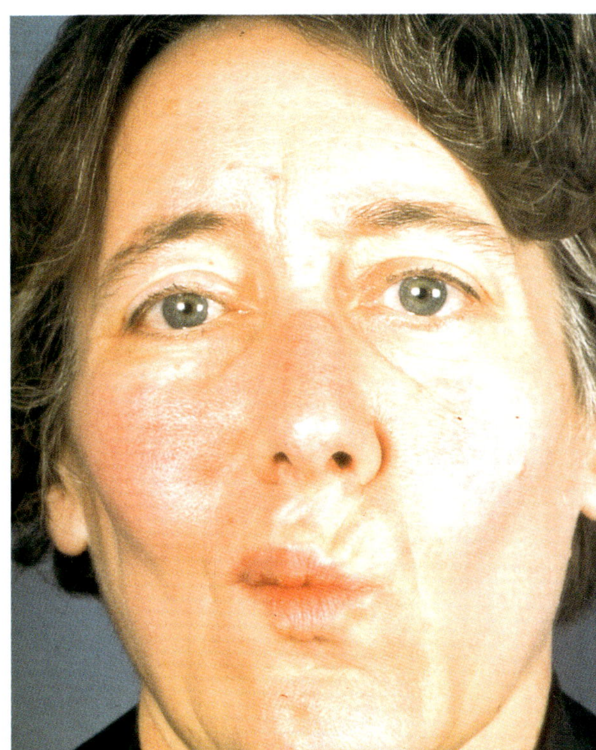

Figure 3.219g Acceptable facial expression

Caudally Pediculated Temporal Transfer

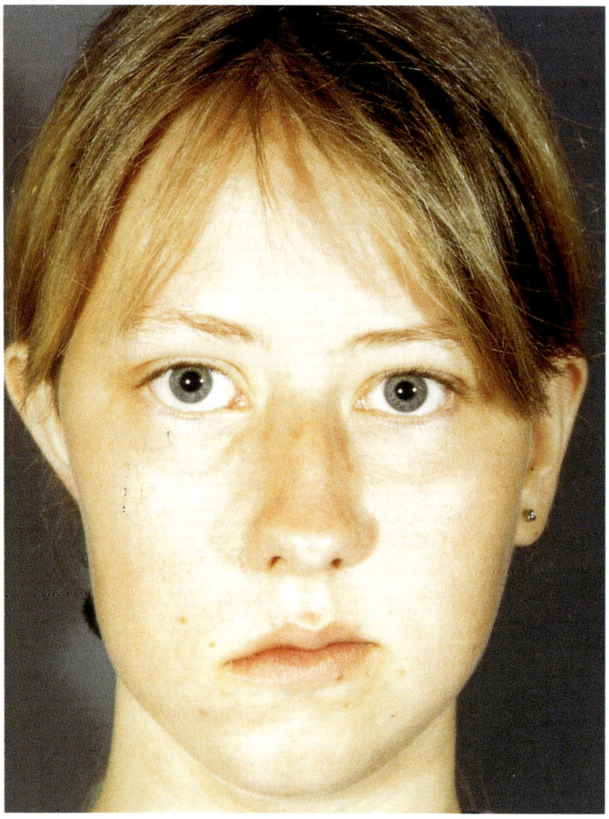

Figure 3.220a Complete and irreversible facial nerve paralysis on the right side

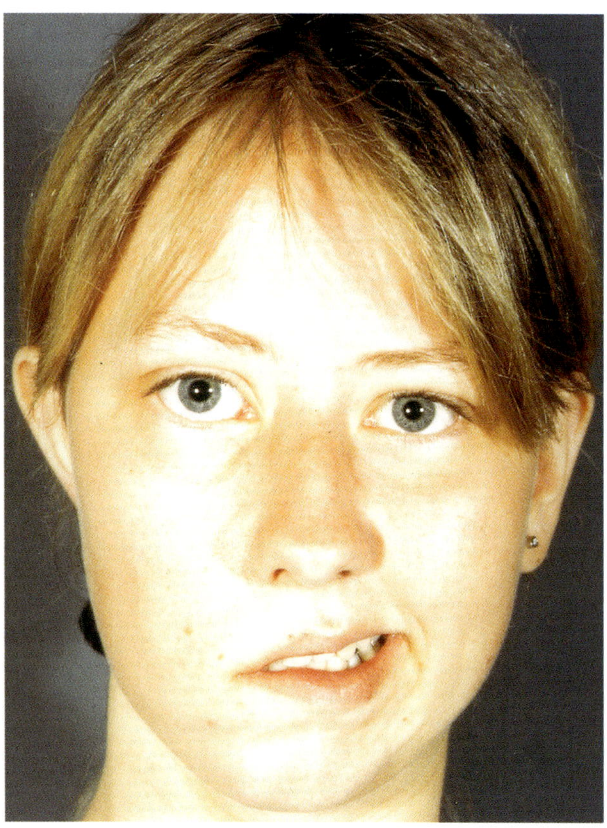

Figure 3.220b Typical defects for facial palsy on the right side

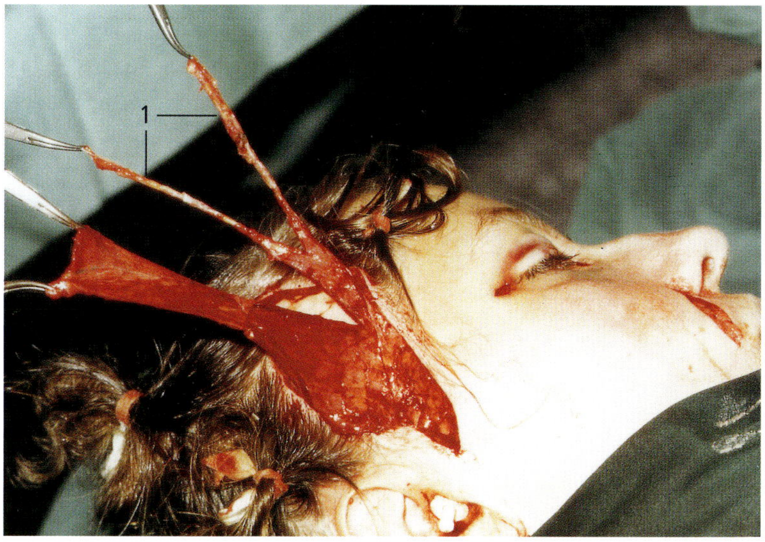

Figure 3.220c Caudally pediculated temporal transfer. Wide fascia strips are planned for the corner of the mouth as well as the nasolabial fold. Two thin strips are used for correcting the eyelid area (1). A prolongation of the muscle is achieved by using temporal fascia.

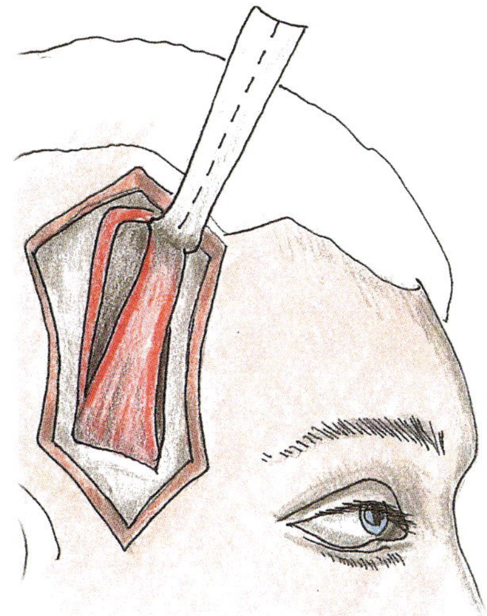

Figure 3.220d Extension of the muscle by surrounding of the temporal fascia

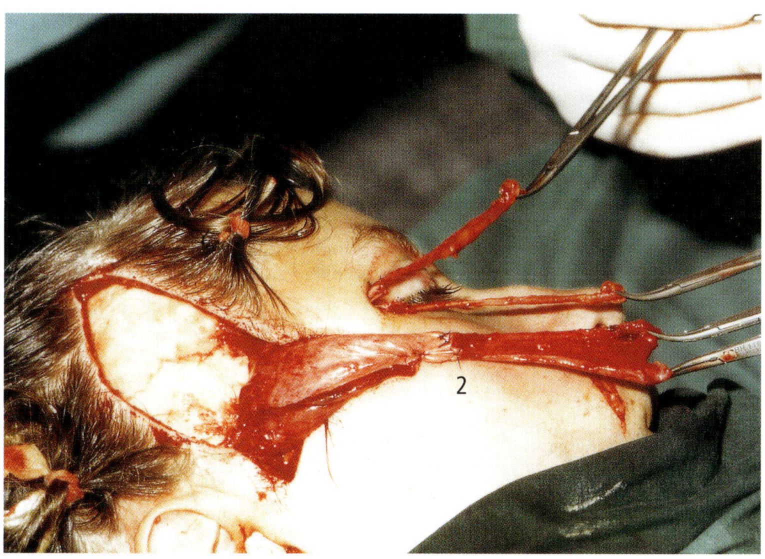

Figure 3.220e Two thin strips are prepared for fixation in the upper and lower eyelid area. The fascia strip easily reaches the mouth area (2).

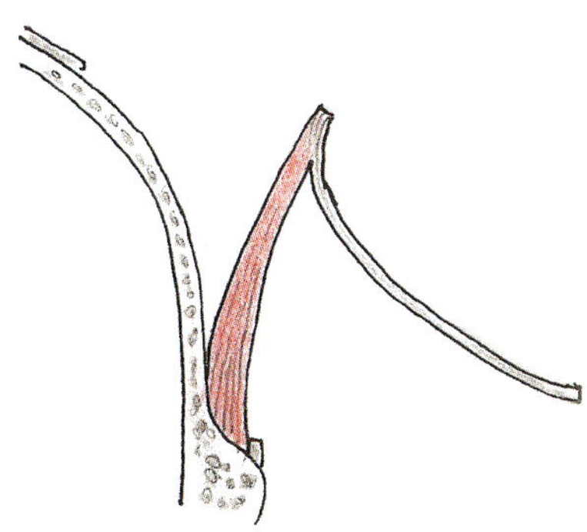

Figure 3.220f In order to achieve a sufficient length, the superficial temporal fascia is used in this way. As such any extension using fascia lata strips is unnecessary.

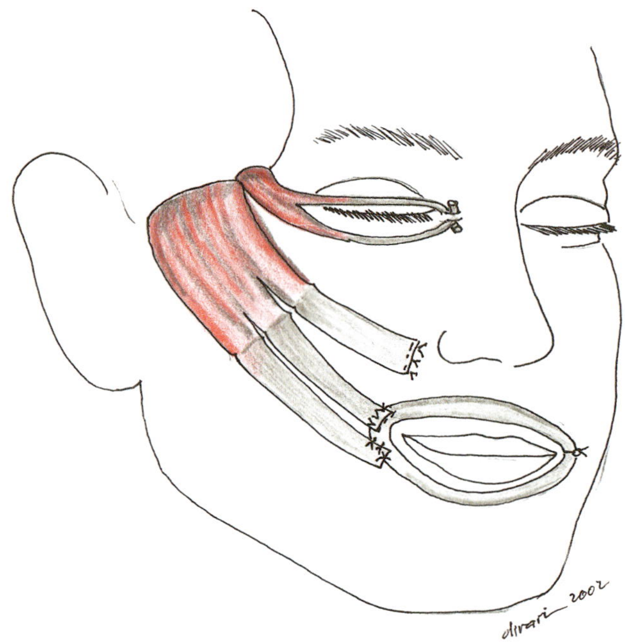

Figure 3.220g Schematic description of the operation

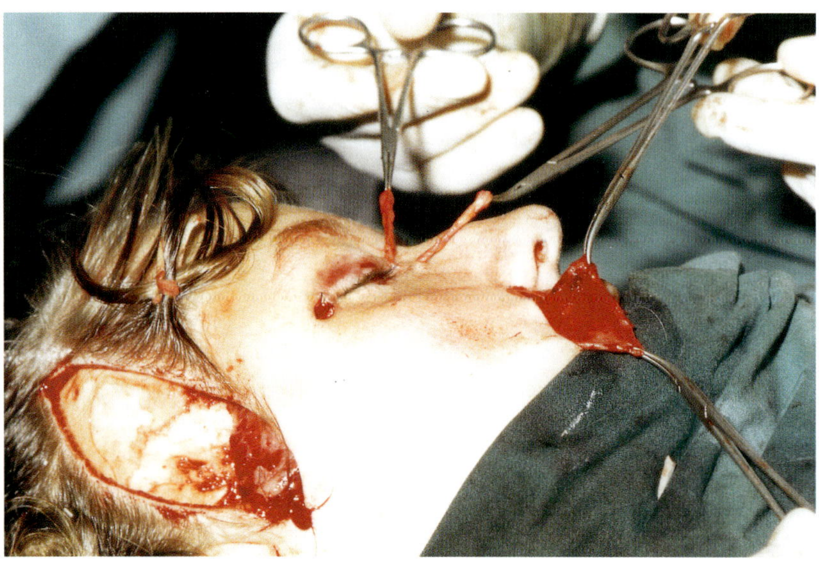

Figure 3.220h Intraoperative image. Two strips in the eyelid area are fixed under the median ligament under moderate strain. The wide fascia strip is fixed at the corner of the mouth and the nasolabial fold.

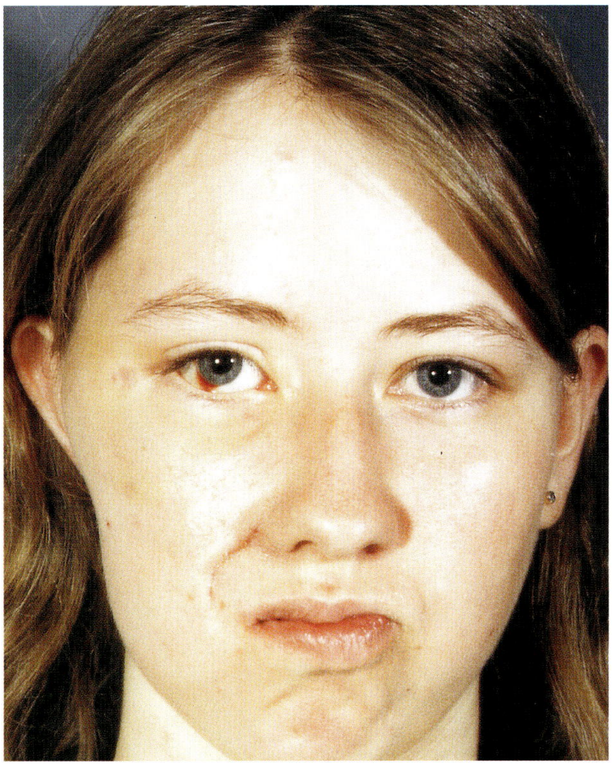

Figure 3.220i Satisfactory facial expression two weeks postoperatively

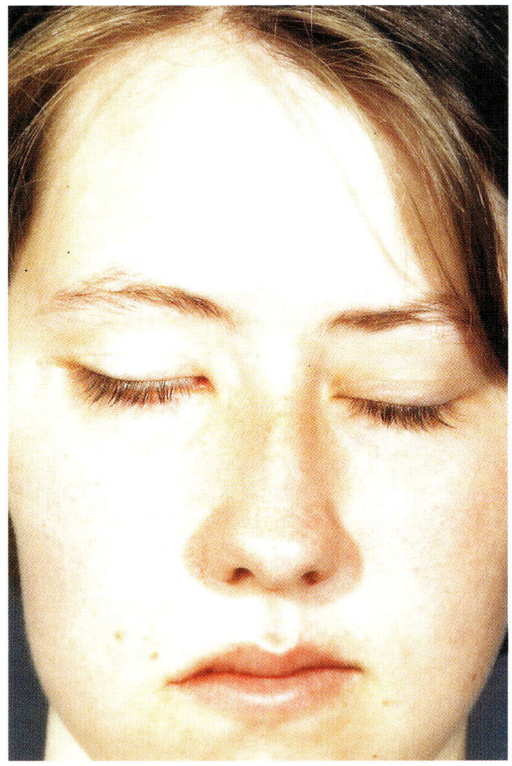

Figure 3.220j Sufficient eyelid closure

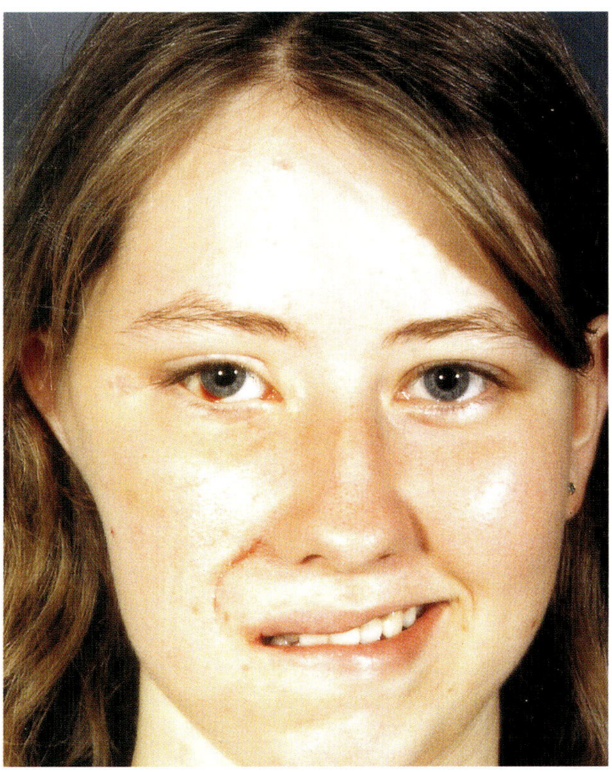

Figure 3.220k The muscle training should already begin on the first postoperative day. The patient shows a considerable psychological improvement. An indentation remains in the temporal fossa.

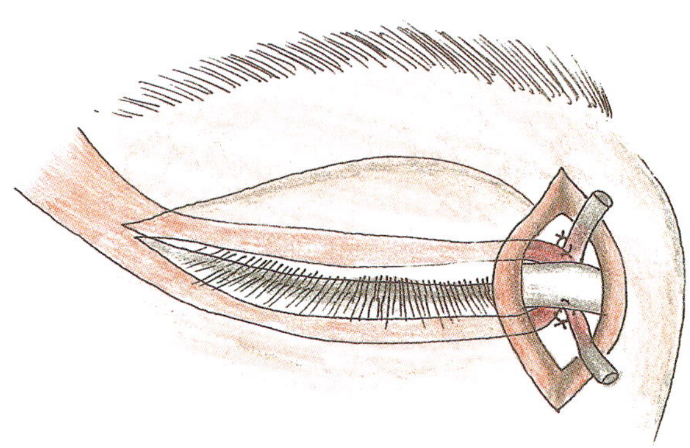

Figure 3.220l Two temporal muscle strips are drawn through the upper and lower eyelid and fixed under the medial ligament.

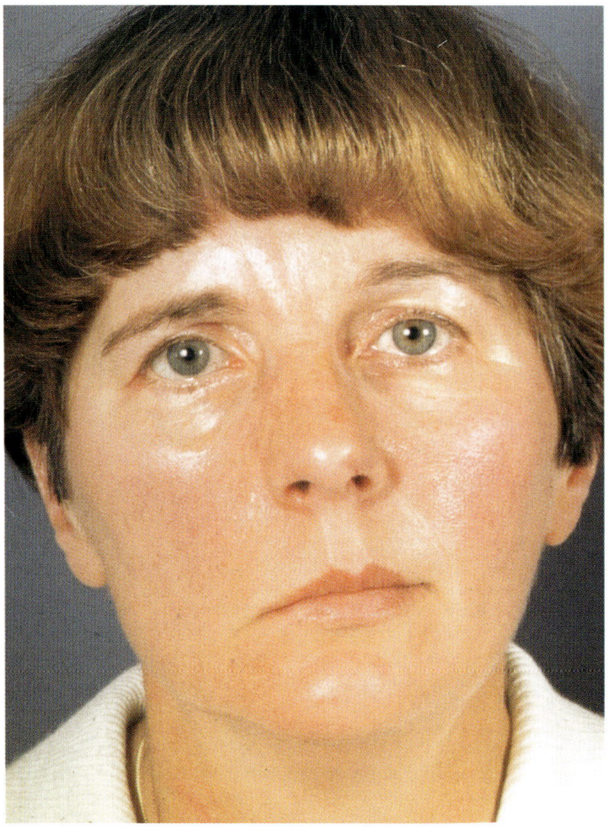

Figure 3.221a Facial nerve paralysis on the right side already lasting four years (cerebellar pontine angle tumor operation).

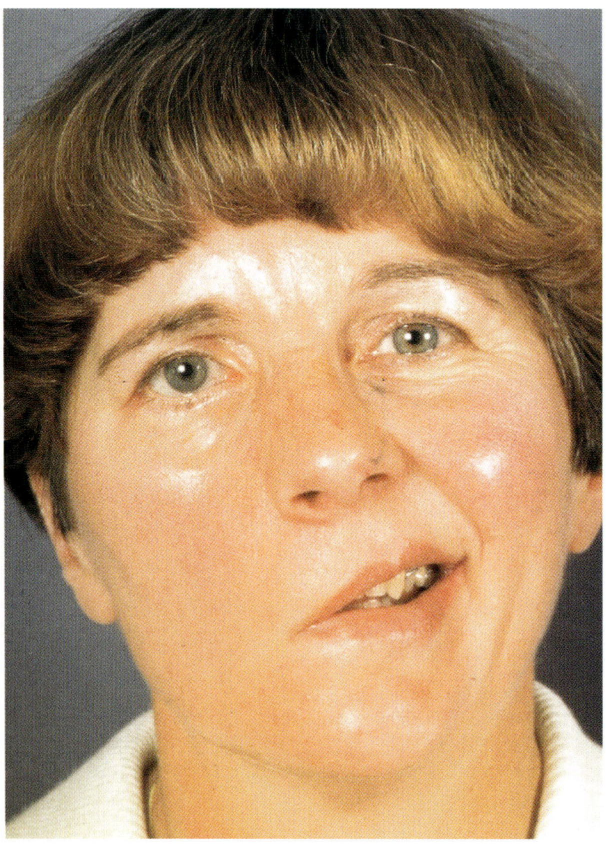

Figure 3.221b Typical facial expression with facial nerve paralysis on the right side

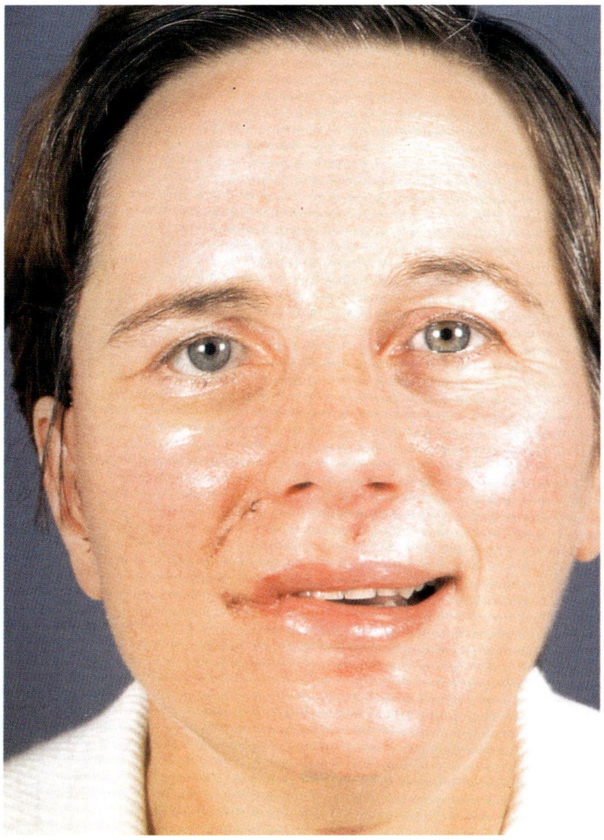

Figure 3.221c Status two weeks after the operation according to McLaughlin. Static suspension of the nasolabial fold with two fascia lata strips which must be overcorrected during the operation. Facelifting on the right side.

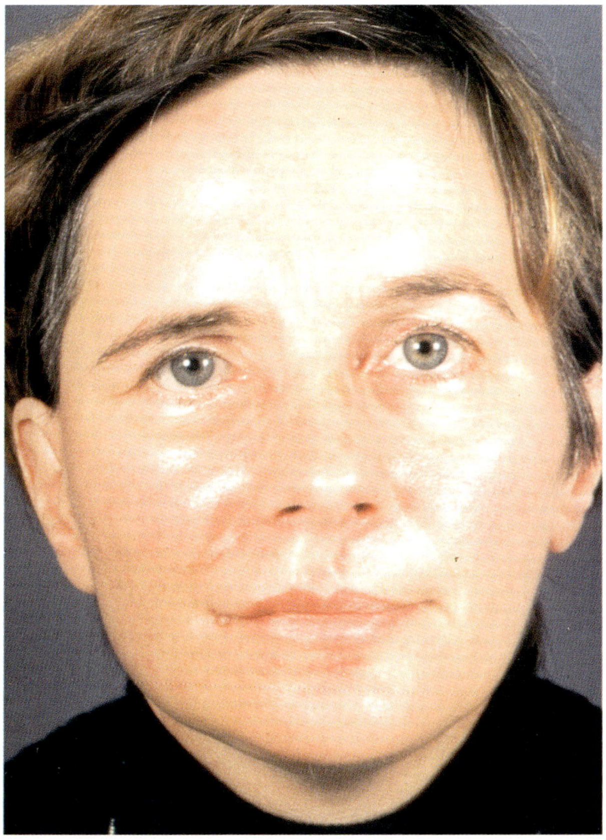

Figure 3.221d Status three years postoperatively

Cross-Face Nerve Grafting (Sural Nerve) and Muscle Grafting (Pectoralis Muscle) (Two-Session Operation)

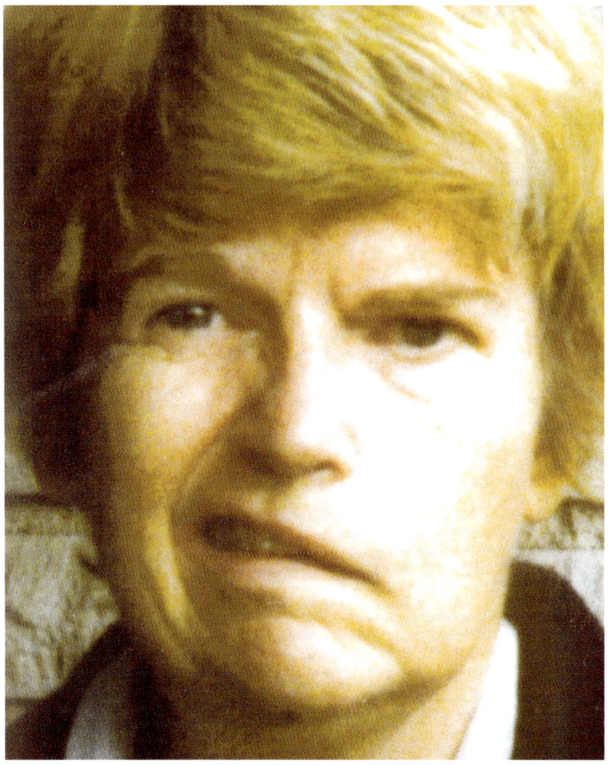

Figure 3.222a 47-year old patient with a complete facial nerve paralysis on the left side already lasting five years. First operation: Cross-face nerve transplantation (sural nerve). Second operation: Microsurgical transplantation of the pectoralis minor muscle six months later.

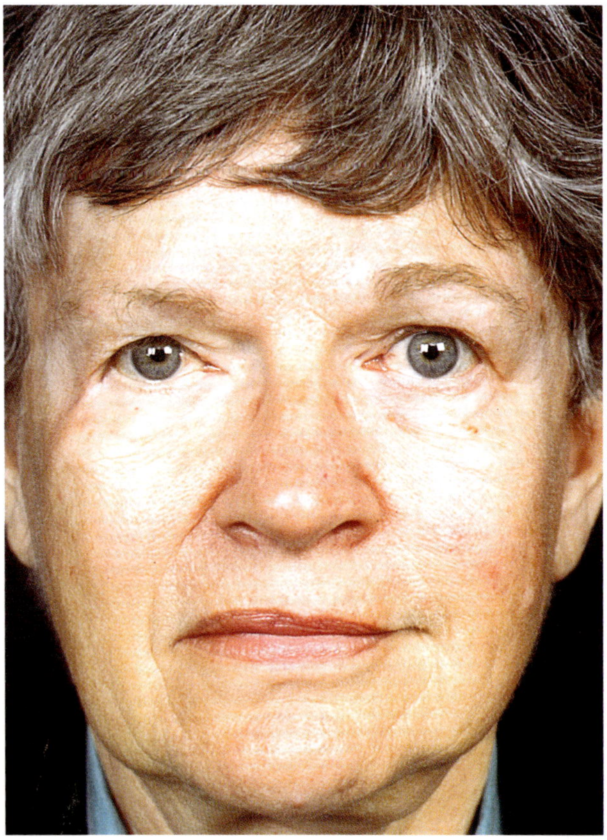

Figure 3.222b Status three years after the operation

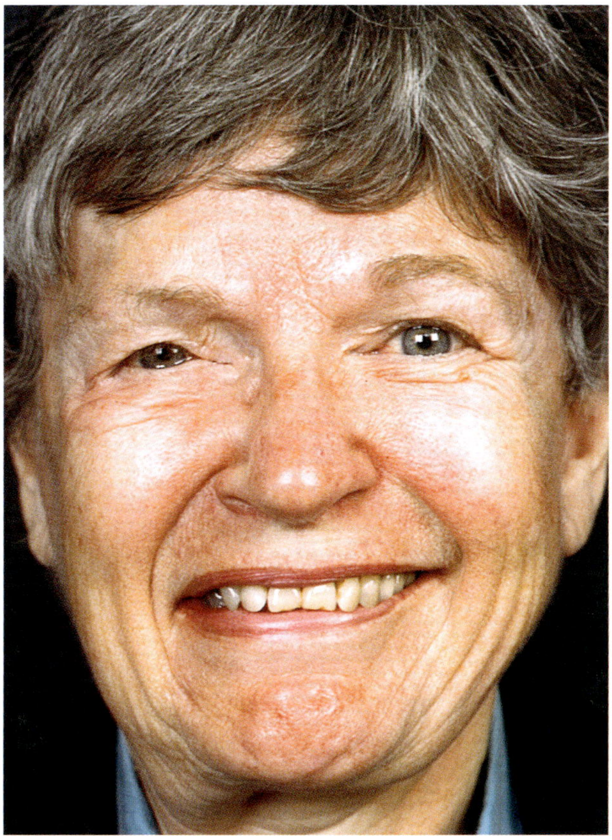

Figure 3.222c Functional result three years postoperatively. With an excellent surgical technique and after intensive training a good outcome can be achieved.

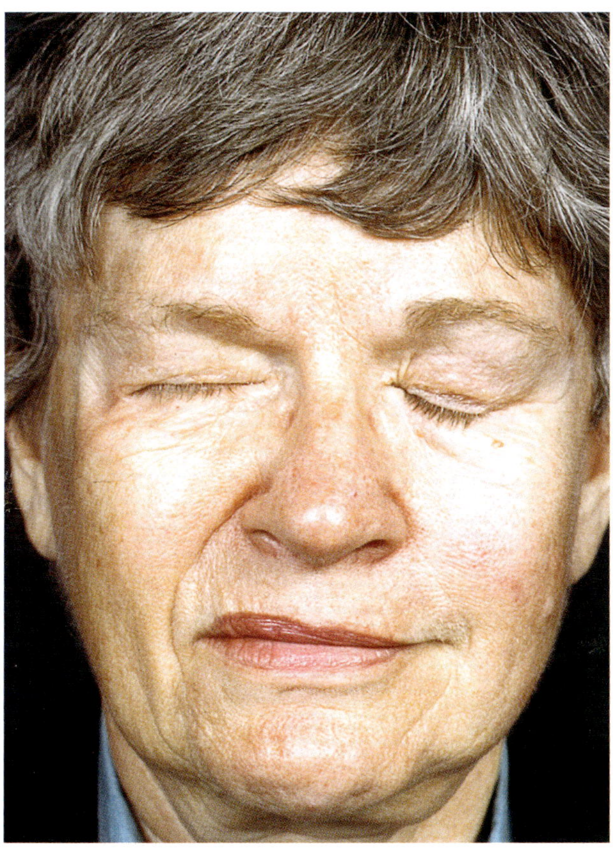

Figure 3.222d The eyelid correction was carried out according to the procedure of Lexer.

Cross-Face Nerve Grafting (Sural Nerve) as Well as Gracilis Muscle Grafting

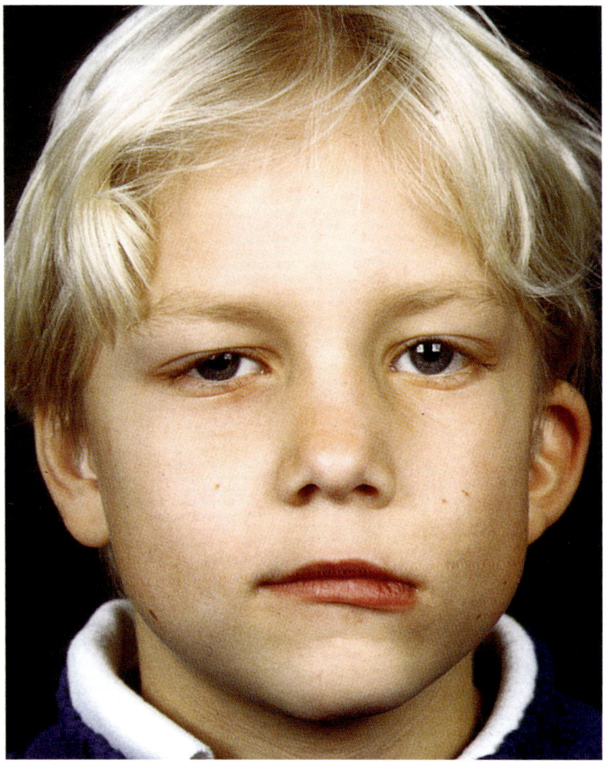

Figure 3.223a 5-year old boy with complete facial nerve paralysis on the left side

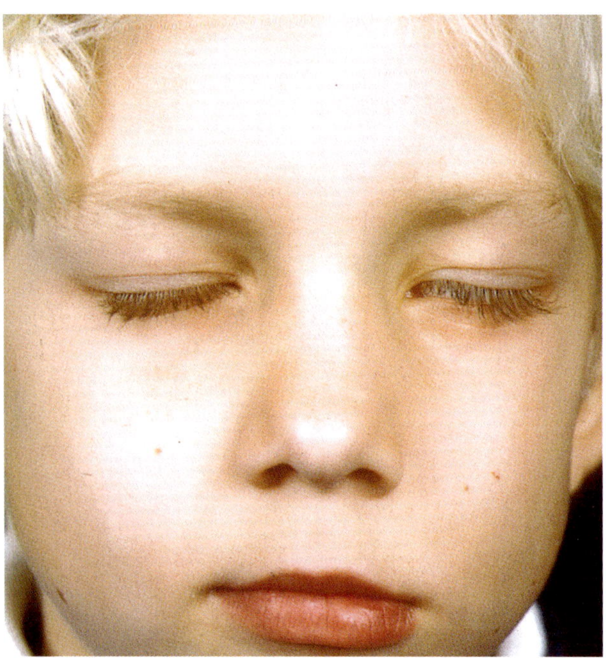

Figure 3.223b Nerve grafting at the age of five years

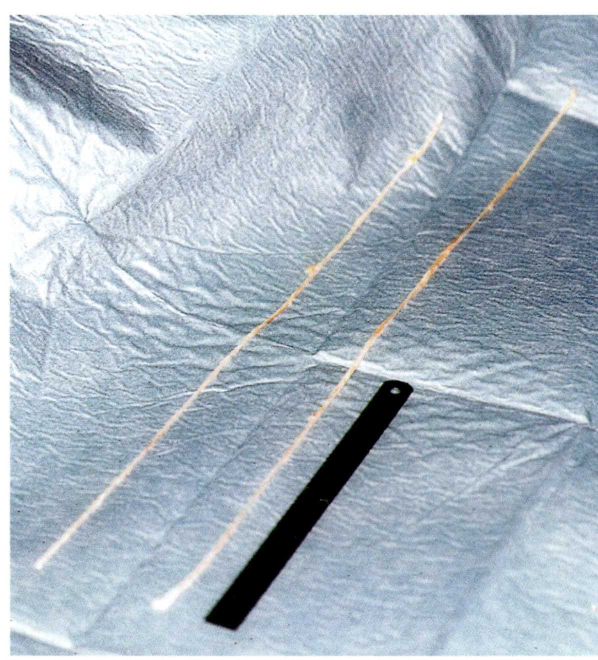

Figure 3.223c Strips of sural nerve

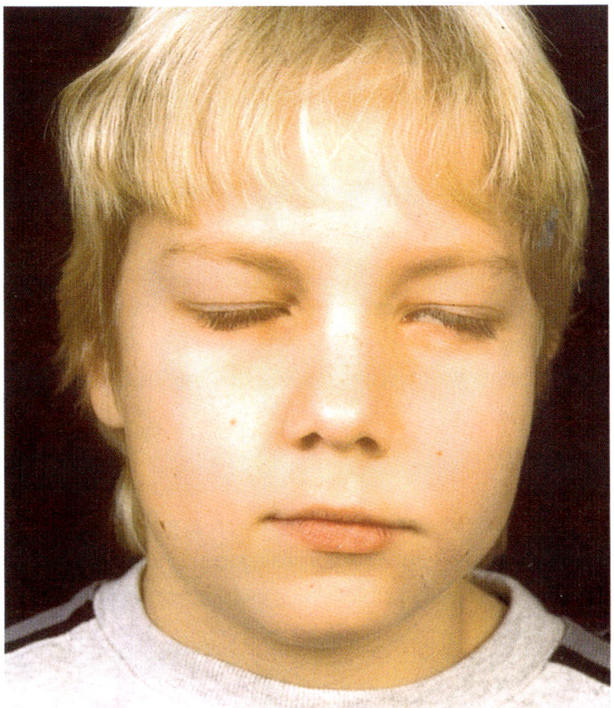

This is a two-session procedure: First the sural nerve was transplanted and anastomosed with nerve branches from the facial nerve of the healthy side. Eight months later the gracilis muscle was implanted as a functional replacement.

Figure 3.223d Result two years after the operation

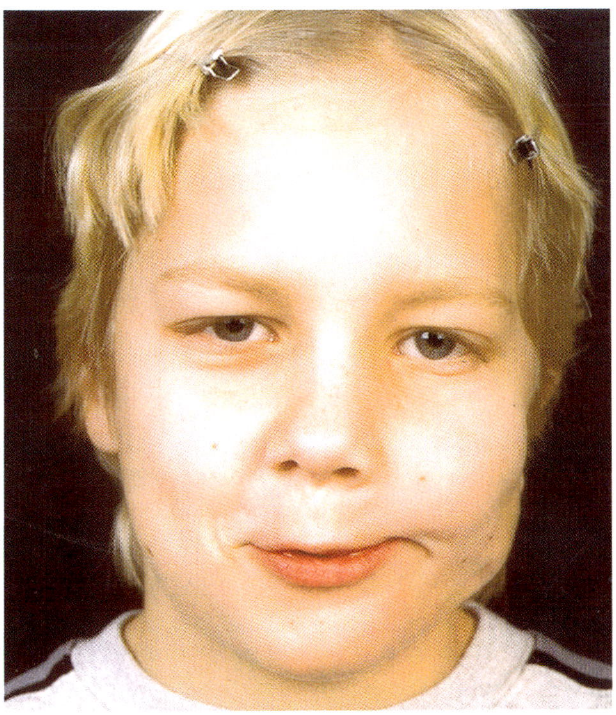

Figure 223d Reanimation of the left facial half with a microsurgical gracilis muscle transfer

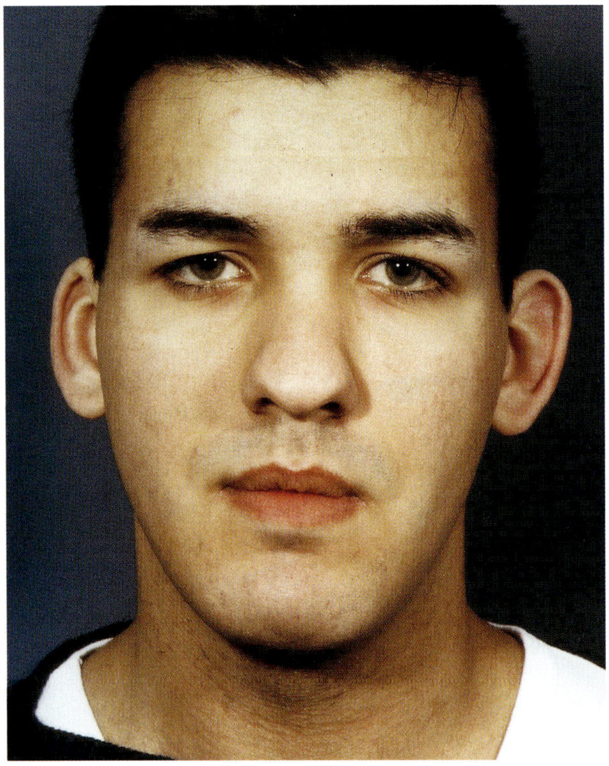

Figure 3.226a Ears protruding asymmetrically and a broad nasal tip. In adults the operation is carried out under local anesthesia.

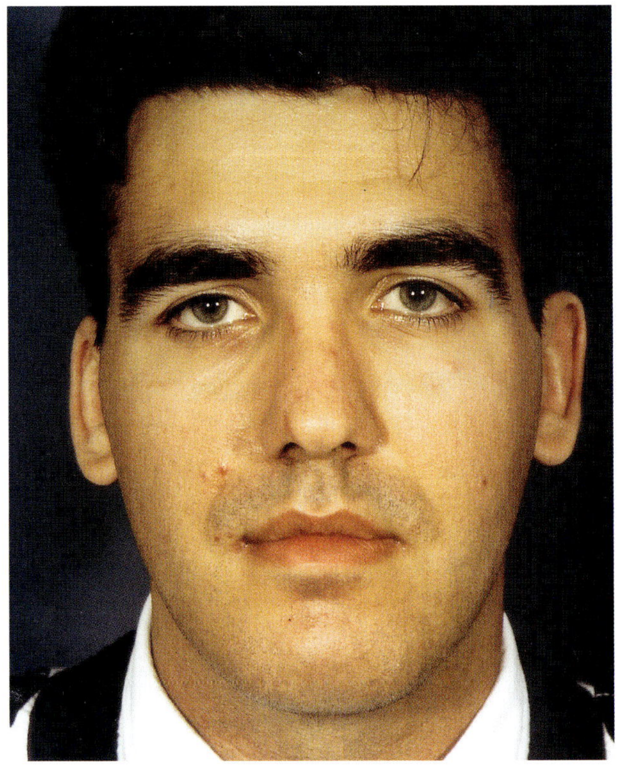

Figure 3.226b Status six months after otoplasty and narrowing of the nasal tip due to reduction of the nasal wing cartilages.

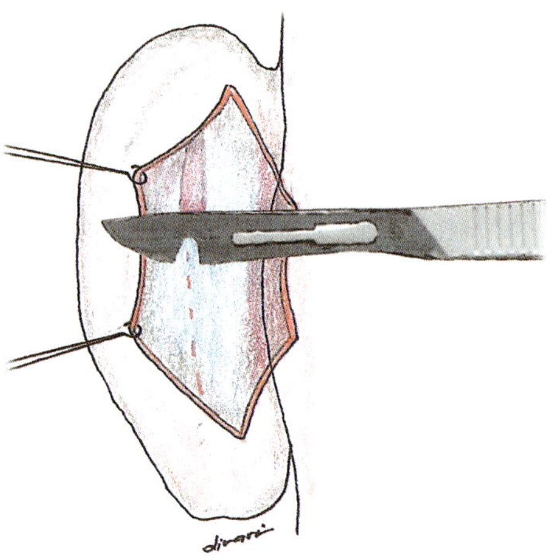

Figure 3.226c Thinning out of the cartilage in the area of the future antihelix.

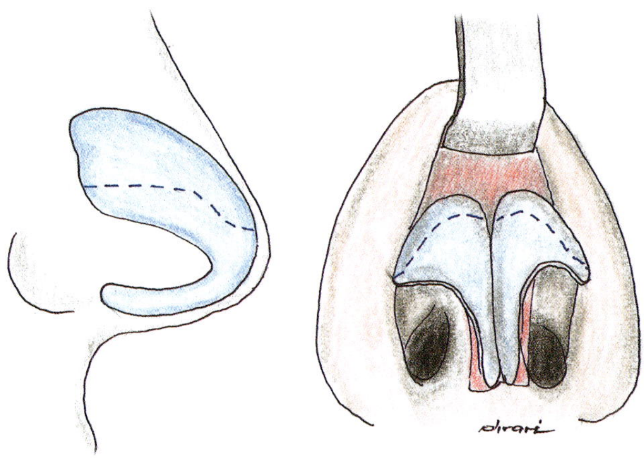

Figure 3.226d The cranial and lateral part of the nasal wing cartilage are resected simultaneously so that the nasal tip is reduced.

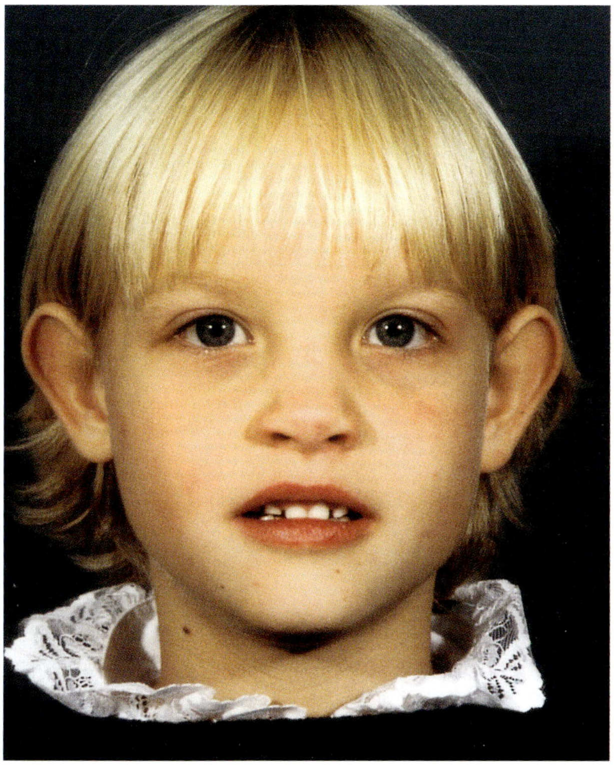

Figure 3.227a Protruding ears

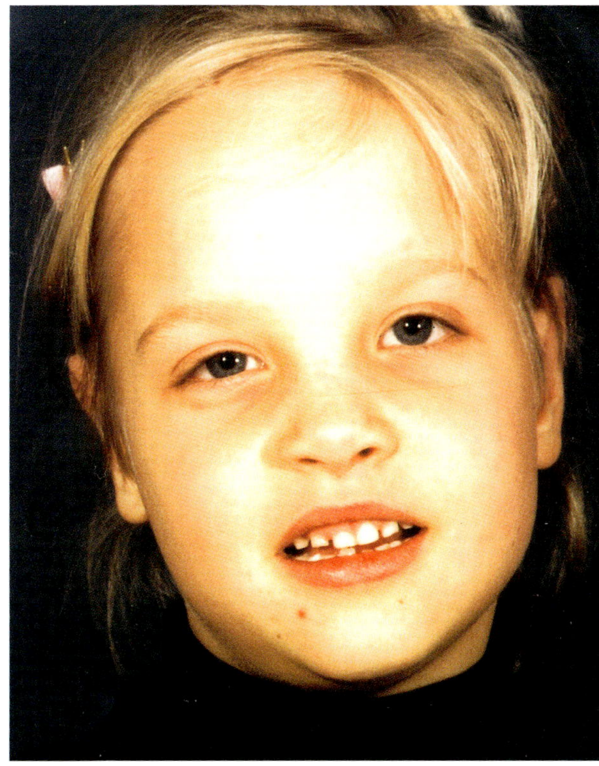

Figure 3.227b Status one year postoperatively

Surgeons who achieve good results with other procedures should stick with their methods (there are more than 20 different procedures)

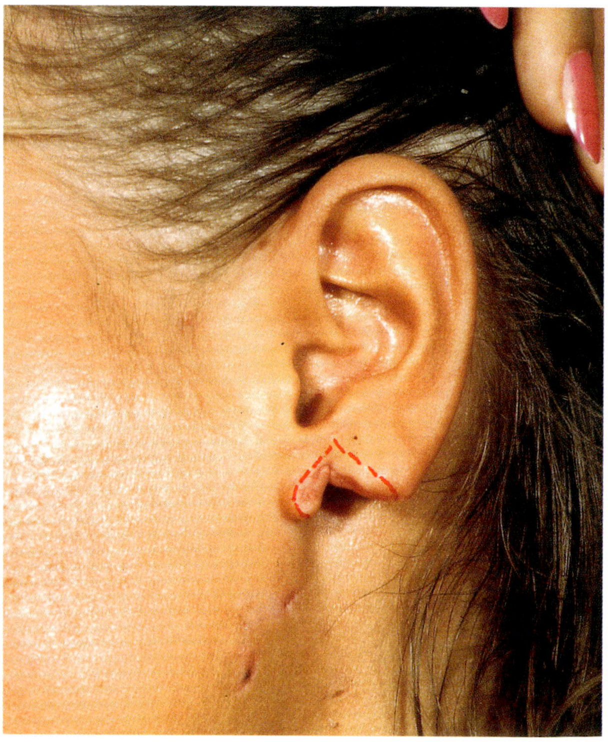

Figure 3.230a Defect of the ear lobe: Here a V-excision and a direct adaptation of the wound edges are adequate.

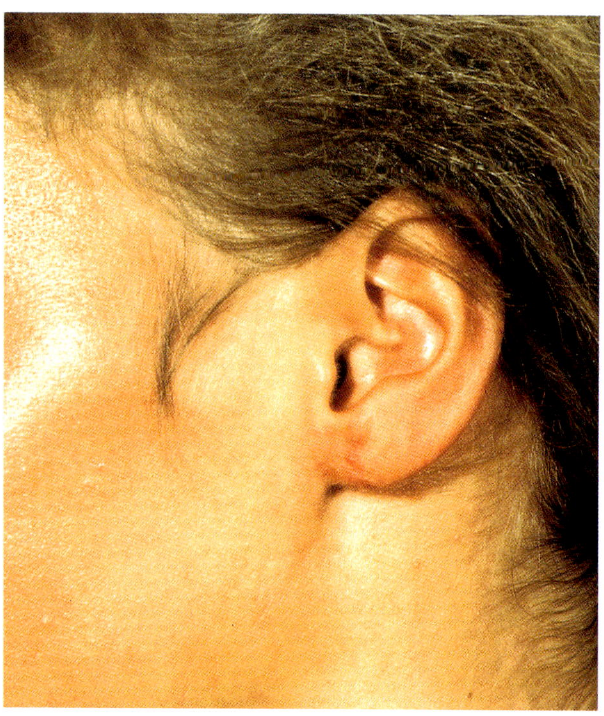

Figure 3.230b Status six months postoperatively

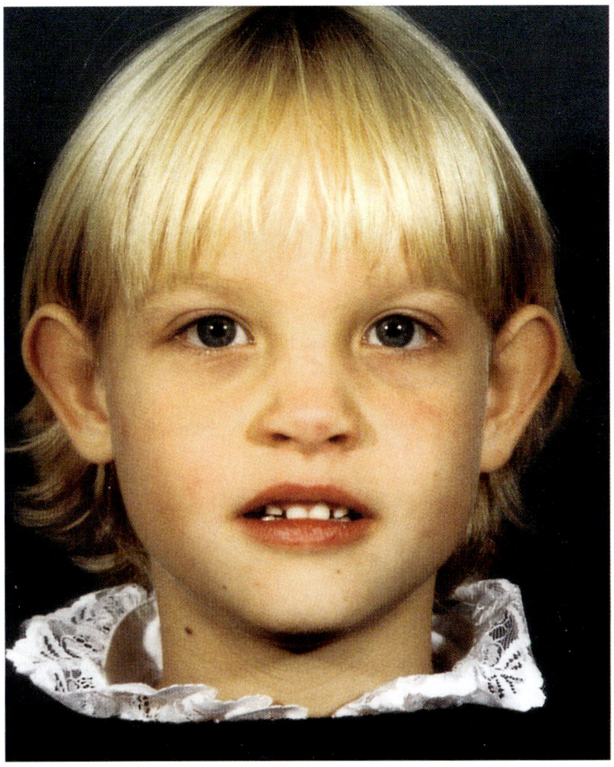

Figure 3.227a Protruding ears

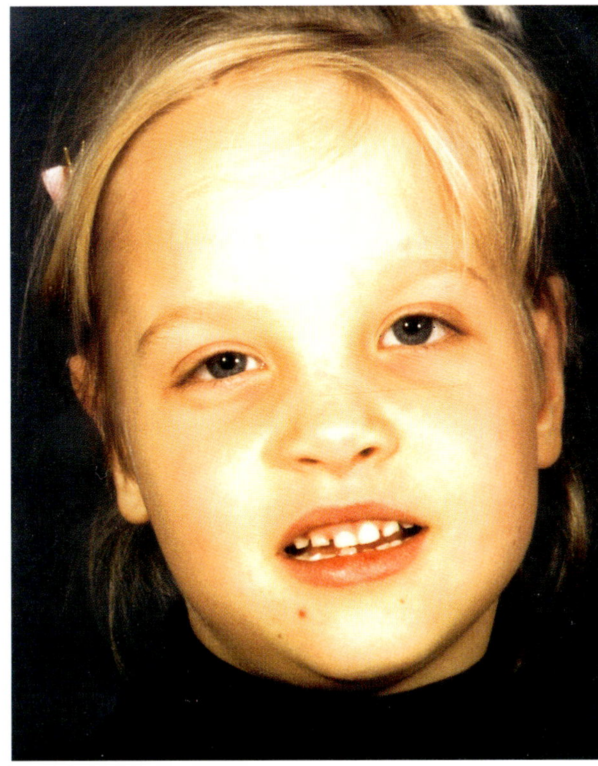

Figure 3.227b Status one year postoperatively

Surgeons who achieve good results with other procedures should stick with their methods (there are more than 20 different procedures)

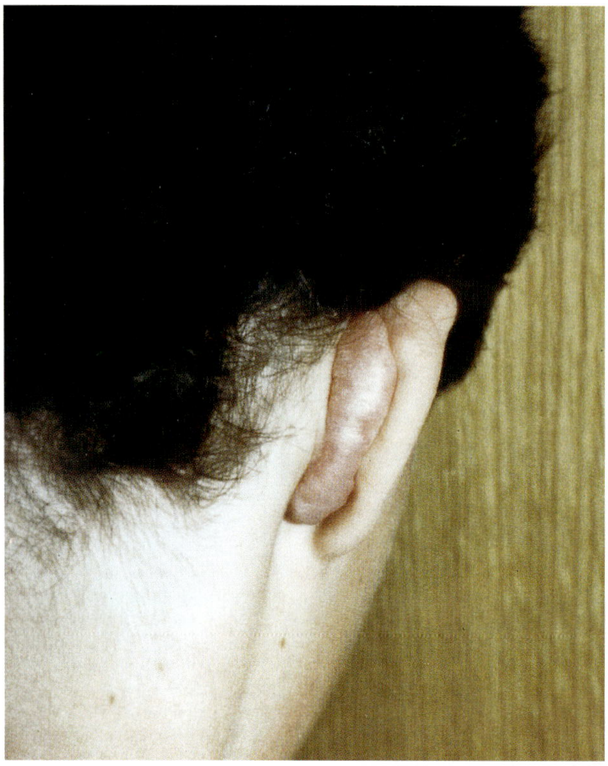

Figure 3.228a Keloid after an otoplasty

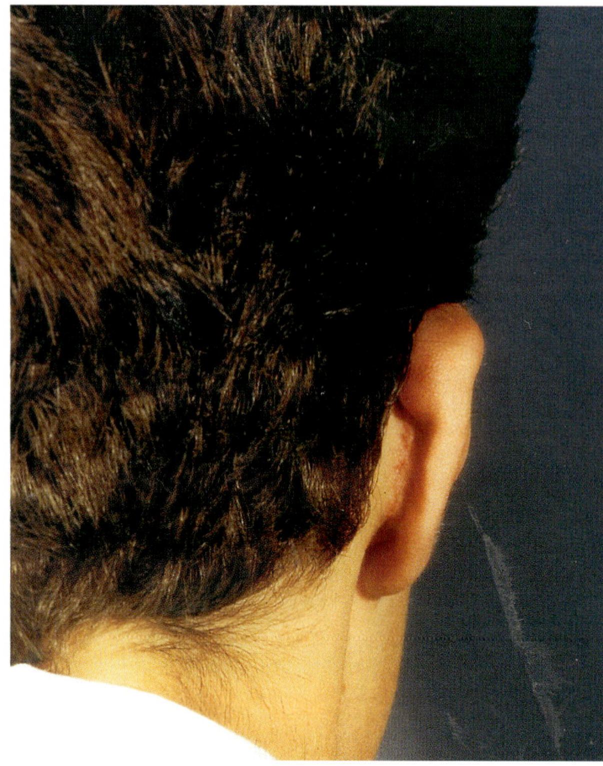

Figure 3.228b Status one year after the excision and irradiation. The irradiation should occur during the first hours after the operation.

b) Ear Concha Defects

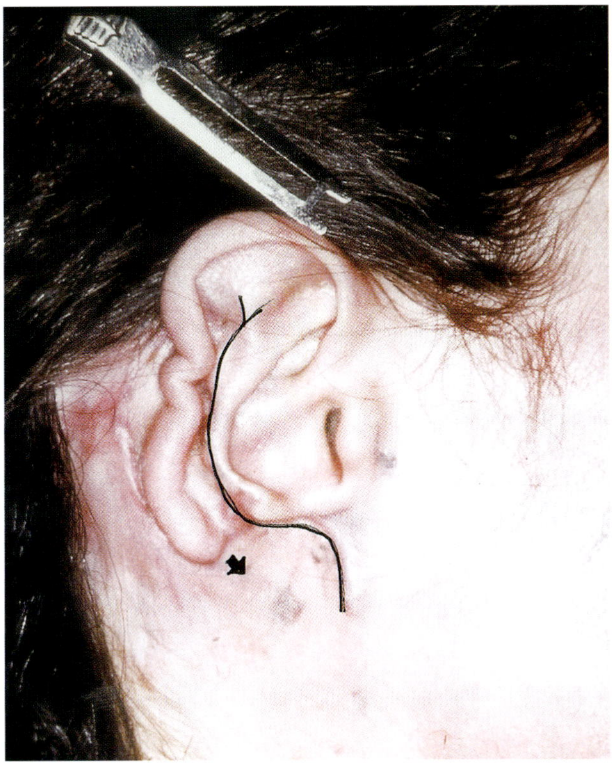

Figure 3.229a A traumatic ear concha defect in reality is not a genuine defect. This deformity arises as a result of an inadequate primary treatment and erroneous wound edge adaptation. The dorsal part is severed up until the cranial basis and mobilized caudally

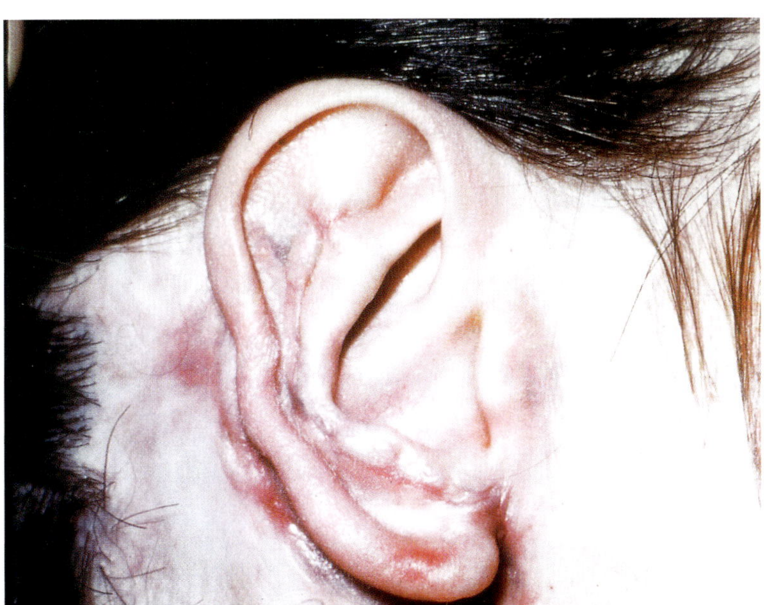

Figure 3.229b Status four weeks after the operation

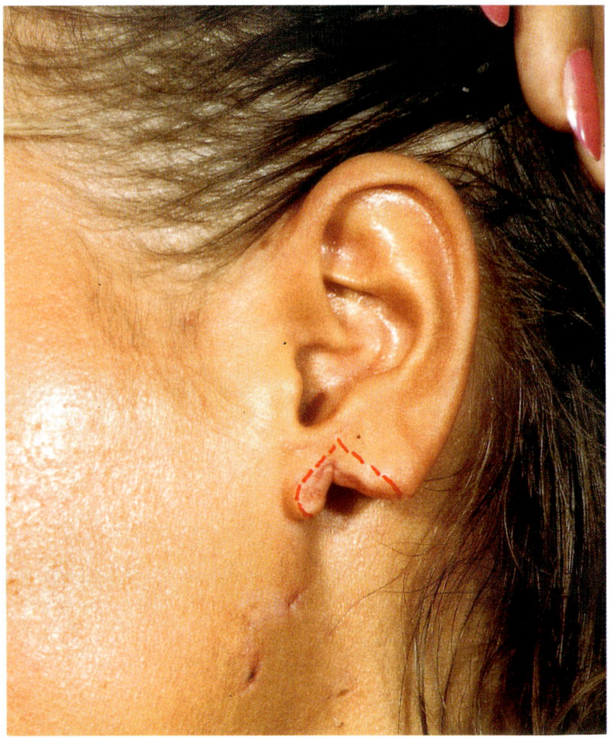

Figure 3.230a Defect of the ear lobe: Here a V-excision and a direct adaptation of the wound edges are adequate.

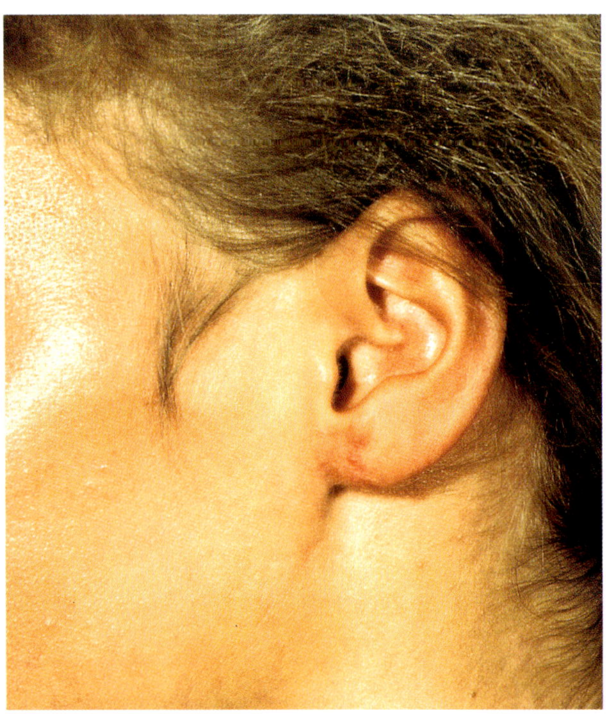

Figure 3.230b Status six months postoperatively

Ear Concha Defect and Pedicle Tube

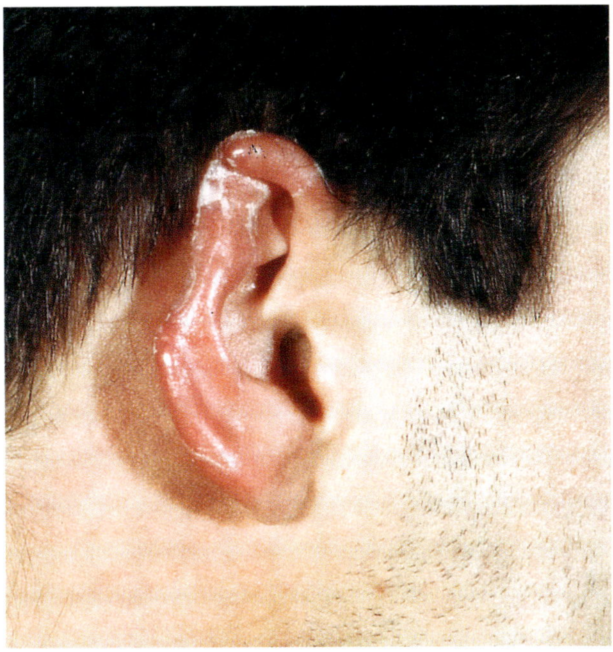

Figure 3.231a Defect of the helix and part of the antihelix

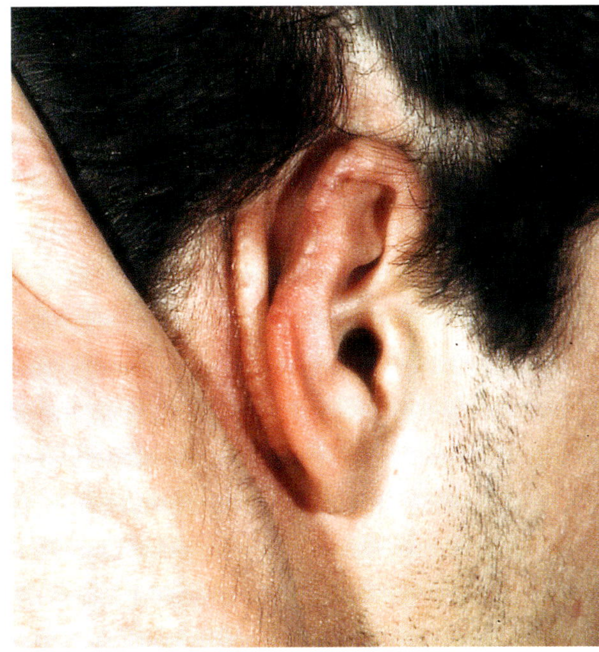

Figure 3.231b Formation of a retroauricular tube pedicle flap, which is first fixed three weeks later at the cranial defect margin and another three weeks later at the lower defect margin.

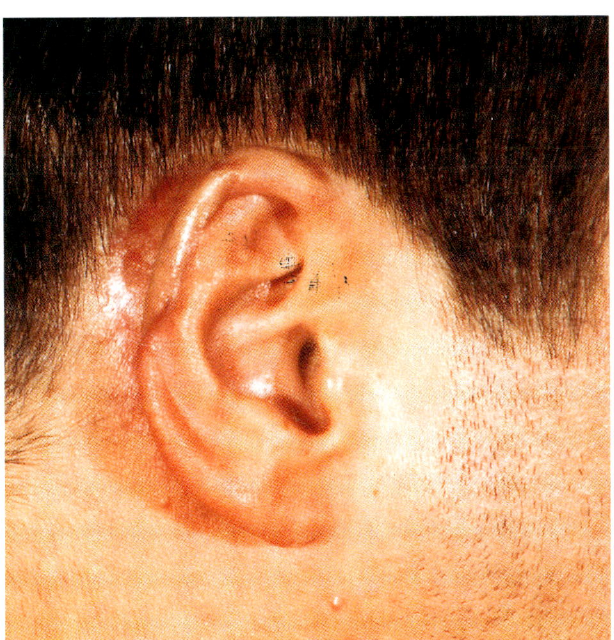

Figure 3.231c Status six months after the operation

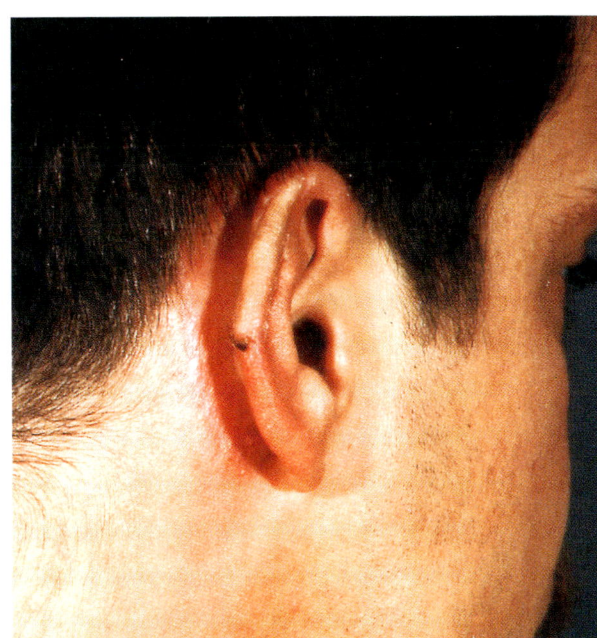

Figure 3.231d Status six months after the operation

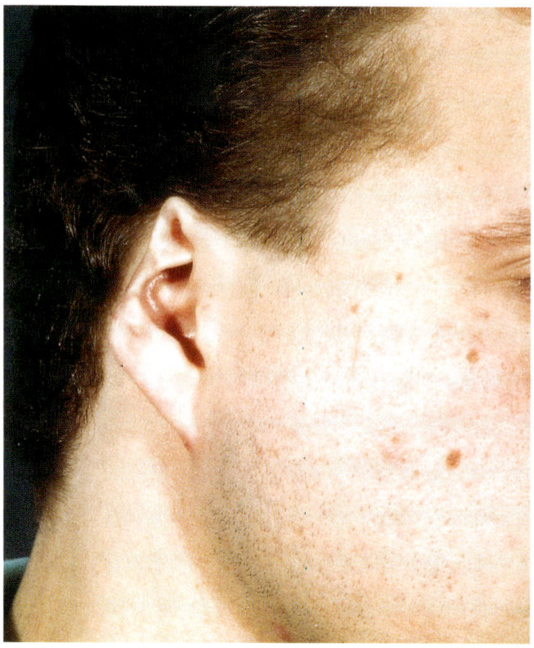

Figure 3.232a Defect of the helix and antihelix

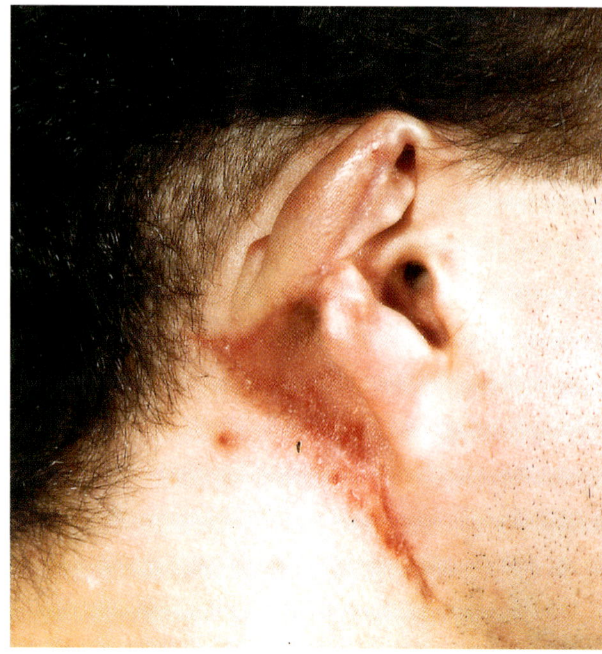

Figure 3.232b A retroauricularly formed tube pedicle flap is fixed onto the cranial defect margin. Three weeks later the flap is expanded and fixed with the caudal defect margin.

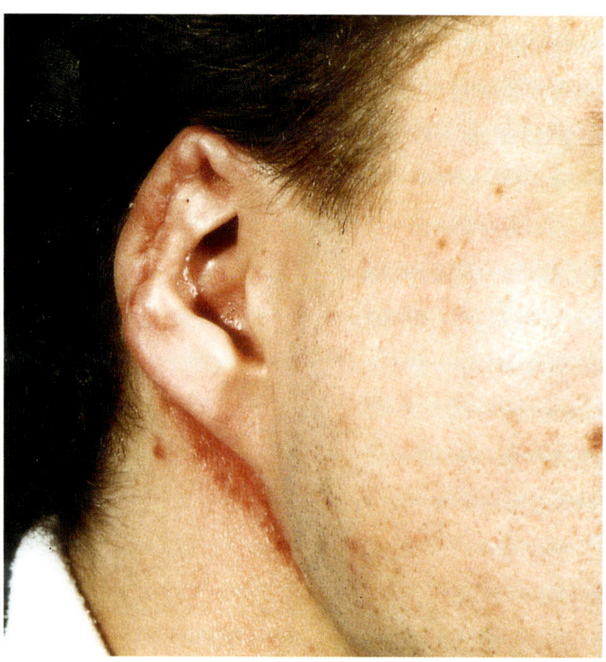

Figure 3.232c Status six weeks after the operation. The result was judged as "satisfactory" by the patient.

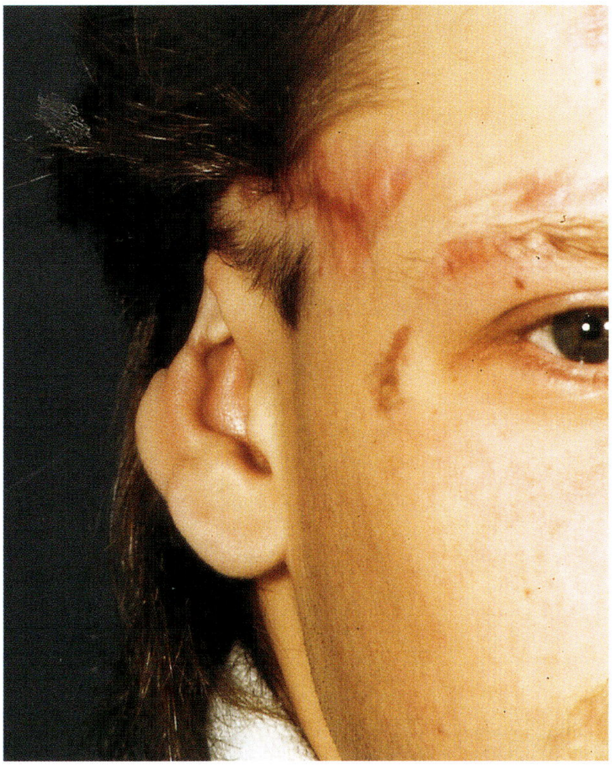

Figure 3.233a Traumatic defect of the right ear concha

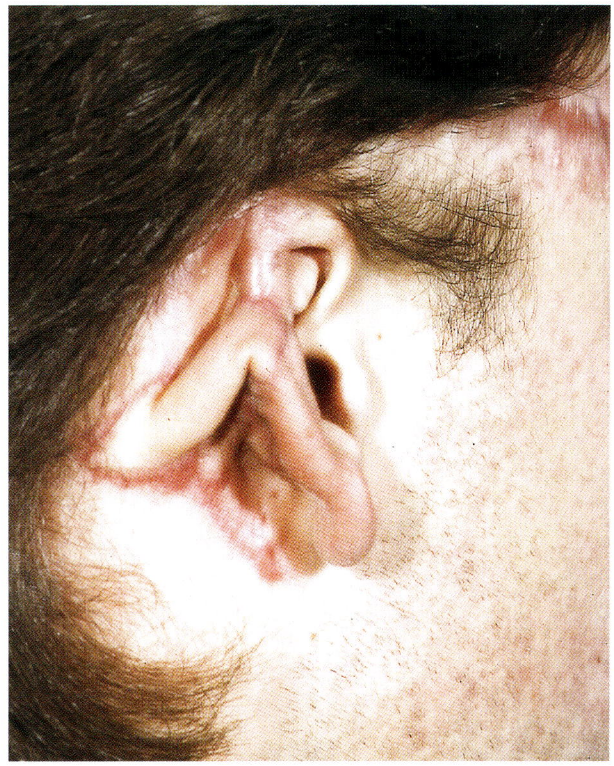

Figure 3.233b The retroauricular tube pedicle flap is fixed first at the caudal and then three weeks later at the cranial defect margin.

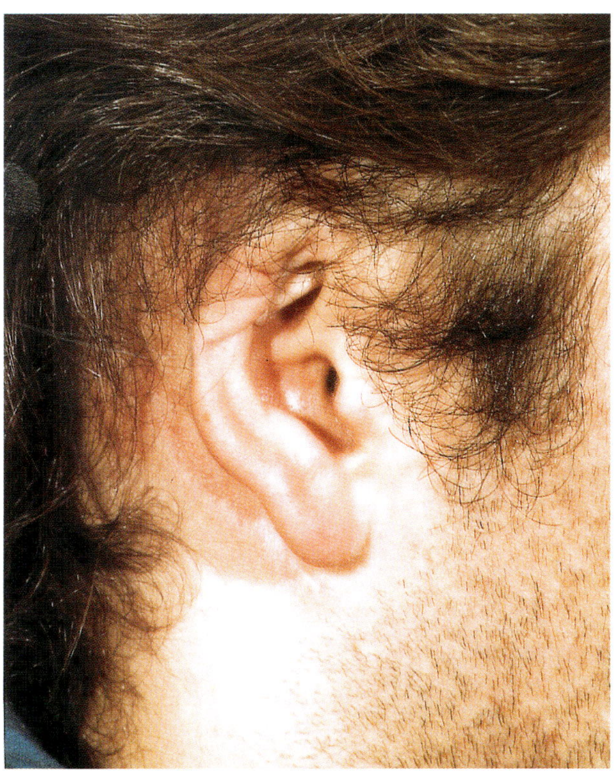

Figure 3.233c Status three years after the operation

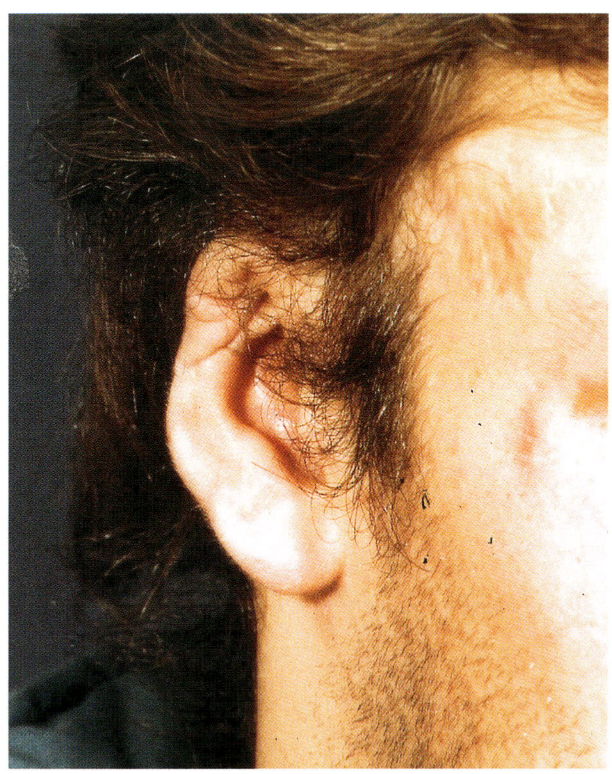

Figure 3.233d Moderate outcome

Ear Concha Defect and Expander

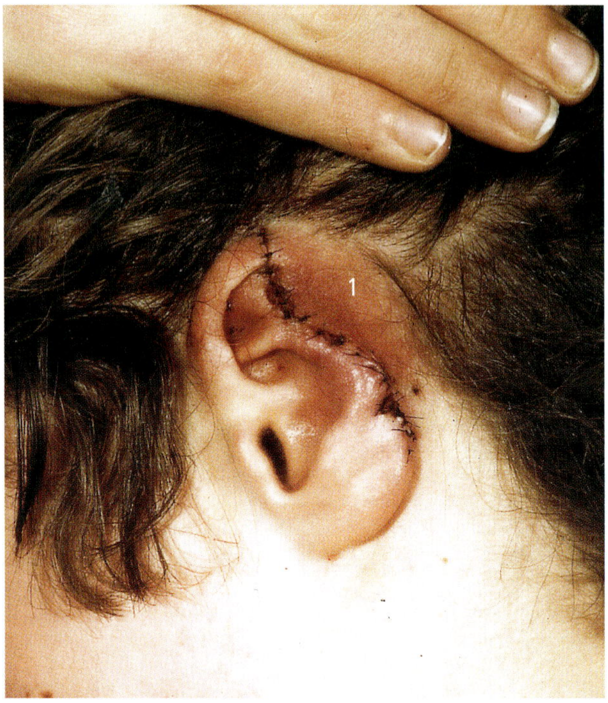

Figure 3.234a Ear concha defect in the upper third. A costal cartilage graft was modeled and implanted subcutaneously (1).

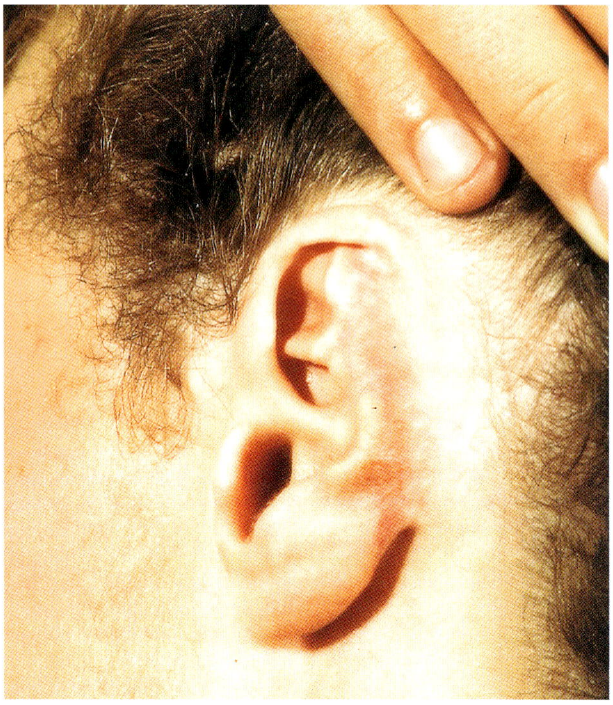

Figure 3.234b Status after healing of the cartilage graft

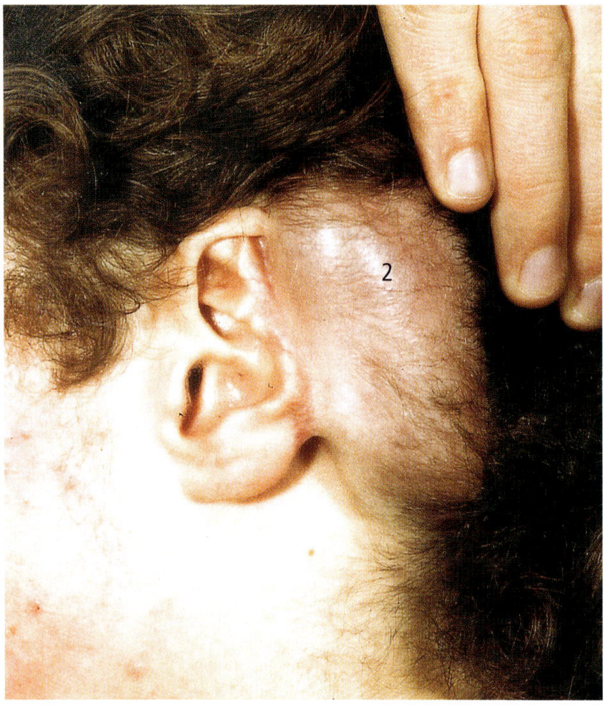

Figure 3.234c In order to acquire sufficient skin, an expander is implanted retroauricularly (2).

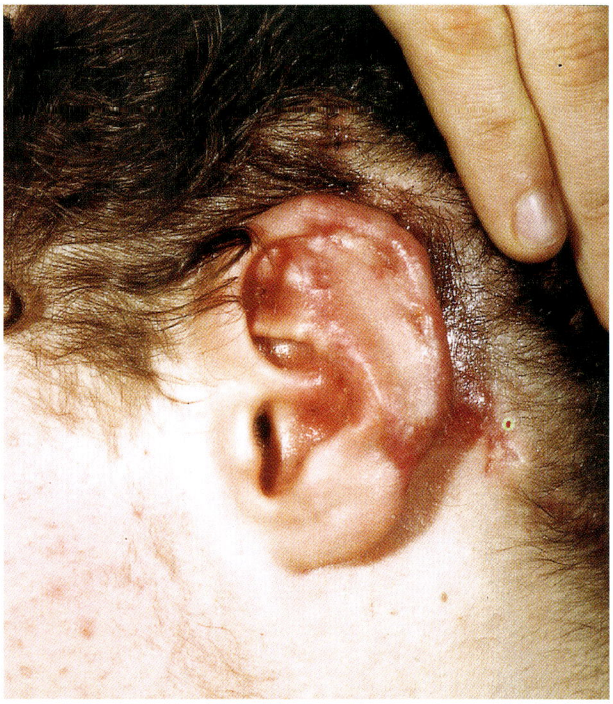

Figure 3.234d The ear concha is reconstructed using the plentily available skin. A good idea and a correspondingly (rarely) good result.

Ear Concha Defect and Cartilage Implant

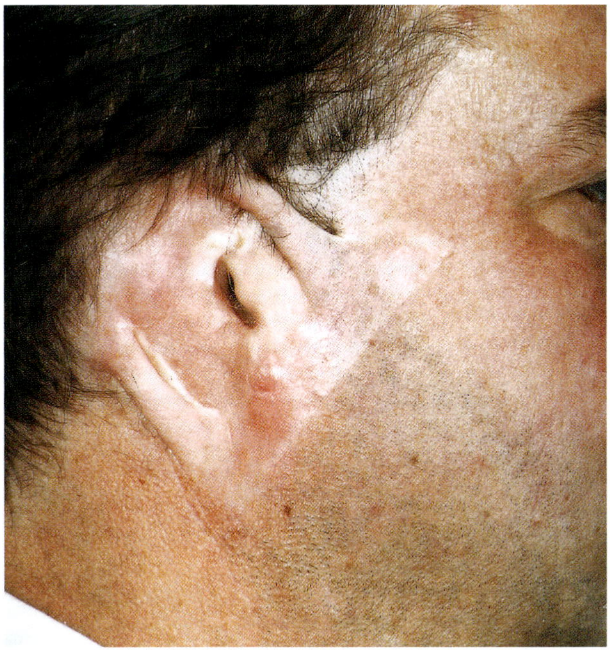

Figure 3.235a Total loss of the ear concha which was operated on four times. Two small tube pedicle flaps are present.

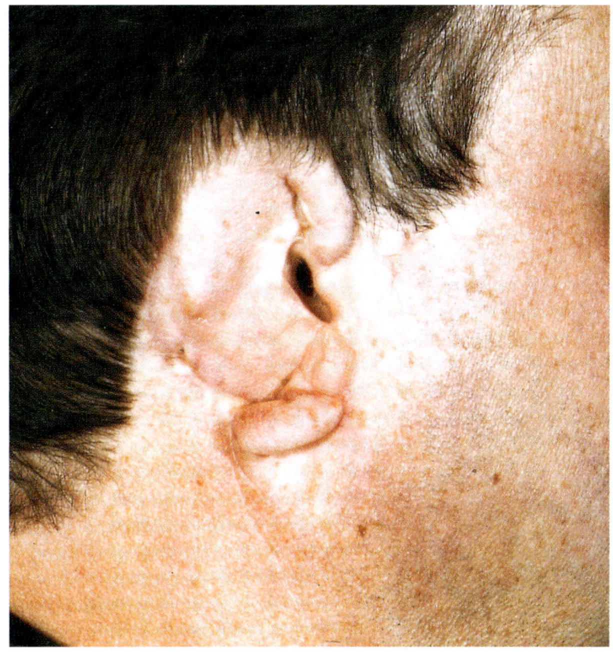

Figure 3.235b A costal cartilage graft is modeled and implanted in the retroauricular area. Two small round pedicle flaps are used for forming the ear lobe and part of the helix.

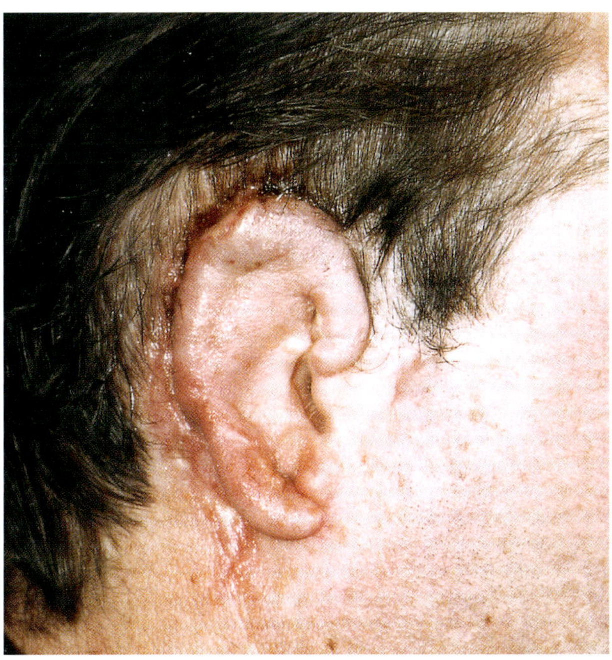

Figure 3.235c After mobilization of the reconstructed ear concha a full skin graft is applied retroauricularly.

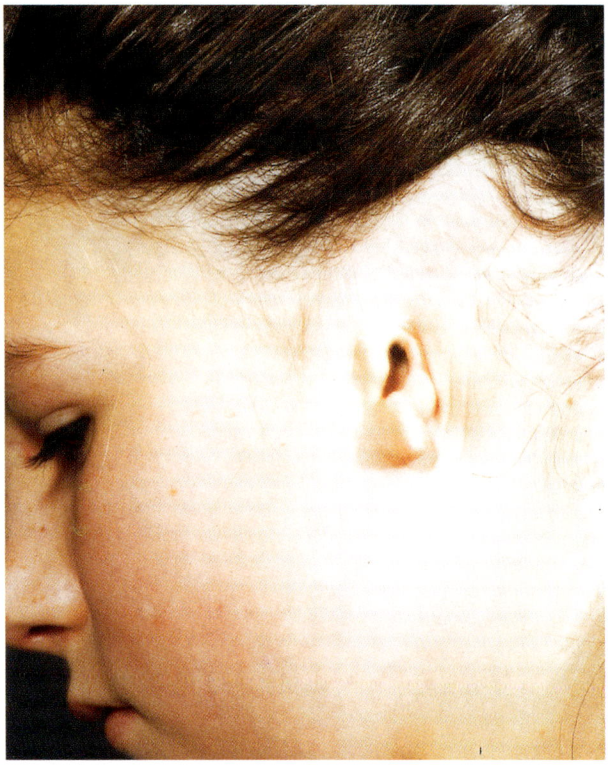

Figure 3.236a Traumatic loss of almost the entire ear concha

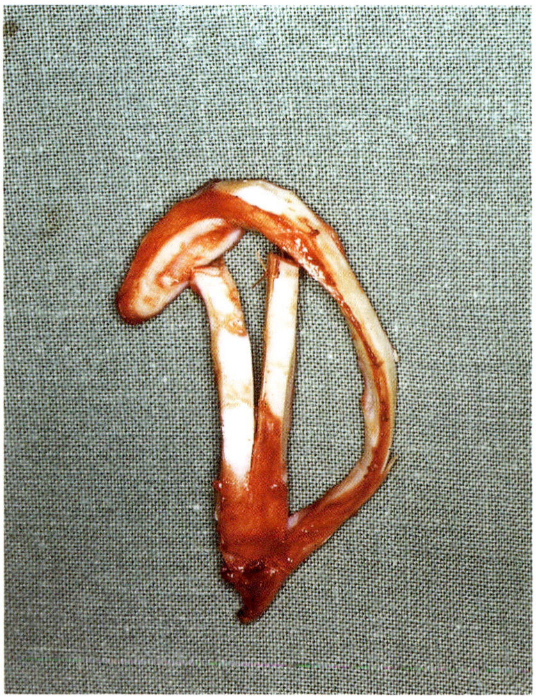

Figure 3.236b Costal cartilage is extracted and modeled

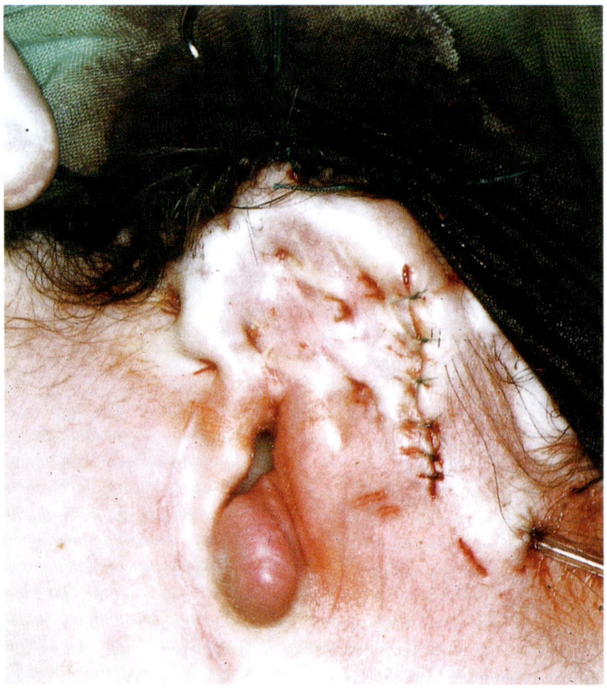

Figure 3.236c The cartilage graft is implanted subcutaneously and fixed. During the first five days a negative air pressure drainage is applied for a better forming of the skin around the cartilage.

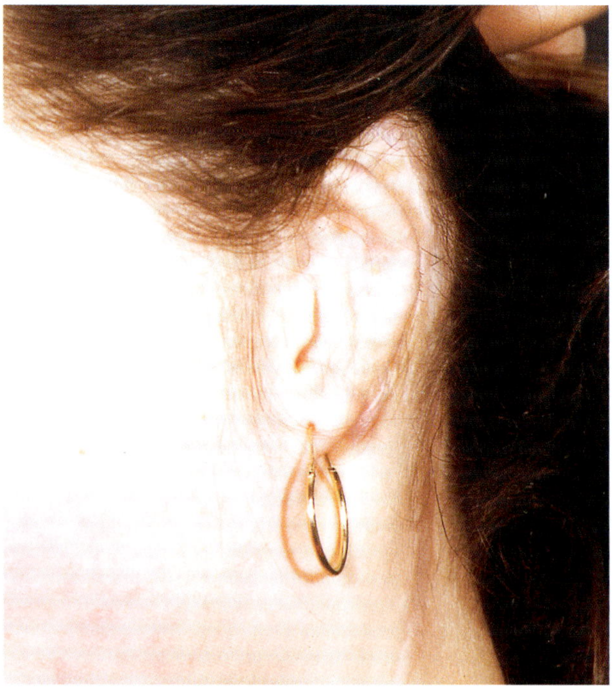

Figure 3.236d Late outcome. The author was never happy about his reconstructed ears, the patients more often so.

Defect Coverage at the Haired Head

The haired skin of the head as well as the skin in the forehead area are inelastic. Rotation flaps or transposition flaps in this area usually leave behind secondary defects which can not be closed directly. Split skin or mesh grafts are often indicated.

By applying expanders some secondary defects can be avoided. However, the expander is indicated only rarely with fresh traumas (see Chapter 2: General Part – Rotation Flap).

The perfusion of the haired skin of the head is considered to be very good. Despite that the dominant arterial supply should be respected when planning the flap.

The main supplying vessels in this area are the superficial temporal, the supraorbital and the occipital arteries that form a dense wickerwork through numerous anastomoses. The skin shows a lack of elasticity and requires special, precision techniques for defect closure.

Transposition Flap

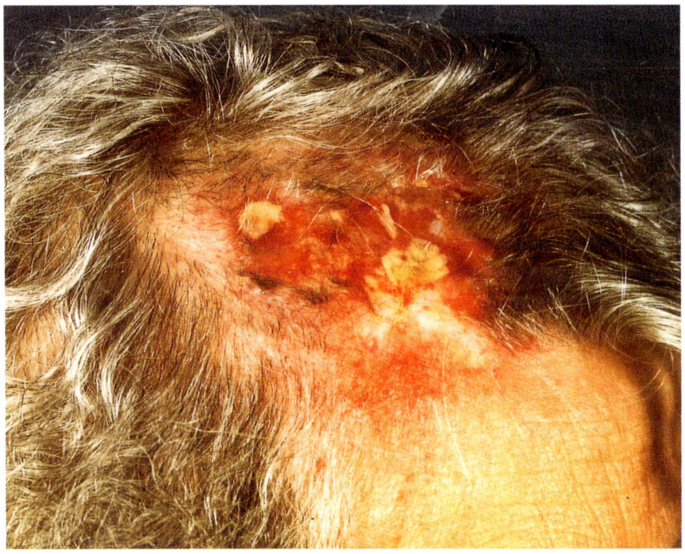

Figure 3.237a Basal cell carcinoma on the haired part of the head with a 72-year old patient.

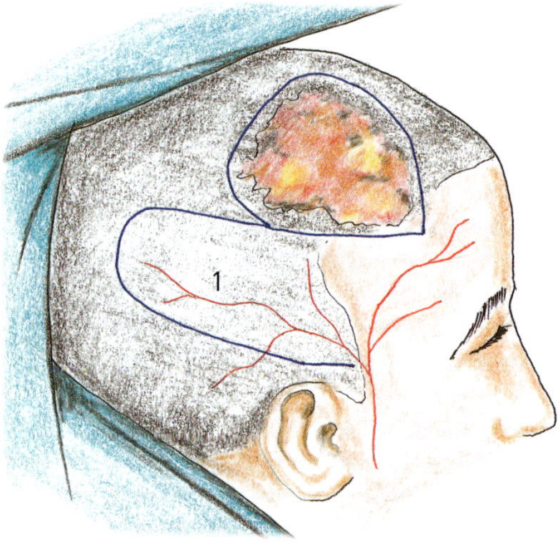

Figure 3.237b After excision of the tumor a transposition flap (1) is planned. It is an axial flap which is supplied via the superficial temporal artery. The haired skin of the head is not elastic; as such the transposition flap must be excised as a considerably larger flap than would be the case with elastic skin in the face or the trunk.

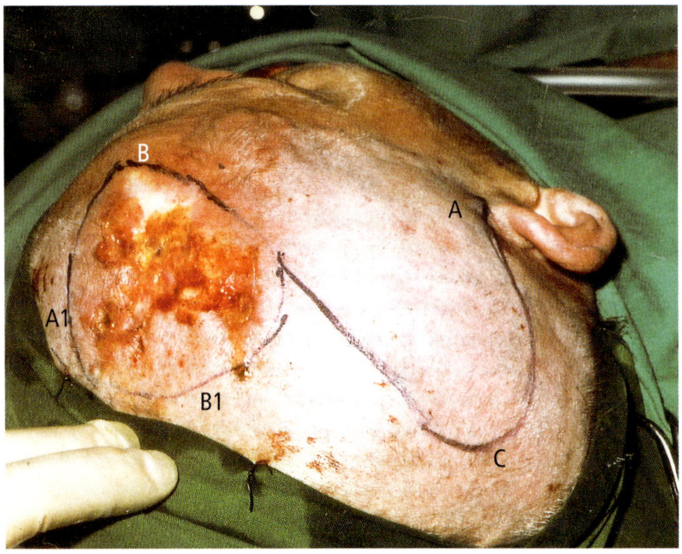

Figure 3.237c During the planning of the flap in the head area the distance from point A to A1 is important and not, as first appears, the distance from point B to B1.

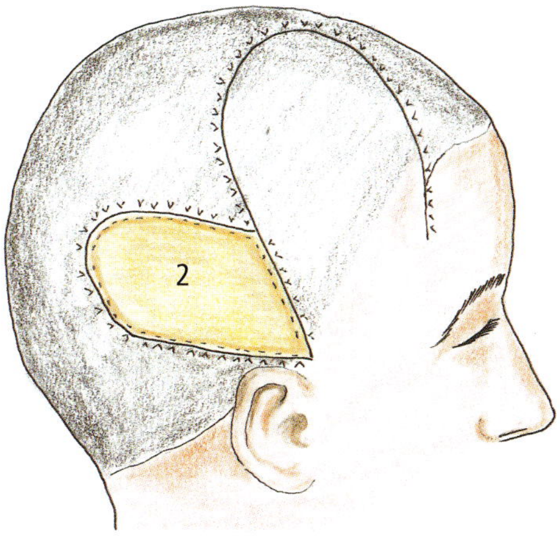

Figure 3.237d The transposition flap is fixed in the defect. Secondary defect (2) is covered with meshed skin.

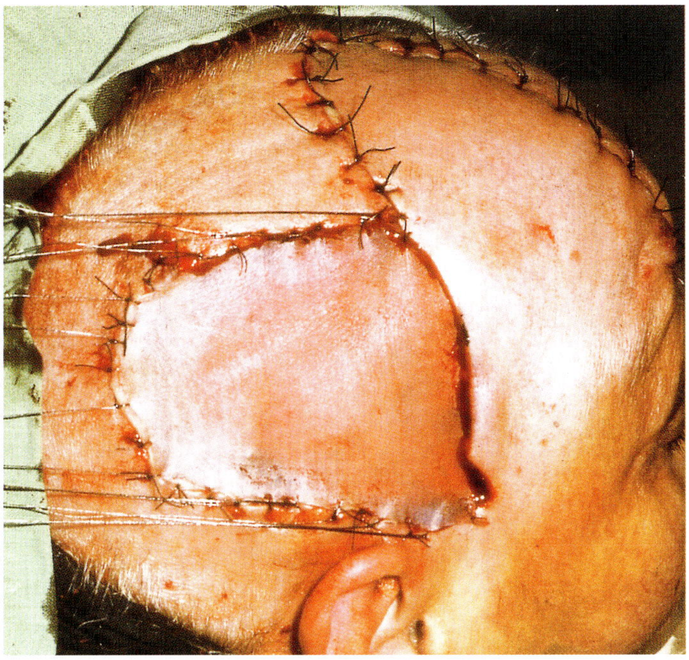

Figure 3.237e Status directly after the operation

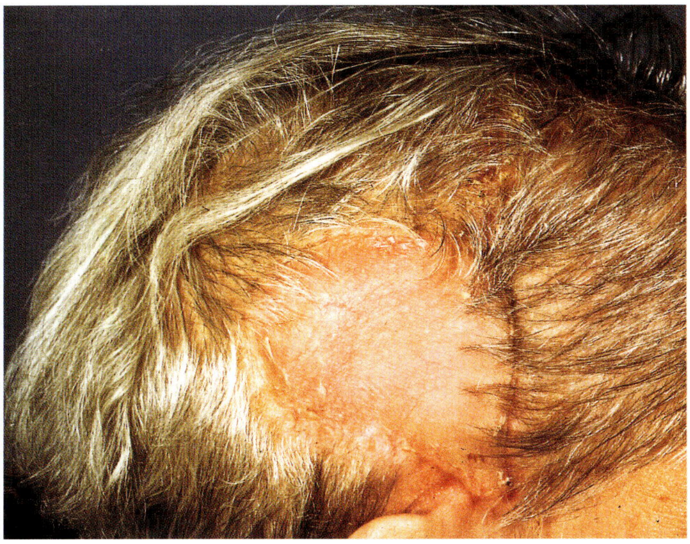

Figure 3.237f Status six months after the operation

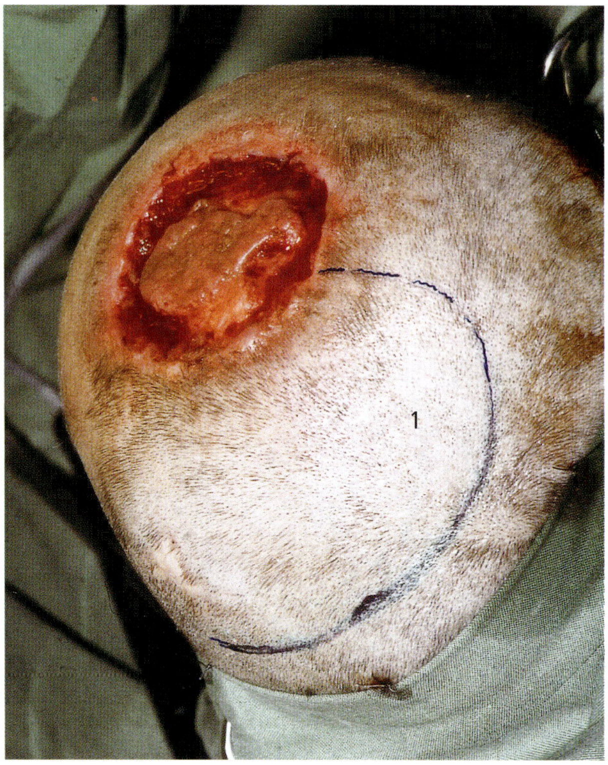

Figure 3.238a Defect in the haired skin of the head. The external lamina has become devitalized. Planning of a local flap (1).

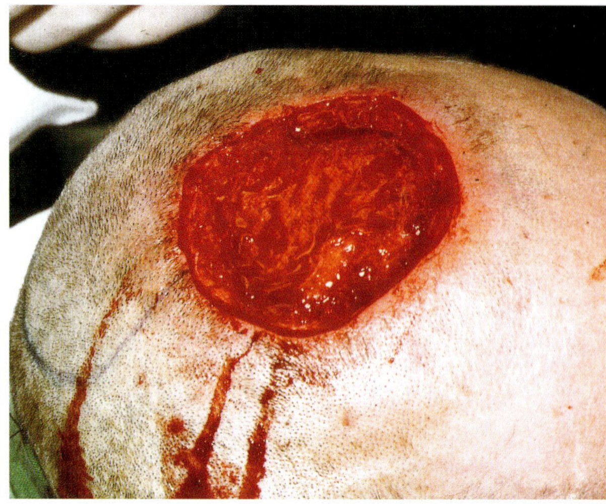

Figure 3.238b After the debridement and chiseling away of the devitalized bone the internal lamina remains well supplied with blood.

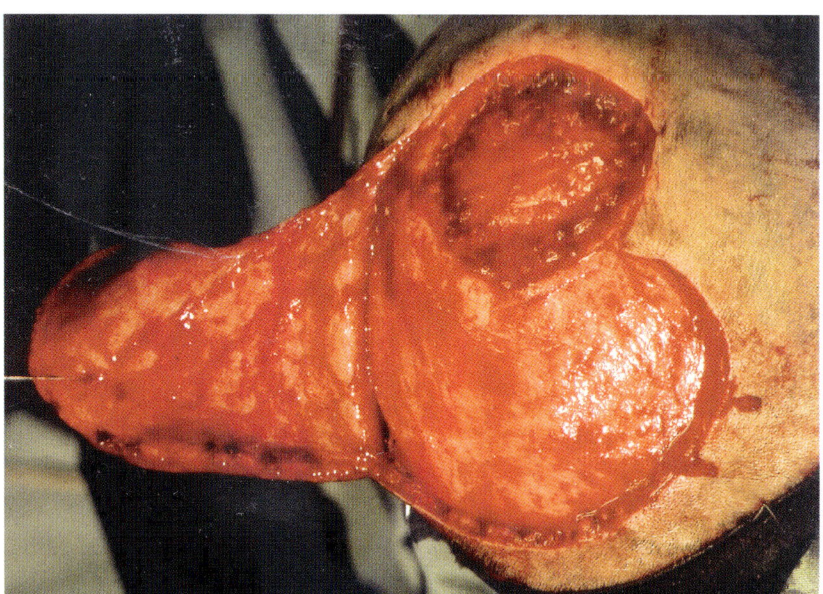

Figure 3.238c **Note** how large a local flap must be in the head area compared to the relatively small defect.

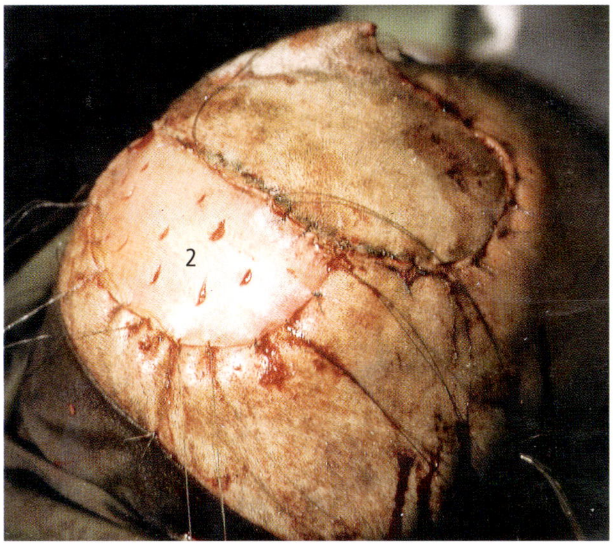

Figure 3.238d Status at the end of the operation: The flap donor site is treated with a mesh graft (2).

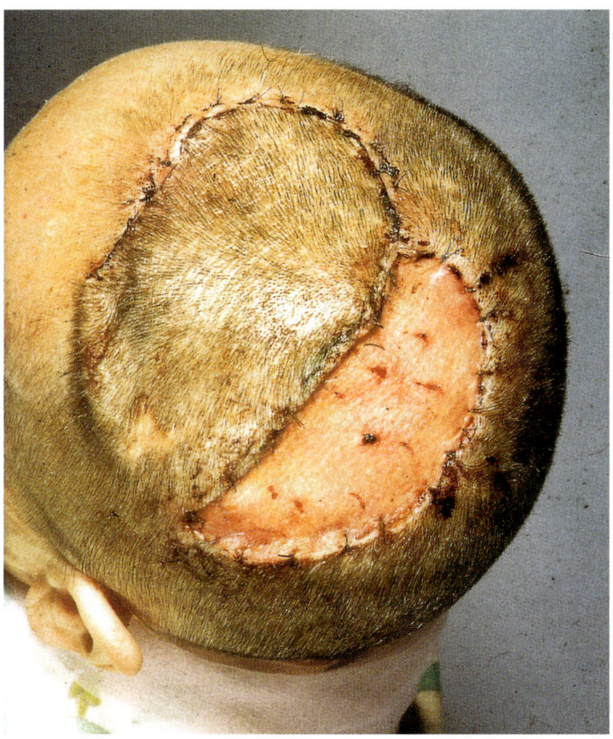

Figure 3.238e Status three weeks after the operation

Rotation Flap

a) Rotation Flap and Mesh Graft

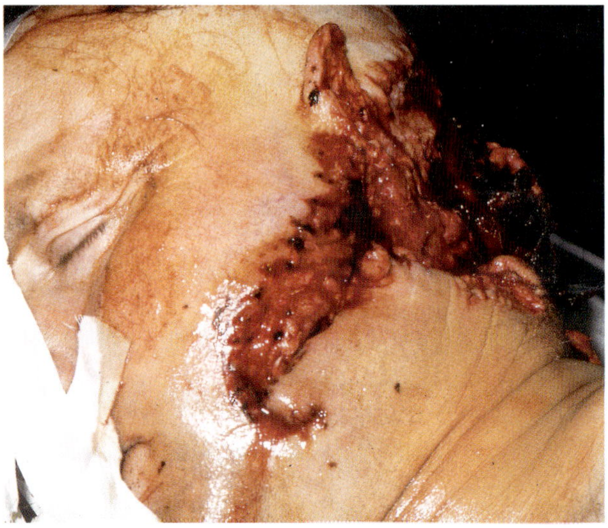

Figure 3.239a Injury due to a circular saw with a defect fracture and CSF fistula of the occipital bone. The facial nerve remained intact despite the extensive soft tissue injury of the left cheek.

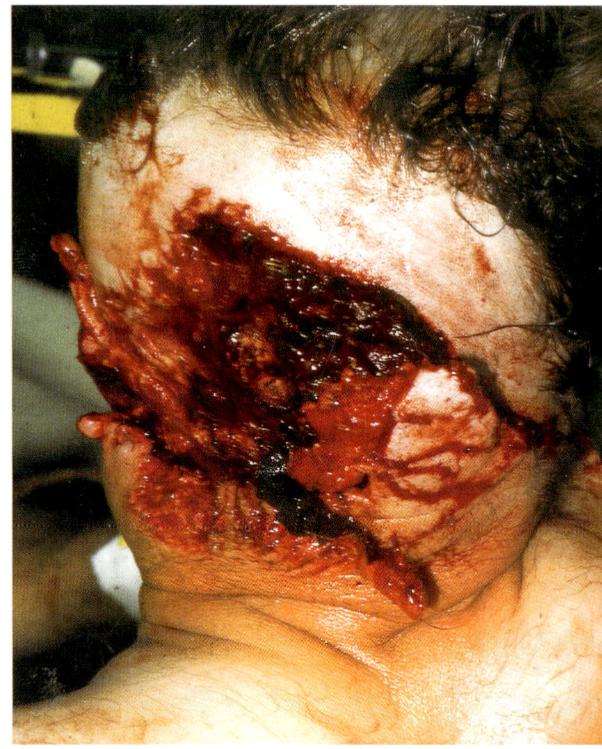

Figure 3.239b A large defect is also present on the haired skin of the head, the soft parts on the throat as well as on the left cheek. The lower two thirds of the ear concha are missing.

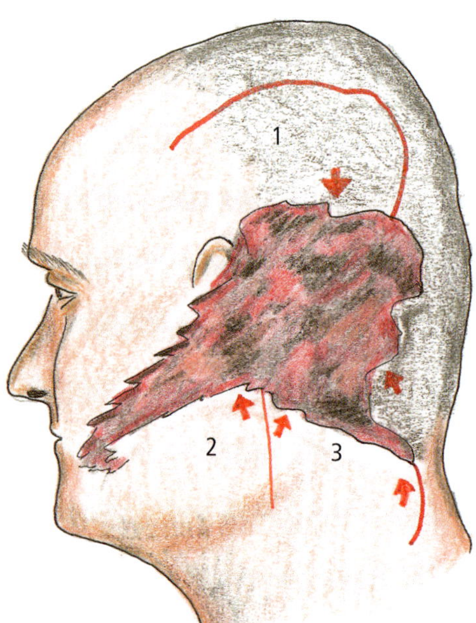

Figure 3.239c A rotation flap is planned from the haired skin of the head (1) in order to cover the defect in the retroauricular area. The cheek could be treated with a direct closure. The throat skin was deeply mobilized in the caudal direction, sagittally divided and rotated in two parts cranially, so that the dorsal part moved cranially and the ventral part moved ventrally (2, 3).

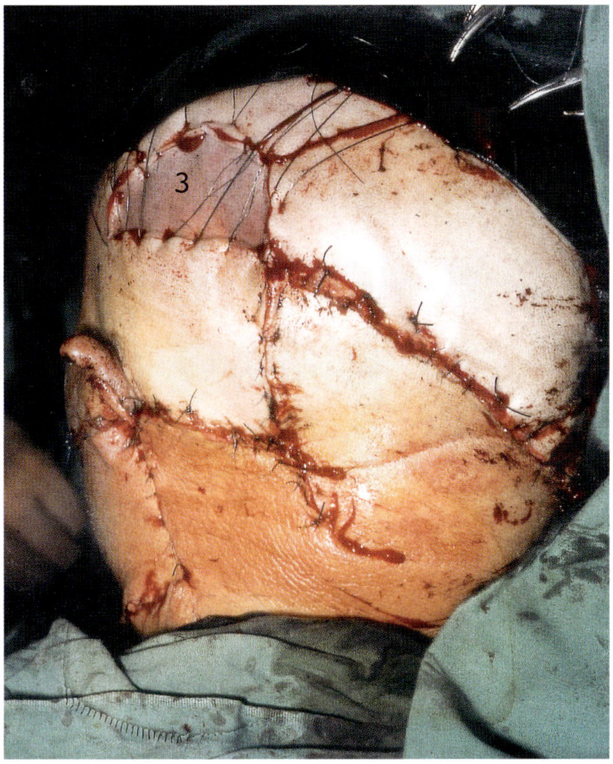

Figure 3.239d Status at the end of the operation: The donor site of the rotation flap covered with a mesh graft (3).

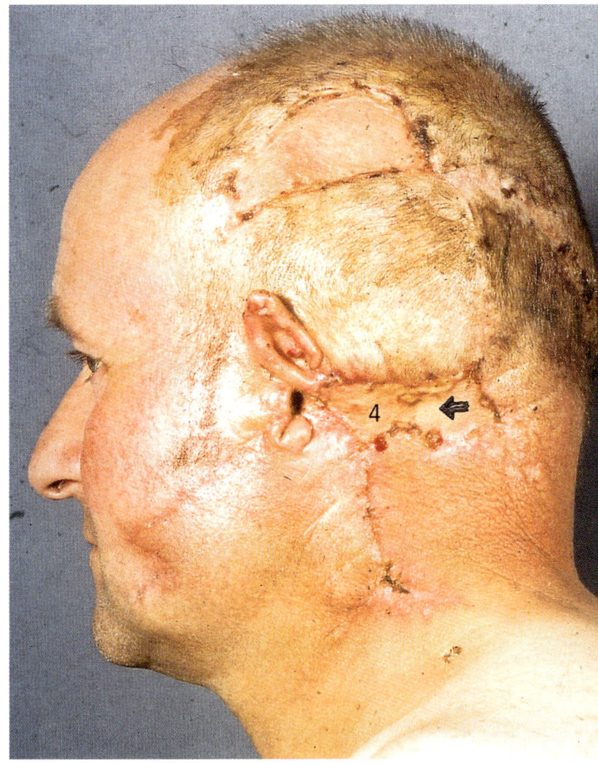

Figure 3.239e Immediately after the operation a flap tip necrosis (throat flap) occurred. This was treated with a mesh graft (see arrow) (4).

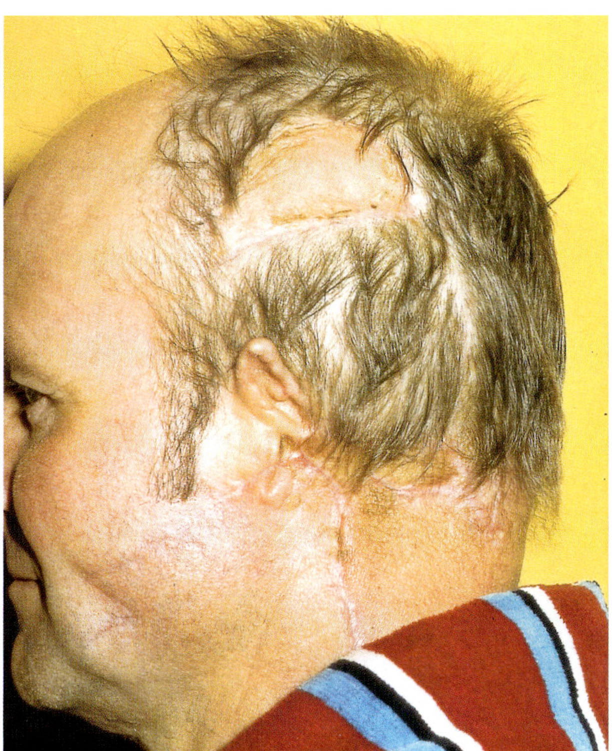

Figure 3.239f Status three months after the accident and operation. The ear concha reconstruction was planned, but was later refused by the patient.

b) Orticochea Flap

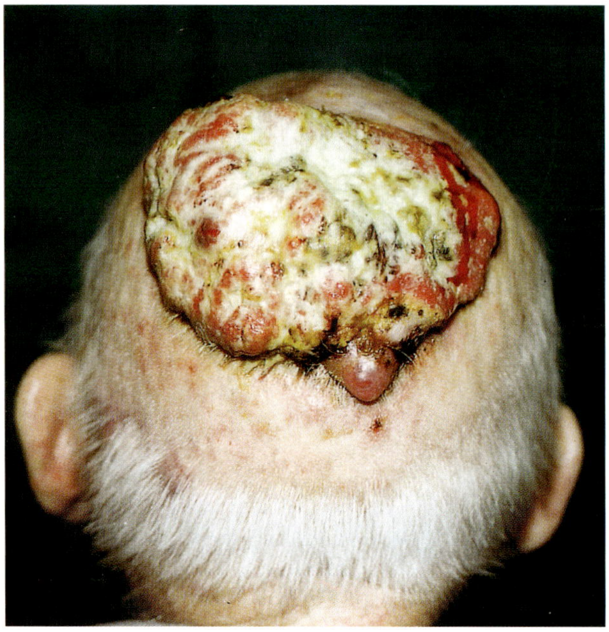

Figure 3.240a Squamous epithelial carcinoma at the haired head. Anamnesis of approximately five years.

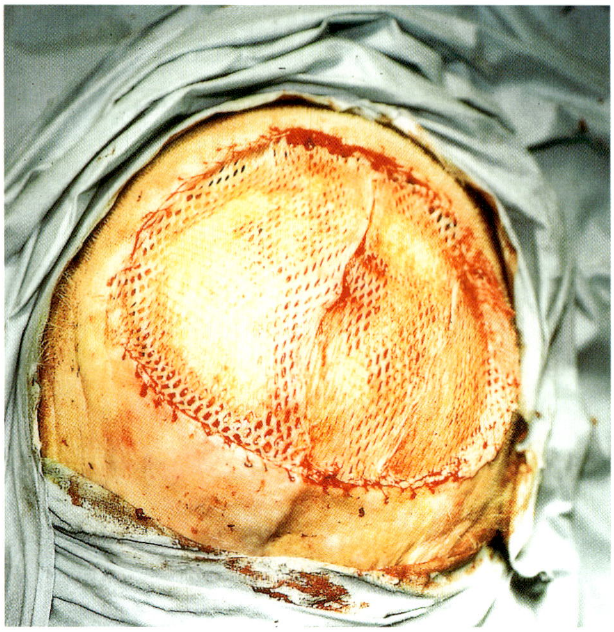

Figure 3.240b After excision of the tumor the defect was covered with a mesh graft up until the results of the histological examination became available.

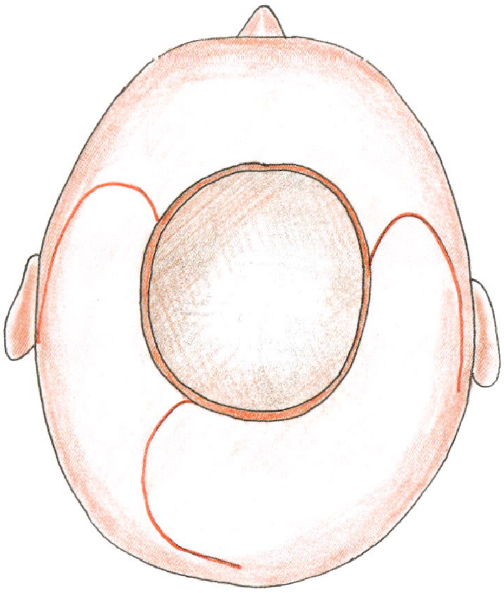

Figure 3.240c Formation of three rotation flaps (according to Orticochea)

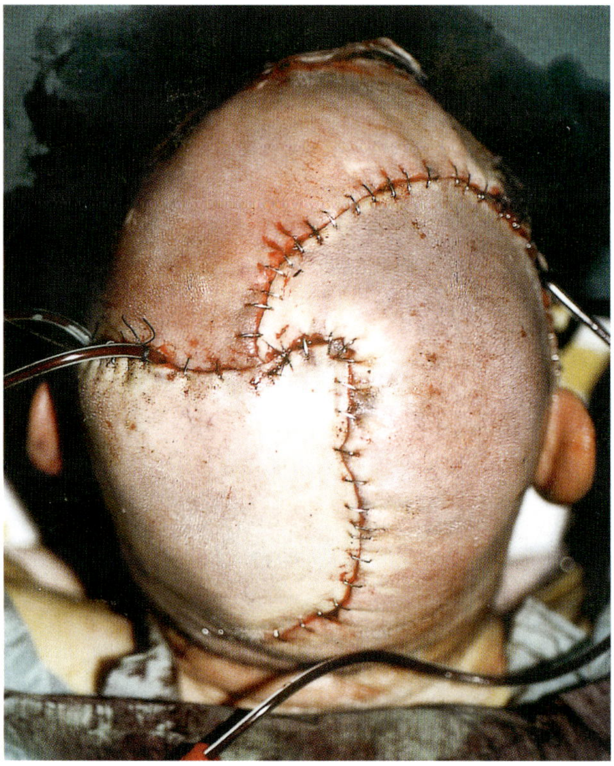

Figure 3.240d The flap donor site is treated with a mesh graft.

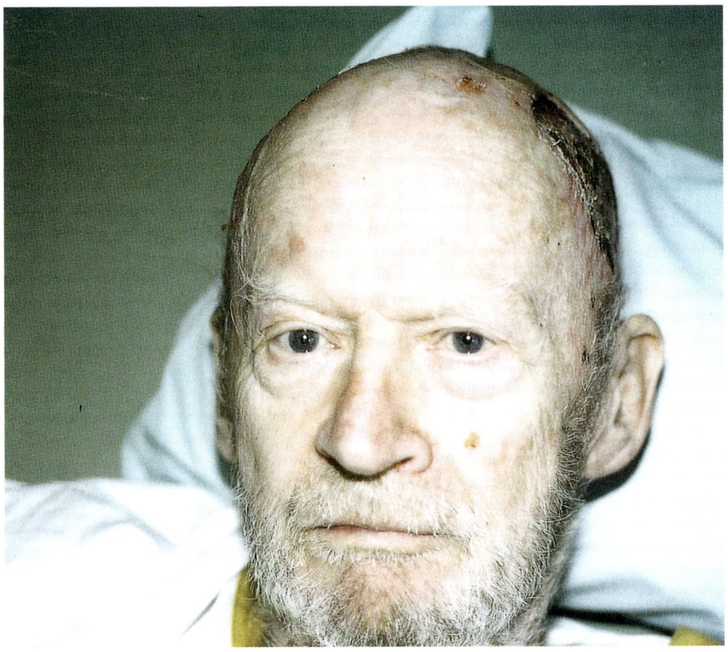

Figure 3.240f Status three weeks after the defect coverage with an Orticochea flap.

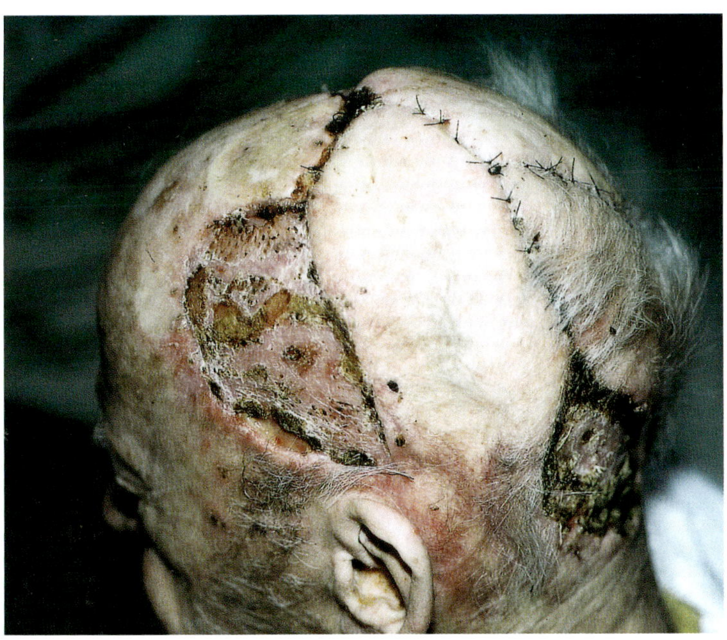

Figure 3.240e The flap donor site is treated with a mesh graft.

Arterial Flaps (Juri Flap)

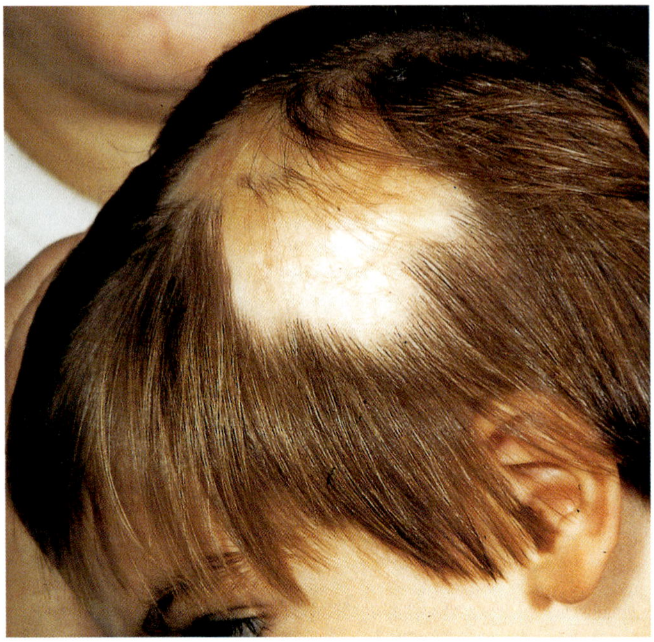

Figure 3.241a Alopecia areata: This is a partial, post-traumatic alopecia in an 8-year old child.

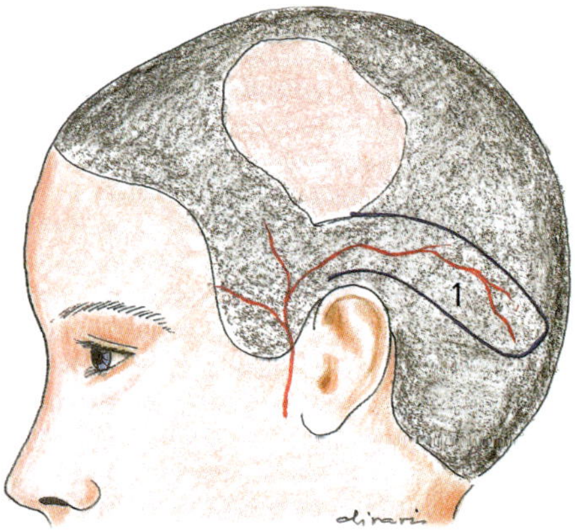

Figure 3.241b An arterial (axial) flap of the haired skin of the head (Juri flap) (1) is planned. The flap can be 2 to 3 cm wide and 12 to 14 cm long. The primary closure of the secondary defect site is achieved by mobilization only in the caudal direction (throat).

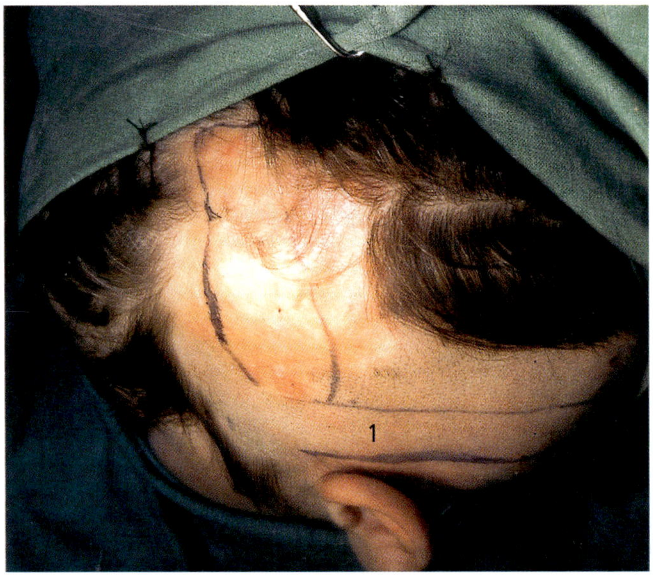

Figure 3.241c The greatest part of the affected alopecia skin is resected. The arterial flap is mobilized (1) and fixed into the defect.

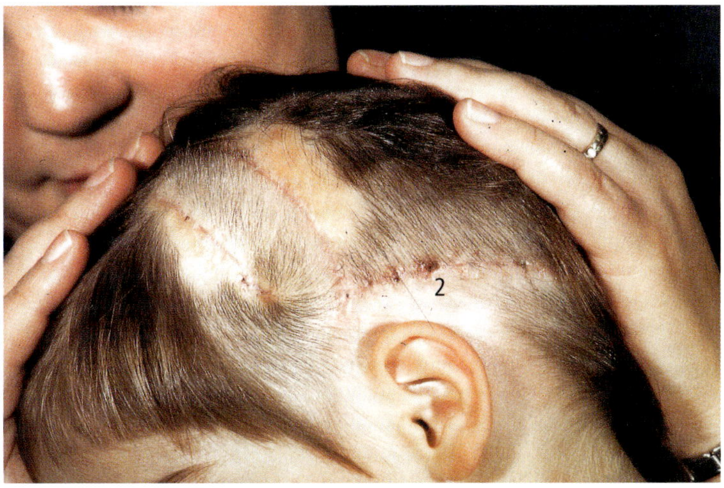

Figure 3.241d The flap donor site (2) is closed primarily after an extensive mobilization only in the caudal direction. This shows the status 12 days after the operation.

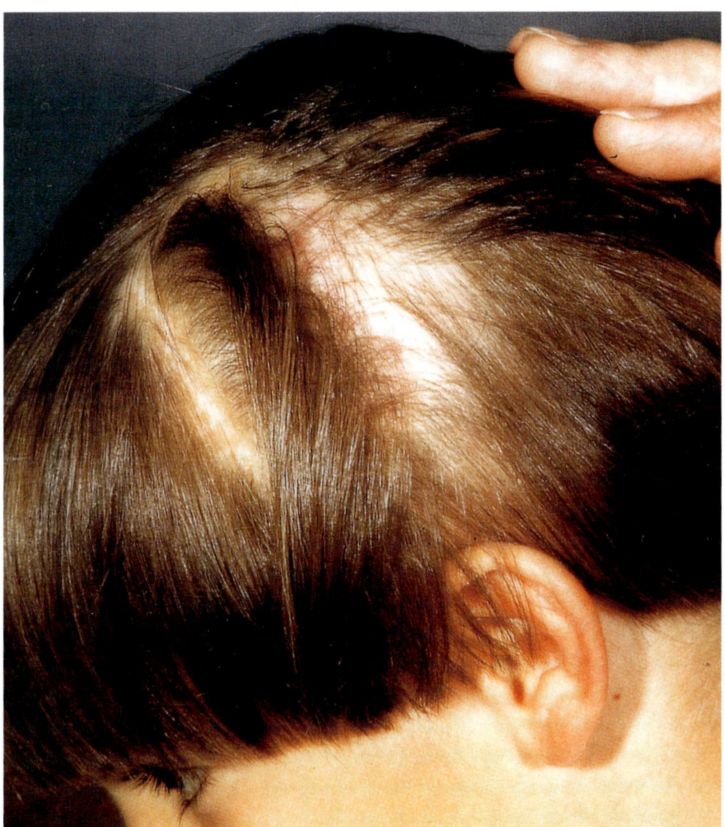

Figure 3.241e Status six months after the operation

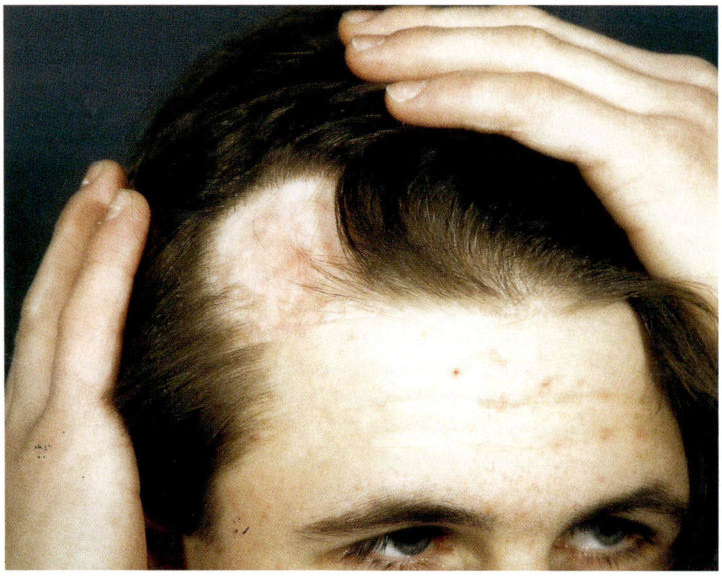

Figure 3.242a Traumatic alopecia

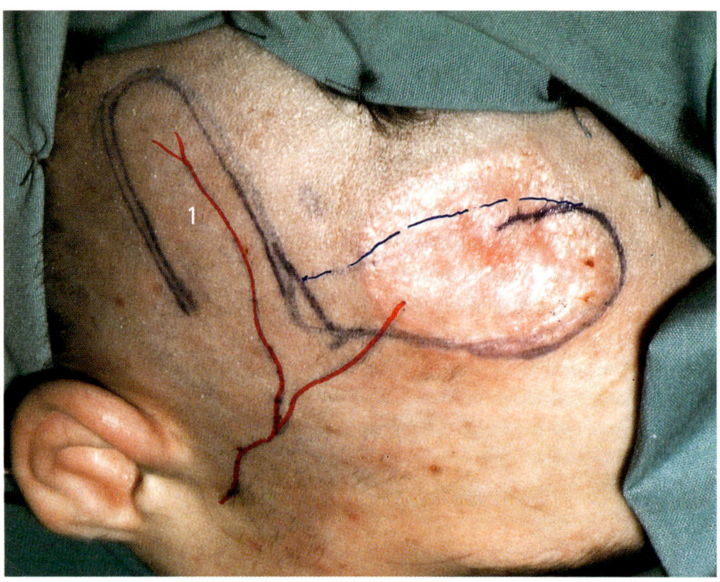

Figure 3.242b An arterial (axial) flap is planned (1) of the haired skin (Juri flap). The flap width may be no more than 2 to 3 cm.

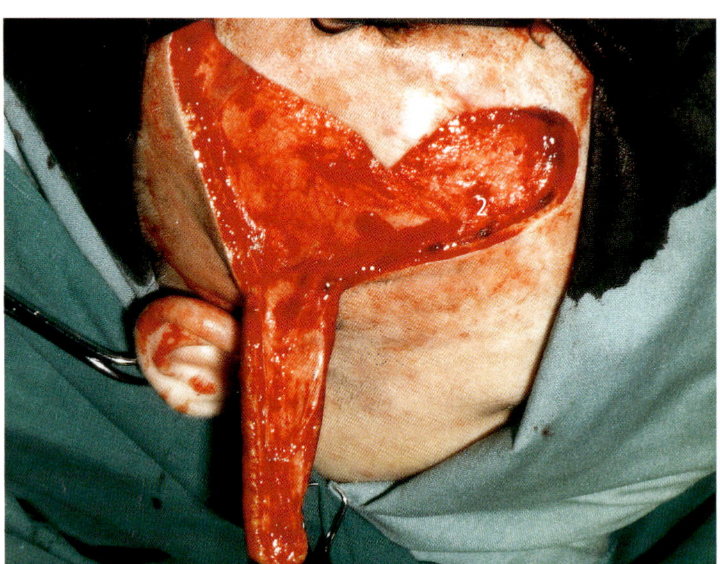

Figure 3.242c In this case the flap is 11 cm long and 3 cm wide. Here we see the situation after excision of the scarred area (2) and mobilization of the flap.

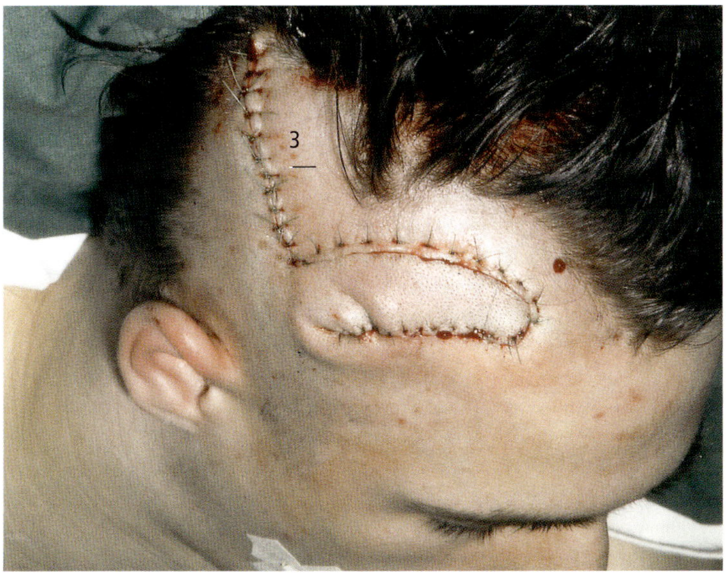

Figure 3.242d Status at the end of the operation

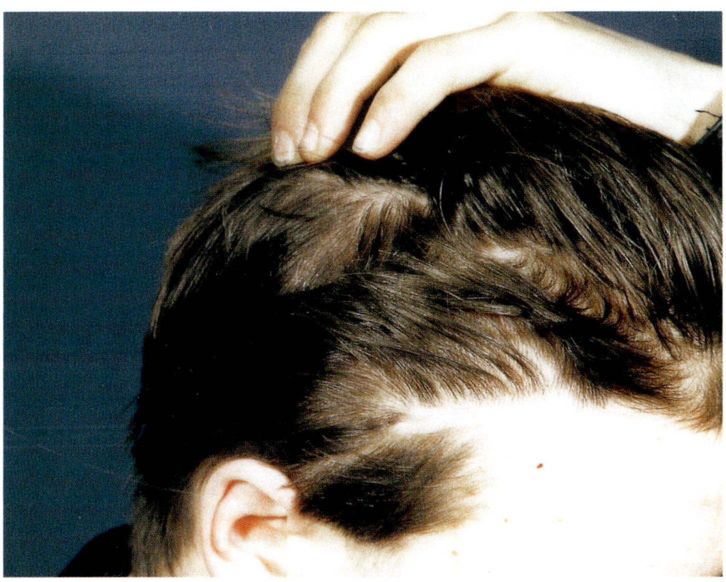

Figure 3.242e Status one year after the operation

Combination of Juri Flaps With an Expander

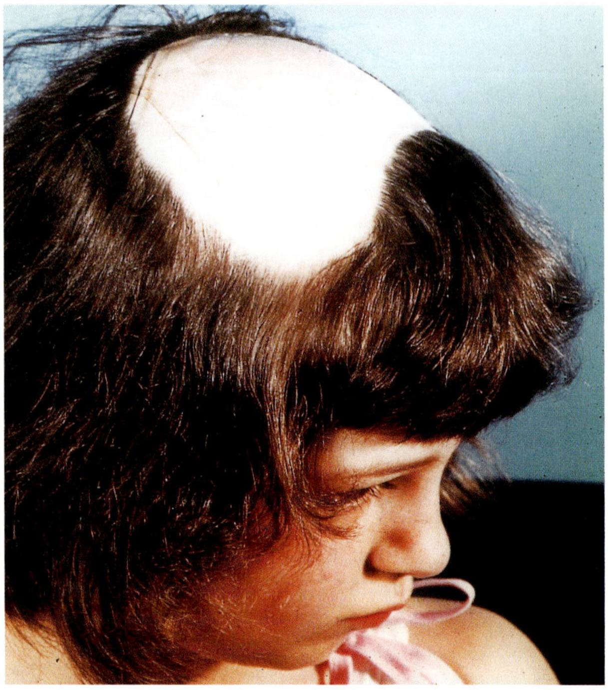

Figure 3.243a Scalp defect on the head due to claw injury from a tiger with tearing of a large part of the haired skin of the head as well as the left ear concha. The patient was initially treated with a mesh graft.

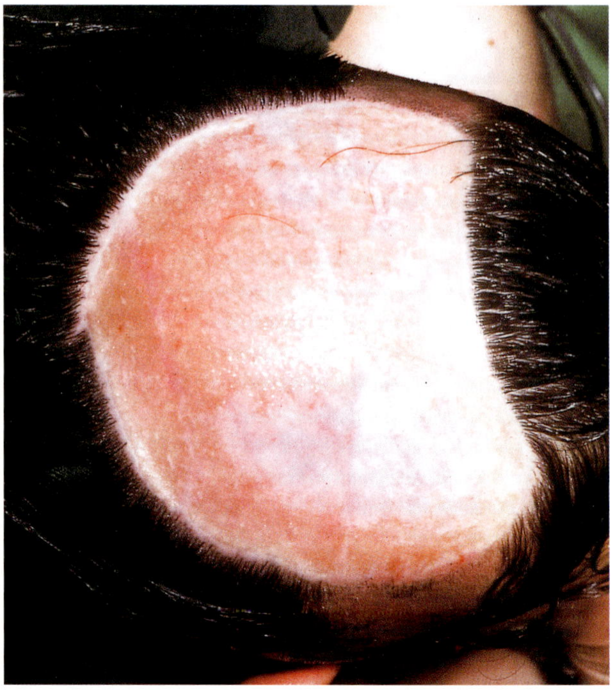

Figure 3.243b It was intended to cover a part of the defect with a pedicular, hairy flap (Juri-flap) and to replace the remainder using an expander. The ear concha should be reconstructed using a cartilage graft.

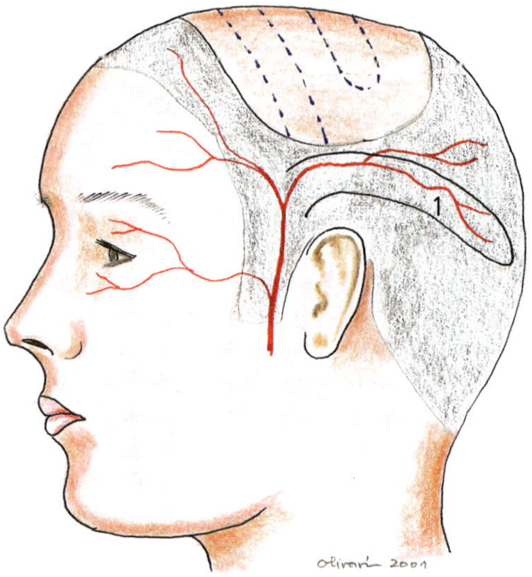

Figure 3.243c The Juri flap is an axial flap (1). Using the Doppler a branch of the superficial temporal artery can be followed dorsally. The flap is 3 cm wide and can be up to 12 to 15 cm long. The circulation is safeguarded. Initially this flap was developed for operations on baldness.

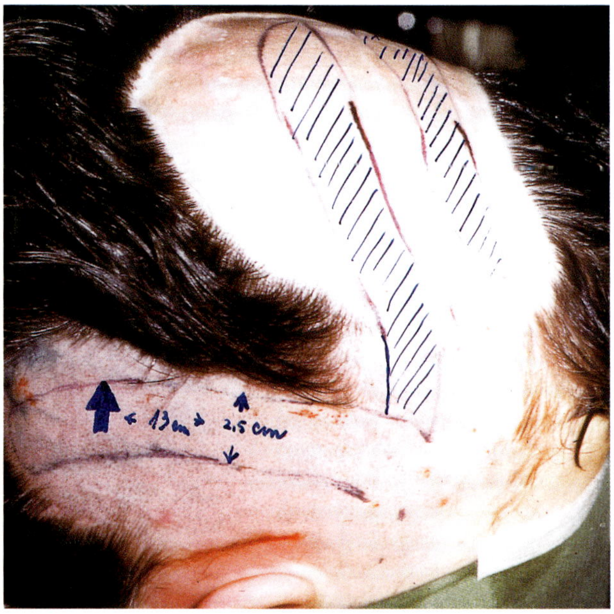

Figure 3.243d With scalp defects the Juri flap is a good procedure alone or in combination with expanders. **Important:** The donor site is primarily closed after extensive undermining in the caudal direction.

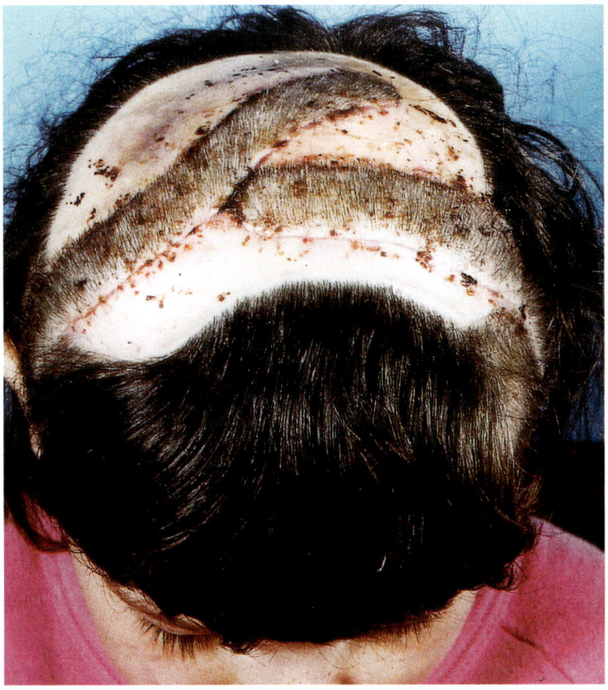

Figure 3.243e Situation two weeks after application of a bilateral Juri flap

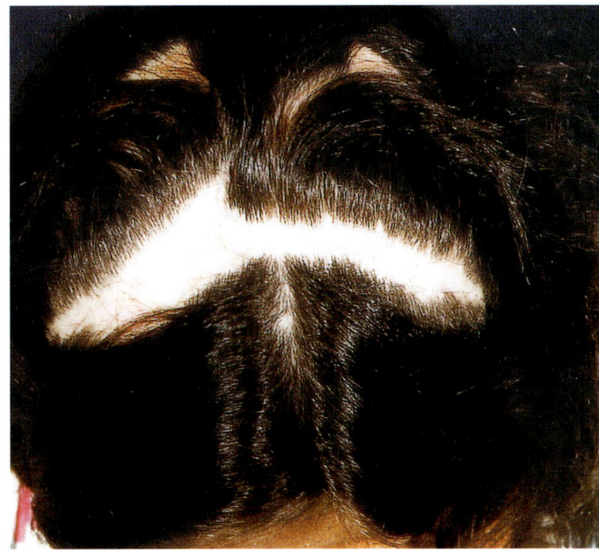

Figure 3.243f Situation six months later, after hairs had already grown from the Juri flap.

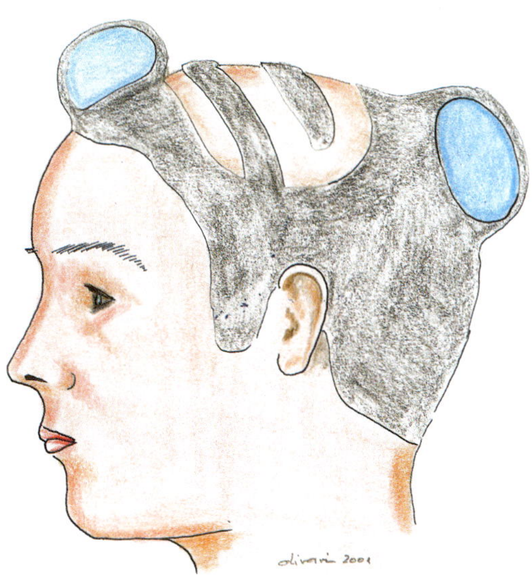

Figure 3.243g Three expanders were implanted in the forehead area to the right and to the left as well as occipitally under the haired skin.

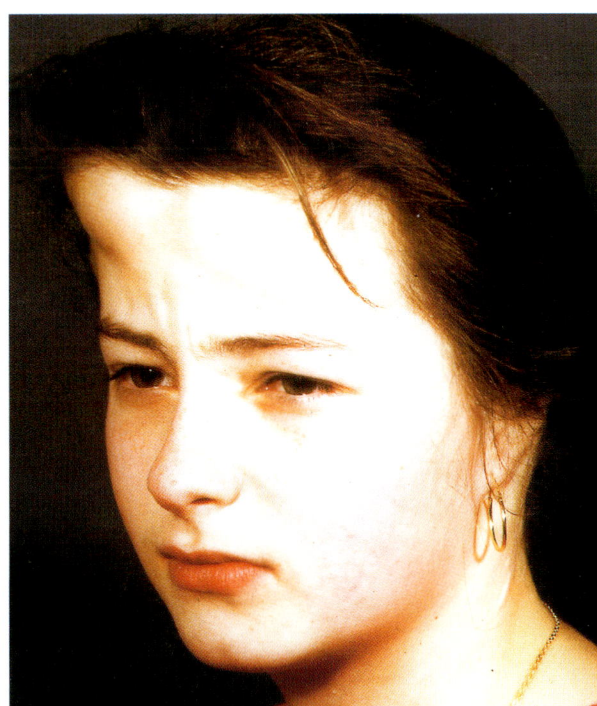

Figure 3.243h Implantation of three expanders

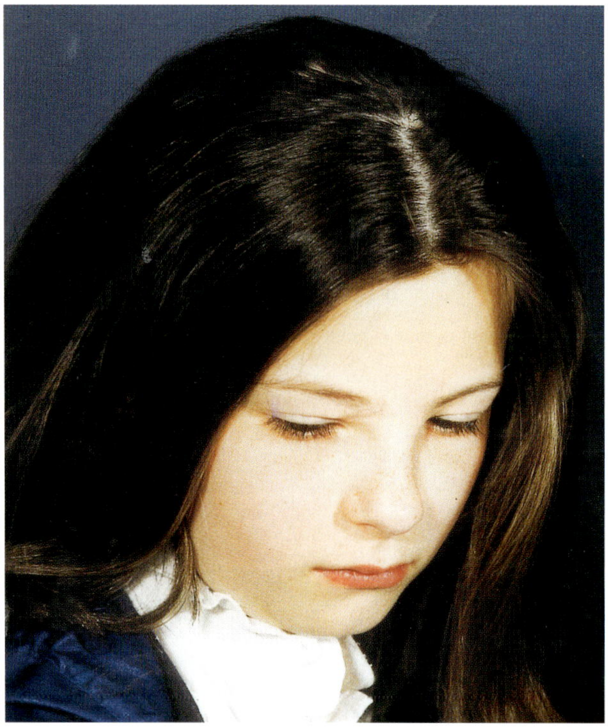

Figure 3.243i Situation after reconstruction of the hair defect with a Juri flap and expander.

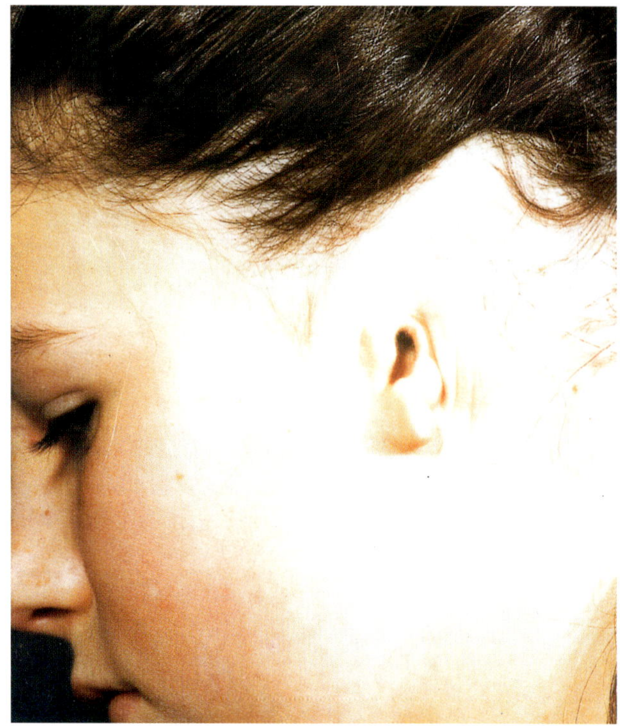

Figure 3.243j During the accident the left ear concha was almost completely torn off.

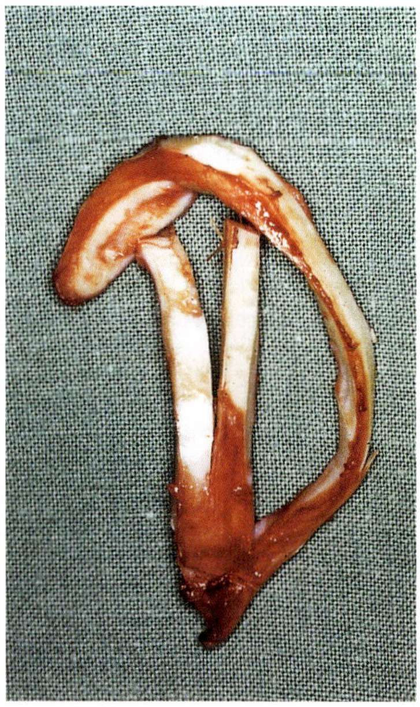

Figure 3.243k In order to reconstruct the ear concha defect, an ear concha was modeled from the costal cartilage.
The scaffold was implanted subcutaneously and corrected twice.

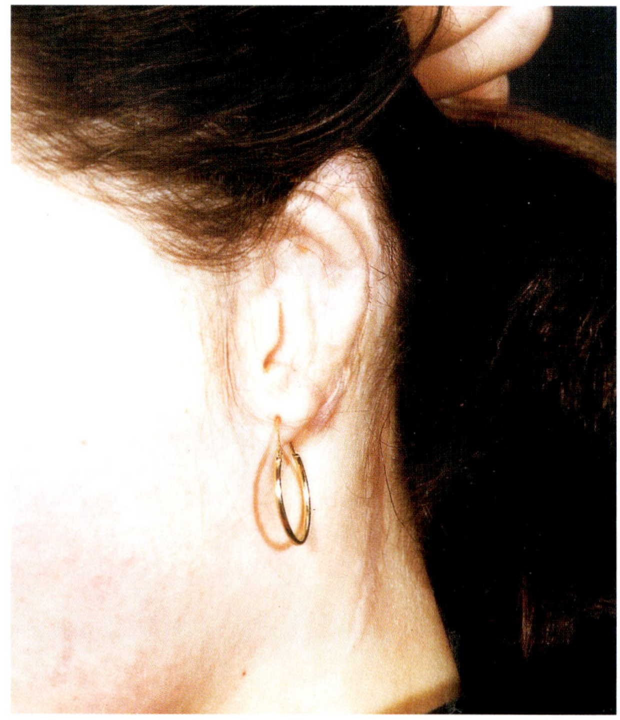

Figure 3.243l Status after the ear concha reconstruction with an acceptable outcome

Juri Operation on a Bald Head

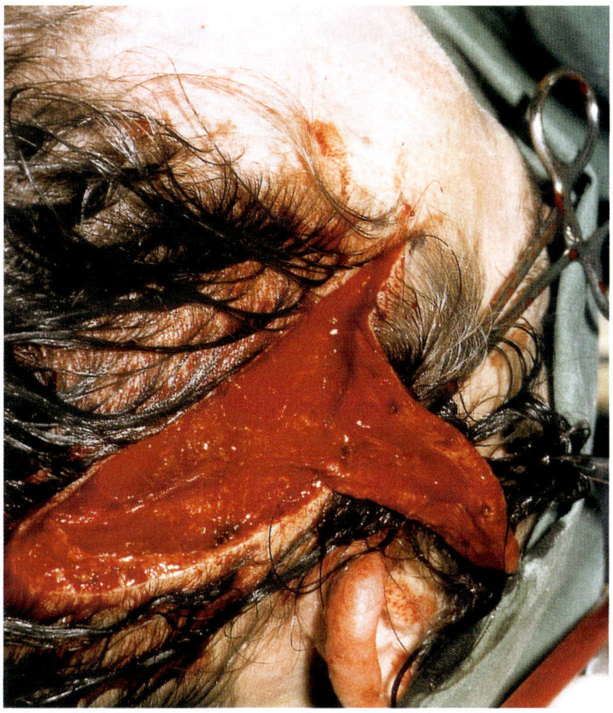

Figure 3.244a Typical bald head in a 41-year old man. An arterial Juri flap that was 3 cm wide and 15 cm long was raised (not previously shaved).

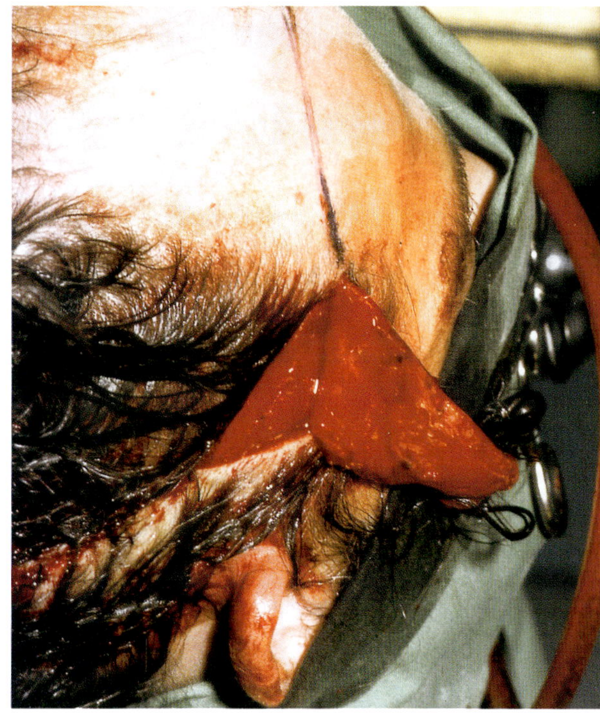

Figure 3.244b After mobilization exclusively in the caudal direction the secondary defect is primarily closed.

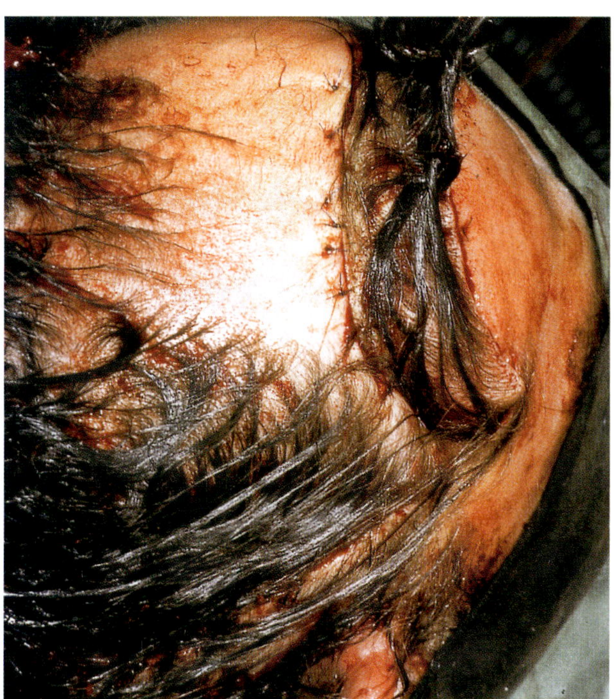

Figure 3.244c A corresponding part of the skin in the balded area is excised and the Juri flap is adapted.

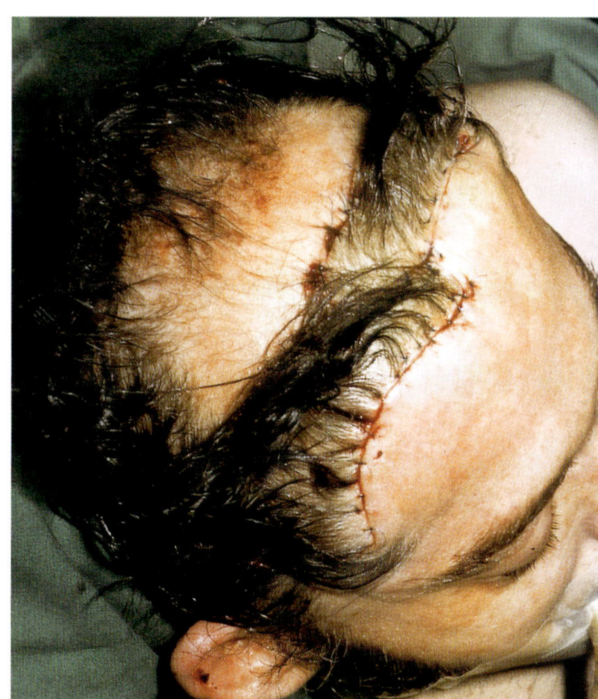

Figure 3.244d Status after fixation of the two flaps of the same length that cross each other in the middle. These hairs can be considered as permanent.

Free Flaps (Radialis Flap)

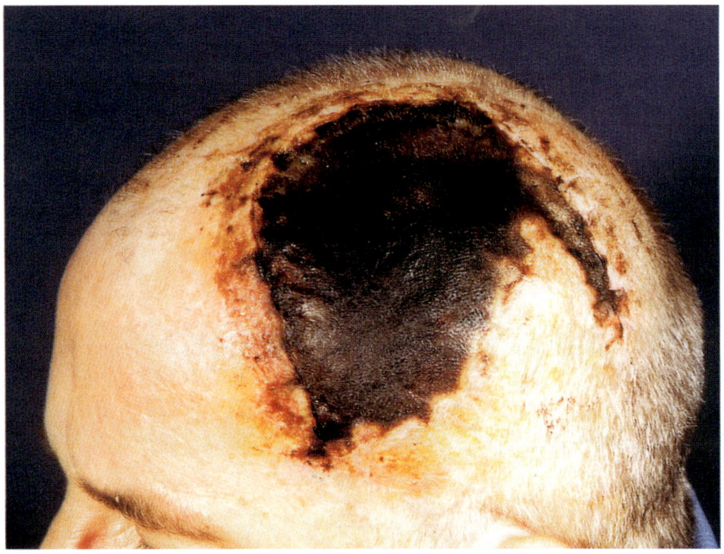

Figure 3.245a Defect at the haired head: After a neurosurgical operation a large-area necrosis of the left parietal area occurred. The superficial temporal artery is presumably damaged.

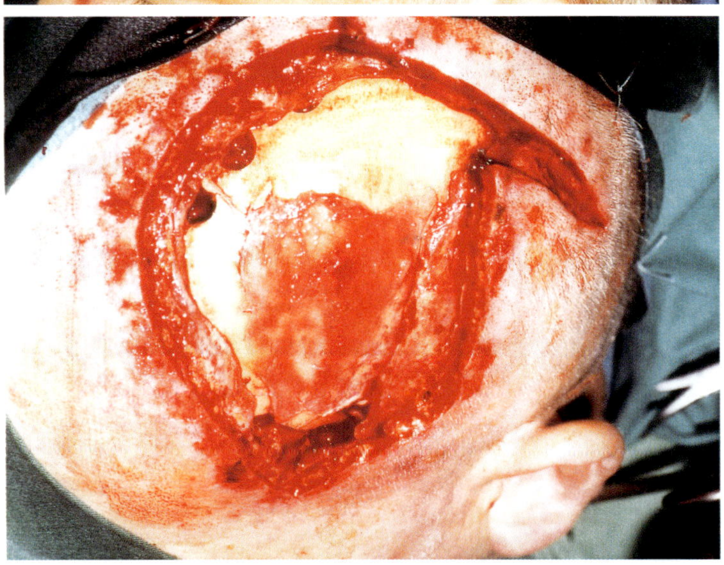

Figure 3.245b The necrotic area is removed

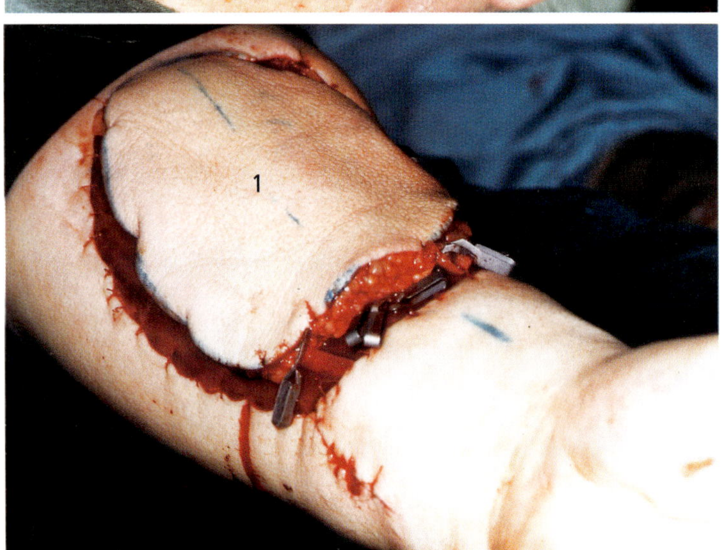

Figure 3.245c A correspondingly large radialis flap is prepared for transplantation (1).

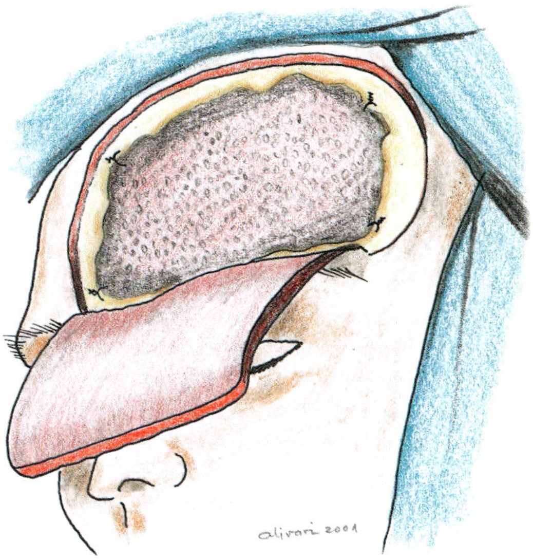

Figure 3.247d The bone graft is precisely modeled, placed with is edge intracranially and epidurally and fixed with only four stitches. The brain (frontal lobe) is covered with a smooth surface. The spongiosa is directed outwards. This allows a more rapid and better revascularization from the skin flap with a reduced resorption tendency of the graft.

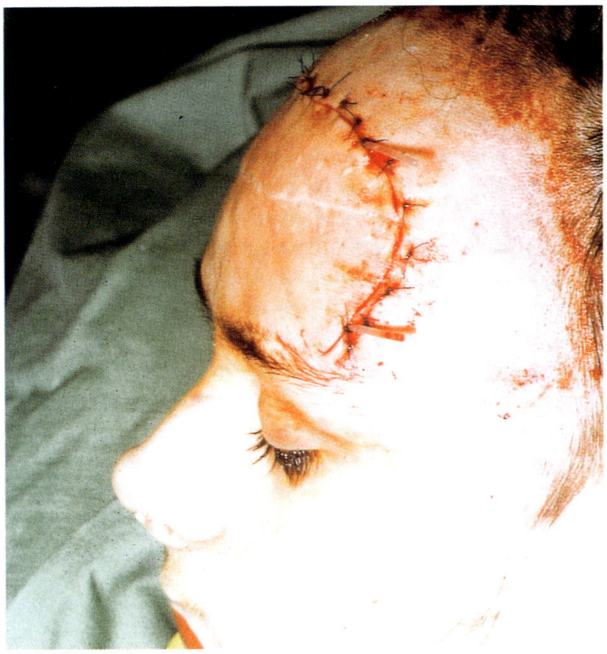

Figure 3.247e Status at the end of the operation

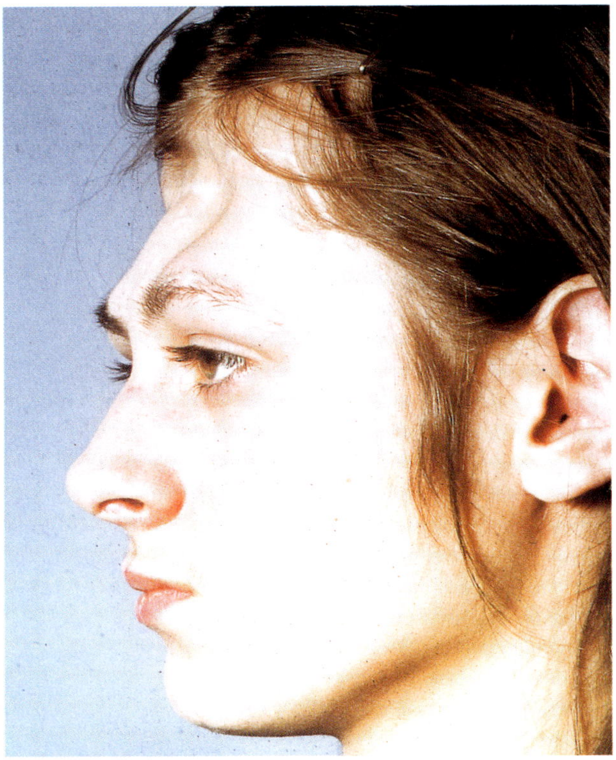

Figure 3.247f Status before the operation

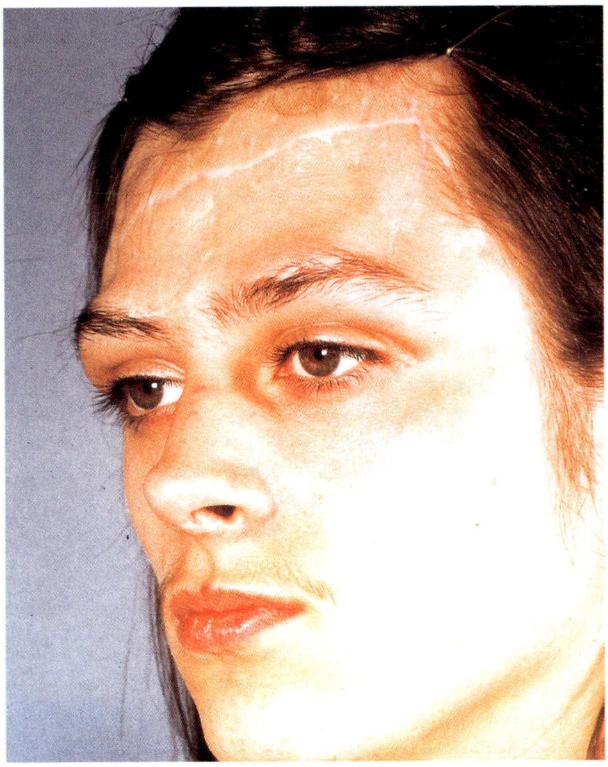

Figure 3.247g Status 18 months after the operation: The bone graft was healed and showed no resorption.

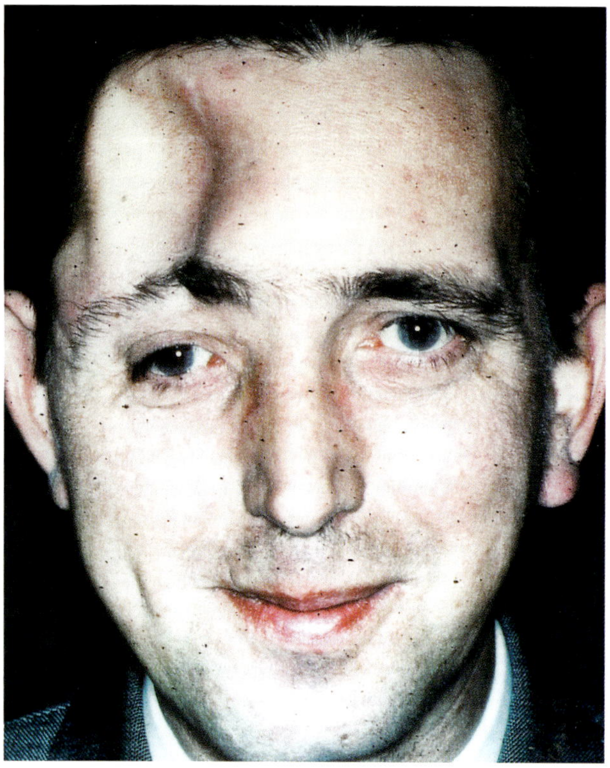

Figure 3.248a Defect of the frontal bone on the right

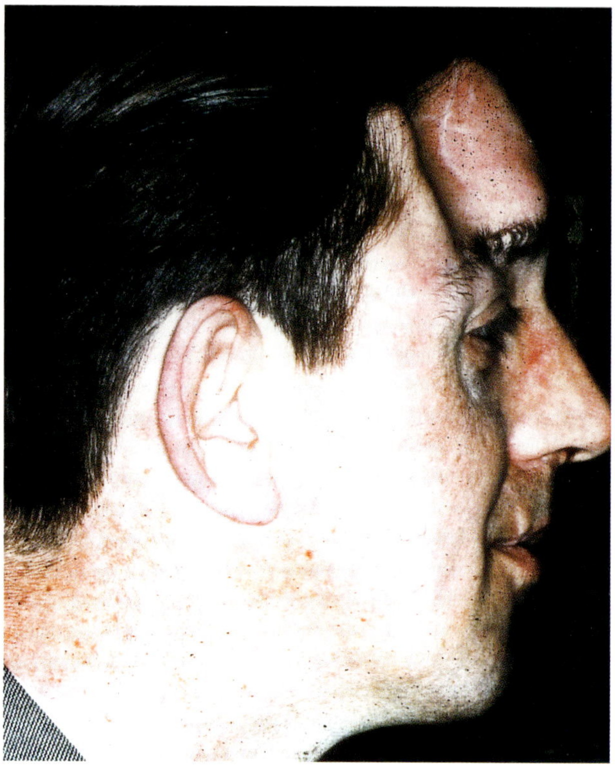

Figure 3.248b The frontal lobe lies directly under the skin as well as the remainder of the frontal muscle.

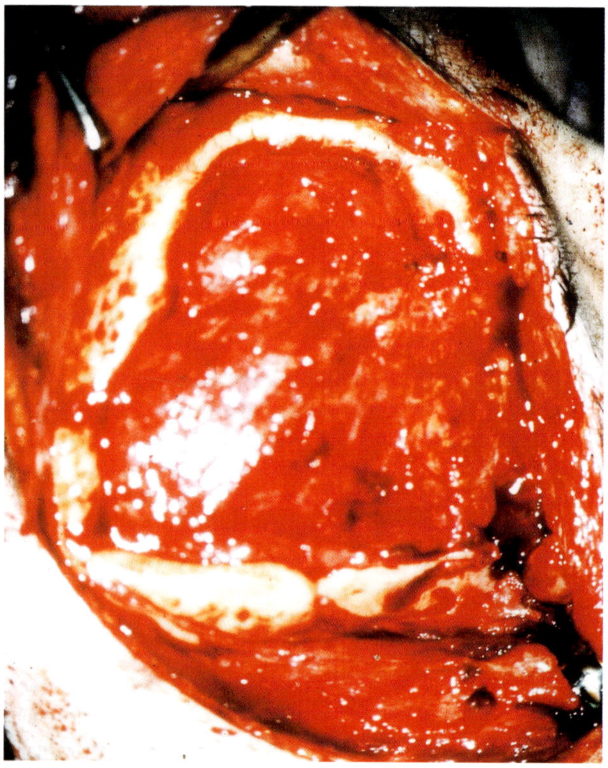

Figure 3.248c The arc-shaped incision is carried out laterocranially in the haired part of the skin. At the bone defect margin preparation is carried out subperiostally.

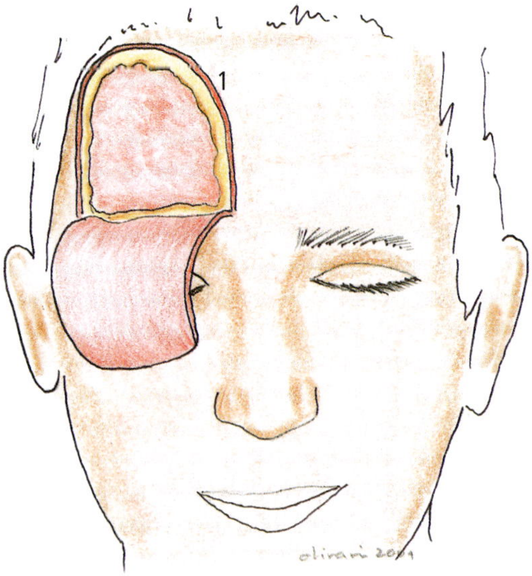

Figure 3.248d The arc-shaped incision is carried out surperiostally, approximately 1 to 2 cm from the defect margin. The bone defect margin is laid open subperiostally (1).

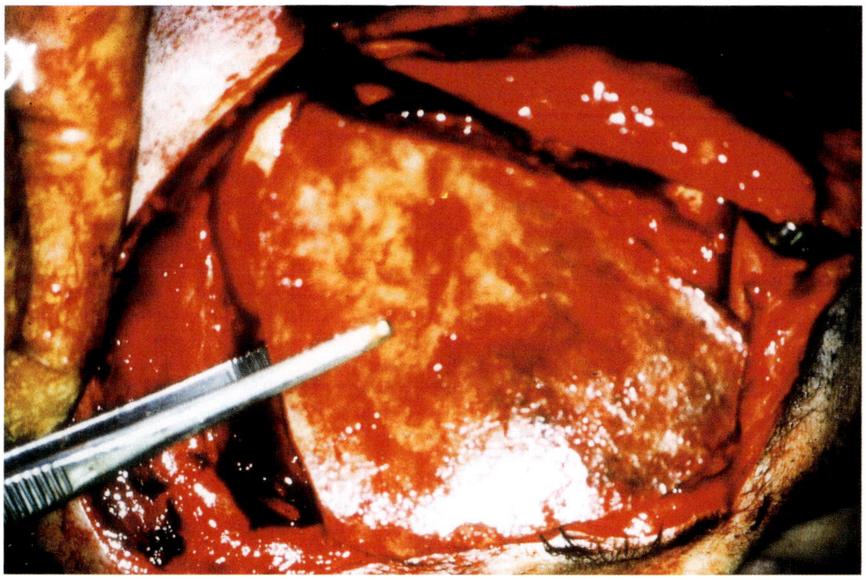

Figure 3.248e The bone graft is withdrawn from the iliac crest, adapted precisely to the defect and fixed.

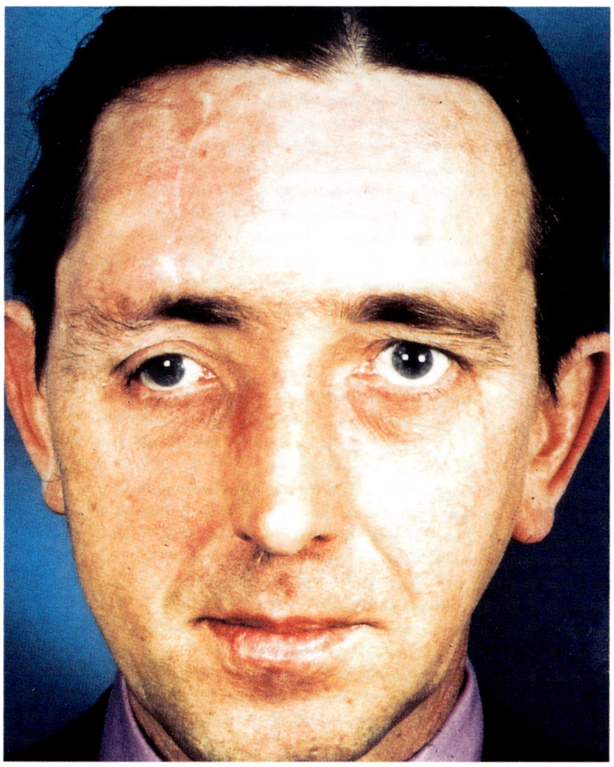

Figure 3.248f Status four years after the operation. No resorption of the graft has occurred.

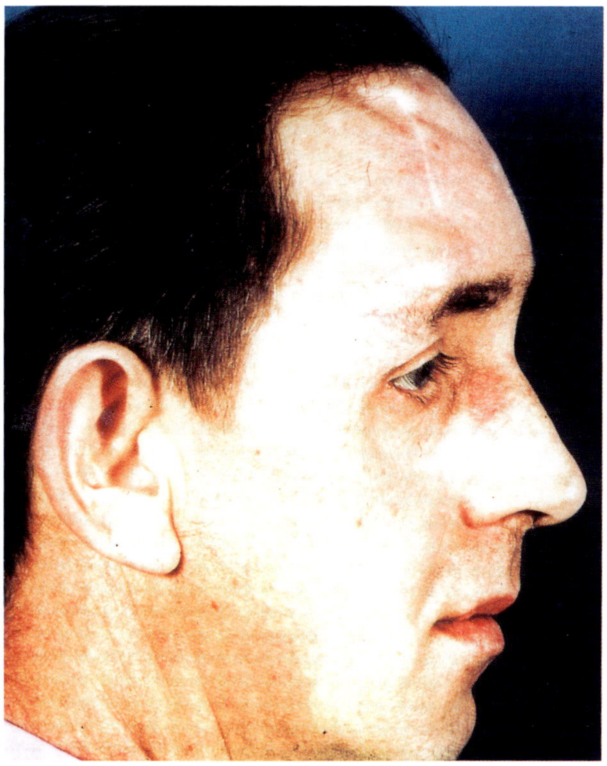

Figure 3.248g Status four years after the operation

CHAPTER 4
Chest and Chest Wall

Breast Cancer

Pathomorphology of Breast Carcinoma

Every surgeon treating breast cancer should have a deep knowledge of the respective pathological changes and oncological treatment principles of the female breast. A permanent interaction with an experienced pathologist is a basic requirement for the appropriate treatment of breast cancer. Furthermore, a close cooperation with an oncologist, as well as a radiologist, is essential. Ideally, all specialties involved jointly decide upon a treatment plan preoperatively.

The author suggests that current consensus recommendations as to diagnostics, treatment, and follow-up protocols of breast cancer should be included routinely.

Diagnosis and Treatment

The diagnosis and required treatment take place as follows:

1) Palpation: Frequently performed by the patient herself.
2) Mammography: Is of vital importance in screening and diagnosis.
3) Ultrasound mammography
4) MR-mammography: Performed when infiltration into adjacent structures is suspected and prior to procedures for treatment of recurrent disease.
5) Needle biopsy for confirmation of diagnosis as well as grading of the severity of disease.
6) Stereotactic marking of tumor before operation.
7) Surgical intervention (quadrantectomy, lumpectomy, or Patey mastectomy), Sentinel node biopsy, and ALND (axillary lymph node dissection) – level I, level II and III are included depend of histopathological finding.
8) Primary breast reconstruction if possible otherwise secondary reconstruction (silicone implant, expander, TRAM, latissimus, DIEP and SIEP).
9) Appropriate stage-adjusted radiotherapy, chemotherapy, and hormonal therapy.

Table 4.1 Histological classification of invasive breast cancer (AFIB, 1992)

- Invasive ductal carcinoma
- Invasive ductal carcinoma with predominant intraductal component
- Invasive lobular carcinoma
- Mucinous carcinoma
- Medullary carcinoma
- Invasive papillary carcinoma
- Tubular carcinoma
- Adenoid-cystic carcinoma
- Secretory (juvenile) carcinoma
- Apocrine carcinoma
- Carcinoma with metaplasia
- Carcinoma with osteoclastic giant cells
- Cystic-hypersecretory carcinoma with invasion
- Carcinoma with endocrine differentiation
- Glycogen-rich carcinoma
- Lipid-rich carcinoma
- Invasive cribriform carcinoma

Histological Classification (Clinical Relevance)

1) Invasive ductal carcinoma
Infiltrating ductal carcinoma accounts for 80 % of all malignant breast lesions and thus is regarded as the prototype of breast cancer. Knowledge on epidemiology, etiology, as well as prognosis of breast cancer refers to this histological type. Histologically solid and glandular growth patterns can be observed with varying degrees of fibrosis. Presenting as irregular lumps these lesions display multiple branches referred to as spiculae. The central aspect of the lesion can undergo complete fibrosis/sclerosis.
2) Invasive lobular carcinoma
Lobular infiltrating carcinoma occurs in 4 to 6 % of cases [Bässler 1978]. Being less aggressive, it demonstrates a slower growth rate, and metastasizes later than the ductal carcinoma.
3) Medullary carcinoma
Although this lesion exhibits a high mitotic index, and significant irregularities as to cell morphology, the level of malignancy is still lower than with the invasive ductal type. 10-year survival rate approaches 84 % [Ridolfi 1977].
4) Mucinous carcinoma
This rare type appears primarily in the elderly female population (1–2 %). It is considered to be associated with a favorable prognosis.
5) Tubular carcinoma
Occurring in 1 to 2 % it is among the highly differentiated breast carcinomas and as such is associated with a very good prognosis.
6) Papillary carcinoma
Infiltrating papillary carcinoma is very rare (0.3–1.5 %). However, it comes along with an suspicious outcome [McDivitt 1968].
7) Adenoid-cystic carcinoma
Having a good prognosis it occurs with a frequency of 1 %.
8) In-situ carcinomas of the breast
In recent years, due to improved diagnostic tools, in-situ carcinomas of the female breast have been diagnosed with an increasing frequency. Ductal carcinoma in-situ represents approximately 12 to 15 % of all newly diagnosed breast carcinomas.

In-situ carcinoma can be classified as follows:
- DCIS: Ductal carcinoma in-situ, representing 80 % of all in-situ carcinomas and
- LCIS: Lobular carcinoma in-situ.

These subgroups not only differ histopathologically but also represent two entirely different entities with regards to diagnostics and treatment. However, one shared histopathological feature is an intact basal lamina and therefore lack of invasive growth.

Ductal Carcinoma In-Situ (DCIS)

DCIS has to be regarded as a direct precursor of an invasive carcinoma and thus needs to be treated as such. Various types are distinguished histopathologically. As to prognosis it seems appropriate to discern between comedo and non-comedo carcinomas. Comedo carcinomas are characterized by an unfavorable grading, high mitotic index, and centrally located necrosis. They seem to display a more aggressive growth pattern associated with a higher recurrence rate when breast-conserving surgery is carried out. Comedo carcinomas frequently exhibit a high proliferation rate. Non-comedo carcinomas are characterized by a more favorable grading, lower mitotic index, and lack of extensive necrosis.

Treatment: Simple mastectomy with primary reconstruction is regarded as an effective prophylactic treatment modality. Thus, all glandular breast tissue can be excised safely including areas which potentially harbour DCIS. ALND is not indicated considering the frequency of lymph node involvement (0–1 %). In selected cases ALND can be discussed (e.g. DCIS with a high risk of invasion). Postoperative radiotherapy of the thoracic wall as well as systemic adjuvant chemotherapy is not indicated. An almost 100 % cure rate can be achieved with mastectomy alone. All newly introduced methods need to be compared with this standard protocol. A multicentric growth pattern is an absolute contraindication for breast-conserving surgery.

■ **Lobular Carcinoma In-Situ (LCIS)**
Similar to DCIS, LCIS is a non-palpable precancerous lesion affecting predominantly premenopausal patients. A characteristic feature is its multicentric growth pattern which involves the unilateral and contralateral breast in 70 % and 28 %, respectively. It is diagnosed with an incidence of 0.8 to 1.5 % in breast biopsies, however, its overall incidence in the female population is not known.

LCIS is not to be underestimated. In approximately 25 % of histologically verified LCIS specimens, those patients not undergoing mastectomy developed invasive carcinoma in the same breast within a period of 5 to 25 years [McDivitt 1969].

Anderson (1977) noted invasive carcinomas in the unilateral and contralateral breast in 15 % and 9.3 %, respectively, following a 10-year observation period.

Treatment: Current treatment protocol recommendations (2nd EORTC-Consensus Conference, 1992) are as follows:

LCIS is not an indication for mastectomy. Subcutaneous mastectomy should only be considered if additional risk factors are present. Performing a bilateral preventive mastectomy is anachronous as well. Just primary tumor excision is recommended without ALND. Additional procedures involving the contralateral breast should be avoided. Furthermore, adjuvant radiotherapy is contra-indicated due to lack of radiation sensitivity of LCIS. Thus, postoperative radiation should be performed exclusively within controlled trials until data as to indication and intensity is available.

9) Paget's disease
Paget's disease is associated with painful oozing, crusted erosions, and ulcerations. Pathological change begins at the nipple with subsequent radial spread. Being a painful lesion distinguishes Paget's disease from other types of breast cancer. Histopathologically, Paget's disease is an intraductal carcinoma, frequently displaying an invasive growth pattern. In advanced stages, involvement of the breast parenchyma can be detected. Early stages (involvement of the nipple-areolar-complex (NAC) only) rarely display lymph node metastases (5–12 %). However, if breast parenchyma is affected lymph node involvement rises to a frequency of 50 to 66 %.

10) Lymphangiosis carcinomatosa
Lymphangiosis carcinomatosa is associated with an infiltrating tumor exhibiting a high grade of malignancy (G3). In accordance with its aggressive growth pattern, lymph node metastases can be found in 86 % irrespective of the tumor size [Citoler 1974]. Prognosis is extremely poor.

Histological Grading

Table 4.2 Grading criteria for breast cancer [Bässler et al. 1992]

Feature	Criteria	Score
Tubule formation	> 75 %	1
	10 – 75 %	2
	< 10	3
Nucleus polymorphism	Low	1
	Moderate	2
	High	3
Rate of mitosis	0-1/HPF (0-10/10 HPF)	1
	1-2/HPF (11-20/10 HPF)	2
	> 2/HPF (>20/10 HPF)	3
	Score	3–9

Score	Grade of malignancy	G-group	Definition
3, 4, 5	Low	G1	Well differentiated
6, 7	Moderate	G2	Moderately differentiated
8, 9	High	G3	Poorly differentiated

HPF = high power field (magnification × 400)

Grading is based upon several parameters including structural differentiation, level of tubular formation, cell size and appearance, as well as the amount of hyperchromasia and mitosis observed, and thus can be classified as follows:

G1 – well-differentiated (displaying a slow growth rate)
G2 – moderately-differentiated
G3 – poorly-differentiated with aggressive growth

Tumor Growth

Tumor growth is calculated according to its so called doubling time. It can vary extremely ranging from 23 (aggressive growth) to 209 days (slow growth) with an average of 100 days. [Gerson-Cohen 1967].

Having doubling times of 23 and 200 days, tumors would need, respectively, 2 and 17 years to reach a size of 1 cm. Thus, growth rate is far more important than tumor size with regards to prognosis.

- Tumors displaying an aggressive and infiltrative growth pattern, with centrally located necrosis, demonstrate axillary lymph node involvement in 75 % of cases and a 10-year survival rate of 29 %.
- In well circumscribed tumors of the same size, without centrally located necrosis, axillary lymph nodes are involved in 30 % of cases with a 10-year survival rate of 61 % [Carter 1978].
- Lymph node involvement is an unfavorable parameter for prognosis.

Hormone Receptors

Estrogen receptor (ER-) positive tumors are associated with a more favorable outcome and a statistically superior survival rate than for ER-negative patients.

Tumor Size

Table 4.3 pT primary tumor [TNM classification (UICC)]

pTx	Primary tumor cannot be assessed	
pT0	No evidence of primary tumor	
pTis	Carcinoma in situ: intraductal carcinoma, LCIS, Paget's disease of the nipple with no associated tumor (Note: Paget's disease associated with a tumor is classified according to the size of the tumor.)	
pT1	Tumor 2 cm or smaller in greatest dimension	
	pT1a	Tumor larger than 0.1 cm but not larger than 0.5 cm in greatest dimension
	pT1b	Tumor larger than 0.5 cm but not larger than 1 cm in greatest dimension
pT1c	Tumor larger than 1 cm but not larger than 2 cm in greatest dimension	
pT2	Tumor larger than 2 cm but not larger than 5 cm in greatest dimension	
pT3	Tumor larger than 5 cm in greatest dimension	
pT4	Tumor of any size with direct extension to (a) chest wall or (b) skin, only as described below (Note: Chest wall includes ribs, intercostal muscles, and serratus anterior muscle, but not pectoral muscle.)	
	pT4a	Extension to chest wall
	pT4b	Edema (including peau d'orange) or ulceration of the skin of the breast or satellite skin nodules confined to the same breast
	pT4c	Both of the above (T4a and T4b)
	pT4d	Inflammatory carcinoma (Lymphangiosis carcinomatosa)

Lymph Node Involvement

Table 4.4 pN – regional lymph nodes [TNM classification (UICC)]

PNx	Regional lymph nodes cannot be assessed	
pN0	No regional lymph node metastasis	
pN1	Metastasis to movable ipsilateral axillary lymph node(s)	
	pN1a	Only micrometastasis (none >0.2 cm)
	pN1b	Metastasis to lymph node(s), any larger than 0.2 cm
	I	Metastasis in 1–3 lymph nodes, any larger than 0.2 cm and all smaller than 2 cm in greatest dimension
	II	Metastasis to 4 or more lymph nodes, any larger than 0.2 cm and all smaller than 2 cm in greatest dimension
	III	Extension of tumor beyond the capsule of a lymph node metastasis, smaller than 2 cm in greatest dimension
	IV	Metastasis to a lymph node 2 cm or larger in greatest dimension
pN2	Metastasis to ipsilateral axillary lymph node(s) fixed to each other or to other structures	
pN3	Metastasis to ipsilateral internal mammary lymph node(s)	

For practical surgical reasons Berg (1955) classified the axillary lymph node into three levels:

Level I Lymph nodes lateral and caudal to the pectoralis minor muscle

Level II Lymph nodes behind the pectoralis minor muscle

Level III Lymph nodes medial and cranial to the pectoralis minor muscle

Scintigraphy of the Lymphatic System

This study is based on the assumption that a tumor primarily metastasizes into the **sentinel lymph node** (SLN). Thus, following injection of a radioactive isotope (^{191m}Tc) the SLN can be visualized and subsequently excised.

In malignant melanomas the SLN is usually the first lymph node involved. However, in breast carcinoma, the SLN is occasionally skipped. Nevertheless, this technique will play a major future role in diagnostics and performance of ALND in breast cancer.

Distant Metastasis (Hematogenic)

Table 4.5 pM – Distant metastasis

pMx	Presence of distant metastasis cannot be assessed
pM0	No distant metastasis
pM1	Distant metastasis present
Optionally, one may further classify:	
pM1a	Metastasis involving only the supraclavicular lymph nodes
pM1b	All others

Table 4.6 Hematogenic metastasis – Distribution

Lungs	63 %
Bone	58 %
Liver	51 %
Pleura	44 %
Skin	20 %
Peritoneum	17 %
Ovaries	13 %
Kidneys	13 %

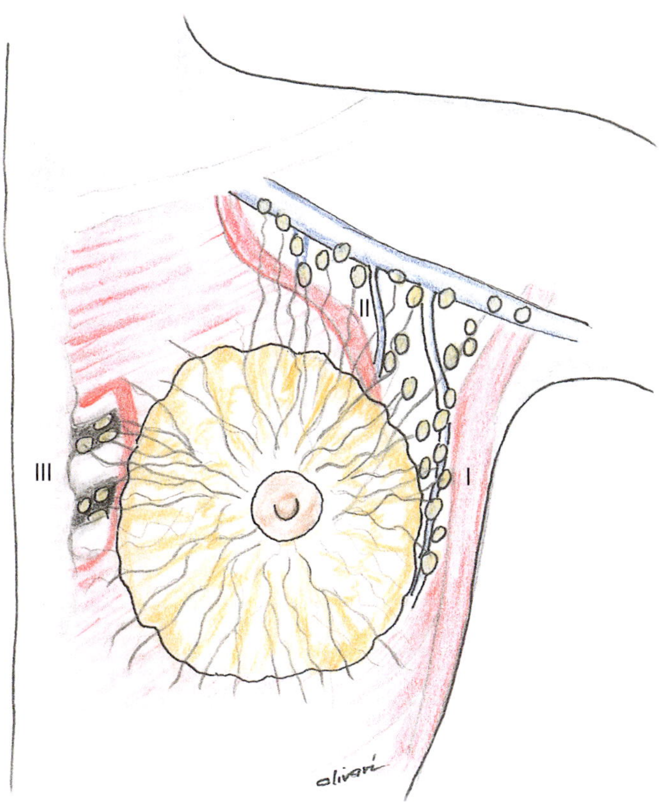

Figure 4.1 Lymphatic drainage of the breast (Level I–III)

Breast Reconstruction

According to recent literature the TRAM and latissimus dorsi flap are the methods of choice for breast reconstruction. Other flaps (SIEP and DIEP) are more and more in use and there is not doubt this method has a future. However, statistical analysis of techniques applied for breast reconstruction does not reflect this recommendation.

In reality approximately 70 to 80 % of all post mastectomy status patients reconstruction is performed with the use of silicone implants with/without expanders. So far, no qualitative deficiencies have been noted with the use of third generation silicone prostheses.

More recently, breast conservation therapy is showing convincing data regarding overall survival. However, if risk factors exist, such as:

- highly malignant tumor
- age >40
- large tumor and little breast volume
- multicentric tumor growth
- R1 resection

then a skin-sparing mastectomy should be performed.

Breast reconstruction may be performed immediately (primary) or later (secondary) = delayed.

1) Primary Reconstruction With Implants

After Patey mastectomy immediately reconstruction: Beginning at the lateral border of the pectoralis muscle meticulous dissection of a subpectoral pocket is performed. Cranial dissection proceeds easily, however, inferiorly and medially the muscle is very thin and reaches the fifth rib.

To achieve a good breast shape it is essential to create an implant pocket reaching the 6th to 7th rib, which requires mobilization of the abdominis oblique, serratus anterior, and fascia of the rectus abdominis muscles. Dissection is challenging and requires technical finesse. If the inferior portion of the implant is placed subcutaneously a correct position has to be claimed. Very often caudal and medial part of pectoralis muscle should be dissected to achieve a good shape. Subcutaneously position of implant in caudal part should be see as normal.

Once the pocket is dissected either an implant (a) or an expander (b) may be placed therein.

a) Since silicone and breast tissue have different specific weights, implant size depends on breast volume and not on the specimen weight following mastectomy.
If the patient has hypertrophic breasts a smaller implant is inserted and reduction of the contralateral breast performed either immediately or at a later stage. However, if a reduction is performed, attention should be paid to remove glandular tissue located centrally and retromammilary, thus, lowering the risk for breast cancer of contralateral breast.
b) The expander is gradually filled and finally replaced by an implant approximately two to three months following initial expander placement. This can be done with a Becker prosthesis.

2) Delayed Reconstruction

In the majority of cases secondary breast reconstruction is performed. Using the lateral aspect of the existing scar following mastectomy a subpectoral pocket is created. Technically dissection is much easier, because in contrast to primary reconstruction, the muscles have already adhered to the subcutaneous tissues.

Similarly, either an implant can be placed immediately or at a later date following pre-treatment with an expander.

3) Primary and Secondary Reconstruction With TRAM Flaps

A de-epithelialized TRAM flap may be used for volume substitution if sufficient amount of skin is existent. However, skin in addition to volume is frequently required in secondary breast reconstruction.

4) Reconstruction With a Latissimus Flap

If skin is deficient, a latissimus island flap is used for reconstruction with additional placement of a silicone implant. Similarly, a deepithelialized flap may be used merely as a volume substitute in cases where sufficient skin in mastectomy area remains.

Lymph Node Involvement

Table 4.4 pN – regional lymph nodes [TNM classification (UICC)]

PNx	Regional lymph nodes cannot be assessed	
pN0	No regional lymph node metastasis	
pN1	Metastasis to movable ipsilateral axillary lymph node(s)	
	pN1a	Only micrometastasis (none >0.2 cm)
	pN1b	Metastasis to lymph node(s), any larger than 0.2 cm
	I	Metastasis in 1–3 lymph nodes, any larger than 0.2 cm and all smaller than 2 cm in greatest dimension
	II	Metastasis to 4 or more lymph nodes, any larger than 0.2 cm and all smaller than 2 cm in greatest dimension
	III	Extension of tumor beyond the capsule of a lymph node metastasis, smaller than 2 cm in greatest dimension
	IV	Metastasis to a lymph node 2 cm or larger in greatest dimension
pN2	Metastasis to ipsilateral axillary lymph node(s) fixed to each other or to other structures	
pN3	Metastasis to ipsilateral internal mammary lymph node(s)	

For practical surgical reasons Berg (1955) classified the axillary lymph node into three levels:

Level I Lymph nodes lateral and caudal to the pectoralis minor muscle

Level II Lymph nodes behind the pectoralis minor muscle

Level III Lymph nodes medial and cranial to the pectoralis minor muscle

Scintigraphy of the Lymphatic System

This study is based on the assumption that a tumor primarily metastasizes into the **sentinel lymph node** (SLN). Thus, following injection of a radioactive isotope (^{191m}Tc) the SLN can be visualized and subsequently excised.

In malignant melanomas the SLN is usually the first lymph node involved. However, in breast carcinoma, the SLN is occasionally skipped. Nevertheless, this technique will play a major future role in diagnostics and performance of ALND in breast cancer.

Distant Metastasis (Hematogenic)

Table 4.5 pM – Distant metastasis

pMx	Presence of distant metastasis cannot be assessed
pM0	No distant metastasis
pM1	Distant metastasis present
Optionally, one may further classify:	
pM1a	Metastasis involving only the supraclavicular lymph nodes
pM1b	All others

Table 4.6 Hematogenic metastasis – Distribution

Lungs	63 %
Bone	58 %
Liver	51 %
Pleura	44 %
Skin	20 %
Peritoneum	17 %
Ovaries	13 %
Kidneys	13 %

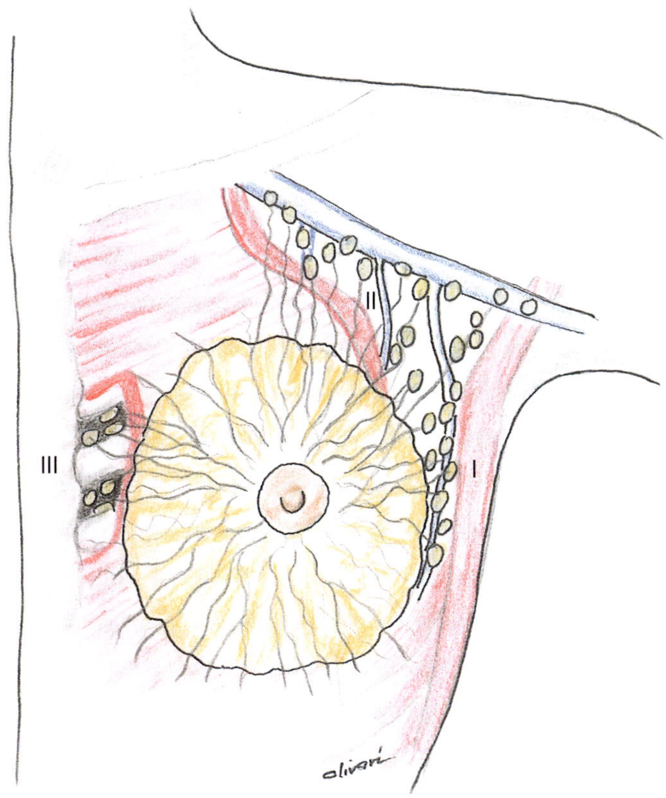

Figure 4.1 Lymphatic drainage of the breast (Level I–III)

Prognosis

Overall prognosis (simplified):
T1, N0, M0, G1, ER-positive = favourable prognosis
T4, N3, M1, G3, ER-negative = poor prognosis
Naturally a myriad of variants exist in-between.

Table 4.7 "Classic" and new prognostic factors with established and questionable clinical relevance

Classic prognostic indicators	New prognostic indicators
TNM-status Tumor size Axillary lymph node involvement Distant metastasis	**Tumor cell detection in bone marrow** **Proliferation and DNA-ploidy** Thymidine-Labelling-Index (TLI) S-Phase-Fraction (SPF) DNA-ploidy Ki-67 (MIBI), PCNA
Morphology Grading (GI-GIII) Histological type Vascular invasion Lymphangiosis carcinomatosa	**EGF-receptor (EGF-R; c-erbB1)** **c-erbB2 (HER-2/neu)-oncogene** P-185 oncogene product Other oncogenes/growth factors: c-erbB3, c-myc, TGF-alpha, TGF-beta, p53, Rb-gene product
Hormone receptors ER PR	
Age at menopause	

Epidemiology

The estimated lifetime probability of developing breast cancer is 9 % in females. 40,000 females are affected annually in Germany. Thus, breast cancer is the most frequent malignant tumor in females.

85 % of breast carcinoma cases occur in patients over the age of 45 years. Here, hormonal interactions play a major role. Female relatives, in particular first-degree relatives, have a threefold increased risk of developing breast cancer.

White females are affected five times more often than Asians. However, the risk of Asian women living in Europe or the United States of America adapts to the incidence of breast cancer observed in European or North American individuals.

A threefold increased risk is displayed for white females when compared to Africans. Furthermore, nullipara are affected three times more often than multipara. Also, women suffering from fibrocystic disease of the breast display an increased risk of suffering from breast cancer.

Precancerous breast lesions, such as ductal or lobular epithelial atypical hyperplasia with apocrine metaplasia increase the relative risk by five times.

Genetics in Breast Cancer (Epidemiology and Molecular Basics)

In the majority of cases breast cancer occurs sporadically, rather than emerging due to a genetic/familial predisposition. A genetic predisposition is observed only in approximately 5 to 10 % of all cases. Four genes play a significant role in this context:

BRCA-1, BRCA-2, p53, and AT which presumably is responsible for Ataxia telangiectasia. These genes belong to the tumor suppressor gene family, which are responsible for cellular protection against malignant transformation. A prerequisite for the development of a malignancy is complete functional loss of a tumor suppressor gene which is represented by two alleles per cell. If a mutated allele is passed on in the gene line spontaneous mutation of the second allele leads to an abolishment of tumor suppression, thus, resulting in malignant cellular transformation. The mutation of the second allele is detectable by loss of heterozygosity testing.

The different tumor suppressor genes are responsible for different manifestations of familial breast cancer. Patients who carry mutations of the BRCA-1 gene have a 50 % risk of suffering from breast cancer up to the age of 50 (approximately 85 % are affected up to the age of 75). Furthermore, the risk for ovarian carcinoma is also significantly higher in this patient subset (approximately 50 % up to the age of 75) [Holinski-Feder, Nestle-Krämling, Untch 1996].

Surgical Treatment

Surgical treatment depends on factors listed above; e.g. indication for breast conservation. Treatment is difficult in a patient with small breasts and a G3 (aggressive) tumor. Also, infiltration of adjacent structures has to be considered together with many other factors.

Thus, prior to performing surgery, several questions need to be answered by;

a) Mammography: Tumor size? Hints as to tumor type? Multicentric growth pattern?
b) Needle biopsy: Tumor group, histology, grading
c) Ultrasound of the breast and axilla: Lymph node enlargement
d) Thorough clinical exam: Liver and thorax (CT or MR

The following operative techniques are available:

1) Lumpectomy, quadrantectomy, sentinel lymph node diagnostic, event. lymph node dissection (level I), plus radiation therapy if lymph nodes are affected or in high risk situations chemotherapy
2) Subcutaneous mastectomy, sentinel lymph node diagnostic, event. lymph node dissection (level I), radiation therapy if lymph nodes are affected or in high risk situations chemotherapy
3) Patey mastectomy with lymph node dissection, usually without radiation therapy, chemotherapy.

Hormone or chemotherapy has to be assessed and administered by an oncologist.

Essential in all surgical procedures is complete tumor resection (R0).

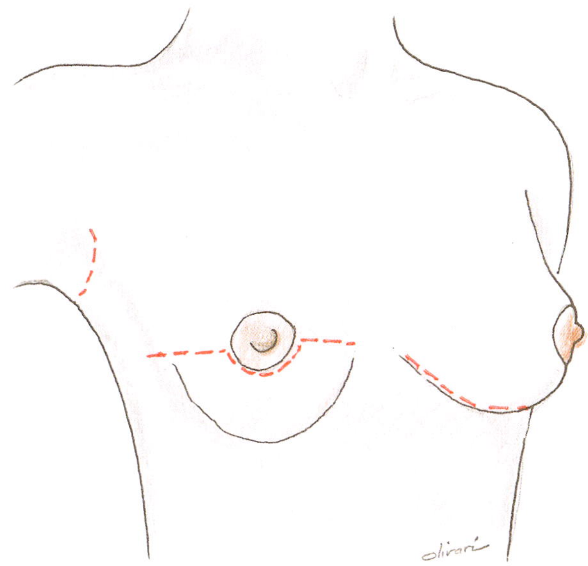

Figure 4.2 Incisions for subcutaneous mastectomy: 1. Transverse incision with inferior arch along the areola, 2. Incision in the inframammary fold (IMF; indicated for small breasts), 3. For large breasts incisions may be placed analogous to those incision used for a breast reduction.

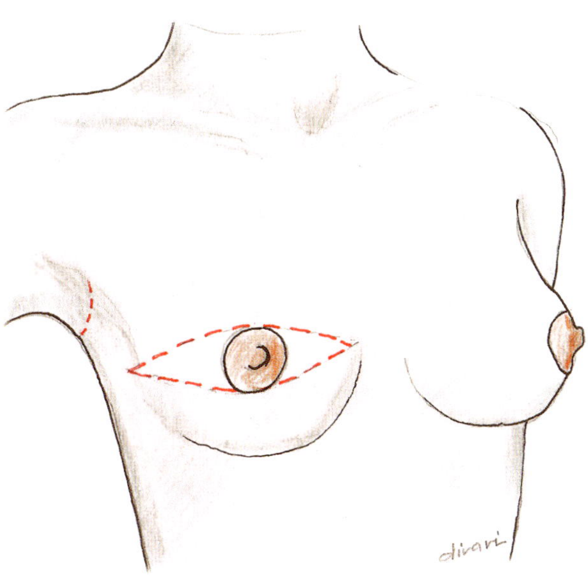

Figure 4.3 Patey incision. Lymph node dissection can be performed through the same or a separately placed incision in the axilla, respectively.

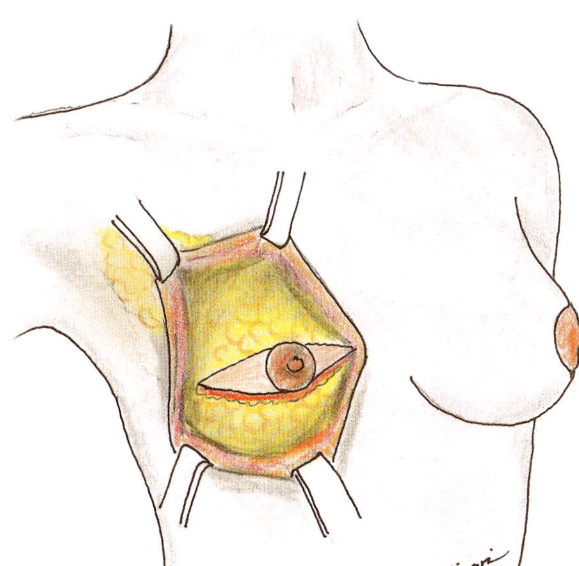

Figure 4.4 **Note** the limited amount of skin resection when performing a modified radical (Patey) mastectomy, thus, facilitating ensuing breast reconstruction. There is no reason to excise the pectoral fascia unless it is infiltrated by tumor.

Breast Reconstruction

According to recent literature the TRAM and latissimus dorsi flap are the methods of choice for breast reconstruction. Other flaps (SIEP and DIEP) are more and more in use and there is not doubt this method has a future. However, statistical analysis of techniques applied for breast reconstruction does not reflect this recommendation.

In reality approximately 70 to 80 % of all post mastectomy status patients reconstruction is performed with the use of silicone implants with/without expanders. So far, no qualitative deficiencies have been noted with the use of third generation silicone prostheses.

More recently, breast conservation therapy is showing convincing data regarding overall survival. However, if risk factors exist, such as:

- highly malignant tumor
- age >40
- large tumor and little breast volume
- multicentric tumor growth
- R1 resection

then a skin-sparing mastectomy should be performed.

Breast reconstruction may be performed immediately (primary) or later (secondary) = delayed.

1) Primary Reconstruction With Implants

After Patey mastectomy immediately reconstruction: Beginning at the lateral border of the pectoralis muscle meticulous dissection of a subpectoral pocket is performed. Cranial dissection proceeds easily, however, inferiorly and medially the muscle is very thin and reaches the fifth rib.

To achieve a good breast shape it is essential to create an implant pocket reaching the 6th to 7th rib, which requires mobilization of the abdominis oblique, serratus anterior, and fascia of the rectus abdominis muscles. Dissection is challenging and requires technical finesse. If the inferior portion of the implant is placed subcutaneously a correct position has to be claimed. Very often caudal and medial part of pectoralis muscle should be dissected to achieve a good shape. Subcutaneously position of implant in caudal part should be see as normal.

Once the pocket is dissected either an implant (a) or an expander (b) may be placed therein.

a) Since silicone and breast tissue have different specific weights, implant size depends on breast volume and not on the specimen weight following mastectomy.
   If the patient has hypertrophic breasts a smaller implant is inserted and reduction of the contralateral breast performed either immediately or at a later stage. However, if a reduction is performed, attention should be paid to remove glandular tissue located centrally and retromammilary, thus, lowering the risk for breast cancer of contralateral breast.
b) The expander is gradually filled and finally replaced by an implant approximately two to three months following initial expander placement. This can be done with a Becker prosthesis.

2) Delayed Reconstruction

In the majority of cases secondary breast reconstruction is performed. Using the lateral aspect of the existing scar following mastectomy a subpectoral pocket is created. Technically dissection is much easier, because in contrast to primary reconstruction, the muscles have already adhered to the subcutaneous tissues.

Similarly, either an implant can be placed immediately or at a later date following pre-treatment with an expander.

3) Primary and Secondary Reconstruction With TRAM Flaps

A de-epithelialized TRAM flap may be used for volume substitution if sufficient amount of skin is existent. However, skin in addition to volume is frequently required in secondary breast reconstruction.

4) Reconstruction With a Latissimus Flap

If skin is deficient, a latissimus island flap is used for reconstruction with additional placement of a silicone implant. Similarly, a deepithelialized flap may be used merely as a volume substitute in cases where sufficient skin in mastectomy area remains.

Conclusion: Primary reconstruction is technically more demanding, however, representing a tremendous benefit for the patient. In primary reconstruction, patients do not have to go through the period of mutilation.

The author favours not only primary breast reconstruction, furthermore, he advocates immediate contralateral breast reduction if indicated. However, the surgeon needs to be sure of achieving a good result.

Lesser experienced surgeons are advised to perform a delayed reconstruction.

Indications for the use of TRAM or latissimus dorsi flaps in breast reconstruction include: thin skin cover, skin deficiency, radiation-induced damage, and removal of pectoralis muscles.

On the Safety of Silicone Implants

Recently, the issue of silicone implant safety has been discussed extensively. Thus, this section is devoted to this topic and focusing on complications caused by their use. Verified complications caused by silicone implants include mainly local symptoms, such as the development of capsular contracture. Furthermore, silicone "bleeding" is a well-described phenomenon. Implants inserted in the 1970s were particularly affected due to their thin shell. Spontaneous gel particle discharge as well as silicone shell breakup was frequently encountered. A dissemination of silicone gel is, however, prevented by the existence of the connective tissue capsule encasing the implant. Exit of silicone into the surrounding tissues with subsequent siliconoma formation is only encountered following direct trauma.

Systemic side effects, such as emergence of rheumatic disorders, are not caused by silicone implants. In multiple, large, retrospective studies, such as the Nurses' Health Study Cohort (including 87501 nurses with a follow-up period of 14 years) no correlation was observed as to the development of autoimmune diseases following exposure to silicone implants.

According to published studies on the safety of silicone implants, the following can be stated:

1) Silicone implants do not cause cancer.
2) Theoretically, silicone implants may delay the diagnosis of breast cancer. However, recent data does not support this statement. A combination of thorough clinical exam with mammography (correctly conducted) and sonography prevents a diagnostic delay. In unclear cases, MRI may bring about clarification.
3) No evidence on the development of autoimmune and rheumatic disorders caused by silicone implants exists.
4) Case reports of the improvement of systemic symptoms following implant removal cannot be considered as evidence for causation (placebo effect).
5) Laboratory tests cannot detect silicone discharge, immune reaction, or toxicity.
6) A correlation of implants to other diseases cannot be proven by laboratory testing.
7) Potential teratogenic or mutagenic properties of silicone have not been shown.
8) The existence of silicone in breast milk has not been demonstrated in patients with implants. However, silicone particles have been proven to exist in cow's milk (from coatings of transmission pipelines) and in bottle milk (from teats).
9) A diffuse spread of silicone is possible if implants are damaged. Particles are subsequently evacuated by lymphatic drainage and thereby the gel can induce a foreign body reaction.

In conclusion, when considering the pros and cons of silicone gel implants, this option can be offered to women who desire breast reconstruction [Gabka 1996].

In the future, breast reconstruction with TRAM, latissimus or other muscle flaps cannot be offered to every patient, not only due to financial reasons but also from the patient's physical build. Furthermore, reconstruction with implants is straightforward with less patient morbidity compared to complex flap transfers.

Secondary Breast Reconstruction With Implants

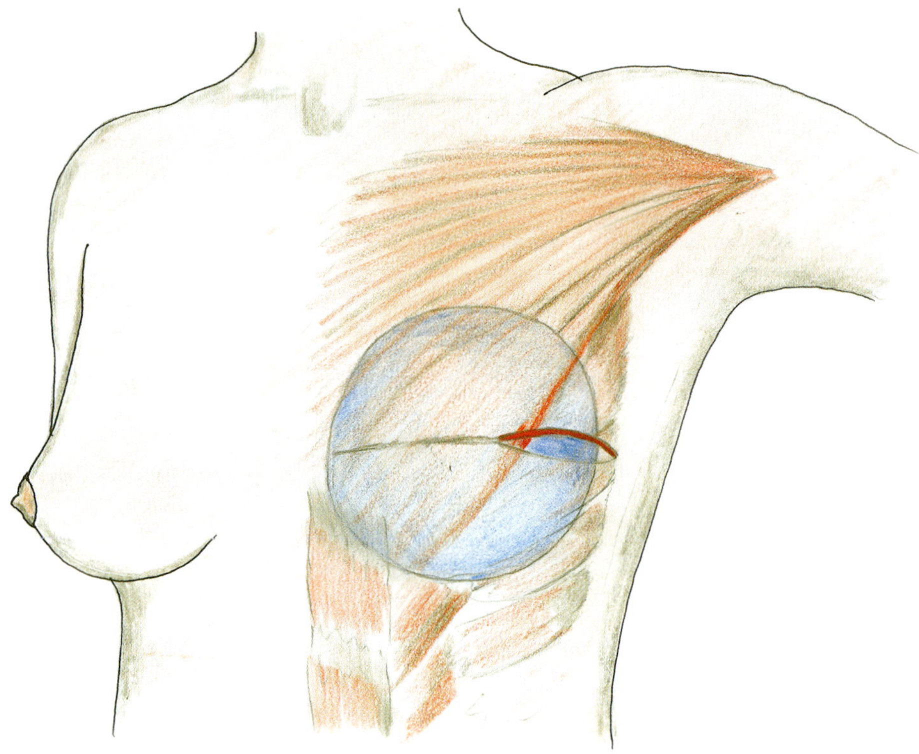

Figure 4.5a Placement of silicone implants for breast reconstruction following mastectomy. The horizontal scar is only excised laterally. Subsequently, a submuscular pocket is created for implant placement. The implant is covered by the pectoralis major muscle craniomedially and by the serratus anterior muscle, sometimes the external oblique muscle, and the rectus fascia caudally and laterally. Often pectoralis major muscle should be dissected in medio-caudal part. If caudal part of inlay is covered only by skin and subcutaneous tissue – this is normal situation. The implant should be positioned slightly inferior to the contralateral breast as it often shifts cranially postoperatively. Wearing a customized brassiere for up to six weeks postoperatively is mandatory for prevention of this phenomenona.

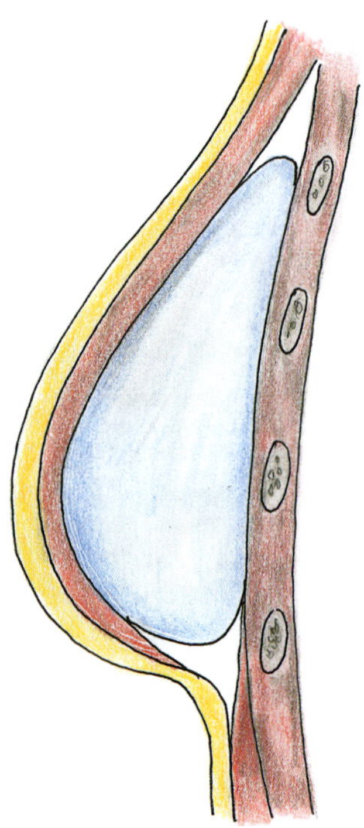

Figure 4.5b Submuscular placement of silicone implants. For technical reasons the lower part of implant mostly cannot be covered entirely by muscle. However, this does not represent a significant disadvantage as the subcutaneous tissue in this area is usually of sufficient thickness to provide for adequate coverage.

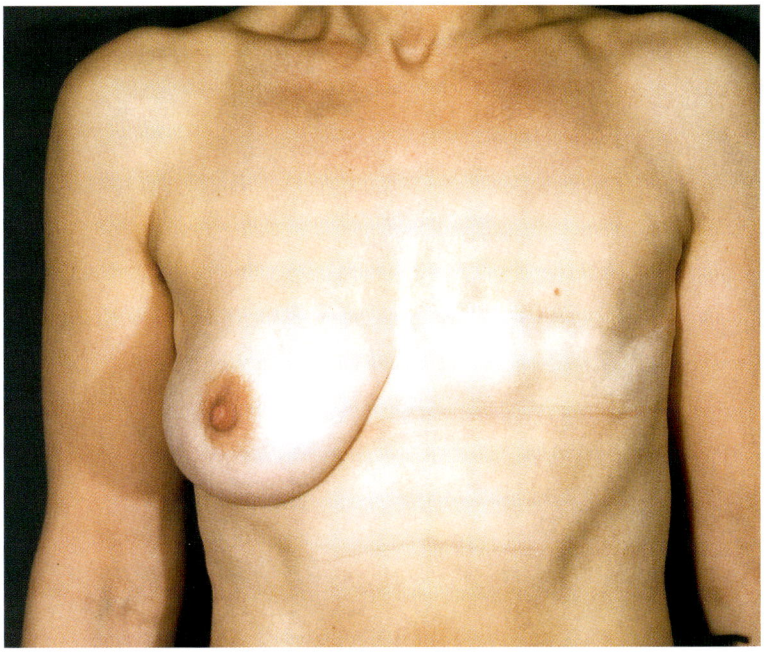

Figure 4.6a Situation after Patey mastectomy three years ago.
Operative plan: Left: Subpectoral augmentation with silicon inlay and NAC reconstruction.
Right: Mastopexy.

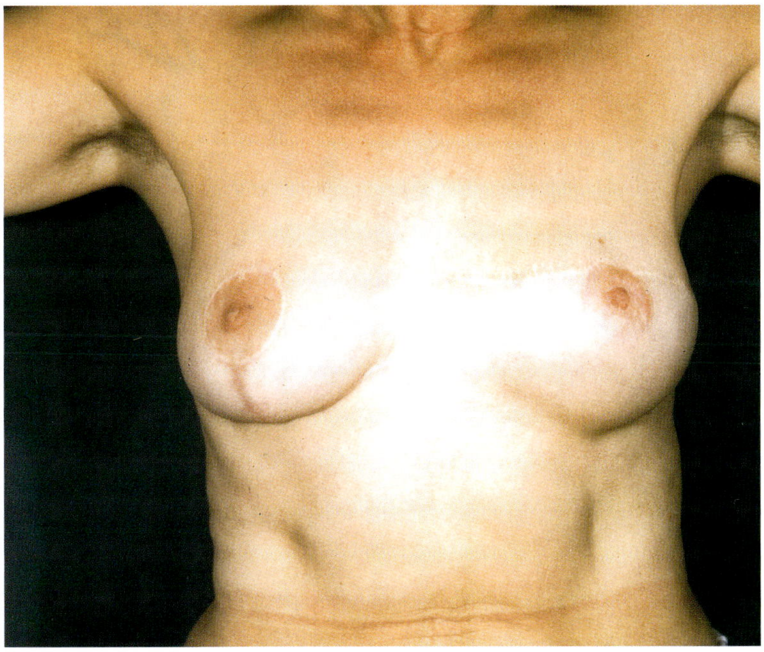

Figure 4.6b Two years postoperatively:
A 280 ccm implant was placed subpectorally via the lateral part of mastectomy scar, the areola tattooed and the nipple reconstructed using tissue from the contralateral nipple.

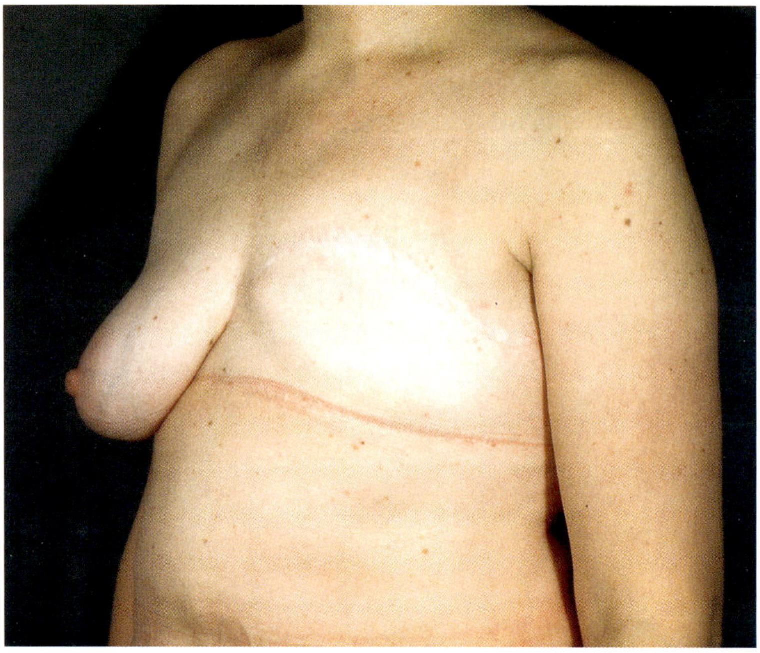

Figure 4.7a Status post left-sided mastectomy four years ago.
Operative plan: Left: Augmentation with a 290 ccm implant and NAC reconstruction.
Right: Limited breast reduction.

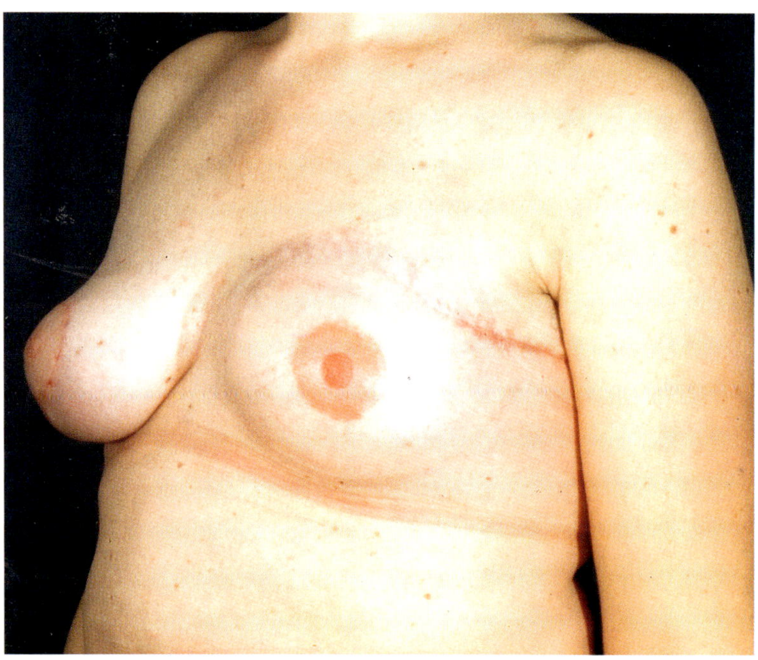

Figure 4.7b Three months postoperatively:
Left: Reconstruction was achieved using a 290 ccm implant for volume replacement. Again, only the lateral aspect of the old mastectomy scar was used for implant placement. NAC reconstruction was accomplished by a combination of nipple-sharing from contralateral side and tattooing of areola.
Right: A total of 180 g were reduced.
(Modified Strömbeck technique)

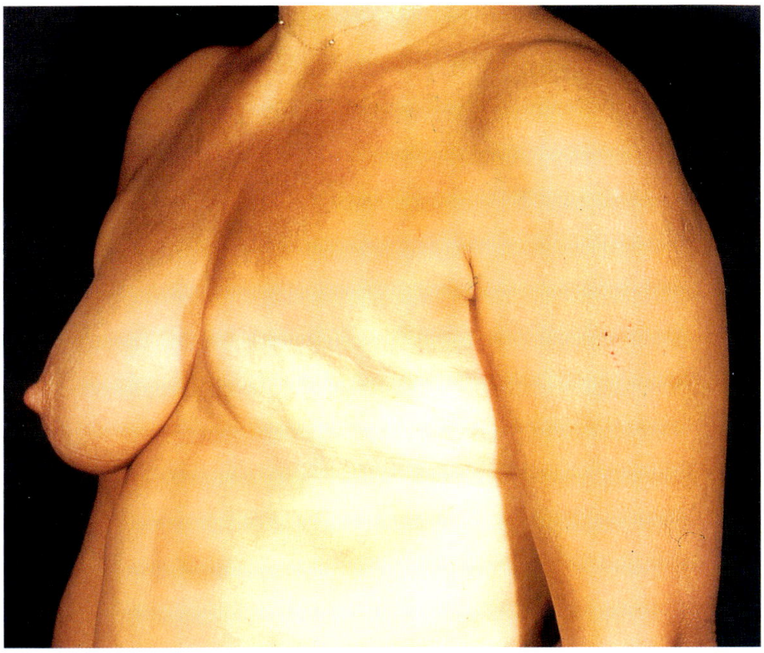

Figure 4.8a Status post left-sided mastectomy four years ago. Good skin quality, which was preserved in sufficient amount by primary surgeon. Treatment: Submuscular placement of a 370 ccm silicone implant.

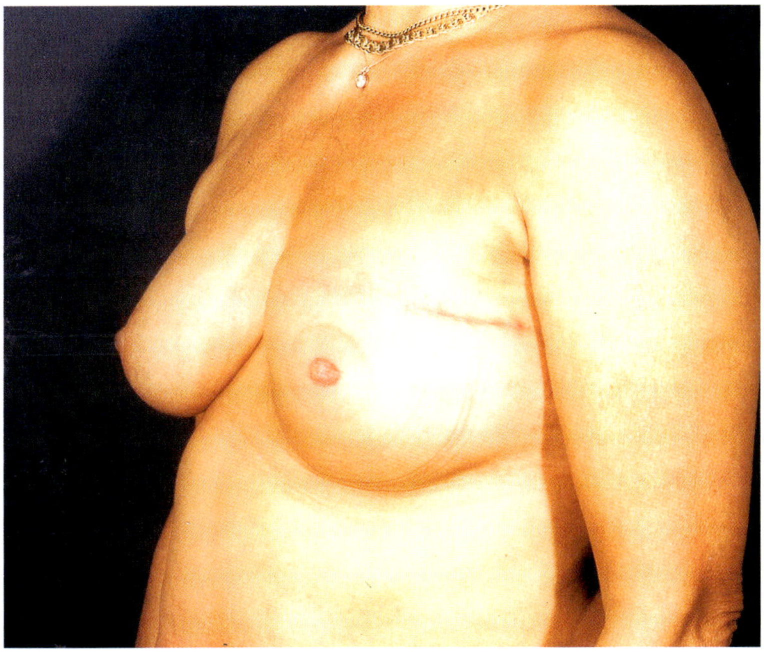

Figure 4.8b Nine months postoperatively: NAC reconstruction was accomplished using a combination of nipple-sharing and tattooing. Sometimes, after six to twelve months tattooing become pale. Redoing of tattoo in local anesthesia is indicated.

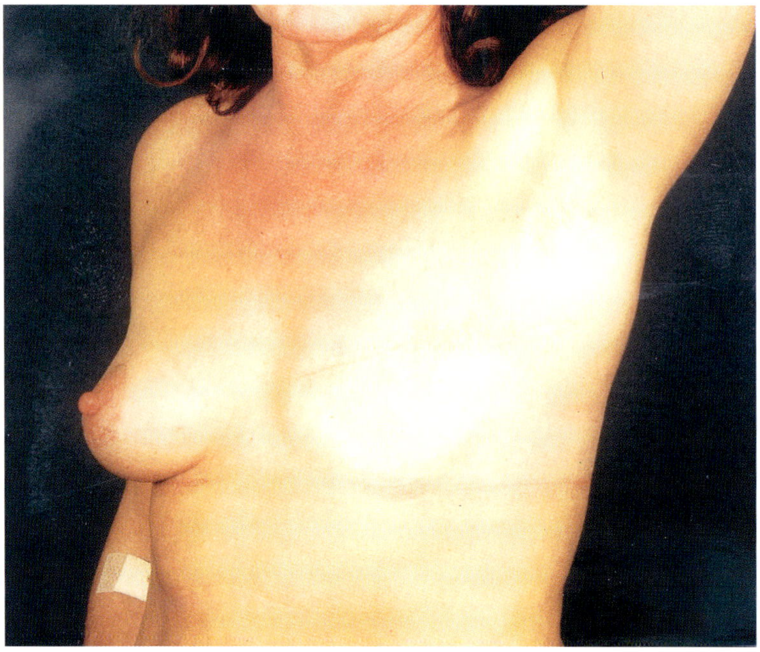

Figure 4.9a Situation after left mastectomy. Good skin quality and adequate amount of soft tissue: Submuscular placement of a silicone prosthesis (270 ccm) through the lateral aspect of the mastectomy scar.

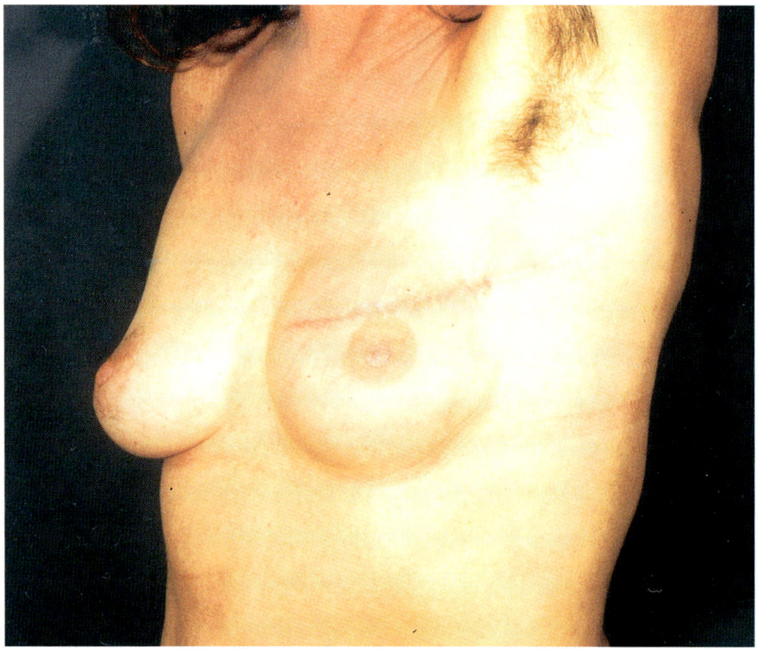

Figure 4.9b Eight months postoperatively: Tattooing of the areola was conducted and the nipple was reconstructed utilizing tissue from the contralateral breast. Tattoo of areola may fade (sometimes) so retattooing can be easily done with local anesthesia.

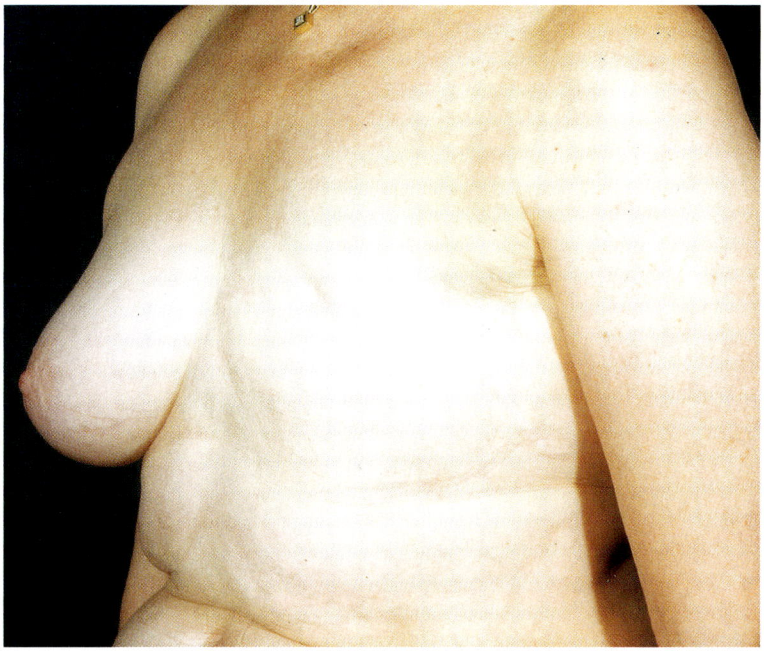

Figure 4.10a Status post left-sided mastectomy six years ago. Treatment: Submuscular placement of a silicone implant (320 ccm).

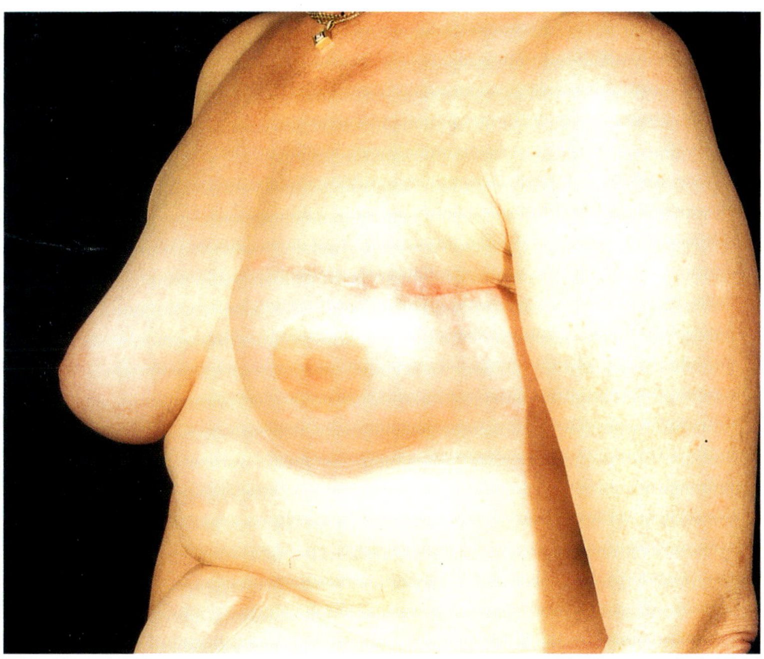

Figure 4.10b Six months postoperatively: The implant has been placed too high, thus, requiring revision. The areola was tattooed and the nipple reconstructed by nipple-sharing.

Breast Conservation Therapy

Conservative Surgery for Small Tumors

Breast conservation surgery, such as segmental mastectomy, lumpectomy, or quadrantectomy with concomitant ALND (level I and II) has become standard care for small breast carcinomas.

30 to 50 % of all breast cancers are treated in this manner and with an increasing frequency.

Indications

Indications for a conservative surgical approach are:

1) Solitary tumor with diameter of 2 cm at most.
2) Safety margin of at least 2 cm. Veronesi described higher rates of recurrence with safety margins of 1 cm.
3) Breast shape needs to be preserved, thus patients with larger breasts are more favoured.
4) The rate of local recurrence must not be higher than following a Patey mastectomy.
5) Postoperative radiotherapy is mandatory.

A higher risk of R1 resections exists with larger tumors (>2 cm). The larger the tumor, the higher the risk (Fisher) that not only is tumor excision incomplete but also that lymph nodes are affected.
Within a 10 year period 22 % patients will suffer from local recurrence if tumor excision is not complete. On the contrary, approximately 6 % of patients will display a similar condition following R0 resection.
The rate of recurrence is inversely proportional to the extent of tumor removal (5 years).

- 15.5 % local recurrence following lumpectomy
- 12 % following segmental mastectomy
- 2.8 % following quadrantectomy with subsequent radiotherapy (Kantorowitz)
- 29 % following quadrantectomy without subsequent radiotherapy

Fisher (1985) observed recurrences in 32 % of patients after 5 years following segmental mastectomy without radiotherapy as opposed to a 7 % if patients had radiotherapy.
Therapeutic consequence: A small tumor (<2 cm) needs to be excised with a 2 cm safety margin. Postoperative radiotherapy is mandatory.
In patients refusing radiotherapy, a mastectomy (Patey) with either primary or delayed reconstruction is a better choice.
Surveying and analyzing the literature reveals that the extent of resection along with patient age and intensity of radiotherapy influences the rate of local recurrence. Thus, more radical resection, along with higher patient age and initiation of high-dose radiotherapy, results in lower rates of local recurrence. However, good breast shape and the parameters mentioned above are inversely related.
Still, many patients perceive breast conservation therapy as an enormous benefit, since they retain their natural breast. However, one year is necessary following radiotherapy for the breast to resume its soft consistency. Lifelong actinic sensitivity remains.

Contraindications

Contraindications for performing breast conservation therapy include:

- incomplete tumor resection histologically
- multicentric growth pattern
- recurrence following primary quadrantectomy and radiotherapy
- small breast, in which a quadrantectomy would result in breast mutilation.

In these cases mastectomy with primary or delayed reconstruction is a better choice.

Cosmetic results following breast conservation therapy depend on several factors including:

1) Breast size
   The smaller the breast the more difficult it is to achieve a good result.

2) Quality/intensity of radiation
   A dose of 50 Gy and more can dramatically affect breast shape. The combination of radio- and chemotherapy has an additive negative effect on breast shape.

Prophylactic chemotherapy is clearly indicated when facing an adequate risk profile since it decreases the risk of recurrence as well as prolongs recurrence-free interval. However, in patients with small tumors (<1 cm), without lymph node involvement, and positive hormone receptor status its administration is limited.

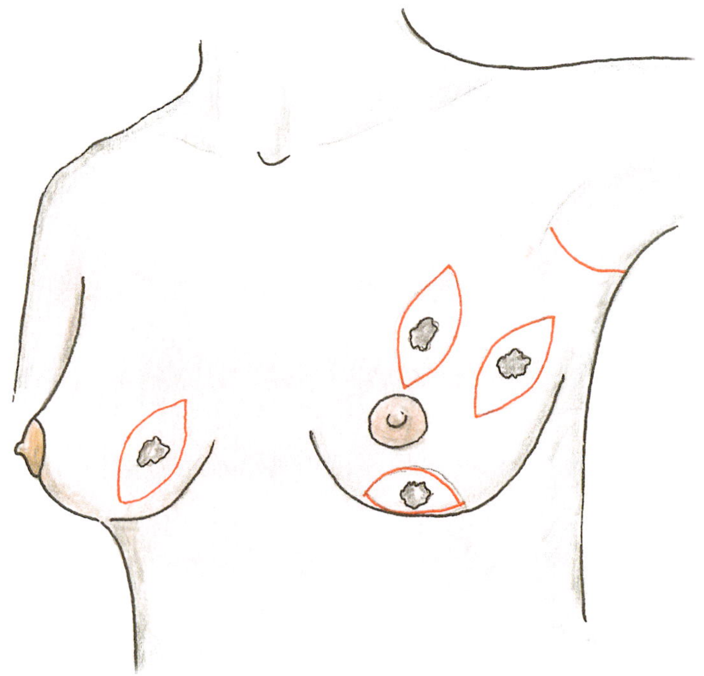

Figure 4.11a Tissue resection in breast conservation therapy of mammary carcinoma has to be performed using a radial approach with a 2 cm safety margin. In the lower quadrants the incision may be placed transversely in the IMF. Broad skin excision is executed only in very superficially located tumors otherwise a narrow strip of skin suffices. For lymphadenectomy a separate incision in axilla is necessary.

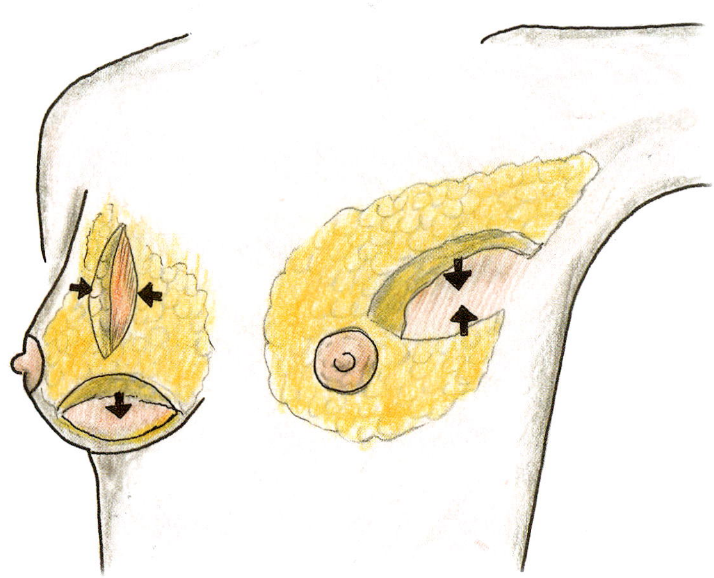

Figure 4.11b The tissue defect is reconstructed through mobilization of adjacent breast gland tissue, which is mobilized off the pectoral fascia. Rarely, small silicone prostheses (60-100 ccm) are necessary for preservation of a natural breast shape, particularly in patients with very small breasts.

Surgical Technique (Conservative Surgery)

Preoperatively, the tumor is stereotactically located by the radiologist. Excision is performed with a 2 cm safety margin.

Often it is assumed that skin has to be excised to a similar extent. However, this is only indicated if the tumor is located near the skin or has already infiltrated it. Usually, it is sufficient to excise a small strip of skin with the specimen.

Axillary LND (10 to 14 lymph nodes; level I) is conducted either through the same or separately placed incision in the axilla.

In general, incisions should be placed radially. Breast tissue defects are subsequently reconstructed by approximation of adjacent tissues which may require dissecting them off the fascia.

If, in a patient with hypertrophic breasts, the tumor is located inferiorly or in the middle portion of the breast, a classic breast reduction with excision of the great part of glandular tissue may be performed. However, it is essential to perform the tumor resection with a wide safety margin. At the same time the contralateral breast may be treated to gain symmetry.

In a small breast, placement of a small implant (60–100 ccm) may be considered in order to prevent a depression.

In cases of extensive defects a TRAM or de-epithelialized latissimus dorsi island flap may be placed for improvement in breast shape.

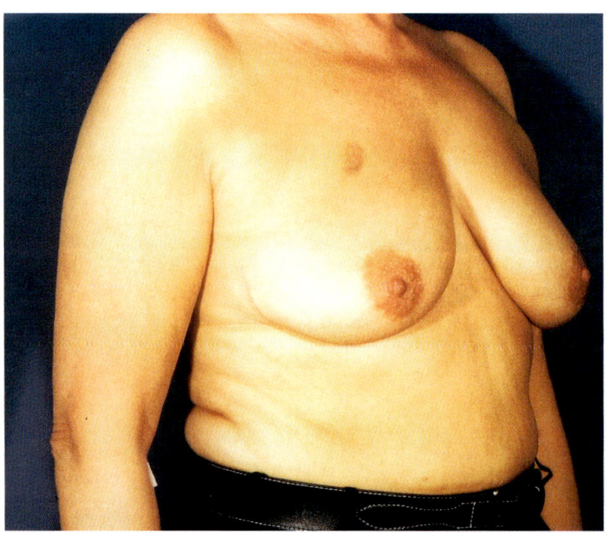

Figure 4.12a The tumor is located in the upper pole of the breast as pictured by the hematoma following needle biopsy. Treatment: Quadrantectomy with mobilization of the remaining breast tissue and subsequent radiation therapy. Unfavorable localization. Lymph node dissection was conducted via a separate incision in the axilla.

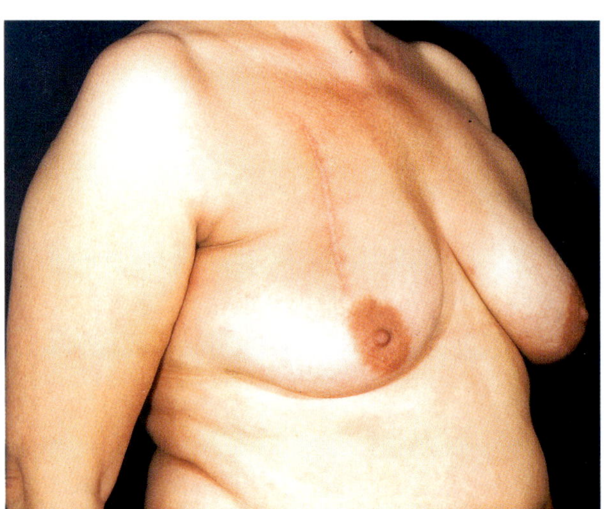

Figure 4.12b Seven years following operative intervention free of recurrence: The localization of the tumor required a disadvantageous scar placement.

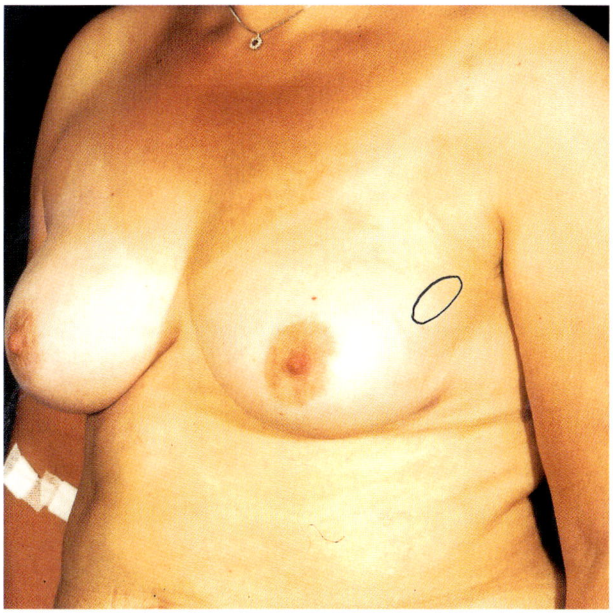

Figure 4.13a Tumor in the left upper outer quadrant (1.8 cm). The tumor is excised with a safety margin of 2,5 to 3 cm. A natural breast contour is preserved by local glandular advancement. Twelve lymph nodes (level I and II) were removed and all were negative for tumor infiltration.

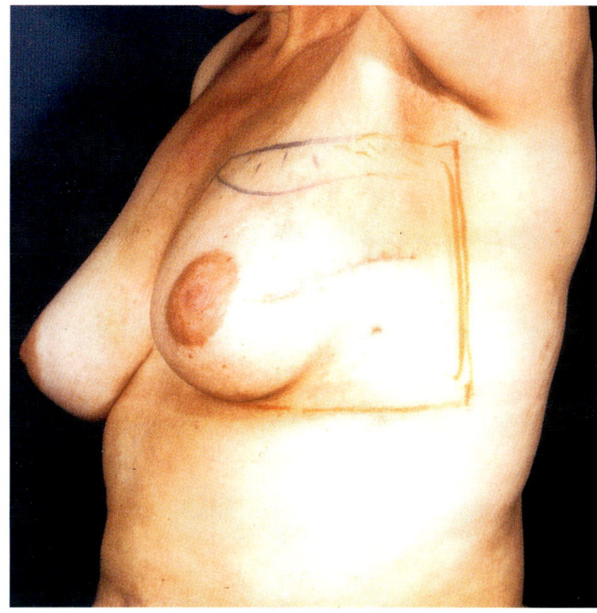

Figure 4.13b Postoperative radiation therapy is conducted over a period of approximately six weeks. During this period the skin is very sensitive and the breast is indurated on palpation.

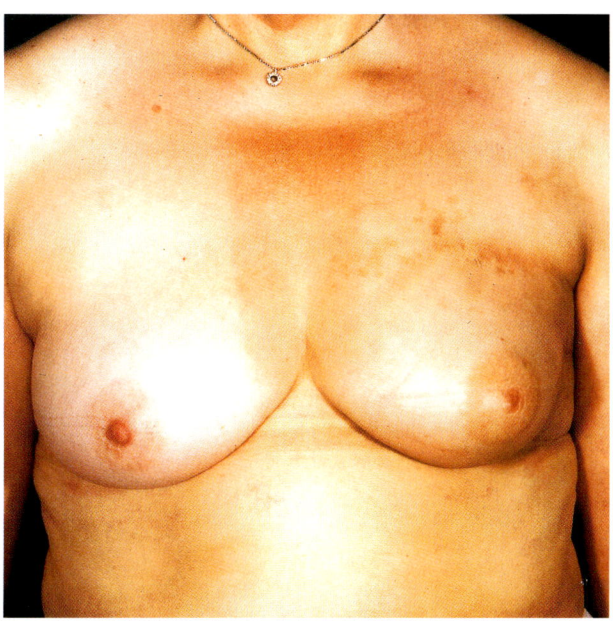

Figure 4.13c Fourteen months following surgery and radiation therapy: A nice breast shape can be observed although a low-grade rigidification of the breast with typical skin findings after irradiation is noted.

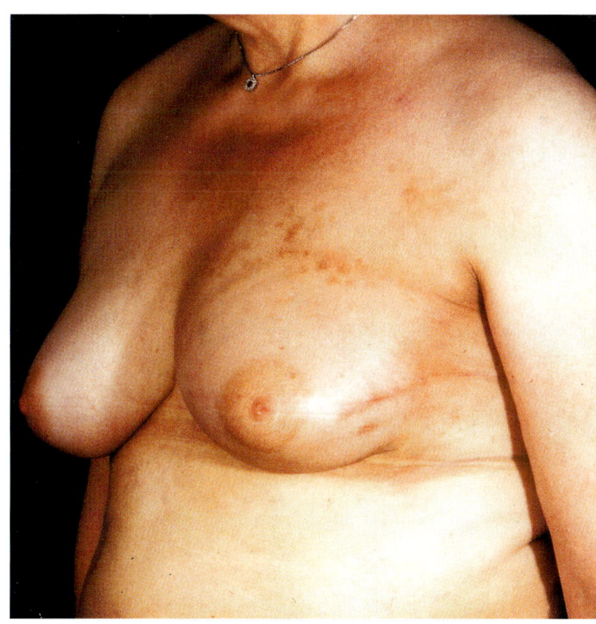

Figure 4.13d Radiated areas demonstrate a higher sensitivity to the sun for years.

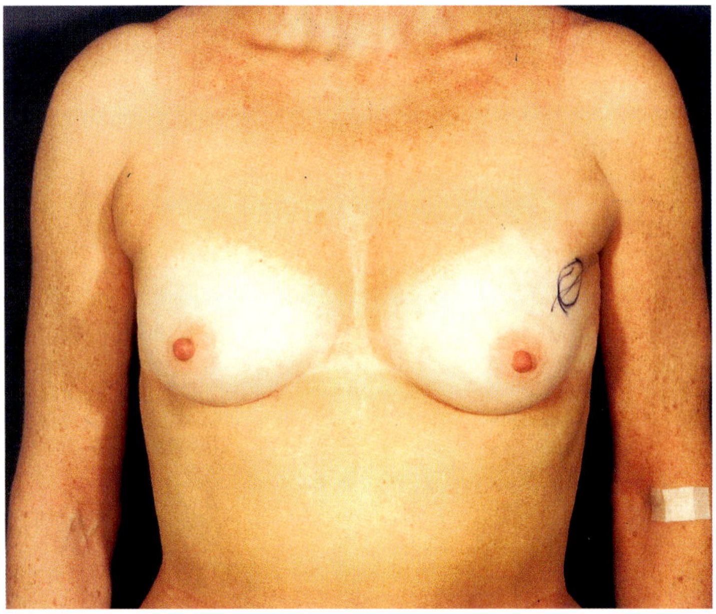

Figure 4.14a Breast carcinoma located in the left upper outer quadrant (diameter: 2 cm). Tumor localization was achieved by stereotactic procedure.

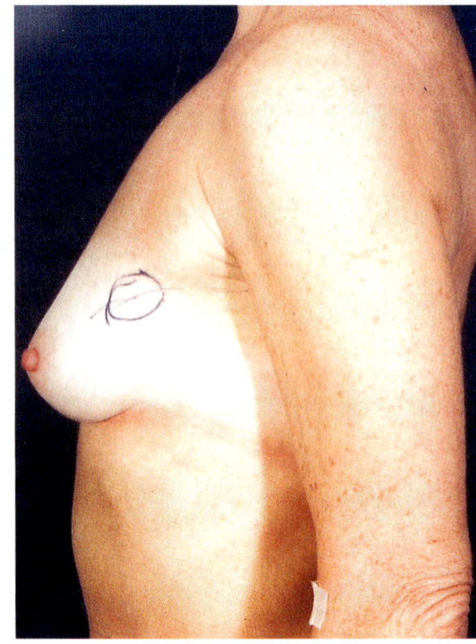

Figure 4.14b Treatment: Tumor excision with a safety margin and reconstruction of the defect by means of glandular mobilization. Postoperatively, radiation therapy was implemented. Ten lymph nodes were removed: Tumor status: pT1 N0 M0.

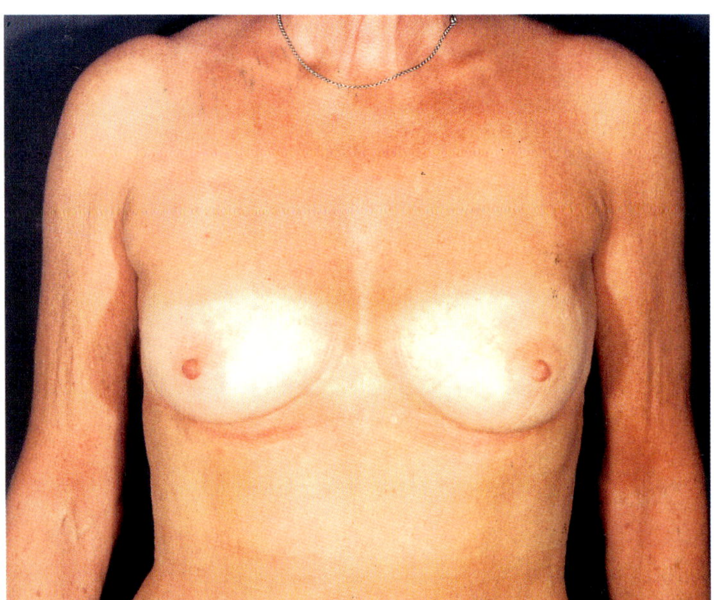

Figure 4.14c Three years postoperatively. The breasts are symmetrical and soft without signs of recurrence.

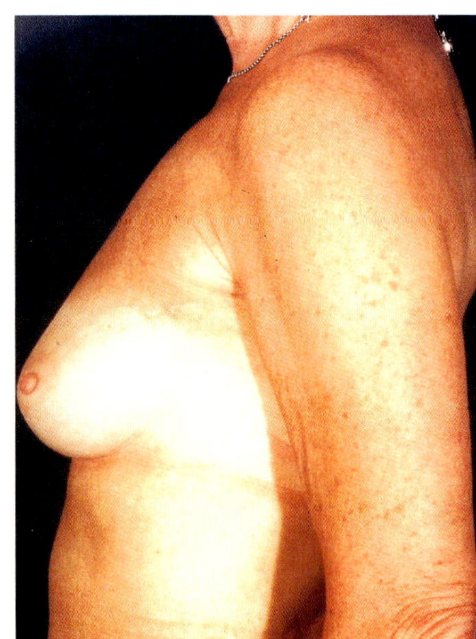

Figure 4.14d Ideal result which hardly can be achieved by other reconstructive methods.

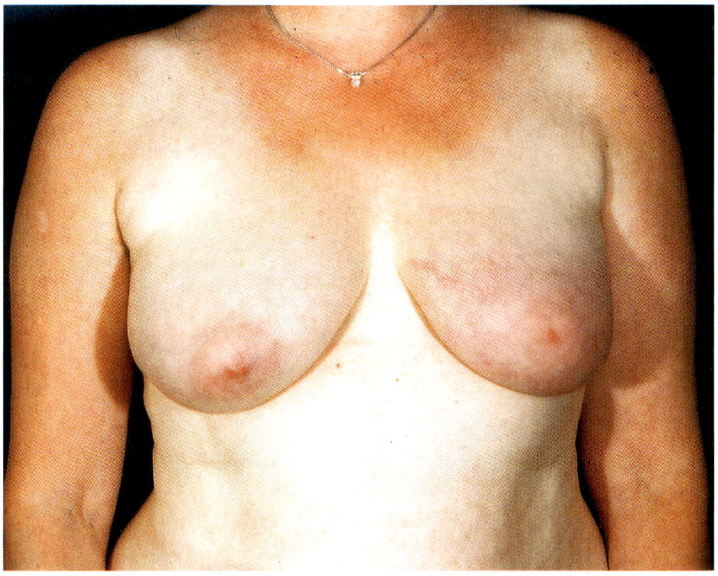

Figure 4.15a Breast cancer (T1 N0 M0) with a tumor size of 2.1 cm is located in the right lower outer quadrant. In this case an inframammary approach is advisable. Tumor was excised with a safety margin of 3 cm. Thirteen lymph nodes were removed by axillary incision.

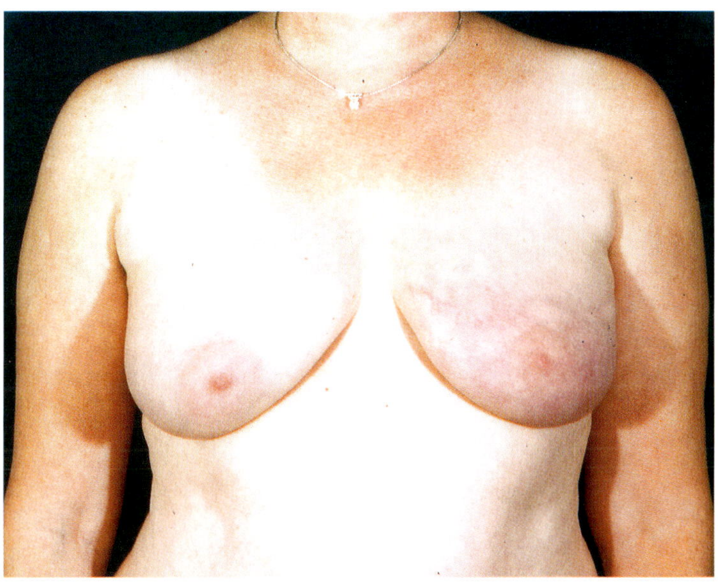

Figure 4.15b Postoperatively: Following excision with subsequent glandular advancement for defect compensation a difference in appearance of the breast can hardly be noted.

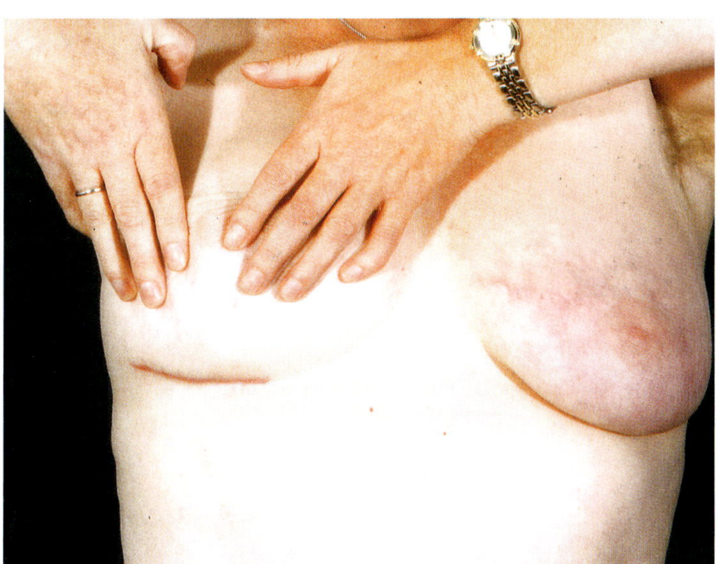

Figure 4.15c Scar located in the IMF

Complications

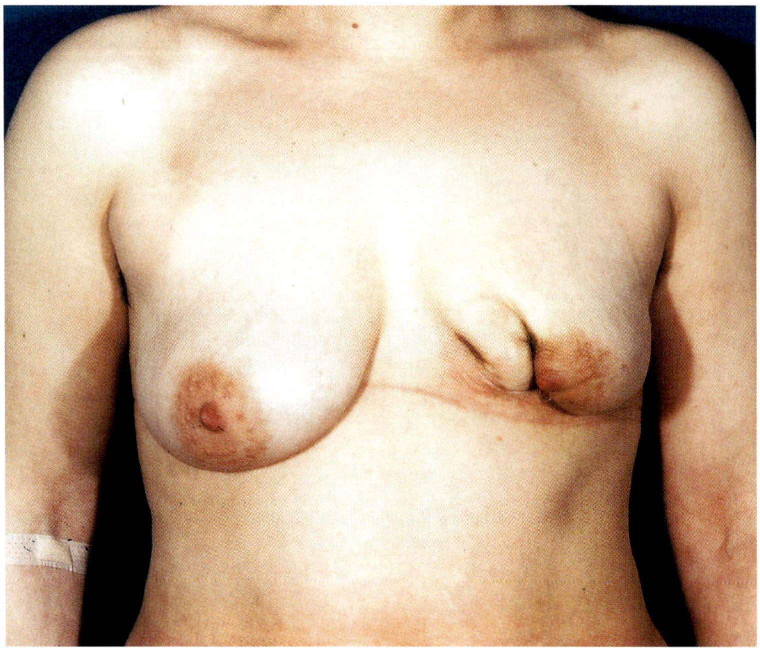

Figure 4.16a While performing breast conservation therapy the primary surgeon excised too much tissue. Subsequent radiation therapy along with a local infection led to this result.

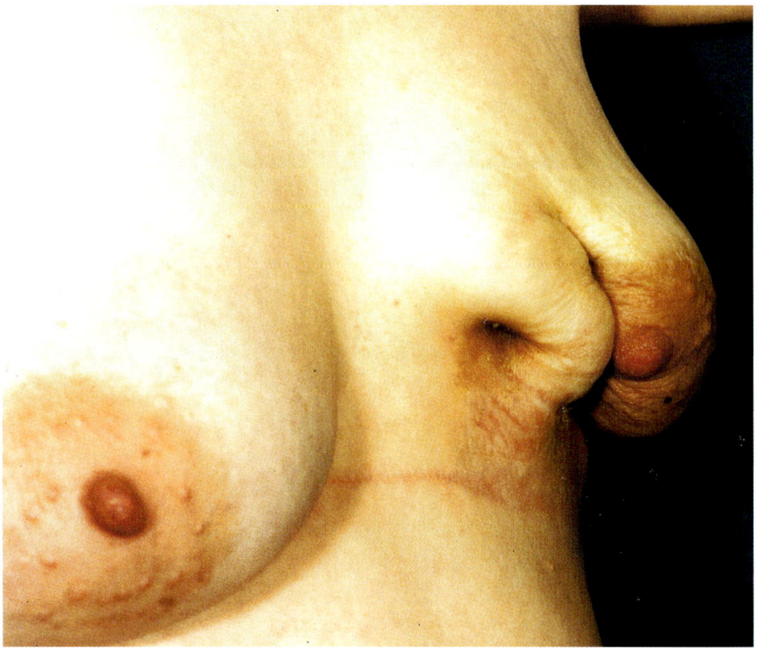

Figure 4.16b Extensive scarring with adherence to the pectoral fascia. Deep pockets exist causing recurrent infections.

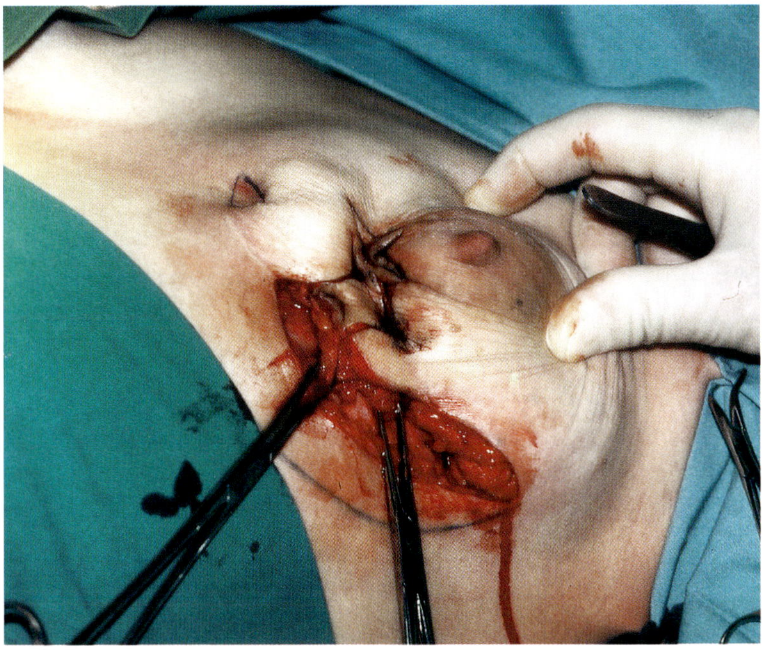

Figure 4.16c Therapy: Lysis of the scars was conducted along with creation of a submuscular pocket for placement of an expander.
Three months later a 290 ccm implant was placed combined with adjustment of contralateral breast.

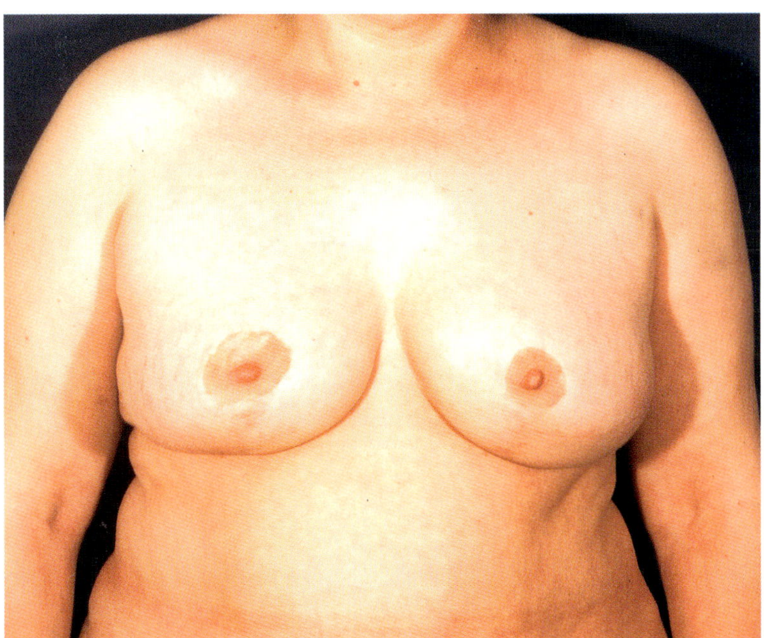

Figure 4.16d Four operations were needed within six months to achieve result. Picture taken seven years postoperatively.

Latissimus Dorsi Flap

History

The myocutaneous latissimus flap is one of the safest and most frequently used flaps in plastic surgery today. Historically, it is a procedure which has been developed and described by two surgeons.

In 1906 Tansini reported on a new method of breast amputation with complete removal of glandular tissues, skin, and muscle with subsequent coverage with a skin flap including the latissimus dorsi muscle. He was already familiar with the axial perfusion pattern of the muscle as well as skin perfusion by means of perforators [Tansini I (1906) Sopra il mio nuovo processo die amputatione della mammela. Riforma medica 12: 757].

However, this method was soon forgotten and the preferred treatment of breast cancer, for many years, was the Rotter-Halsted technique of radical mastectomy, which, due to Halsted's enormous authority, superseded all other techniques. The latissimus flap was not performed for more than 60 years.

From 1970 to 1974 the author was engaged in the treatment of radiation ulcers following mastectomy and radiotherapy at the University Hospital in Cologne, Germany.

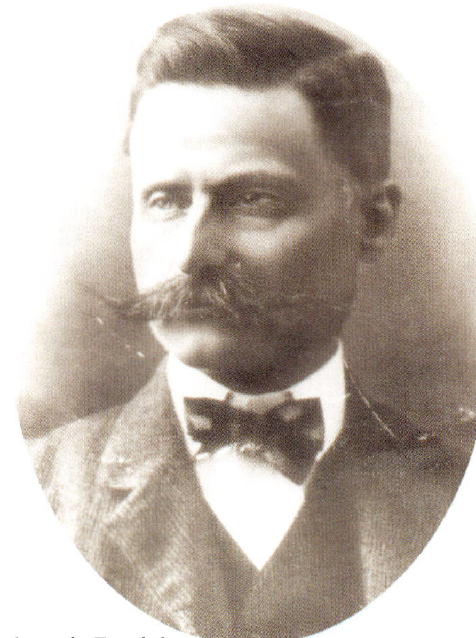

Figure 4.17a Ignazio Tansini

Due to the increased implementation of radiotherapy for the treatment of breast cancer, radiation-induced damaged was encountered much more often. Traditional reconstructive techniques resulted in limited success rate.

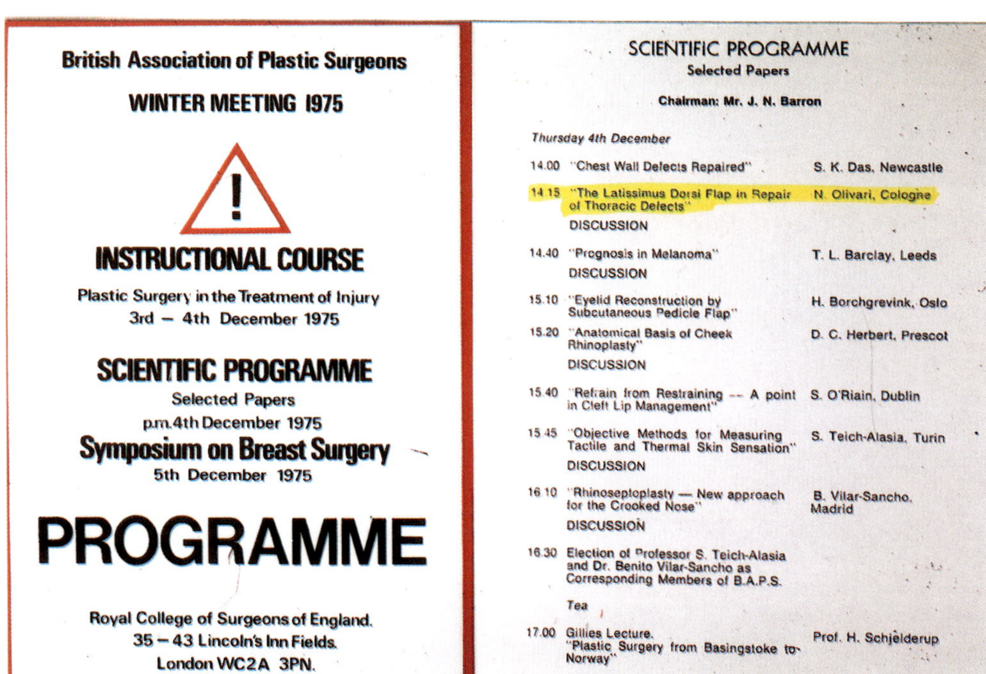

British Association of Plastic Surgeons
WINTER MEETING 1975

INSTRUCTIONAL COURSE
Plastic Surgery in the Treatment of Injury
3rd – 4th December 1975

SCIENTIFIC PROGRAMME
Selected Papers
p.m. 4th December 1975

Symposium on Breast Surgery
5th December 1975

PROGRAMME

Royal College of Surgeons of England.
35 – 43 Lincoln's Inn Fields.
London WC2A 3PN.

SCIENTIFIC PROGRAMME
Selected Papers

Chairman: Mr. J. N. Barron

Thursday 4th December

14.00	"Chest Wall Defects Repaired"	S. K. Das, Newcastle
14.15	"The Latissimus Dorsi Flap in Repair of Thoracic Defects"	N. Olivari, Cologne
	DISCUSSION	
14.40	"Prognosis in Melanoma"	T. L. Barclay, Leeds
	DISCUSSION	
15.10	"Eyelid Reconstruction by Subcutaneous Pedicle Flap"	H. Borchgrevink, Oslo
15.20	"Anatomical Basis of Cheek Rhinoplasty"	D. C. Herbert, Prescot
	DISCUSSION	
15.40	"Refrain from Restraining — A point in Cleft Lip Management"	S. O'Riain, Dublin
15.45	"Objective Methods for Measuring Tactile and Thermal Skin Sensation"	S. Teich-Alasia, Turin
	DISCUSSION	
16.10	"Rhinoseptoplasty — New approach for the Crooked Nose"	B. Vilar-Sancho, Madrid
	DISCUSSION	
16.30	Election of Professor S. Teich-Alasia and Dr. Benito Vilar-Sancho as Corresponding Members of B.A.P.S.	
	Tea	
17.00	Gillies Lecture. "Plastic Surgery from Basingstoke to Norway"	Prof. H. Schjelderup

6

Figure 4.17b Programme of the BAPS Winter Meeting 1975

THE LATISSIMUS FLAP

By NEVEN OLIVARI

Universitätskliniken Köln, Plastische Chirurgie, 5 Köln 41, Robert-Koch-Strasse 10, West Germany

SKIN transposition flaps are the simplest means of covering defects of the anterior chest wall. But when the defects are large and/or the region has been irradiated, the blood supply of the flap may be inadequate and, even after delay operations, necrosis may occur. By incorporating the latissimus dorsi muscle in the flap, however, adequate circulation is assured and no delays are necessary. The increased thickness is also an advantage to provide stability in certain cases.

The latissimus dorsi is a large triangular muscle which has a broad origin from the lower thoracic and lumbar vertebrae and the posterior crest of the ilium, sweeps round into the axilla and is inserted into the lower end of the bicipital groove of the humerus. The nerve to the latissimus dorsi comes from the posterior cord of the brachial plexus and in the lower part of its course is accompanied by the terminal branches of the subscapular artery. Both nerve and blood supply enter the undersurface of the upper part of the muscle and are thus not interfered with when the muscle is freed from its origin and the structures underneath it to allow its incorporation in the flap. The whole thickness of the muscle is mobilised and detached distally; attempts to spare some of it to retain function simply lead to atrophy from denervation. The muscle is more firmly attached to the skin because of perforating blood vessels than to the underlying chest wall.

Figure 4.17c Olivari's publication in the *British Journal of Plastic Surgery* in January 1976. For the first time the term 'latissimus flap' was used.

Not only was there poor healing of split thickness skin grafts (STSG), but the performance of pedicled skin flaps was unsuccessful too, as they almost invariably displayed a poor marginal perfusion of the distal third, with eventual necrosis resulting (see Figure 4.19).

Random pattern flaps, particularly when located near an irradiated area display an inadequate perfusion. Performing an omental flap necessitates an additional laparotomy and strong cranial tension on the omentum. Since most areas that exhibit signs of radiation-induced damage are infected, a laparotomy presents an additional unnecessary risk. Moreover, in patients with thoracic wall defects with rib removal, the omental flap is useless since it does not result in thoracic wall stabilization.

In his search for an adequate flap, with which large defects could be covered, Olivari discovered the latissimus dorsi muscle with its axial perfusion pattern. Subsequently, he recognized there was an option to raise the muscle including the overlying skin for coverage of thoracic wall defects. In 1974 he introduced this procedure, not being familiar with the work of Tansini (1906), and giving it the title of "latissimus flap". The first presentation, following 17 procedures, was at the BAPS Winter Meeting in the *Royal College of Surgeons of England* on December 12, 1975. The first publication was in 1976 in the *British Journal of Plastic Surgery* and subsequently in the German journal *Der Chirurg*.

Within one year, this technique had been adopted by Mühlbauer and Olbrisch in Germany, as well as by many other surgeons worldwide. With increasing frequency this island flap technique was being used for breast reconstruction. Additionally, it was used as a free flap for defect coverage in the head and neck area, and the upper and lower extremities. The first free latissimus flap transfers were performed by Marko Godina in 1978.

Anatomy

Being the largest muscle in humans, the latissimus dorsi muscle has a broad origin from the dorsal processes of the 7th to 12th thoracic vertebrae as well as all lumbar vertebrae. Furthermore, the muscle originates from the inferior three ribs as well as from the medial half of the iliac crest and sacrum via the thoracodorsal fascia. Muscle fibres running horizontally cover the inferior margin of the scapula. All parts converge and form a small, flat tendon which inserts at the minor tubercle of the humeral crest, thus forming the dorsal boundary of the axilla. The thoracodorsal nerve, deriving from the brachial plexus (C6–C8), innervates the muscle.

Embryologically the latissimus dorsi muscle presumably corresponds to the panniculus carnosus seen in mammals.

Fundamental in reconstructive surgery is knowledge of vascular anatomy: The subscapular artery, being a branch of the axillary artery, gives off the cir-

Indications for the Myocutaneous Latissimus Flap

- Volume substitution following breast conservation therapy
- Defect coverage following radical mastectomy
- Breast reconstruction following mastectomy with removal of the pectoralis muscle and skin deficiency. A silicone implant is necessary in this indication
- Coverage of full-thickness thoracic wall defects following rib and sternum resections
- Breast reconstruction with a deepithelialized latissimus flap without insertion of a silicone implant
- Free latissimus flap with which large defects can be covered, predominantly used for coverage of lower extremity defects

Contraindications

If the thoracodorsal vessels are not available, either following ligation or radiation damage, island and free flaps are not feasible. However, a pedicled myocutaneous flap is possible if an intact serratus arcade is present.

Planning the Operation

During preoperative examination the innervation and function of the latissimus muscle needs to be evaluated. In many cases damage to the axillary region has been caused by radiation or previous surgery so putting the thoracodorsal vessels at risk. Muscle function and thus innervation is verified clinically. Additionally, Doppler sonography is helpful in evaluating vessel presence and patency.

Occasionally visualization of the thoracodorsal vessels is not possible intra-operatively due to extensive fibrosis. Based on our clinical experience we assumed the presence of sufficient collateralization in such cases. However, it is worthwhile preserving the serratus branches as well as, if possible, the CSA. Routinely performed preoperative angiography is not necessary [Olivari 1979]. This applies to the original pedicled latissimus flap.

Planning the incision is best performed the day before surgery with the patient in a standing position. The operative procedure is rather simple with clear anatomy and has limited patient morbidity with a procedure length of approximately two hours and 15 minutes.

Surgical Technique

Original Pedicled Latissimus Flap

Indications include extensive thoracic wall defects or absence of the TDA. The flap is designed in a manner to match the defect in size and shape. In general, a somewhat longer flap is designed than apparently required following measurement. A flap that is too short can present significant technical problems and is more likely to fail.

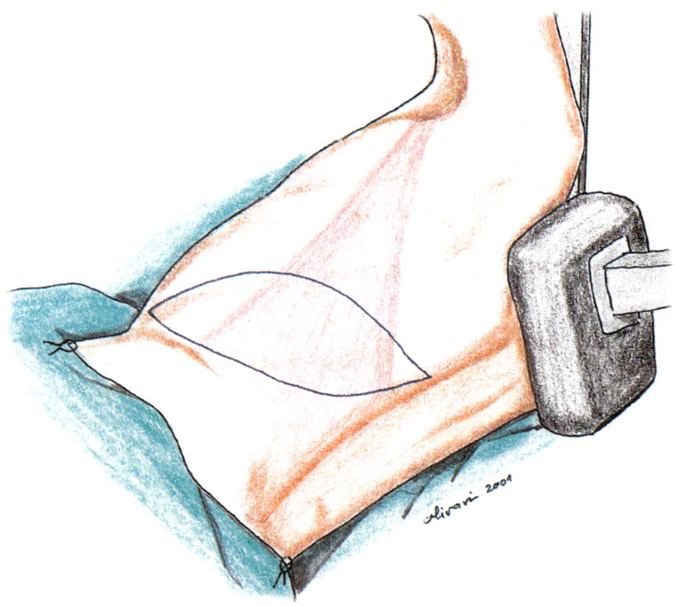

Figure 4.20 Positioning of the patient for latissimus dorsi musle flap transfer. The lateral position is advantageous when performing ipsilateral reconstruction of thorax defect or breast reconstruction. Thus, the flap can be raised and the defect covered without patient repositioning. Using both latissimus dorsi muscles requires repositioning of the patient.

THE LATISSIMUS FLAP

By Neven Olivari

Universitätskliniken Köln, Plastische Chirurgie, 5 Köln 41, Robert-Koch-Strasse 10, West Germany

Skin transposition flaps are the simplest means of covering defects of the anterior chest wall. But when the defects are large and/or the region has been irradiated, the blood supply of the flap may be inadequate and, even after delay operations, necrosis may occur. By incorporating the latissimus dorsi muscle in the flap, however, adequate circulation is assured and no delays are necessary. The increased thickness is also an advantage to provide stability in certain cases.

The latissimus dorsi is a large triangular muscle which has a broad origin from the lower thoracic and lumbar vertebrae and the posterior crest of the ilium, sweeps round into the axilla and is inserted into the lower end of the bicipital groove of the humerus. The nerve to the latissimus dorsi comes from the posterior cord of the brachial plexus and in the lower part of its course is accompanied by the terminal branches of the subscapular artery. Both nerve and blood supply enter the undersurface of the upper part of the muscle and are thus not interfered with when the muscle is freed from its origin and the structures underneath it to allow its incorporation in the flap. The whole thickness of the muscle is mobilised and detached distally; attempts to spare some of it to retain function simply lead to atrophy from denervation. The muscle is more firmly attached to the skin because of perforating blood vessels than to the underlying chest wall.

Figure 4.17c Olivari's publication in the *British Journal of Plastic Surgery* in January 1976. For the first time the term 'latissimus flap' was used.

Not only was there poor healing of split thickness skin grafts (STSG), but the performance of pedicled skin flaps was unsuccessful too, as they almost invariably displayed a poor marginal perfusion of the distal third, with eventual necrosis resulting (see Figure 4.19).

Random pattern flaps, particularly when located near an irradiated area display an inadequate perfusion. Performing an omental flap necessitates an additional laparotomy and strong cranial tension on the omentum. Since most areas that exhibit signs of radiation-induced damage are infected, a laparotomy presents an additional unnecessary risk. Moreover, in patients with thoracic wall defects with rib removal, the omental flap is useless since it does not result in thoracic wall stabilization.

In his search for an adequate flap, with which large defects could be covered, Olivari discovered the latissimus dorsi muscle with its axial perfusion pattern. Subsequently, he recognized there was an option to raise the muscle including the overlying skin for coverage of thoracic wall defects. In 1974 he introduced this procedure, not being familiar with the work of Tansini (1906), and giving it the title of "latissimus flap". The first presentation, following 17 procedures, was at the BAPS Winter Meeting in the *Royal College of Surgeons of England* on December 12, 1975. The first publication was in 1976 in the *British Journal of Plastic Surgery* and subsequently in the German journal *Der Chirurg*.

Within one year, this technique had been adopted by Mühlbauer and Olbrisch in Germany, as well as by many other surgeons worldwide. With increasing frequency this island flap technique was being used for breast reconstruction. Additionally, it was used as a free flap for defect coverage in the head and neck area, and the upper and lower extremities. The first free latissimus flap transfers were performed by Marko Godina in 1978.

Anatomy

Being the largest muscle in humans, the latissimus dorsi muscle has a broad origin from the dorsal processes of the 7th to 12th thoracic vertebrae as well as all lumbar vertebrae. Furthermore, the muscle originates from the inferior three ribs as well as from the medial half of the iliac crest and sacrum via the thoracodorsal fascia. Muscle fibres running horizontally cover the inferior margin of the scapula. All parts converge and form a small, flat tendon which inserts at the minor tubercle of the humeral crest, thus forming the dorsal boundary of the axilla. The thoracodorsal nerve, deriving from the brachial plexus (C6–C8), innervates the muscle.

Embryologically the latissimus dorsi muscle presumably corresponds to the panniculus carnosus seen in mammals.

Fundamental in reconstructive surgery is knowledge of vascular anatomy: The subscapular artery, being a branch of the axillary artery, gives off the circumflex scapular artery (CSA) as well as the thoracodorsal artery (TDA). The latter continues inferiorly with the corresponding nerve and vein along the lateral border of the latissimus dorsi. The mean length of the thoracodorsal vessels is 9cm with a diameter of 2.7 mm for the artery and a vein of 3.4 mm. They run 3 cm medial to the lateral border of the muscle. Prior to entering the muscle the TDA gives off a branch to the serratus anterior muscle.

Due to the existence of multiple musculocutaneous perforators the muscle can be used as a pedicled, island, and free flap.

Mediocaudally the muscle is additionally perfused by perforators derived from the intercostal arteries. If the TDA is not available, such as following damage from ALND and radiotherapy, a pedicled latissimus flap may still be possible, a phenomenon we observed in our clinic. Collateral circulation is presumably provided from the serratus branch.

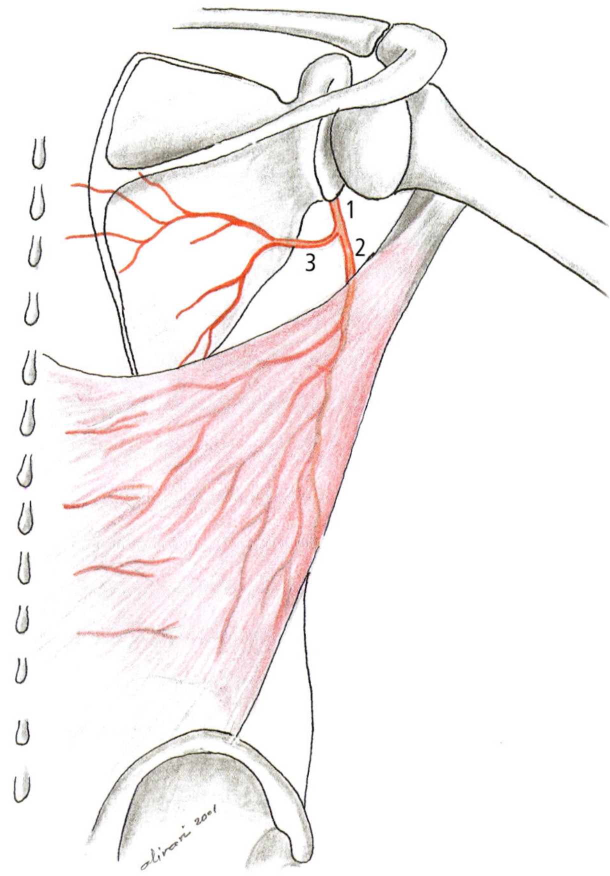

Figure 4.18a Blood supply. The subscapular artery (1) being a branch of the axillary artery bifurcates and forms the circumflex scapular (CSA) (3) and thoracodorsal artery (TDA) (2), the latter being the dominant vessel to the latissimus dorsi muscle. Prior to entering the latissimus dorsi muscle the TDA gives off branches to the serratus anterior and teres major muscle, respectively. Additionally, the latissimus dorsi muscle is perfused via intercostal arteries, thus allowing theoretically a medial pedicle when utilizing this muscle for reconstruction. However, a medially pedicled latissimus dorsi muscle is rarely applied in the clinical use. Venous congestion may occur when conducting the turnover technique.

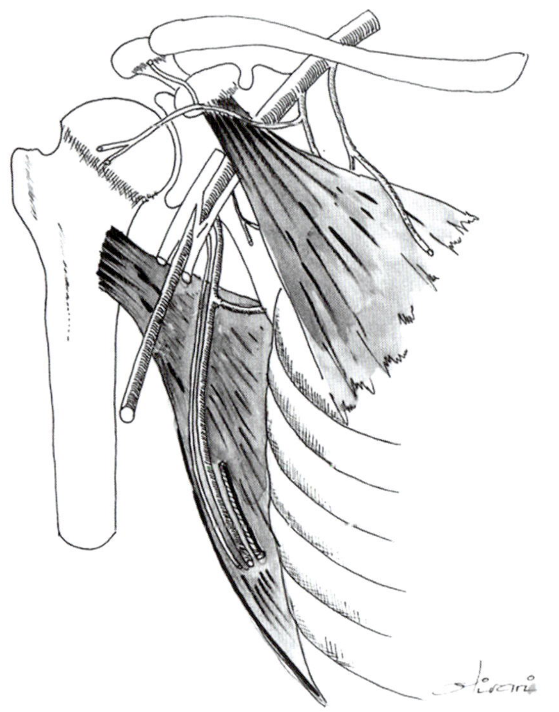

Figure 4.18b Important: A countless number of perforators pierce the muscle and supply the overlying skin. Thus, the latissimus dorsi muscle flap is the safest of all flaps, regardless of whether used as a pedicled, island or free flap. If required, skin extending 5 to 10 cm beyond the muscle margin may be raised and transposed safely.

At the hilum, the neurovascular structures divide into two bundles running parallel to the upper and lateral borders of the muscle. This allows the creation of two independent flaps.

Muscle function of the latissimus dorsi muscle includes arm adduction and extension, as well as dorsal-medial rotation.

The teres major muscle is a synergist of the latissimus dorsi muscle and is located under the cranial border of the latissimus dorsi. Both muscles can move the shoulders dorsally and caudally. Furthermore, they help with forced expiration as well as cough. Loss of latissimus dorsi function does not result in a detectable functional impairment because the teres major muscle takes over its function. However, decreased shoulder strength may be observed in athletes.

Two clinical cases which provoked the author for the development of the latissimus dorsi flap for thoracic wall reconstruction following radiation-induced injury.

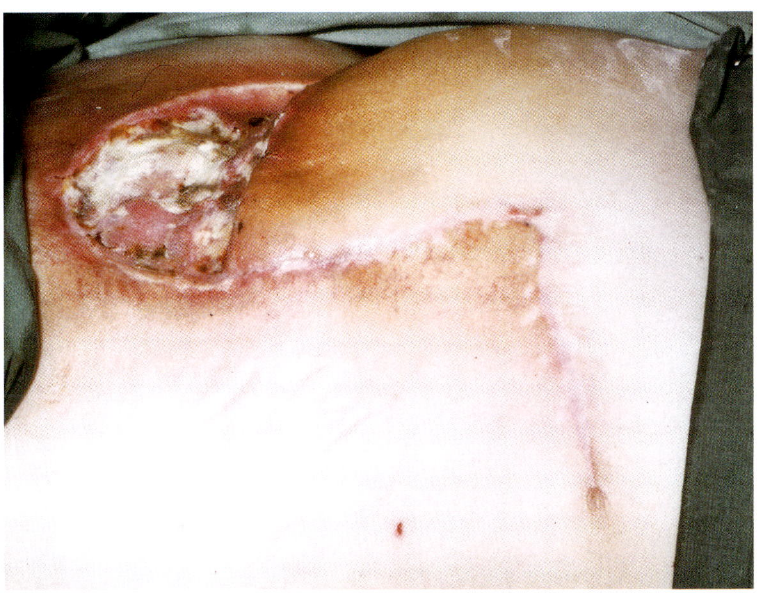

Figure 4.19a Transposition skin flap for coverage of radiation-induced dermatitis (1971). The distal (important) third was necrotic.

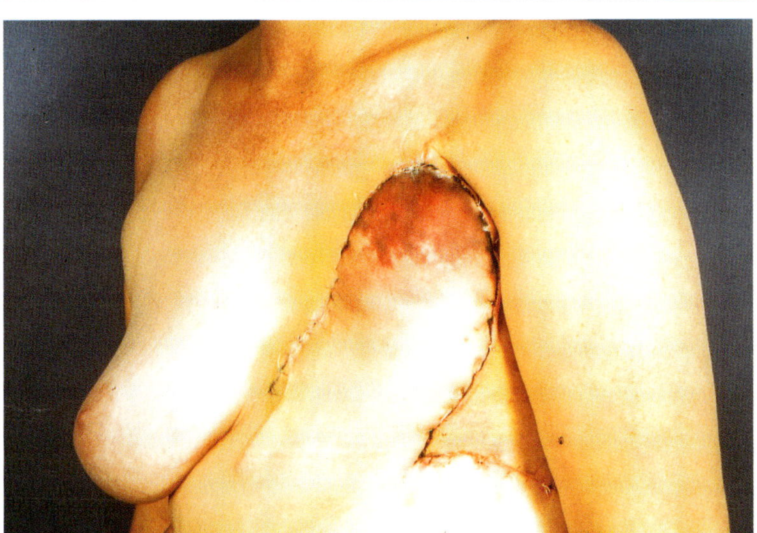

Figure 4.19b Random pattern flap (1972) for reconstruction of a radiation-induced defect. The distal third displays clinical signs of necrosis.

Indications for the Myocutaneous Latissimus Flap

- Volume substitution following breast conservation therapy
- Defect coverage following radical mastectomy
- Breast reconstruction following mastectomy with removal of the pectoralis muscle and skin deficiency. A silicone implant is necessary in this indication
- Coverage of full-thickness thoracic wall defects following rib and sternum resections
- Breast reconstruction with a deepithelialized latissimus flap without insertion of a silicone implant
- Free latissimus flap with which large defects can be covered, predominantly used for coverage of lower extremity defects

Contraindications

If the thoracodorsal vessels are not available, either following ligation or radiation damage, island and free flaps are not feasible. However, a pedicled myocutaneous flap is possible if an intact serratus arcade is present.

Planning the Operation

During preoperative examination the innervation and function of the latissimus muscle needs to be evaluated. In many cases damage to the axillary region has been caused by radiation or previous surgery so putting the thoracodorsal vessels at risk. Muscle function and thus innervation is verified clinically. Additionally, Doppler sonography is helpful in evaluating vessel presence and patency.

Occasionally visualization of the thoracodorsal vessels is not possible intra-operatively due to extensive fibrosis. Based on our clinical experience we assumed the presence of sufficient collateralization in such cases. However, it is worthwhile preserving the serratus branches as well as, if possible, the CSA. Routinely performed preoperative angiography is not necessary [Olivari 1979]. This applies to the original pedicled latissimus flap.

Planning the incision is best performed the day before surgery with the patient in a standing position. The operative procedure is rather simple with clear anatomy and has limited patient morbidity with a procedure length of approximately two hours and 15 minutes.

Surgical Technique

Original Pedicled Latissimus Flap

Indications include extensive thoracic wall defects or absence of the TDA. The flap is designed in a manner to match the defect in size and shape. In general, a somewhat longer flap is designed than apparently required following measurement. A flap that is too short can present significant technical problems and is more likely to fail.

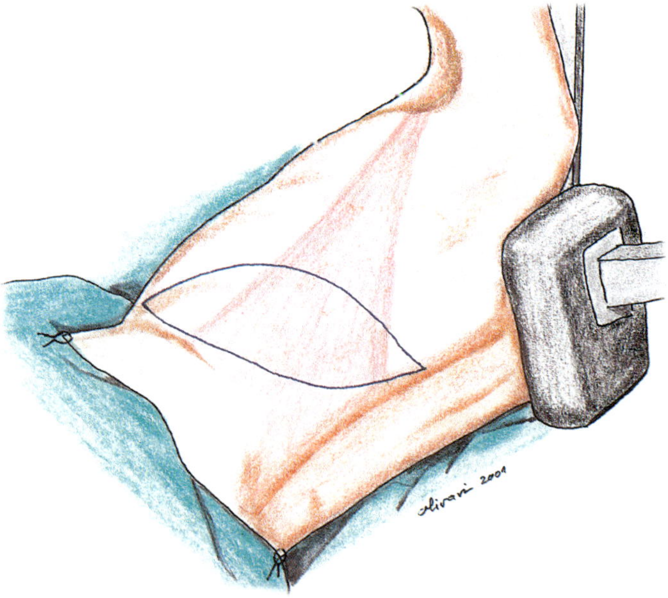

Figure 4.20 Positioning of the patient for latissimus dorsi musle flap transfer. The lateral position is advantageous when performing ipsilateral reconstruction of thorax defect or breast reconstruction. Thus, the flap can be raised and the defect covered without patient repositioning.
Using both latissimus dorsi muscles requires repositioning of the patient.

The flap is raised starting laterally. The muscle, with the overlying skin, is bluntly dissected off the thoracic wall. This layer contains virtually no fibrous bands and is almost avascular. Cranially, the latissimus dorsi muscle has to be separated from the teres major muscle. Furthermore, the latissimus dorsi muscle needs to be detached from the serratus posterior and anterior muscles as well as from the lumbodorsal fascia.

Skin and muscle are incised distally according to defect size. The flap base can be designed rather narrow for two reasons: 1) Flap perfusion is via the muscle, 2) A base too broad will cause an unpleasant fold in the axilla.

The flap is transferred into the defect. Following mobilization the donor site in most cases can be closed primarily. STSG may be necessary if larger flaps are raised.

Latissimus Dorsi Island Flap

Indications include coverage of thoracic wall defects as well as cervical defects and breast reconstruction in combination with silicone implants.

The desired flap size is designed spindle-shaped. The flap displays an oblique orientation extending from the 7th to the 9th thoracic vertebra medially to the lateral edge of the iliac crest laterally. This orientation (mediocranial to laterocaudal) allows the use of larger flaps with primary donor site closure and a much more favorable postoperative scar than the axial flaps presented by Bostwick and McGraw (Figure 4.39). Dissecting the flap off the thoracic wall is rather simple and is mostly performed bluntly. Isolation of the muscular pedicle off the subcutaneous tissue is much more demanding and requires sharp dissection.

Due to the presence of extensive musculocutaneous perforator vessels meticulous hemostasis is of utmost importance. Cranially, the trapezius muscle must not be injured.

A long tunnel is necessary to reach the axilla which requires patient dissection. Often an additional axillary incision in necessary for visualization of the thoracodorsal vessels and for transection of the insertion of the latissimus dorsi muscle if indicated. By doing this an axillary "bulge" is prevented and flap mobility is enhanced.

Deepithelialized Latissimus Island Flap

This flap is used for breast reconstruction without silicone implants.

Flap design and surgical technique are similar to the steps described with the latissimus dorsi island flap. However, since volume is key the island is designed as large as possible. Thus, the island flap extends beyond the muscle margin anteriorly for about 10 cm and thus includes dermoadipose tissue from the lateral abdominal wall. This portion includes abundant well perfused adipose tissue although not overlying the muscle. Furthermore, the flap extends the muscle medially as displayed in Figure 4.52.

The significant difference of this flap when compared to the regular latissimus island flap is that it is de-epithelialized. ***Deepithelialization needs to be performed prior to raising the flap*** or else technical difficulties will be encountered.

Following flap mobilization ***an additional axillary incision is mandatory.*** The thoracodorsal vessels are visualized and the thoracodorsal nerve transected for prevention of subsequent muscular movement of the reconstructed breast. The muscular insertion at the humerus is transected and subsequently sutured to the thoracic wall so preventing traction on the thoracodorsal vessels. (Figure 4.53e).

A flap size of 30 × 9 cm, with a volume of 200 to 300 ccm, can be raised easily depending on the abundance of subcutaneous tissues.

Free Latissimus Dorsi Flap

The free latissimus dorsi flap is an island flap which can be transferred to almost any region of the body using microsurgical techniques. Thus, defects from head to toe may be covered. It is the most frequently used free flap. Advantages include technical ease, a long vascular pedicle (6–13 cm) and large arterial diameter (1.8–4.0 mm). No other free flap is as robust as the latissimus dorsi flap.

Transfer is possible as a myocutaneous and muscle flap, respectively. Due to the course of the TDA with early division into two main branches, two free muscle transfers of smaller size can be raised from each latissimus dorsi muscle.

Due to its volume when transferred as a free myocutaneous flap, it is occasionally too thick, e.g. for reconstruction of head and facial defects. However, when transferred as a free muscle flap with STSG the resultant volume reduction may allow reconstruction in these areas. Furthermore, coverage of plantar defects with myocutaneous latissimus flaps poses problems due to the existence of a thick subcutaneous fat layer. Because of shear forces occurring upon movement, bursa formation and ulcerations may be encountered.

Clinical experience has shown that in these cases free muscle transfer with STSG cover is more robust.

Dissection is similar to the steps described for the latissimus island flap. The thoracodorsal vessels are identified and dissected up to the CSA. A second team outlines the defect and visualizes the recipient vessels. Then, the thoracodorsal artery and vein are transected with subsequent microvascular anastomosis to the recipient vessels.

a) The Pedicled Latissimus Dorsi Flap

The pedicled latissimus dorsi flap is a typical axial, arterial, myocutaneous flap.

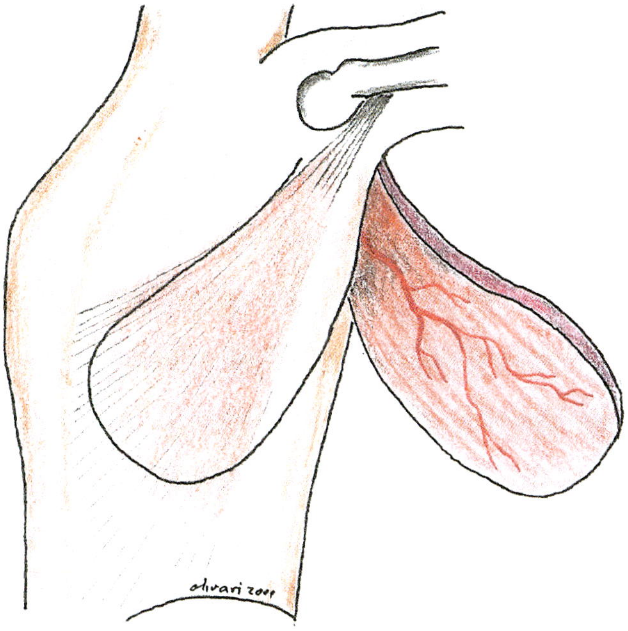

Figure 4.21a Pedicled latissimus dorsi muscle flap for reconstruction of thoracic wall defects. When transferring the flap its versatility becomes evident.

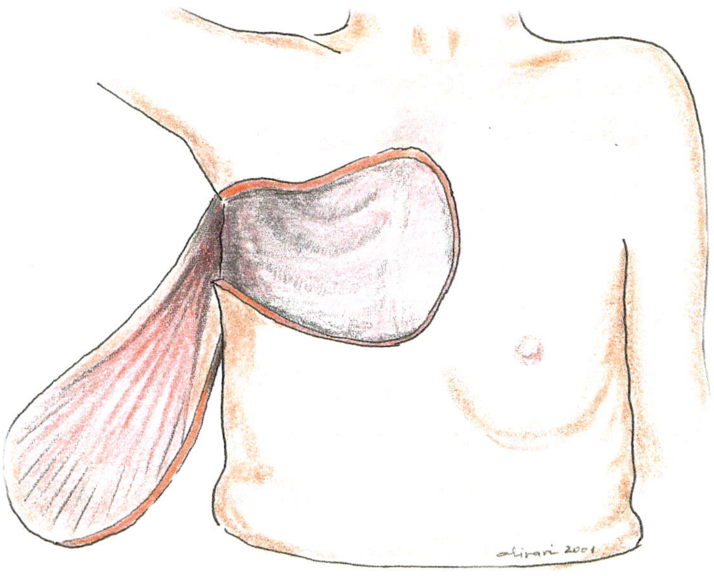

Figure 4.21b On the anterior thoracic wall defects extending beyond the midline can be covered.

First Latissimus Flap (of New Age)
(Published 1976, *British Journal of Plastic Surgery*)

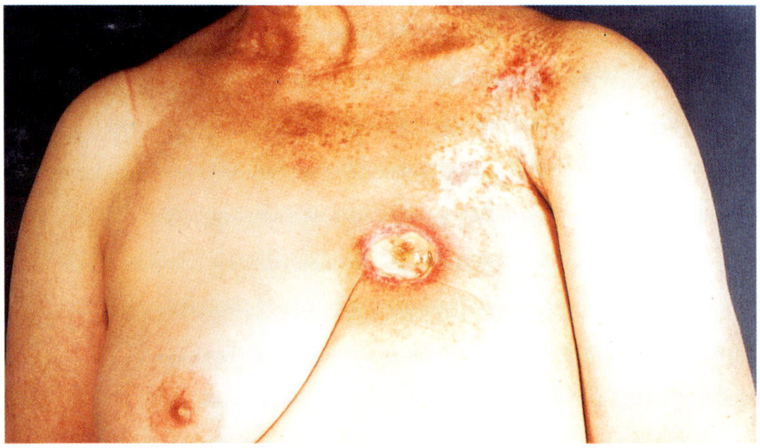

Figure 4.22a First patient. Radiation ulcer and radiodermatitis following mastectomy and radiation therapy. History: Five years.

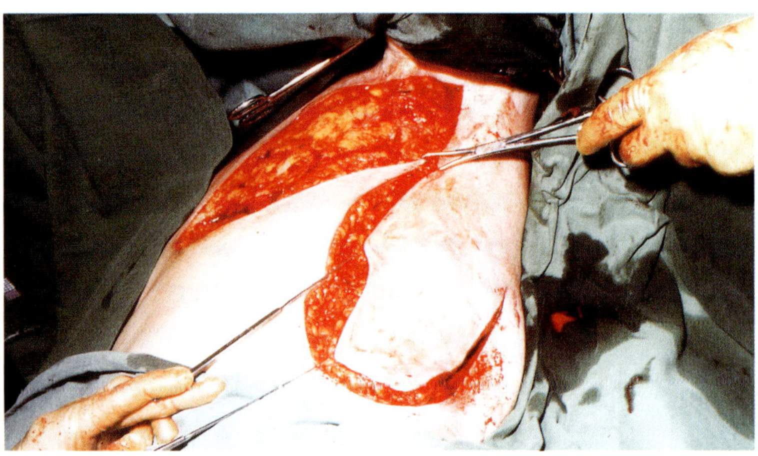

Figure 4.22b First latissimus flap (July 2, 1974). Operative plan: Radical debridement is performed with subsequent mobilization of the myocutaneous latissimus dorsi flap.

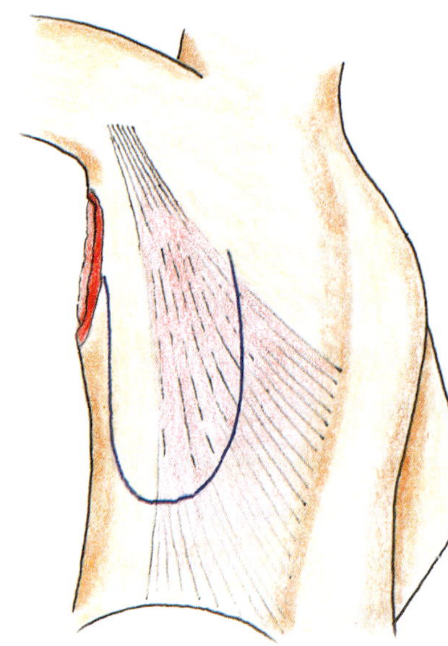

Figure 4.22c Note, that the anterior part of the flap does not cover the latissimus dorsi muscle.

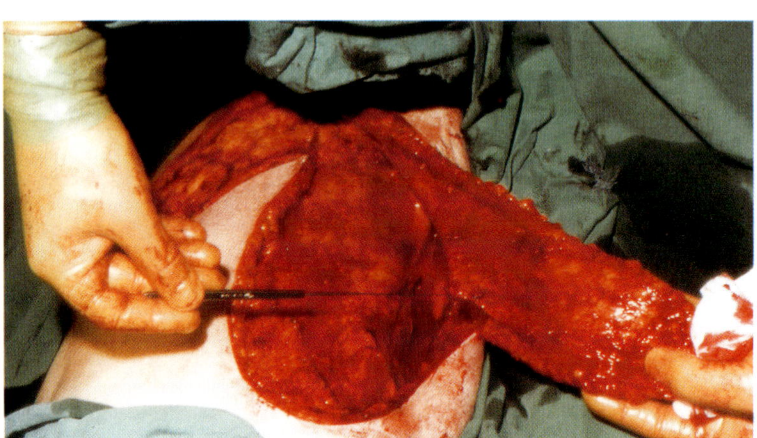

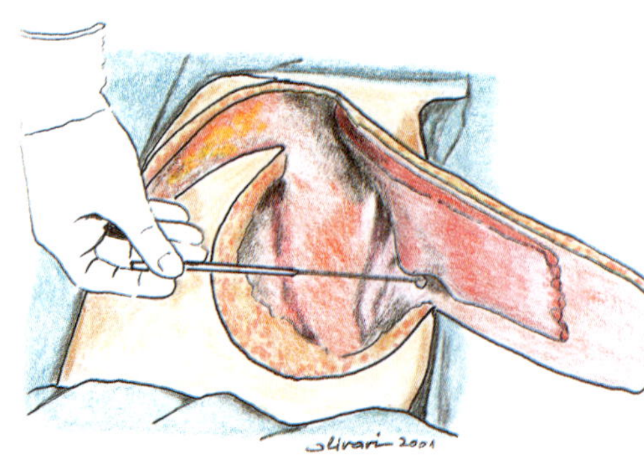

Figure 4.22d,e The distal part of the flap does not contain muscle. However, perfusion of the flap is excellent. (d) Intra operative image (July 2, 1974)

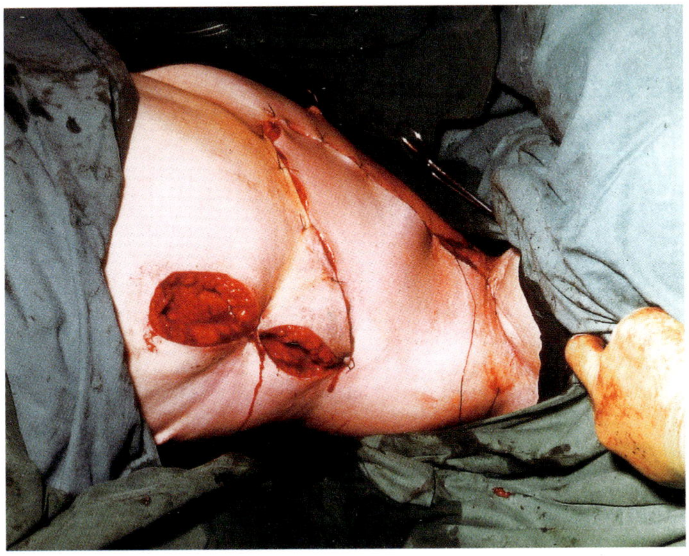

Figure 4.22f At the end of the procedure the flap (18 × 12 cm) is optimally perfused. This was a unique surgical experience for the author (July 2, 1974).

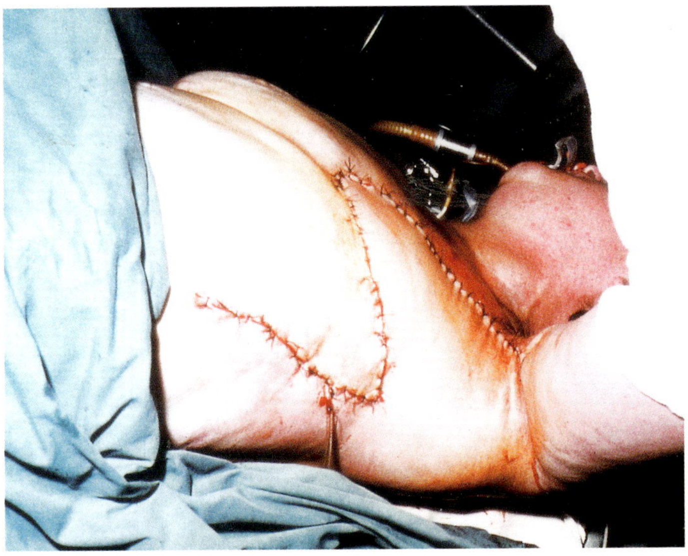

Figure 4.22g End of surgery: The donor site was closed primarily.

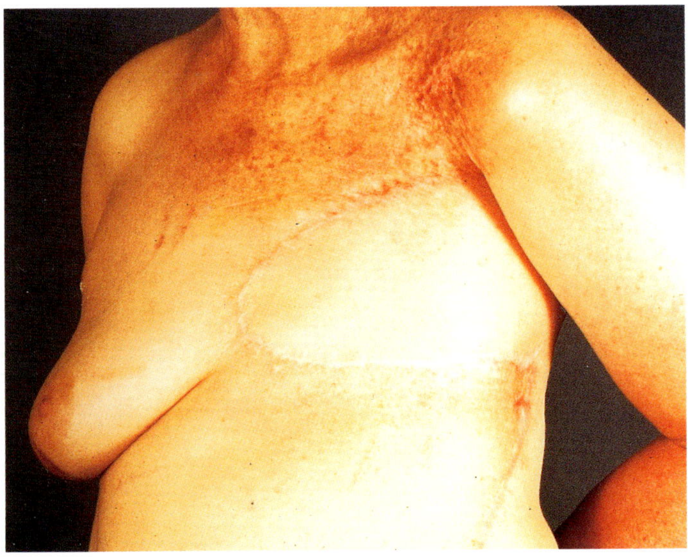

Figure 4.22h Six months postoperatively

Advanced Breast Cancer

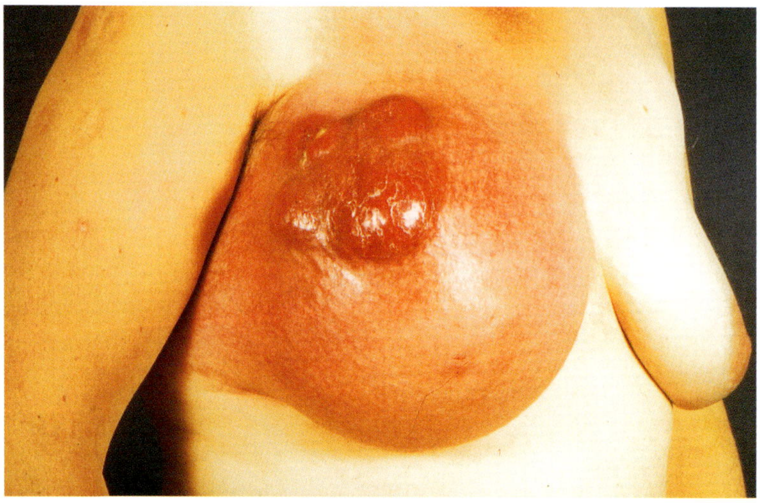

Figure 4.23a Advanced breast cancer of the right breast which is about to perforate the skin (July 2, 1975). Indications for performing an operation:

- Reduction of tumor volume
- Prevention of perforation with subsequent infection
- Facilitation of oncologic treatment and care
- Improvement of quality of life

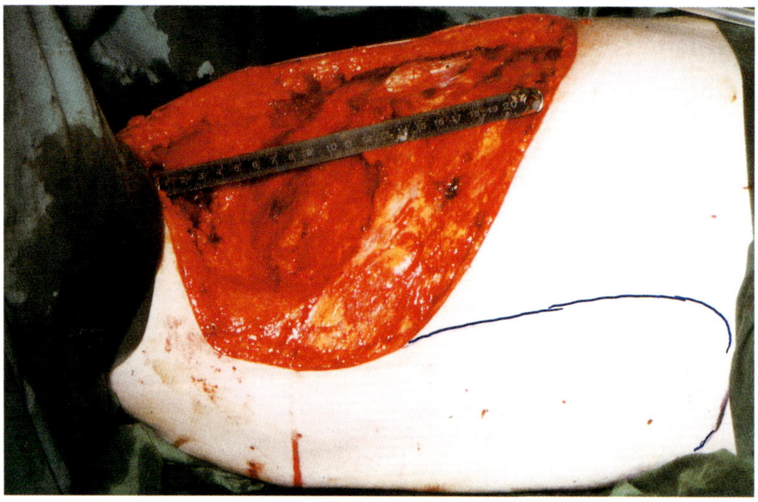

Figure 4.23b This procedure is of course palliative. Tumor resection is conducted along with axillary and subclavian lymph node dissection. Furthermore, the pectoral major and minor muscles as well as the serratus anterior muscle are removed. A defect was of 20 × 20 cm in size.

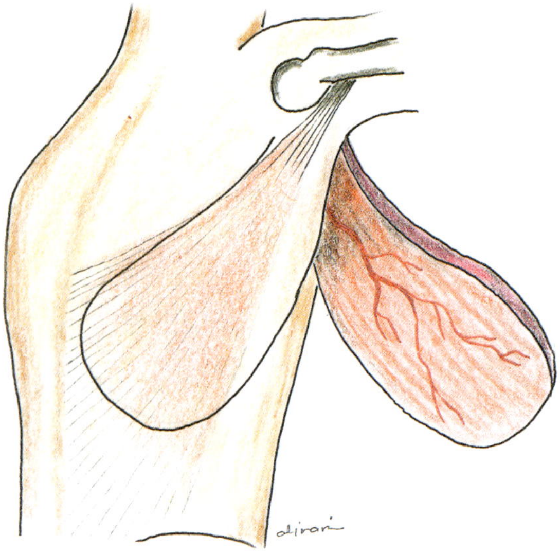

Figure 4.23c Design of a pedicled latissimus dorsi flap

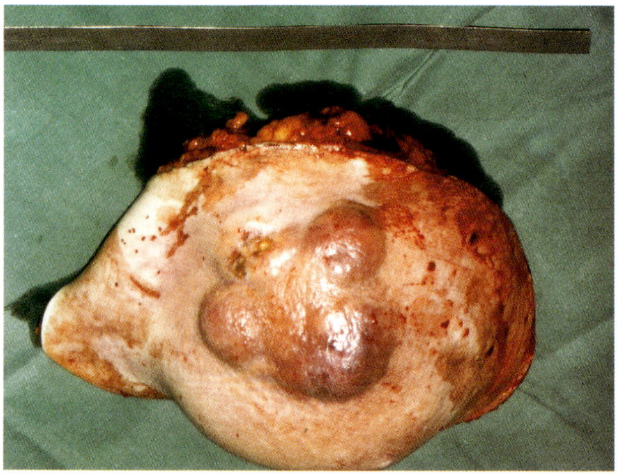

Figure 4.23d Removed tumor

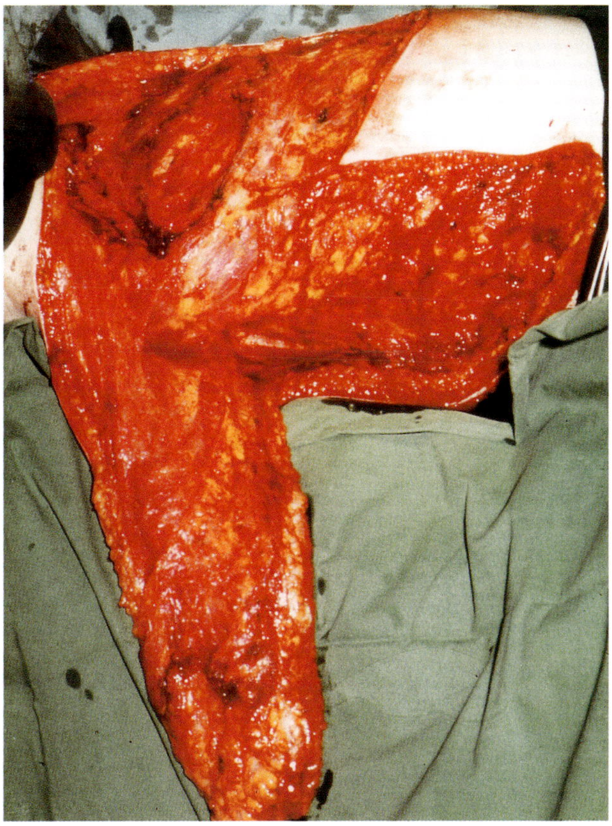

Figure 4.23e The pedicled latissimus flap is raised. The donor site is mobilized dorsally beyond the spinal column so primary closure was possible.

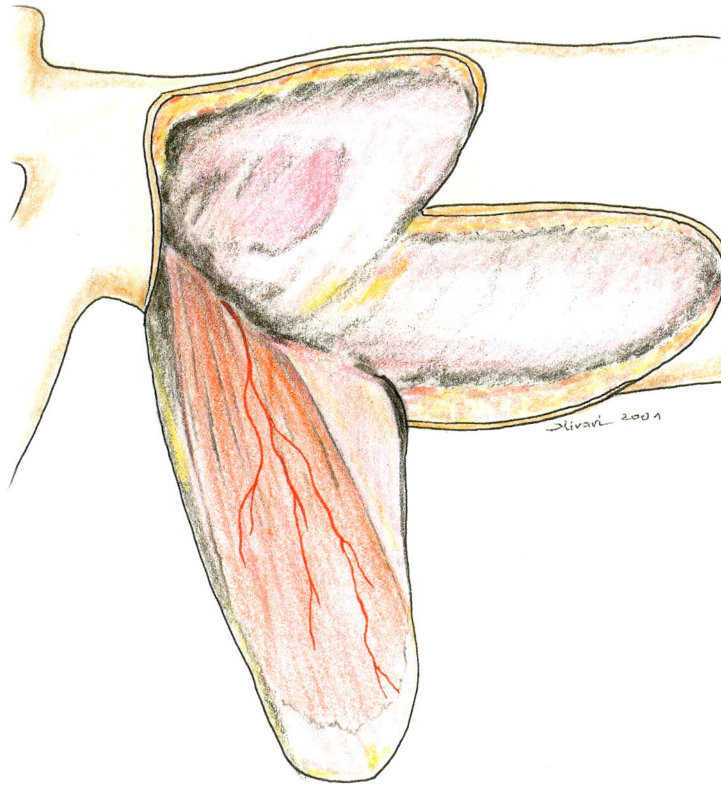

Figure 4.23f For primary donor site closure after considerable mobilization

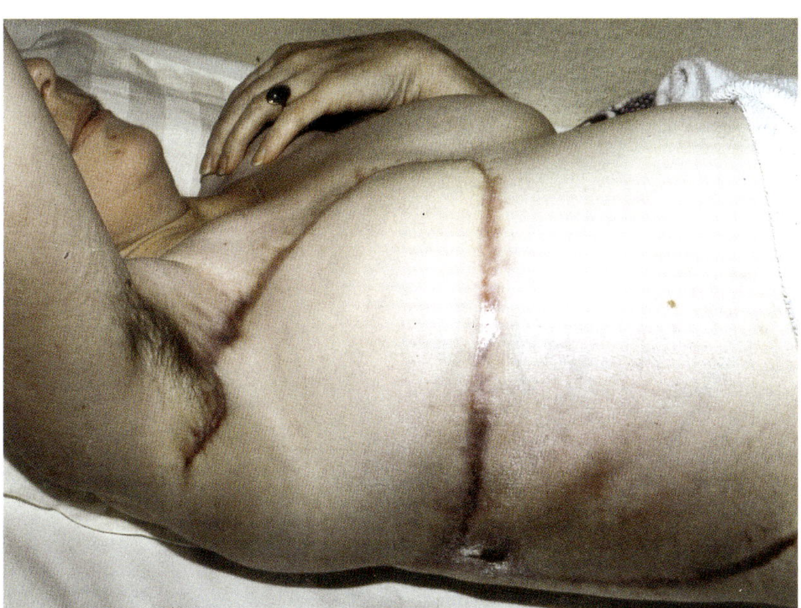

Figure 4.23g Picture taken two months following surgery (September 7, 1975). At this point the patient was in oncologic care. The operation performed was merely a palliative procedure. However, it facilitated oncologic treatment (chemotherapy) and care and considerably improved the patient's quality of life.

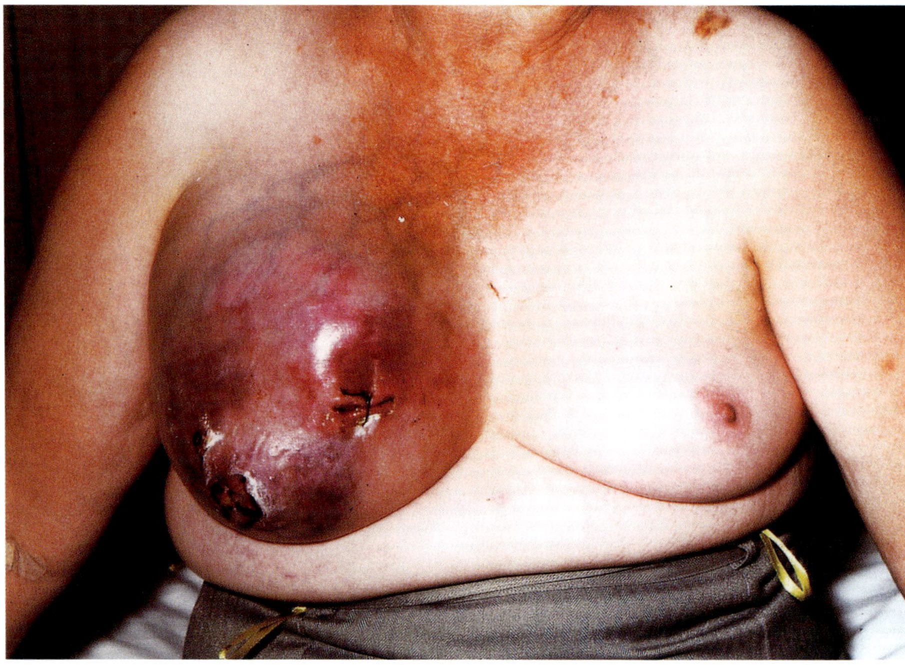

Figure 4.24a Advanced breast cancer.
A palliative procedure is planned for:
– Reduction of tumor
– Prevention of perforation with subsequent infection
– To make possible of oncologic treatment and care
– Improvement of quality of life

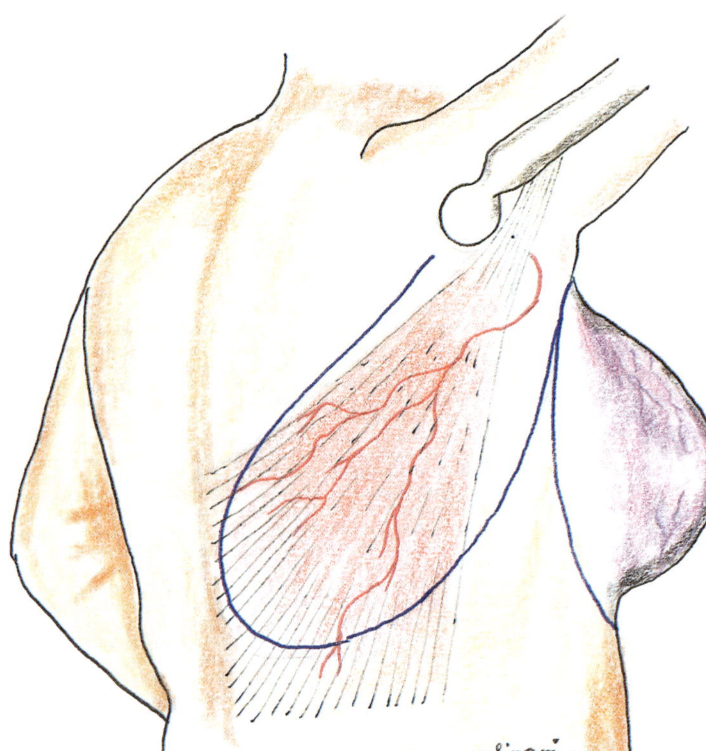

Figure 4.24b Operative plan: A pedicled latissimus flap (25 × 18 cm) is designed.

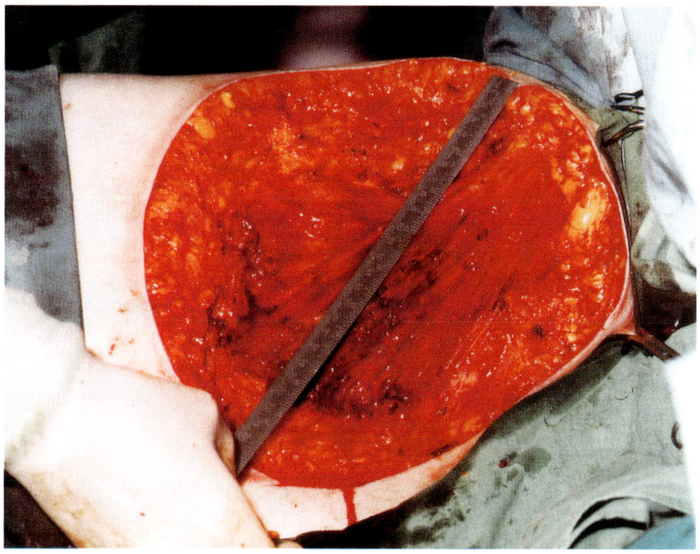

Figure 4.24c Tumor resection is performed with removal of pectoral major and minor muscles as well as axillary and subclavian lymph node dissection. The resultant defect has a size of 25 × 23 cm.

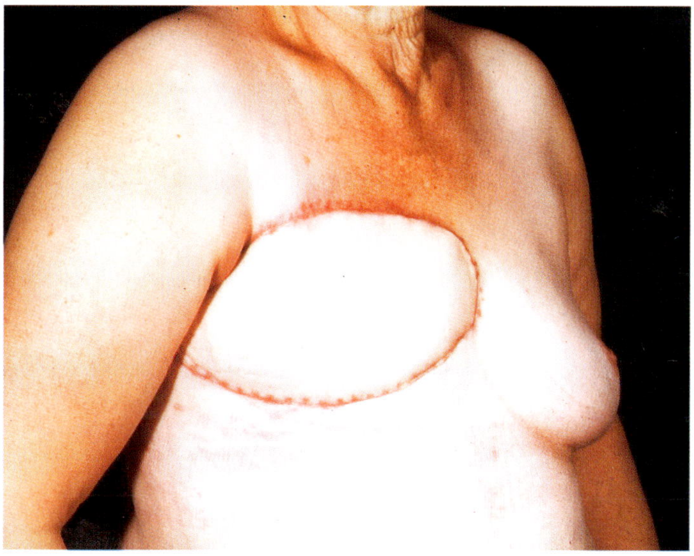

Figure 4.24d Three months postoperatively. Oncologic treatment had been initiated on postoperative day 6.

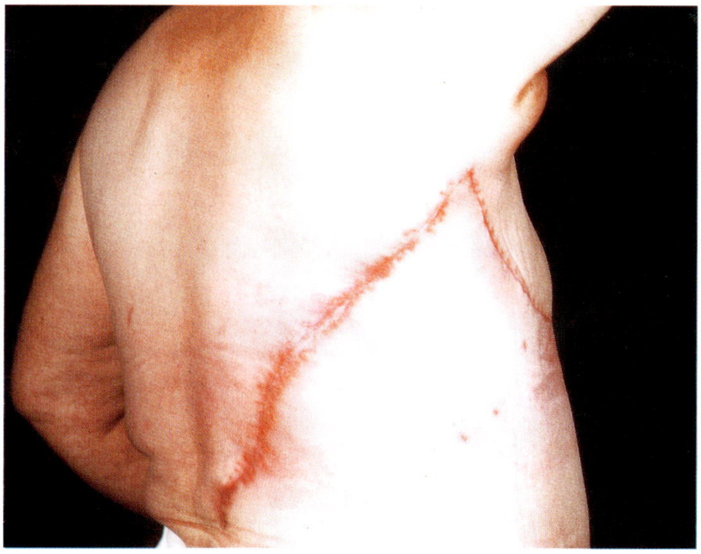

Figure 4.24e Primary closure is possible sometimes even with flaps of this size. A prerequisite for primary closure is extensive mobilization frequently extending beyond the spinal column. However, primary closure may not always be possible. Then, the donor site may be grafted with STSG (split thickness skin grafts). This STSG extends hospitalization and is significantly more painful.

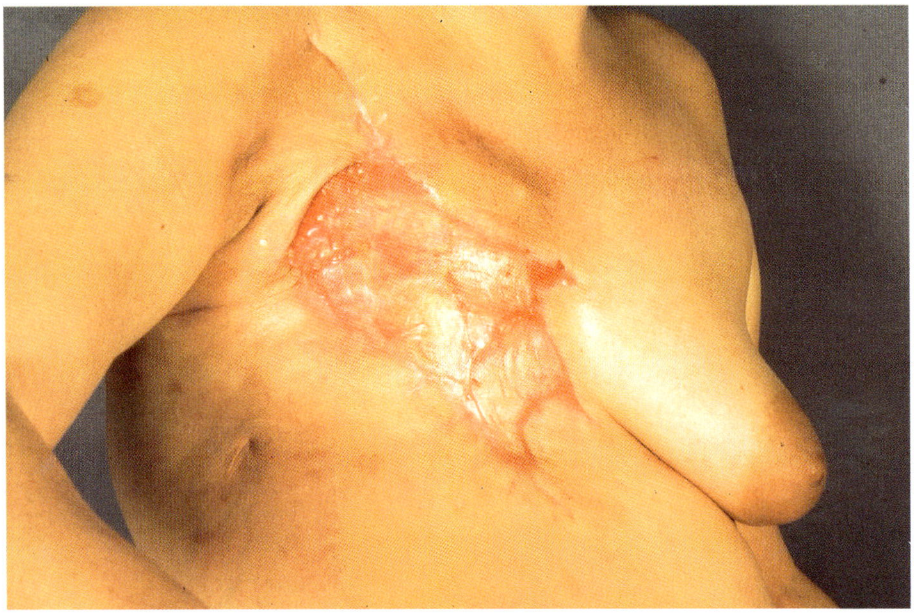

Figure 4.25a Status post mastectomy with postoperative skin necrosis. The defect was covered with STSG which to some extent directly overly the ribs, thus, causing substantial pain.

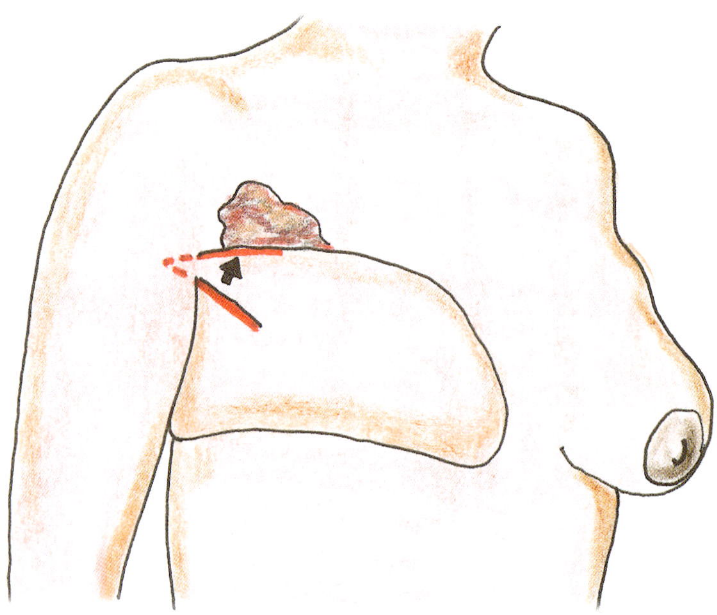

Figure 4.25b Following transposition of a pedicled latissimus flap a pre axillary defect remained which was covered with a medially pedicled random pattern flap originating from the latissimus flap.

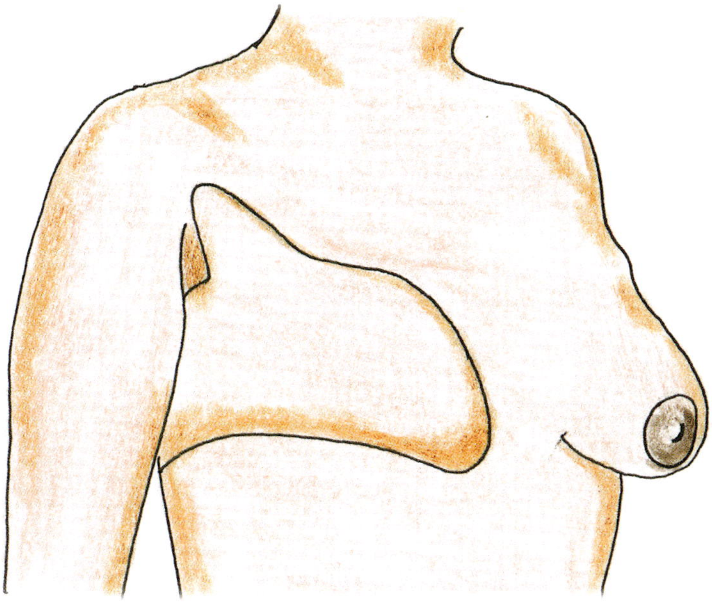

Figure 4.25c End of surgery

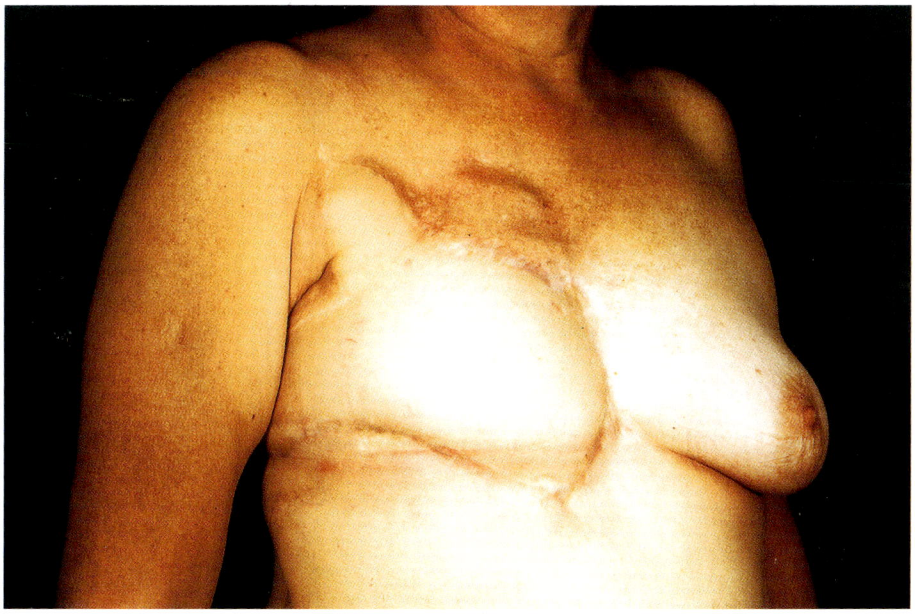

Figure 4.25d Two years postoperatively

Complicated Case – Life-Saving Operation!

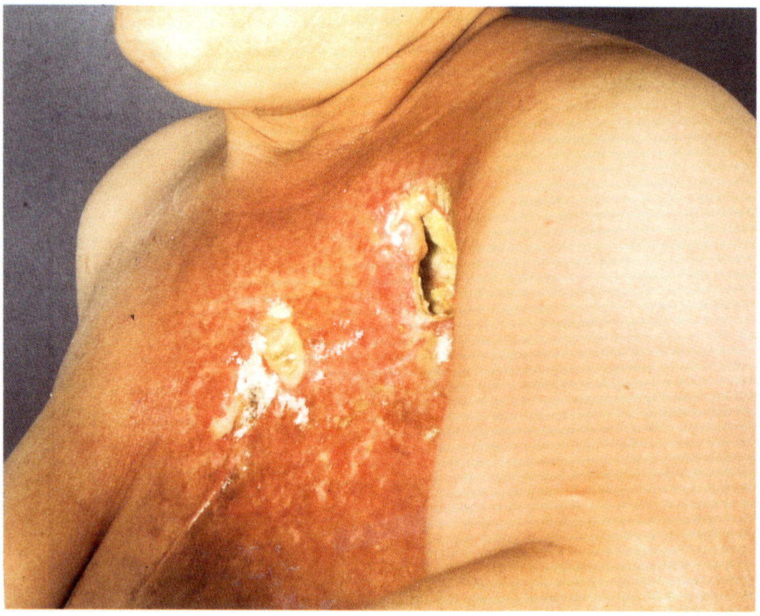

Figure 4.26a Advanced radiation injury of the left breast and axilla. Multiple infected deep ulcerations. The patient complains of high-grade lymphedema of the left upper extremity. Overall, patient was clinically in a very critical condition.

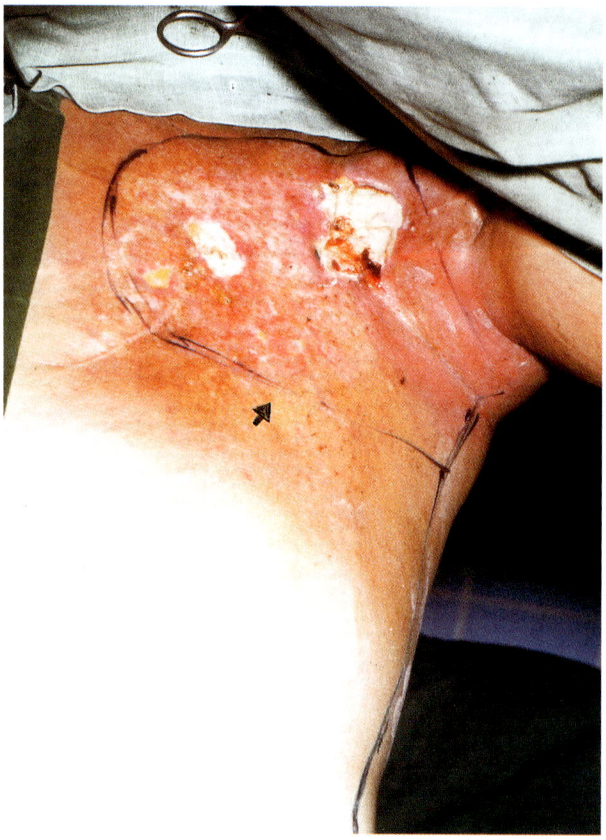

Figure 4.26b Initially, debridement was performed. However, the inferior margin of the radiated area was not excised (arrow). In the following years (1976) we had to learn that radical excision of irradiated area is essential for primary wound healing.

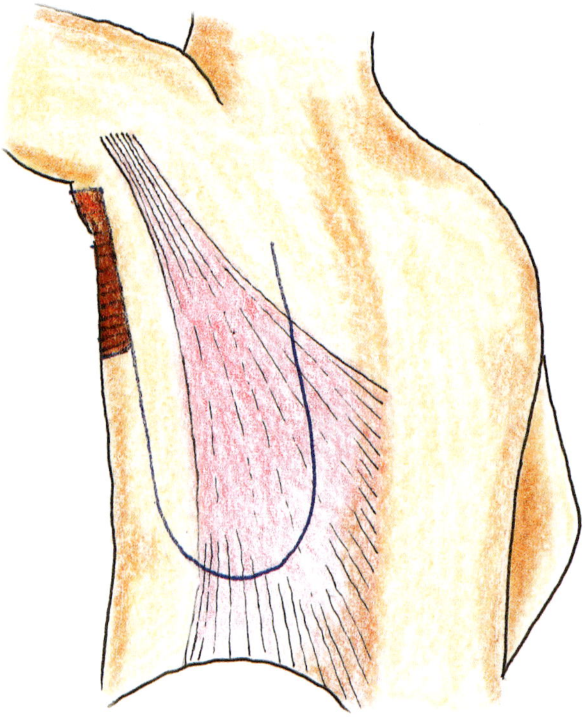

Figure 4.26c Design of the classic latissimus dorsi flap

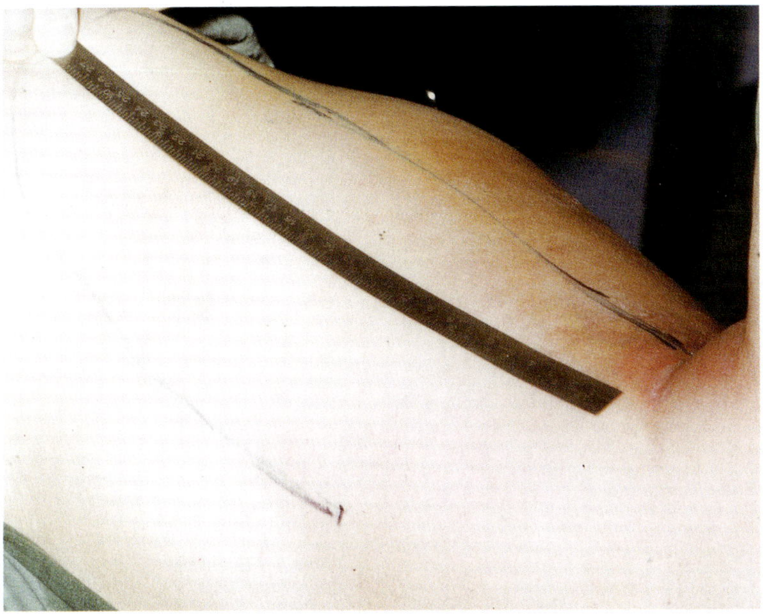

Figure 4.26d Design of the pedicled axial latissimus flap, which was used frequently for such cases. The flap is 30 cm long and has a width of 18 cm.

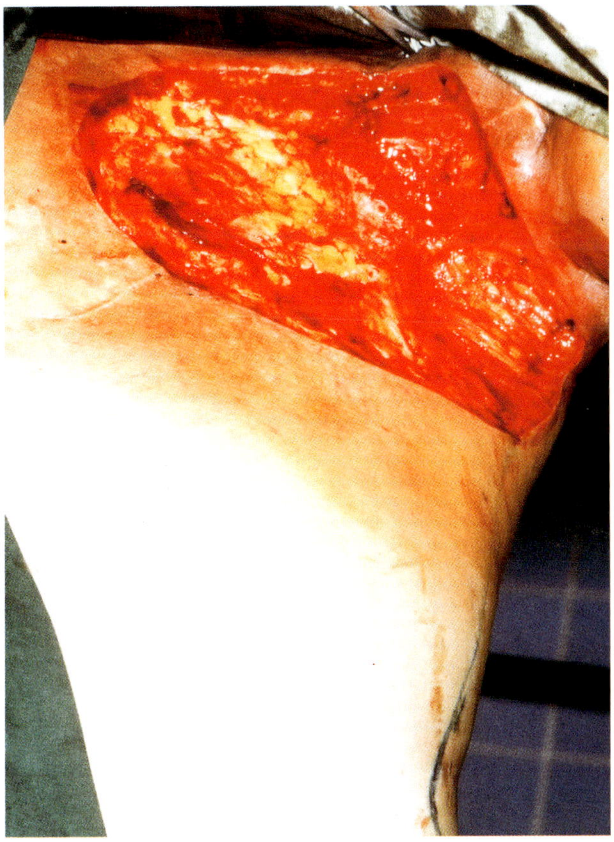

Figure 4.26e Appearance post excision of major necrotic wound. However, areas displaying signs of radiodermatitis were not removed inferiorly. Defect size: 24 × 17 cm.

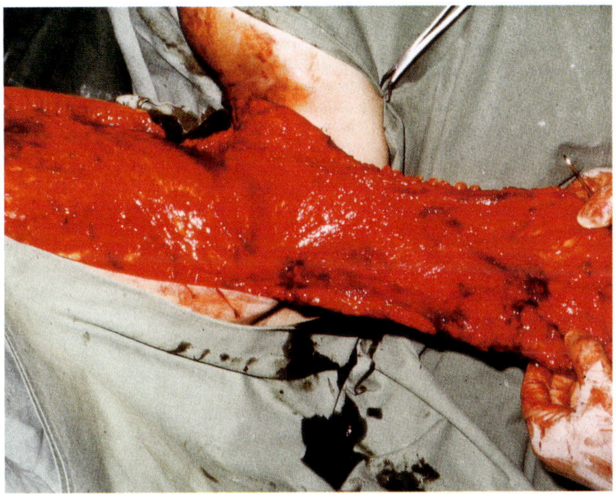

Figure 4.26f Reconstruction is achieved with the latissimus dorsi flap. The thoracodorsal artery was not present. However, its absence is not a contraindication to using this flap if a broad skin base is designed and if the serratus arcade is intact.

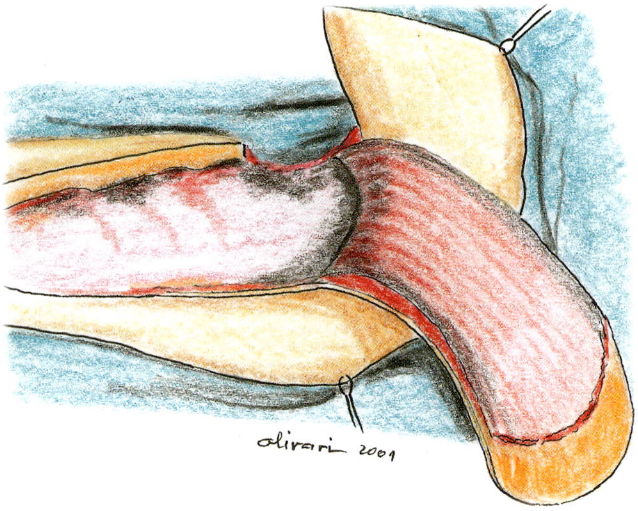

Figure 4.26g Raising the latissimus dorsi flap with a broad skin pedicle.

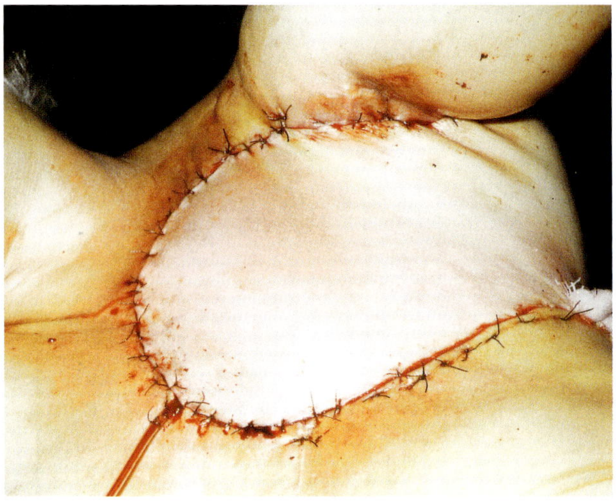

Figure 4.26h At the end of the procedure the flap displays an excellent perfusion.

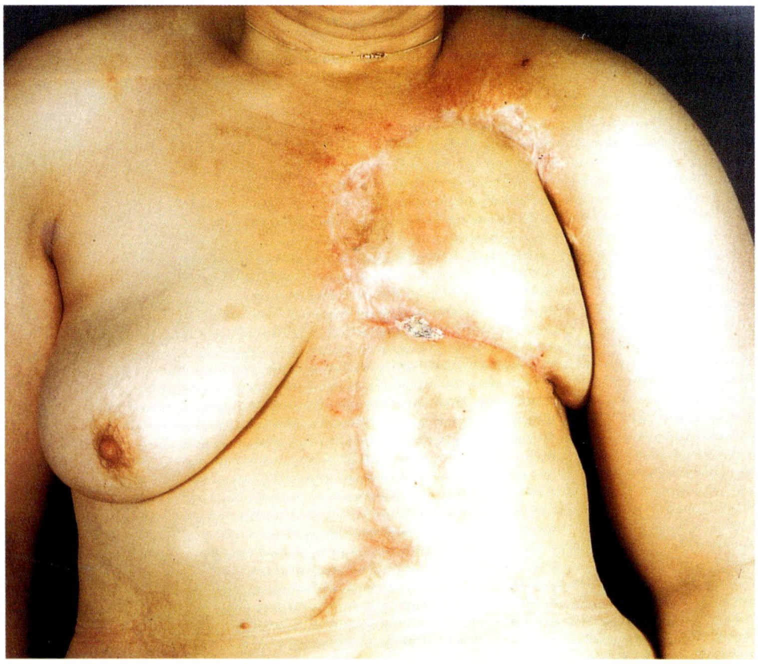

Figure 4.26i Due to soft tissue necrosis inferiorly a secondary procedure needed to be conducted with defect coverage using a local random pattern flap based inferiorly. Of note, the flap itself did not exhibit any signs of vascular impairment.

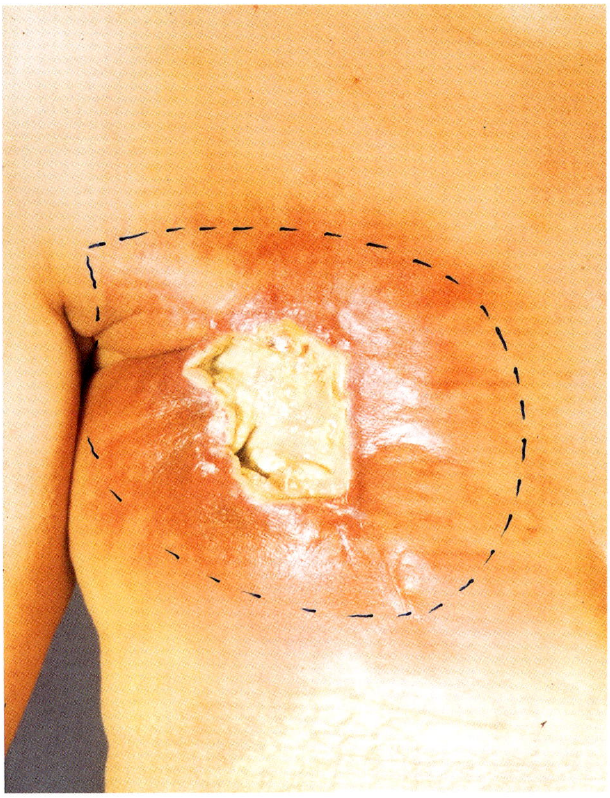

Figure 4.27a Radiation ulcer following mastectomy and postoperative radiation therapy. History: Six years. Symptoms included pain, recurrent infections, and foul odor. **Note:** Size of planned excision.

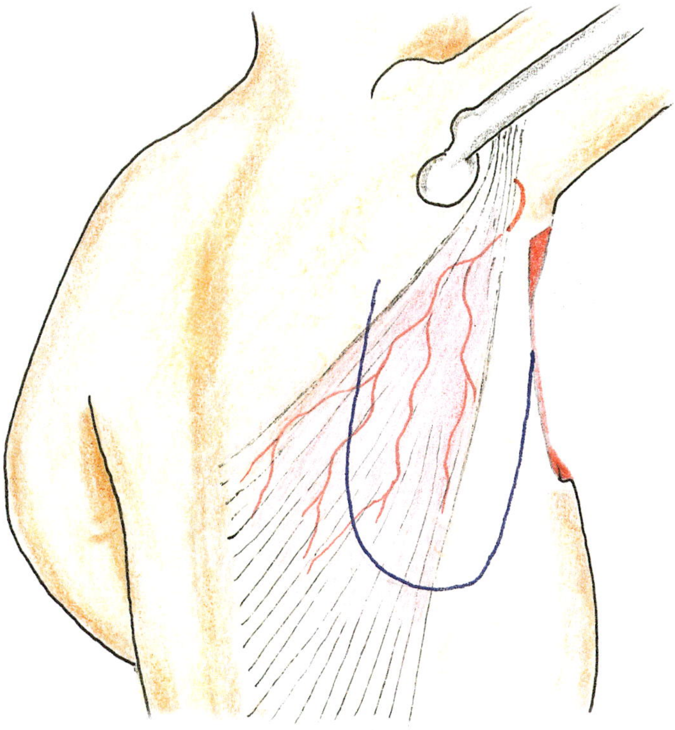

Figure 4.27b Design: Pedicle axial latissimus flap was used for reconstruction.

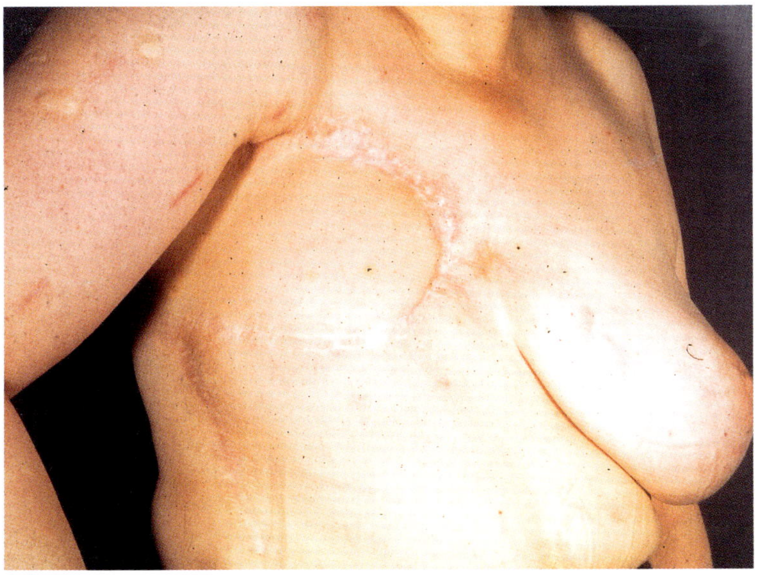

Figure 4.27c Picture two years postoperatively. Primary donor site closure was achieved.

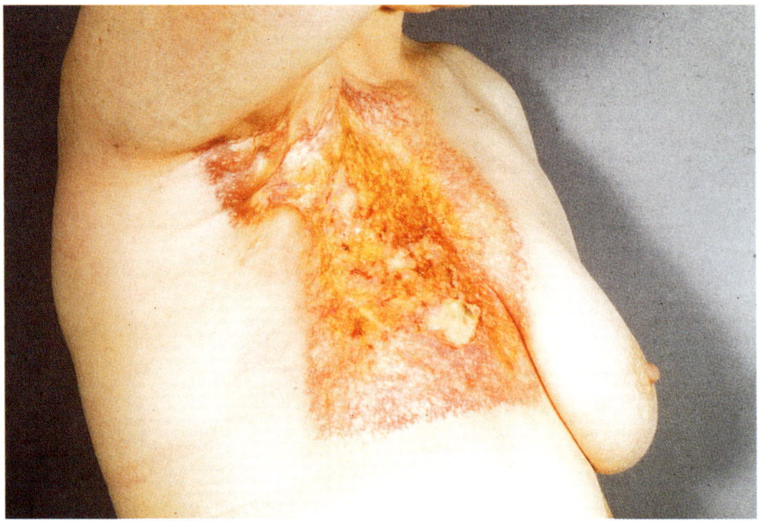

Figure 4.28a Radiodermatitis with multiple painful ulcerations eight years following mastectomy and irradiation therapy. Question: Is it possible to close the secondary defect primarily in this clinical case?

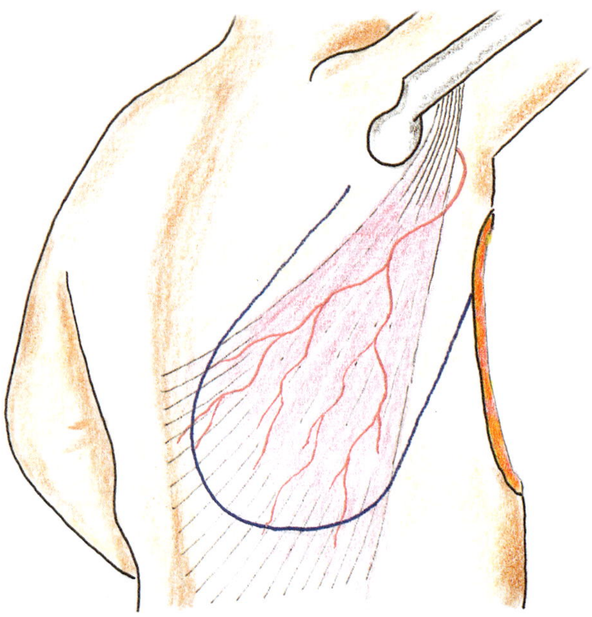

Figure 4.28b Schematic illustration: Relationship of the latissimus flap to the defect. If in doubt is it advisable to design a larger flap. Too small flap may be catastrophic. Here the flap displayed a size of 27 × 18 cm.

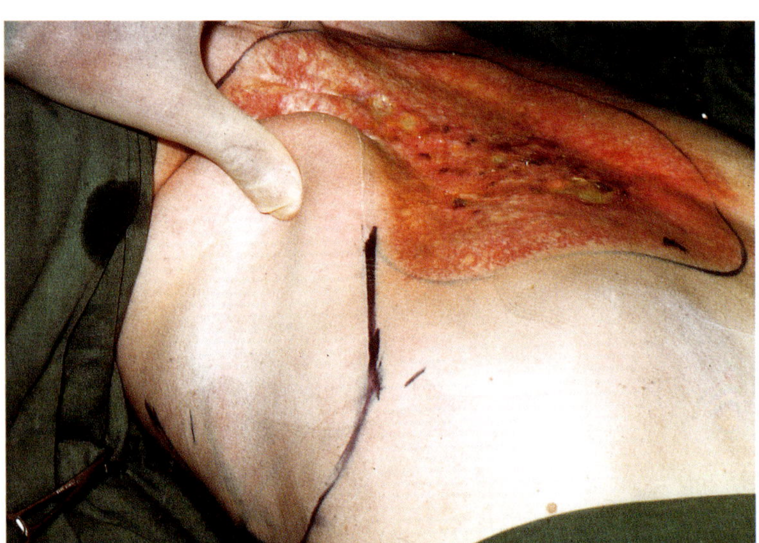

Figure 4.28c Evaluation whether the donor site can be closed primarily or whether a mesh graft is necessary for coverage.

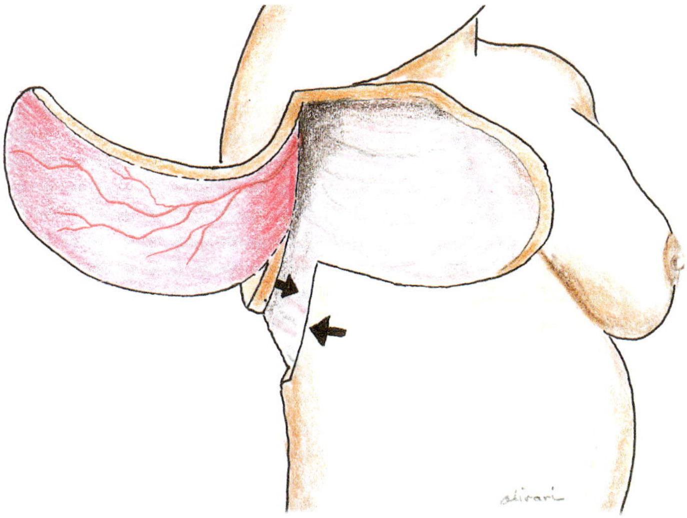

Figure 4.28d Mobilization of the latissimus flap following radical debridement. Simultaneously, extensive mobilization at the donor site is conducted extending beyond the spinal column.

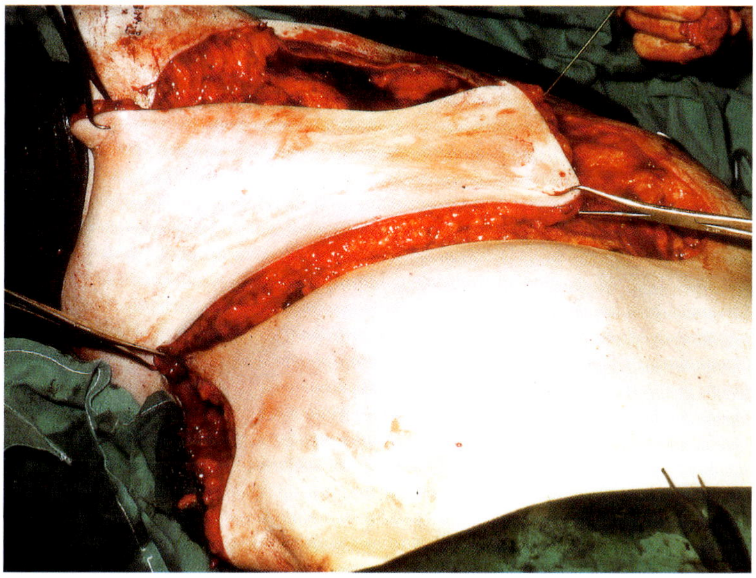

Figure 4.28e In this case, the secondary defect can be closed primarily. In situations where tension is too high it is advisable to use mesh graft.

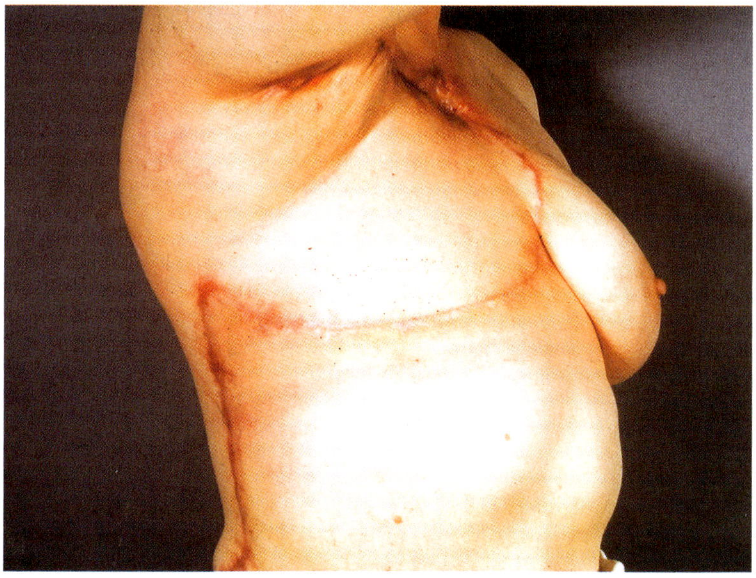

Figure 4.28f Three months postoperatively. Not quite tension-free closure at donor site with primary healing.

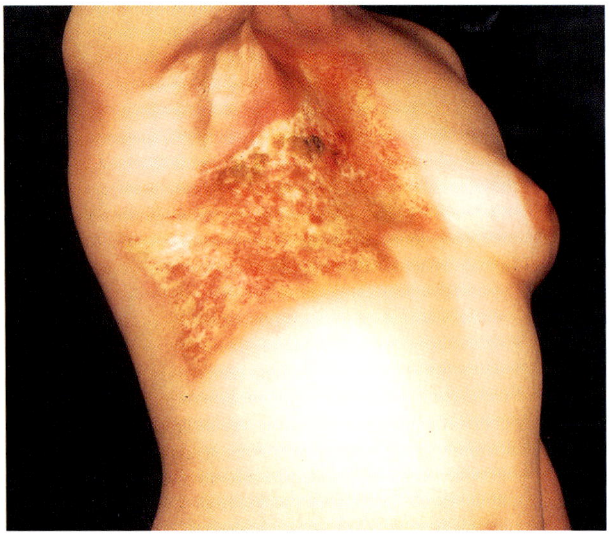

Figure 4.29a Radiodermatitis and ulcerations five years following mastectomy and radiation therapy. Patient suffered from an extremely indurated thoracic wall with concomitant breathing problems.

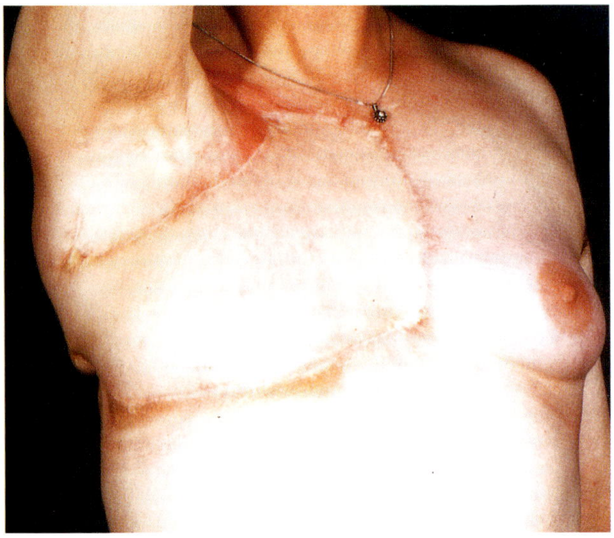

Figure 4.29b Two years postoperatively

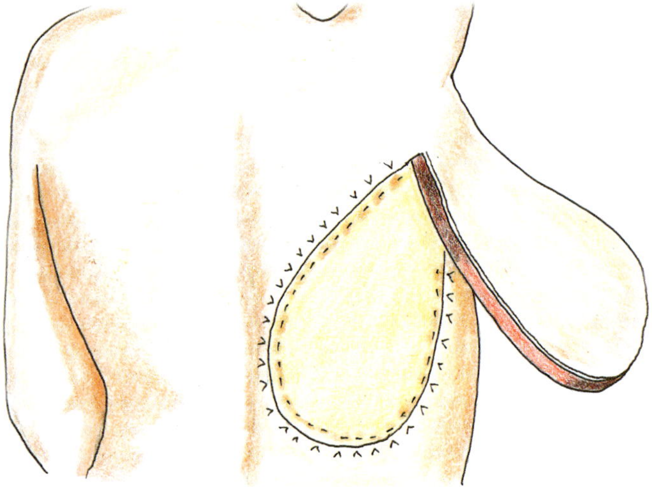

Figure 4.29c A pedicled latissimus flap (25 × 17 cm) was designed for reconstruction. The donor site was covered with mesh graft.

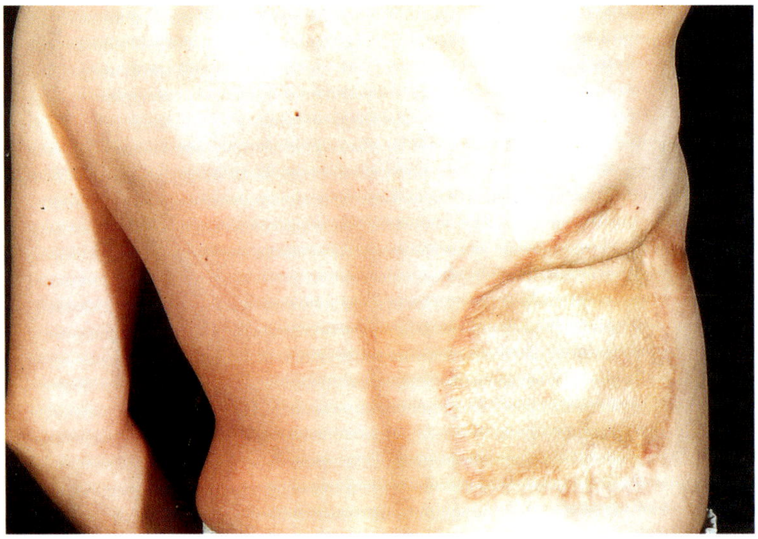

Figure 4.29d Two years postoperatively: Donor site covered with mesh graft.

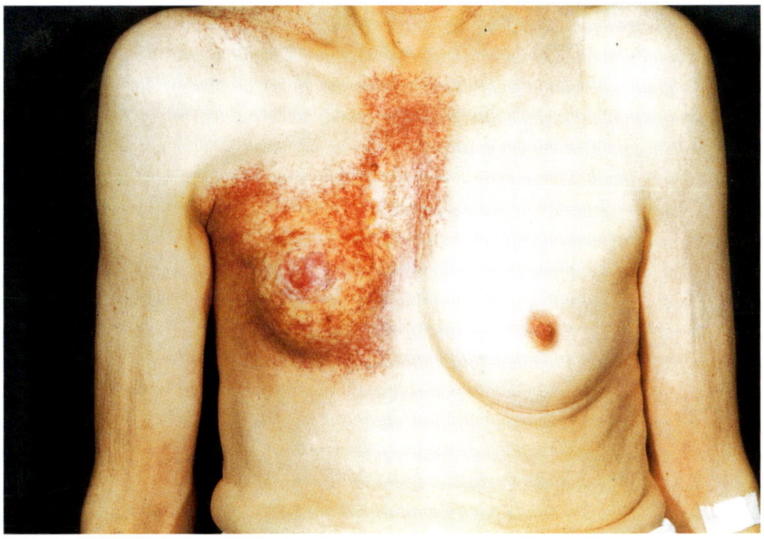

Figure 4.30a Status post quadrantectomy and postoperative radiation therapy of the right breast. The patient suffered from extensive radiation-induced fibrosis and an extremely indurated and painful breast.

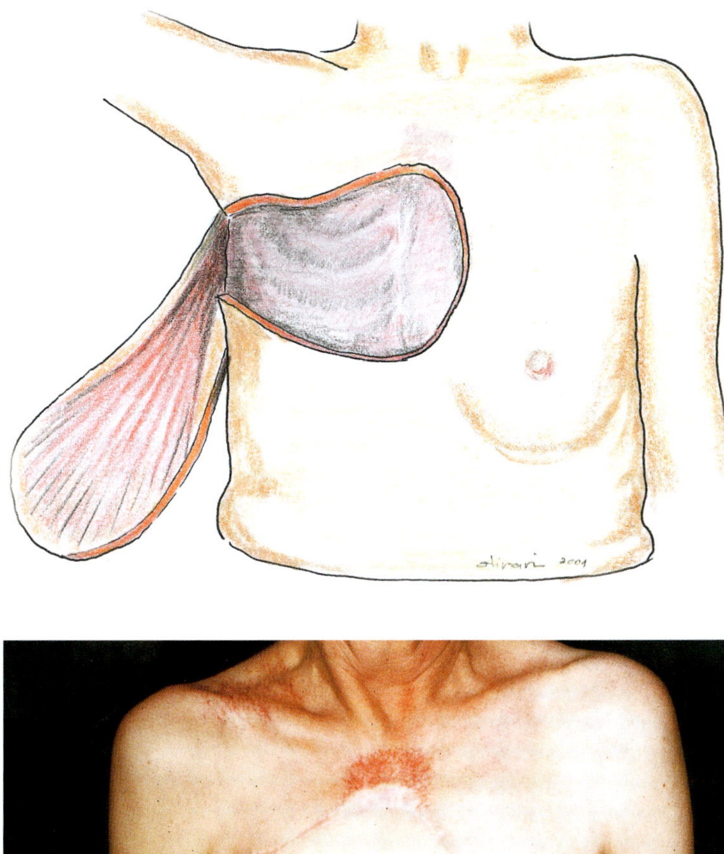

Figure 4.30b Wide excision was performed. The histopathological report revealed the existence of a carcinoma in the irradiated breast. A pedicled latissimus dorsi flap was chosen for reconstruction.

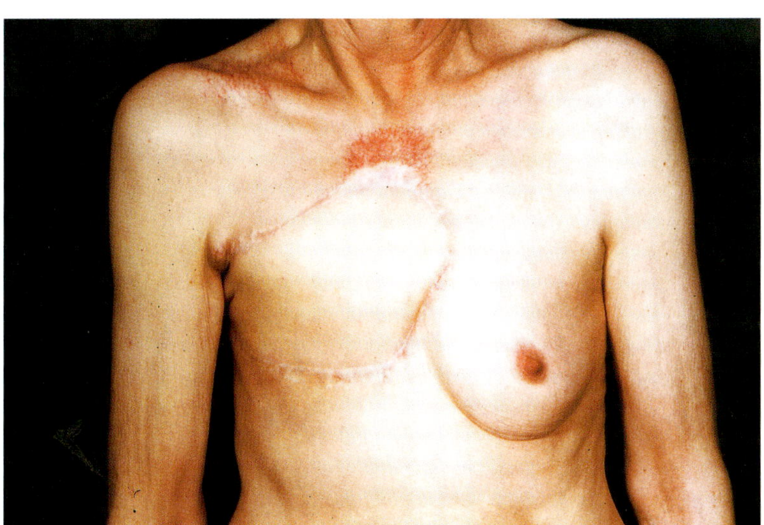

Figure 4.30c Situation one year postoperatively

Axillary Defect and Latissimus Dorsi Flap

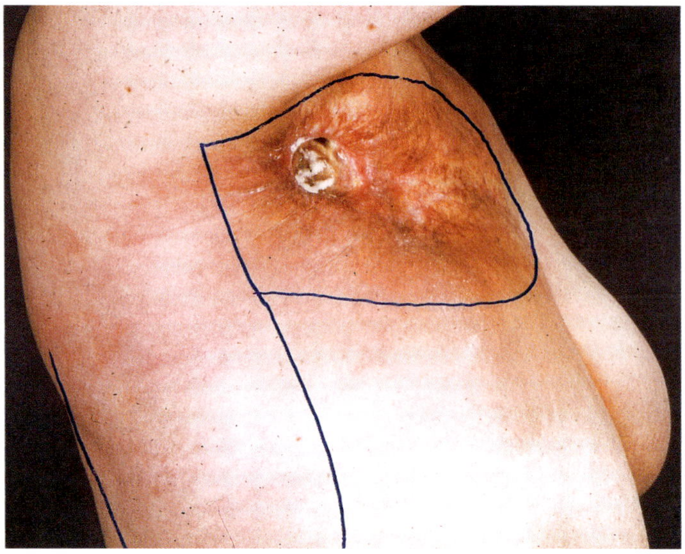

Figure 4.31a Radiodermatitis and ulcer in the right axilla and part of the thoracic wall. Complaints included recurrent purulent infections along with persistent pain and lymphedema of the right upper extremity.

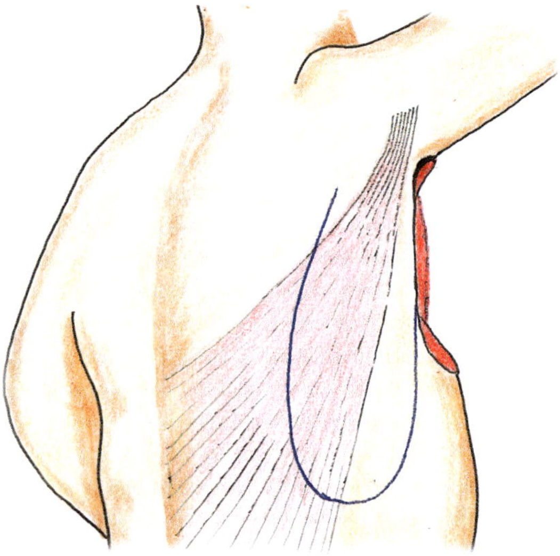

Figure 4.31b It is essential to excise the entire irradiated area. No necrotic tissue should remain. Rib excision may be required to achieve healthy deep wound margins.

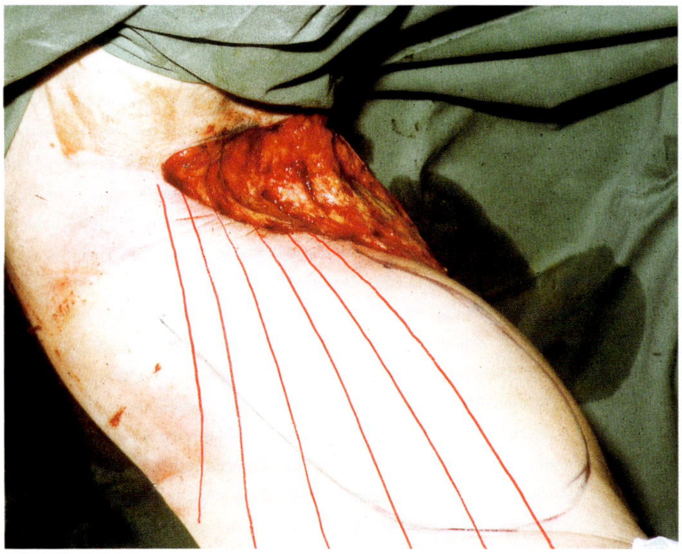

Figure 4.31c Anteriorly, small part of the flap consists only of skin and subcutaneous tissue. Dorsally it is a myocutaneous flap.

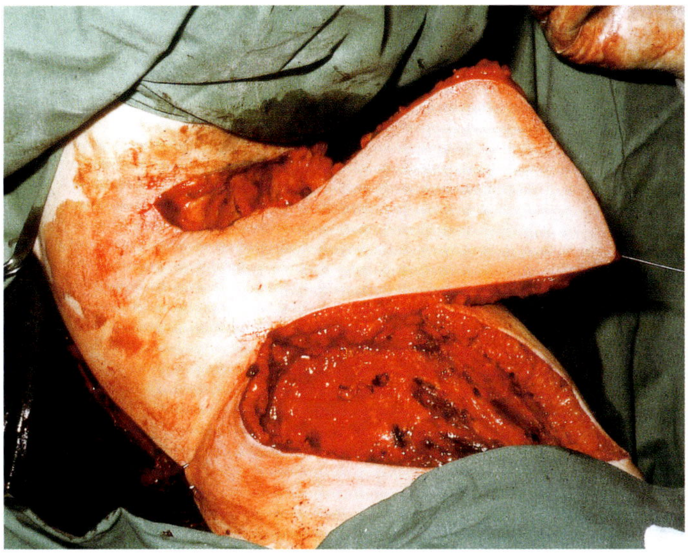

Figure 4.31d The pedicled latissimus flap is mobilized and fitted into the defect.

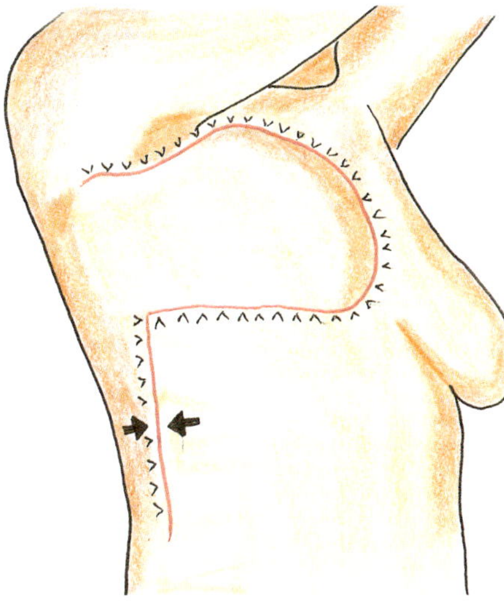

Figure 4.31e The latissimus flap is very suitable for defects located in the axilla. The donor site in this case can be closed primarily. Mobilization is performed predominantly in dorsal direction.

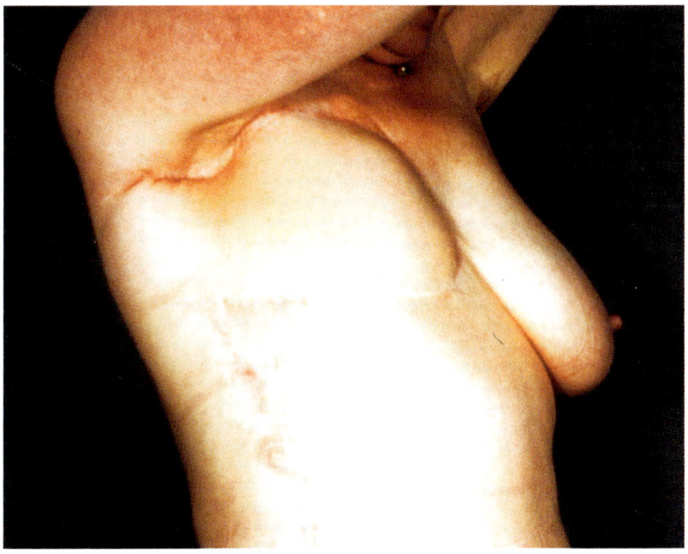

Figure 4.31f Four-and-a-half years postoperatively. The patient is pain-free. Reduction of upper arm circumference (4 cm) is noted documenting relief of complaints caused by lymphedema. Lymphatic drainage improved significantly following excision of inflamed axillary tissue.

Largest Latissimus Dorsi Flap

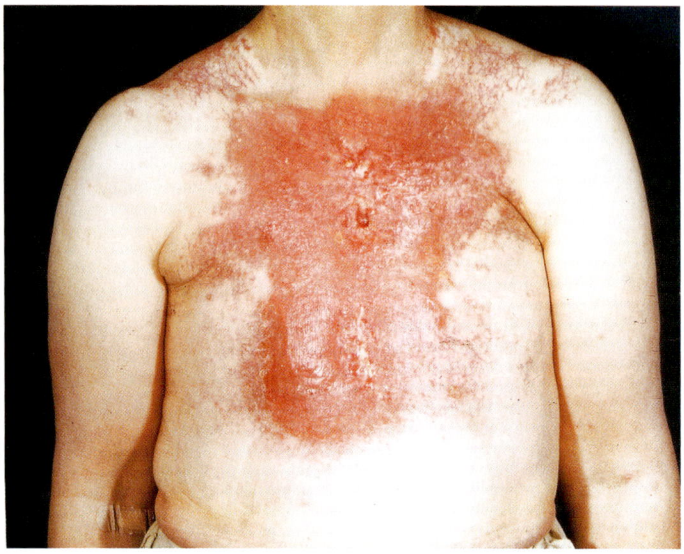

Figure 4.32a Extensive radiodermatitis with multiple ulcerations taking up the entire anterior thorax. Intoxication with subsequent renal damage due to abuse high pain medication.

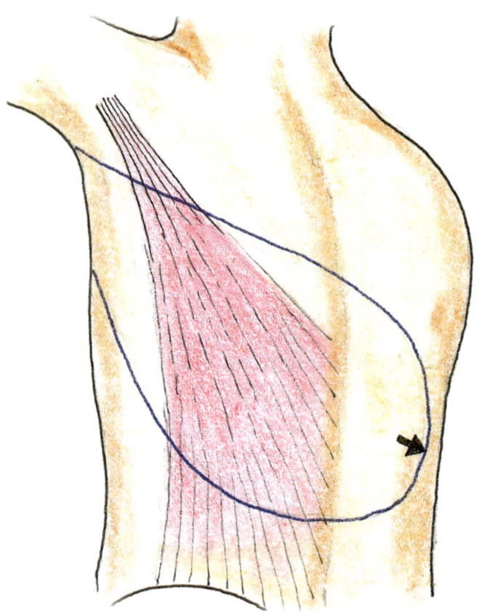

Figure 4.32b A pedicle latissimus dorsi flap (38 × 26 cm) is designed. This is the largest published latissimus dorsi flap. The flap is raised extending beyond the midline of the back. The distal part of the flap displays a random pattern perfusion without an axial component. However, it is a safe flap for extremely large defects.

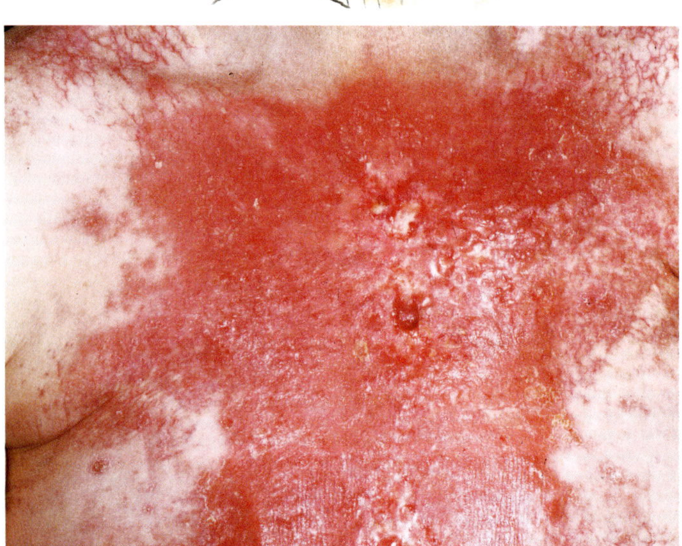

Figure 4.32c Close-up view of the area displaying ulcerations as well as signs of radiodermatitis.

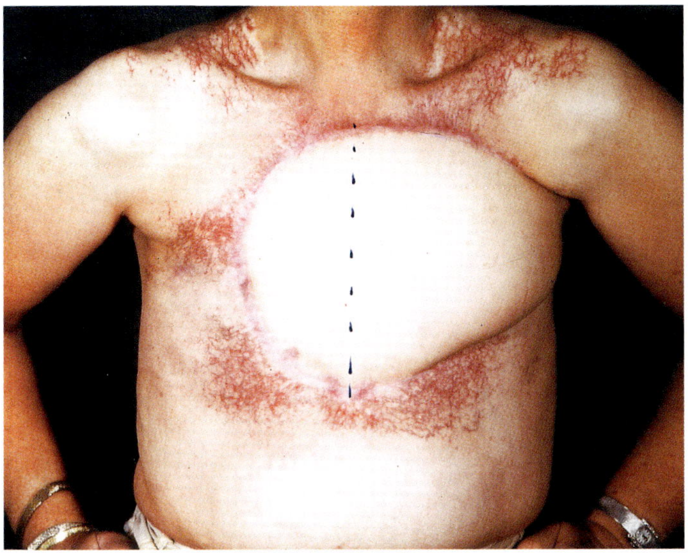

Figure 4.32d Eight months postoperatively. The latissimus flap extends far beyond the midline covering the contralateral thoracic wall. Flap size: 38 x 26 cm.

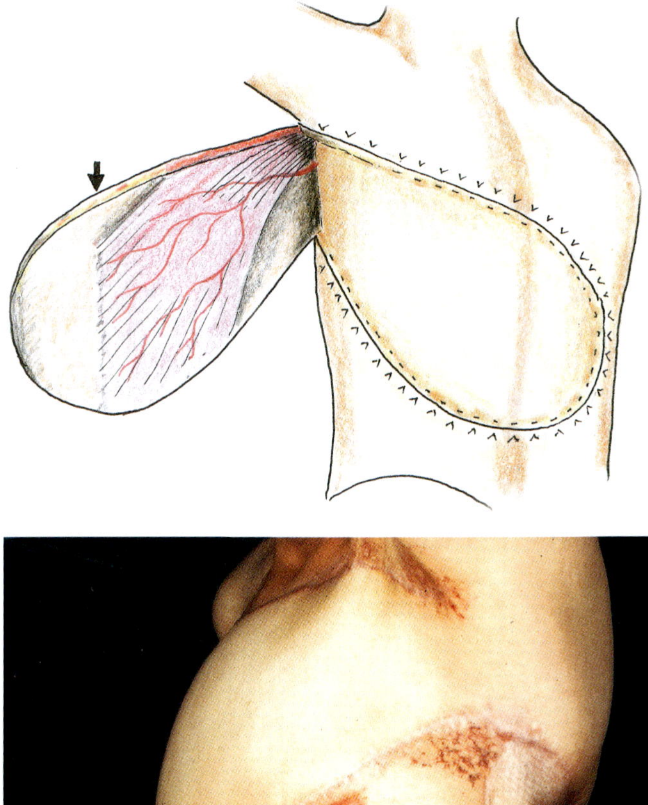

Figure 4.32e A latissimus flap extending far beyond the midline (in this particular case 15 cm) is considered safe. The donor site covered with mesh graft.

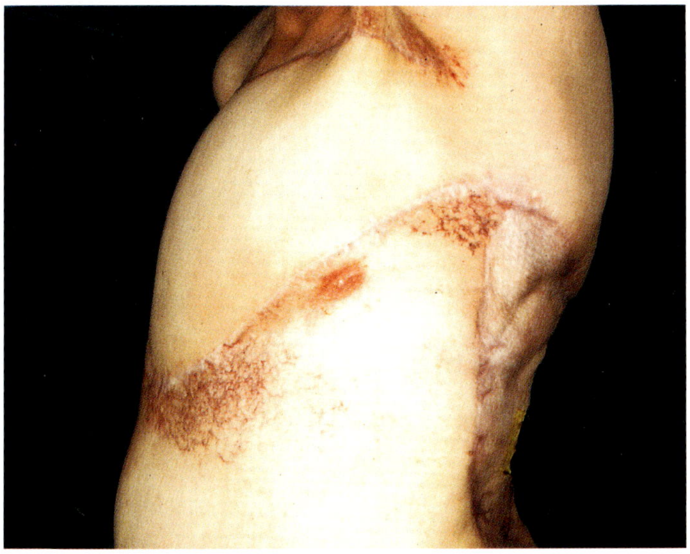

Figure 4.32f Situation eight months postoperatively. The patient is pain-free.

Pedicled Latissimus Dorsi Flap for Coverage of Defects of the Thoracic Wall (Including Rib Defects)

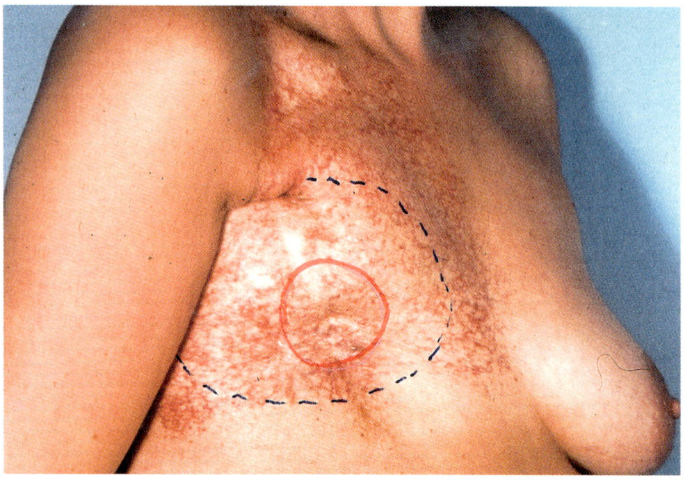

Figure 4.33a Situation five years following mastectomy and postoperative radiation therapy. Diagnosis: Radiodermatitis and small ulcerations, local recurrence of breast cancer (red circle).

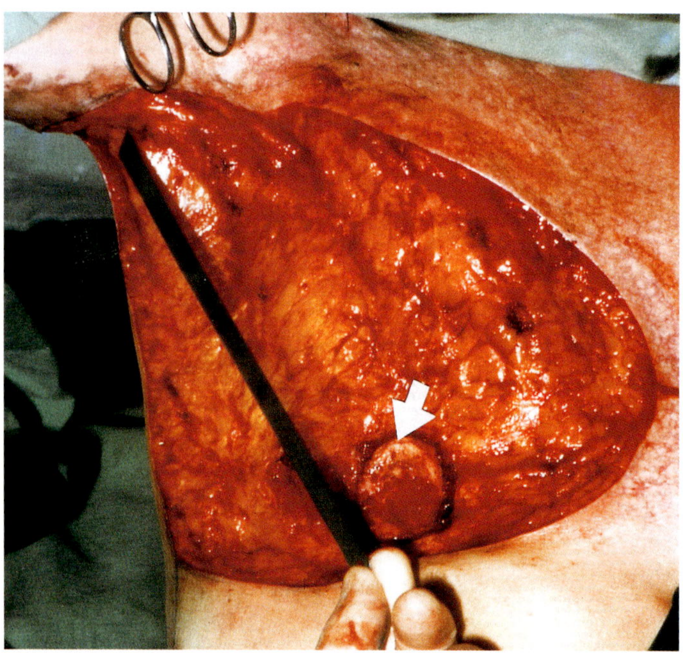

Figure 4.33b Status post excision of irradiated and damaged tissues. Immediate histopathological sectioning revealed breast cancer recurrence extending into the intercostal space. Thus, a full thickness thoracic wall resection including four ribs was performed.

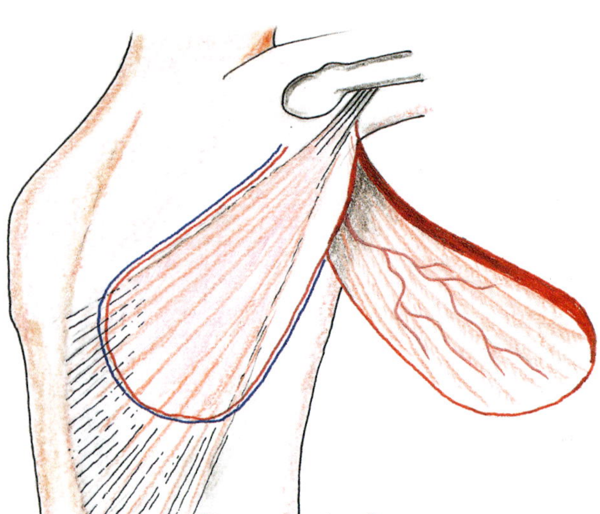

Figure 4.33c A standard pedicled myocutaneous latissimus flap is designed.

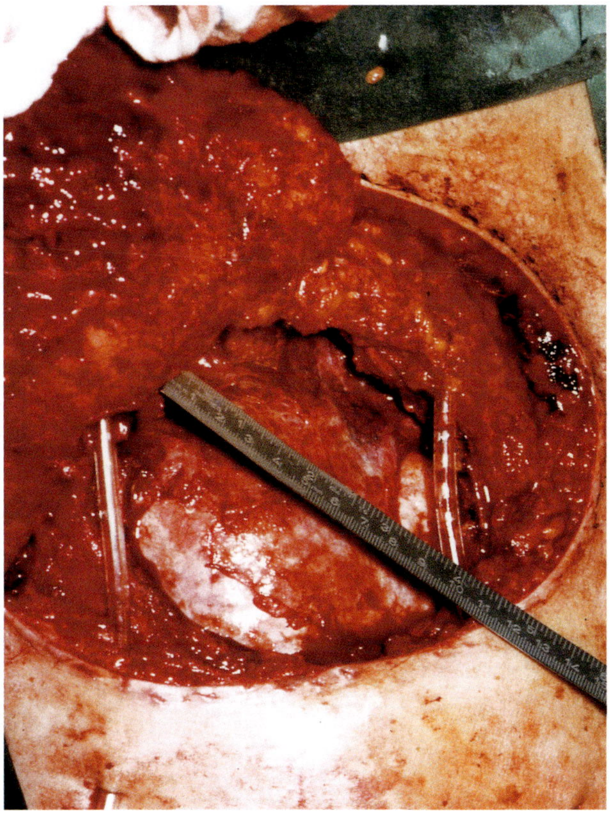

Figure 4.33d Status post tumor and thoracic wall resection (including four ribs). The visceral pleura is exposed.

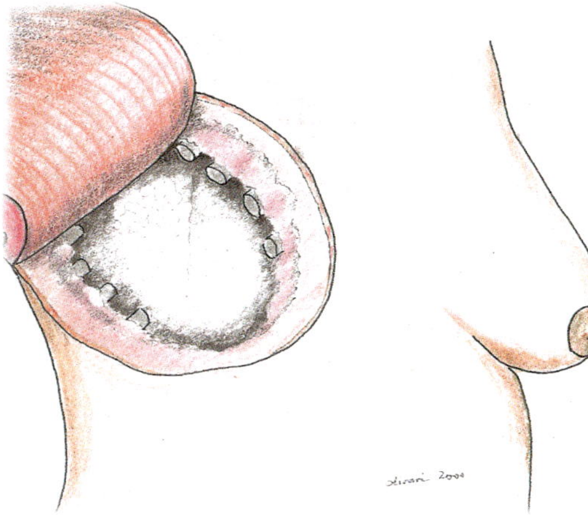

Figure 4.33e Reconstruction of the open thoracic wall with a latissimus flap

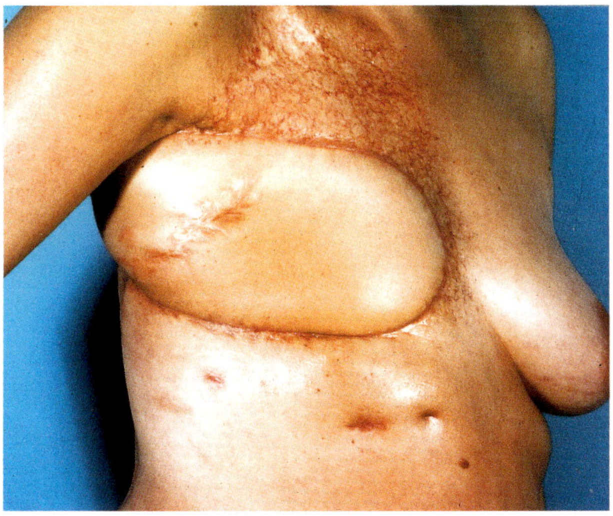

Figure 4.33f The patient had no relapse at nine years after operation.

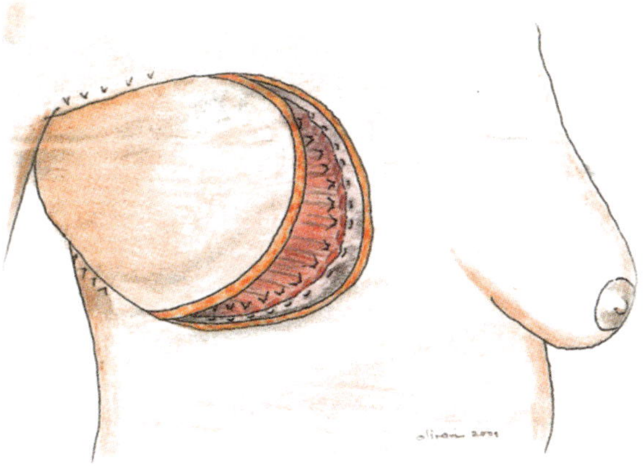

Figure 4.33g Important: First, the latissimus dorsi muscle is meticulously sutured to the intercostals muscles for sealing the thoracic cage. Then the skin is closed. The scar seen on the flap is caused by a trauma many years ago. Vacuum drainage is applied for approx. six to ten days in order to promote adherence of the visceral pleura to the latissimus dorsi muscle.

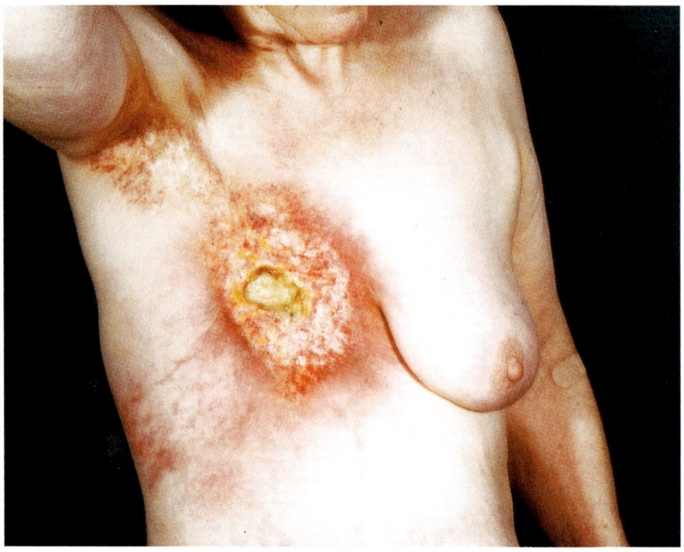

Figure 4.34a Radiation ulcer with necrosis of four ribs, chronic infections, and intense persistent pain. Status post mastectomy and postoperative radiation therapy eight years ago. Radiation injuries frequently occur eight to ten years following treatment.

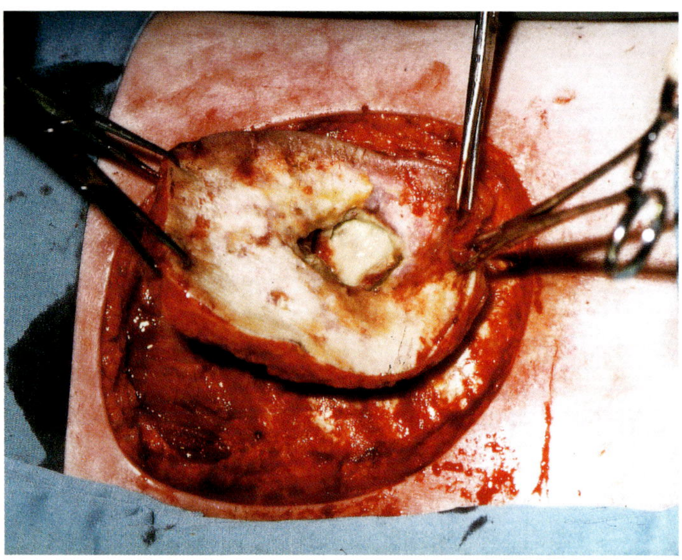

Figure 4.34b Operative plan: First radical excision of necrotic tissue and infected tissue including four ribs is performed.

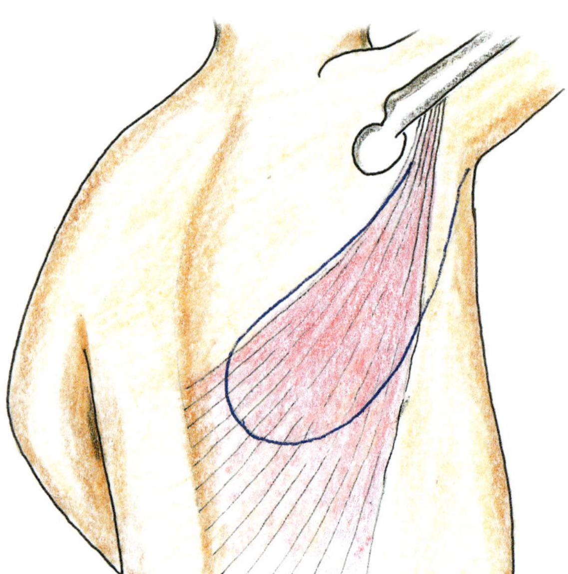

Figure 4.34c Thoracodorsal artery was no longer present due to the high-dose radiation therapy conducted. Thus, designing the latissimus flap as an island flap was not indicated.

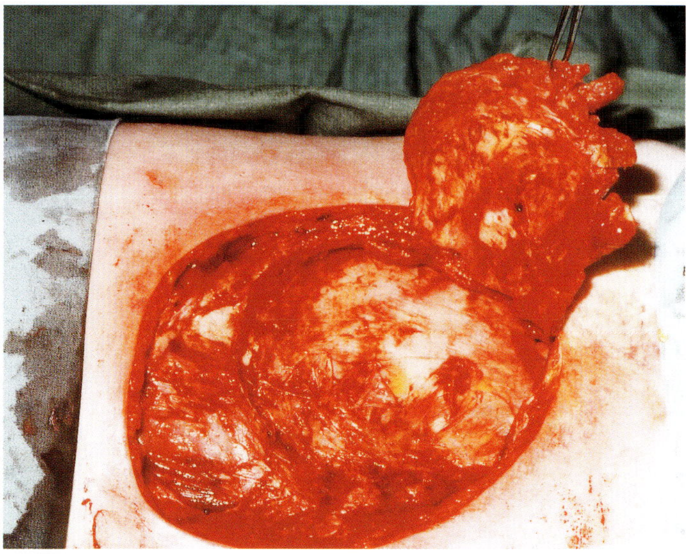

Figure 4.34d Four ribs including the intercostals are removed. The underlying visceral pleura is firmly adherent to the thoracic wall demonstrating adhesion of lung following radiation.

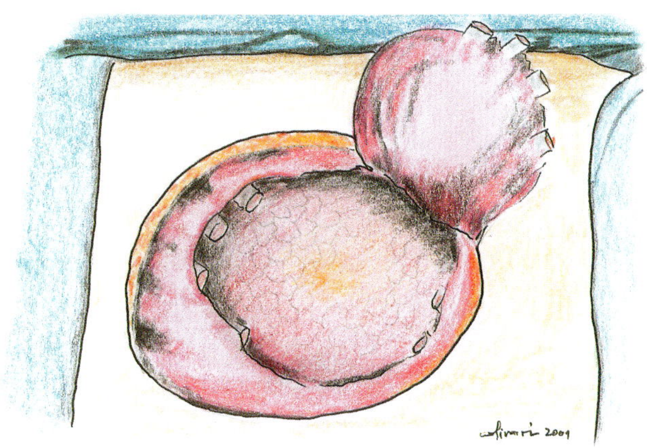

Figure 4.34e Following radical excision of necrotic tissue including ribs clean wound margins are seen along with exposed visceral pleura.

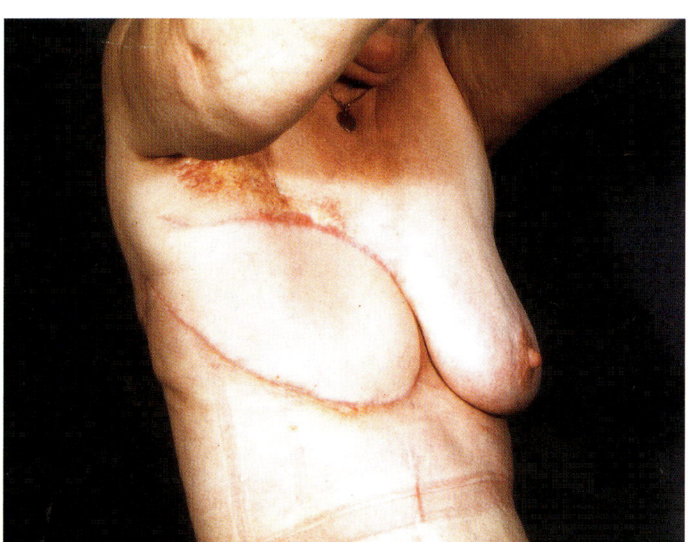

Figure 4.34f Appearance five months postoperatively. The donor site was closed primarily.

Latissimus Dorsi Flap Transfer as a Life-Saving Procedure

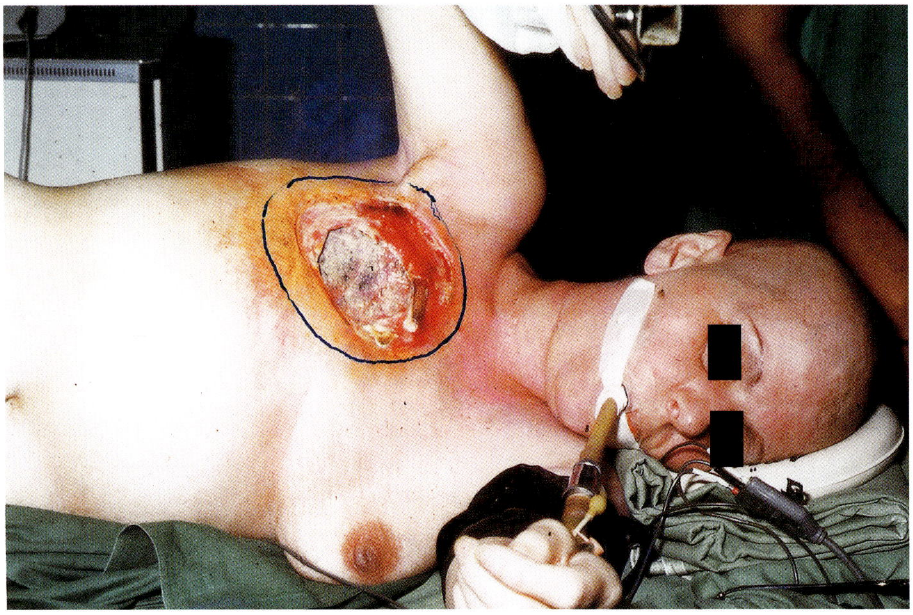

Figure 4.35a A patient post mastectomy and cobalt radiation therapy (presumably overdosed). Initially, the skin exhibited signs of necrosis, then, sequestrae in four ribs were noted. Finally, the patient was transferred to the operating room in clinically critical condition with multiple perforations of the visceral pleura.

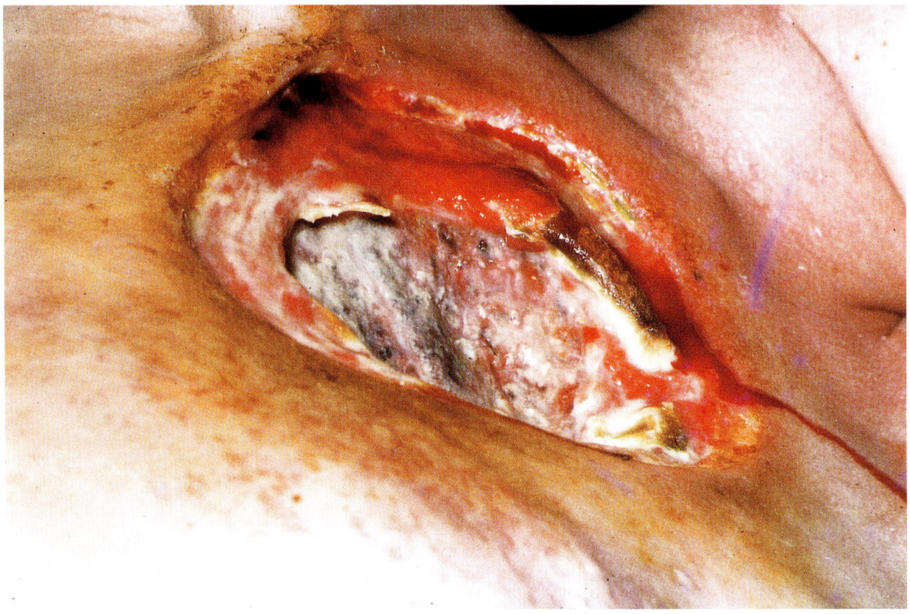

Figure 4.35b Rib edges can be seen with exposed visceral pleura. Multiple perforations on the surface of lung cause whistling sounds. The entire area is infected.

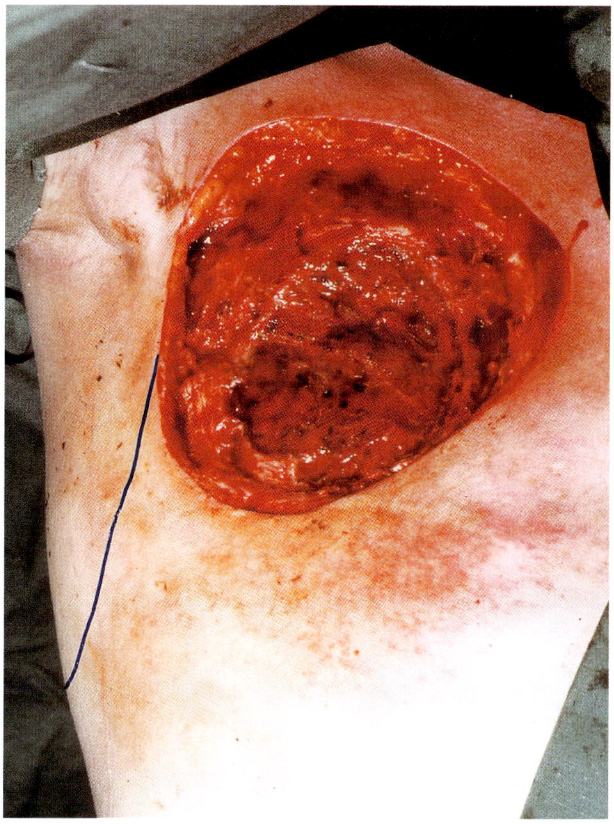

Figure 4.35c The most essential step of this procedure is complete excision of the necrotic tissue. Rib edges were removed and tissue displaying signs of vascular impairment were widely excised. The infected lung surface was debrided until healthy tissue was visualized. Even with the use of fibrin glue it was not possible to seal up the existent lung fistulas.

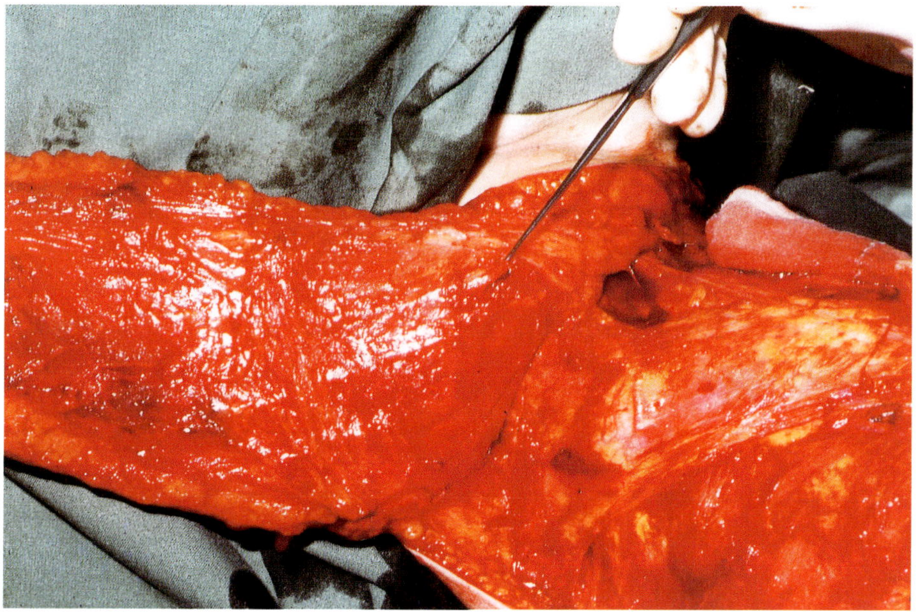

Figure 4.35d Despite massive irradiation the thoracodorsal artery was present.

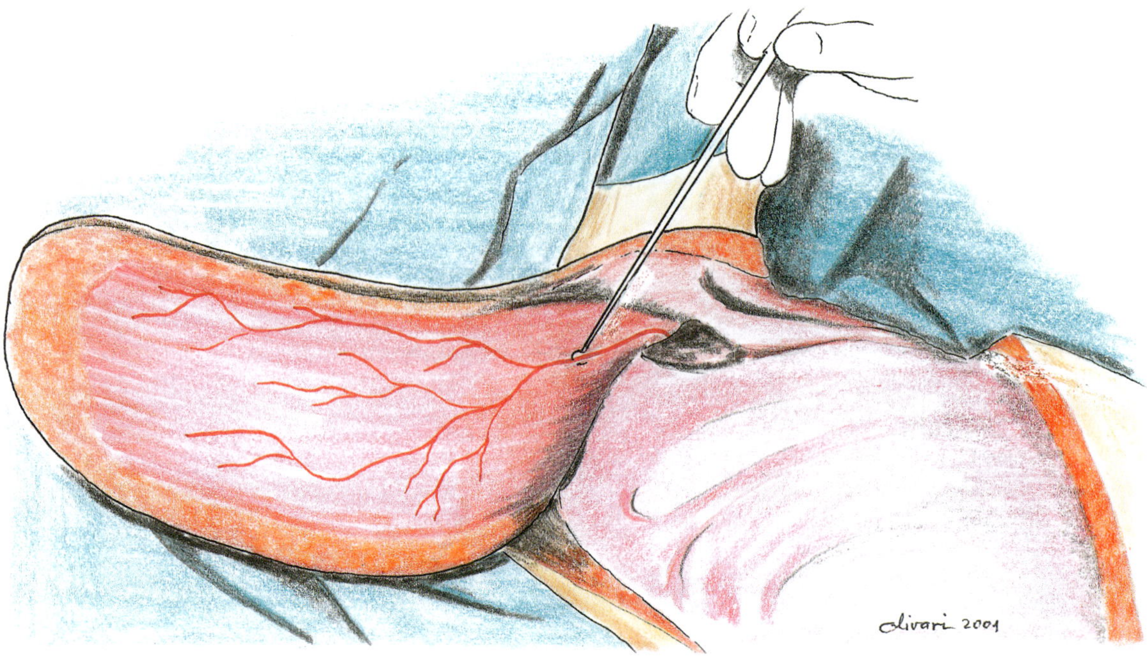

Figure 4.35e With the thoracodorsal artery present the flap displays excellent perfusion despite high-dose irradiation.

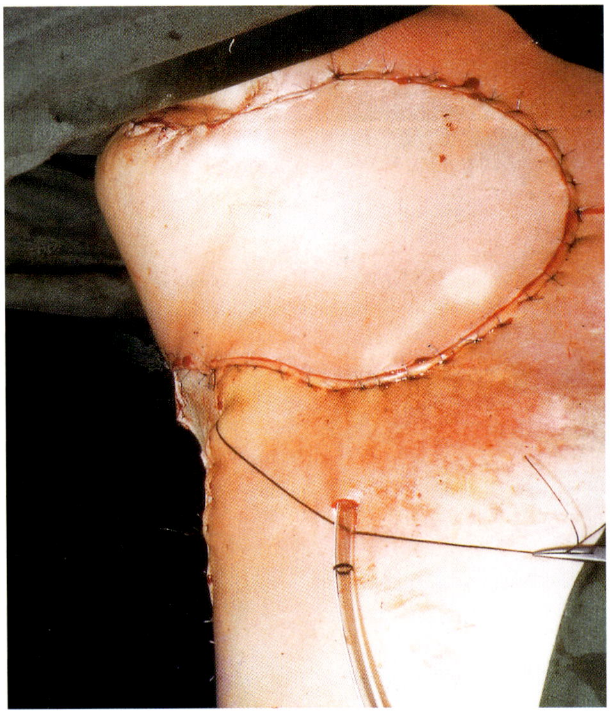

Figure 4.35f Due to existent lung fistulas positive pressure was noted between the flap and lung following reconstruction. After two weeks of closed pleural drainage (Buelau's method) the lung surface adhered to the latissimus dorsi muscle. One-third of the donor site could be closed primarily, the remaining two-thirds requiring mesh graft.

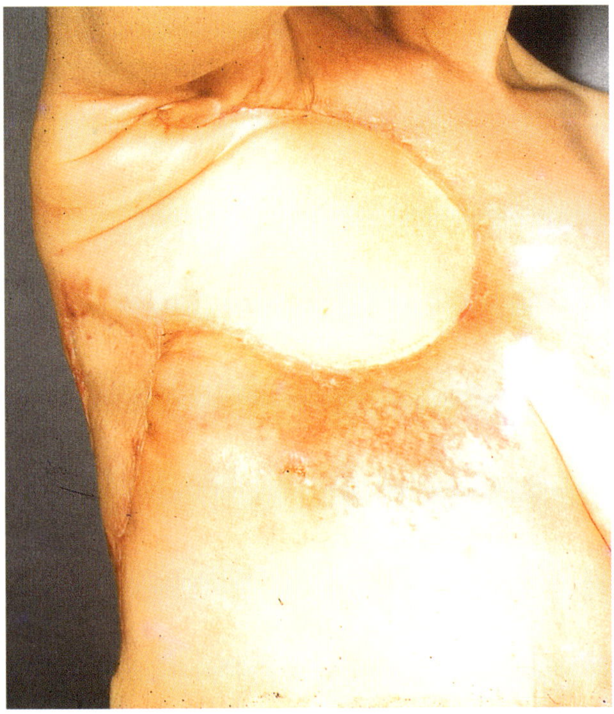

Figure 4.35g Picture taken eight months postoperatively. Evident recovery of patient. The patient gained eight kilograms of weight.

Pedicled Latissimus Dorsi Flap And Thoracic Wall Defects (Caused by Use of Intra-arterial Local Chemotherapy)

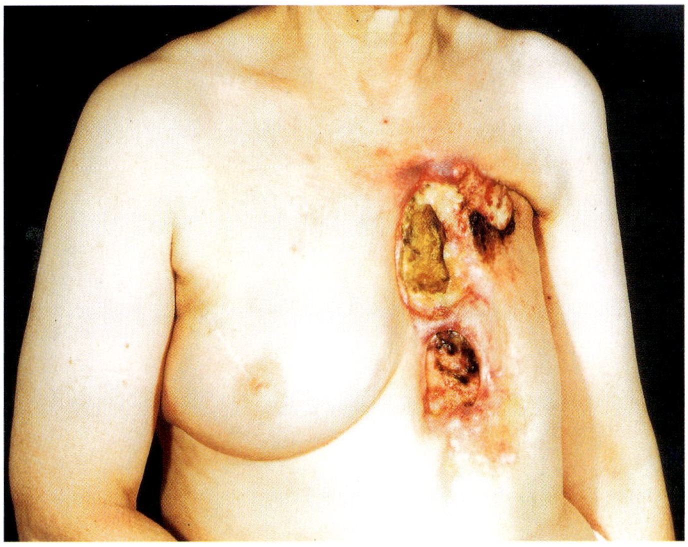

Figure 4.36a Special indication – Diagnosis: Status post mastectomy of the left breast. Local recurrence affecting the thoracic wall. Treatment consisted of selective intra arterial chemotherapy with resultant extensive necrosis and infection.

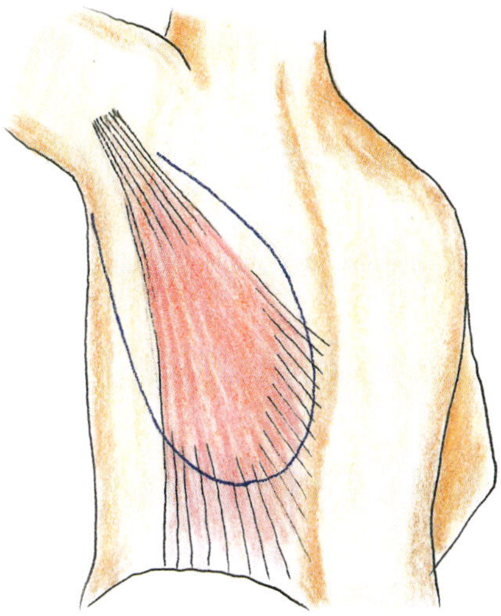

Figure 4.36b Following radical debridement, reconstruction is performed with a pedicled latissimus flap. Due to flap dimension the donor site is grafted with mesh graft.

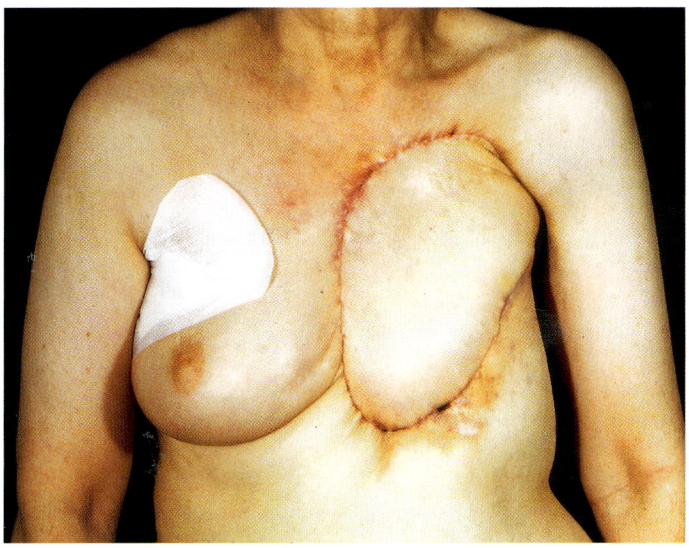

Figure 4.36c Four weeks postoperatively. At this point the patient was readmitted to the oncological service.

Pedicled Latissimus Flap – Long-Term Results

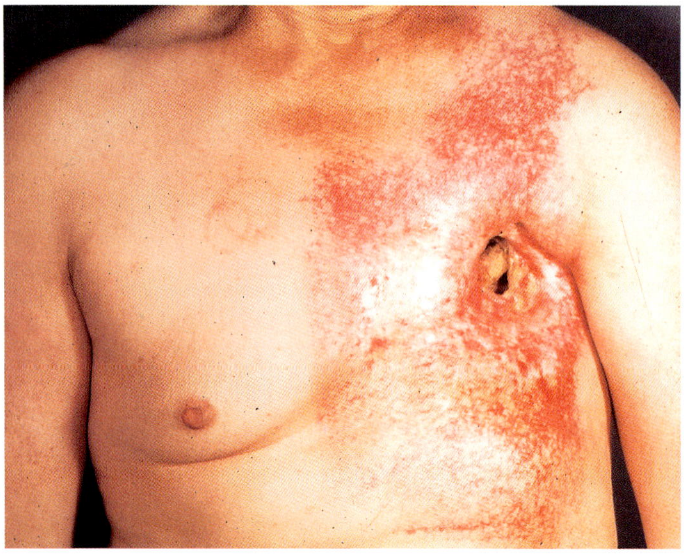

Figure 4.37a Status post mastectomy and radiation therapy. Left-sided radiodermatitis and radiation ulcer. Three ribs are necrotic. Pleura and pericardium are infected.

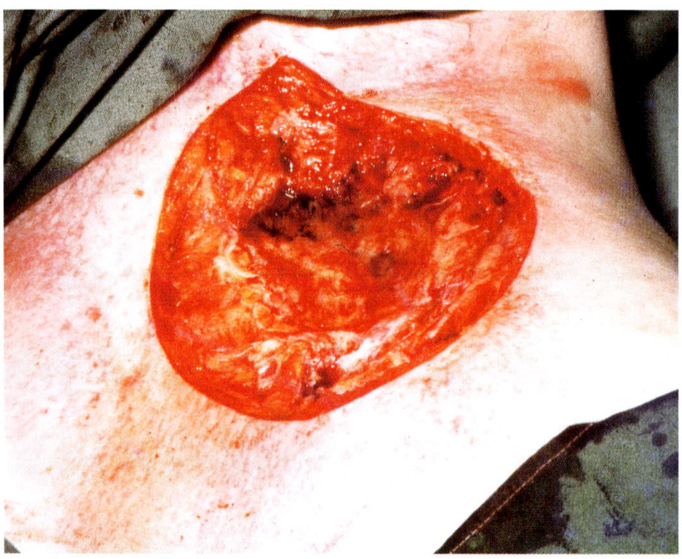

Figure 4.37b Debridement of the affected area. Three ribs are removed. The TDA was not available following mastectomy with subsequent radiation therapy.

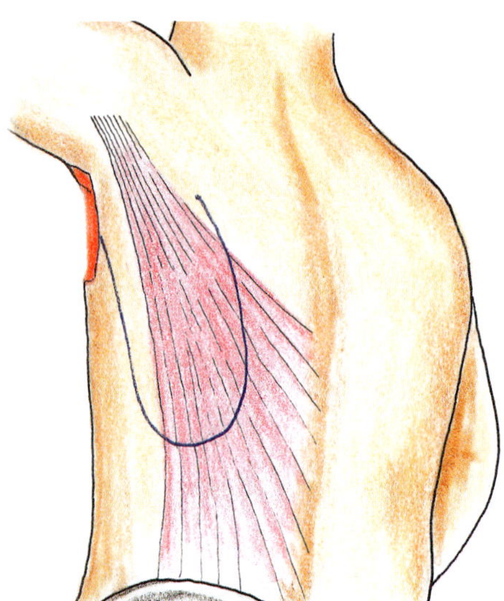

Figure 4.37c Design of a pedicled latissimus flap

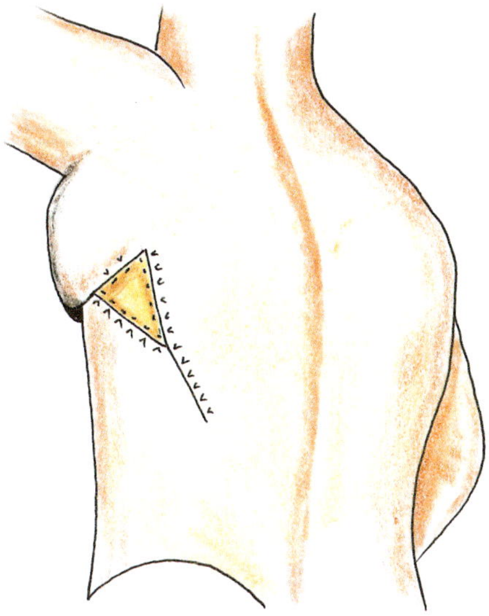

Figure 4.37d The donor site is closed primarily except a small area cranially requiring split skin graft.

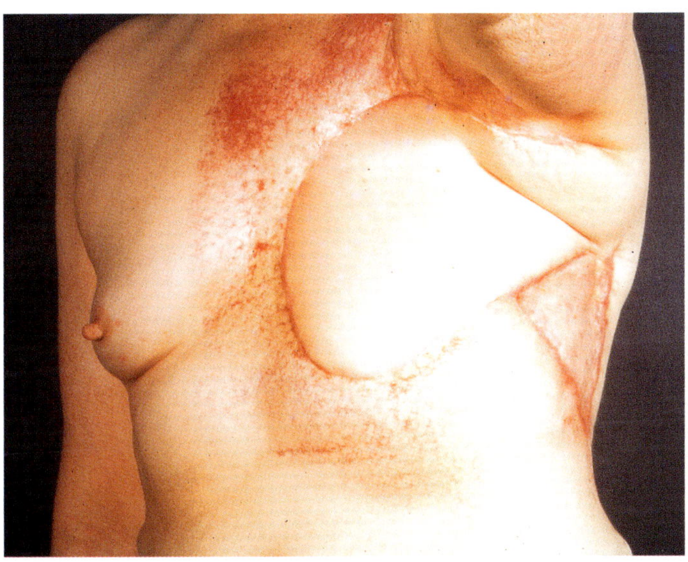

Figure 4.37e One year postoperatively

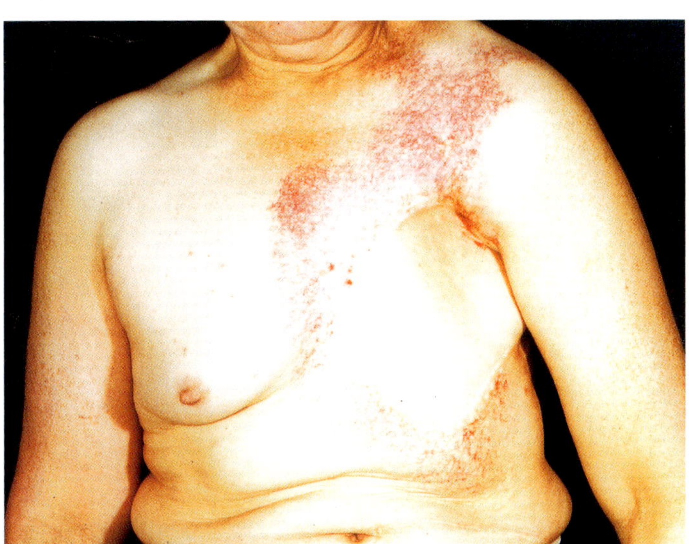

Figure 4.37f Eleven years postoperatively

Pedicled Latissimus Flap and Design Modifications

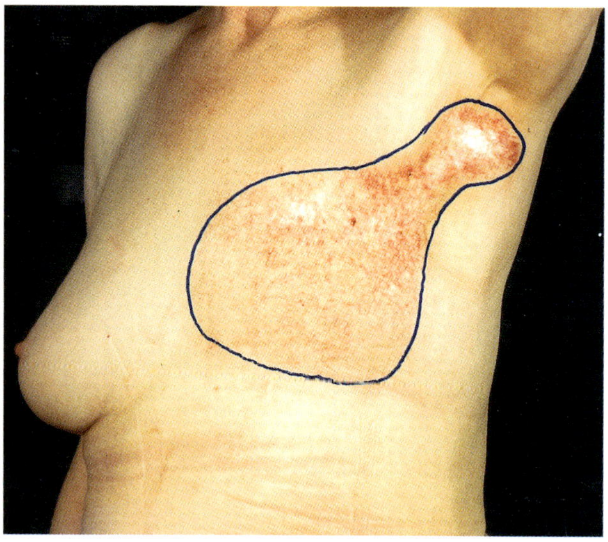

Figure 4.38a Status post mastectomy and radiation therapy. Radiodermatitis of the left axilla and thoracic wall. A pear-shaped defect results following excision.

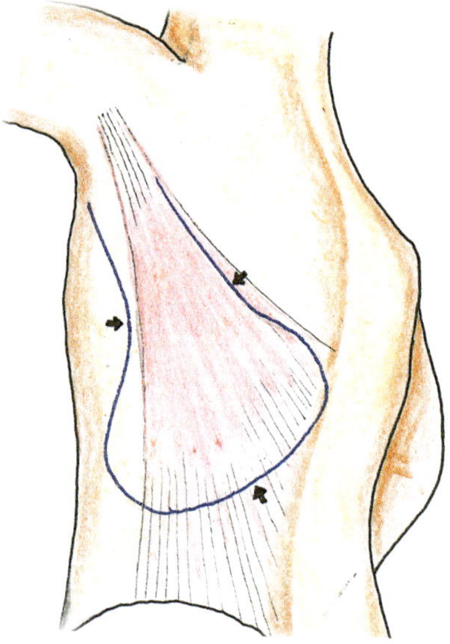

Figure 4.38b A pear-shaped flap is designed with a narrow base for coverage of the axilla and a broad tip for the anterior thorax

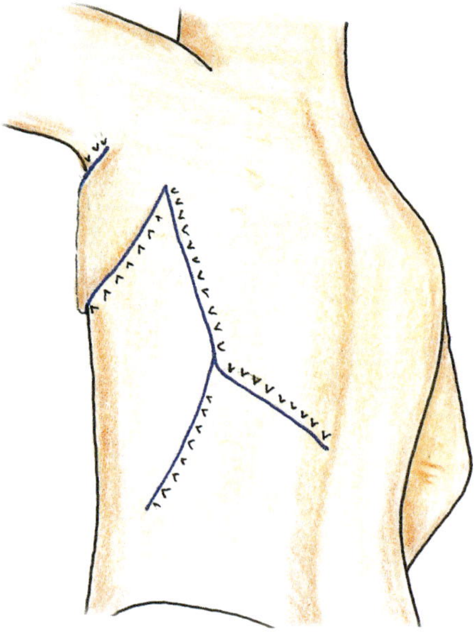

Figure 4.38c Primary closure of donor site

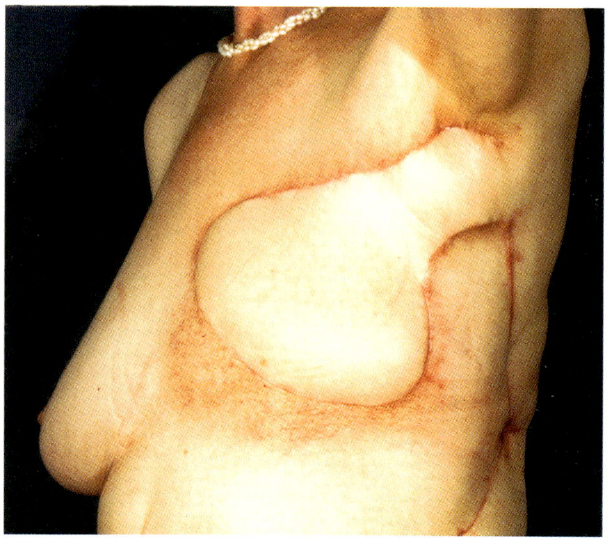

Figure 4.38d Three months postoperatively. The latissimus flap is versatile allowing a design fitting the individual needs.

b) Latissimus Dorsi Island Flap

Reconstruction of Thoracic Wall Defects

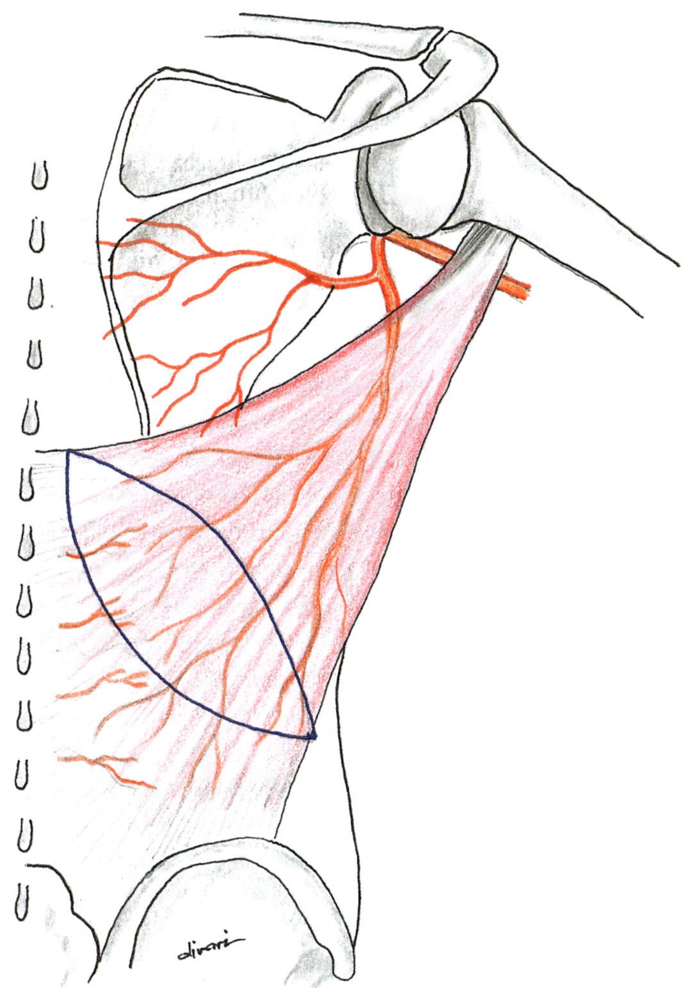

Figure 4.39 Note the orientation of the skin island, which allows design of larger flaps with a larger arc of rotation as well as aesthetically more appealing scars. Flap direction is from cranially-medially to laterally-caudally. The donor site can usually be closed primarily without considerable tension.

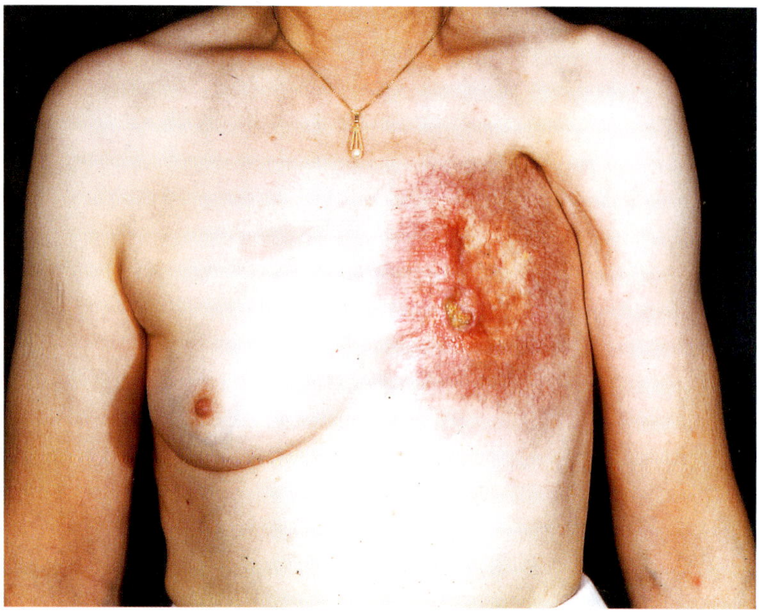

Figure 4.40a Radiodermatitis and ulcerations following mastectomy and radiation therapy. History: Six years. Symptoms: Chronic infections, pain, and shortness of breath.

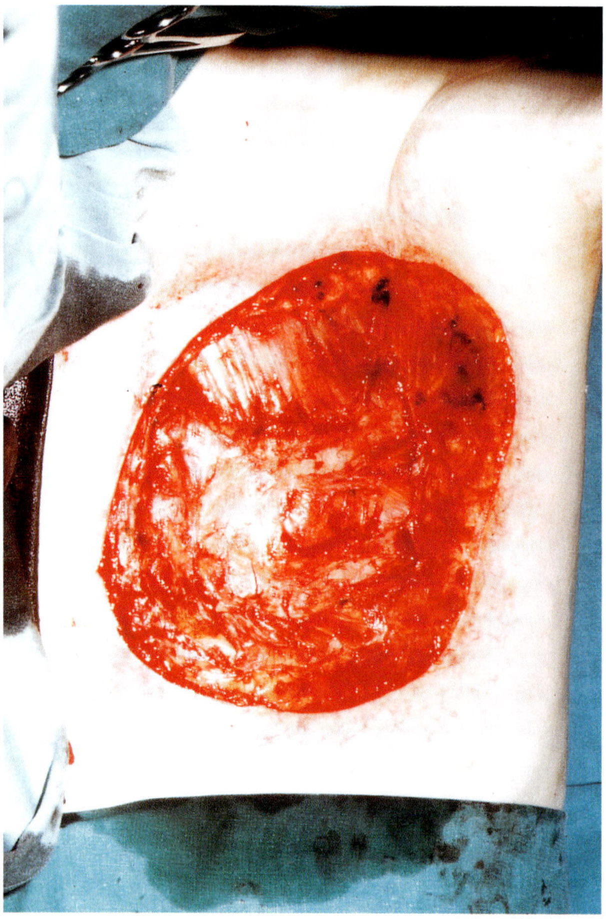

Figure 4.40b Radical debridement is essential for uneventful wound healing. Ribs were not involved. Due to an existing lobular carcinoma in situ of the right breast a subcutaneous mastectomy was performed.

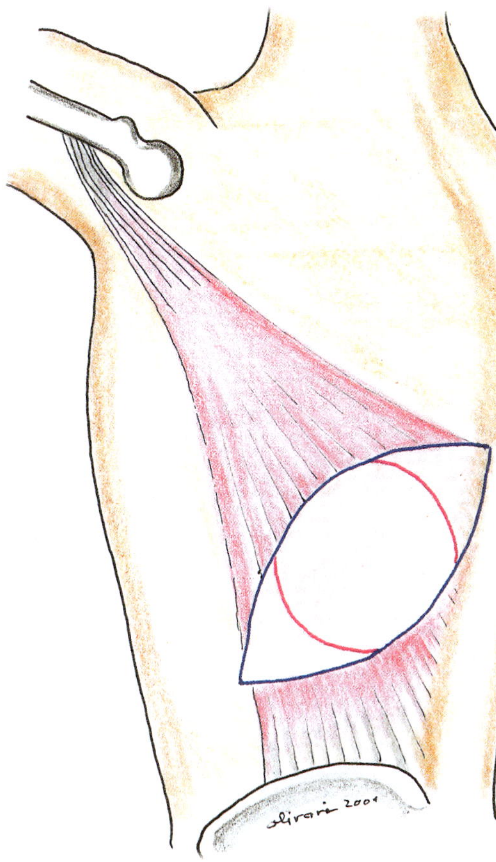

Figure 4.40c The latissimus island flap is dissected. Note the position and orientation of the flap. The "spindle-shaped" island allows for an easy primary closure of the donor site. Following creation of a subcutaneous tunnel the flap is transposed anteriorly for coverage.

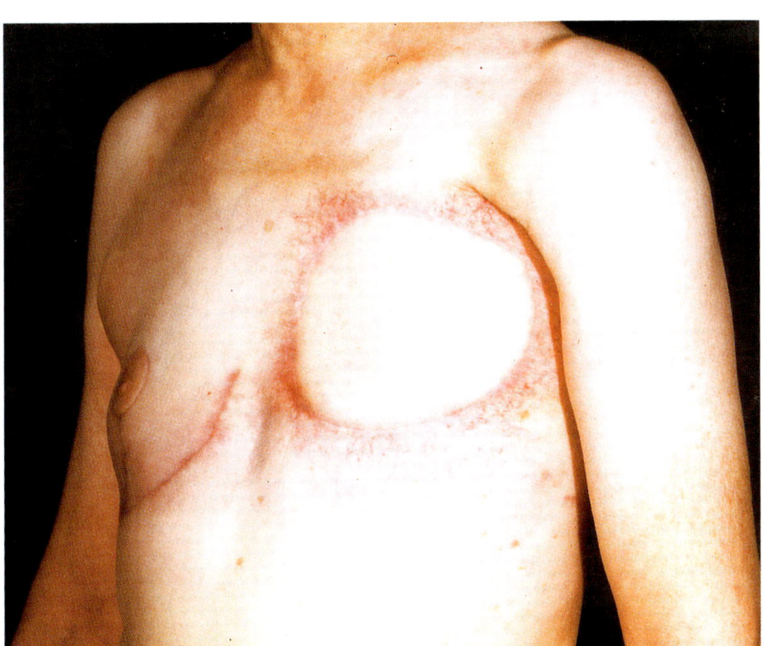

Figure 4.40d Fourteen months postoperatively. Right breast: Status post subcutaneous mastectomy. The patient was free of local and distant metastases at this point but did not wish to have a breast reconstruction performed.

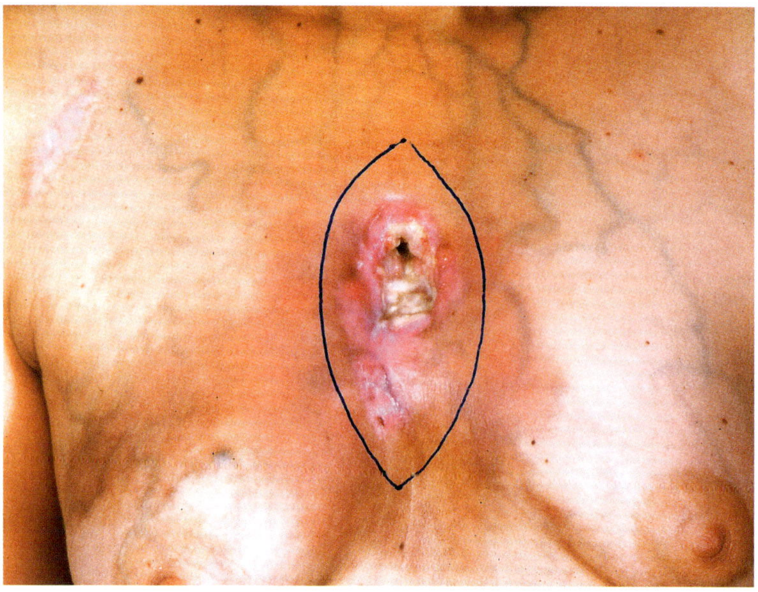

Figure 4.41a Hodgkin's disease – status post radiation and chemotherapy. The sternum, four ribs, as well as tissue in the anterior mediastinum are partially necrotic. Infection and necrosis existed for one year. The patient lost seven kilograms of body weight. Her general condition was progressively deteriorating.

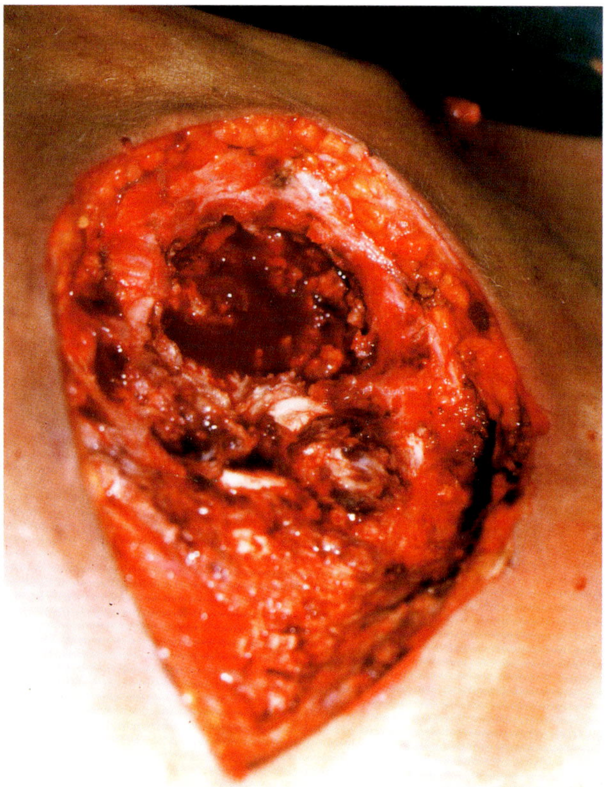

Figure 4.41b Partial resection of the sternum (inferior two-thirds) as well as bilateral partial resection of four ribs has been performed. Debridement of the anterior mediastinum has been done. Meticulous dissection is mandatory due to the complex anatomy and the damage done by the chronic infection.

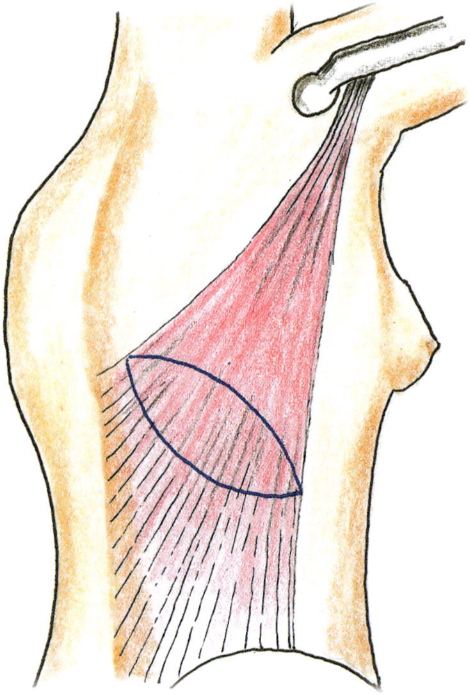

Figure 4.41c Design of latissimus island flap. **Note** flap direction!

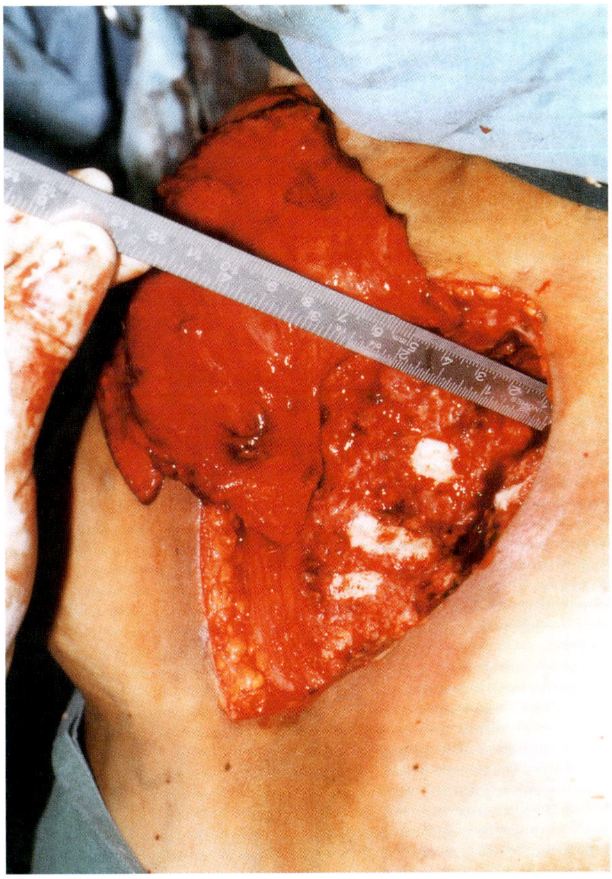

Figure 4.41d Situation after removal part of sternum and several ribs. A 20 × 9 cm defect of the anterior chest with a depth of 6 cm is the result of the preceding debridement.

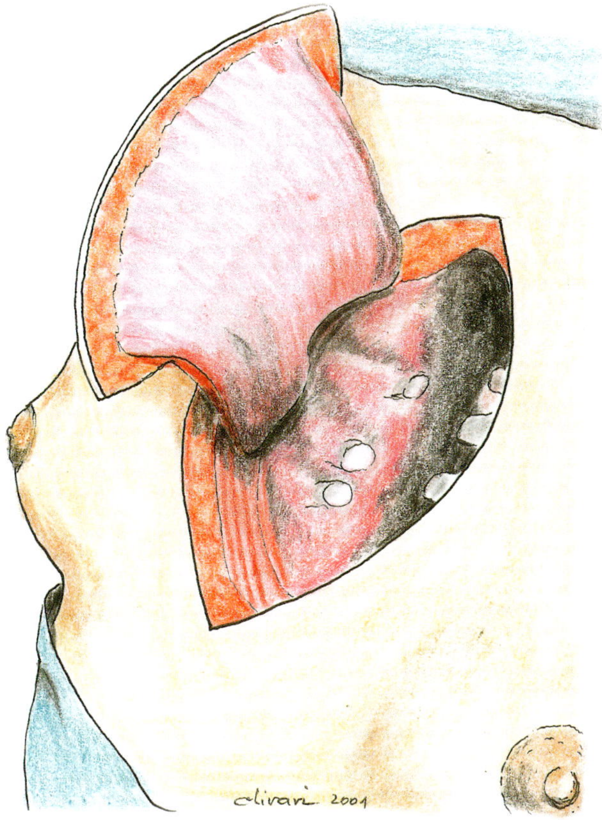

Figure 4.41e After elevation the latissimus island flap is passed through a subcutaneous tunnel from the right side for defect coverage of the anterior chest.

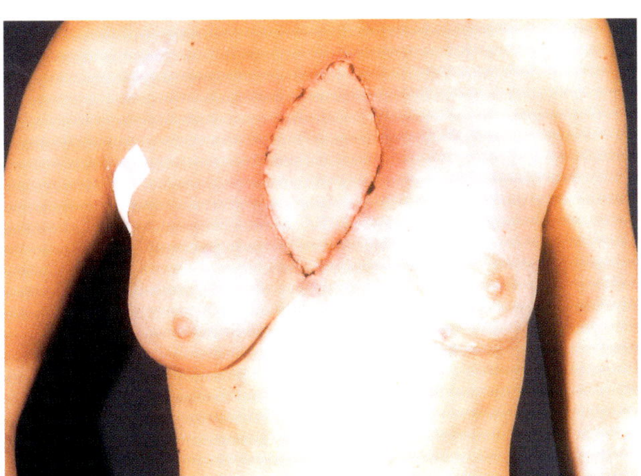

Figure 4.41f Two weeks postoperatively. Rapid recovery following treatment. The patient gained five kilograms of body weight within three months.

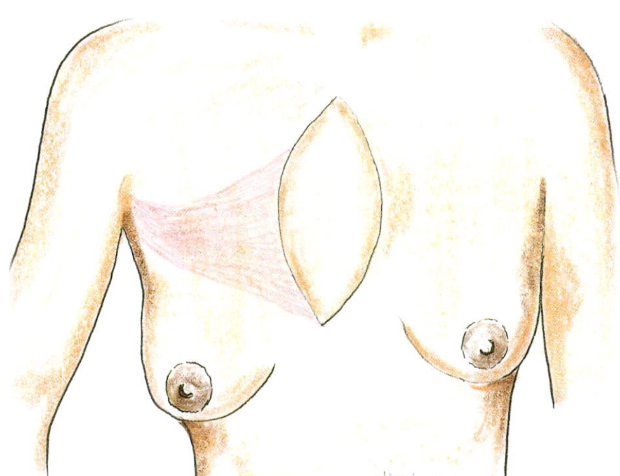

Figure 4.41g Schematic illustration of the latissimus island flap

Tumor Recurrence Located Intercostally and Latissimus Island Flap

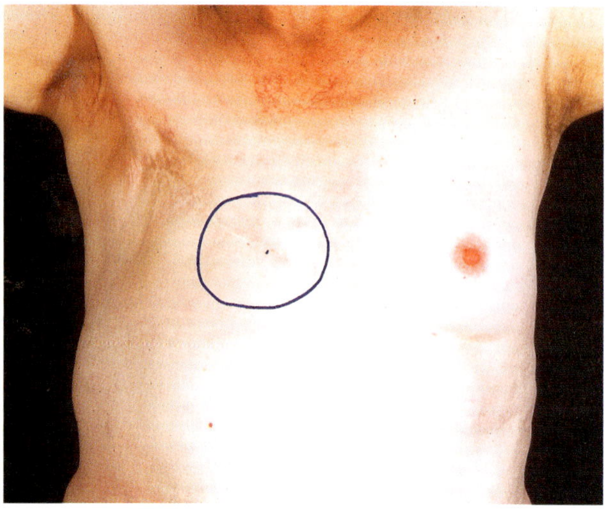

Figure 4.42a Local recurrence of breast cancer located intercostally

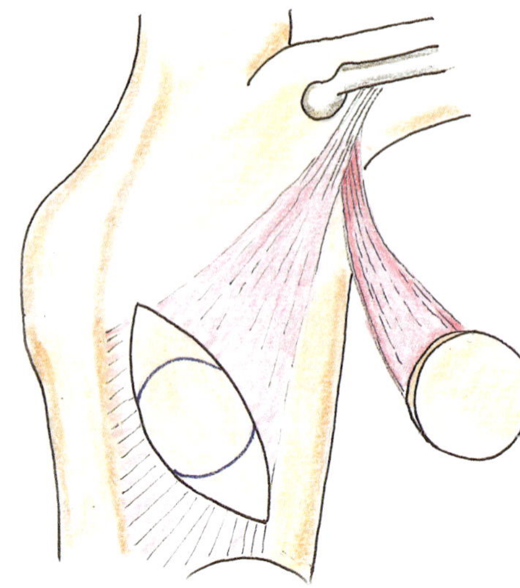

Figure 4.42b Plan for coverage with a latissimus island flap

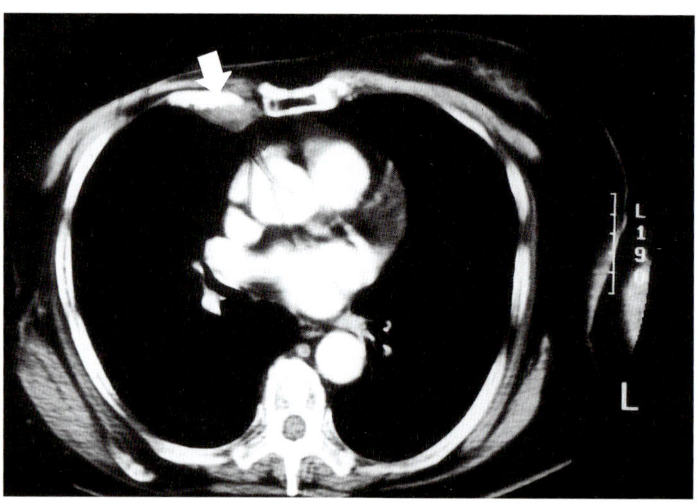

Figure 4.42c Local recurrence (CT scan) located intercostally growing towards the sternum and mediastinum (arrow).

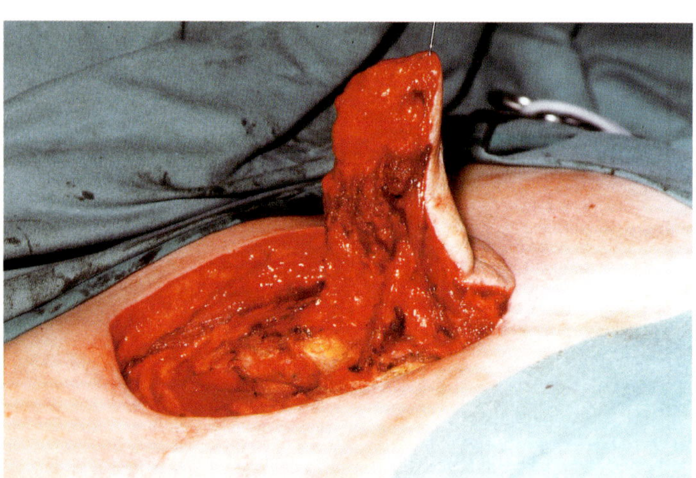

Figure 4.42d En-bloc resection including three ribs and a portion of the sternum. The visceral pleura remained intact.

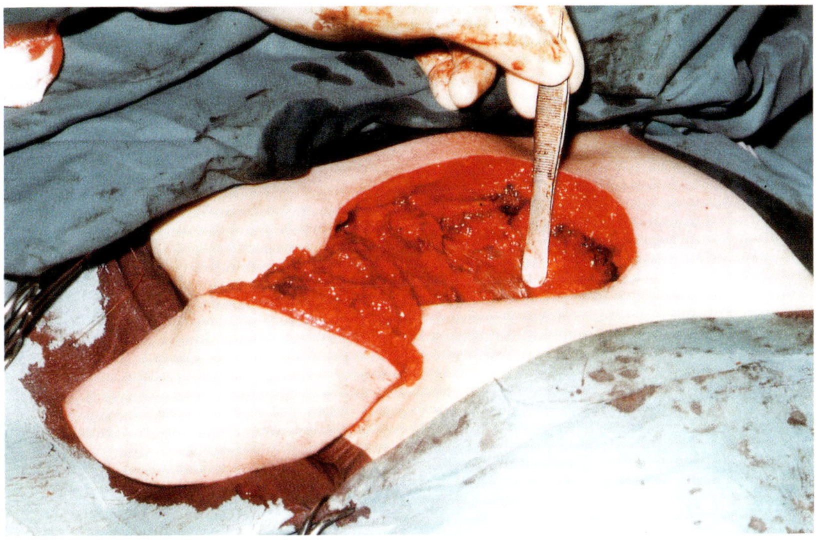

Figure 4.42e The latissimus island flap is brought through a subcutaneous tunnel and closed in two layers.
Note the depth of the defect. First, the latissimus dorsi muscle is sutured to the defect margins with 2 × 0 Vicryl in order to close the thoracic cavity. Finally, the skin is closed.

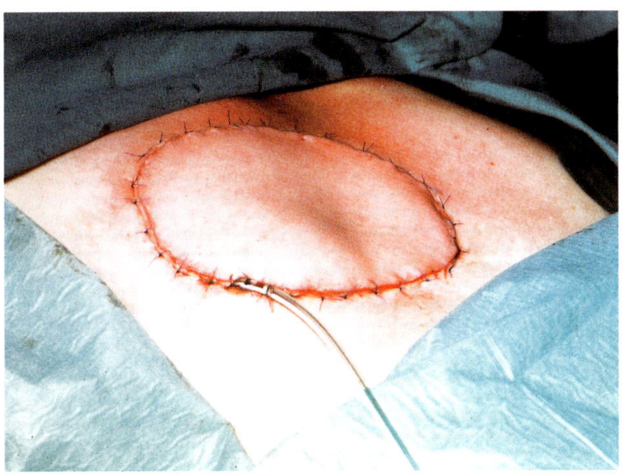

Figure 4.42f Following skin closure

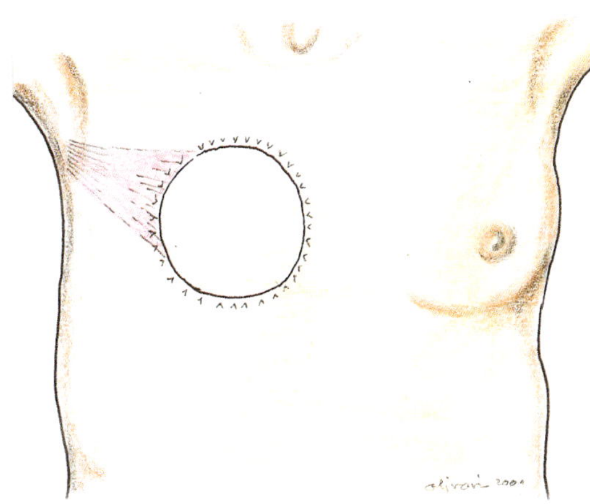

Figure 4.42g The island flap in place

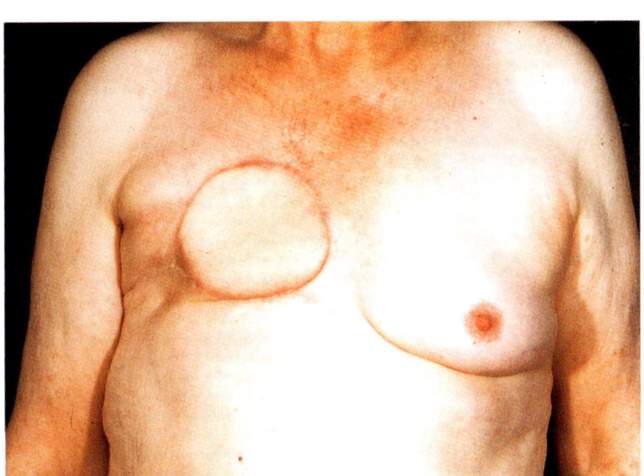

Figure 4.24h Six months postoperatively

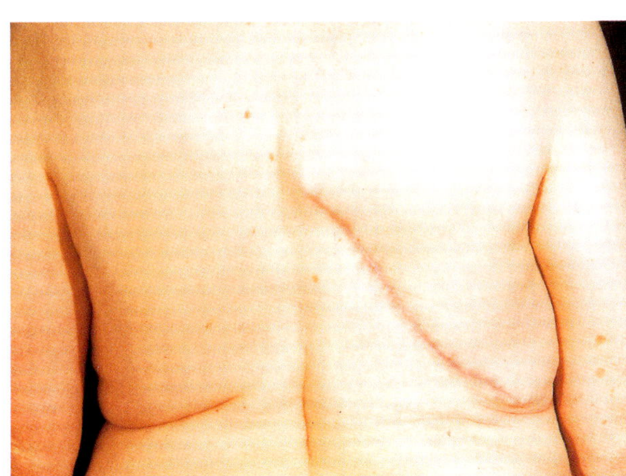

Figure 4.42i **Note** the orientation of the scar!

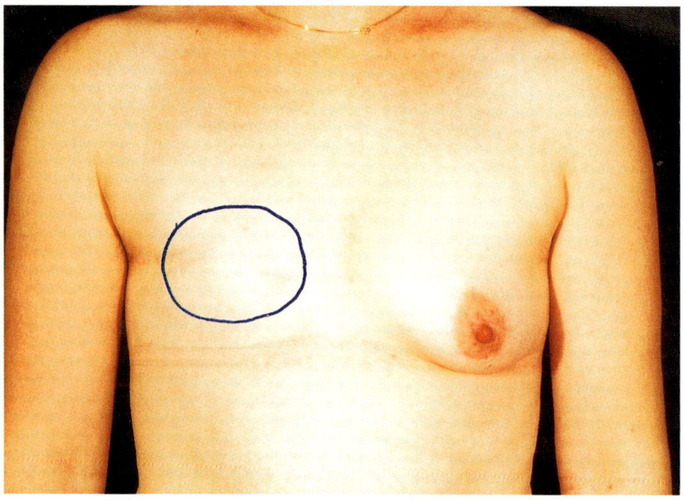

Figure 4.43a Status post mastectomy for breast cancer of the right breast. Presently has local recurrence located intercostally with extensive thoracic wall infiltration.

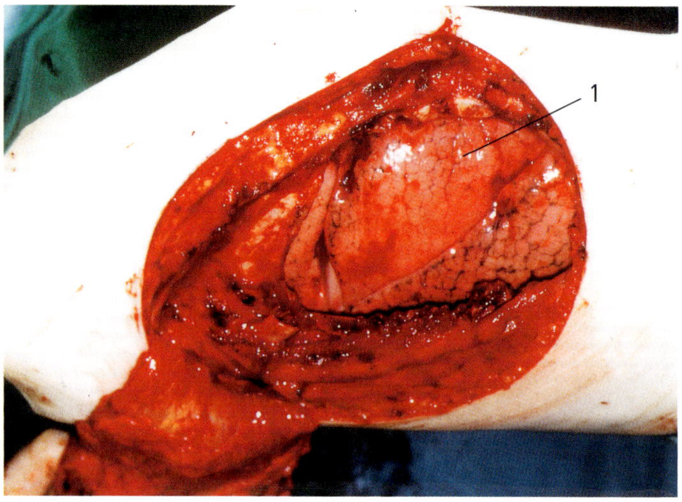

Figure 4.43b Full thickness resection of the thoracic wall including five ribs. The lung is exposed. No infiltration of the pleura (1).

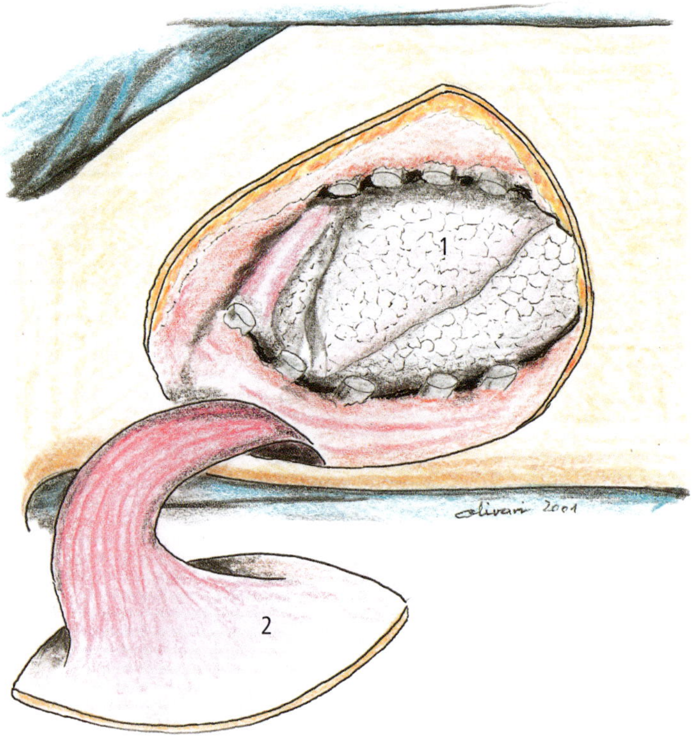

Figure 4.43c A latissimus island flap (2) is brought through a subcutaneous tunnel for defect coverage. First the muscle is meticulously sutured to the intercostals with 2 × 0 Vicryl. Subsequently, tension-free skin closure is achieved using 3 × 0 Trofilene. Two suction drains are placed. A Buelau suction followed for ten days.

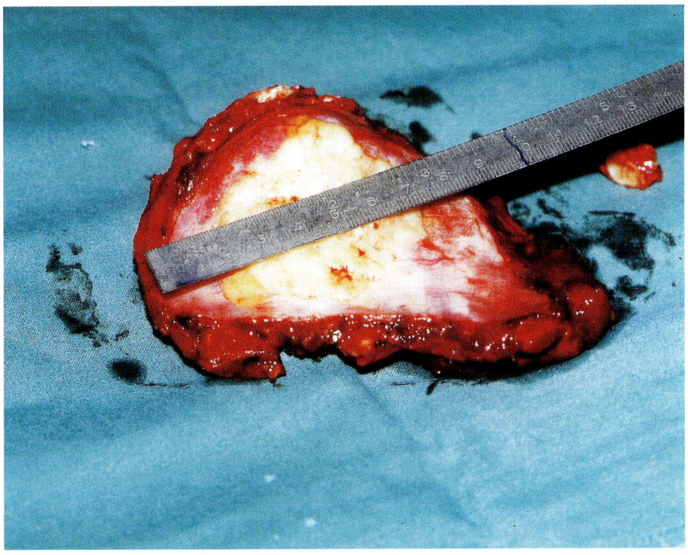

Figure 4.43d En-bloc resection of the tumor including five ribs

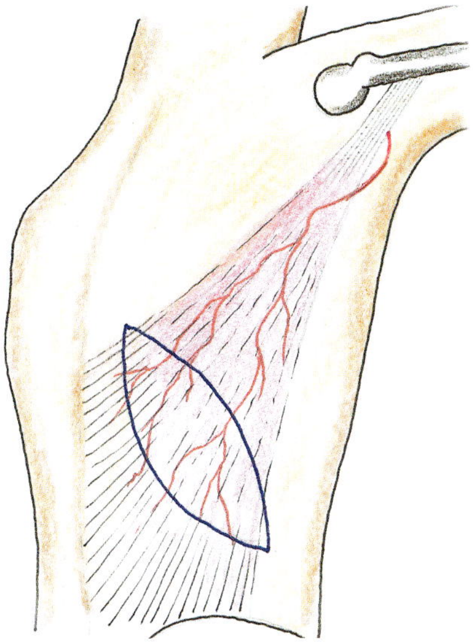

Figure 4.43e Schematic illustration of proposed latissimus island flap. Additional stabilization of the thoracic wall using synthetic materials is not necessary.

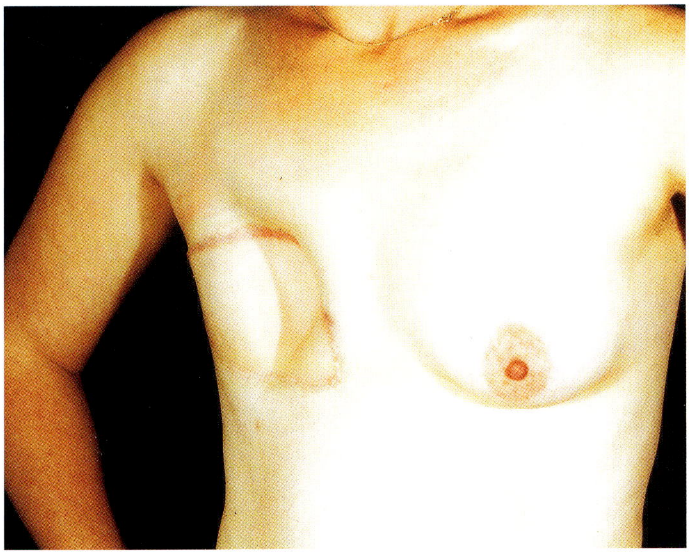

Figure 4.43f Seven months postoperatively.
Note: Paradoxical thoracic wall excursions during breathing. However, this has no functional impact. By-and-by the latissimus dorsi muscle undergoes fibrosis, thus, limited these paradoxical excursions.

Bilateral Latissimus Dorsi Island Flaps for Thoracic Wall Recurrences. Extreme Case!

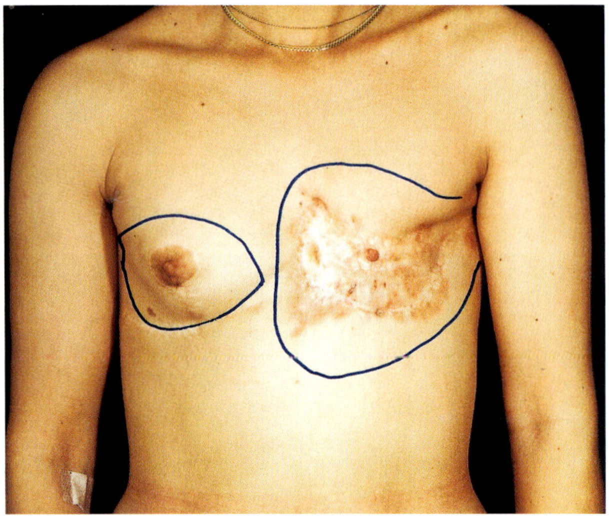

Figure 4.44a Wide local recurrence of a left-sided breast carcinoma with infiltration of multiple intercostal spaces. Right breast: Carcinoma recurrence following quadrantectomy. Treatment: Left-sided thoracic wall resection including five ribs as well as sternum and right-sided mastectomy (see markings).

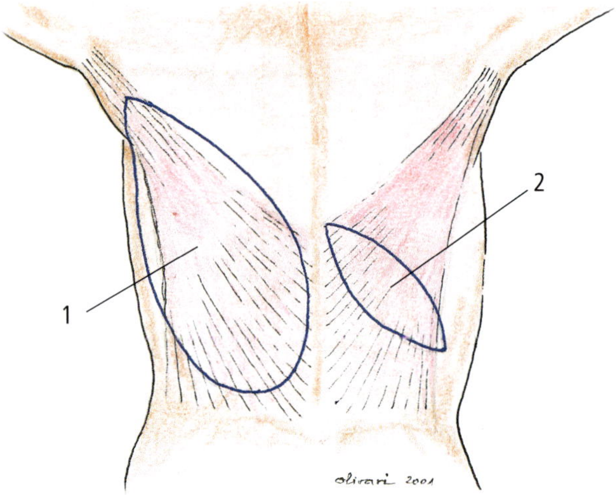

Figure 4.44b Flap design: Left: Large latissimus island flap (1) Right: Small latissimus island flap (2)

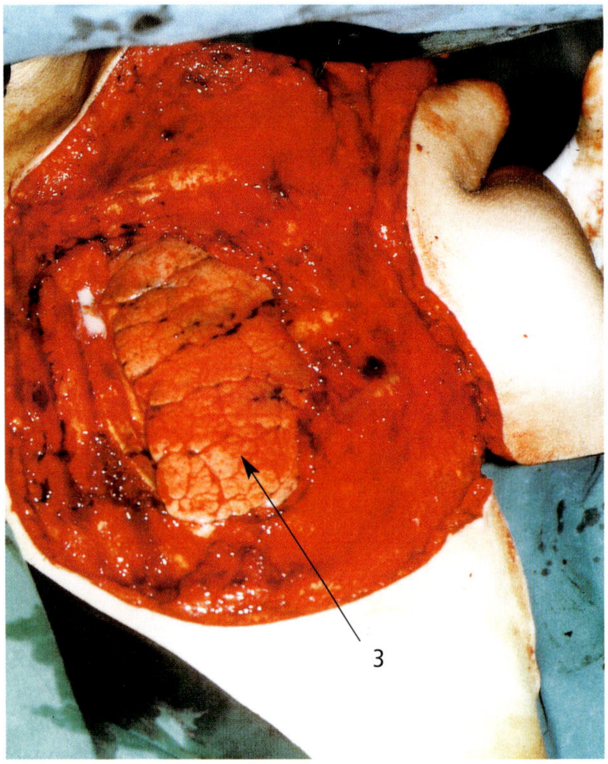

Figure 4.44c The thoracic wall is resected (five ribs) along with parts of the sternum. The lung surface is exposed (3).

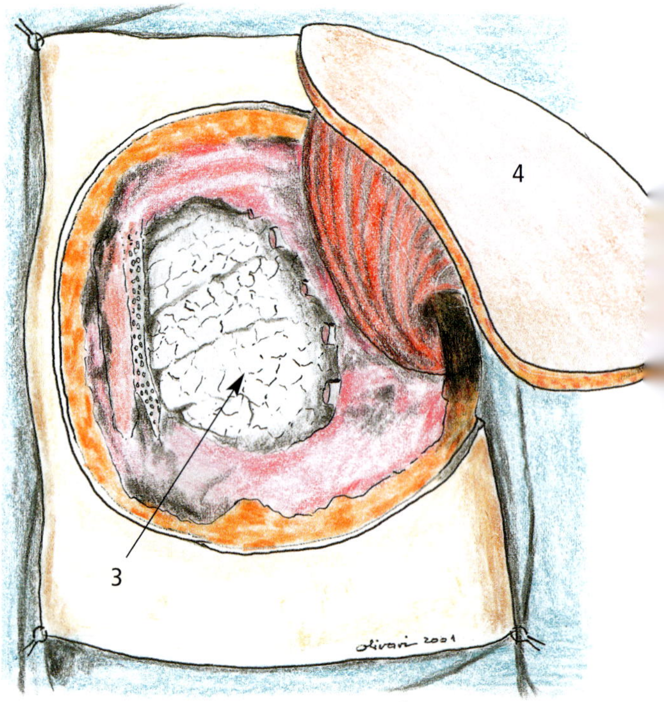

Figure 4.44d Mobilization of the latissimus island flap for defect coverage.

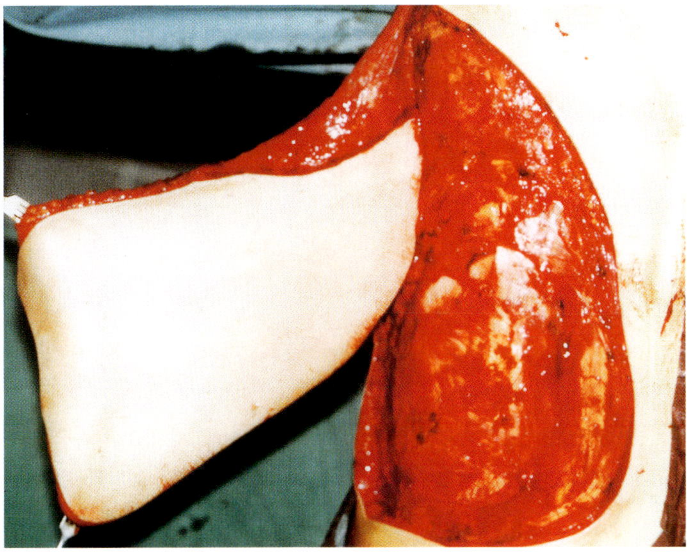

Figure 4.44e A large latissimus flap left is mobilized and prepared for transfer as an island flap. Simultaneously a smaller latissimus island flap is prepared contralaterally.

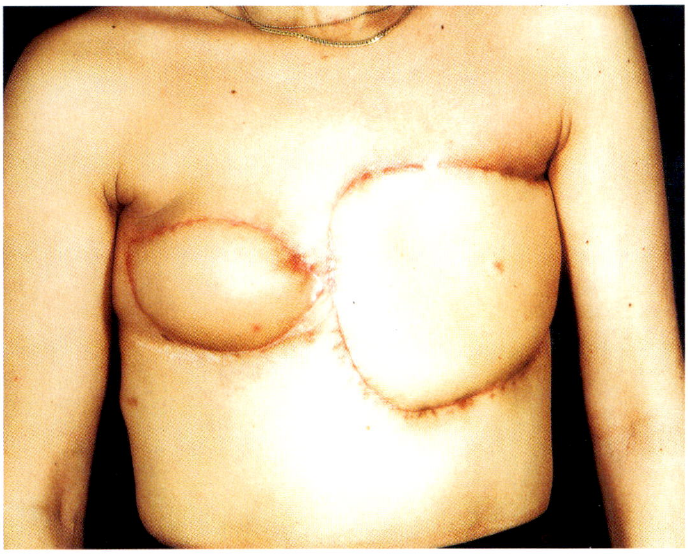

Figure 4.44f Three months postoperatively. The patient was transferred to the oncology service two weeks postoperatively.

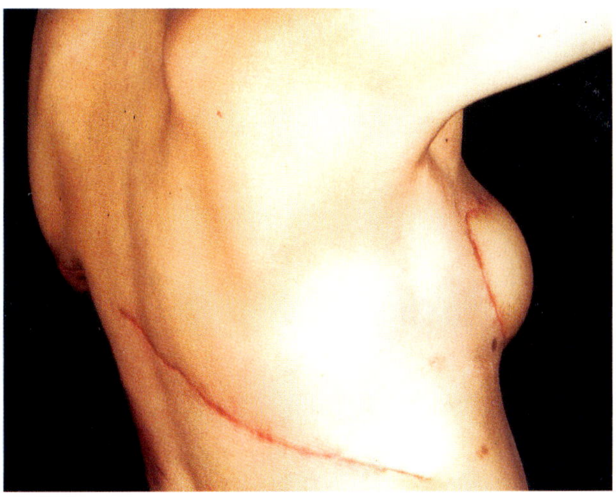

Figure 4.44g The donor site of the right-sided latissimus island flap is inconspicuous with a favorable orientation.

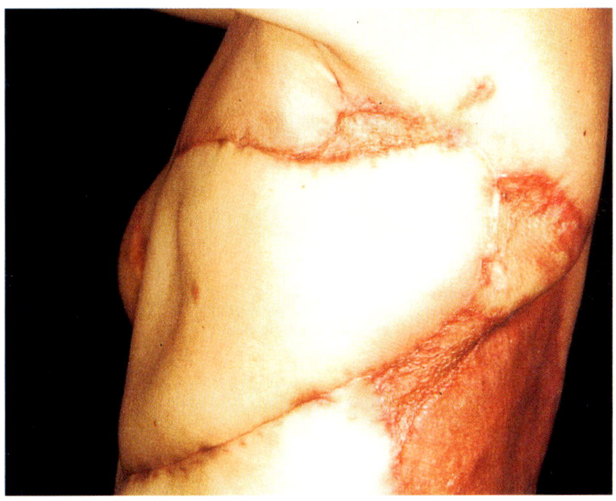

Figure 4.44h The donor site of the larger left side had to be covered with a STSG due to flap dimensions. Comment: This is about maximum of possibility in covering defects of thorax wall in case of recurrence of cancer.

Latissimus Dorsi Island Flaps for Breast Reconstruction With Implants (Silicone Gel Inlay)

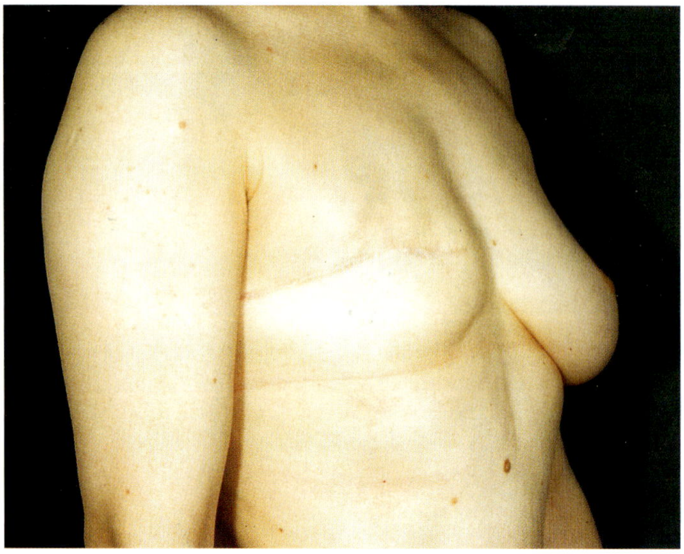

Figure 4.45a Status post mastectomy (Patey)

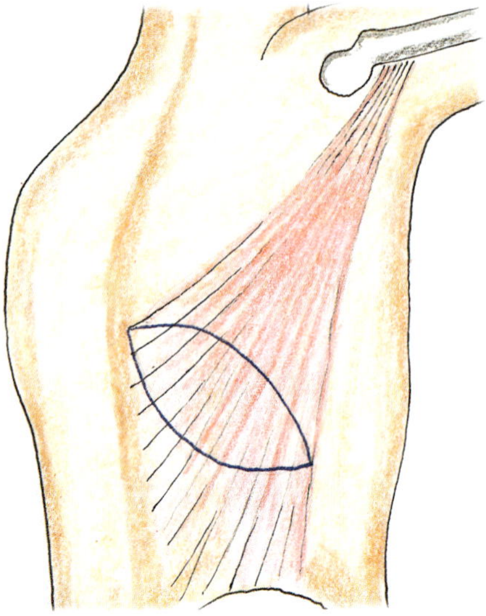

Figure 4.45b Mobilization of a latissimus dorsi island flap. **Note:** Flap orientation!

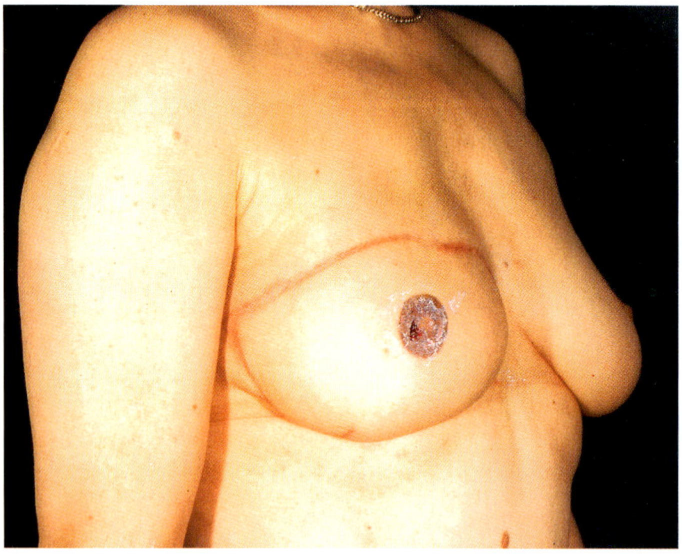

Figure 4.45c Eight months postoperatively

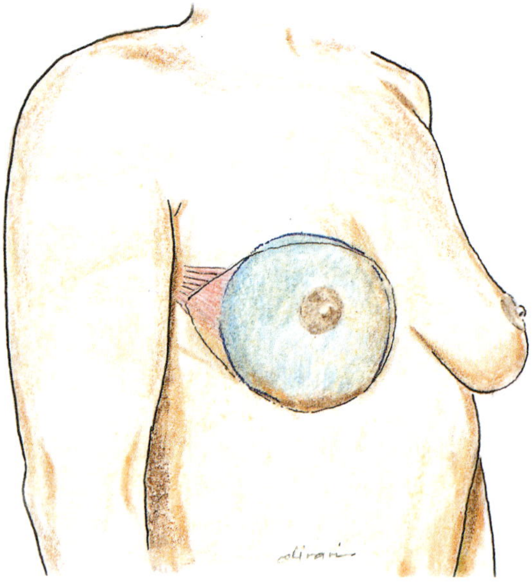

Figure 4.45d The flap is positioned horizontally so that the inferior border creates the IMF.

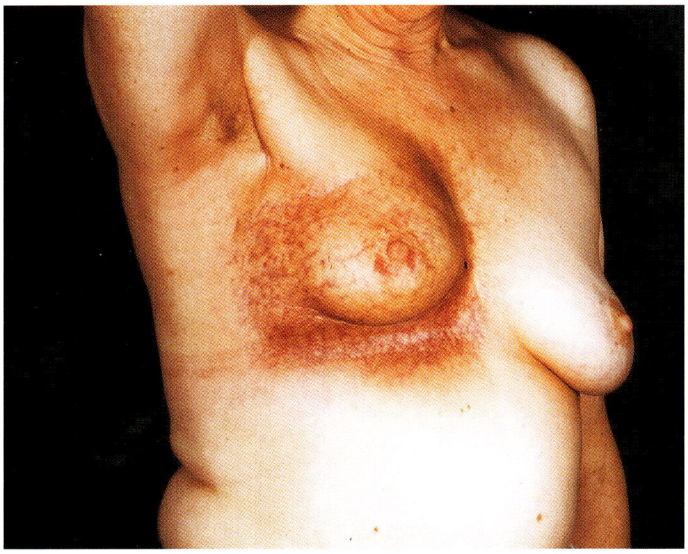

Figure 4.46a Status post quadrantectomy and postoperative radiation therapy for breast cancer ("breast conservation therapy").
Diagnosis: Radiodermatitis, radiation-induced fibrosis, residual tumor in irradiated area.

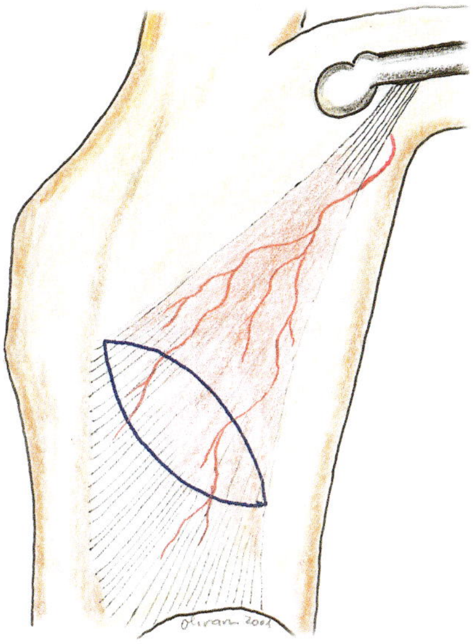

Figure 4.46b Note: Flap orientation from cranial-medial to caudal-lateral!

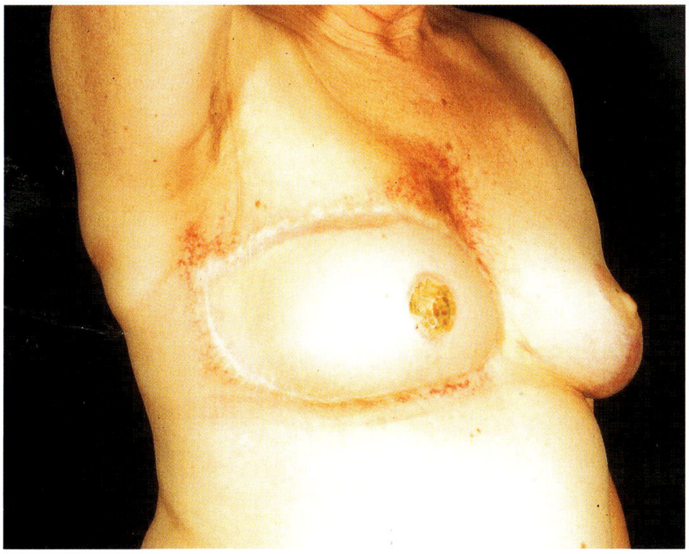

Figure 4.46c Situation three years postoperatively. The entire area was excised. Histopathological exam revealed residual tumor. Reconstruction is performed with a latissimus dorsi island flap and a silicone gel implant (270 ccm).

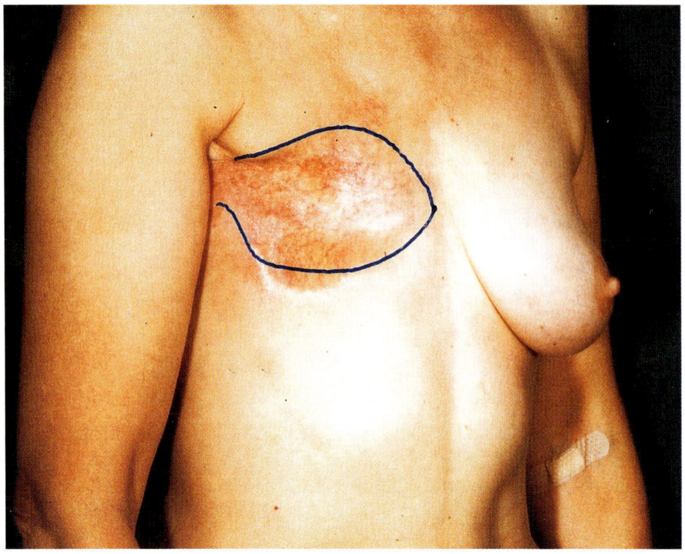

Figure 4.47a Status post mastectomy and radiation therapy five years ago. The pectoral muscles (major and minor) are not present.

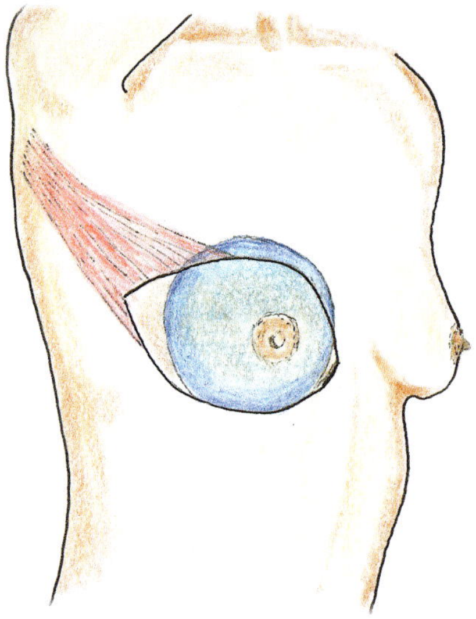

Figure 4.47b A large latissimus island flap is designed anticipating the large defect following radical excision of the existing radiodermatitis. The implant is covered almost entirely by the flap.

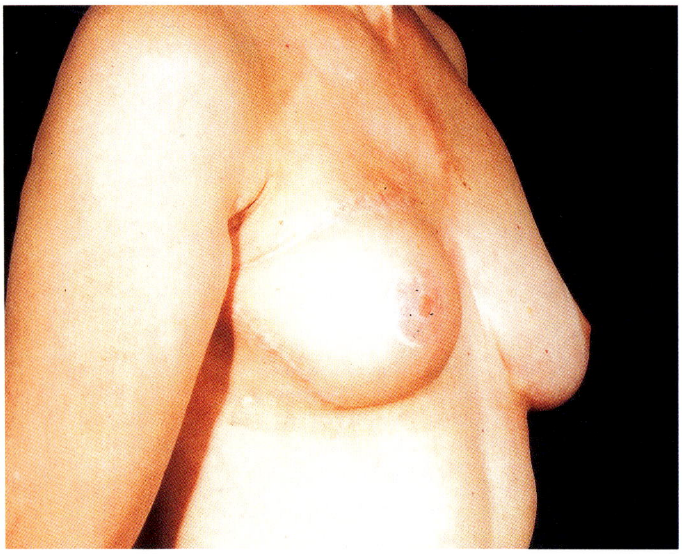

Figure 4.47c Five years postoperatively. The inferior margin of the horizontally positioned flap creates the IMF.

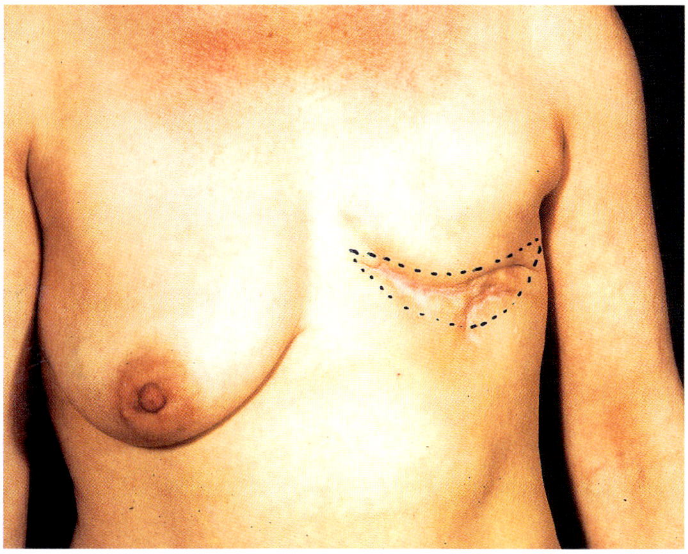

Figure 4.48a Status post mastectomy with extensive cicatrisation

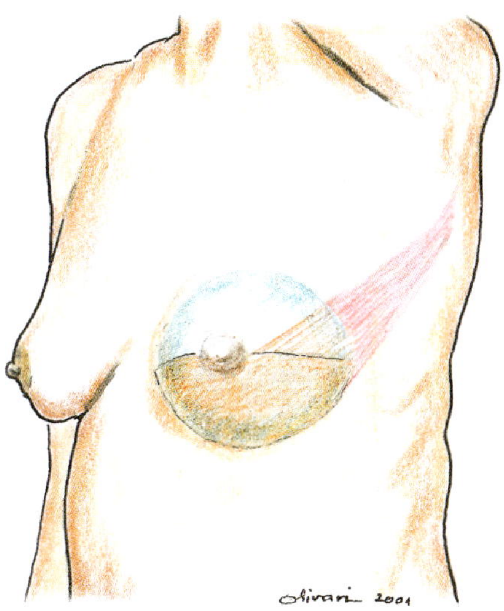

Figure 4.48b Following scar excision reconstruction was performed with a horizontally orientated latissimus dorsi island flap. The lower margin of the flap formed the IMF. The silicone gel implant is in symmetrical position.

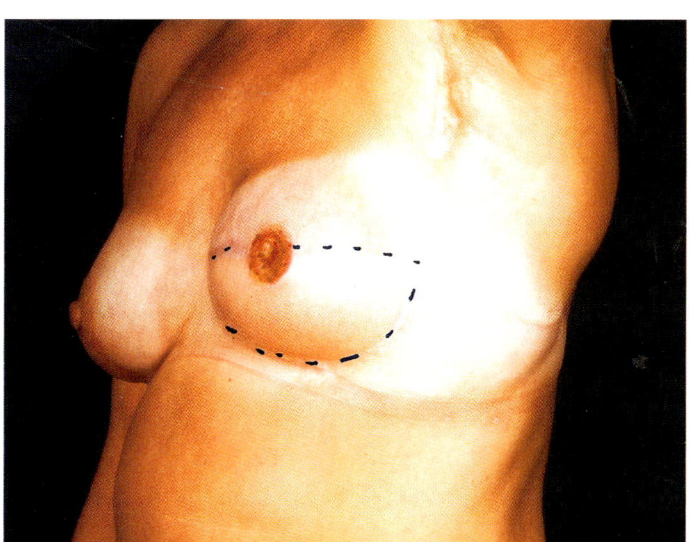

Figure 4.48c Two years postoperatively.
Note the orientation of the island flap! The areola was tattooed and nipple reconstruction performed by nipple-sharing.

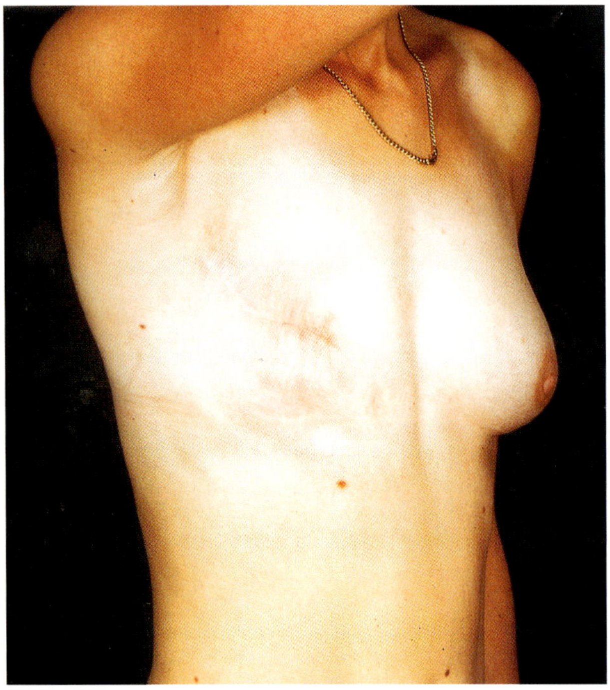

Figure 4.49a Status post radical mastectomy for breast cancer with removal of the pectoral major muscle.

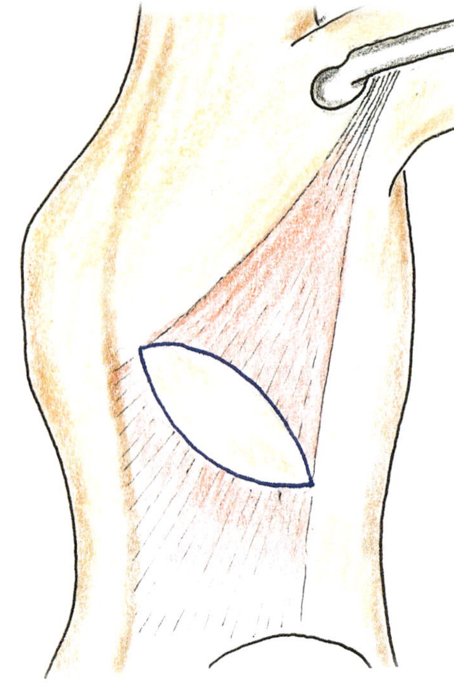

Figure 4.49b Design of a latissimus island flap. **Note** the orientation of the flap!

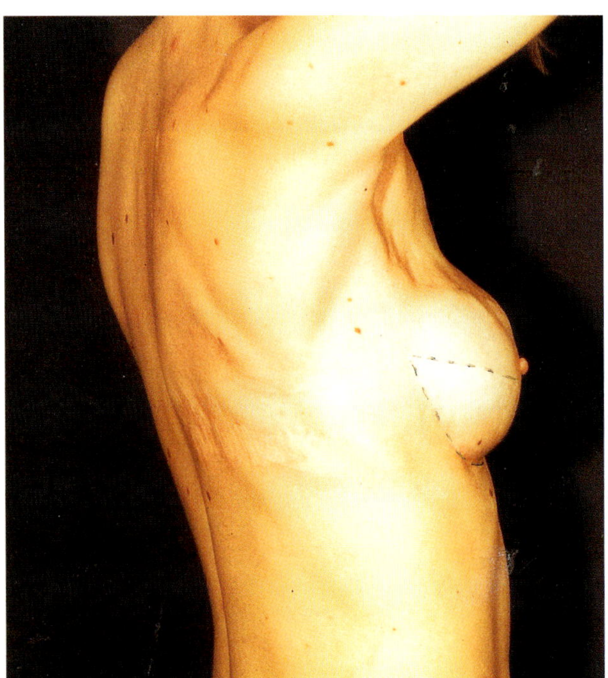

Figure 4.49c One year postoperatively. Note the horizontal flap orientation. The inferior margin forms the IMF! Very acceptable scar at donor site!

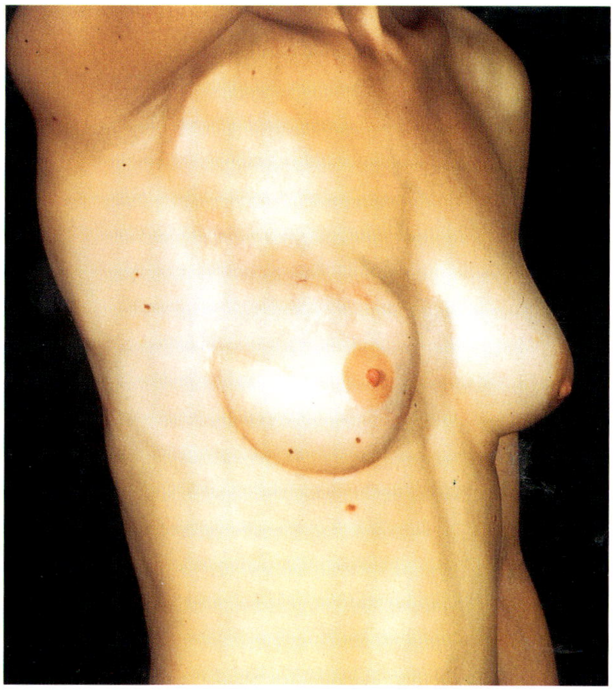

Figure 4.49d Note the position of the silicone implant. The lower part is supported by the strong tissue of the latissimus dorsi flap. The areola was tattooed and the nipple reconstructed applying the nipple-sharing technique.

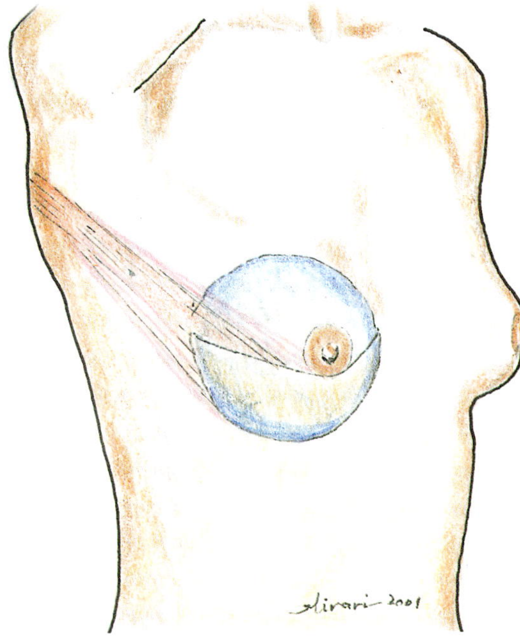

Figure 4.49e Location of the implant in relation to the latissimus island flap.

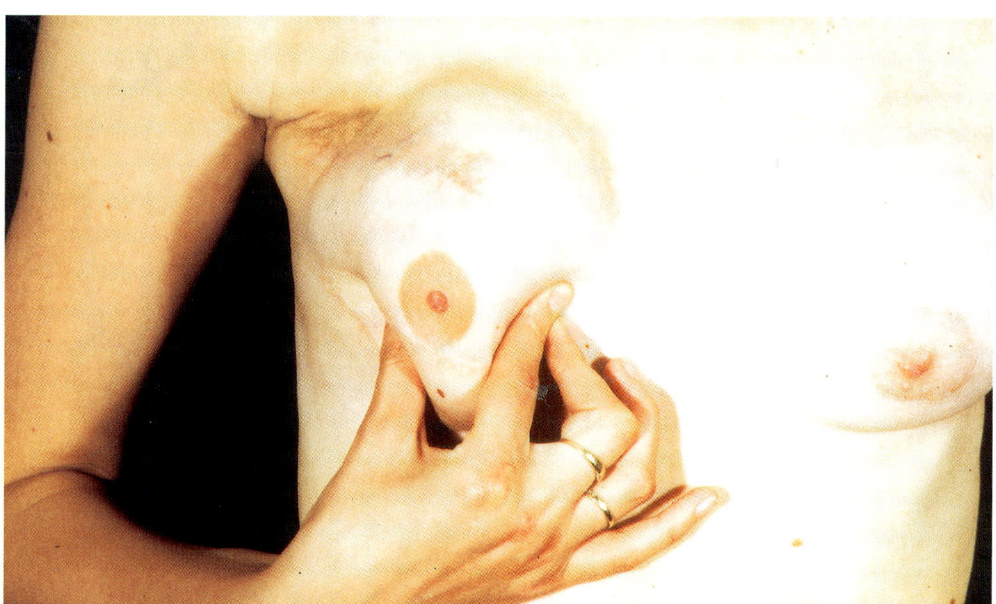

Figure 4.49f One year postoperatively. Using silicone gel implants with a textured surface dramatically lowered the rate of capsular contracture.

d) Deepithelialized Latissimus Dorsi Island Flap for Breast Reconstruction Without Implants

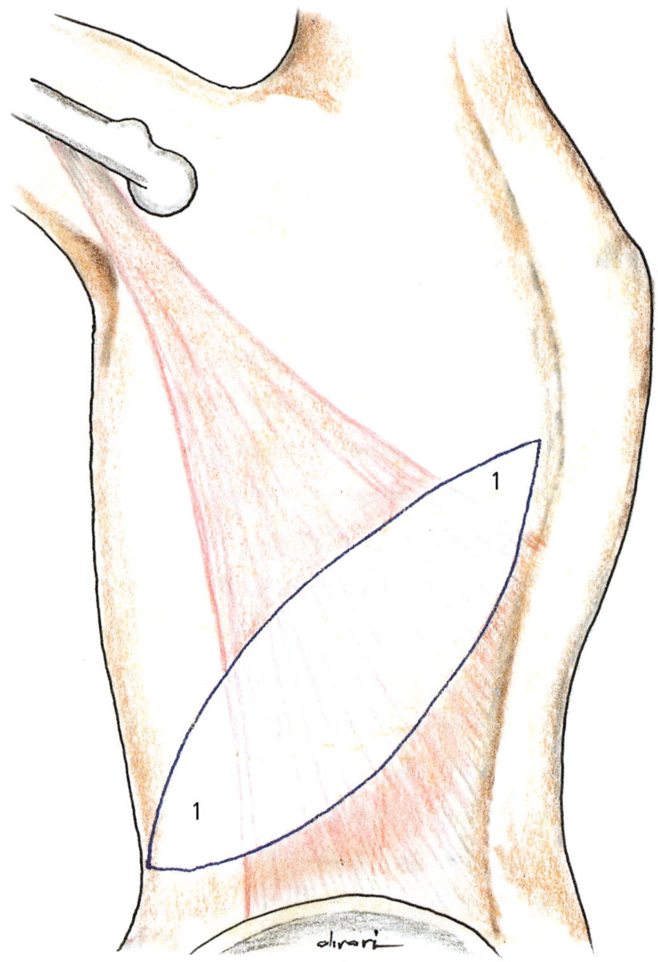

Figure 4.50a Ideal flap orientation when using large latissimus island flaps. Anteriorly and medially the skin island does not cover the latissimus muscle and thus is not directly over the muscle, but displays excellent perfusion. This flap following deepithelialization allows breast reconstruction without the use of implants if there is a sufficient amount of skin in area of mastectomy. The island flap should be positioned as low as possible for achievement of larger volumes. The donor site can be closed easily in this location.

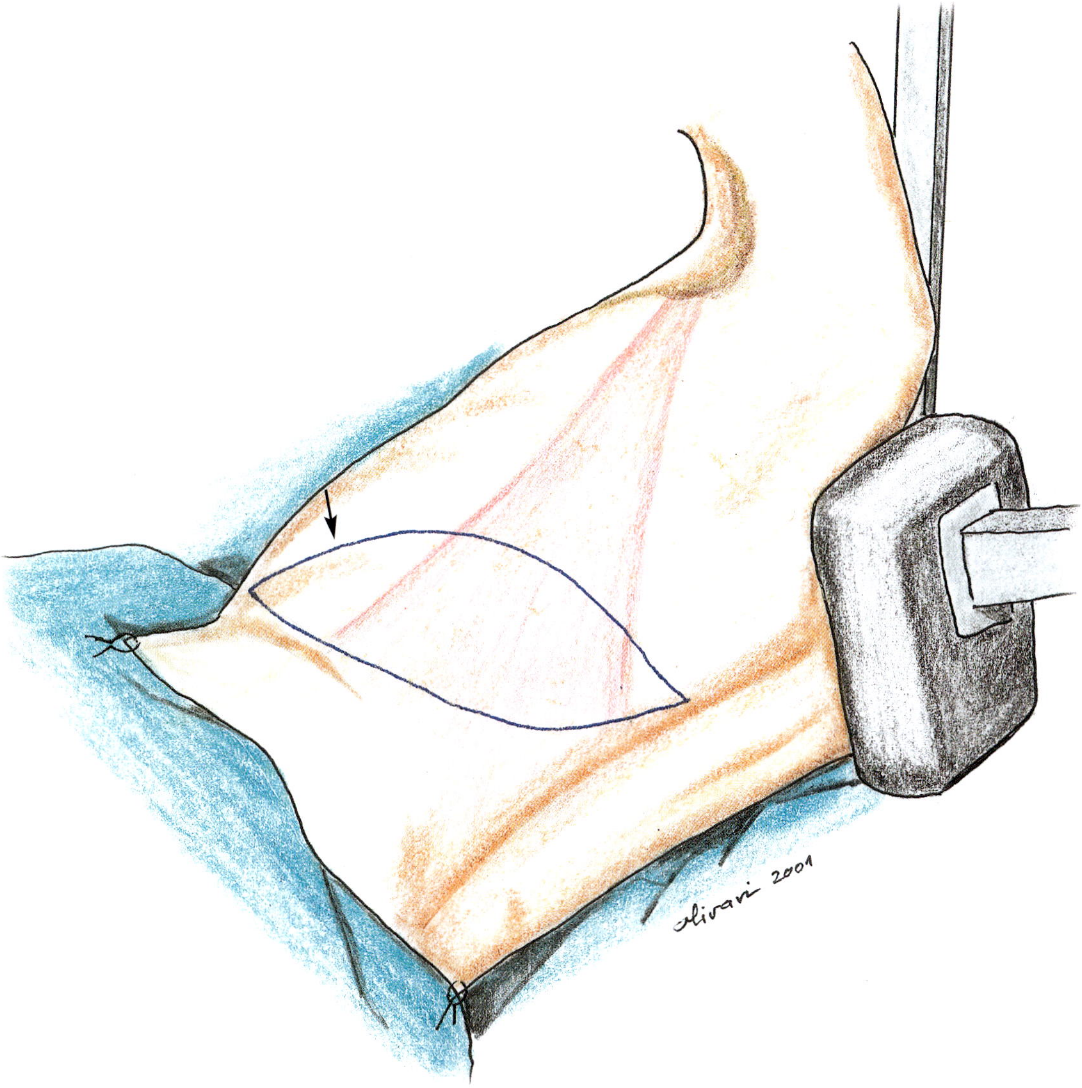

Figure 4.50b Patient positioning during surgery: The lateral position allows flap mobilization and breast reconstruction without the need to reposition the patient intraoperatively. Simple tilting of the operating table (approx. 30 degrees) allows for an easy access anteriorly and posteriorly. The illustration displays the design of a deepithelialized latissimus island flap. Note how far the flap extends beyond the muscular margin, particularly anteriorly (arrow).

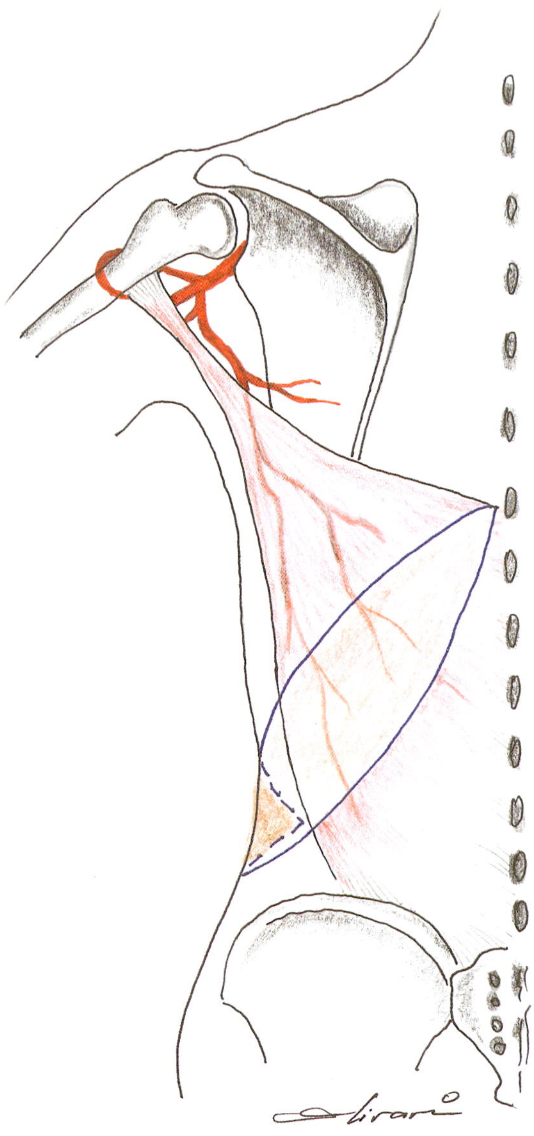

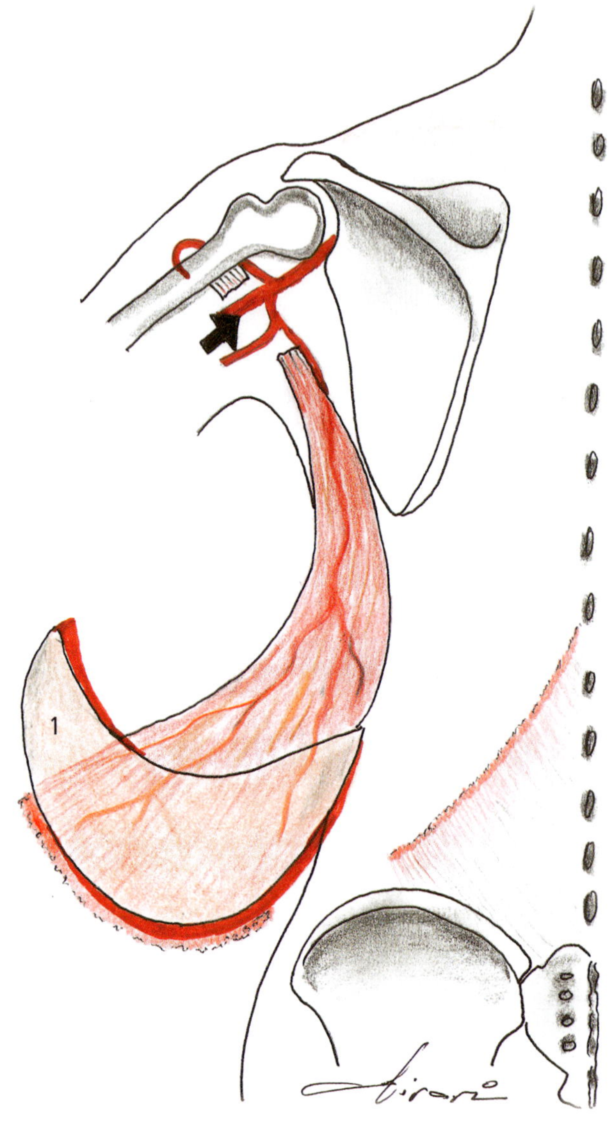

Figure 4.51a Creation of a deepithelialized latissimus flap. **Note** that the flap partially extends beyond the margins of the muscle. In fact, the lateral part of a TRAM-flap is included (1) and gets its blood supply from the latissimus dorsi muscle.

Figure 4.51b Following deepithelialization of the island skin the muscle is mobilized. The muscle insertion (arrow) at the humerus is transected for better flap mobility. The transected muscle is sutured to the thoracic wall (serratus muscle) to prevent tension along the thoracodorsal vessels.

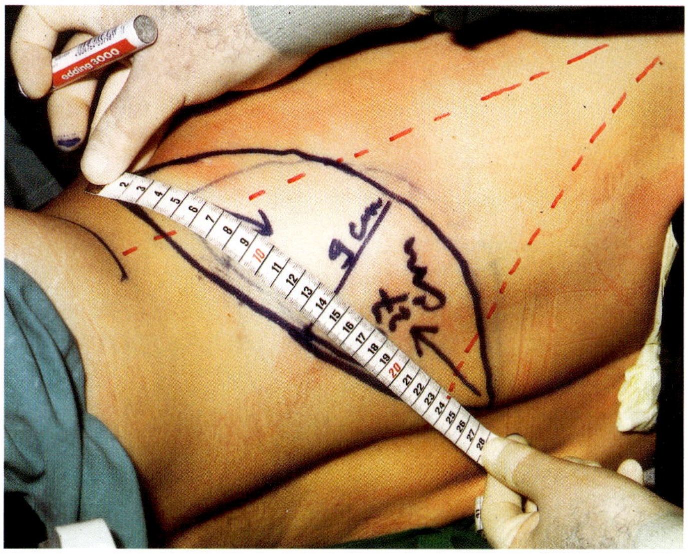

Figure 4.52a When performing skin incisions according to the illustration one third of the flap is in reality random pattern flap. A flap measuring 27 × 9 cm is easy to raise. A tension-free closure of the donor site can be performed.

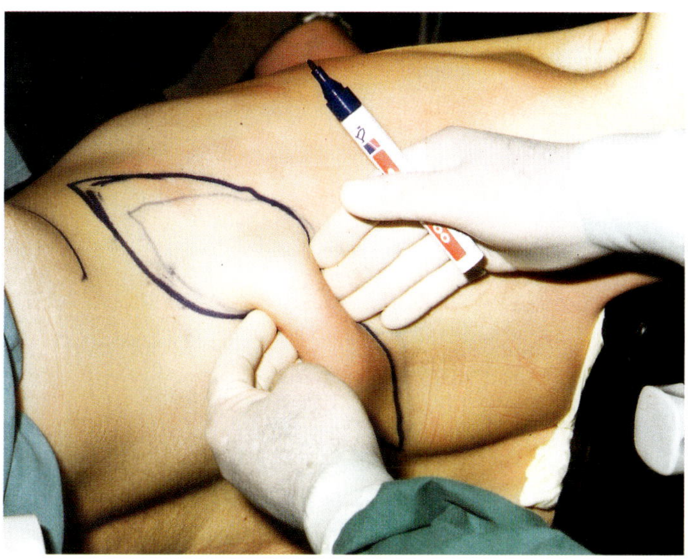

Figure 4.52b Illustrated is a test demonstrating the ease with which a tension-free closure of the donor site can be accomplished. Using tissue from this region provides more volume for breast reconstruction procedures. Thus, breast reconstructions are often possible without the use of implants.

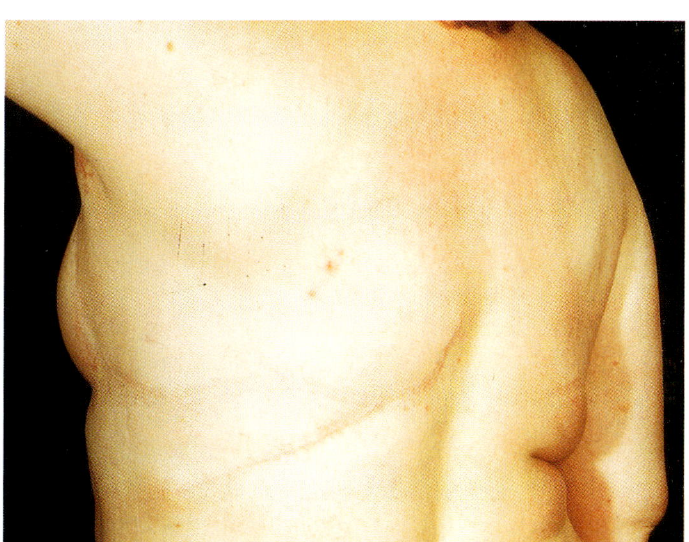

Figure 4.52c The orientation of the incision allows the use of large flaps and leaves acceptable scars. Drawback: Tunneling the flap is technically more demanding.

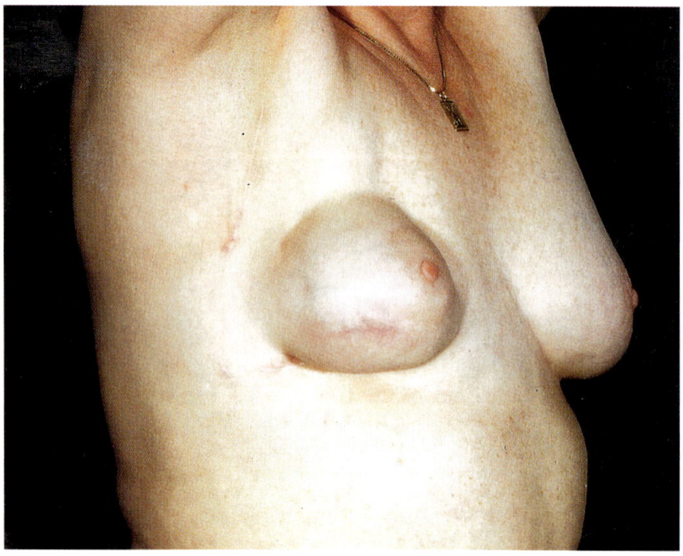

Figure 4.53a "Breast cripple" following subcutaneous mastectomy and reconstruction with silicone implants. Capsular contracture and a very thin skin overlying the implant are illustrated. The breast was previously operated on twice.

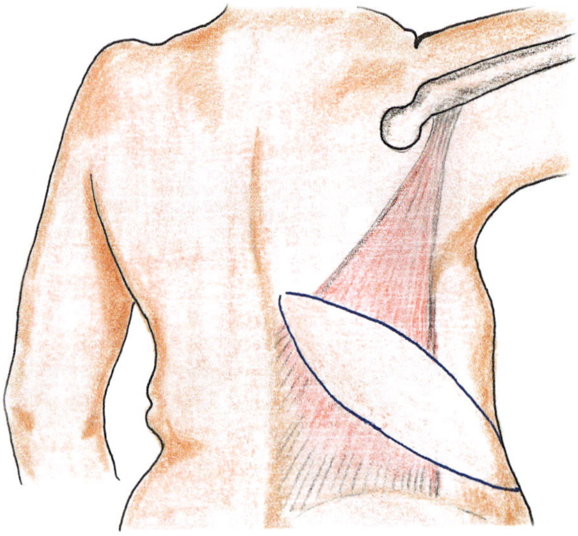

Figure 4.53b Plan: Removal of the silicon gel implant and reconstruction with a deepithelialized latissimus island flap.

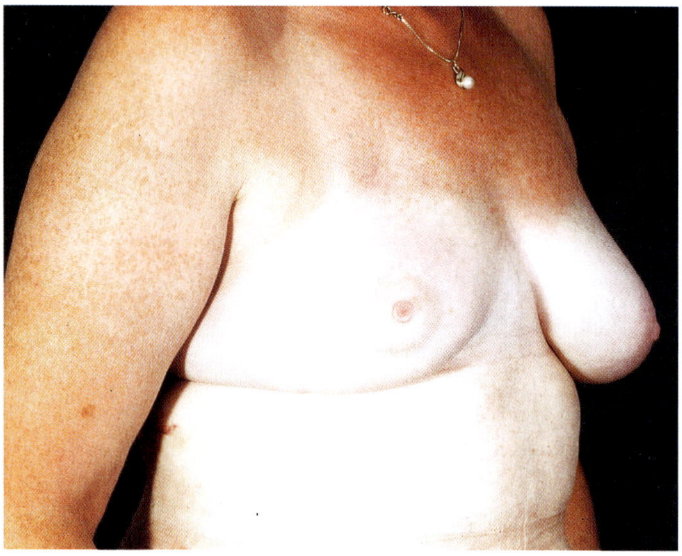

Figure 4.53c Sixteen months postoperatively: The volume observed was provided by the deepithelialized island flap alone without the use of an implant.

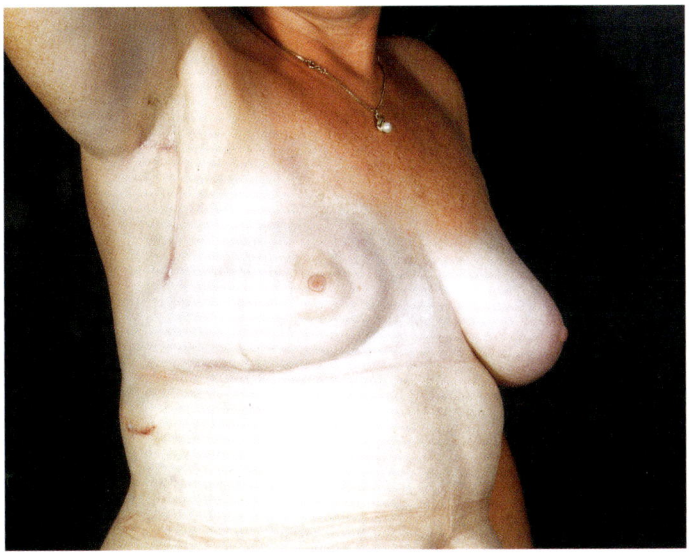

Figure 4.53d Sixteen months postoperatively. Nice breast shape, soft consistency.

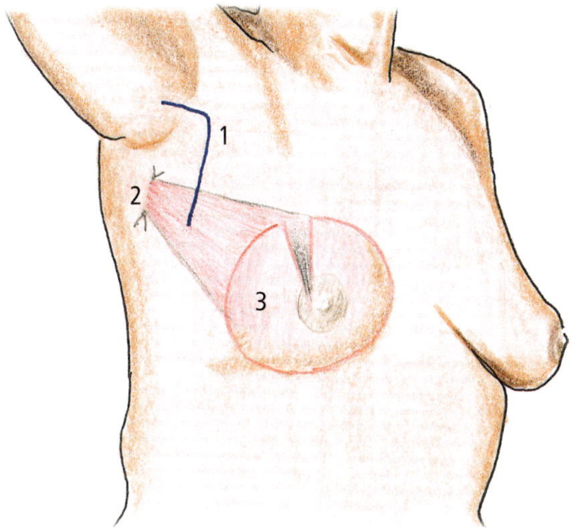

Figure 4.53e An additional incision (1) is necessary in the axilla in order to transect the muscular insertion at the humerus. The latissimus dorsi muscle is sutured to the pectoralis muscle margin (2) which prevents tension along the thoracodorsal vessels. The flap is formed cone-shaped.

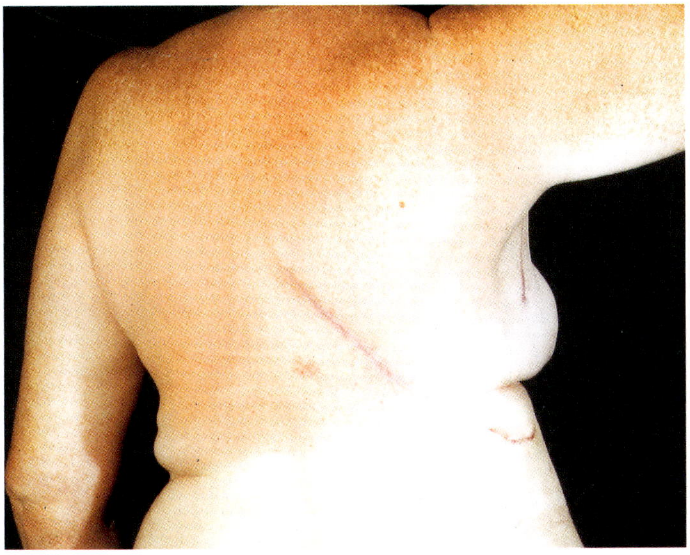

Figure 4.53f Sixteen months postoperatively with an acceptable scar when flap design displays the orientation illustrated.

Bilateral Breast Reconstruction With Deepithelialized Latissimus Dorsi Island Flaps Without Implants

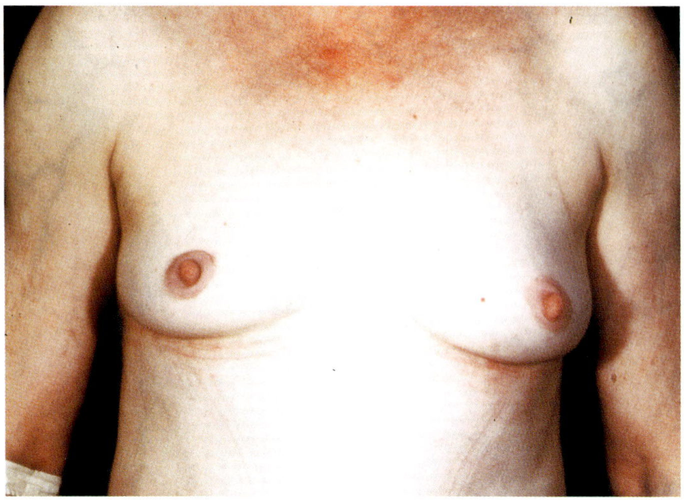

Figure 4.54a 62-year old patient with multicentric DCIS bilaterally. Plan: Subcutaneous mastectomy bilaterally and primary reconstruction with de-epithelialized latissimus dorsi island flaps without implants. The patient smoked 60 cigarettes daily. She rejected the use of implants.

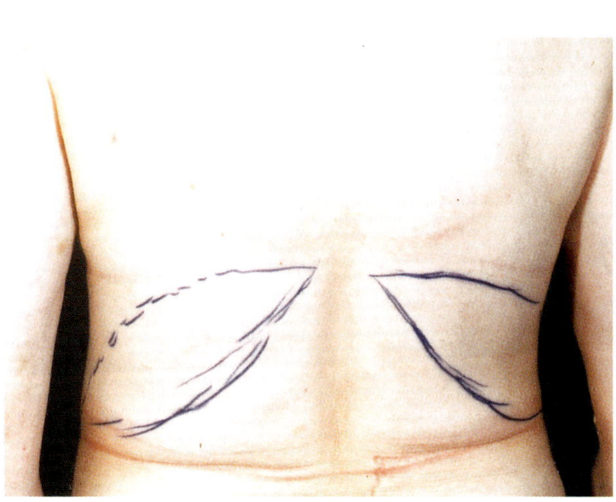

Figure 4.54b **Note** the position and orientation of the island flaps.

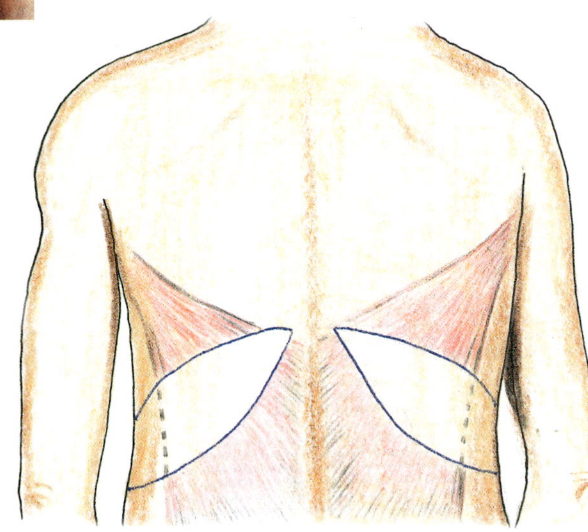

Figure 4.54c Positioning of bilateral flap

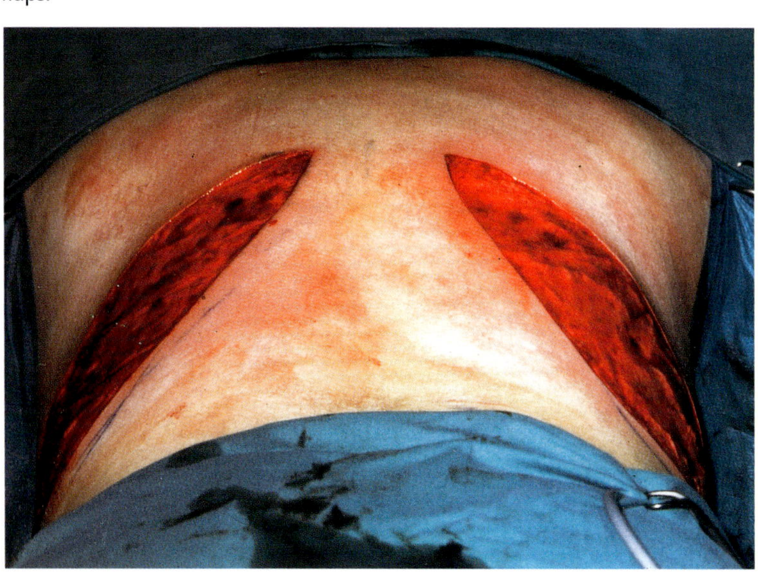

Figure 4.54d First the flap is de-epithelialized and then raised. Deepithelializing a raised flap is technically more difficult.

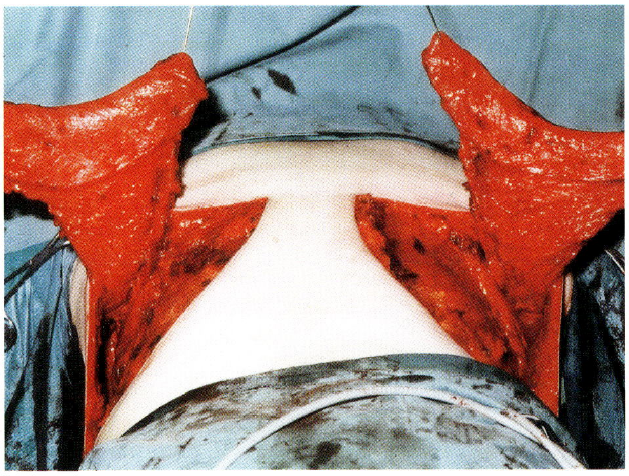

Figure 4.54e Mobilization of the flaps bilaterally

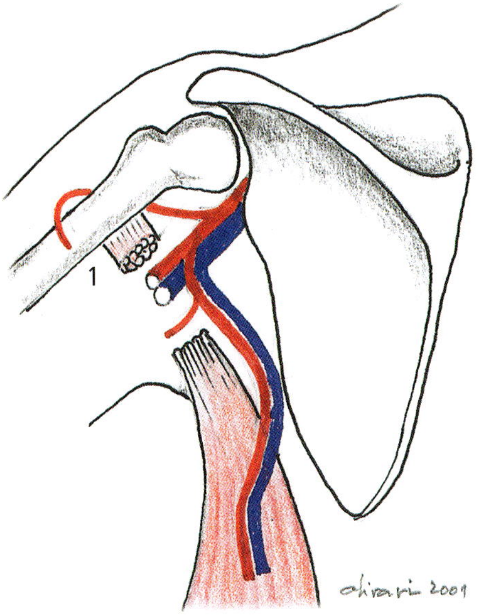

Figure 4.54f The muscular insertion at the humerus is transected (1) and fixed to thorax wall. This prevents tension on thoracodorsal vessels and removes an undesirable fold in axilla and allows easier "breast molding".

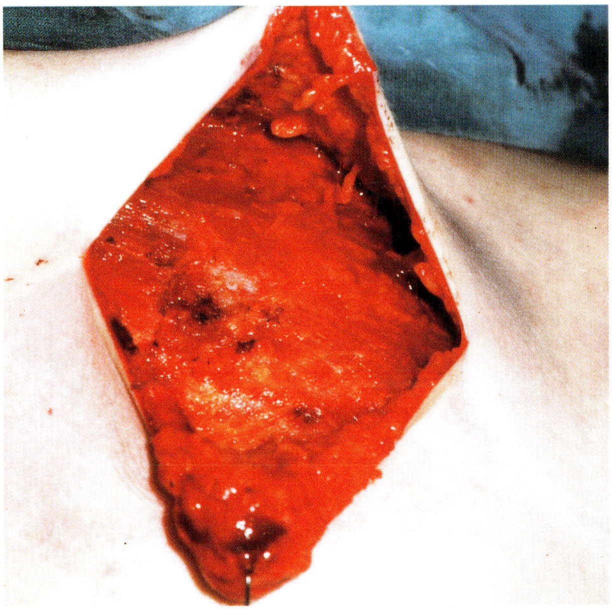

Figure 4.54g Subcutaneous mastectomy on the right side is finished.

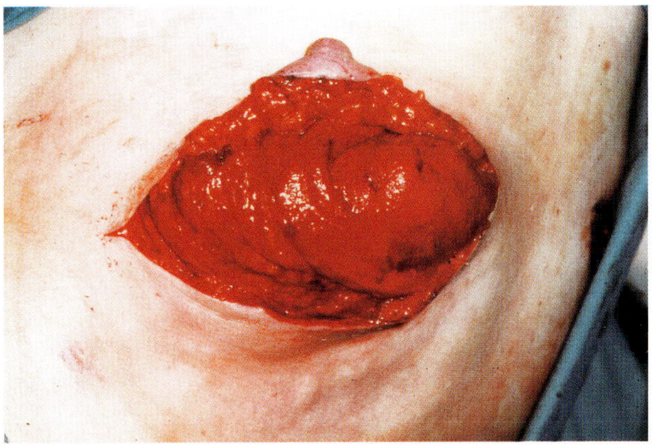

Figure 4.54h The deepithelialized latissimus island flap is transferred anteriorly and shaped to fill the cavity created following subcutaneous mastectomy.

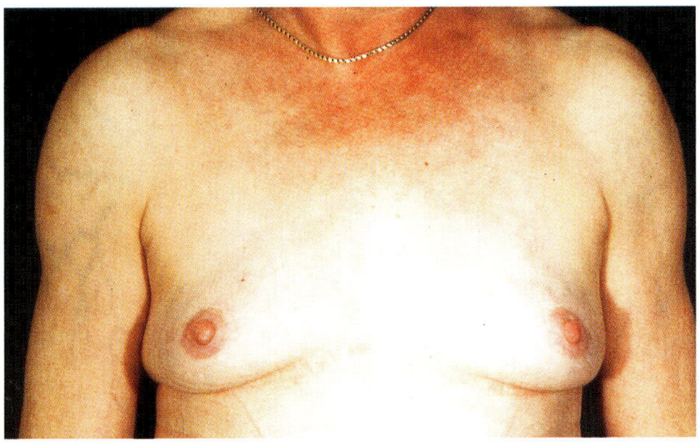

Figure 4.54i Two years postoperatively with an acceptable result

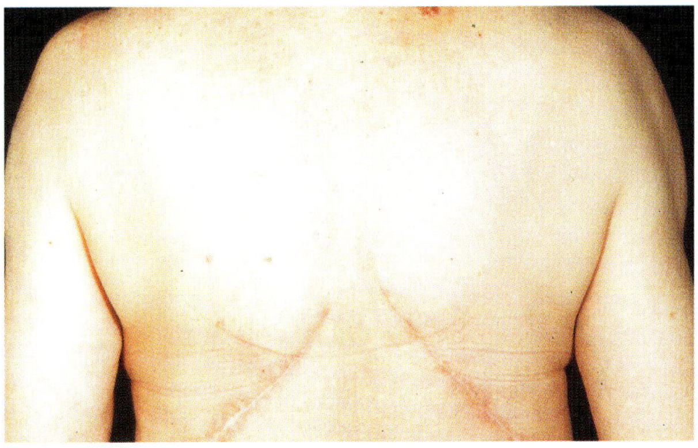

Figure 4.54j Favorable orientation of the donor scars

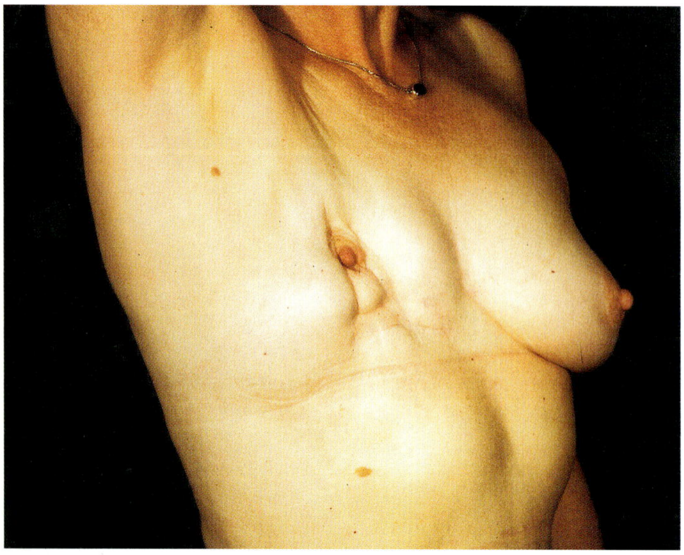

Figure 4.55a Unacceptable result following quadrantectomy and irradiation for breast cancer. There is a very noticeable tissue deficit.

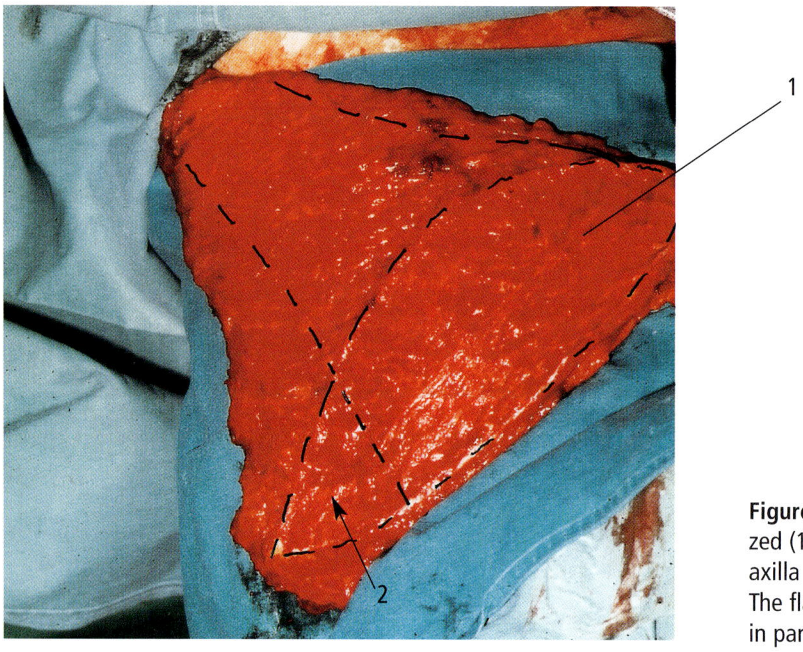

Figure 4.55b The latissimus flap is deepithelialized (1). Muscle and fat are dissected up to the axilla to obtain as much volume as possible. The flap extends far beyond the muscle margin, in particular ventrally (2).

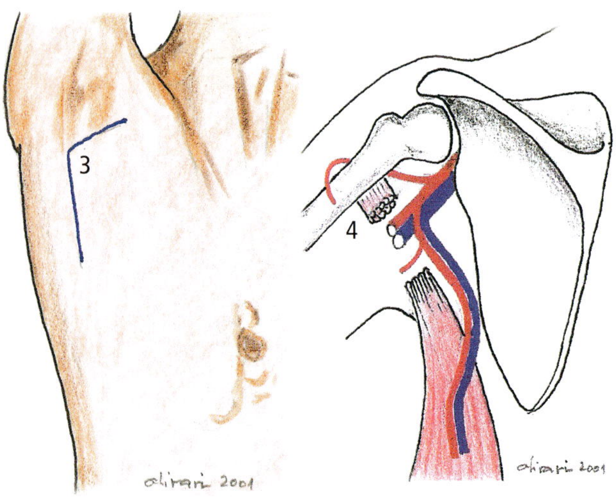

Figure 4.55c An additional incision in the axilla (3) is necessary to divide the latissimus dorsi muscle from the humerus and allows better control over the vascular pedicle (4). The muscular insertion is then sutured to the serratus or pectoralis margin preventing traction on the thoracodorsal vessels.

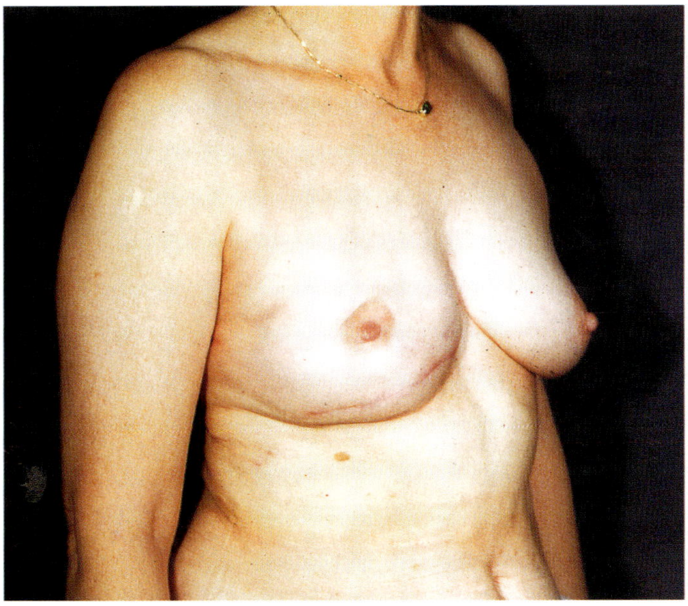

Figure 4.55d Five months following breast reconstruction with a deepithelialized latissimus island flap. Sufficient volume could be obtained without the use of implants. Depending on existing adipose tissue a volume of 200 to 350 ccm can be obtained.

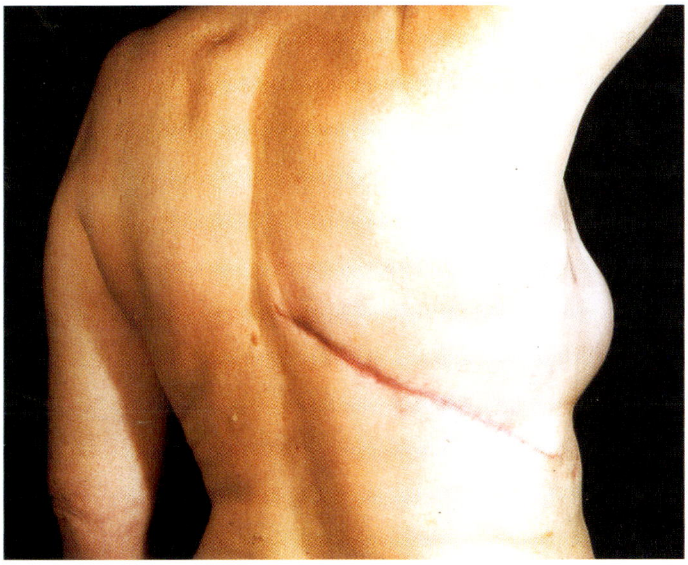

Figure 4.55e The donor site with a "tension-free" closure

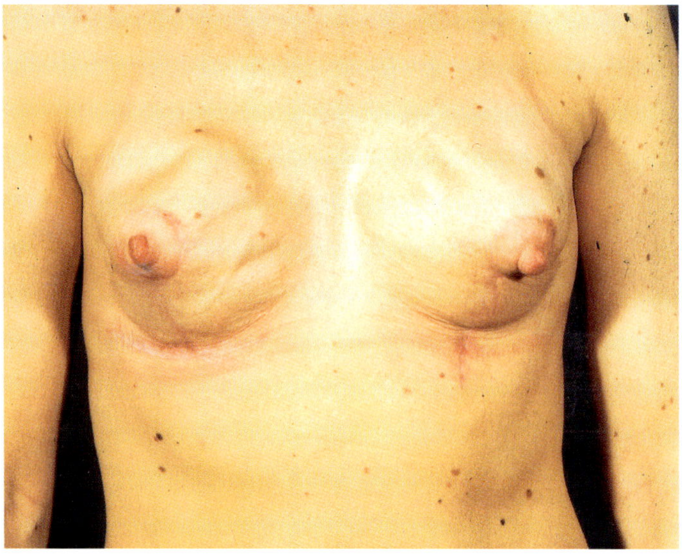

Figure 4.56a Status post subcutaneous mastectomy and reconstruction with implants following three revisions. The skin overlying the implant is very thin with impending perforation of the skin frequently seen following use of saline implants subcutaneously.

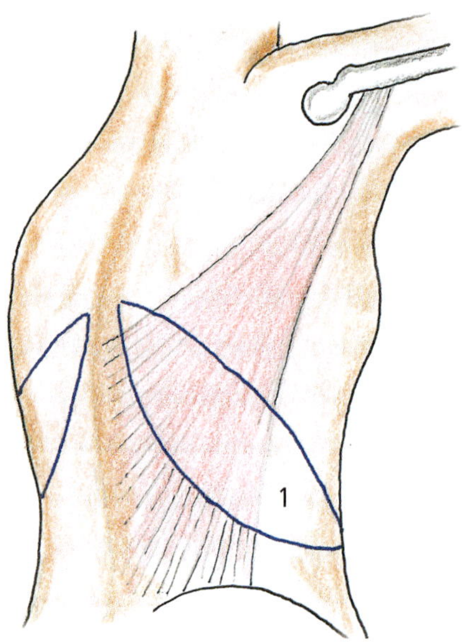

Figure 4.56b Preoperative plan with deepithelialized latissimus flap.

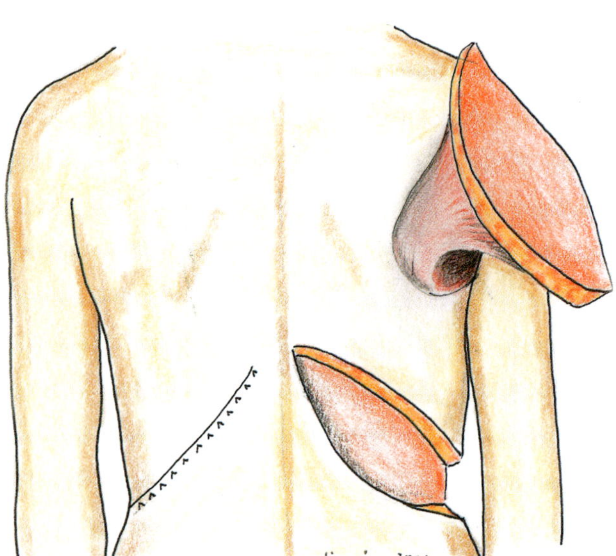

Figure 4.56c First, the flap is deepithelialized then raised. Tension-free closure of the donor site is easily possible with the flap orientation illustrated.

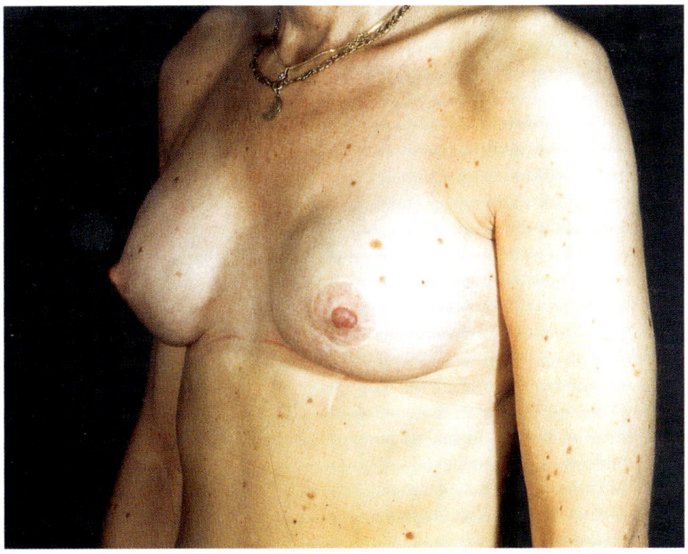

Figure 4.56d Two years postoperatively. Reconstruction was achieved with a deepithelialized latissimus flap without an implant.

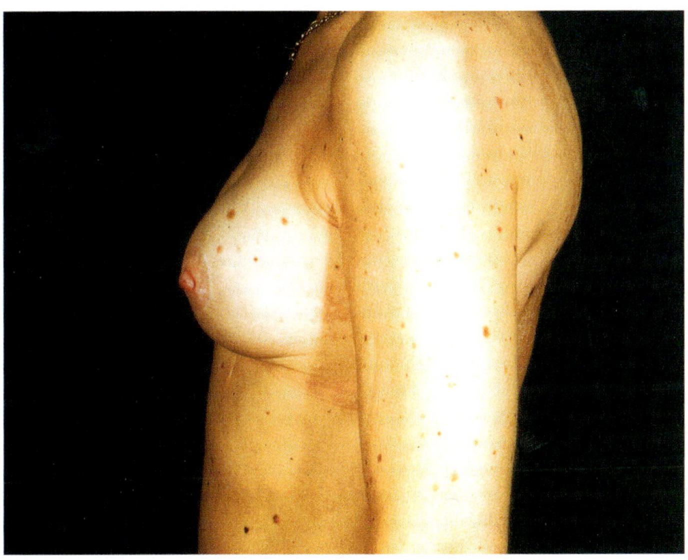

Figure 4.56e 250–350 ccm of tissue volume are easily available for reconstruction obviating the use of implants. The reconstructed breast is soft.

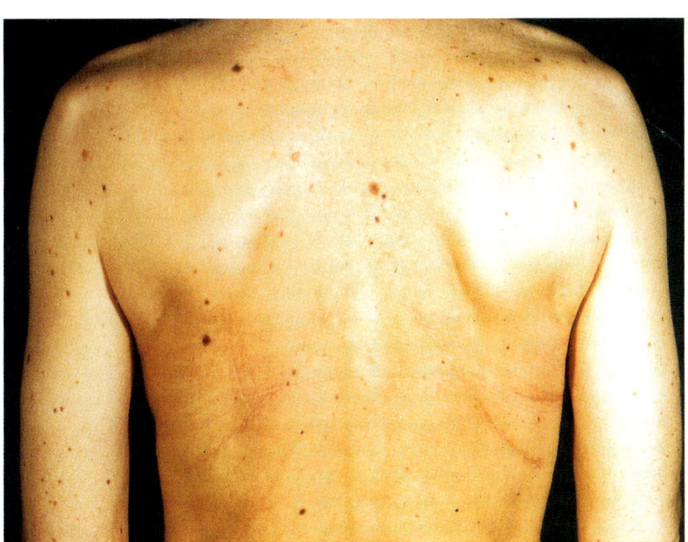

Figure 4.56f Donor site two years postoperatively. Scars of this quality can only be achieved when the flap is designed to have an orientation according to the technique described above.

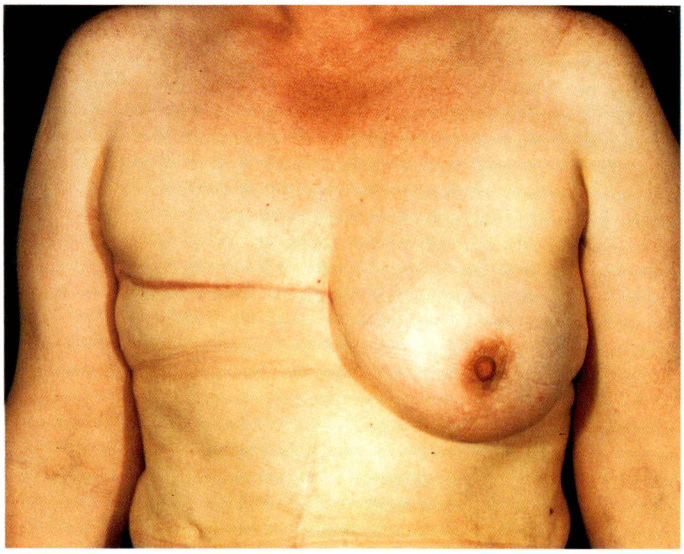

Figure 4.57a Two years following right mastectomy for breast cancer with a new cancer in the left breast. Plan: First, a subcutaneous mastectomy of the left breast is performed with bilateral reconstructions with deepithelialized latissimus flaps without implants.

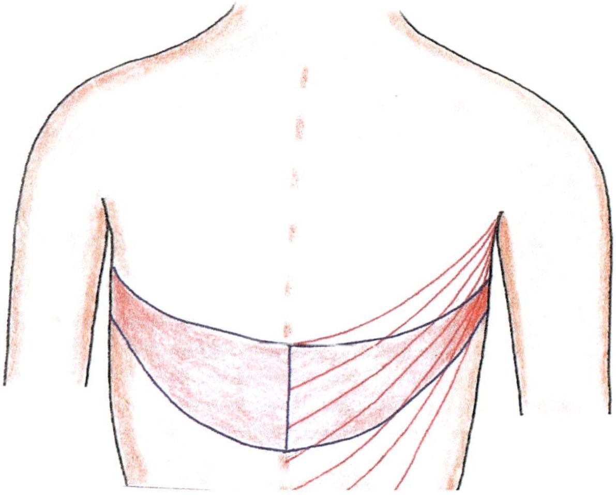

Figure 4.57b First, the marked area is deepithelialized and the myocutaneous latissimus flap is raised and transferred anteriorly through a subcutaneous tunnel.

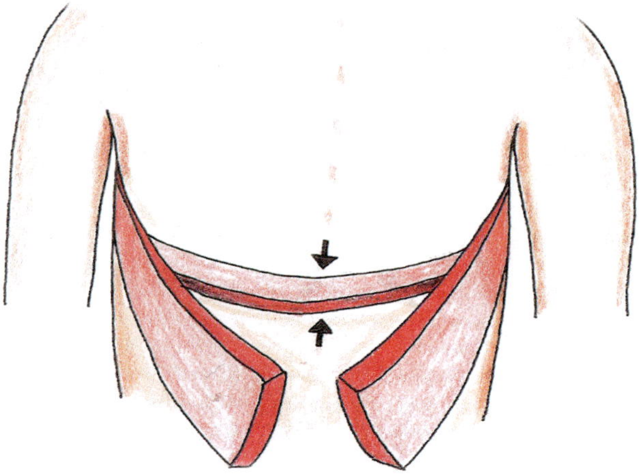

Figure 4.57c Atypical orientation of the donor site which is possible only when ample adipose tissue is available.

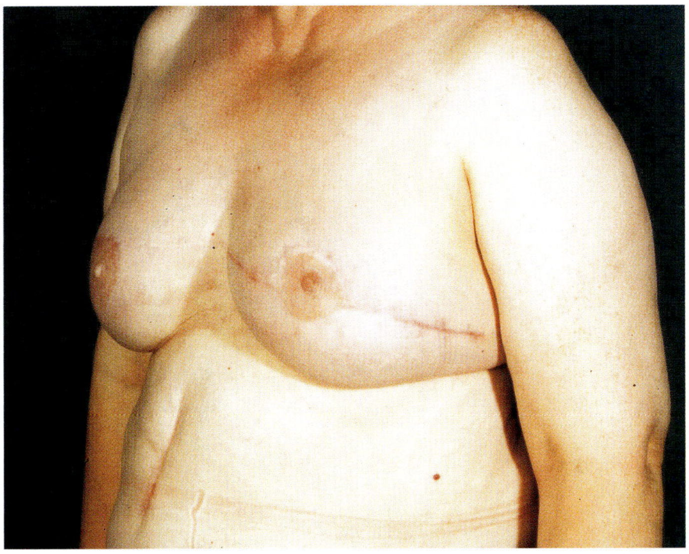

Figure 4.57d One year following breast reconstructions with deepithelialized latissimus flaps without implants. The NAC was reconstructed three months following the first operation.

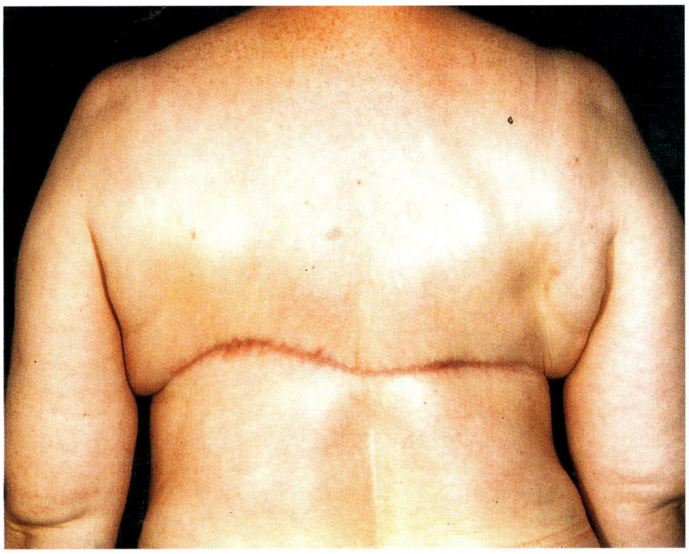

Figure 4.57e This technique can be performed in exceptional cases in overweight patients only. The author prefers the oblique flap orientation described earlier.

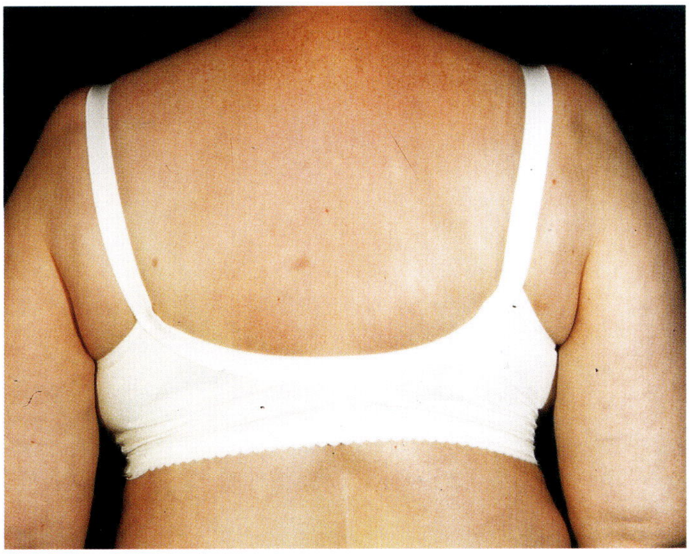

Figure 4.57f The scar has an unfavorable appearance. However, it can be covered easily by a bra. This method is not very advisable.

e) Free Latissimus Dorsi Flap

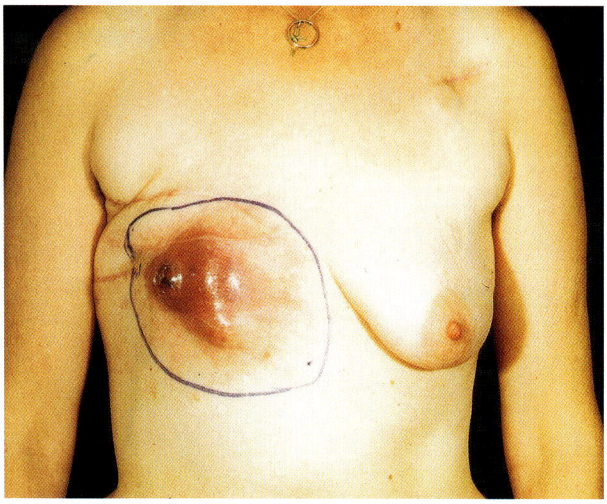

Figure 4.58a Free latissimus flap: Recurrent breast cancer with infiltration of the thoracic wall/intercostals. En-bloc tumor resection including four ribs is planned.

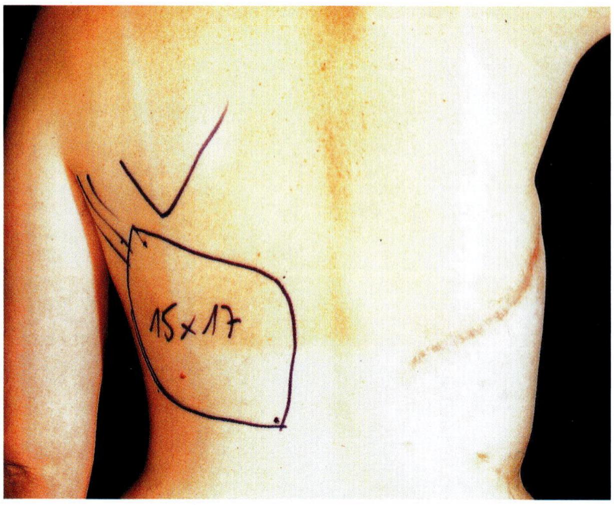

Figure 4.58b Since the ipsilateral latissimus dorsi flap was used during mastectomy, a 17 × 15 cm flap from the contralateral side was used for reconstruction as a free flap.

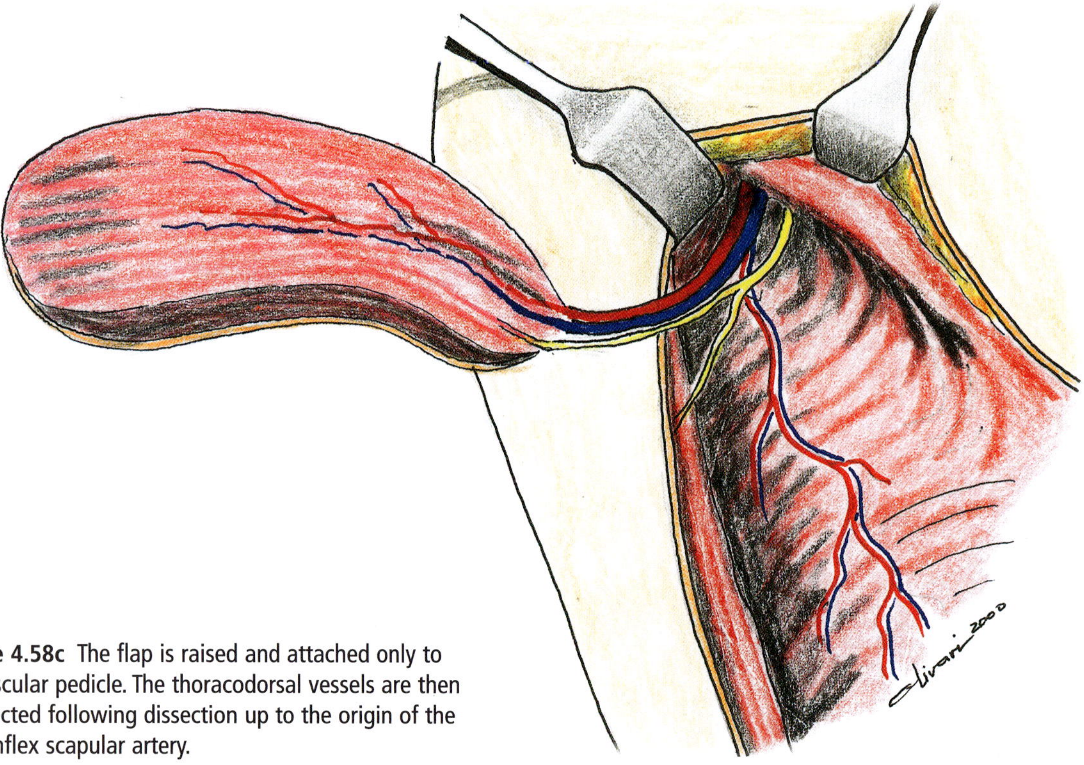

Figure 4.58c The flap is raised and attached only to its vascular pedicle. The thoracodorsal vessels are then transected following dissection up to the origin of the circumflex scapular artery.

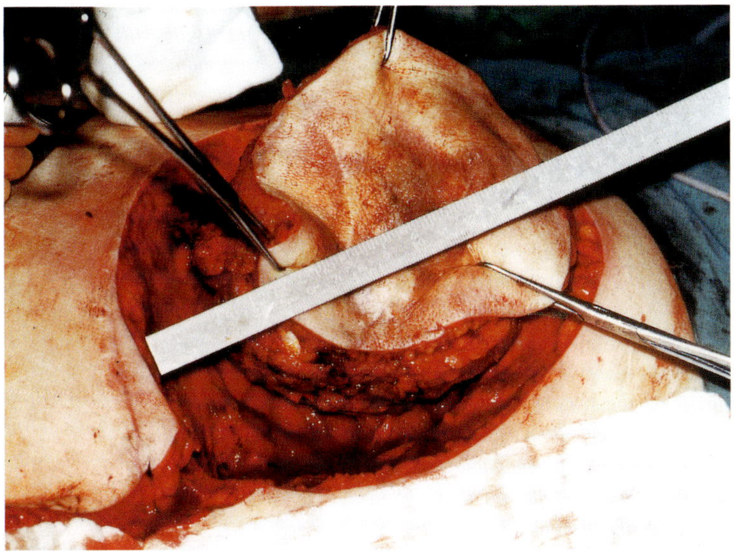

Figure 4.58d En-bloc resection of the tumor including four ribs. The visceral pleura was not involved.

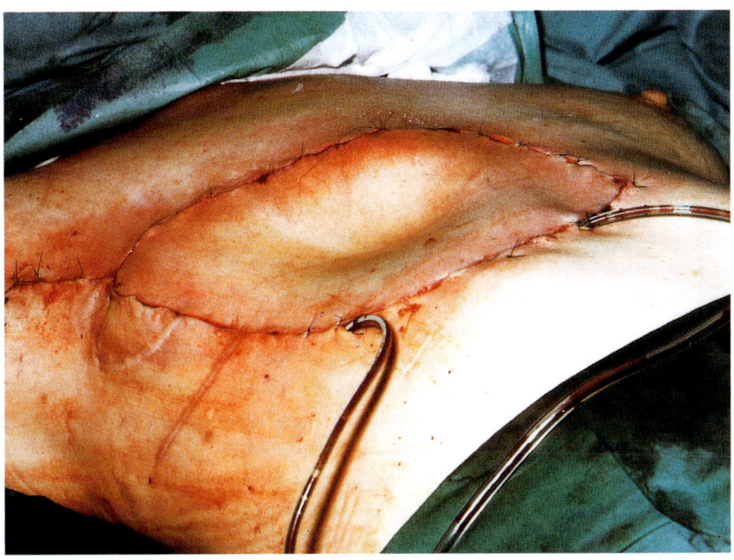

Figure 4.58e Paradoxical thoracic wall excursions are noted at the end of surgery. However, the lung appeared normal. The muscle undergoes fibrosis and becomes stiffer with time and paradoxical excursion decreases. Thoracic wall support with synthetic material may be considered in patients with impaired lung function or larger defects involving four or more rib segments. The danger of infection increases with the use of synthetic materials.

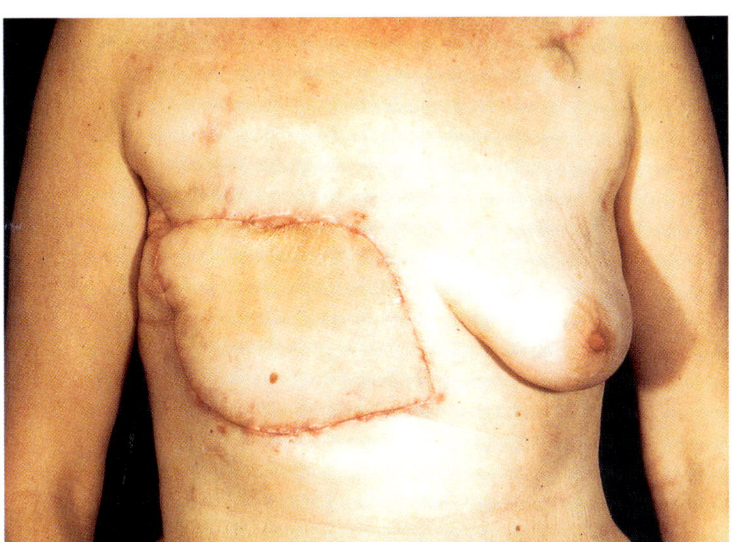

Figure 4.58f Two weeks postoperatively at the time of transfer to the oncology service for further treatment.

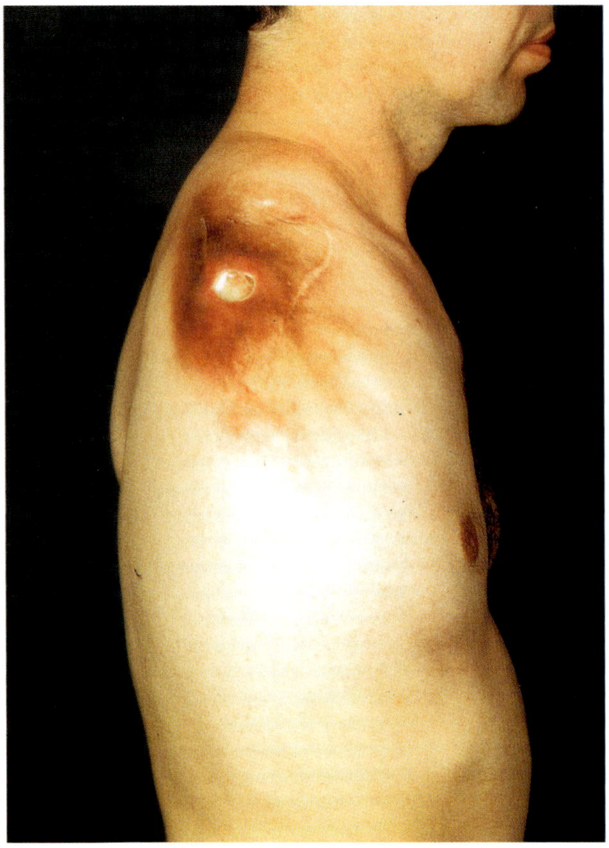

Figure 4.59a Defect at the right shoulder following amputation and postoperative radiation therapy for osteosarcoma. The patient suffered from an infected radiation ulcer with surrounding painful radiodermatitis.

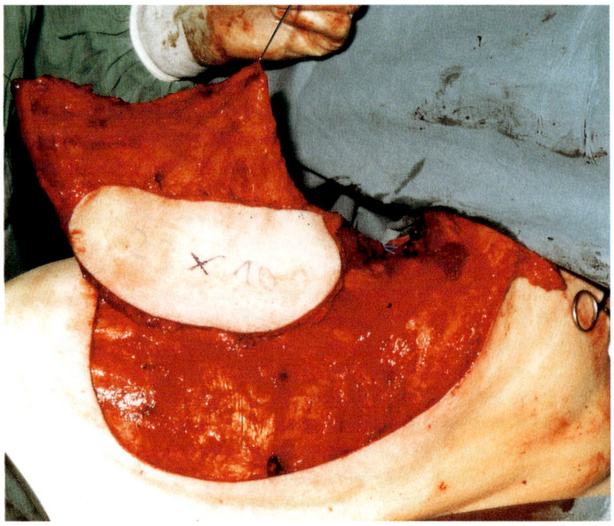

Figure 4.59b The ipsilateral thoracodorsal artery was not available, thus, a free contralateral latissimus dorsi flap was dissected. The skin island measured 23 × 10 cm. Ample muscular tissue was included for padding.

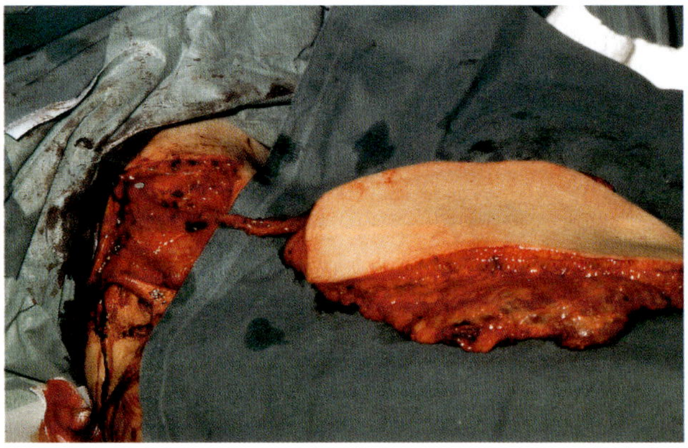

Figure 4.59c The irradiated, damaged, and painful area including the avascular part of the scapula were excised with subsequent microsurgical anastomosis of the latissimus flap.

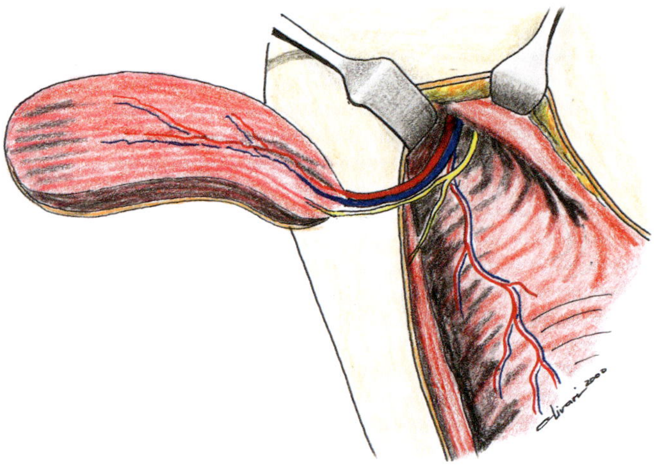

Figure 4.59d Free latissimus flap from contralateral prepared for transfer

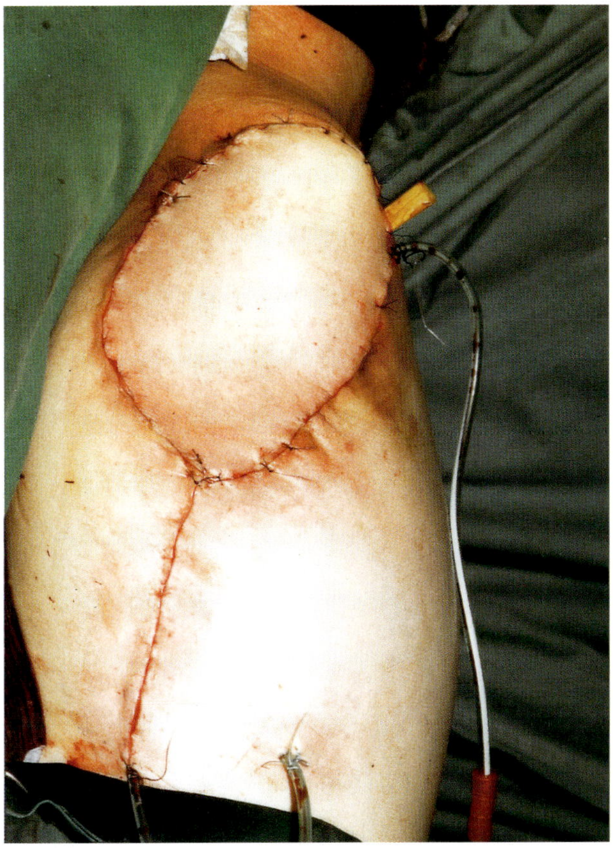

Figure 4.59e At the end of surgery, following micro-anastomosis

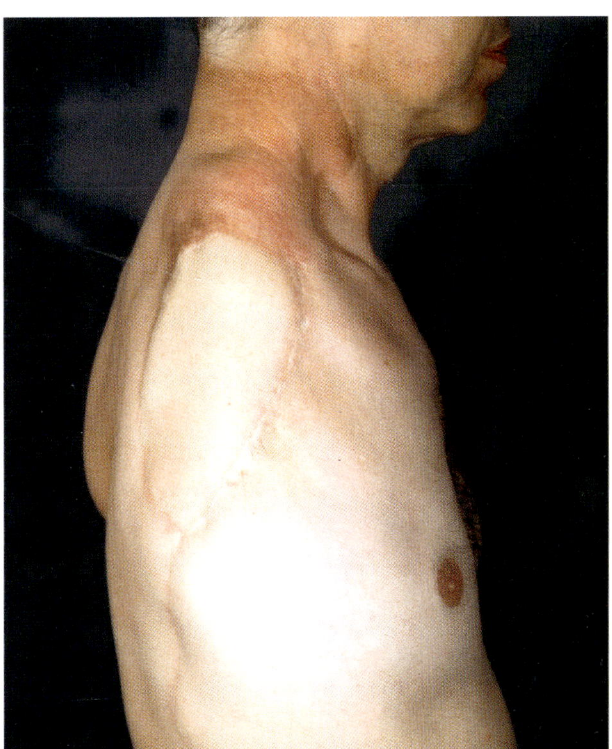

Figure 4.59f Seven years postoperatively

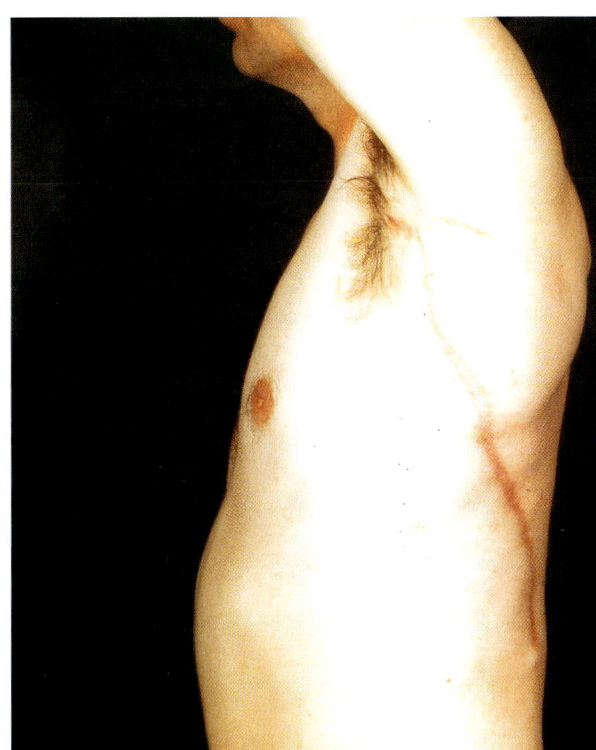

Figure 4.59g The donor site was closed primarily

f) Latissmus Dorsi Flap: Donor Site and Scar Formation

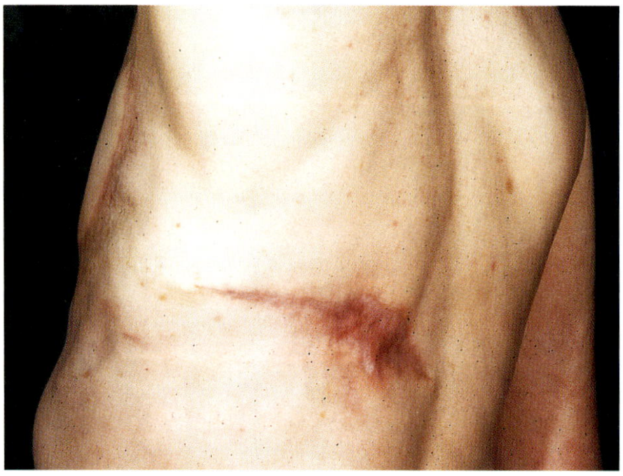

Figure 4.60a Poor scar formation resulting from an unfavorable donor site six months postoperatively. Insufficient volume for breast reconstruction.

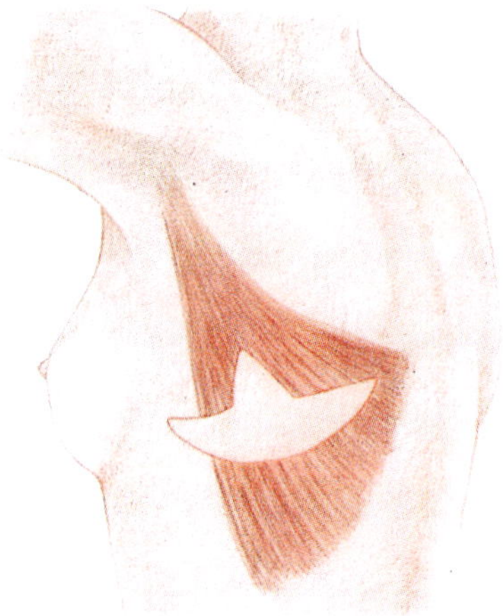

Figure 4.60b McGraw method (fleur-de-lis)

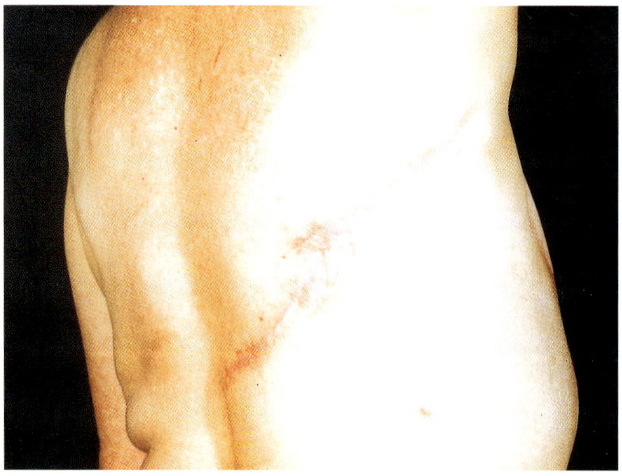

Figure 4.60c Broad scar formation one year postoperatively

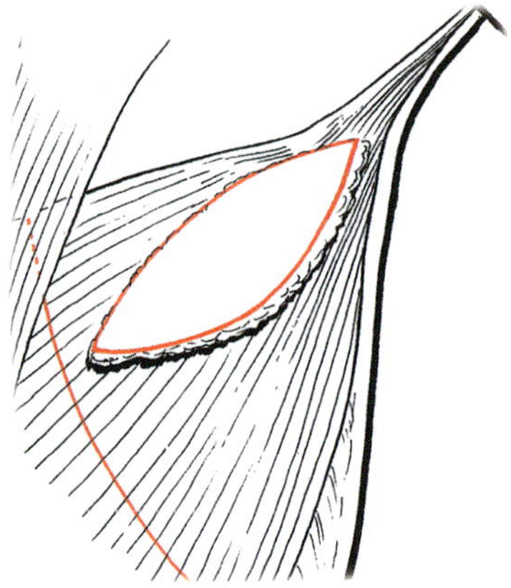

Figure 4.60d Most frequently described latissimus island flap

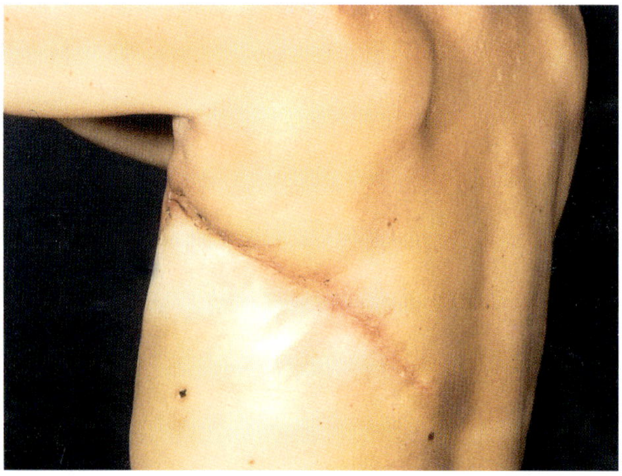

Figure 4.60e Poor scar formation at the donor site three months postoperatively

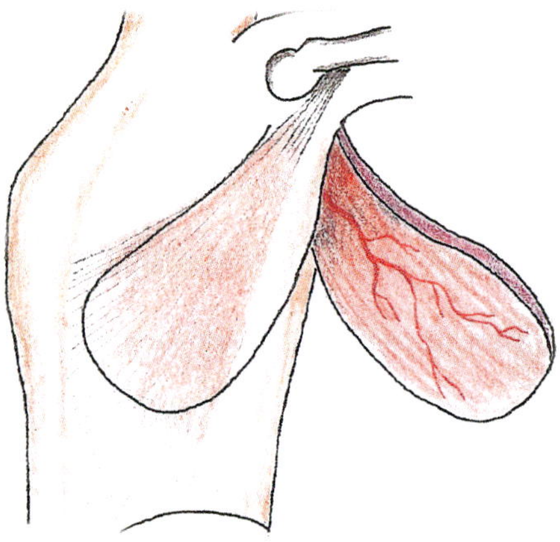

Figure 4.60f Olivari method (I) (Tansini): Pedicled latissimus flap

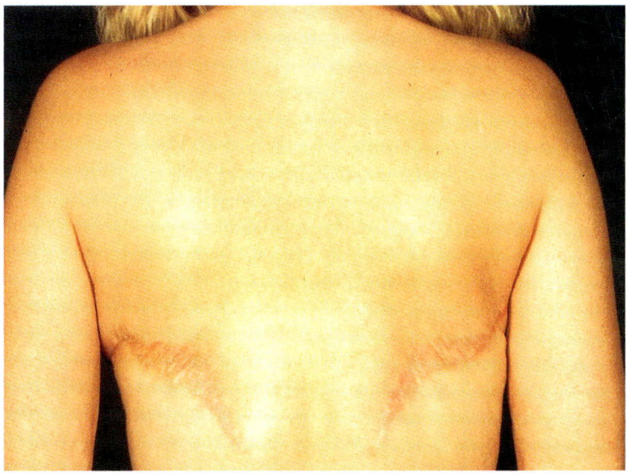

Figure 4.60g Poor scar formation resulting from an unfavorable flap design one year postoperatively.

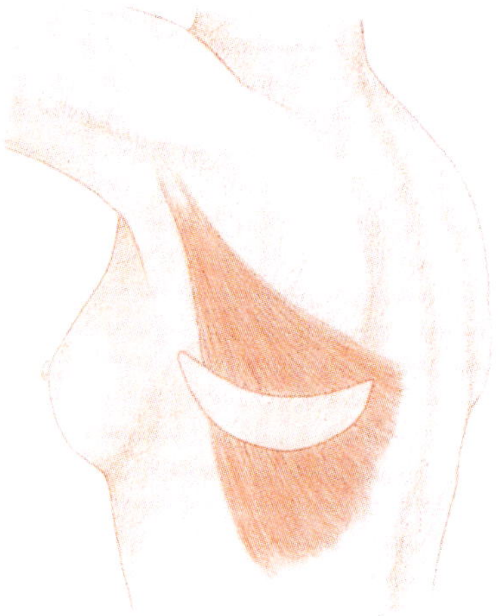

Figure 4.60h Bostwick method

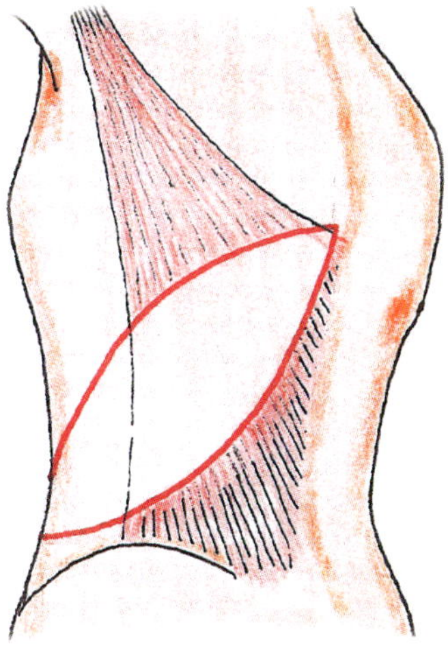

Figure 4.60i Favorable scar orientation following latissimus island flap transfer. Drawback: Scar is visible is bathing suite.

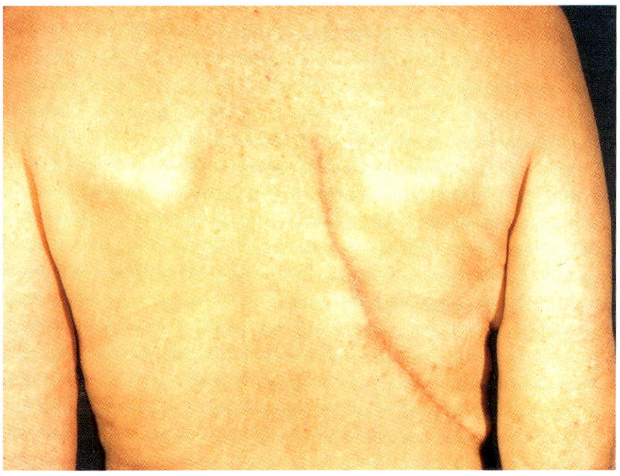

Figure 4.60j Olivari method (II): Three months postoperatively

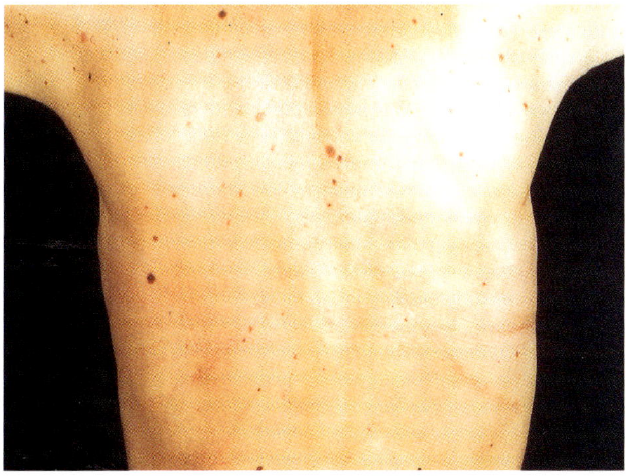

Figure 4.60k Favorable scar orientation. Preferred design for bilateral latissimus island flaps two years postoperatively for breast reconstruction without prosthesis.

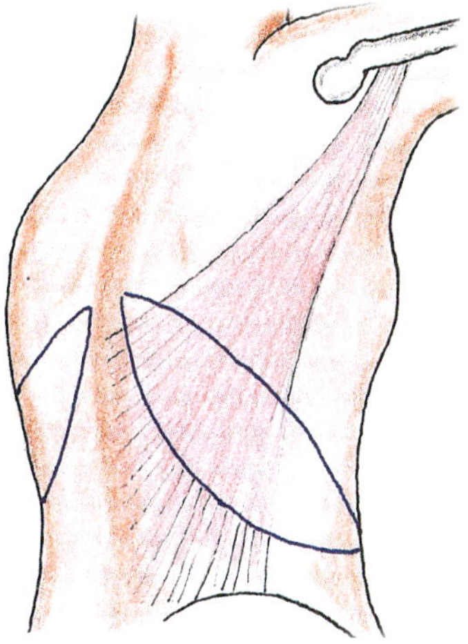

Figure 4.60l Olivari method (II): Island flap

Statistics

Table 4.8 Total number of operations (pedicled, island, and free latissimus flaps)

Clinic	Time period	Number of patients
University Hospital Cologne	1974–1982	188
Dreifaltigkeits-Hospital Wesseling	1982–1997	455
	Total	643

607 patients were female (94.4 %) and 36 male (5.6 %).

Table 4.9 Flap types (latissimus)

Flap type	Number	Percent
Free flaps	61	9.5 %
Island flaps	104	16.2 %
Island flaps with implants	147	22.9 %
Deepithelialized island flaps	225	35.0 %
Pedicled flaps	106	16.4 %
Total	643	

Table 4.10 Indication for surgery (N=643)

Indication	Percent
Breast reconstruction	50.2 %
Local/thoracic wall tumor recurrence (Ca)	23.6 %
Radiation dermatitis – radiation ulcer	14.2 %
Lower extremity defects (free flaps)	9.5 %
Other indications	2.7 %
Total	100.0 %

Table 4.11 Flap innervation one year postoperatively (N=68)

Flap innervation	Percent
Innervation intact	7.3 %
Marginal innervation present	66.3 %
No innervation	26.4 %
Total	100.0 %

In a series of 195 operations, on average, the time for the operation was 2.15 hours (range: 1.40–2.45). 80 patients required blood transfusions (41 %). The average amount of blood given was 500 ccm. The remaining 115 patients (59 %) did not require blood transfusion.

Table 4.12 Complications (N=195)

Complication	Number	Percent
Marginal necrosis	6	3.0 %
Hematoma	7	3.5 %
Total flap loss (infection)	1	0.5 %

Table 4.13 Donor site complications (N=195)

Complication	Number	Percent
Seroma	16	8.2 %
Infection	1	0.5 %
Dehiscence	2	1.0 %

Primary donor site closure was possible in 81 % of all patients. The remaining 19 % required meshed STSG for coverage.

Table 4.14 Scars along the secondary defect (N=195)

Scar width	Number	Percent
>1 cm	16	8.2 %
0.5–1 cm	131	67.1 %
<0.5 cm	48	24.7 %

TRAM Flap

TRAM flap was first described by Holmström as a free flap 1979 and 1982 popularized by Hartrampf and Sheflan as unilateral pedicle flap. Original Holmström flap is superior to Hartrampf flap due to clear better blood supply.

1) Unilateral Pedicled TRAM Flap
[Hartrampf, Sheflan 1982]

This is a myocutaneous transverse rectus abdominis flap. In order to reduce donor site morbidity only a middle muscular portion should be included as pedicle. Preferentially the TRAM is used for breast reconstruction but may also be utilized for the coverage of thoracic wall defects.

The one main vessel in this flap is the superior epigastric artery which derives from the internal mammary artery (IMA).

The unilateral pedicled TRAM flap (see Figure 4.62b), as originally described by Hartrampf, is in fact the most hazardous TRAM flap. Flap perfusion which is provided by the superior epigastric artery, is secured by a network of multiple anatomoses with the dominant inferior epigastric artery in the middle of the rectus abdominis muscle.

This vascular network displays a wide variation in its development. Because the inferior epigastric artery has a larger diameter it is considered to be the dominant vessel. However, this dominant vessel is transected when performing a pedicled TRAM flap. Thus, perfusion of the (frequently large) flap is not provided by the dominant vessel but rather via a network of small vessels which have given off perforators to the skin, from a variable development. This explains the relatively high complication rate (10–20 %), particularly with regards to partial necrosis.

Studies by Taylor demonstrate that the vascular connections between the superior epigastric and inferior epigastric arteries are highly variable. In the majority of cases two vascular networks exist (57 %), a further 29 % have a scarce network, and only 14 % have three vascular networks.

Thus, a strict patient selection needs to be conducted. Exclusion criteria include smoking, obesity, and elderly patients (age >60 years). The unilateral pedicled TRAM flap has les than 50 % of its regular blood supply. Since the contralateral portion is actually a random pattern flap, only a small medial portion of it should be included in the flap (Zone 2) (Figure 4.62a).

The complication rate rises dramatically if more than 60 % of the flap is required.

The perforators are located lateral to the umbilicus in the medial portion of the rectus muscle extending caudally to the arcuate line. This flap is no longer used in our clinic.

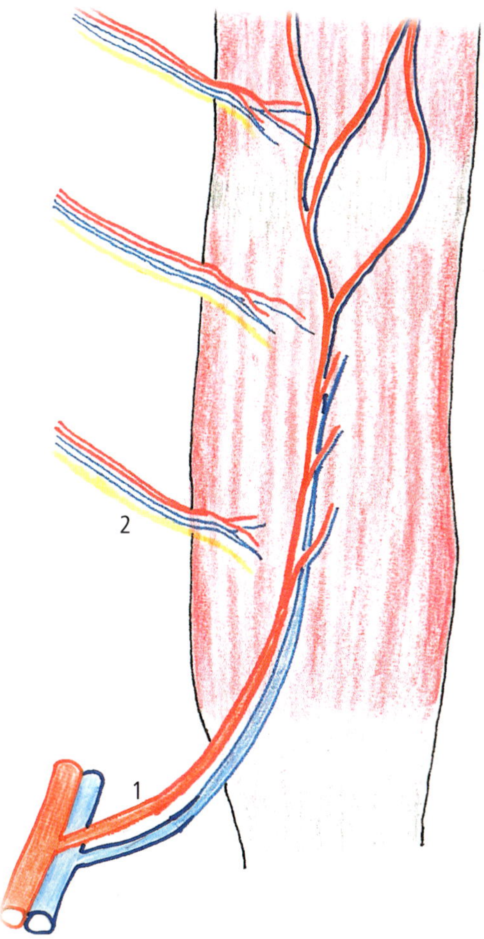

Figure 4.61 Blood supply (dorsal view). Dorsal: The inferior epigastric artery (1) is a branch of the iliac artery and enters the rectus abdominis muscle dorsally. Several branches enter the muscle of which a few perforating branches reach the skin. Additional blood supply is provided by the intercostal vessels. The rectus abdominis muscle is innervated by intercostal nerves. These vessels and nerves are transected during transfer of a **pedicled** TRAM flap. Opinion of some authors that if one take only middle part of muscle, its function stay intact, is an illusion.

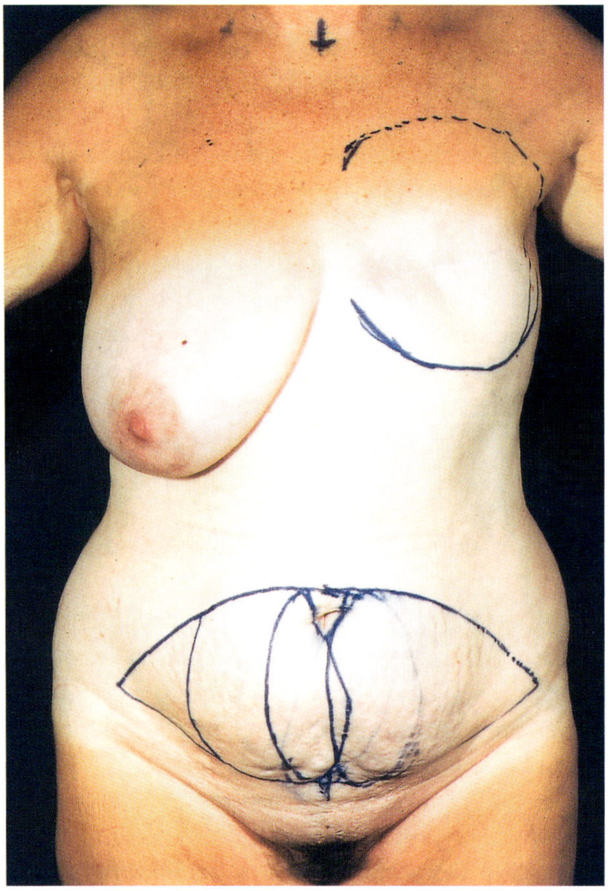

Figure 4.68a Status post mastectomy: A contralateral free TRAM flap is planned. Following identification of perforators the inferior epigastric artery and vein are visualized and dissected caudally in order to preserve a long vascular pedicle.

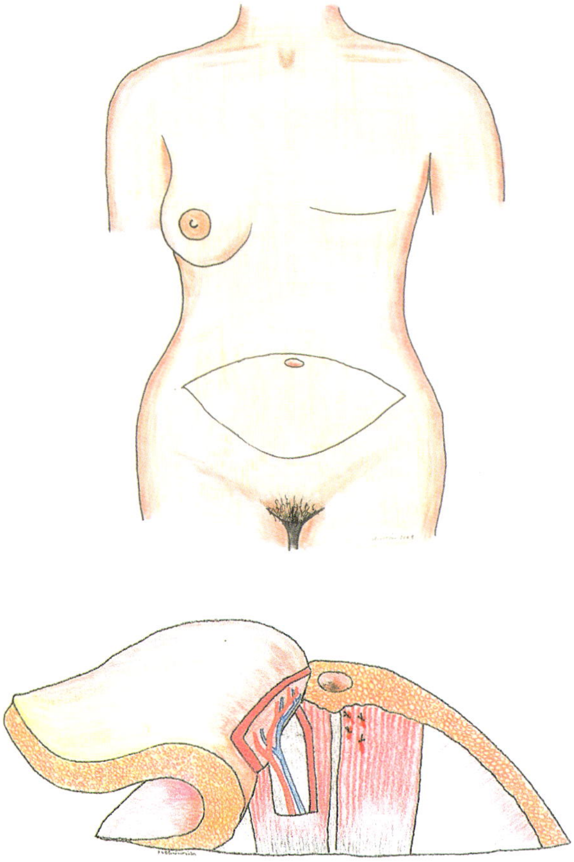

Figure 4.68b Only a small muscular cuff is included in the flap and sufficient muscle strips are preserved bilaterally which allows for an easy closure as well as decreased hernia formation. It is safer to use a small patch of Prolene mesh as well. If a DIEP flap is used there is no need for any Prolene mesh.

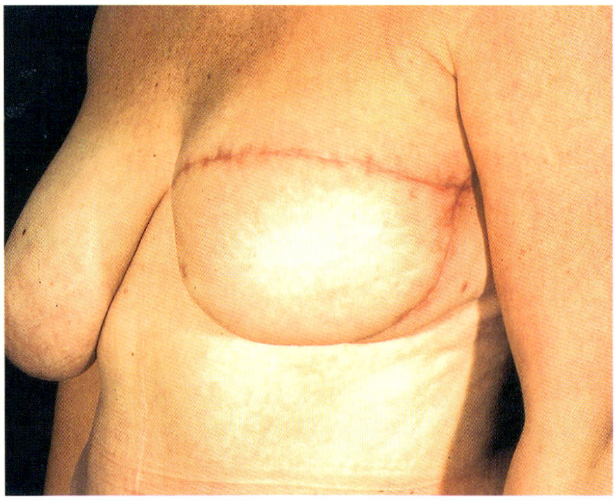

Figure 4.68c Four weeks postoperatively

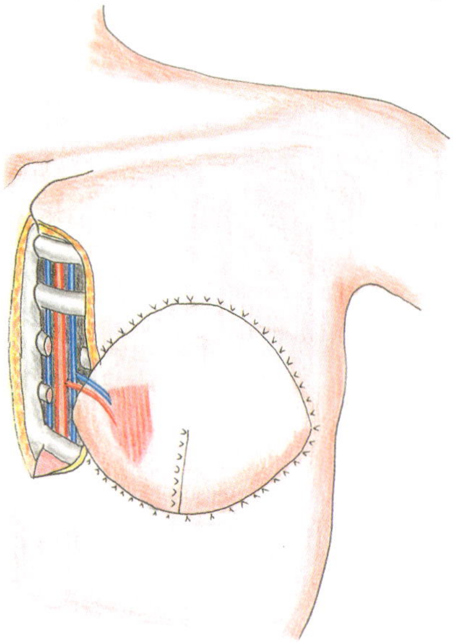

Figure4.68d The free TRAM flap is anastomosed to the IMA whenever possible. This facilitates breast modeling and preserves the thoracodorsal vessels.

TRAM Flap

TRAM flap was first described by Holmström as a free flap 1979 and 1982 popularized by Hartrampf and Sheflan as unilateral pedicle flap. Original Holmström flap is superior to Hartrampf flap due to clear better blood supply.

1) Unilateral Pedicled TRAM Flap [Hartrampf, Sheflan 1982]

This is a myocutaneous transverse rectus abdominis flap. In order to reduce donor site morbidity only a middle muscular portion should be included as pedicle. Preferentially the TRAM is used for breast reconstruction but may also be utilized for the coverage of thoracic wall defects.

The one main vessel in this flap is the superior epigastric artery which derives from the internal mammary artery (IMA).

The unilateral pedicled TRAM flap (see Figure 4.62b), as originally described by Hartrampf, is in fact the most hazardous TRAM flap. Flap perfusion which is provided by the superior epigastric artery, is secured by a network of multiple anatomoses with the dominant inferior epigastric artery in the middle of the rectus abdominis muscle.

This vascular network displays a wide variation in its development. Because the inferior epigastric artery has a larger diameter it is considered to be the dominant vessel. However, this dominant vessel is transected when performing a pedicled TRAM flap. Thus, perfusion of the (frequently large) flap is not provided by the dominant vessel but rather via a network of small vessels which have given off perforators to the skin, from a variable development. This explains the relatively high complication rate (10–20 %), particularly with regards to partial necrosis.

Studies by Taylor demonstrate that the vascular connections between the superior epigastric and inferior epigastric arteries are highly variable. In the majority of cases two vascular networks exist (57 %), a further 29 % have a scarce network, and only 14 % have three vascular networks.

Thus, a strict patient selection needs to be conducted. Exclusion criteria include smoking, obesity, and elderly patients (age >60 years). The unilateral pedicled TRAM flap has les than 50 % of its regular blood supply. Since the contralateral portion is actually a random pattern flap, only a small medial portion of it should be included in the flap (Zone 2) (Figure 4.62a).

The complication rate rises dramatically if more than 60 % of the flap is required.

The perforators are located lateral to the umbilicus in the medial portion of the rectus muscle extending caudally to the arcuate line. This flap is no longer used in our clinic.

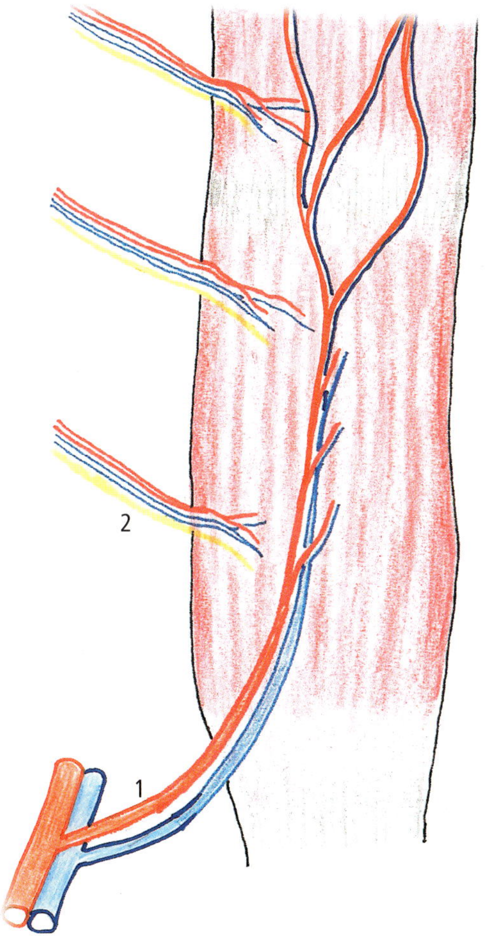

Figure 4.61 Blood supply (dorsal view). Dorsal: The inferior epigastric artery (1) is a branch of the iliac artery and enters the rectus abdominis muscle dorsally. Several branches enter the muscle of which a few perforating branches reach the skin. Additional blood supply is provided by the intercostal vessels. The rectus abdominis muscle is innervated by intercostal nerves. These vessels and nerves are transected during transfer of a **pedicled** TRAM flap. Opinion of some authors that if one take only middle part of muscle, its function stay intact, is an illusion.

Unilateral Pedicled TRAM Flap

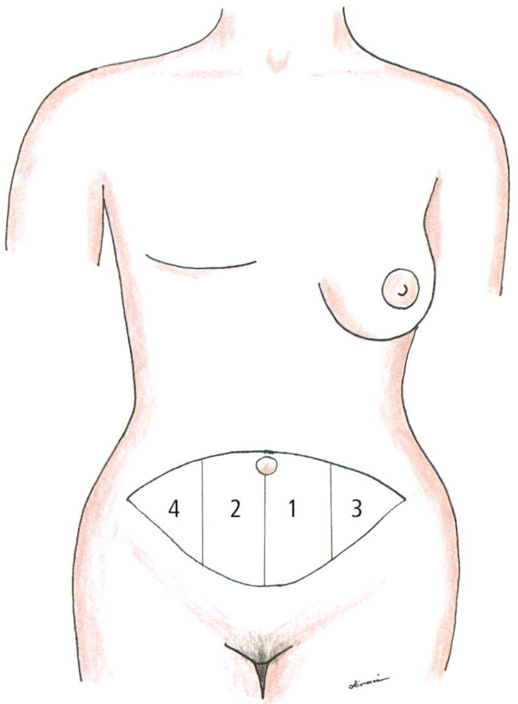

Figure 4.62a The skin island of the **pedicled** TRAM flap can be divided into four zones. Zone 1 and 3 are located ipsilateral to the pedicle, whereas zone 2 and 4 are located contralaterally. The best perfusion pattern is displayed by zone 1. Zone 2 has a good blood supply, zone 3 is characterized by a fair blood supply, and zone 4 is frequently excised primarily during a **pedicled** TRAM flap transfer due to an unreliable blood supply.

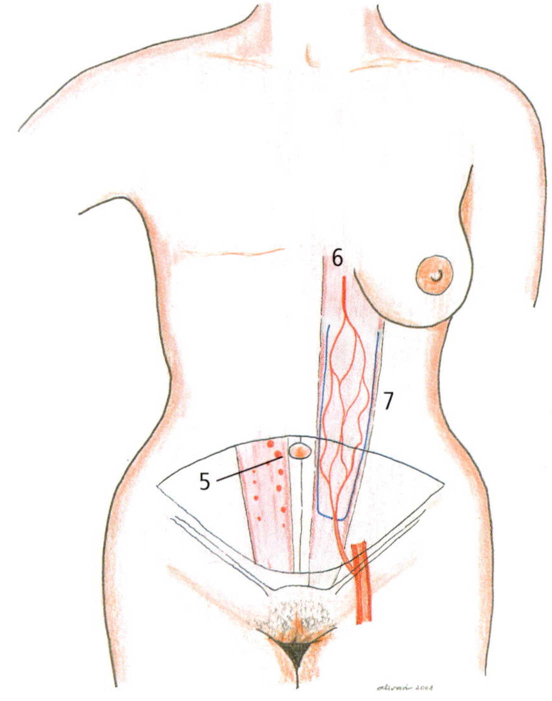

Figure 4.62b Perforator distribution: The strongest perforators are located periumbilically (5). In a **pedicled** TRAM flap vascularization is provided by the superior epigastric artery (6) through anastomoses within the rectus abdominis muscle (7). The superior epigastric artery is not the dominant vessel when a conventional TRAM flap is utilized.

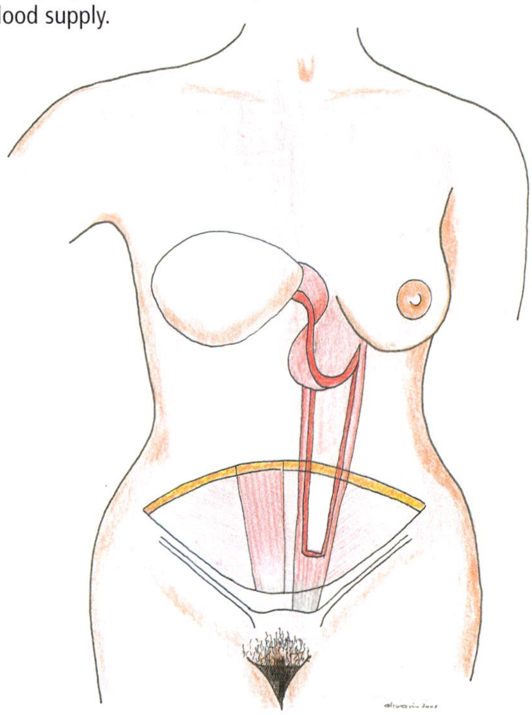

Figure 4.62c The complete muscle is not included in a pedicled TRAM flap transfer. The medial and lateral margins are excluded, thus allowing for an easier closure. Full muscle function is *not* preserved in pedicle TRAM.

2) Bilateral Pedicled TRAM Flap

The bilateral pedicled TRAM flap displays a better perfusion pattern. Thus, a larger portion of skin and adipose tissue can be used for breast reconstruction. Complication rates from necrosis are markedly reduced. However, donor site complications rise significantly. Abdominal wall hernias, laxity, and functional deficits (e.g. sit-ups) occur more frequently. In younger females who plan to get pregnant this may lead to significant problems. The assumption that the lateral portion of the rectus abdominis muscle conserves function is of theoretical interest only since clinical evidence to date does not show this. Blood supply is additionally reduced by tunnel needed to bring the flap in position.

Rectus muscle function is lost following a pedicled TRAM flap.

Unilateral and bilateral pedicled TRAM flaps are contraindicated in the following clinical settings:

a) Radiation within the range of the IMA
b) Smoking
c) Very slim patients without sufficient amount of subcutaneous fat
d) Young patients wishing to get pregnant

3) Free TRAM Flap [Holmström 1979]

Here, blood supply is via the inferior epigastric artery which is the dominant vessel to the flap. Thus, the free TRAM flap displays a marked improvement with regards to perfusion pattern when compared to the pedicled TRAM flap. Flap dimensions may be increased. The entire TRAM region may be included except the contralateral tip. Only a small muscular portion is included in free transfer. The remaining muscle is left behind, thus preserving abdominal wall strength and so resulting in a reduced incidence of hernias. The vascular pedicle is long. As a result of the better blood supply, risk factors may be reduced (smoking, obesity, scars in the upper abdomen).

The rate of necrosis is low; marginal necroses are almost unknown. However, total flap losses are dramatic (2–6 %). Every total necrosis is a heavy burden for patient and surgeon alike. In our clinic (1993–1996) we observed a total of five flap losses, representing 4.7 % (N=106). In the last decade complication rate such as total necrosis decreased to less than one percent.

Two sets of host vessels are utilized for microvascular anastomosis:

a) Thoracodorsal artery and vein
   The artery has a large diameter (2–2.5 mm) and is easy to visualize. A major drawback is that the latissimus dorsi flap may not be used anymore in the case of flap loss. This, however, may be pivotal.
   A few authors recommend anastomosis to the serratus branch of the TDA, thus preserving the TDA. However, this branch often displays a very small lumen resulting in a higher risk of necrosis. When using the TDA, the shaping of the breast is somewhat more difficult. Some lateralization could happen.
b) Internal mammary artery and vein
   First the course of the artery needs to be outlined by Doppler studies. Then, two ribs are partially resected along the sternal border with subsequent visualization of the IMA and accompanying veins. Anastomosis is performed end-to-side or end-to-end. With this technique shaping the breast is facilitated markedly. Furthermore, the latissimus flap can still be used if there is TRAM flap necrosis.

A drawback of free TRAM flap transfer to IMA is its technical complexity. The operation is prolonged by approximately 15 minutes. *When performing a free TRAM flap we clearly prefer the internal mammary artery and vein as the vessels for anastomosis.*

DIEP Flap
Recently and more increasingly the **deep inferior epigastric perforator flap** (DIEP) is performed preserving completely the rectus abdominis muscle, thus preserving its function. No herniated and no bulging after DIEP is described. There is no doubt that this flap will more and more replace a standard free TRAM flap.

Free TRAM Flap [Holmström 1979]

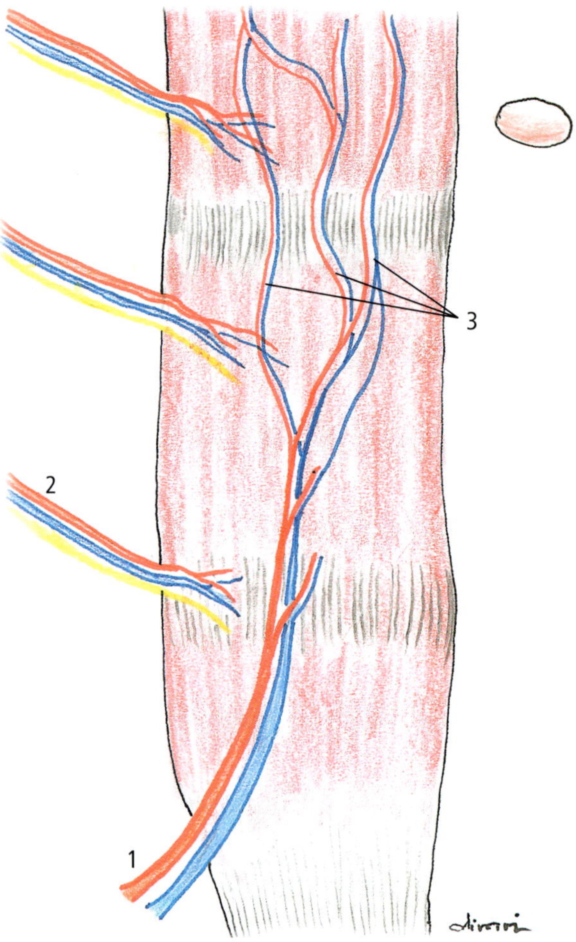

Figure 4.63a Blood supply of rectus muscle (dorsal site). The inferior epigastric artery is the dominant vessel to the rectus abdominis muscle (1). The intercostal vessels enter the muscle laterally and are interrupted in TRAM operation. The perforators which are important for the TRAM flap are located periumbilically.

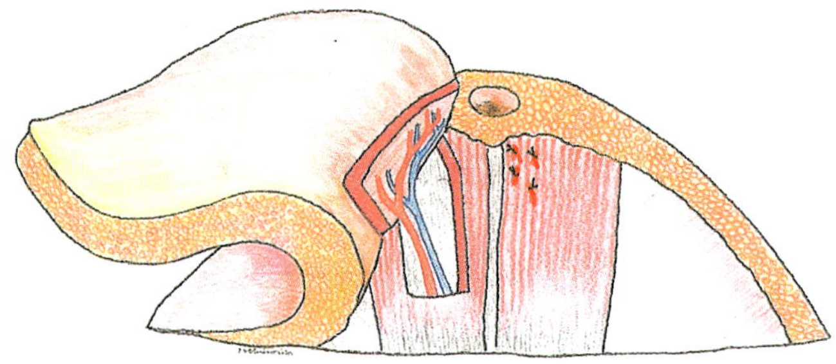

Figure 4.63b Free unilateral TRAM flap dissection. Dissection is started contralaterally in order to locate the perforators, which are almost exclusively positioned symmetrically, thus facilitating orientation. The vascular pedicle should be kept as long as possible (8–10 cm). The lumen of the inferior epigastric artery is 3.5 mm and accompanying veins 3 to 4.5 mm, respectively.

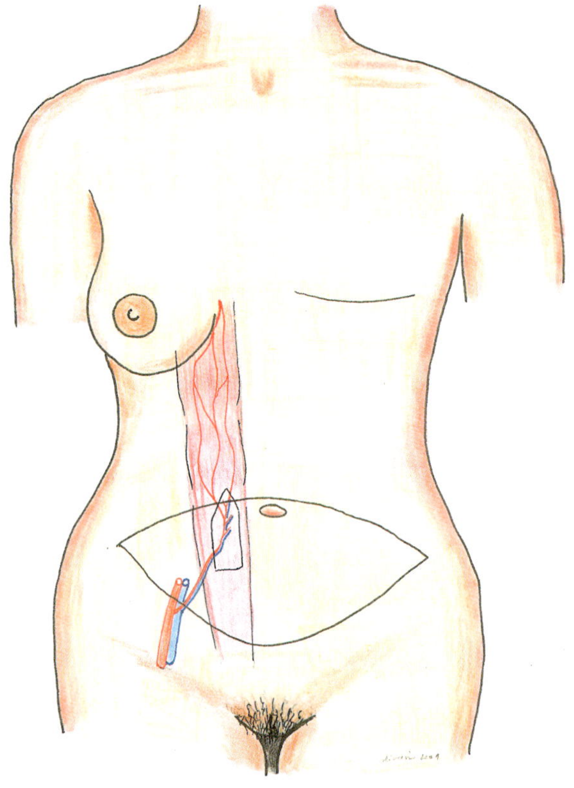

Figure 4.63c The **free TRAM** flap includes a small cuff of rectus abdominis muscle which contains the inferior epigastric vessels.

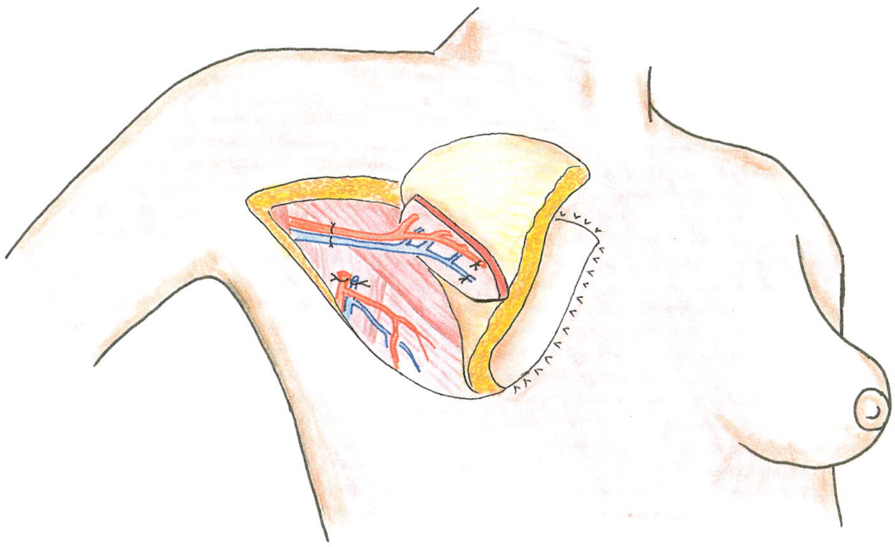

Figure 4.64a The **free TRAM** flap is anastomosed to the thoracodorsal vessels. The free TRAM flap displays a remarkably better blood supply than the pedicled TRAM flap because it incorporates the dominant vessel (inferior epigastric artery and vein).

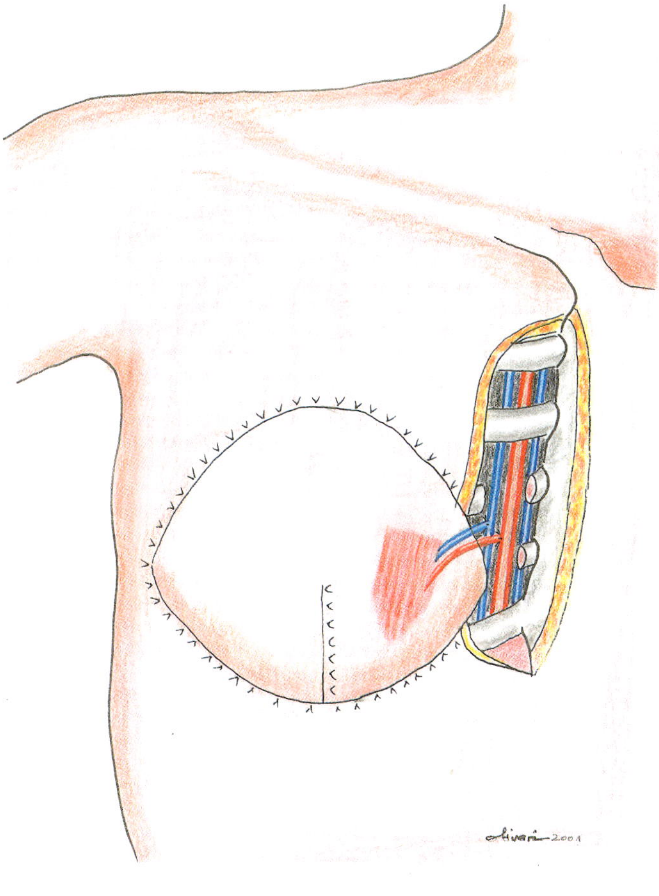

Figure 4.64b The anastomosis between the inferior epigastric artery and the mammary internal artery is usually performed end-to-side. The use of the IMA as the host vessel considerably facilitates shaping of the breast. Furthermore, the thoracodorsal vessels are preserved. In case of TRAM flap necrosis an available latissimus flap is a blessing to patient and surgeon.

4) Bilateral Free TRAM Flap

All facts listed for the unilateral TRAM flap apply here. One has the option to use only half of the TRAM flap for breast reconstruction. However, due to its excellent perfusion the flap may be used to its most lateral extent.

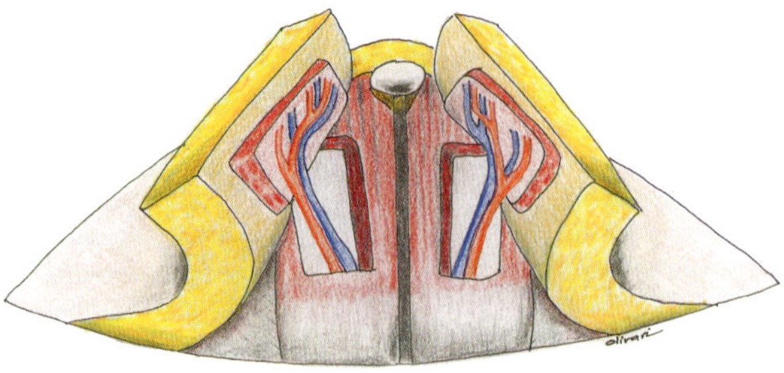

Figure 4.65b Dissection in **bilateral free TRAM** flap transfer. A meticulous dissection for locating the perforators is essential since the contralateral side is not available as a control. As usual, the vascular pedicle should be kept as long as possible (8–10 cm).

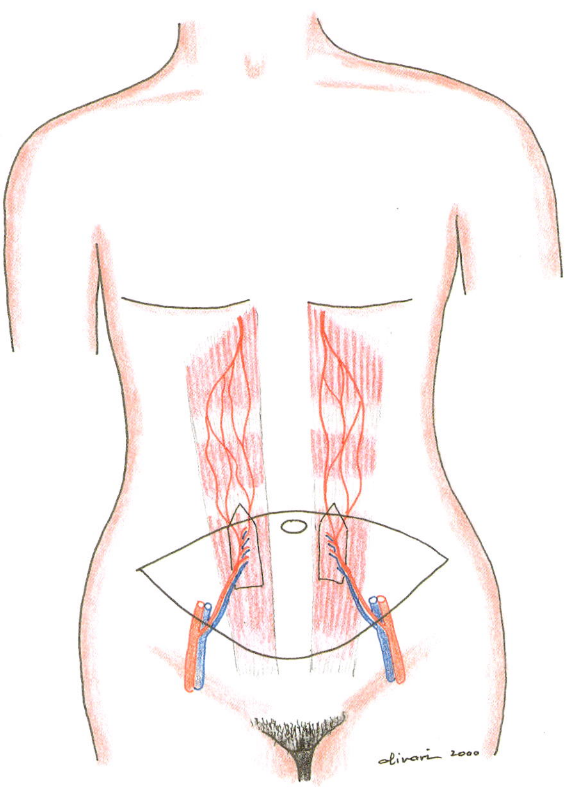

Figure 4.65a Design of a **bilateral free TRAM** flap. Only a small muscular cuff of the rectus abdominis muscle incorporating its perforating vessels is utilized for transfer. The vascular pedicle is kept as long as possible.

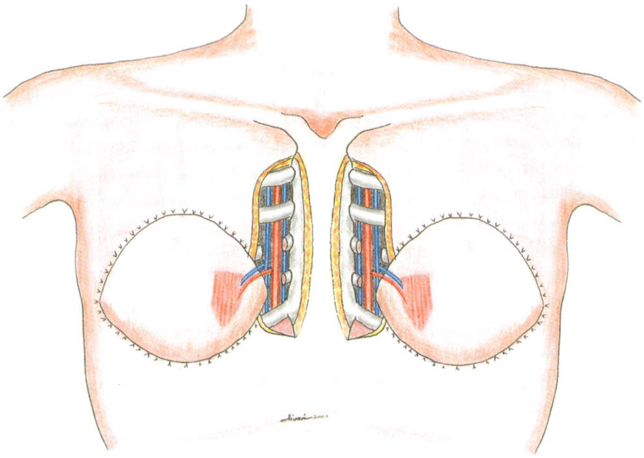

Figure 4.65c The IMA is a recipient vessels provider with advantages including preservation of the thoracodorsal vessels, and shaping the breast is facilitated. Preoperative Doppler study of the IMA is recommended.

5) "Turbo" TRAM Flap

The "Turbo" TRAM flap is a unilateral pedicled flap with an additional vascular supply from an additional microsurgical anastomosis of the inferior epigastric vessels with either the thoracodorsal or internal mammary vessels (preferred) (see Figures 4.66a, b). Flap perfusion is very reliable. In our clinic this flap is performed mainly in high-risk patients. In a series of 57 "Turbo" flaps partial or total necrosis was not observed at all. Problems as to abdominal wall weakness are similar to the data presented for the unilateral pedicled TRAM flap.

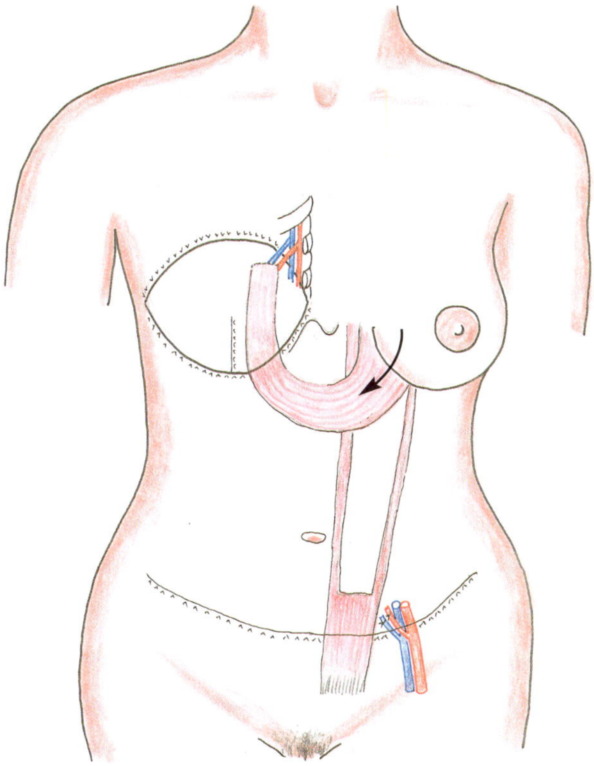

Figure 4.66a "Turbo"-TRAM with anastomosis of the inferior epigastric artery to the internal mammary artery.

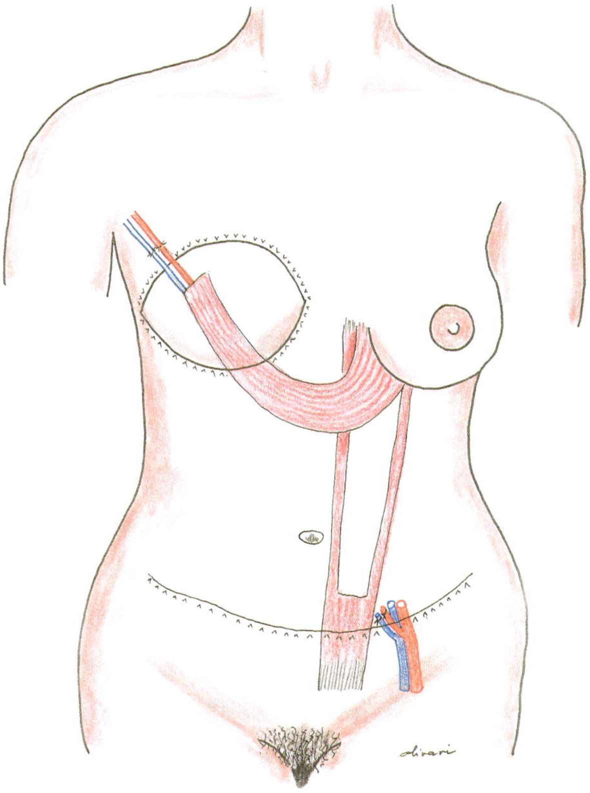

Figure 4.66b "Turbo"-TRAM with anastomosis to the thoracodorsal artery. In pedical and "turbo" TRAM abdominal wall defect is closed using a non-absorbable Prolene mesh.

Figure 4.66a,b Illustrated are unilateral pedicled TRAM flaps which are additionally anastomosed either to the TDA or the IMA (preferably) for better perfusion. This type of flap has been shown to be very reliable in our clinic with the least number of complications. On the one hand flap perfusion is provided by its muscular pedicle via the superior epigastric artery; on the other hand an additional blood supply is established by means of a microvascular anastomosis with the TDA and IMA, respectively. During the last years the "Turbo"-TRAM flap was performed increasingly in our clinic, especially for more risky patients. Problems with abdominal wall laxity is the same as in unilateral pedicle TRAM.

6) DIEP (Deep Inferior Epigastric Perforator) or Muscle Sparing TRAM Flap

This is a free TRAM flap in which inferior epigastric artery is used without a part of the rectus muscle. Artery with perforators is prepared through the muscle without harvesting it. This method is increasing in use. Results are similar with standard free TRAM but without harvesting abdominal wall. Operation time is prolonged by about 30 minutes. In most plastic surgical units this method in the moment is the most used TRAM flap.

Evaluation of the TRAM Flap Techniques

Advantages

Following completion of wound healing the TRAM flap displays the best cosmetic results. Breast shape is natural, soft and eventually gains the same complexion as the contralateral healthy breast. Problems such as foreign body reactions or capsular contractures are not encountered (no silicone prosthesis required). It represents a definite solution.

Disadvantages

The unilateral pedicled TRAM flap is accompanied by a partial necrosis and fat necrosis rate of approximately 15 to 25 % resulting in induration or cyst formation.

In the literature, free TRAM flap has been described as having a 2 to 6 % complication rate – in our clinic: 4.6 %. Partial necrosis rarely occurs. In situations following total flap loss it is advantageous if the TDA has been preserved for a latissimus flap transfer. The reconstructed breast lacks sensibility.

Conclusion

The unilateral pedicled TRAM is a risky procedure and thus should only be performed in selected patients.

The bilateral pedicled TRAM is much safer, however, it results in functional impairment of the abdominal wall. Long-term sequelae have not been fully evaluated yet.

The free TRAM flap displays an excellent perfusion pattern. Thus, larger flaps may be used for reconstruction. Abdominal wall defects are limited. Used as DIEP flap leave no defects of abdominal wall at all. Total flap loss rates of 2 to 6 % impose a heavy burden on patients and surgeons alike. Nevertheless, the free TRAM should be preferred whenever indicated. Complications rate have been decreased in recent years to 1 %.

In patients with an unfavorable history (smoking, obesity, etc.) the "Turbo" flap has proven of value. Complication rates are much lower than in other TRAM flaps. Double blood supply is great advantage.

In the last eight years we discovered the deepithelialized latissimus dorsi flap as a good alternative to the TRAM flap if skin quality after mastectomy it allows (see p. 530). Many patients benefit from this procedure due to its safety, short operative duration, and technical ease (see chapter Latissimus Flap).

Optimal method for breast reconstruction is: Skin sparing mastectomy and immediately reconstruction with free deepithelialized TRAM or DIEP flap. In our clinic mastectomy and reconstruction is done by a plastic surgeon. It makes procedure easier and save a time.

Donor Site (Complication)

A 1-year follow-up in 46 patients showed after free TRAM the following abdominal wall problems following either primary closure of the fascia or placement of an absorbable Vicryl net:

- 5 hernias (10.9 %)
- 6 abdominal wall laxity (13 %)

Subsequently, fascial closure was managed in 21 patients using non-absorbable Prolene mesh. One year postoperatively, none of these patients complained of hernias or laxity. Since then this technique has been considered the standard care at our clinic. 10 % of patients in both groups were not able to perform a "sit-up". Since DIEP is used no problems of donor site are found.

a) Free TRAM Flap for Breast Reconstruction

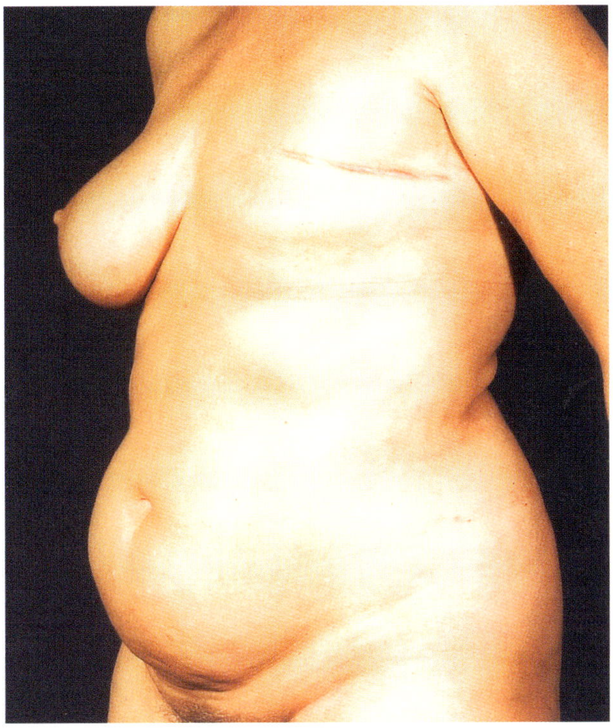

Figure 4.67a Status post mastectomy for breast cancer

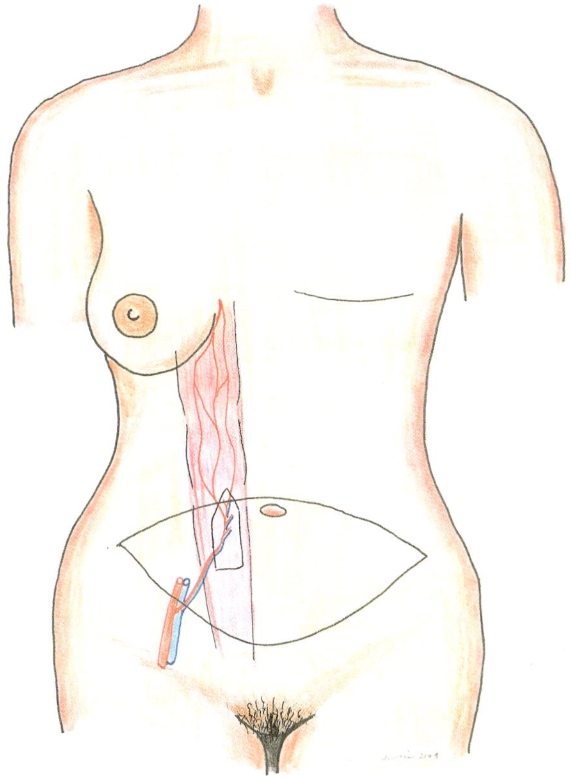

Figure 4.67b Design of a contralateral free TRAM flap for reconstruction

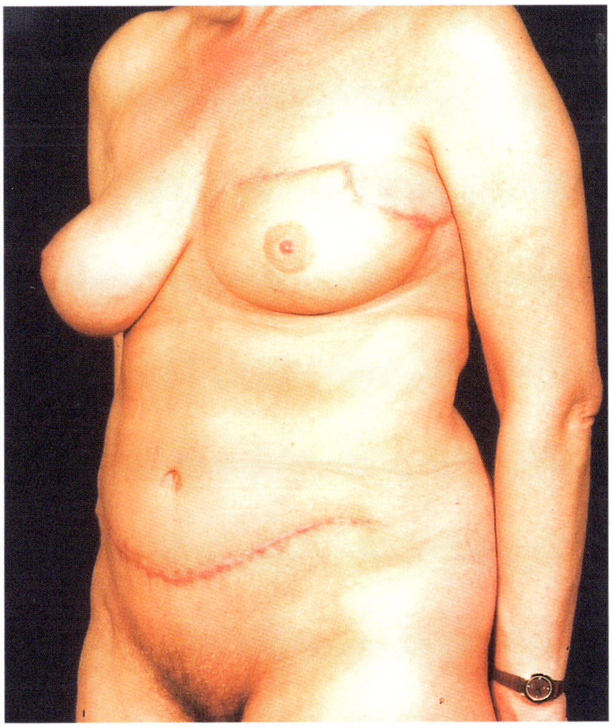

Figure 4.67c Eight months postoperatively: In addition to breast reconstruction the patient enjoyed the improved abdominal appearance.

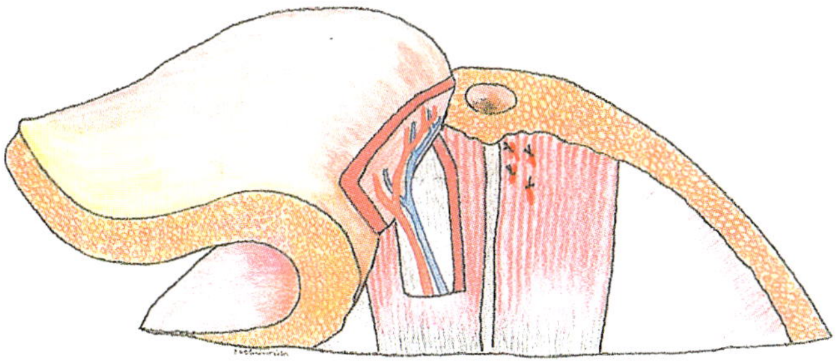

Figure 4.67d Dissection is started contralaterally. Perforating vessels are marked since they exhibit a symmetrical distribution pattern, thus, facilitating orientation. Finally, the vascular pedicle including its corresponding small muscular cuff is dissected.

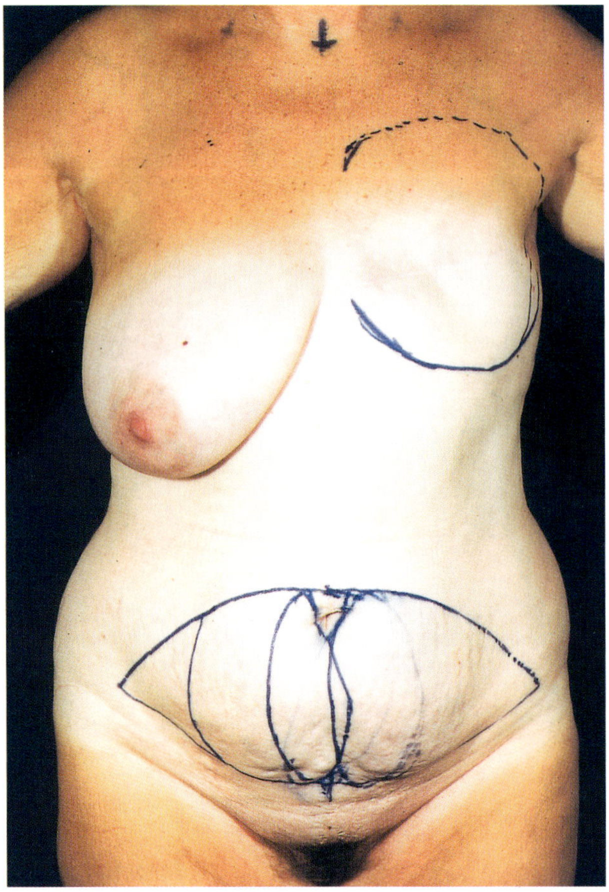

Figure 4.68a Status post mastectomy: A contralateral free TRAM flap is planned. Following identification of perforators the inferior epigastric artery and vein are visualized and dissected caudally in order to preserve a long vascular pedicle.

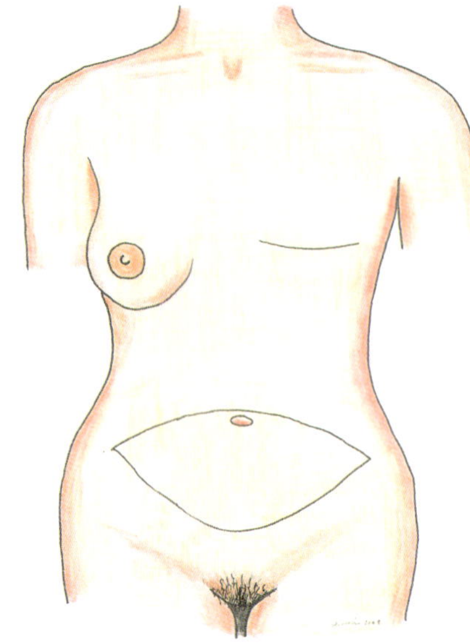

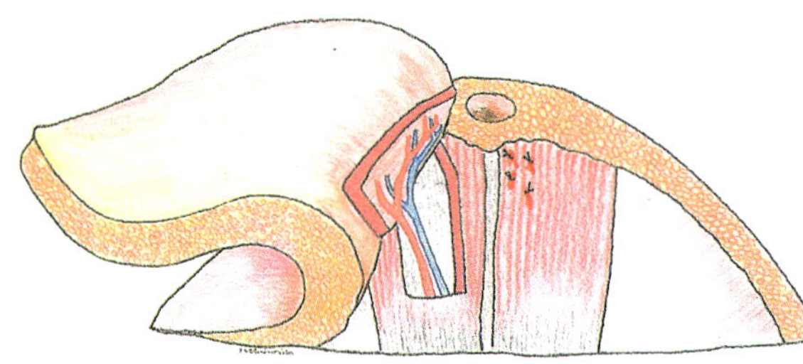

Figure 4.68b Only a small muscular cuff is included in the flap and sufficient muscle strips are preserved bilaterally which allows for an easy closure as well as decreased hernia formation. It is safer to use a small patch of Prolene mesh as well. If a DIEP flap is used there is no need for any Prolene mesh.

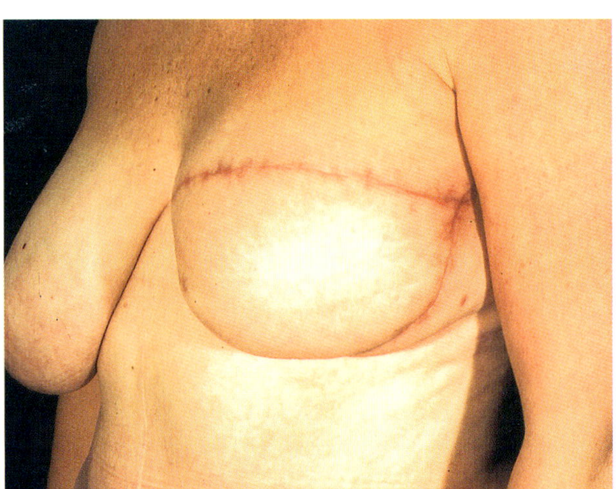

Figure 4.68c Four weeks postoperatively

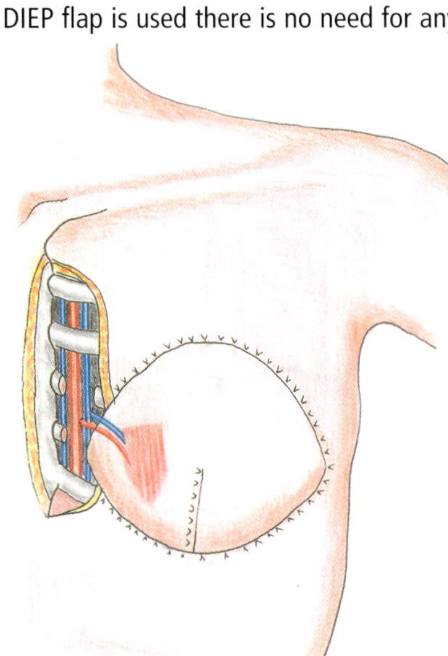

Figure4.68d The free TRAM flap is anastomosed to the IMA whenever possible. This facilitates breast modeling and preserves the thoracodorsal vessels.

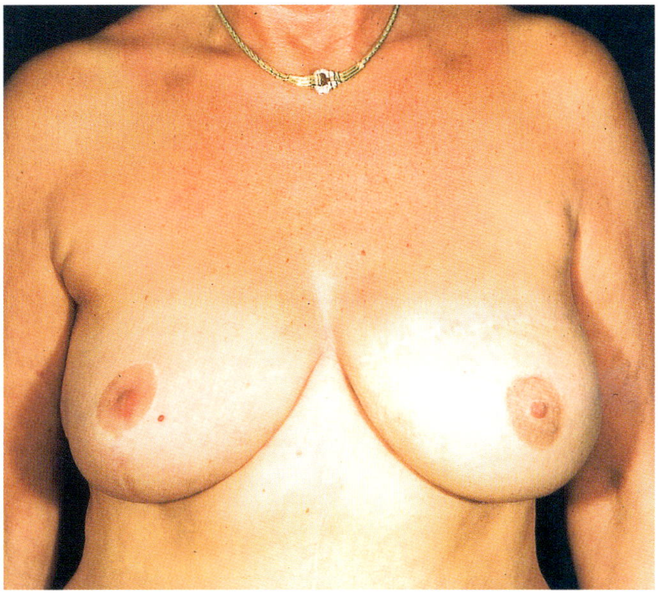

Figure 4.68e Situation three years postoperatively. Three months following free TRAM flap transfer the hypertrophic contralateral breast was reduced and NAC reconstruction performed. The areola was tattooed and the nipple was created using peripheral areolar tissue from the contralateral breast.

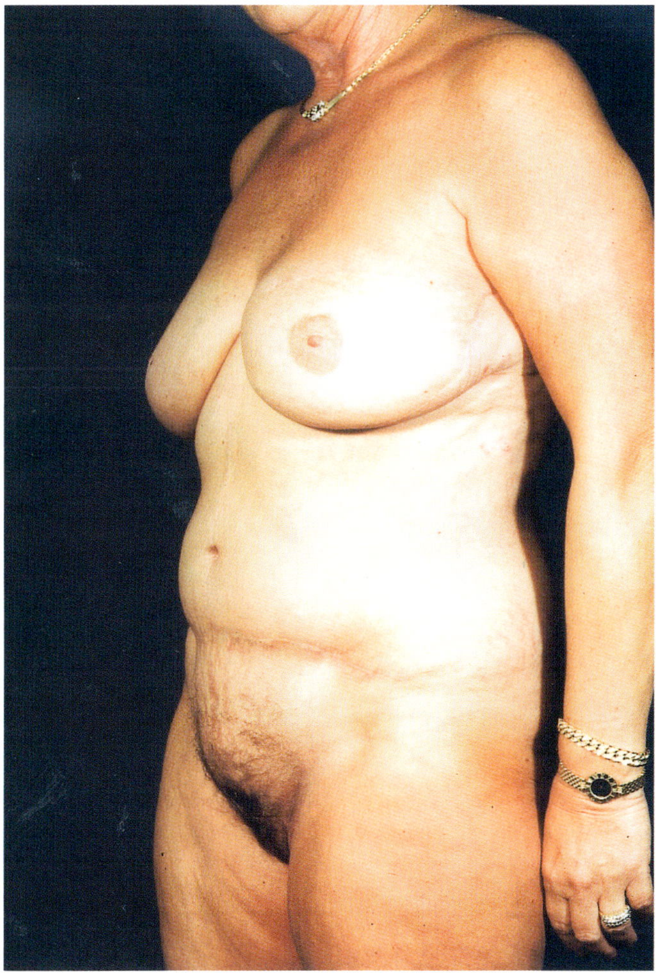

Figure 4.68f Three years postoperatively. The abdomen has a considerably improved shape without hernia formation.

Primary Breast Reconstruction With Free TRAM Flap

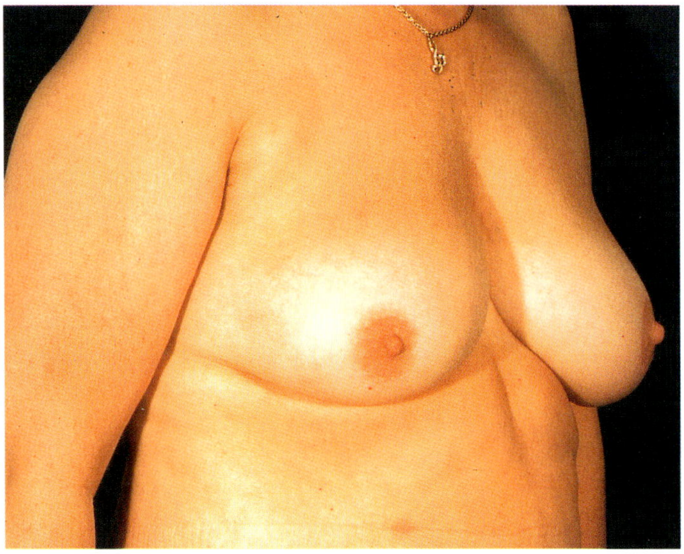

Figure 4.69a Breast cancer of the right breast. Plan: Mastectomy (Patey) and primary reconstruction with a free TRAM flap.

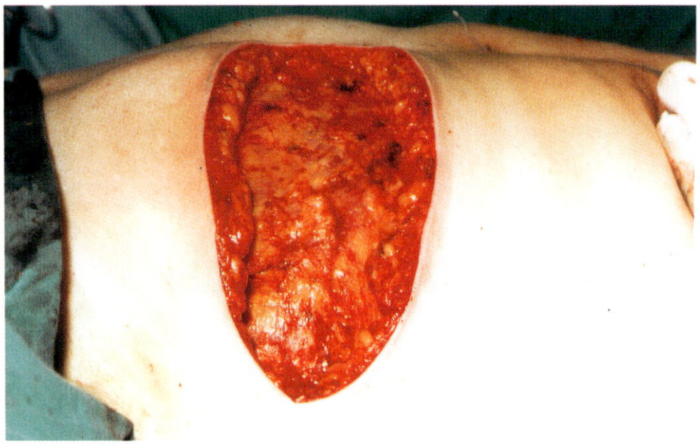

Figure 4.69b Status post mastectomy and axillary LND (Level I)

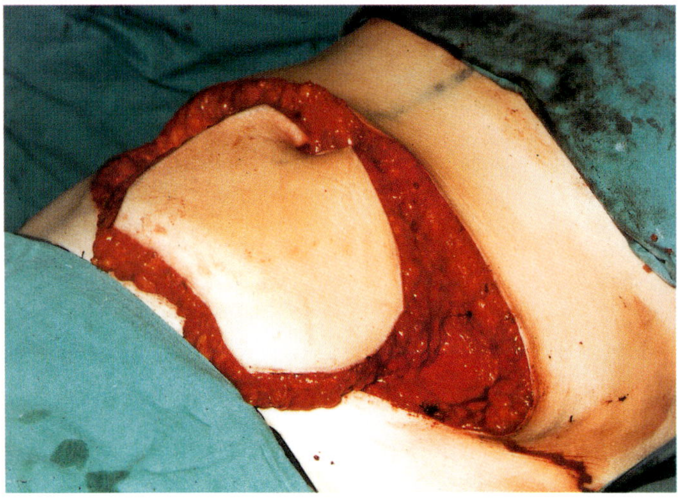

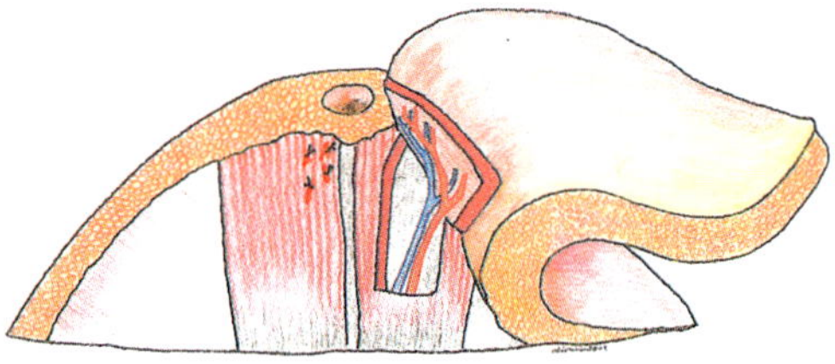

Figure 4.69c A contralateral free TRAM flap is dissected (see illustration).

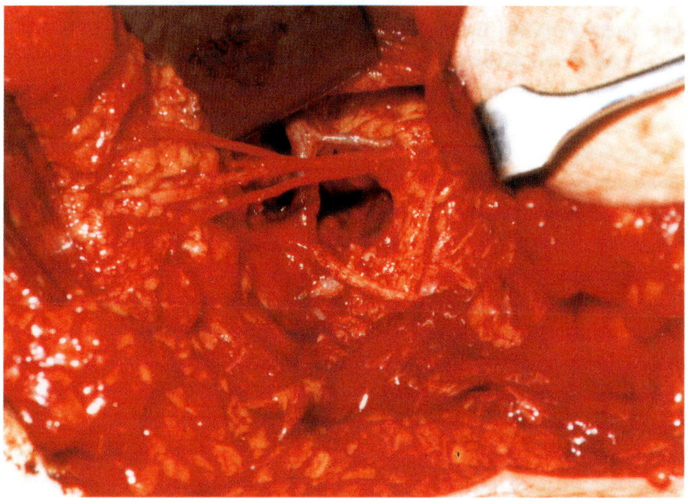

Figure 4.69d The inferior epigastric artery is dissected down to its origin from the femoral artery. Thus, a sufficiently long vascular pedicle is available. The inferior epigastric artery and vein are anastomosed to the thoracodorsal vessels. Anastomosis to the IMA was not possible.

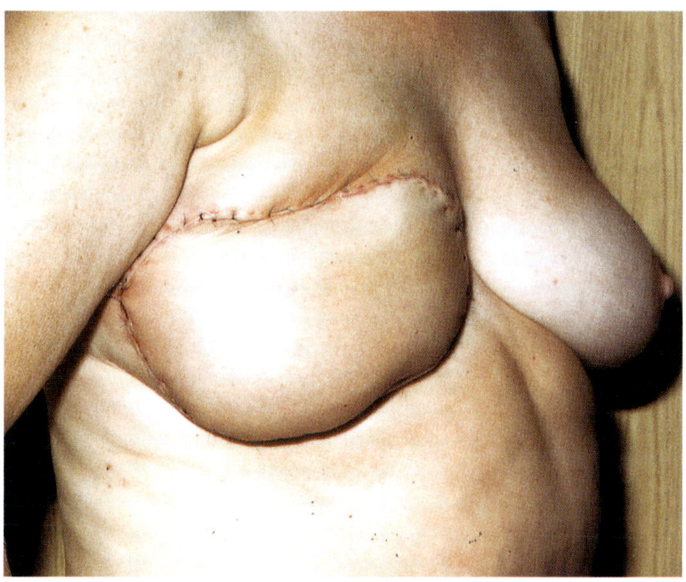

Figure 4.69e Four weeks postoperatively: Anastomosing the inferior epigastric artery to the TDA results sometimes in a "lateralization" of the TRAM flap.

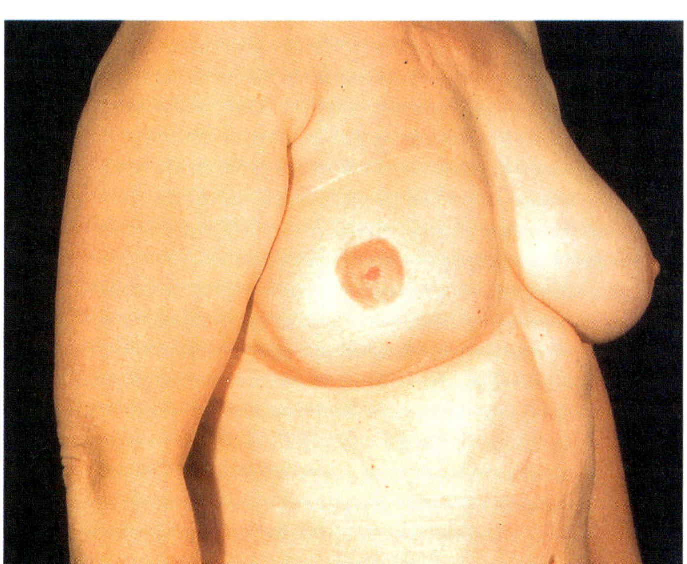

Figure 4.69f Two years postoperatively

Bilateral Free TRAM Flap

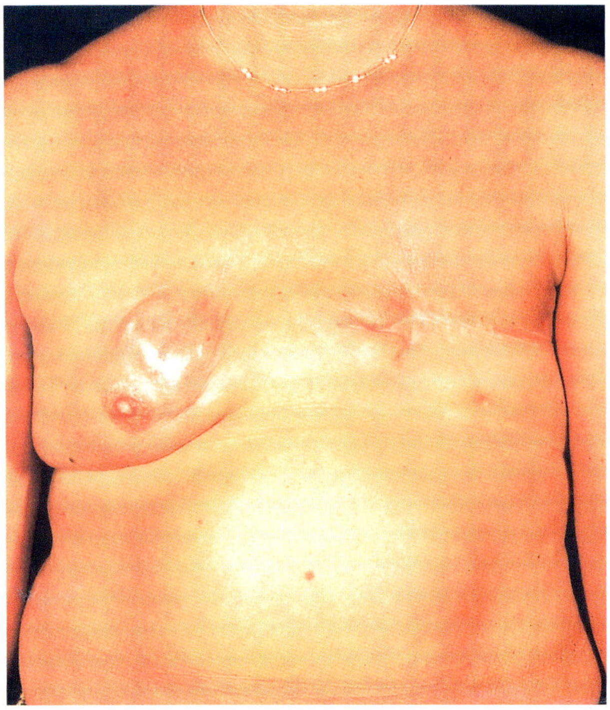

Figure 4.70a Status post mastectomy (left) and subcutaneous mastectomy (right) with subcutaneous silicone-gel implant placement. Followed by that four operations were performed unsuccessfully.

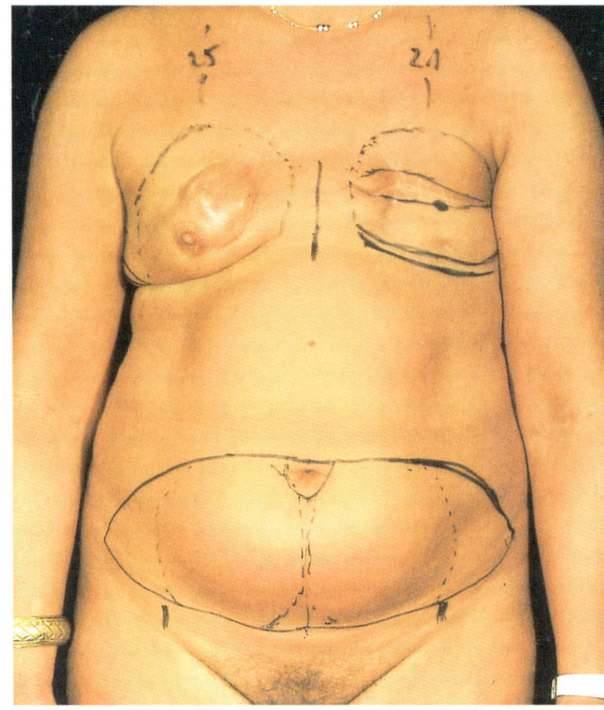

Figure 4.70b Two free TRAM flaps are designed

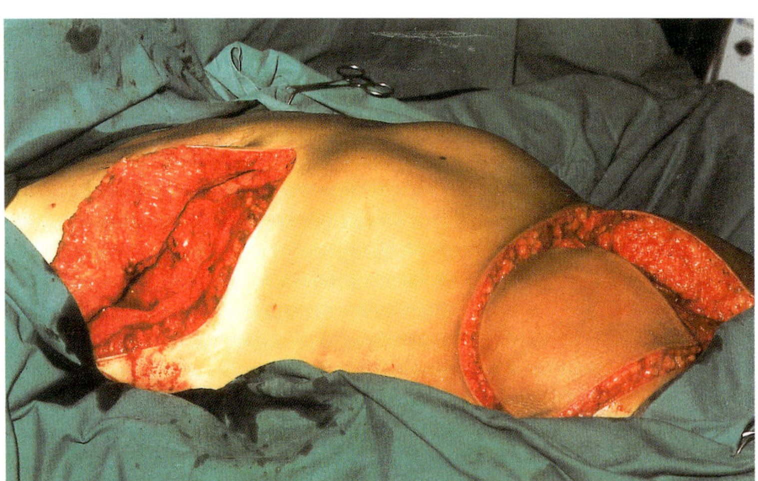

Figure 4.70c The right breast is reconstructed with a **free deepithelialized TRAM** flap serving merely as a volume substitute due to the existence of sufficient amount of skin. The left breast is reconstructed with a cranially and caudally **deepithelialized free** TRAM flap with skin island in its middle portion only.

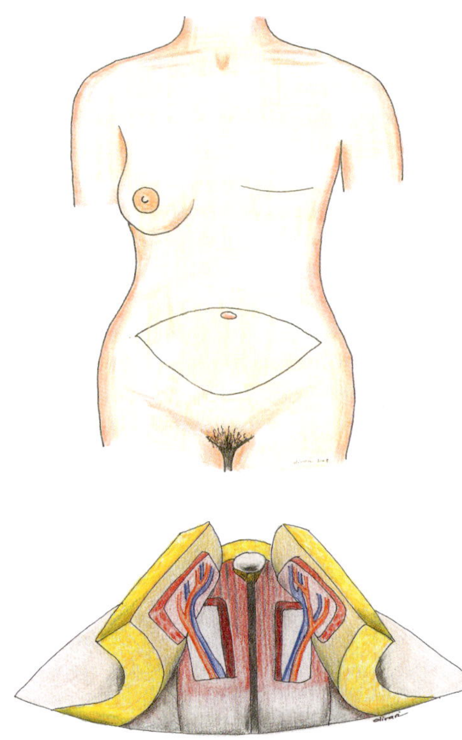

Figure 4.70d Schematic illustration of a bilateral free TRAM flap

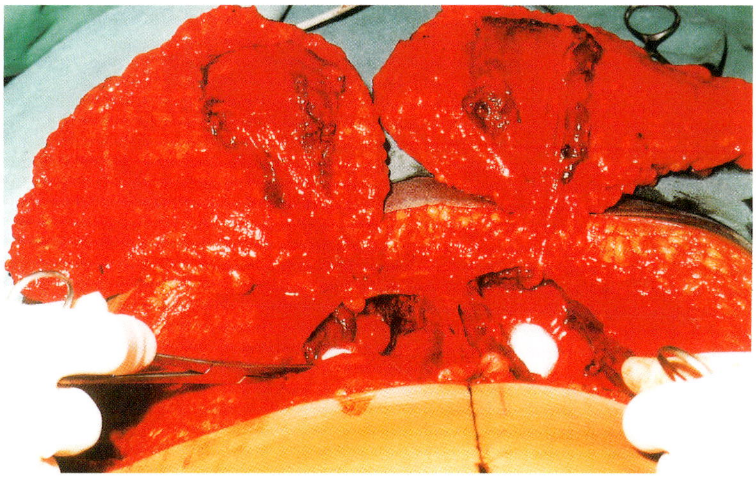

Figure 4.70e The inferior epigastric artery and vein are dissected and prepared for anastomosis.

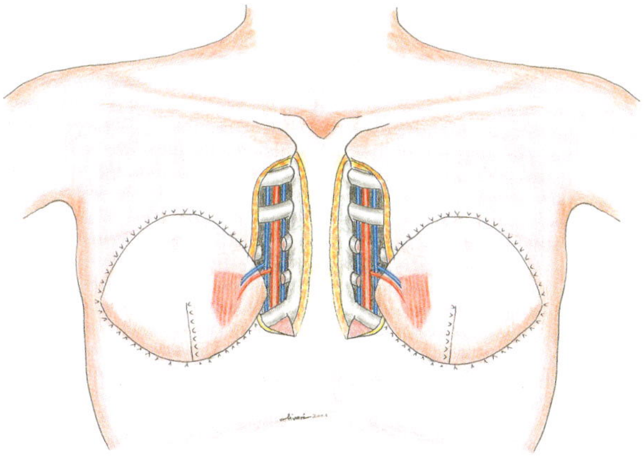

Figure 4.70f Anastomosis is performed to the IMA bilaterally

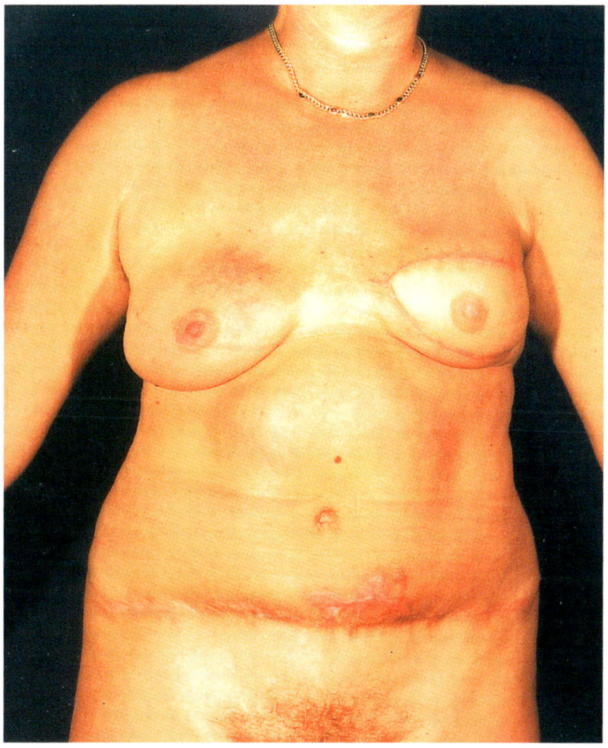

Figure 4.70g Situation six months postoperatively: The right breast has been reconstructed with a deepithelialized free TRAM flap. Breast reconstruction on the left side has been conducted with a partially deepitheliazed free TRAM flap which has been partly used as a skin substitute.

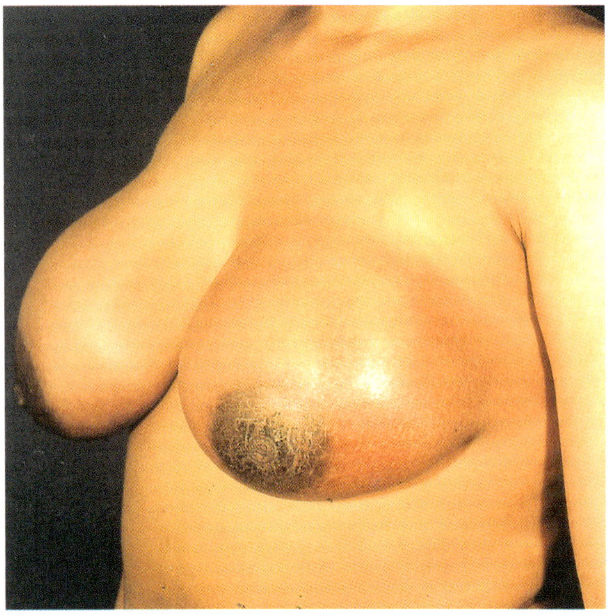

Figure 4.71a Bilateral free TRAM for primary breast reconstruction. Pronounced siliconoma caused by massive injections of industrial silicone. A subcutaneous mastectomy was not possible because the silicone has already infiltrated skin and breast tissue.

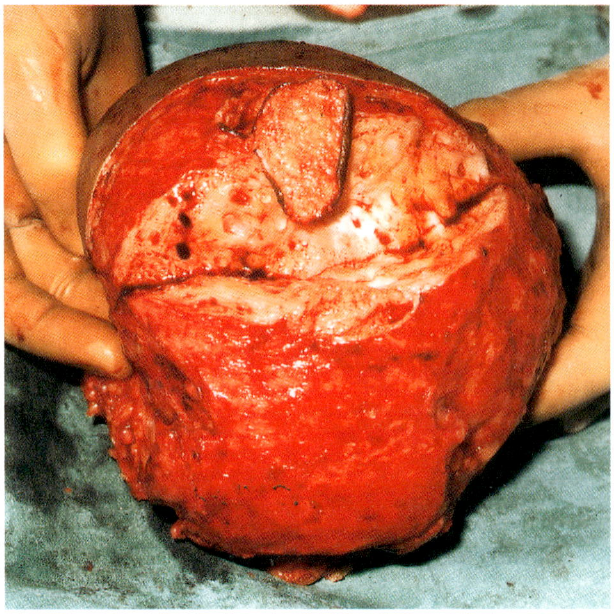

Figure 4.71b The silicone has infiltrated the entire breast including skin and muscle.

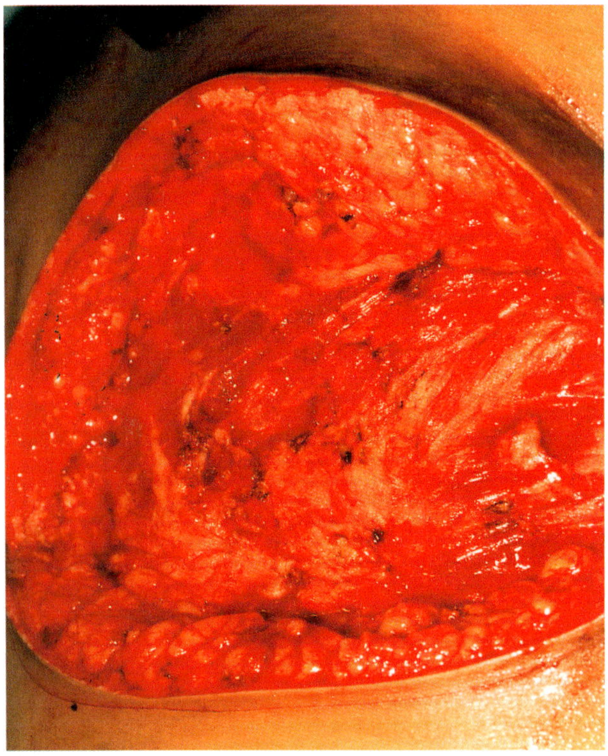

Figure 4.71c Wide removal of the breast and a portion of the pectoralis muscle due to silicone infiltration.

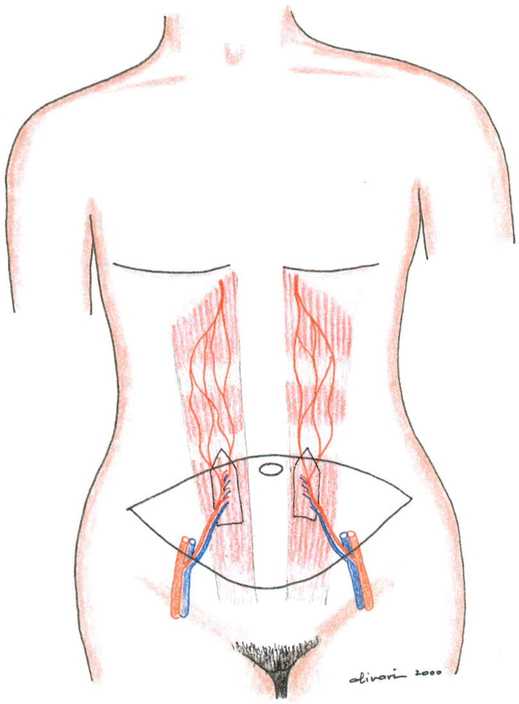

Figure 4.71d Operative plan: Bilateral mastectomy with primary reconstruction using free TRAM flaps.

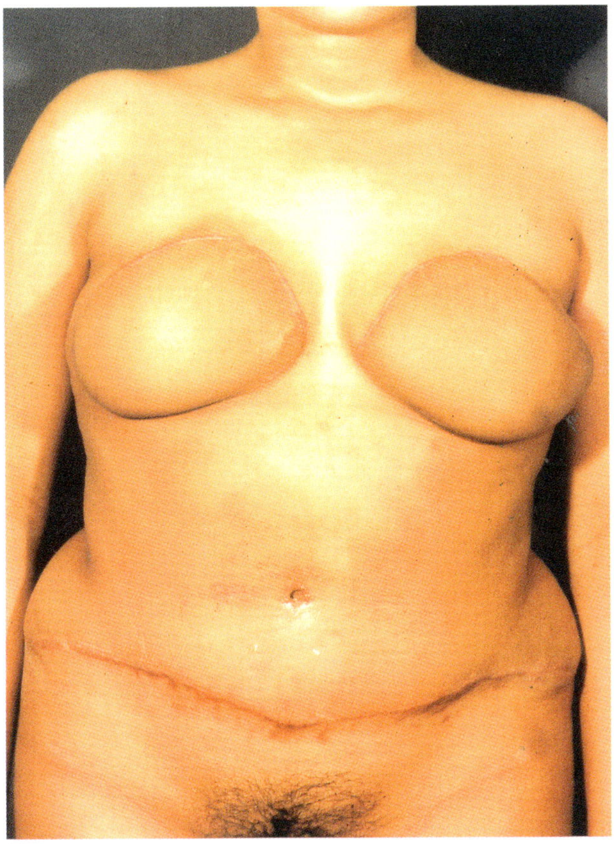

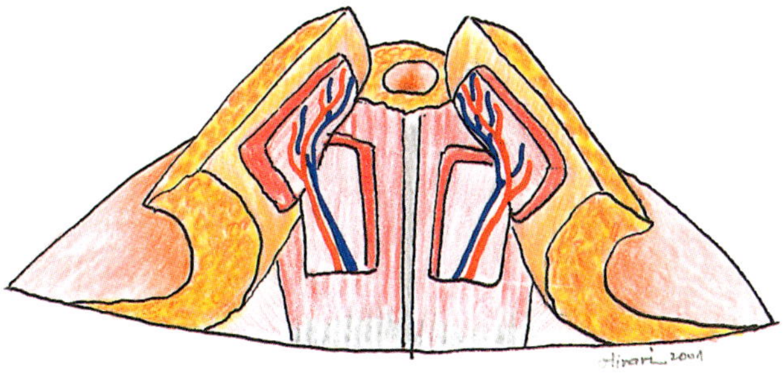

Figure 4.71e Primary reconstruction is performed with two free TRAM flaps. The inferior epigastric artery and vein are anastomosed to the IMA and its accompanying veins bilaterally (see illustration).

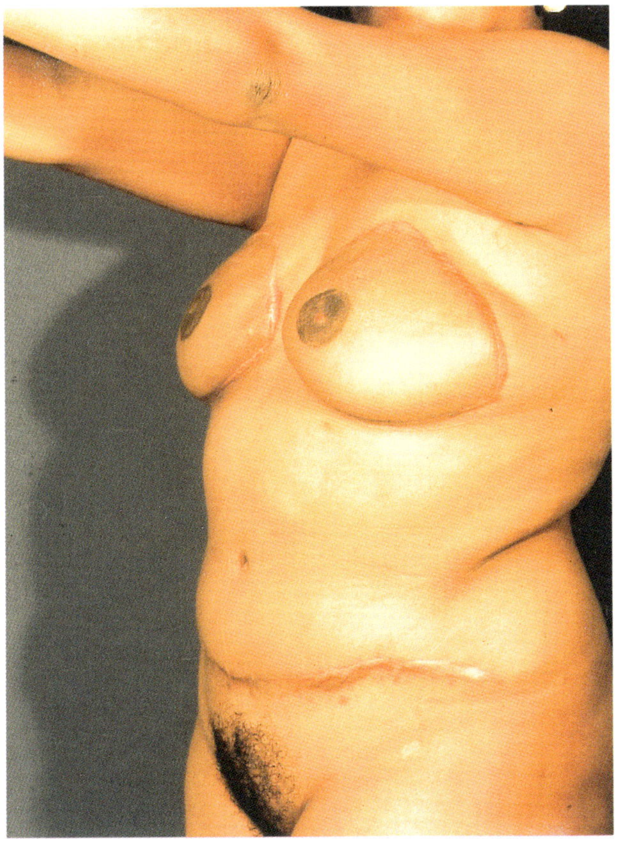

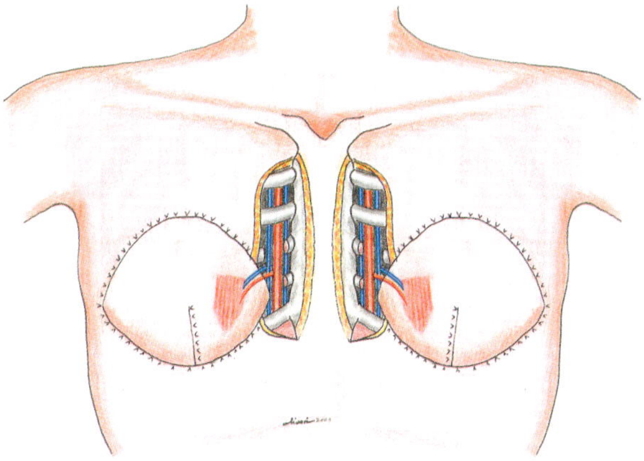

Figure 4.71f Situation six months postoperatively. Due to the patient's dark skin type hypertrophic scarring was encountered. Scheme: The IMA was used for anastomosis bilaterally.

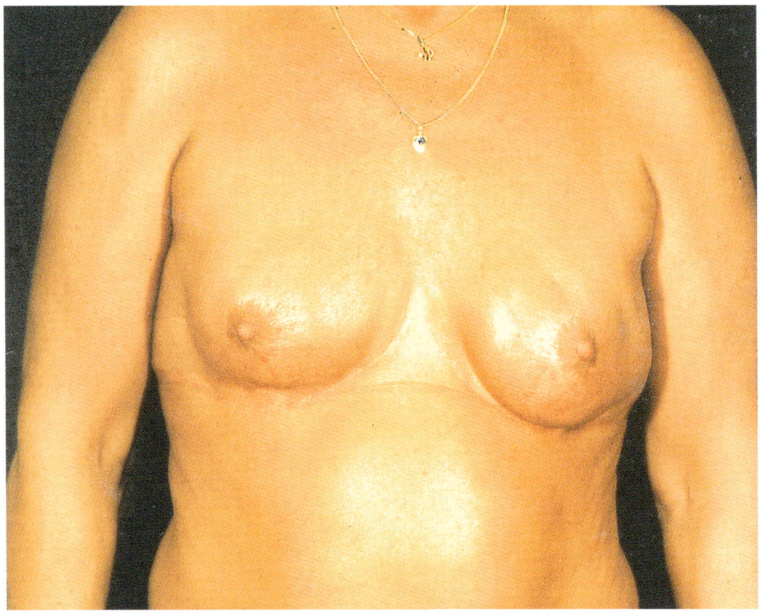

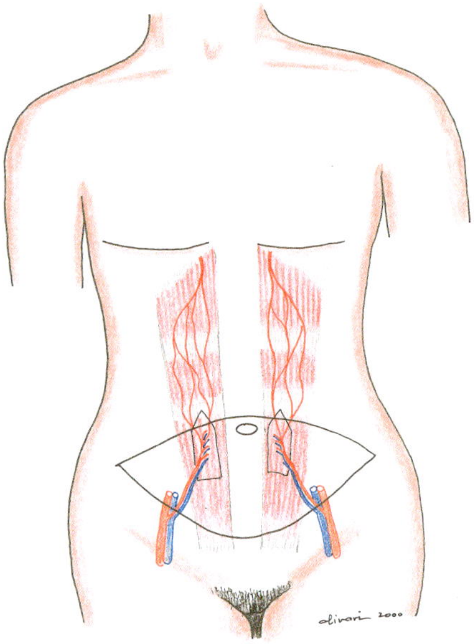

Figure 4.72a Status post subcutaneous mastectomy with multiple capsular contractures and implant exchanges. The patient rejected the further use of implants and requested autologous breast reconstruction.

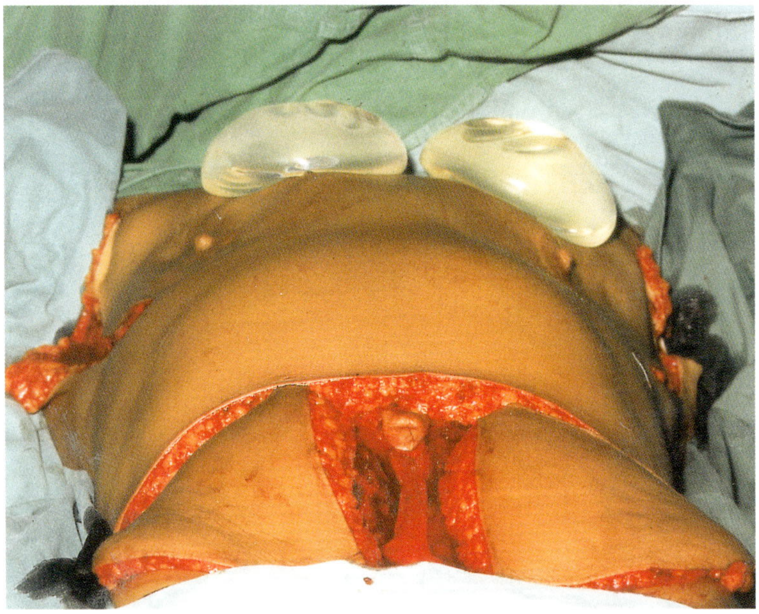

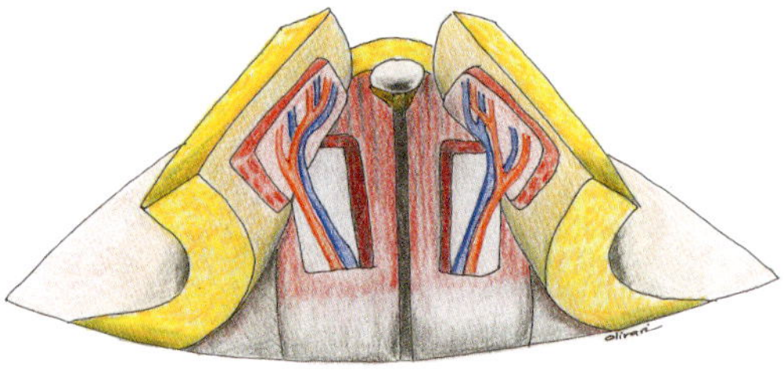

Figure 4.72b Implants have been removed and two free TRAM flaps are dissected and deepithelialized. Meticulous dissection with identification of perforators and their location is essential in bilateral free TRAM flap transfer.

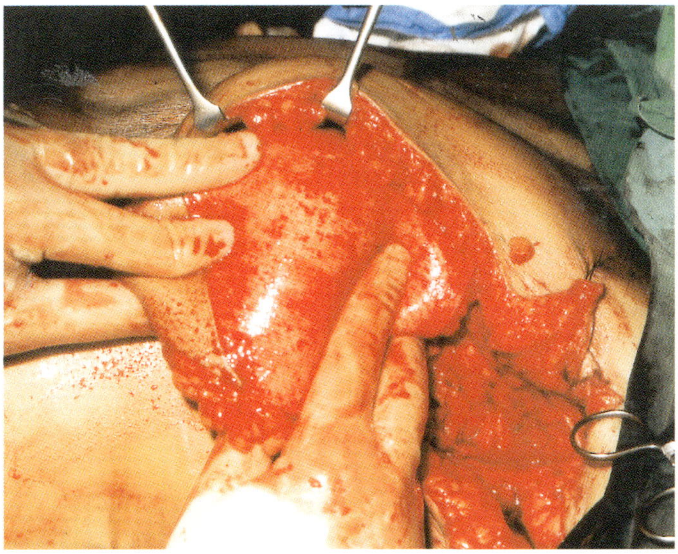

Figure 4.72c Almost the entire flap is deepithelialized. Only a small island is left behind as a monitor.

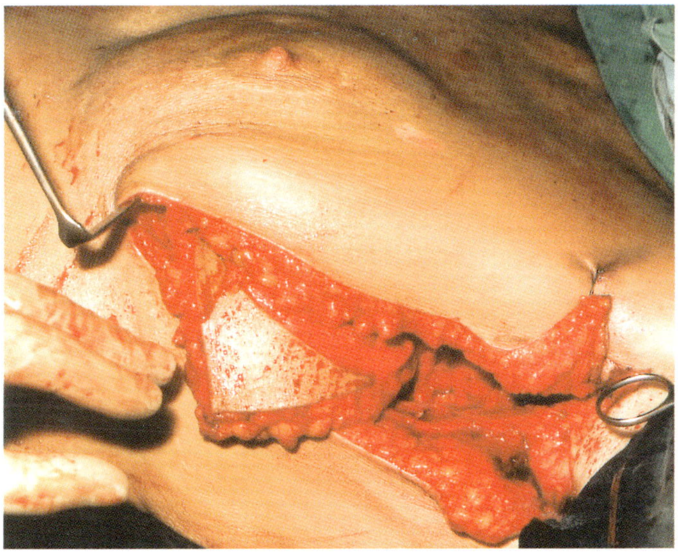

Figure 4.72d Anastomosis of the TRAM exceptionally with TDA.

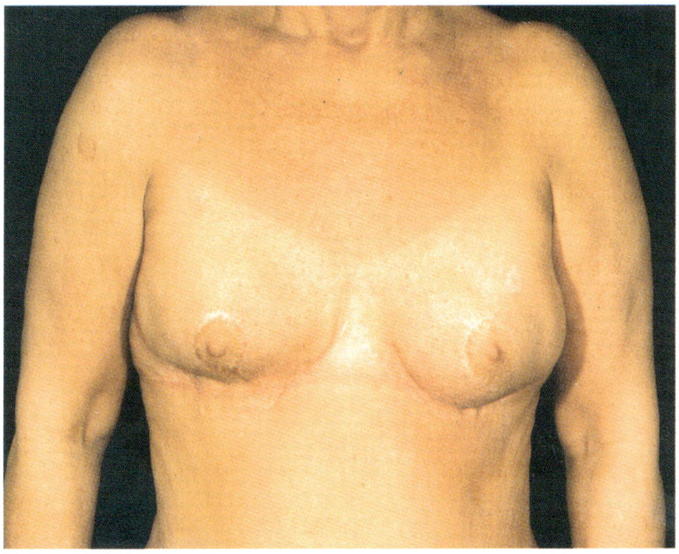

Figure 4.72e Picture three months postoperatively

b) Free TRAM Flap for Thoracic Wall and Breast Reconstruction

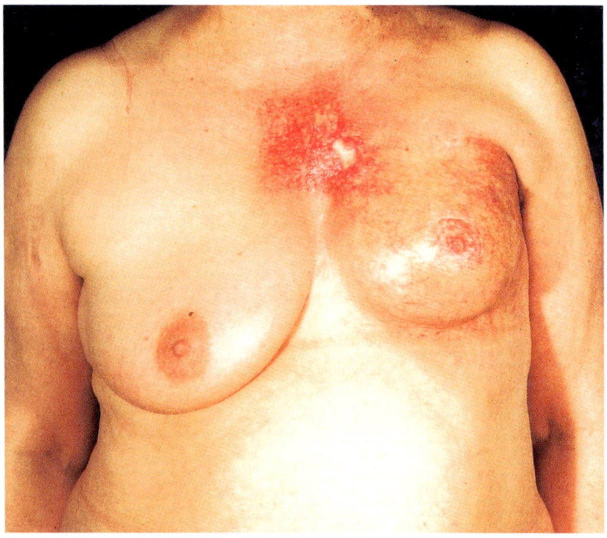

Figure 4.73a Radiation ulcer, radiodermatitis, and extreme fibrosis of the left breast following "breast conservation" and radiation therapy. The patient has major complaints and additionally suffers from an extremely indurated remnant breast. A pedicled TRAM flap is contraindicated due to the history of radiation therapy (internal mammary artery is damaged by irradiation).

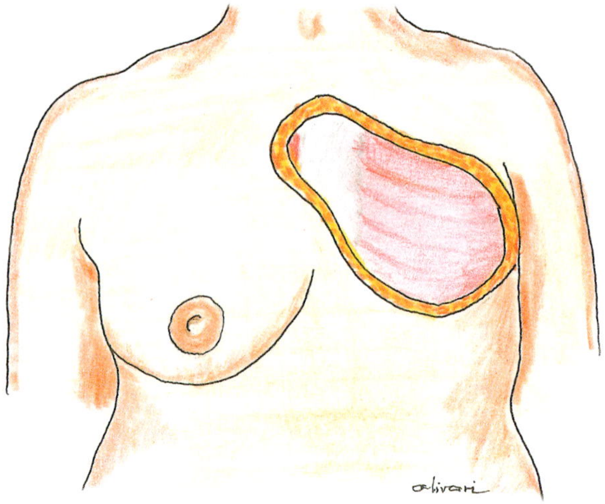

Figure 4.73b Excision of remnant breast including irradiated tissues extending beyond the sternum

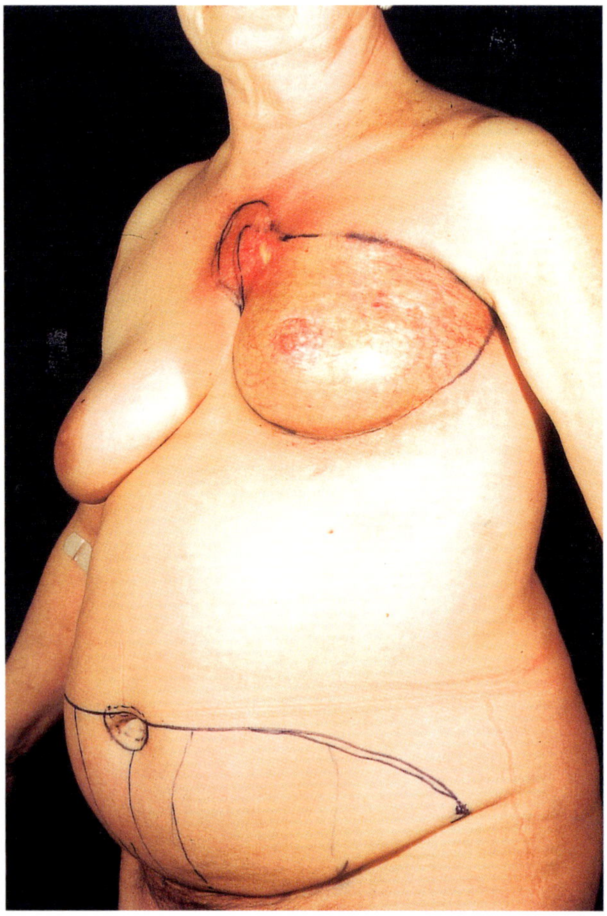

Figure 4.73c Operative plan: The IMA cannot be used due to the history of radiation. A large free TRAM flap is planned for breast reconstruction as well as coverage of the sternal defect.

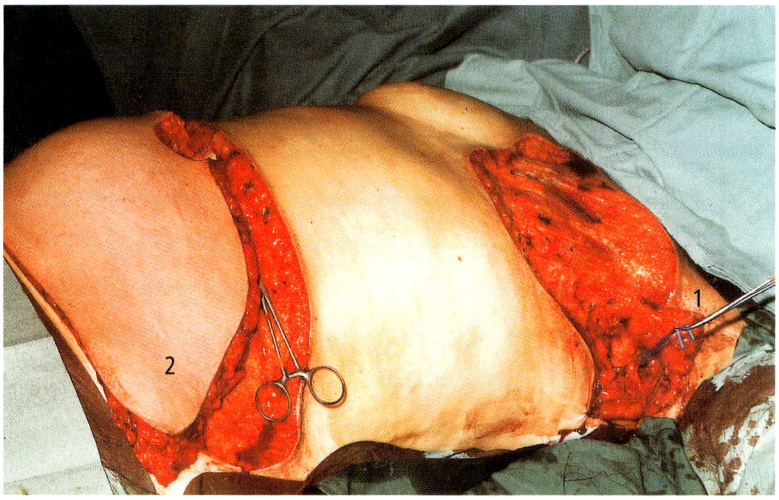

Figure 4.73d The irradiated area has been excised and the thoracodorsal vessels identified (1). A free TRAM flap (2) has been dissected.

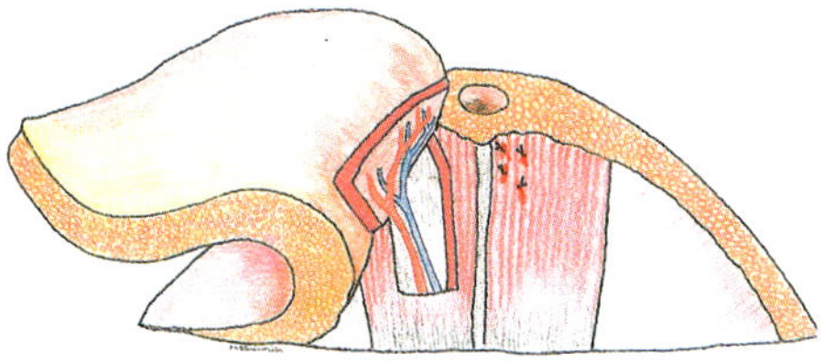

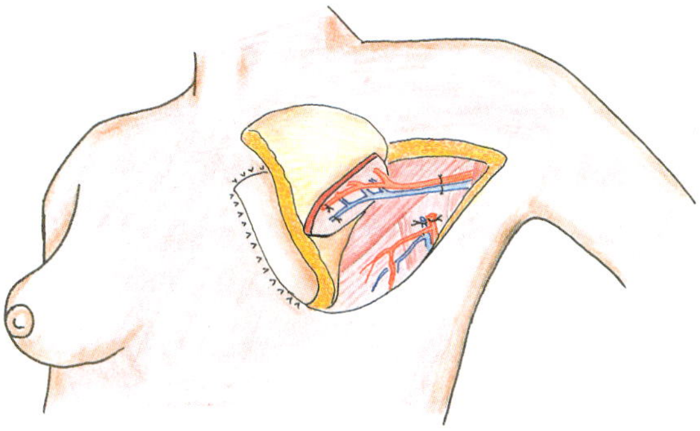

Figure 4.73e The inferior epigastric artery and vein are anastomosed to the thoracodorsal vessels.

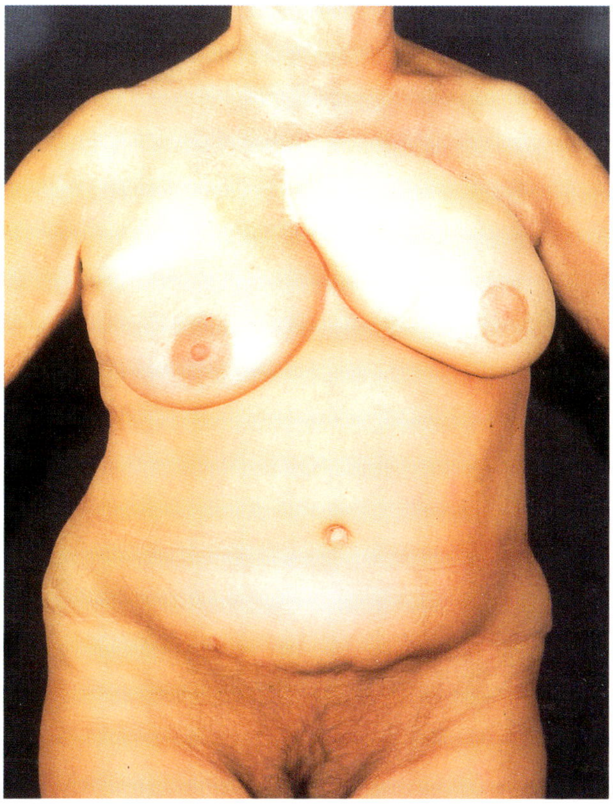

Figure 4.73f Picture two years postoperatively

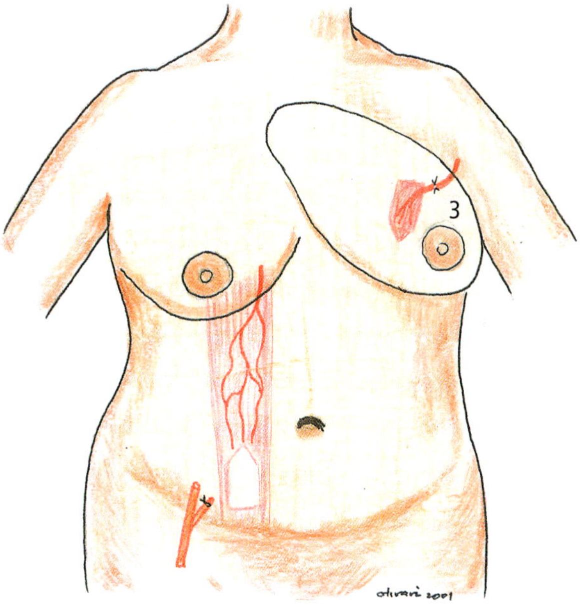

Figure 4.73g Due to radiation damage to the IMA the thoracodorsal vessels were used for anastomosis (3).

c) Turbo TRAM Flap for Large Thoracic Wall Defects

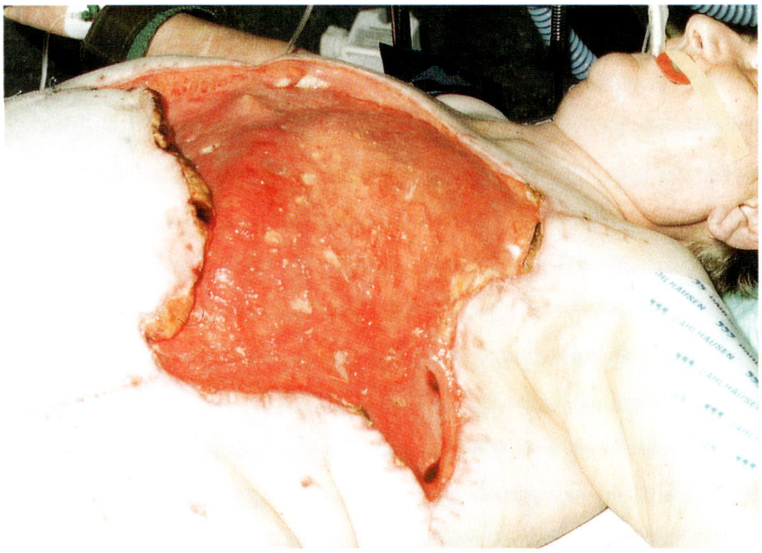

Figure 4.74a A mastectomy was performed in this 74-year old patient due to of breast cancer (T4). Complication: Extensive necrosis and infection. The primary surgeon (gynecologist) had tried to reduce the defect size by pulling up the abdominal wall cranially which resulted in further tissue necrosis.

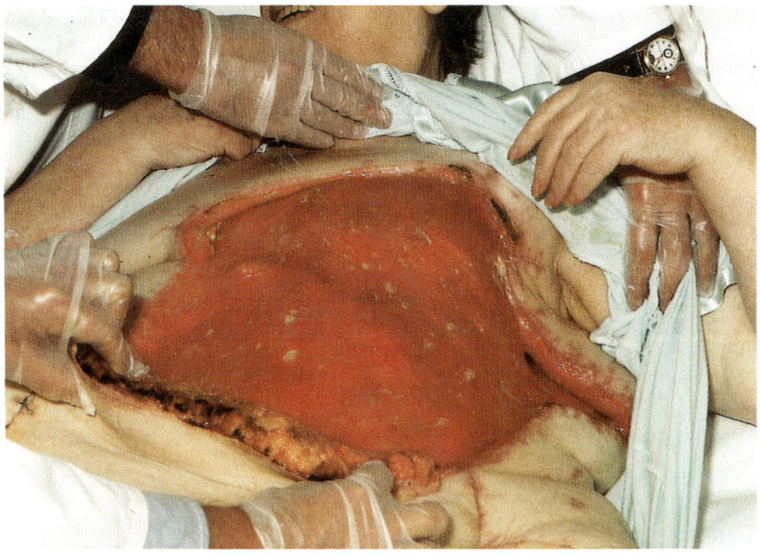

Figure 4.74b Defect size constituted an area of 68 × 38 cm. An additionally aggravating factor was the patient's obesity and age.

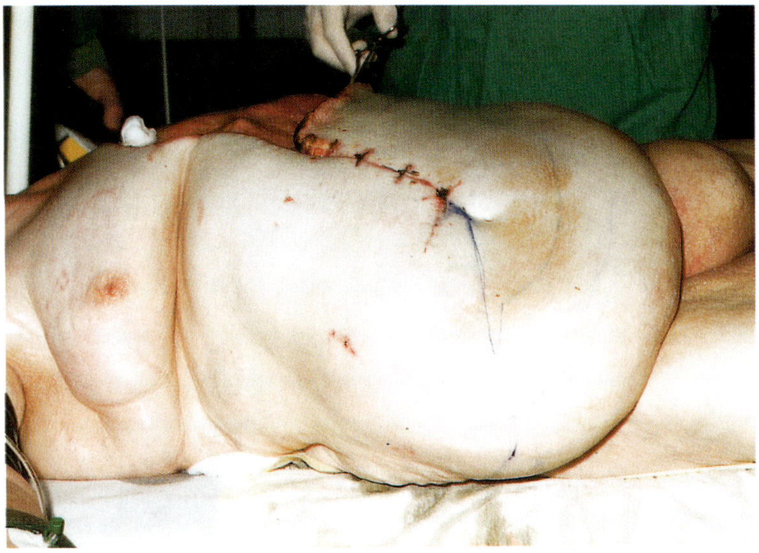

Figure 4.74c Plan: First cleaning of open area, excision of necrotic skin and coverage with meshed graft.

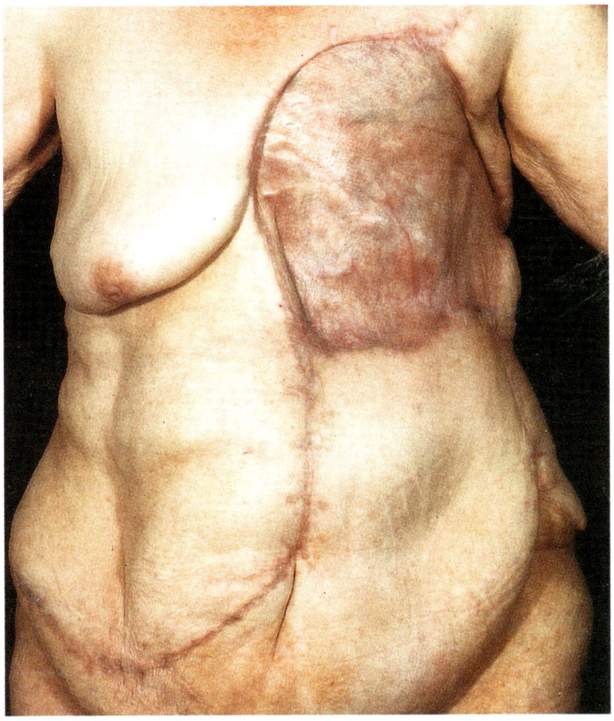

Figure 4.74d Following treatment of the infected surface and wound coverage with mesh graft a Turbo TRAM flap is planned three months later. Mesh graft covered areas undergo contraction thus reducing defect size. Performing a pedicle TRAM flap would be too risky considering the patient's age (74 years) and preexisting obesity.

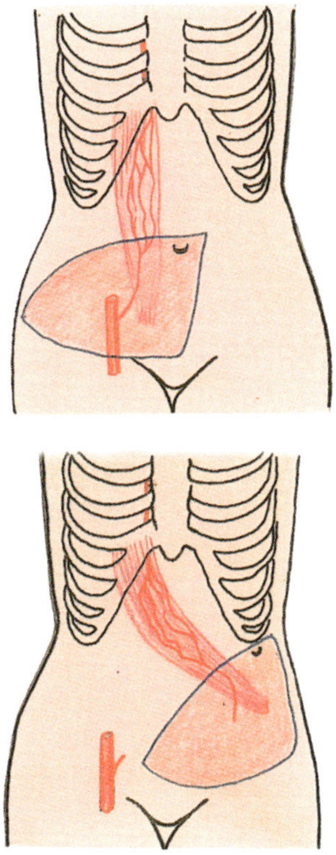

Figure 4.74f A unilateral pedicled Turbo TRAM (right) flap is mobilized. The inferior epigastric artery is kept as long as possible.

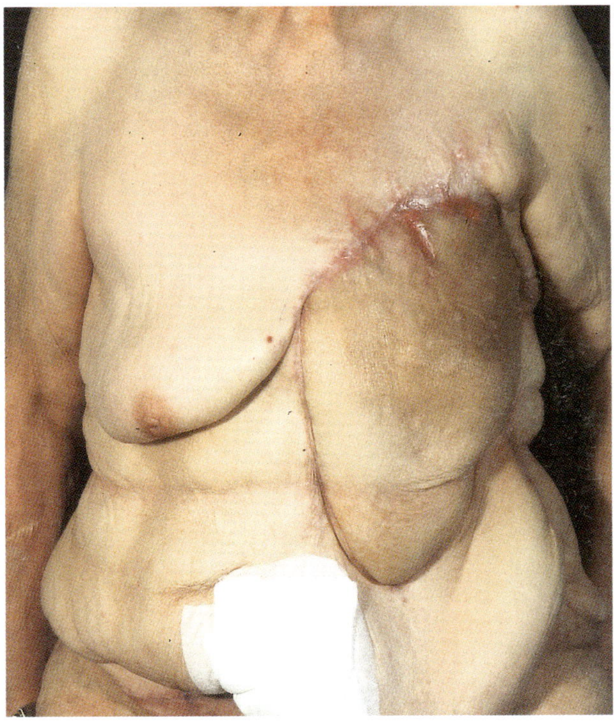

Figure 4.74e Six weeks after closure of defect with "turbo" TRAM flap

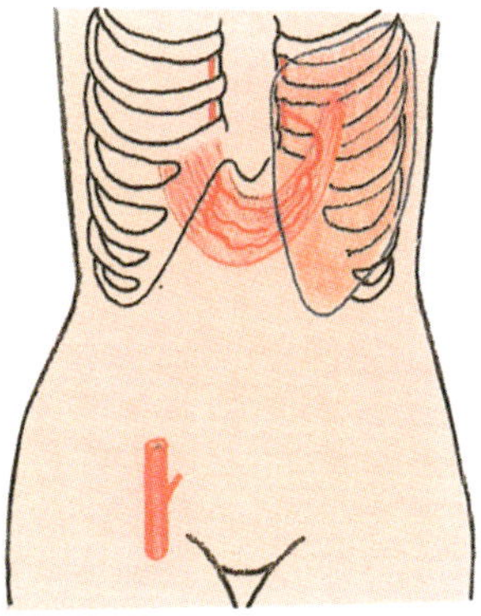

Figure 4.74g It is basically unilateral pedicle TRAM flap. Additionally, an anastomosis is performed between the inferior epigastric artery and the IMA for improved blood supply.

d) Complications Following TRAM Flap Transfers

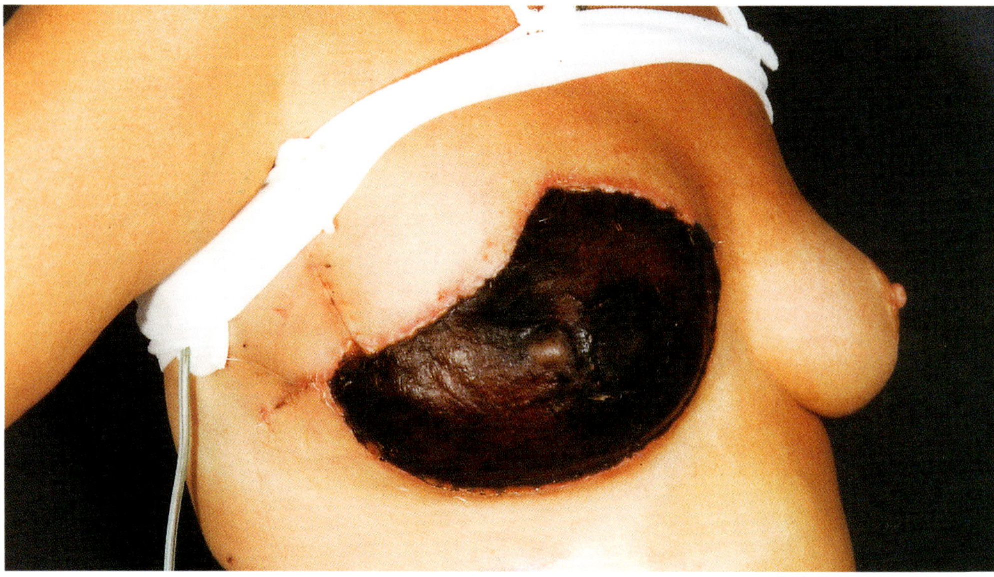

Figure 4.75a Worst complication following free TRAM flap transfer: A total flap loss rate has been described in literature to range between 2 to 7 %. In a series of 111 free TRAM flaps we observed five (4.7 %) total flap losses (problems at the anastomosis = 4, infection = 1). Statistically, this number is acceptable. However, every flap loss has an extremely strong impact on the patient and surgeon as well. Luckily, mostly the internal mammary artery was used as the host vessel, thus, the TDA was still available which allowed rescue situation for closure of defect with a latissimus dorsi flap. In free TRAM flap transfers the IMA should be used for anastomosis whenever possible in order to preserve the TDA which allows reconstruction with a latissimus dorsi flap as an alternative.

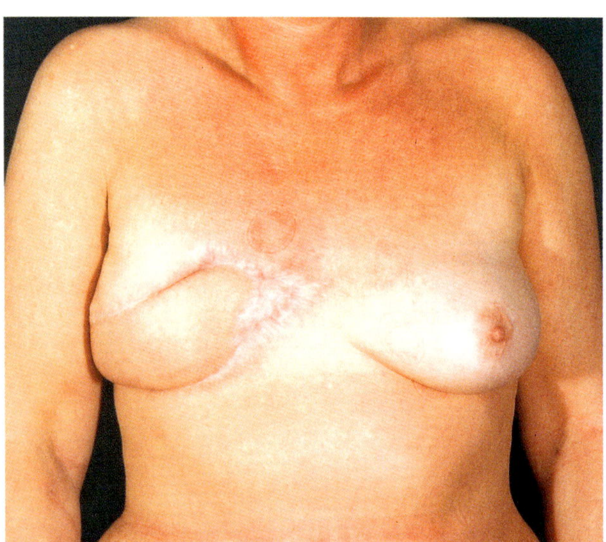

Figure 4.75b Situation after removal of necrotic TRAM flap and closure of defect with a latissimus dorsi flap.

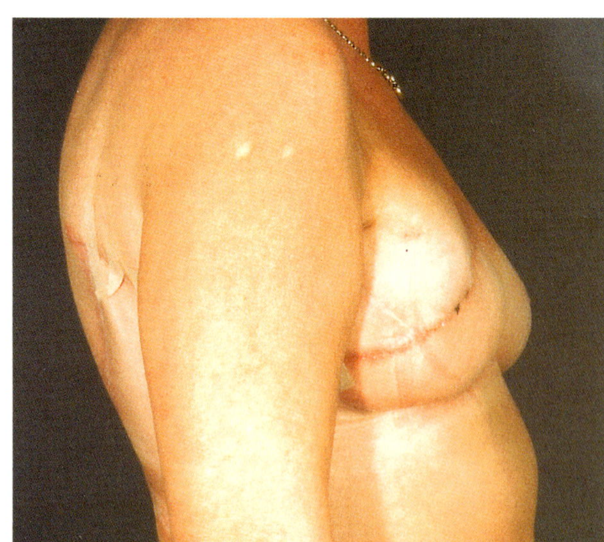

Figure 4.75c Lateral view. Further reconstruction is planned

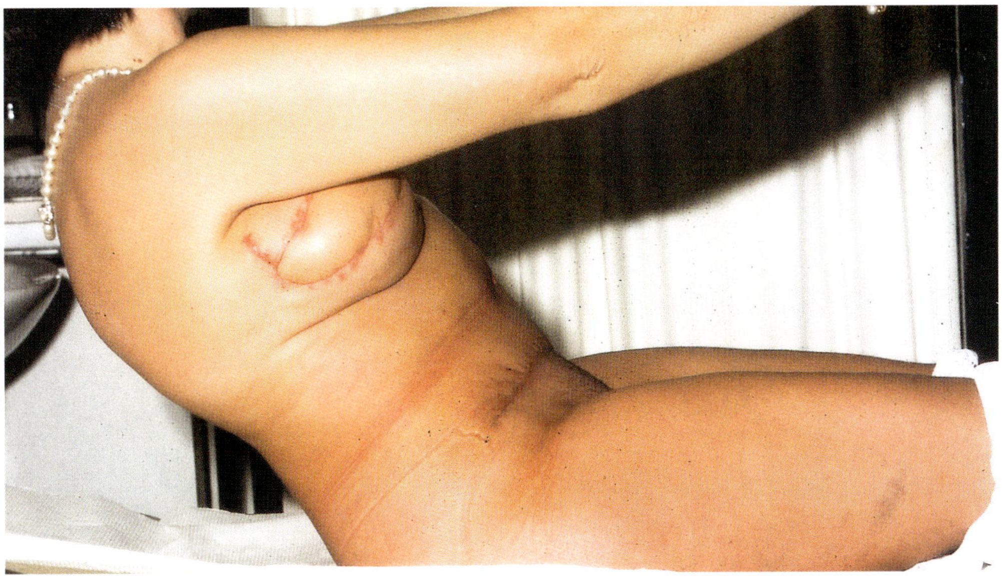

TRAM-Donor Site

Figure 4.76 Donor site: A follow-up of our patients one year postoperatively revealed the following abdominal wall problems in 46 patients whose donor sites were closed either directly or by use of absorbable Vicryl mesh shows: Five hernias (10.9 %), six relaxations (13 %) of abdominal wall. Subsequently, non-absorbable Prolene meshes were used for fascial closure in 21 patients. One year postoperatively none of these patients complained of hernias or relaxation. 10 % of patients in either group were not able to perform sit-ups postoperatively. In last five years only Prolene non-absorbable nets were used, except in DIEP flap.

Breast Reconstruction – Statistics

Table 4.15 Breast reconstruction (N=1967)

Operation	Quantity	%
Mastectomy and primary reconstruction	777	39.5
Secondary reconstruction	796	40.5
Breast conserving therapy – Quadrantectomy	153	7.8
Latissimus flap with implant placement	75	3.8
TRAM/deepithelialized latissimus	166	8.4
Total	1967	100

Table 4.16 Local recurrence (N=910). Comparison: Primary vs. secondary reconstruction. Follow-up: 4.6 years.

	Primary	Secondary
Reconstruction	343 (100 %)	567 (100 %)
Local recurrence	10 (2.9 %)	17 (2.9 %)

Primary reconstruction does not influence the rate of local recurrence. Surgical procedures for breast reconstruction have changed in recent years. Data for 2002 are as follows:

Table 4.17 Breast reconstruction 2002 (N=266)

Operation	Quantity	%
Primary breast reconstruction	54	20.4
– Breast conserving therapy	28	52.0
– Patey mastectomy and primary reconstruction	26	48.0
Secondary breast reconstruction	212	79.6

The deepithelialized latissimus flap was used in 51 patients, the TRAM and DIEP in 36 patients. The trend is as follows: In primary breast cancer, breast conserving therapy is performed with increasing frequency, if staging allows so. Our data further demonstrates that a considerable number of reconstructions are still performed using silicone implants.

It is an illusion to suggest that all reconstructions should be performed with autologous tissue (TRAM/latissimus). Allowing for all surgical enthusiasm one should still remember that TRAM and latissimus flaps are complex and challenging procedures. Breast reconstruction with silicone implants may be indicated in patients with abundant skin of good quality and pectoralis muscle still present. There is no doubt breast reconstruction with autologous tissue will play an increasing role in the future.

Free Gluteus Maximus Muscle Flap for Breast Reconstruction

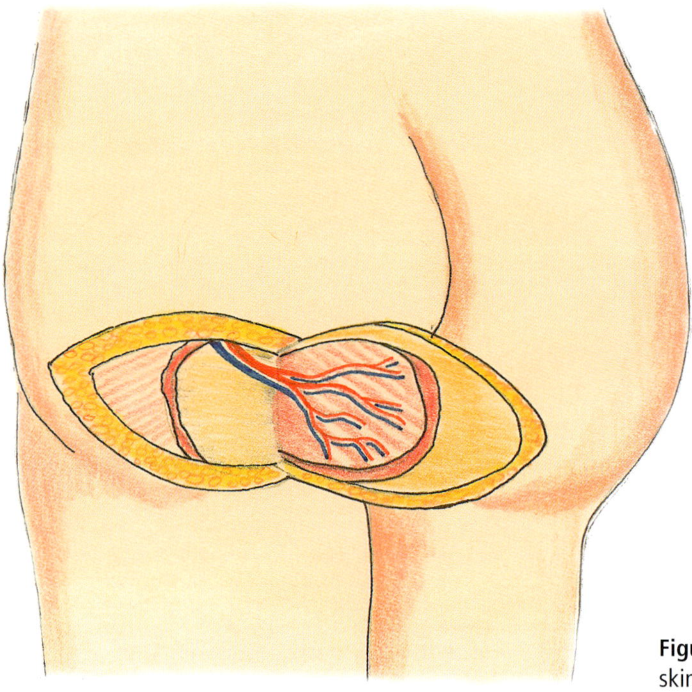

Figure 4.77 A large spindle-shaped portion of gluteal skin-fat flap is raised with a cuff of the gluteus maximus muscle. The flap is pedicled on the inferior gluteal artery.
The vascular pedicle is long enough with an adequate diameter. This technique is rarely used because the donor site is not always aesthetically pleasing. Additionally, intraoperative repositioning of the patient is required. Thus, in our experience TRAM and latissimus flap are better solutions. Certainly some authors shows a quite nice results with this technique.

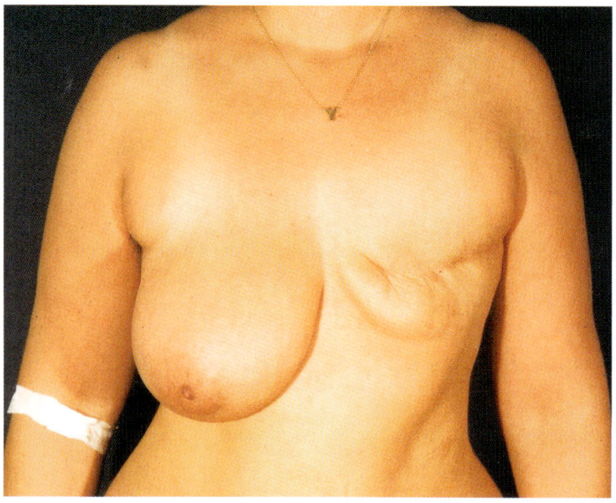

Figure 4.78a Status post mastectomy for cancer

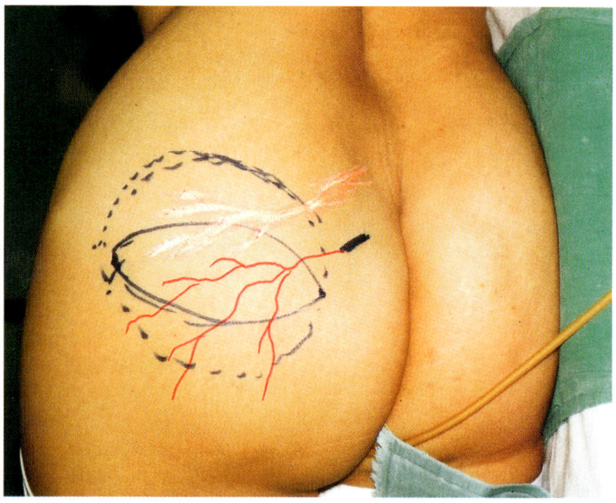

Figure 4.78b Plan: The inferior gluteal artery is identified

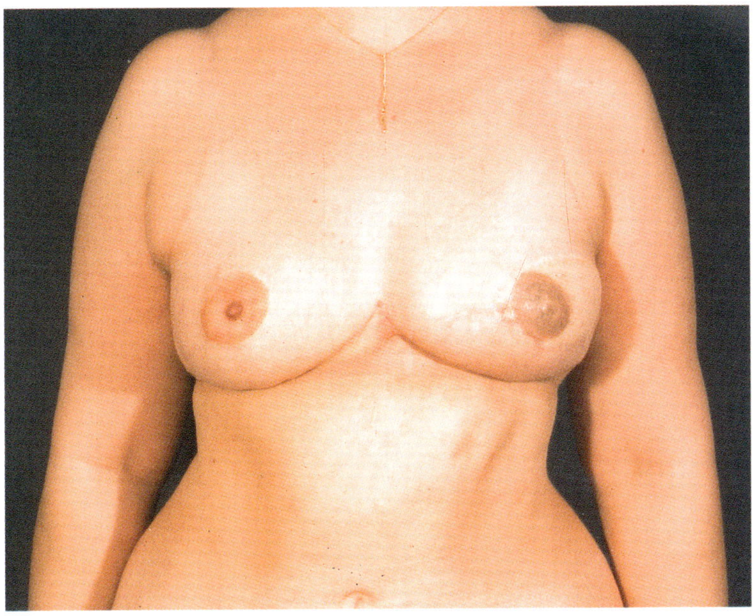

Figure 4.78c One year postoperatively (three operations)

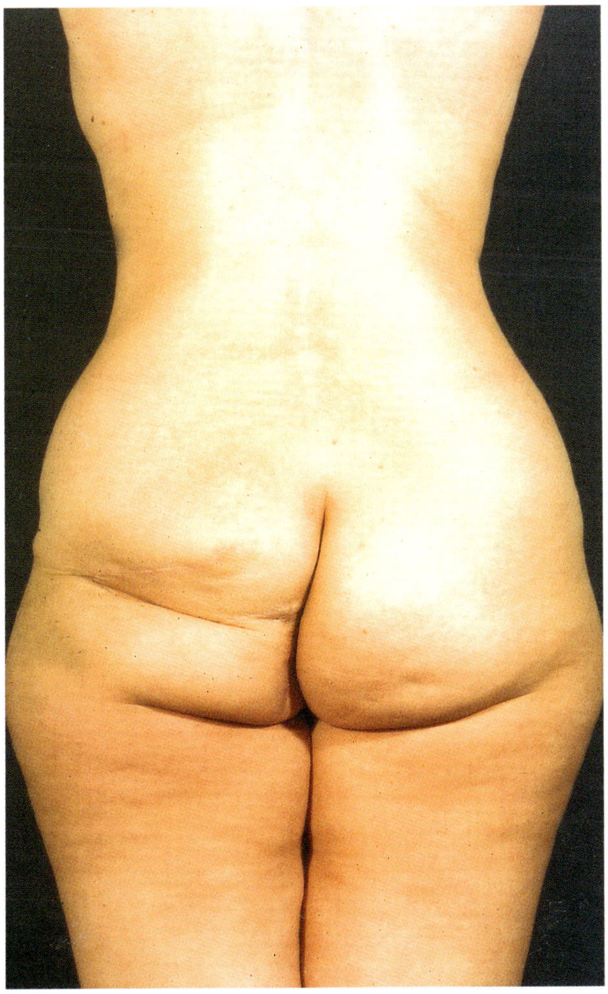

Figure 4.78d The donor site displays an aesthetically unpleasing appearance. Some authors report on having more favorable results when the inferior portion of the gluteus maximus muscle is raised with the flap. The author does not prefer this procedure as a routine. This method should be reserved to specialists in selected cases only. The incision should be placed more inferiorly in the gluteal crease or more cranially for better appearance of the donor site. Other authors (Shaw, Papp, a.o.) presented very nice results with this method.

Free Tensor Fascia Lata Flap for Defect Coverage in the Axilla

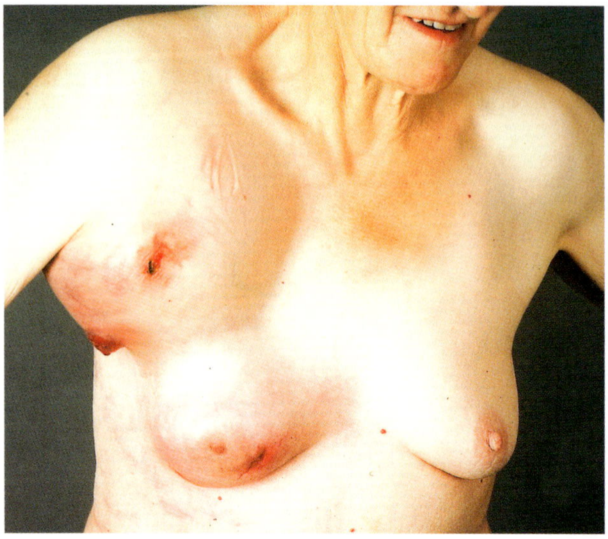

Figure 4.79a Advanced sarcoma in the right axilla with infiltration of the latissimus flap arcade, pectoralis muscles and breast. The patient complains of axillary pain due to infiltration of the axillary plexus.

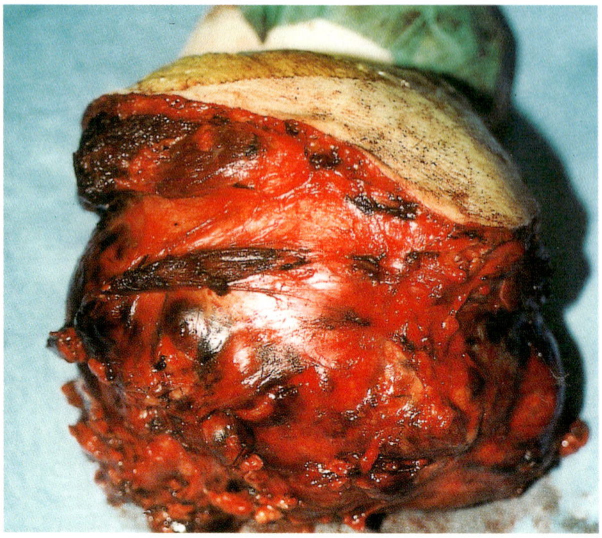

Figure 4.79b Excised tumor. Due to intended postoperative radiation therapy a local flap with meshed STSG is not indicated. Latissimus was not available. There was a good indication for a free tensor fascia lata flap.

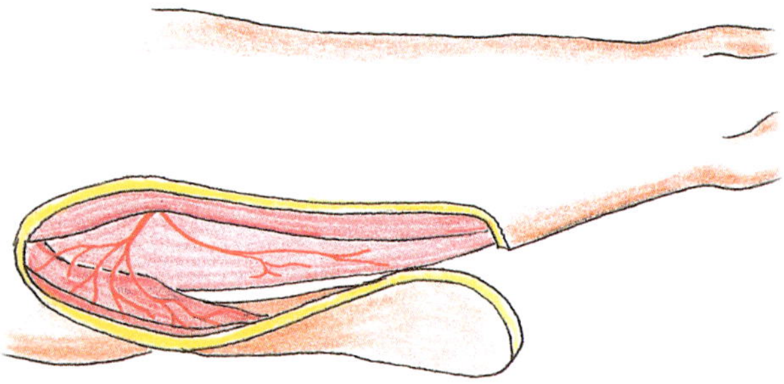

Figure 4.79c Blood supply to the TFL muscle, fascia and overlying skin is provided by a branch of the lateral circumflex femoral artery. The pedicle may have a length of approximately 8 cm with a diameter of 2 mm. The vessel can be located approximately 8 to 10 cm inferior to the anterior superior iliac spine between the rectus femoris and lateral vastus muscles.

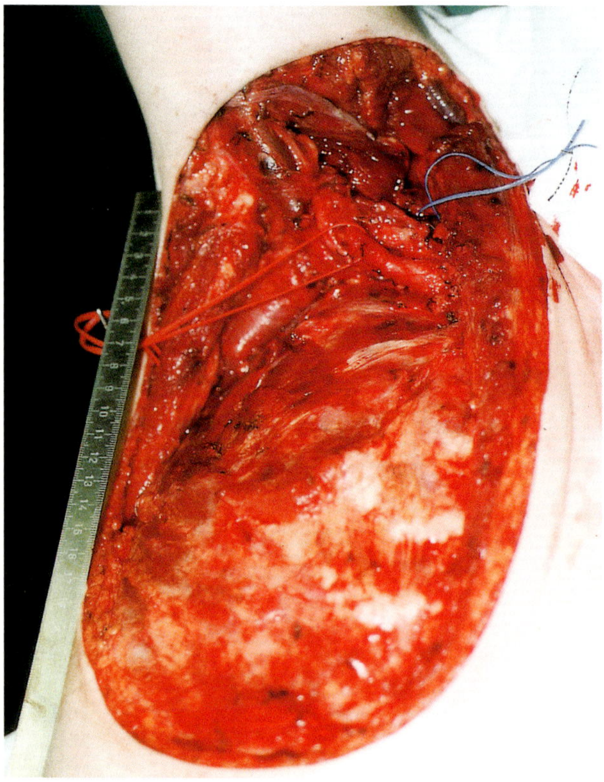

Figure 4.79d Right axilla following tumor removal. The vessels are prepared for anastomosis. The branch of the lateral circumflex femoral artery will be anastomosed to the anterior circumflex humeral artery and the vein to the axillary vein in an end-to-side fashion.

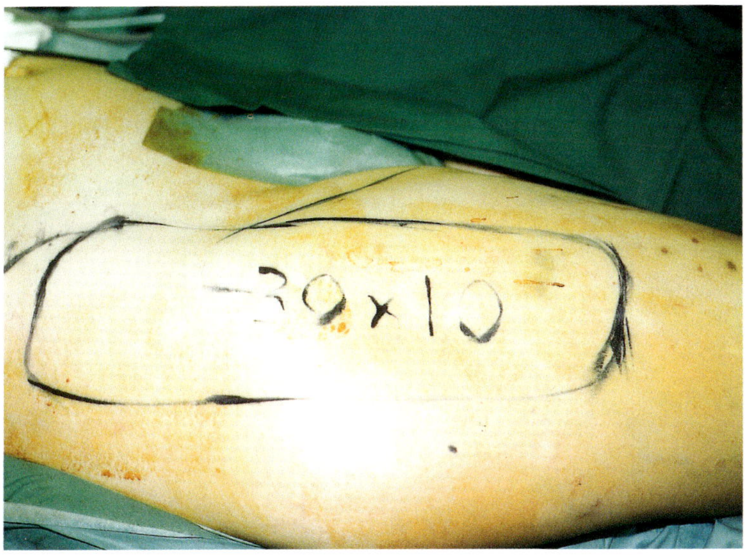

Figure 4.79e A 30 × 10 cm myocutaneous TFL flap is designed

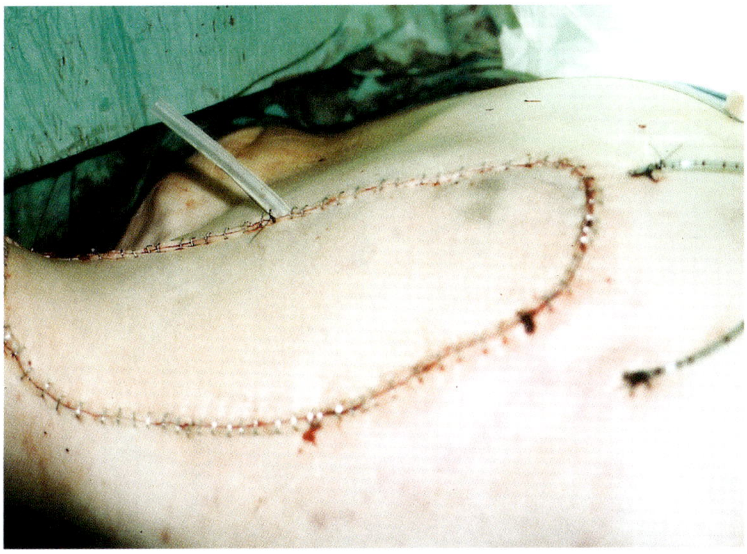

Figure 4.79f At the end of the procedure

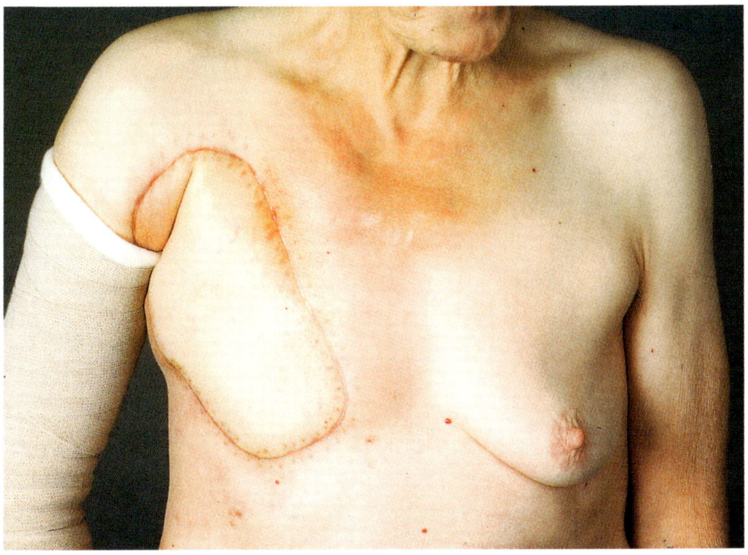

Figure 4.79g Four weeks postoperatively. The patient was on the oncological service at this point.

Scapular and Parascapular Flaps

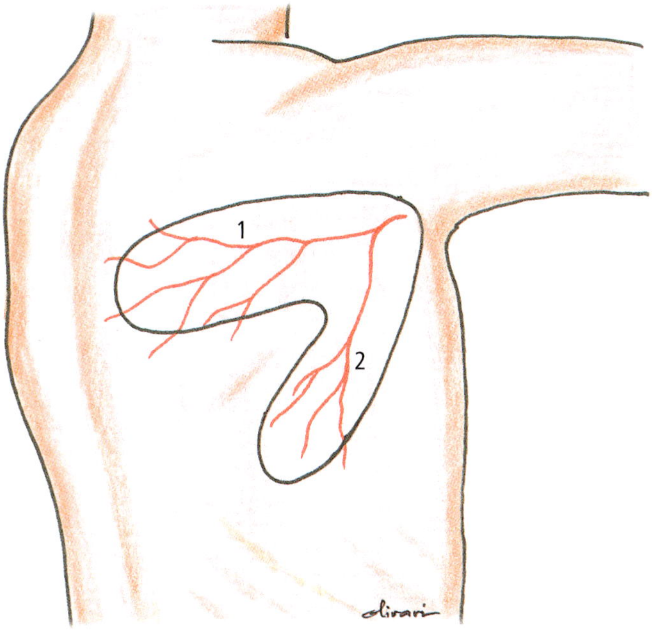

Figure 4.80a Blood supply: The horizontal branch (1) of the circumflex scapular artery (CSA) supplies the scapular flap, whereas the inferior branch supplies the parascapular flap (2). Both branches are necessary for the boomerang flap.

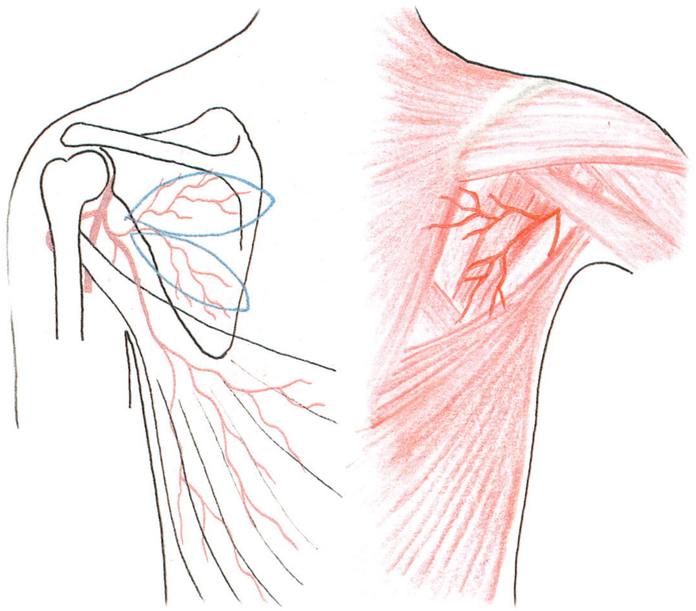

Figure 4.80b Topographic anatomy of scapular and latissimus dorsi flaps. The spine, lateral margin and inferior angle of the scapula are outlined for orientation.

Indication: Reconstruction of shoulder and axillary defects when used as island flaps. When used as free flaps head and neck reconstruction as well as hand and lower extremity reconstruction can be performed.

Advantages: Easy surgical access. The skin displays a good color and is mostly hairless. Primary donor site closure can be achieved. No functional impairments remain. When used as a combined flap (boomerang flap) larger defects may be covered.

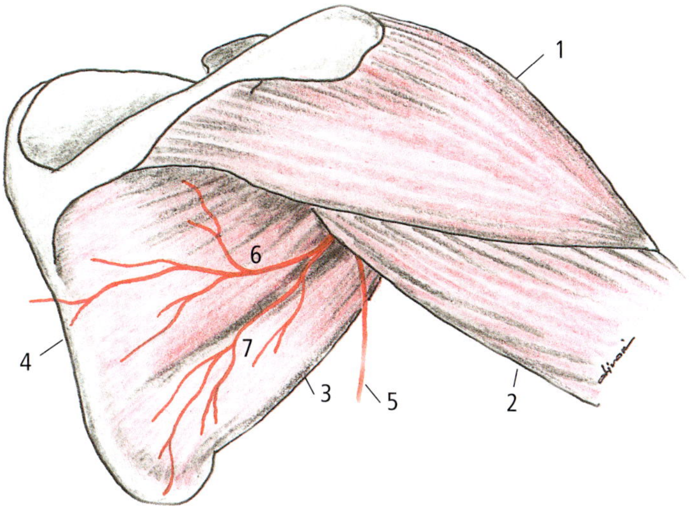

Figure 4.80c Anatomy of the fasciocutaneous scapular as well as the subscapular flap. The CSA is located between the teres minor and major muscles lateral to the scapula. In free transfers the vascular pedicle is dissected up to the TDA.
1) Deltoid muscle
2) Triceps muscle
3) Teres minor muscle
4) Teres major muscle
5) TDA
6) Horizontal branch of the CSA
7) Inferior branch of the CSA

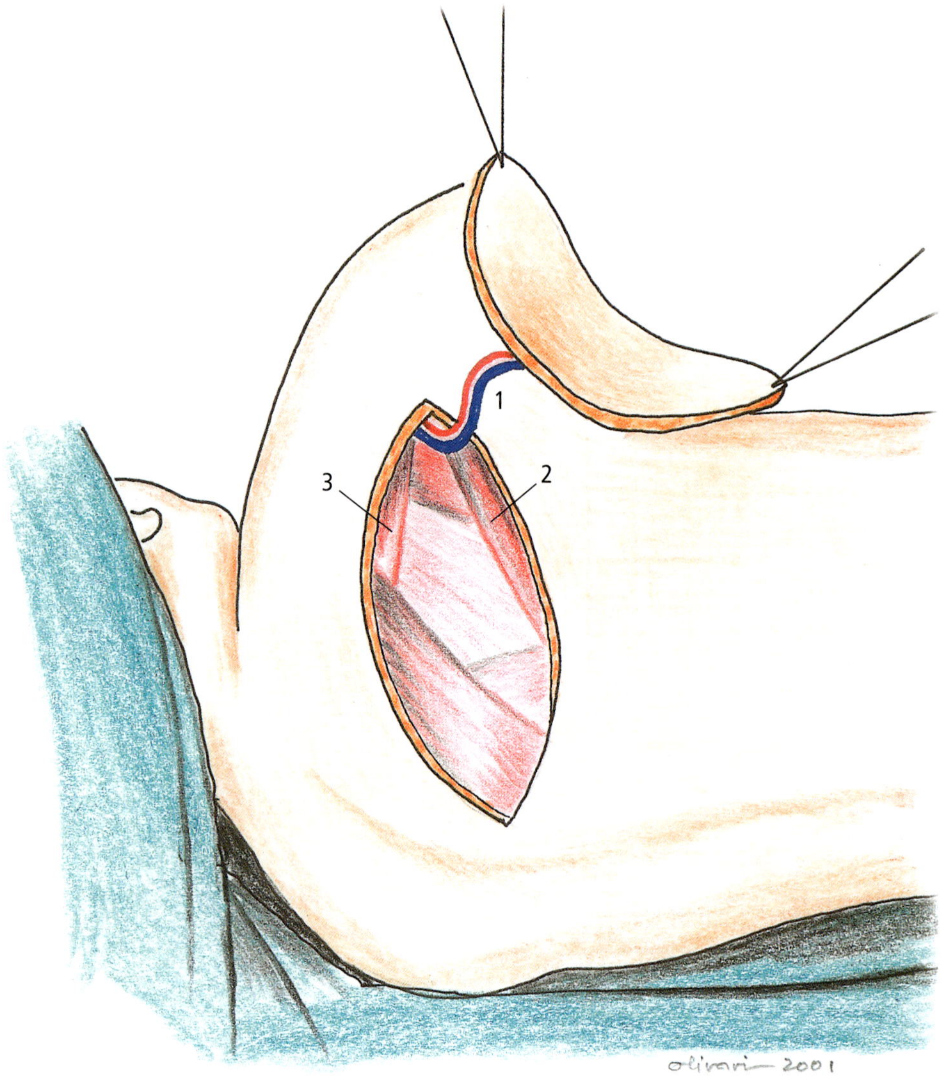

Figure 4.81 Free fasciocutaneous scapular flap: The vascular pedicle (1) (circumflex scapular artery and vein) is dissected up to the TDA which is located ventrally under the triceps muscle between the teres major (2) and minor (3) muscles. In free flap transfers the vascular pedicle is transected at the origin of the TDA.

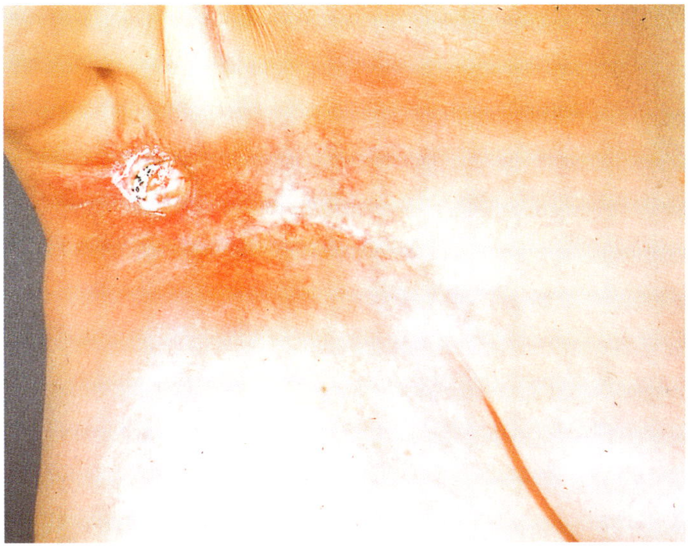

Figure 4.82a Radiation ulcer and radiodermatitis in the right axilla following mastectomy and radiation therapy.

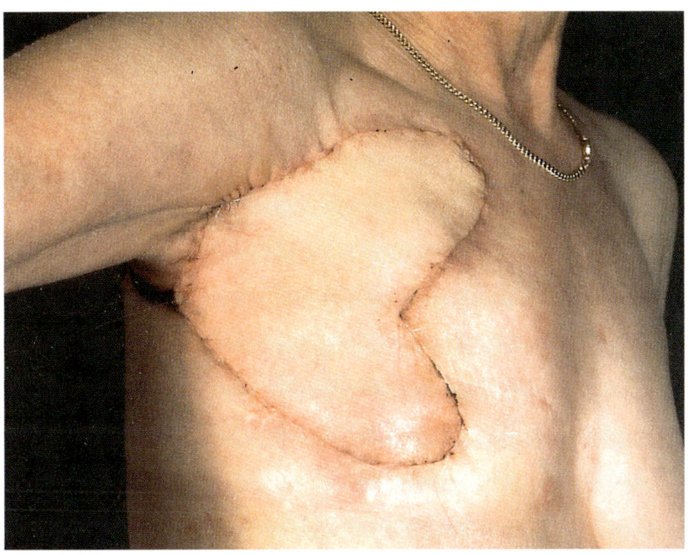

Figure 4.82b Three weeks postoperatively. Reconstruction with a combined scapular/parascapular island flap (boomerang flap)

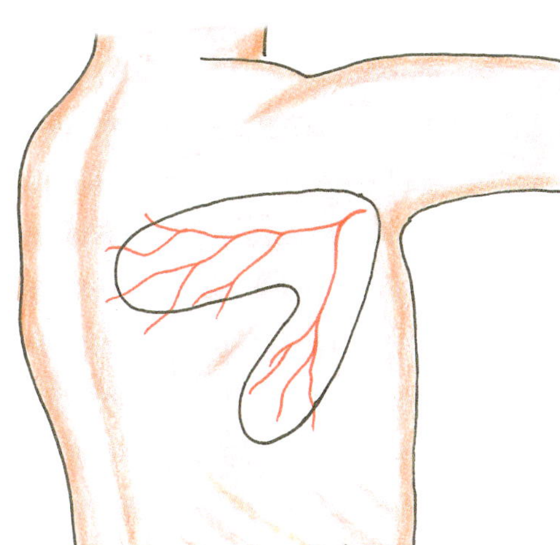

Figure 4.82c The scapular and parascapular flap are raised as a boomerang island flap for reconstruction.

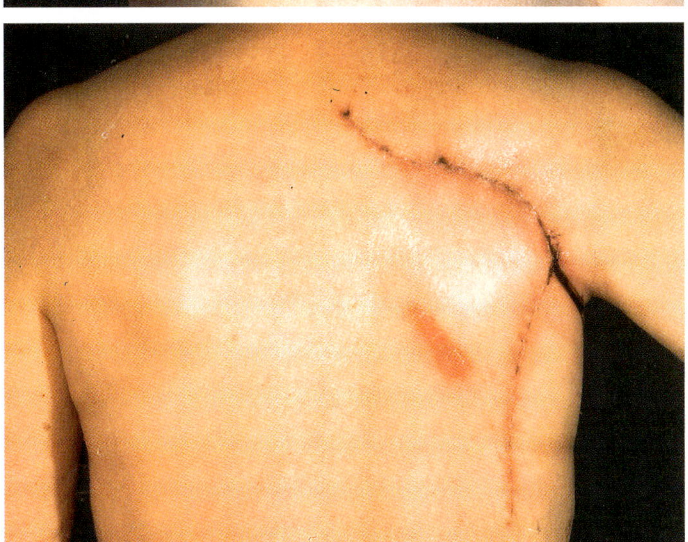

Figure 4.82d The donor site was closed primarily

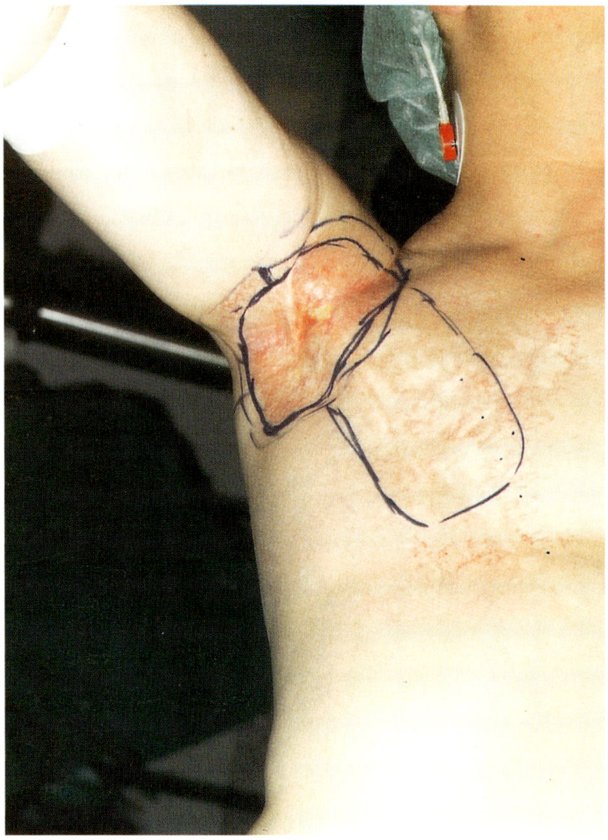

Figure 4.83a Status post mastectomy and radiation therapy. Radiation damage of the right axilla with resultant lymphatic congestion of right arm and chronic pain.

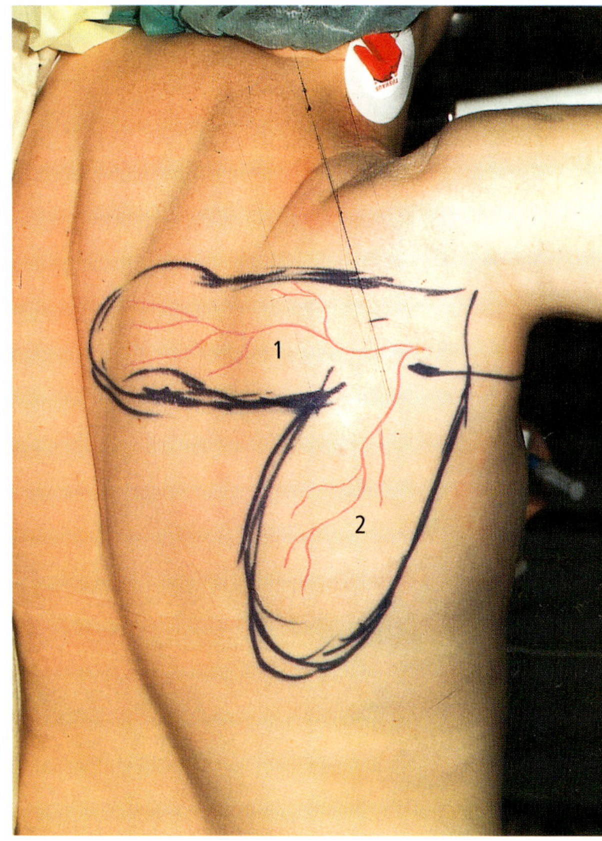

Figure 4.83b Design of a scapular "boomerang" island flap: Scapular (1) and parascapular (2) flap

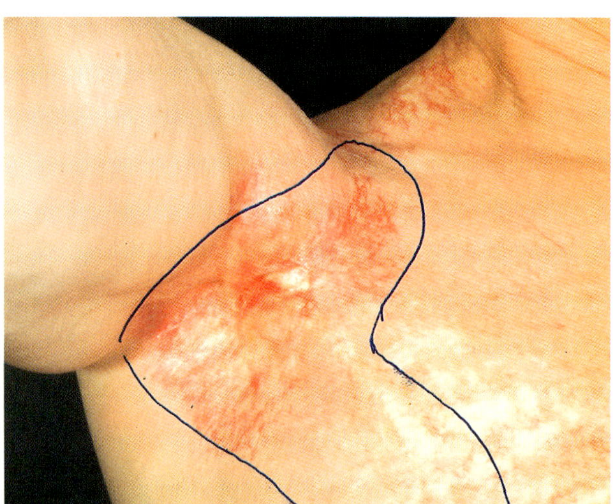

Figure 4.83c Excision of necrotic and fibrotic tissues

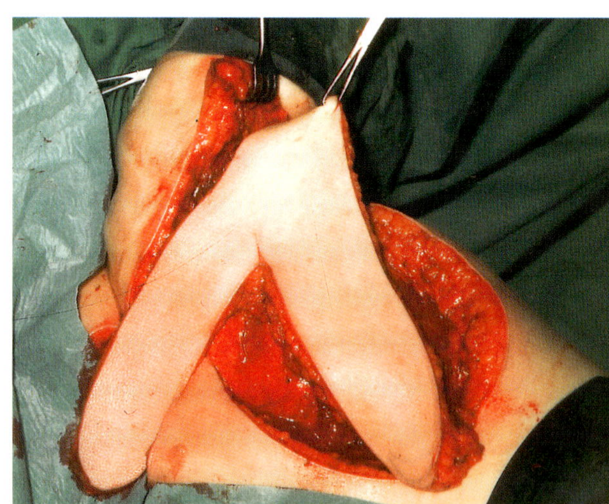

Figure 4.683d In the lateral position the boomerang flap is raised and rotated into the axillary defect. The CSA needs to be meticulously dissected.

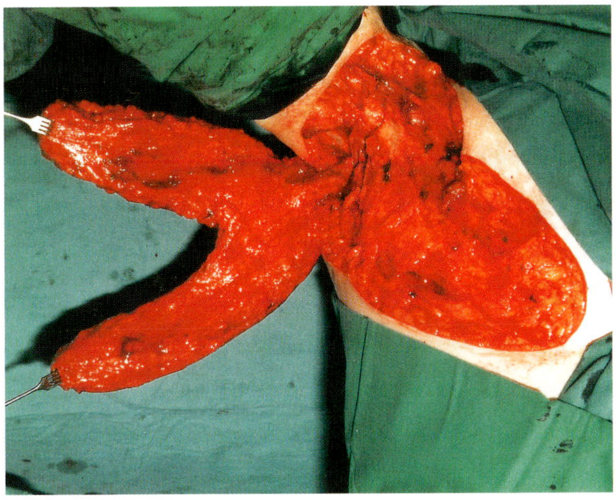

Figure 4.83e The boomerang flap has been mobilized and brought into the axillary defect as an island flap. The flap is only attached to its vascular pedicle.

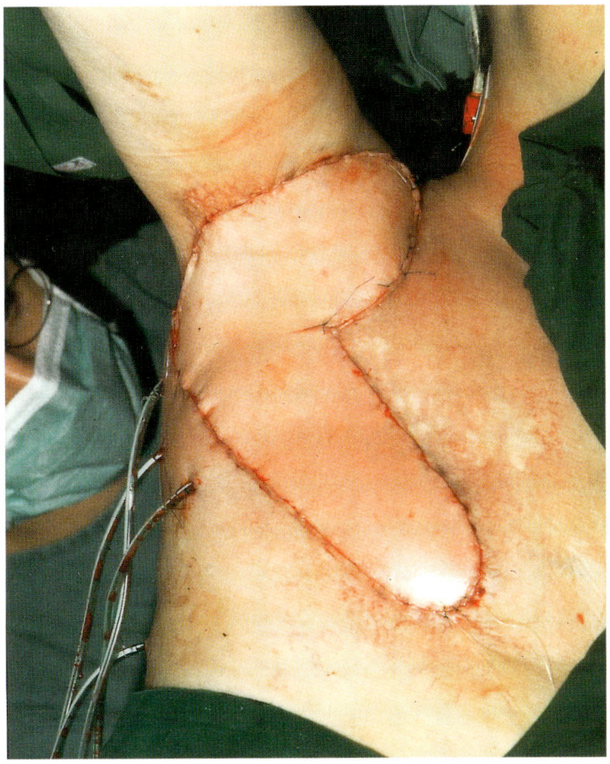

Figure 4.83f At the end of surgery. Note: Excellent flap perfusion following meticulous dissection and careful transposition.

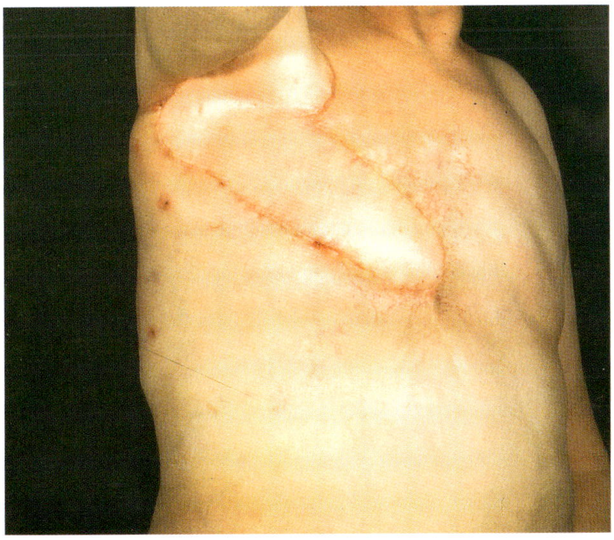

Figure 4.83g Two months postoperatively

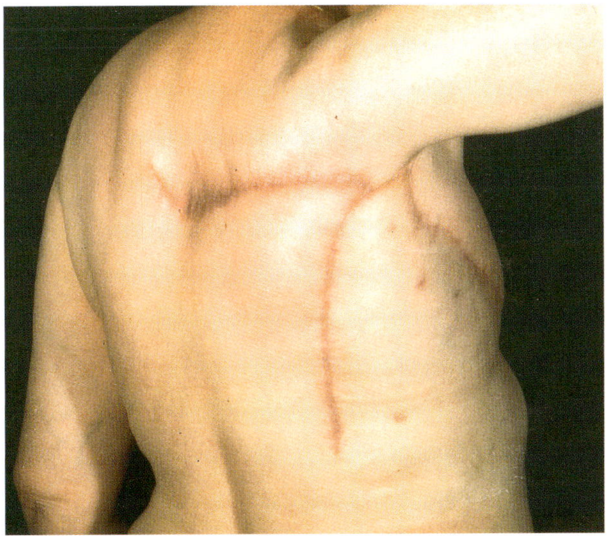

Figure 4.83h Primary donor site closure. The scars are clearly visible.

Combined Scapular and Latissimus Flap for Open Thoracic Wall Defects

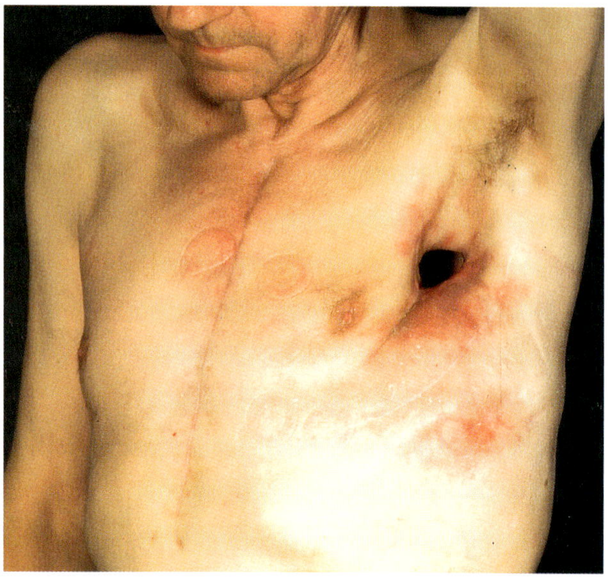

Figure 4.84a Status post left-sided lung resection with resultant open thoracic wall defect and chronic empyema. Superficial closure with a local flap would be technically easy but would not solve the problem. The goal of the operation is to obliterate the empyema cavity and also the chest wall defect.

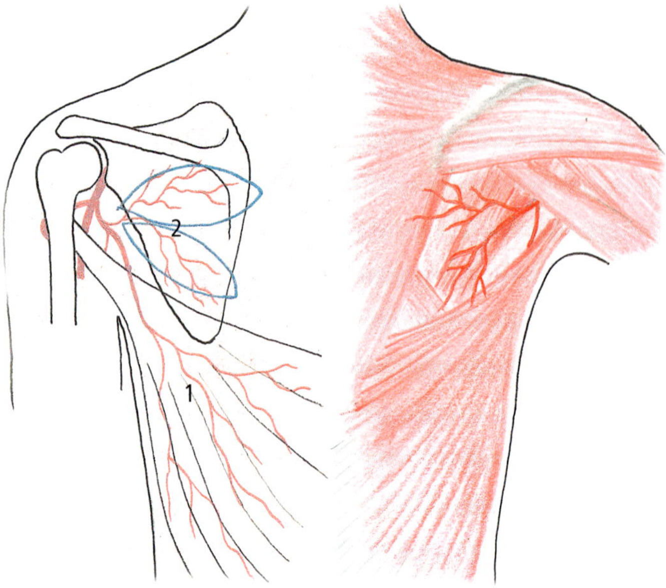

Figure 4.84b Anatomy of the latissimus (1) and scapular (2) flap

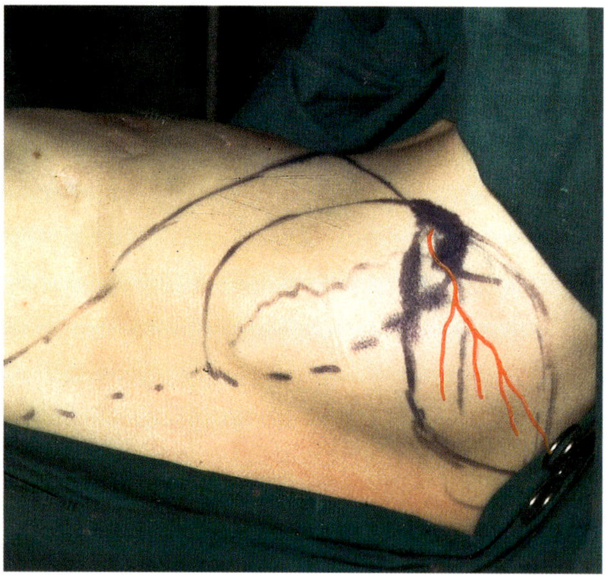

Figure 4.84c Plan: The infected thoracic cavity is cleansed thoroughly and subsequently sealed with an antibiotic fluid. Intravenous antibiotic therapy is used concomitantly. Planning of latissimus muscle flap, for obliteration of the empyema cavity and scapular island flap for closure of thoracic wall defect.

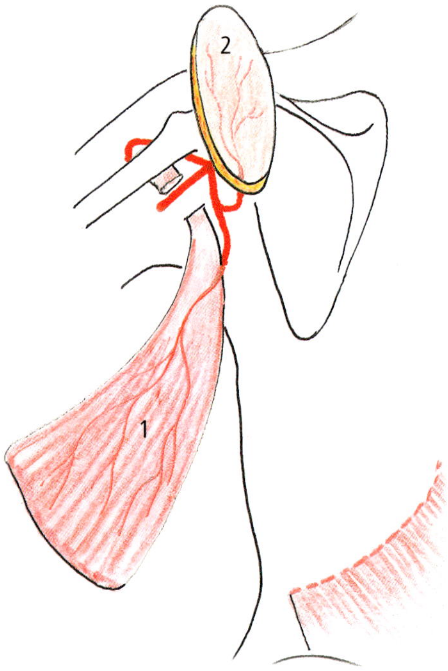

Figure 4.84d The latissimus dorsi muscle is placed as a muscle "filler" into the thoracic cavity (1) attached only to the thoracodorsal vessels. The thoracic wall defect is subsequently covered by a scapular flap (2) which is supplied by the circumflex scapular vessels.

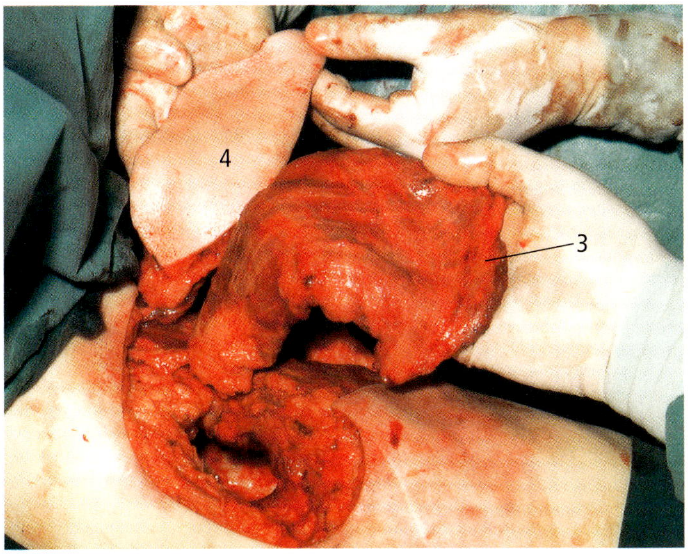

Figure 4.84e Mobilization of the latissimus dorsi muscle (3) which is attached only to the thoracodorsal vessels. The image shows the situation shortly prior to placement of the muscle into the thoracic cavity. Simultaneously, the scapular flap is mobilized as an island flap (4).

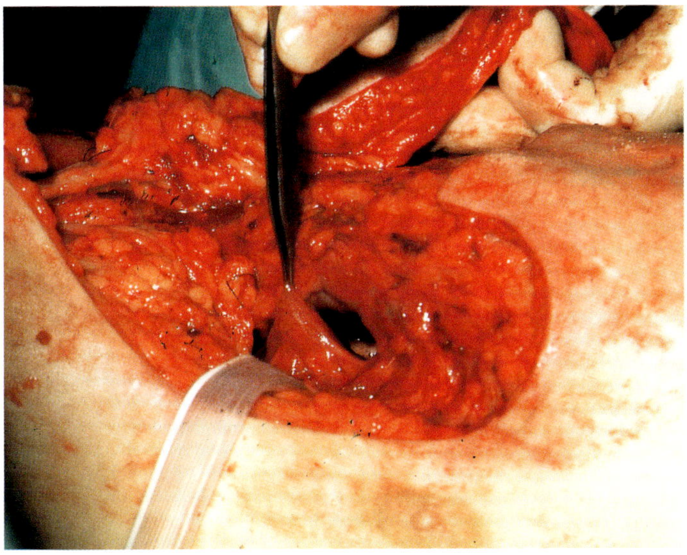

Figure 4.84f The latissimus dorsi muscle is placed into the thoracic cavity, thus, eliminating dead space and simultaneously transferring excellently vascularized tissue. Finally, the thoracic wall defect is covered by a scapular island flap.

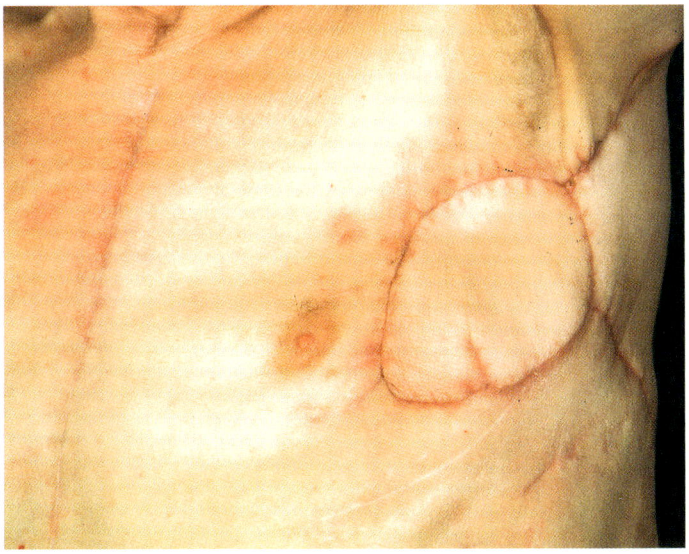

Figure 4.84g Situation six weeks postoperatively

Pectoralis Island Flap

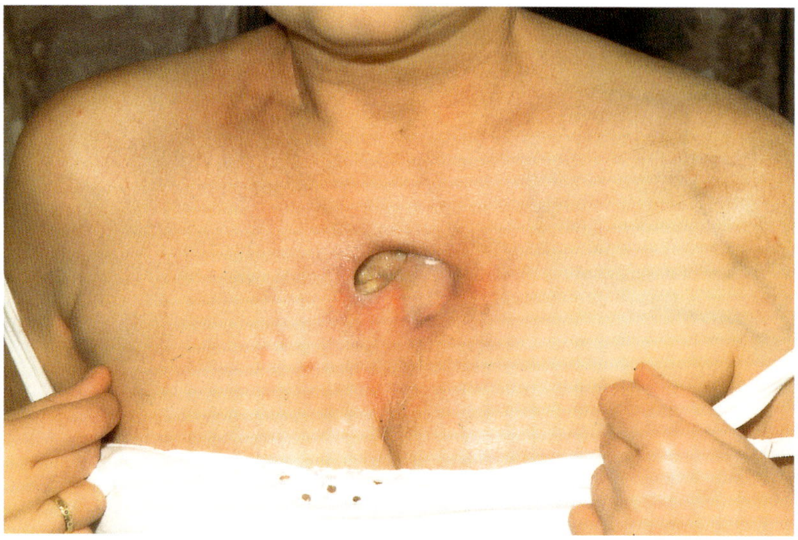

Figure 4.85a Status post radiation therapy of Hodgkin's disease with resultant ulceration and partial necrosis of the sternum. Excision of necrotic tissue including a portion of the sternum is performed. Reconstruction is planned with a pectoralis island flap.

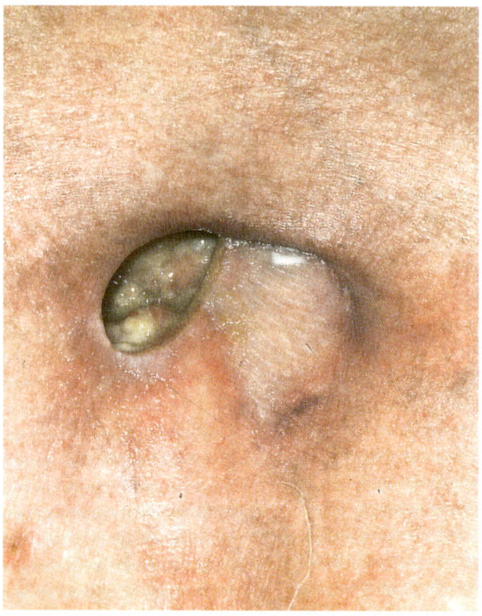

Figure 4.85b Close-up of the defect before excision

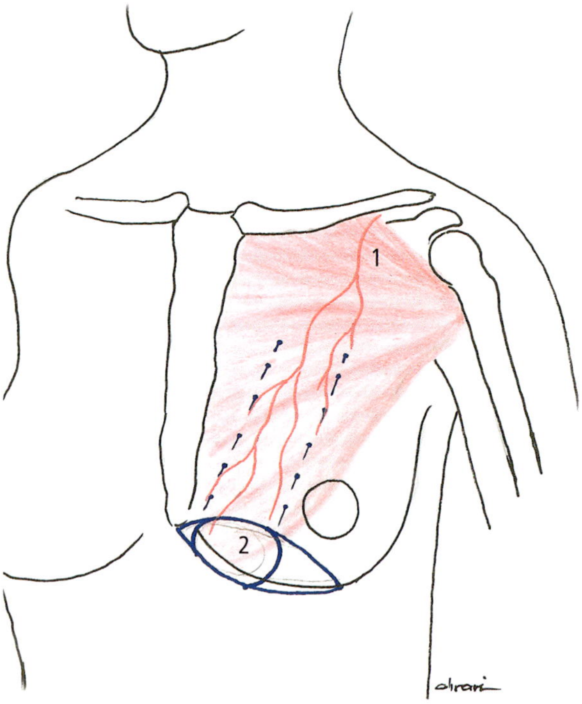

Figure 4.85c Blood supply to the pectoralis major muscle is supplied by the thoracoacromial artery and vein (1). In females it is cosmetically more appealing to harvest the flap from the IMF (2). In doing so, half of the skin island is located above and the other half below the IMF.

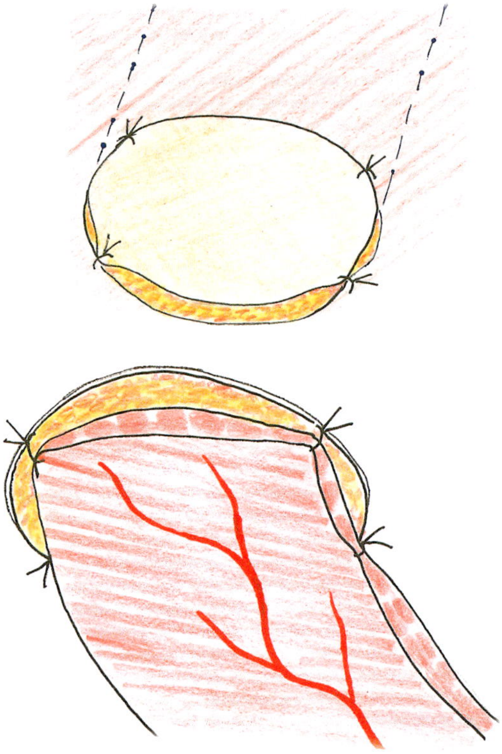

Figure 4.85d The island flap is sutured to the muscle with a few sutures to prevent injury to the supplying vessels during manipulation and transfer. The muscular pedicle is isolated from the subcutaneous as well as underlying tissues in a combination of blunt and sharp dissection.

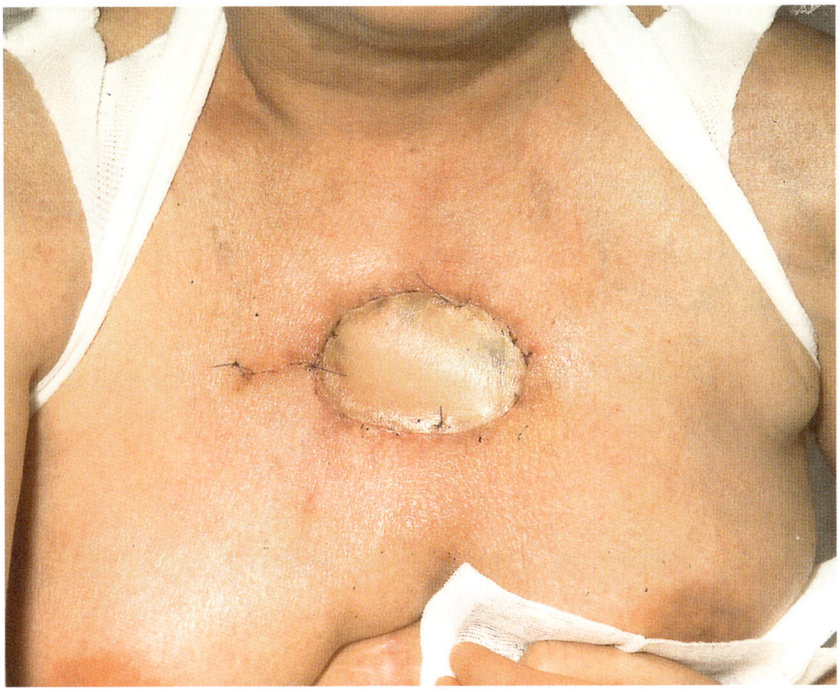

Figure 4.85e The pectoralis island flap is transferred through a subcutaneous tunnel for defect coverage and sutured into place. The muscular pedicle should not be under tension.

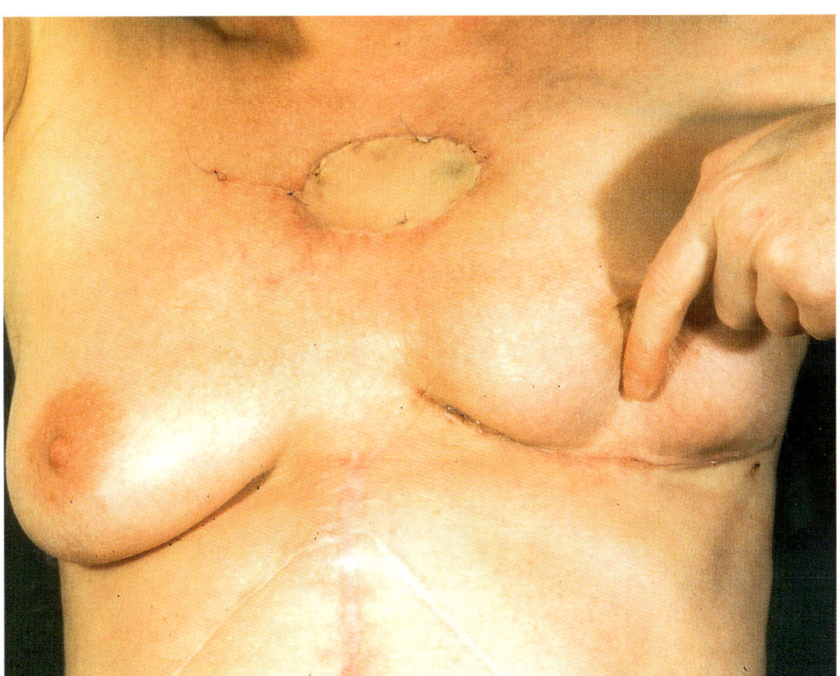

Figure 4.85f Three weeks postoperatively. Note the favorable position of the scar in the IMF.

Myocutaneous Trapezius Flap

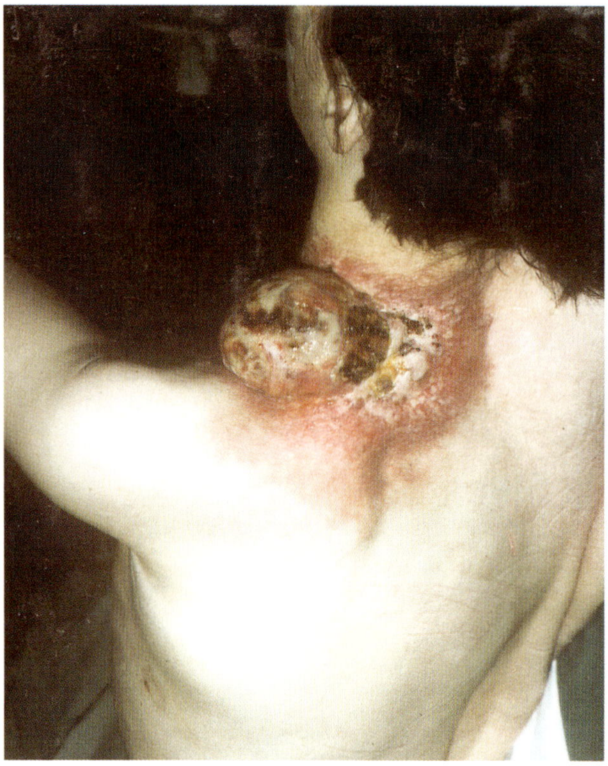

Figure 4.86a Status post mastectomy and radiation therapy: Radiation-induced squamous cell carcinoma of the left cervical and shoulder area nine years following irradiation.

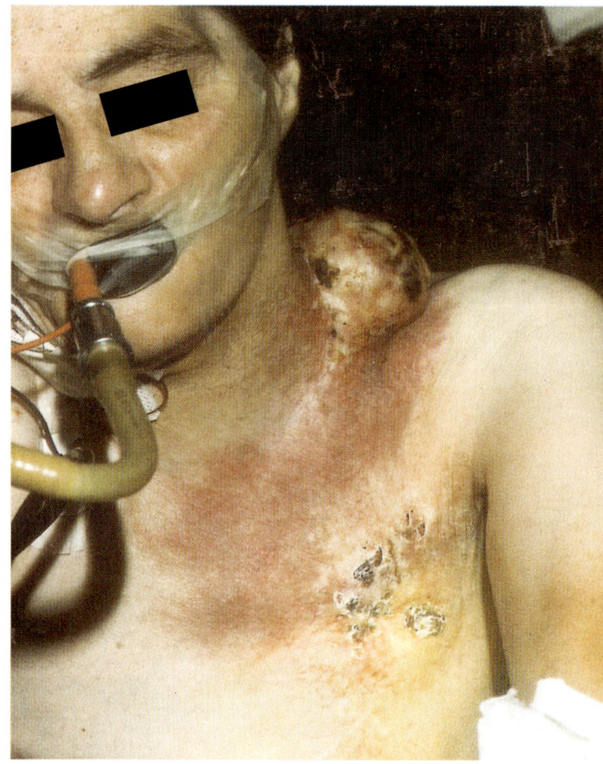

Figure 4.86b Radiation damage of the tissues adjacent to the tumor.

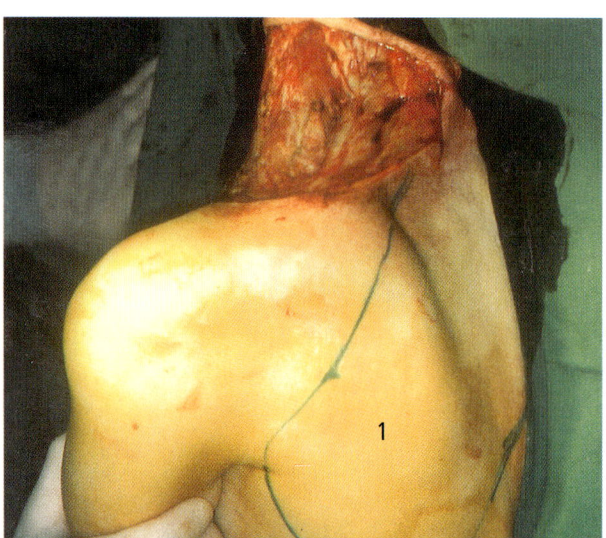

Figure 4.86c Radical excision of the tumor is performed first and a myocutaneous trapezius flap is designed. The distal part of the flap does not contain muscle (1).

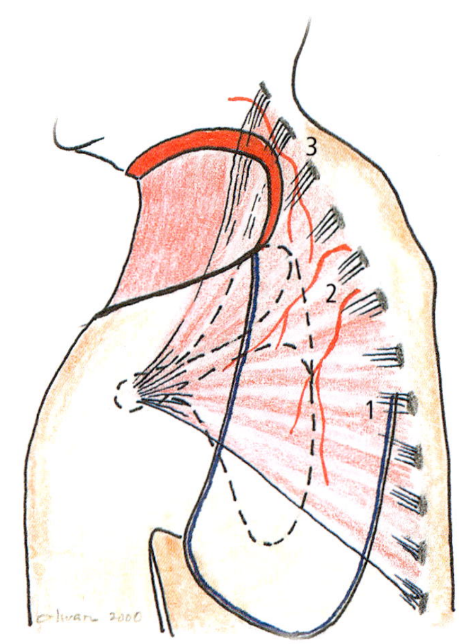

Figure 4.86d Design of a trapezius flap. Blood supply to the trapezius muscle (1) is by means of the transversal colli (cutaneous branches) (2) and occipital arteries (3).

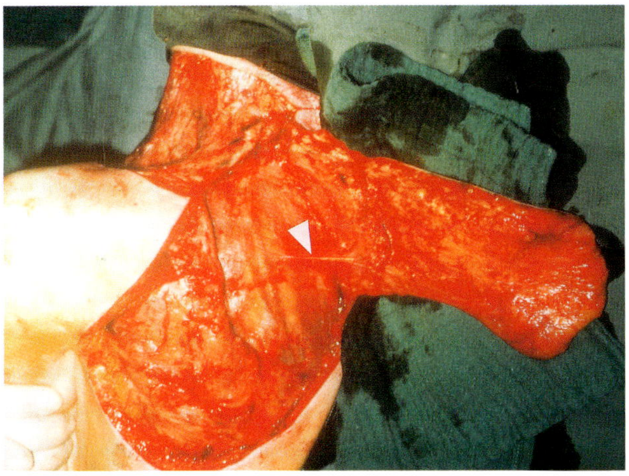

Figure 4.86e The flap is raised. Arrow: The transversal colli artery is preserved.

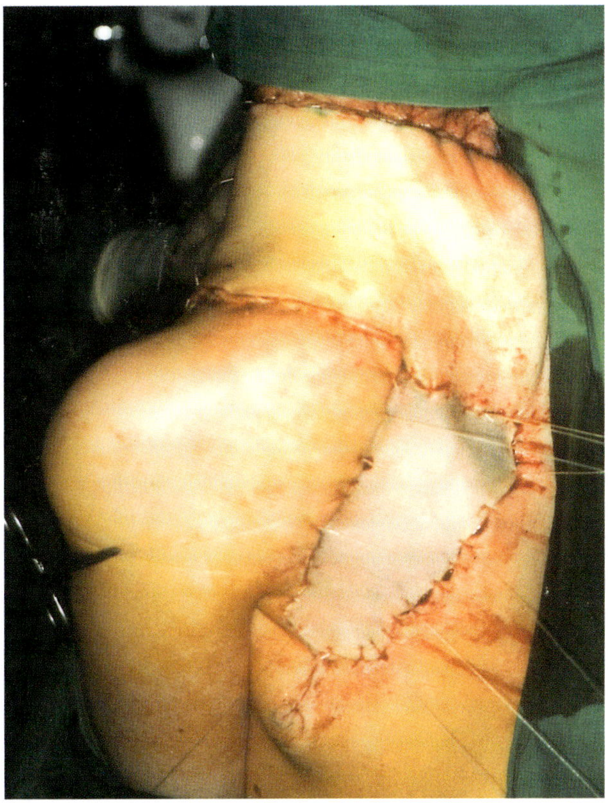

Figure 4.86f Split thickness skin graft is necessary for donor site closure.

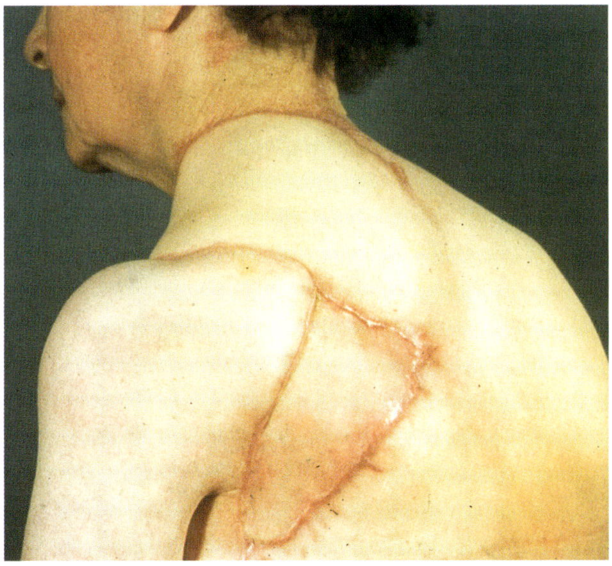

Figure 4.86g One year postoperatively

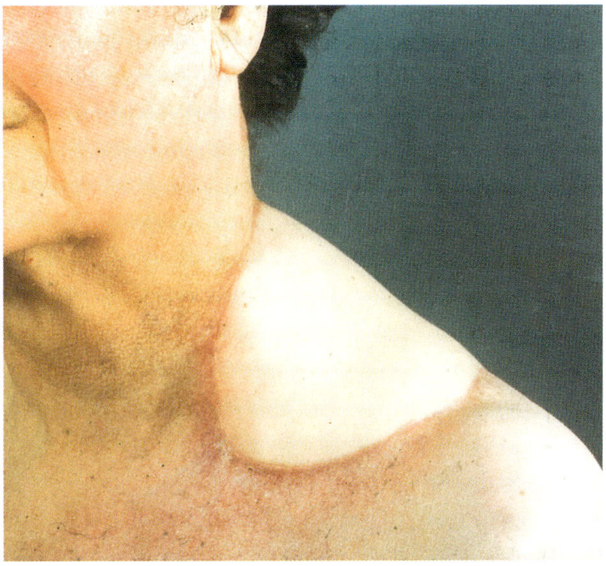

Figure 4.86h Close-up

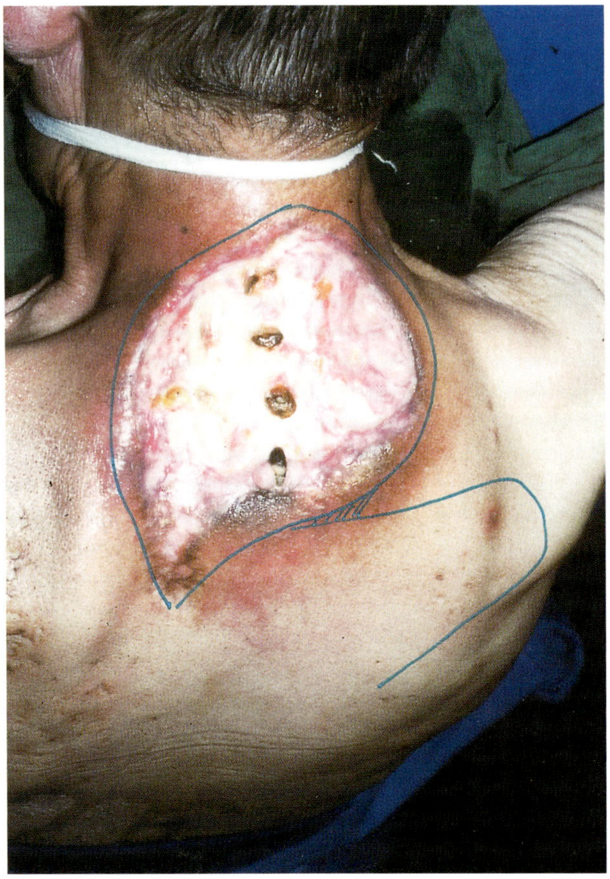

Figure 4.87a Diagnosis: Radiation ulcer, Bechterew syndrome. Symptoms: Persistent pain and infection. Design of a myocutaneous trapezius flap following extensive debridement with resection of four dorsal processes of the cervical spine. Risky flap because it contains some irradiated tissue.

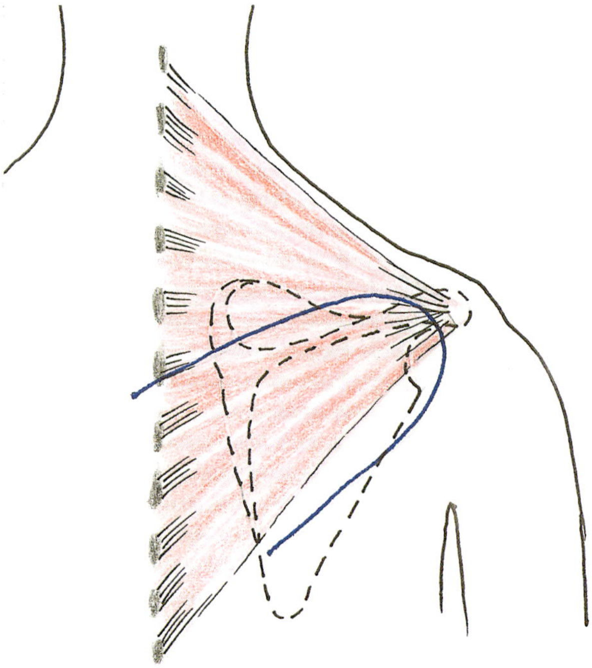

Figure 4.87b The trapezius flap has a medial pedicle and displays a latero-cranial orientation.

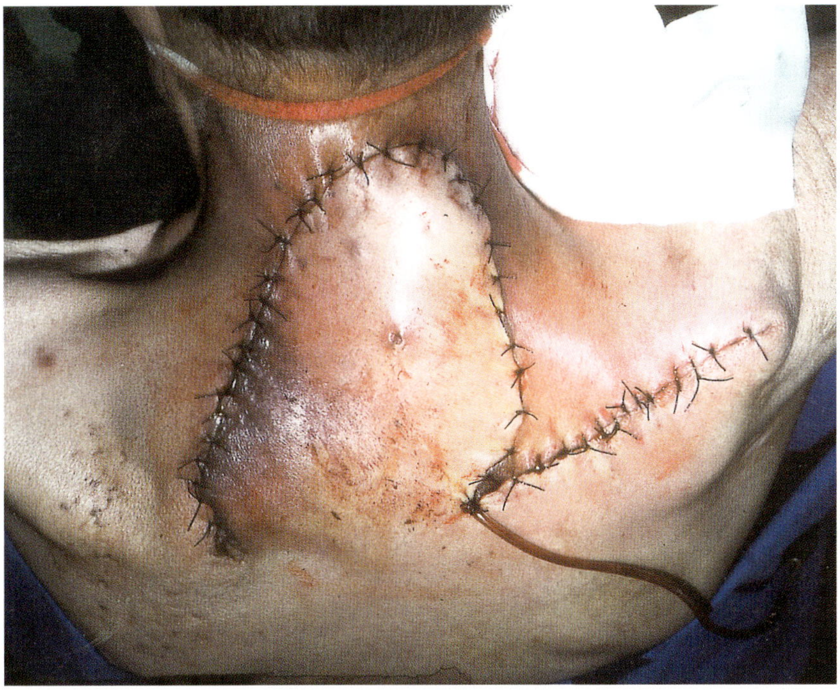

Figure 4.87c Following extensive debridement with resection of four dorsal processes of the cervical spine the trapezius flap is used for defect coverage. The donor site is closed primarily after extensive inferior mobilization.

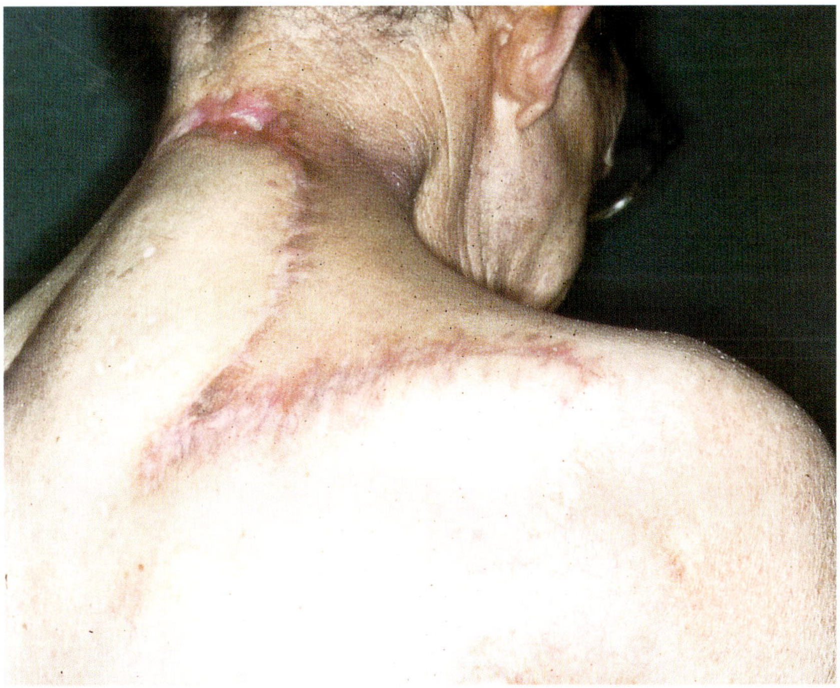

Figure 4.87d Eleven months post-operatively. This was a risky procedure since the flap contained irradiated tissue. A pedicled or free latissimus flap would have been a very good alternative.

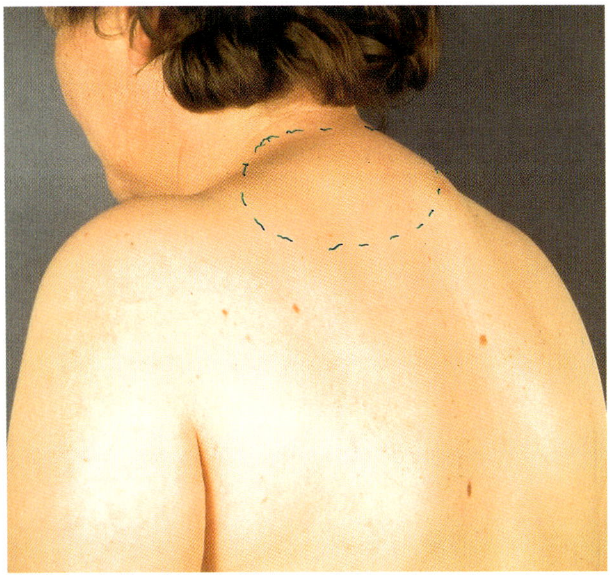

Figure 4.88a Myosarcoma of the nape of the neck (T1 N0 M0 G2)

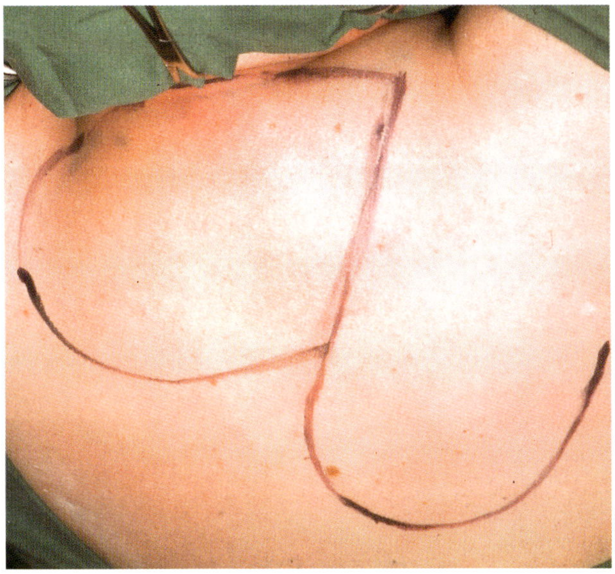

Figure 4.88b Operative plan

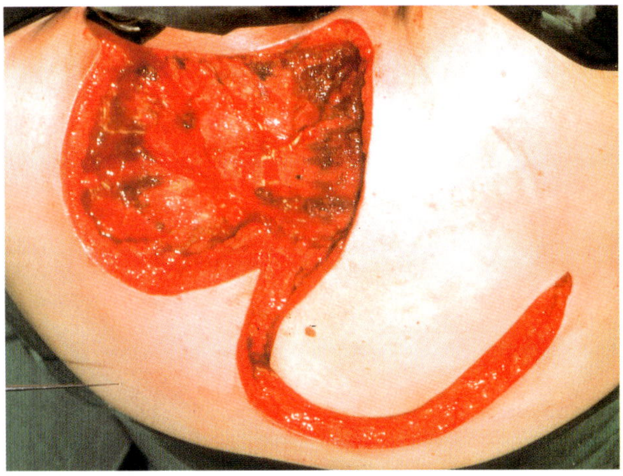

Figure 4.88c En-bloc excision of skin and tumor with a wide safety margin. A myocutaneous trapezius flap is designed and raised.

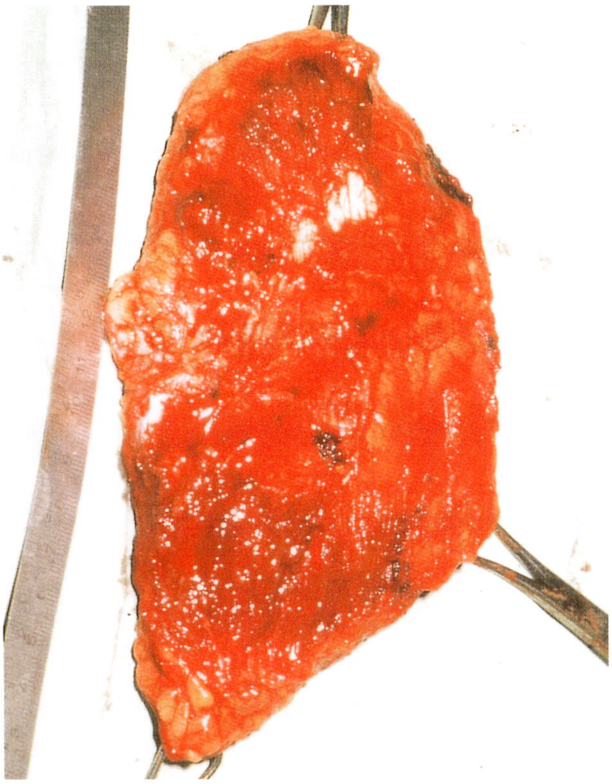

Figure 4.88d 17 × 14 × 8 cm large specimen. Border of defect are free of tumor. Postoperative radiation therapy is planned.

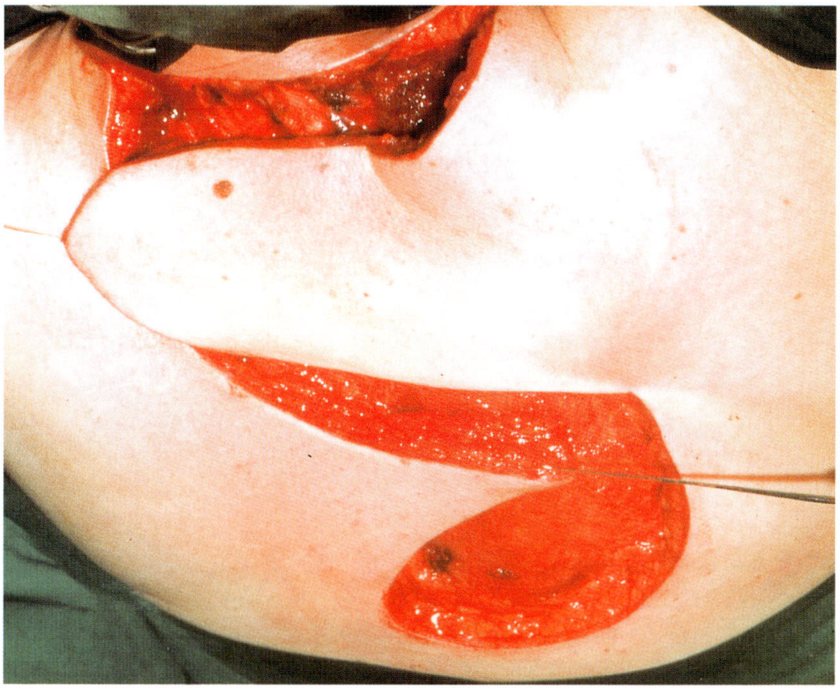

Figure 4.88e Flap transfer into the defect: Donor site margins need to be mobilized extensively to achieve a primary closure.

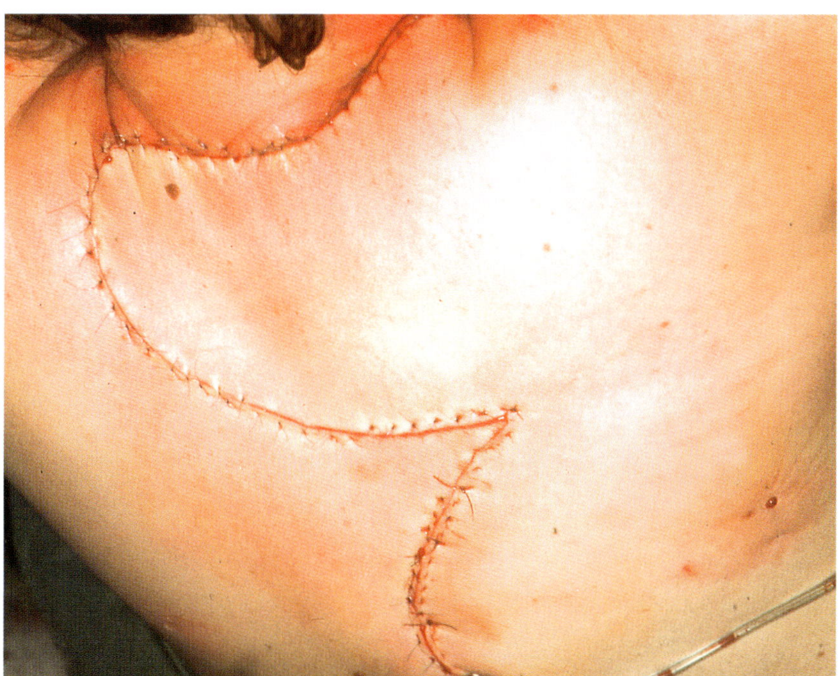

Figure 4.88f Appearance at time of closure

Breast Reduction

Breast hypertrophy, macromastia, or gigantomastia are often hereditary conditions, and are frequently evident in puberty. Breasts may enlarge during pregnancy, however, reduction of breast volume during pregnancy has also been observed.

Macromastia and gigantomastia not only cause orthostatic complaints but also frequently cause psychological problems which may be grave during adolescence.

Complaints may include:

1) Back/neck pain, malposition
2) Pressure marks in the shoulder region (brassiere)
3) Eczema in the inframammary fold
4) Pressure on the brachial plexus

Psychological problems present as insecurity, and sense of inferiority. Additionally, affected patients avoid participating in sports. Thus, breast reduction surgery should be advocated generously and with early performance in order to circumvent manifestation of psychological pathology. Patients must be informed that nursing of child after operation could be impossible.

Breast reduction is a safe procedure in competent hands.

Two separate techniques need to be distinguished:

1. Standard reduction (inverse T-incision)
   Introduced by Strömbeck and modified by many others this technique is precise, safe, and easy to learn. It is easy to achieve a pleasing breast shape, even in very large breasts. The only drawback is the long scar along the inframammary fold.
2. Vertical reduction
   Introduced by Lassus, this technique has also had many modifications. This more demanding technique has been popularized by Lejour. The beginner should apply this technique for correction of breast ptosis only. With increased experience larger breasts may be reshaped by this method. Within the last 10 years 70 % of all our patients (ever increasing frequency) have been treated with the vertical reduction technique.

Both techniques considerably reduce NAC-sensitivity. Furthermore, breast feeding is possible in only 50 % of cases (Strömbeck). Probably less.

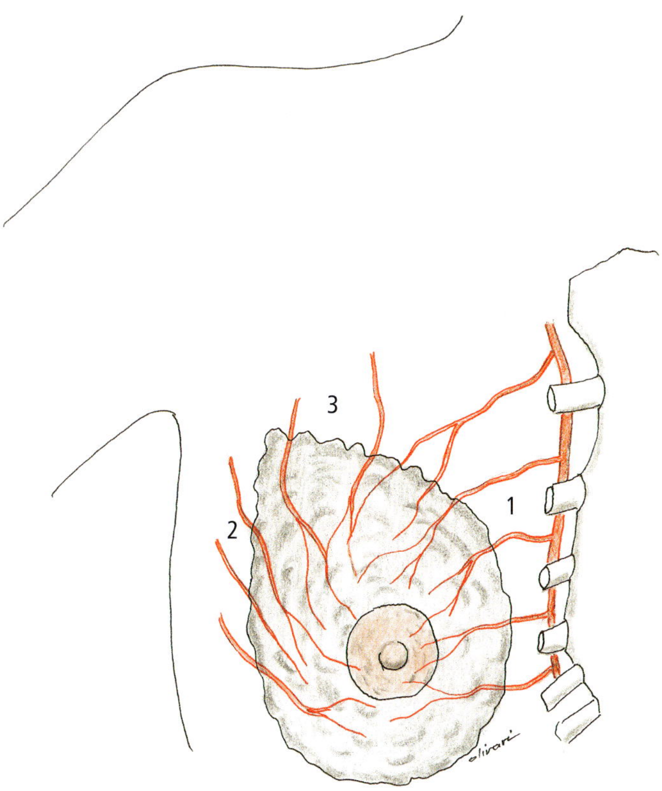

Figure 4.89 Perfusion of the breast: The dominant blood supply to the breast derives from medial branches of the internal mammary artery (1). Laterally, blood supply is provided by branches of the intercostal arteries (2). Cranially, branches of the lateral mammary artery and thoracoacromial artery supply the breast (3). According to the author's experience medial and mediocranial blood supply is optimal. Thus, only a mediocranial pedicle has been used for many years in breast reduction, regardless of the chosen incision (inverted T; vertical incision). Of note, during the last 15 years of his practice Strömbeck used a mediocranial pedicle as well.

a) Standard Breast Reduction

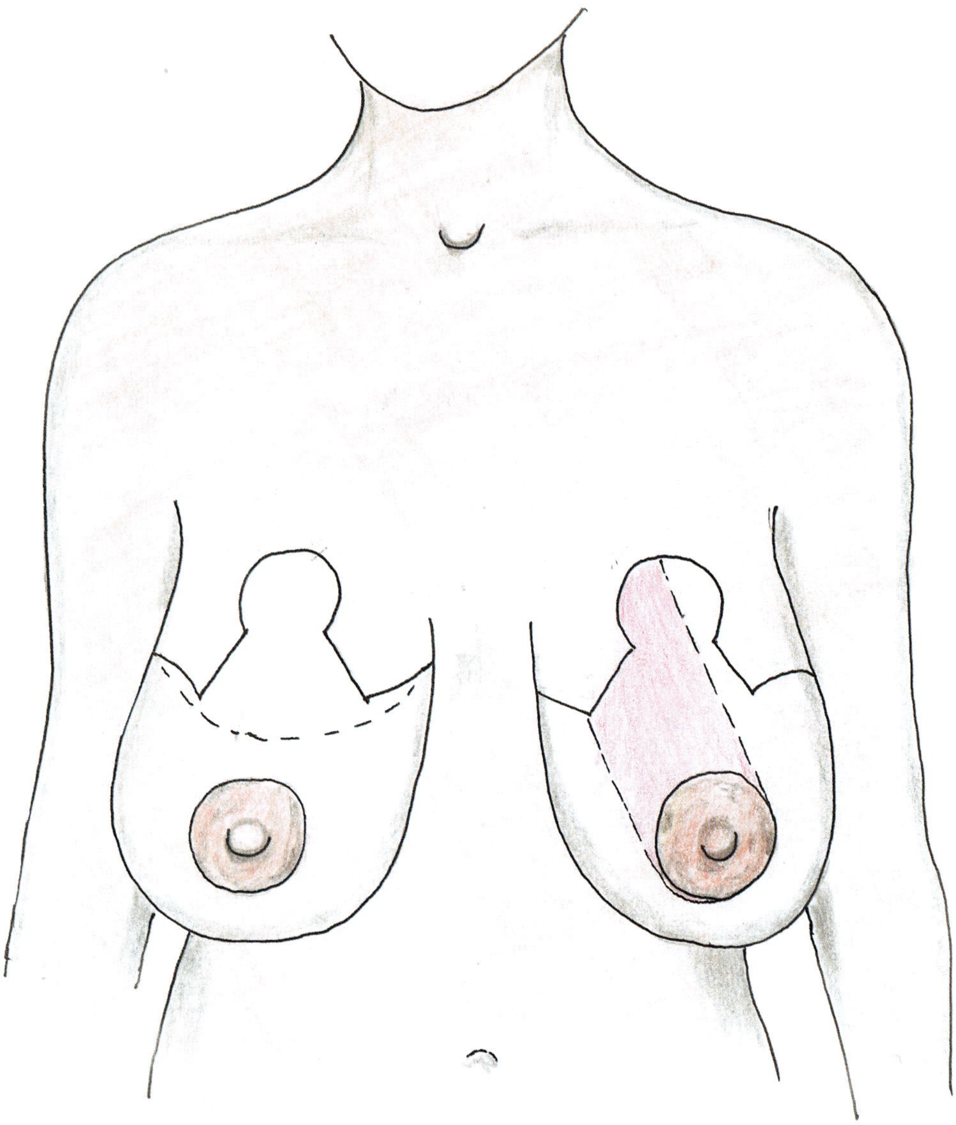

Figure 4.90 Standard breast reduction – Strömbeck modification:

a) The distance from the sternal notch to the upper border of the future areola is 21 to 23 cm. The heavier the breast the longer must this distance be. If in doubt, a longer distance should be chosen.
b) The distance from median to medial border of the future areola measures 8 to 10 cm.
c) The vertical incision should have a length of 6 cm.
d) The length of the areola circumference should be 14 cm (Areola diameter 4.5 cm $\times$ 3.14 = 14.13 cm or if the diameter is 4 cm = 12.56 cm).
e) The incision in the IMF should not exceed the length of the IMF medially and laterally. Following removal of subcutaneous tissue during surgery or liposuction the fold shortens considerably.
f) The connecting incisions between the vertical and inframammary incision distinguish a good from an excellent surgeon. The sum of both incisions should slightly increase the length of the inframammary incision or else tension at point G will be too high.

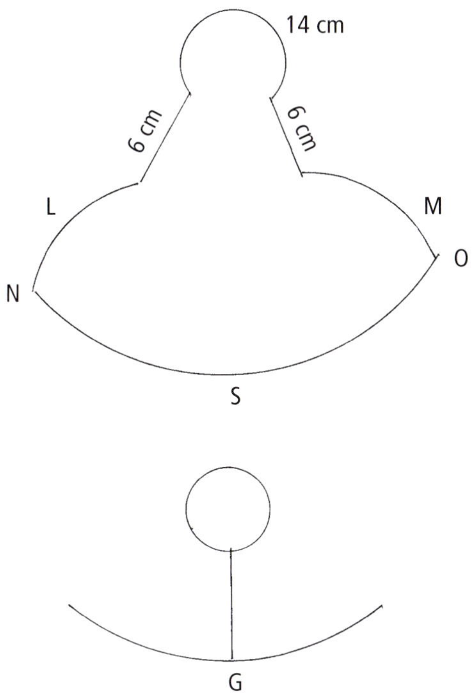

Figure 4.91a Point G should be tension-free, thus the sum of L and M should be more than S. Dog ear formation needs to be prevented which can be achieved by removing excessive fat at point N and O, either by open excision or by liposuction. Skin closure is always started laterally and medially respectively and ends at point G. One must never begin skin closure at point G. First subcutaneous stitches are conducted with 3 × 0 Vicryl then a continuous intracutaneous suture is performed either with 3 × 0 Trofilene.

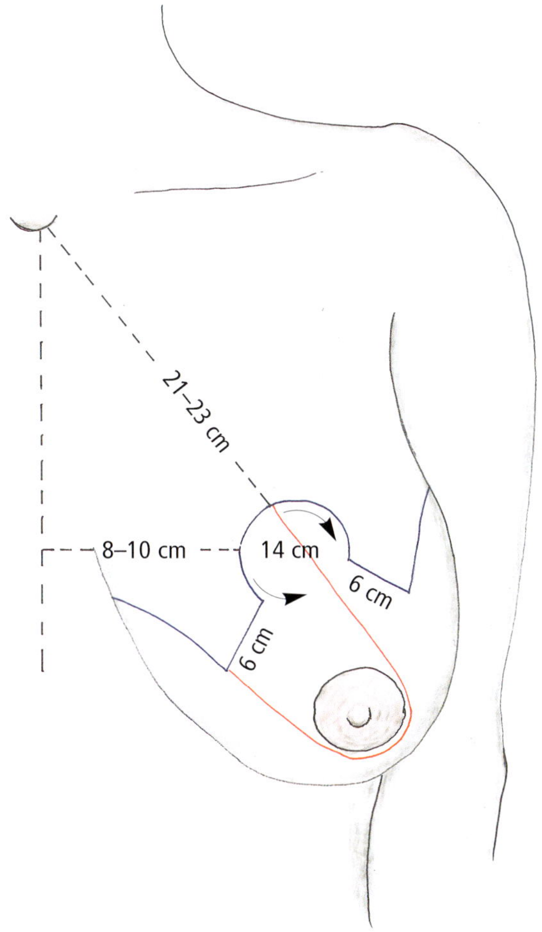

Figure 4.91b Markings in standard reduction (in standing position)

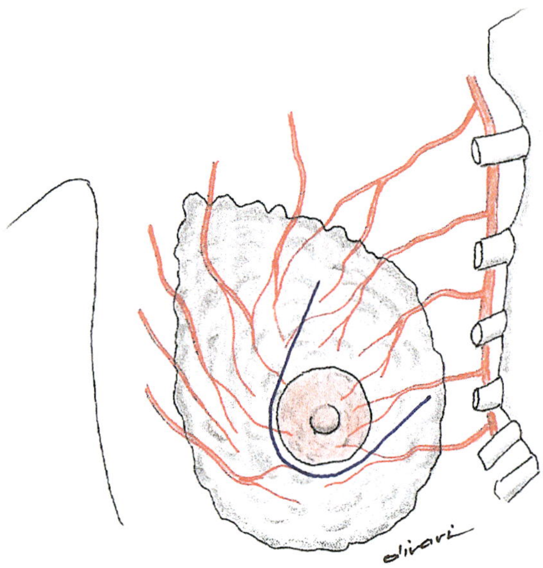

Figure 4.92a Blood supply to the areola via a medio-cranial pedicle (predominantly by branches from the internal mammary artery.)

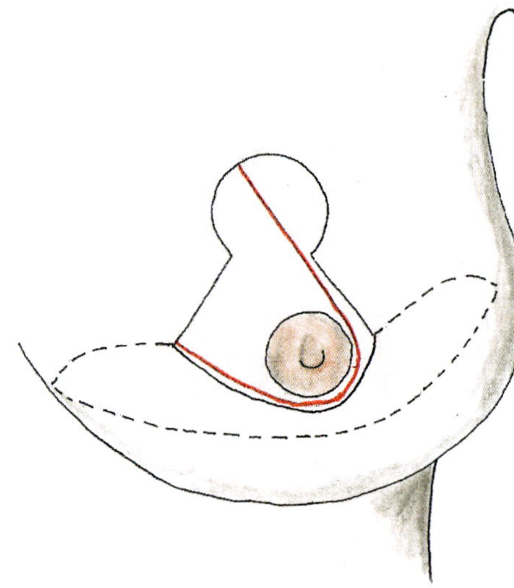

Figure 4.92b Operative plan (see preoperative markings)

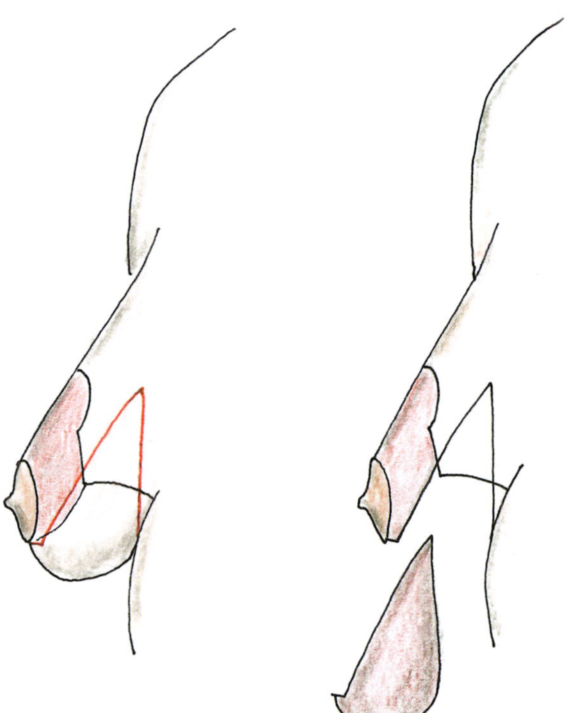

Figure 4.92c First deepithelialization of the periareolar area is conducted then excision of glandular tissue is performed beginning at the thoracic wall (pectoralis fascia). The cut surface at the remaining glandular tissue needs to be smooth is order to prevent small tissue necroses.

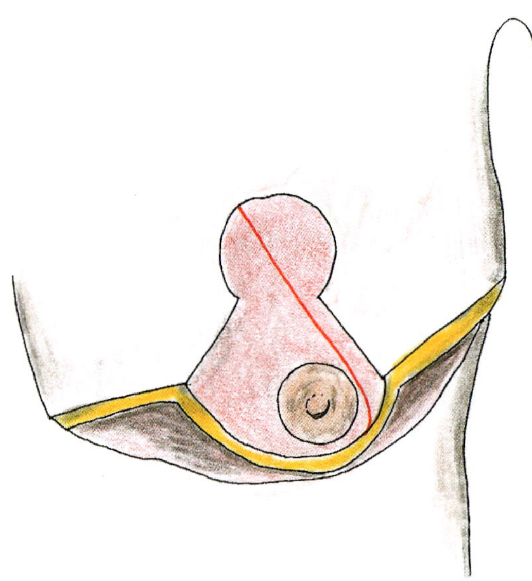

Figure 4.92d Following resection the areola has a medio-cranial pedicle.

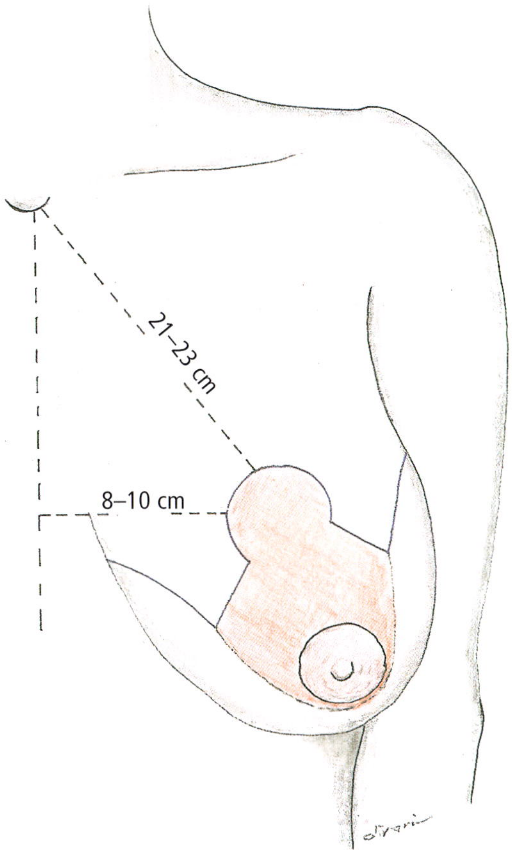

Figure 4.93a Red area is to be deepithelialized.

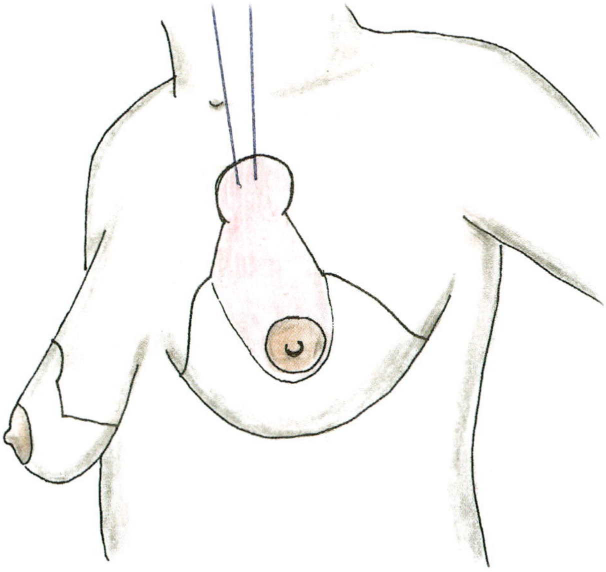

Figure 4.93b The inframammary incision has to be shorter than the length of the IMF.

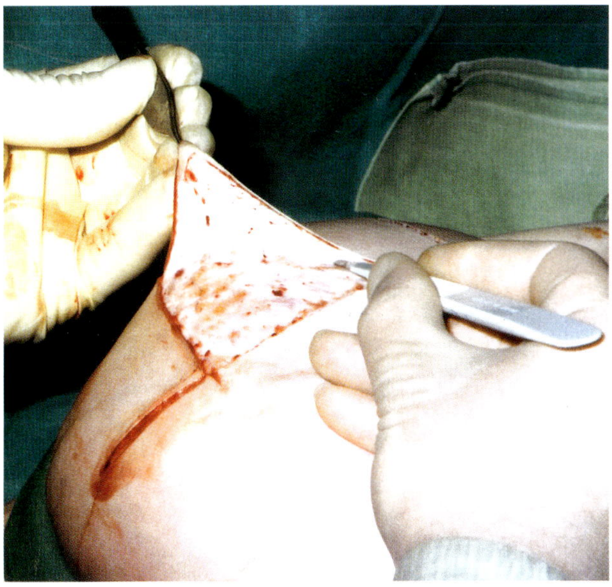

Figure 4.93c Deepithelialization needs to be performed with the breast under considerable tension. It is done with a scalpel since use of dermatomes may lead to epithelial cysts.

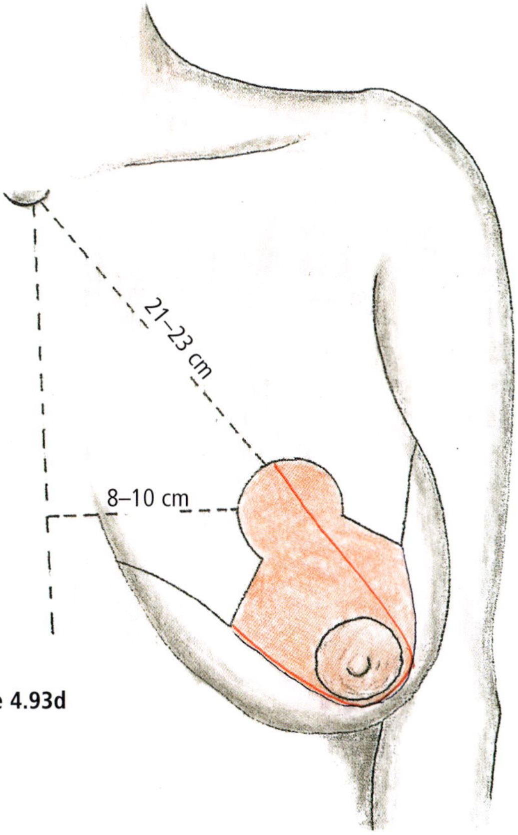

Figure 4.93d

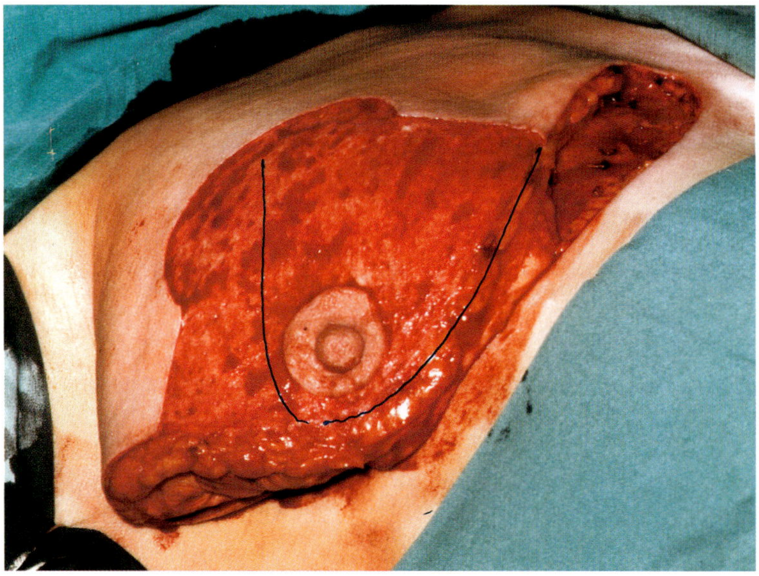

Figure 4.94a Right breast: Status post deepithelialization and resection of breast tissue. Design of the medio-cranial pedicle.

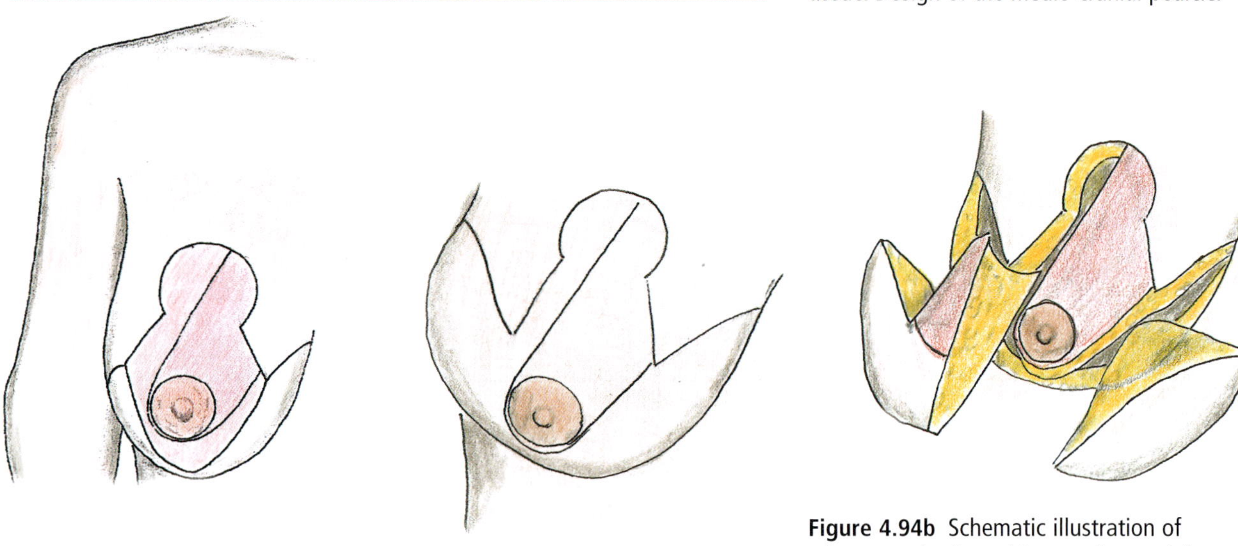

Figure 4.94b Schematic illustration of a breast reduction with a medio-cranial pedicled areola.

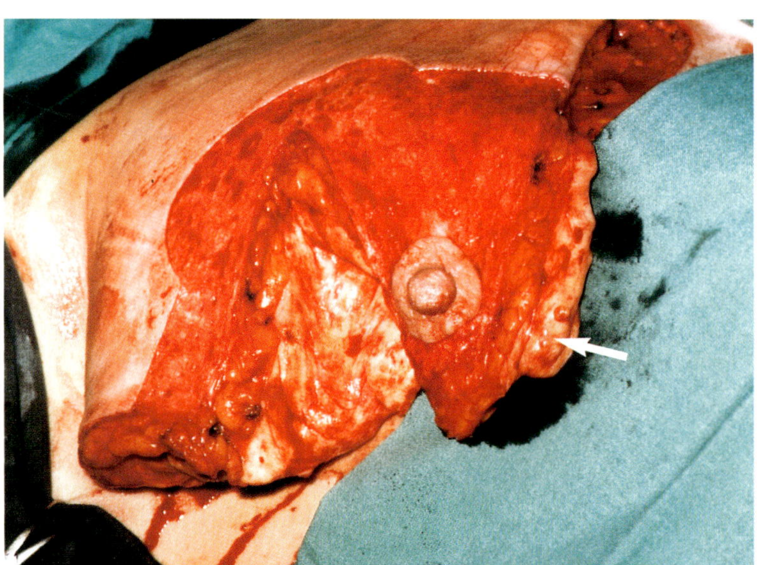

Figure 4.94c Mobilization of the medio-cranially pedicled flap. The flap should not be too thick as this prevents mobilization. Vascular impairment may result if tension is too high. Here the flap is still too thick and thus needs further thinning (arrow).

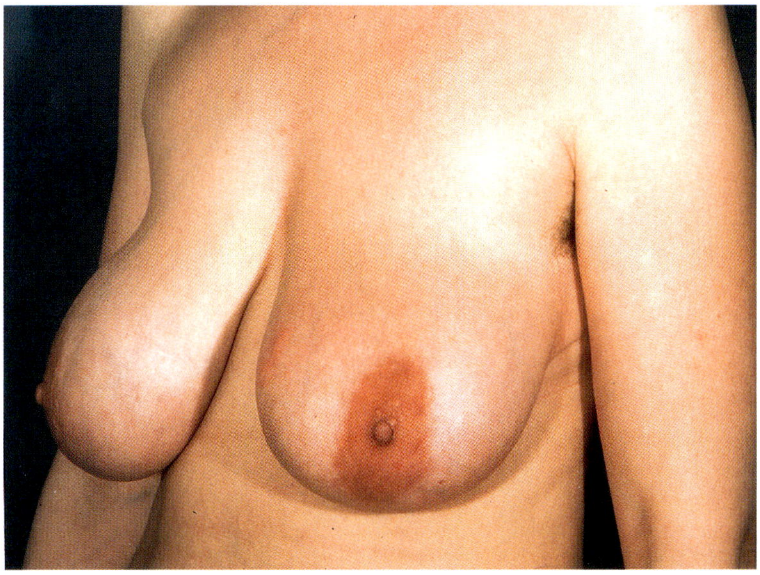

Figure 4.95a Bilateral breast ptosis and hypertrophy. Removal of 870 g per breast.

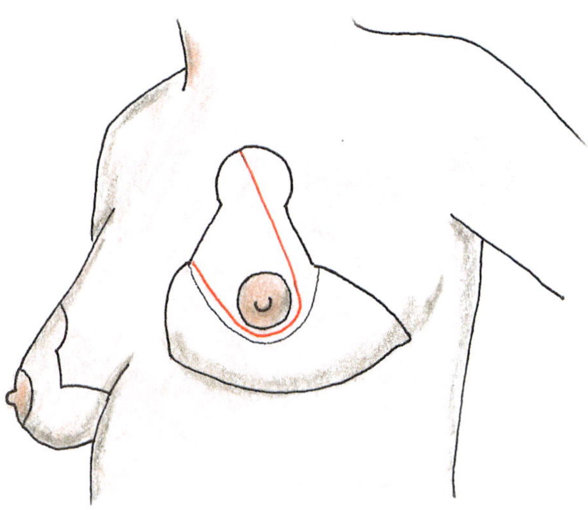

Figure 4.95b Planning a breast reduction with a medio-cranial pedicle

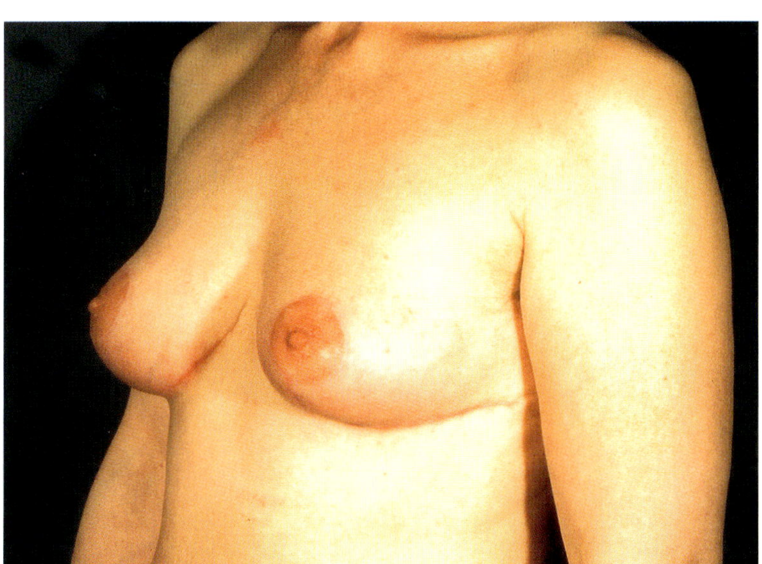

Figure 4.95c Eight months postoperatively: Nice shape but relatively long scars

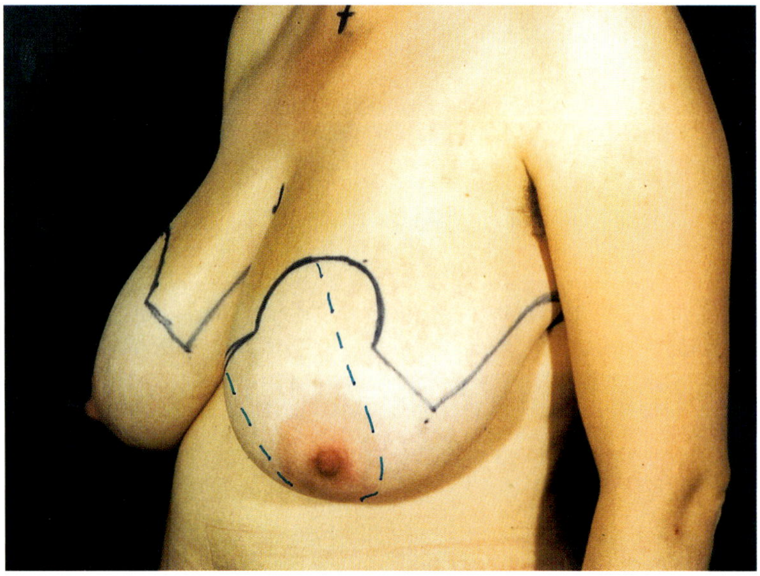

Figure 4.96a Hypertrophy and ptosis. Typical markings always done in standing position. The dotted line illustrates the medio-cranial pedicle of the flap containing the NAC.

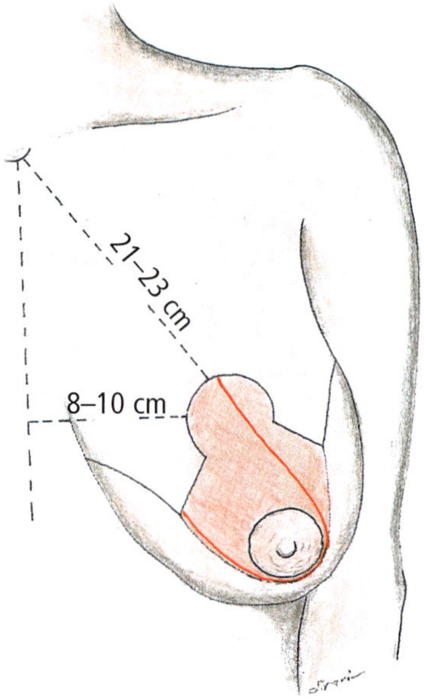

Figure 4.96b Preoperative plan

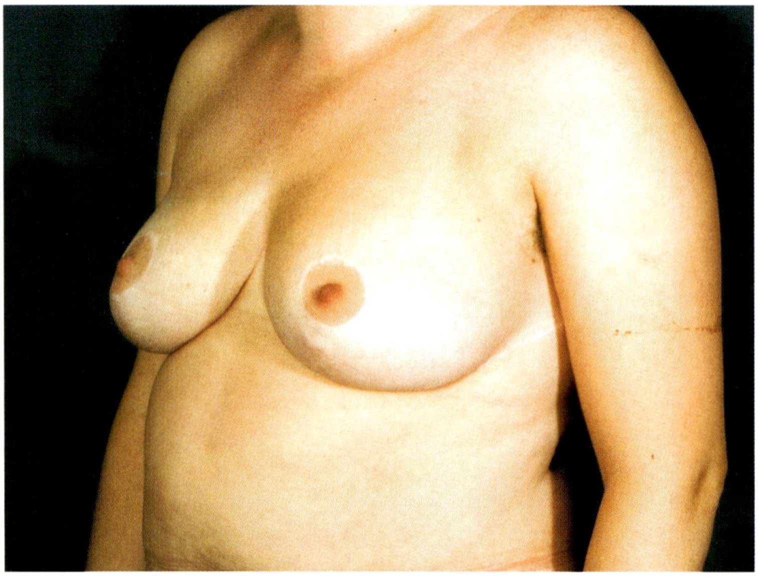

Figure 4.96c Late result – two years postoperatively. 900 g were excised per breast. The scars are inconspicuous.

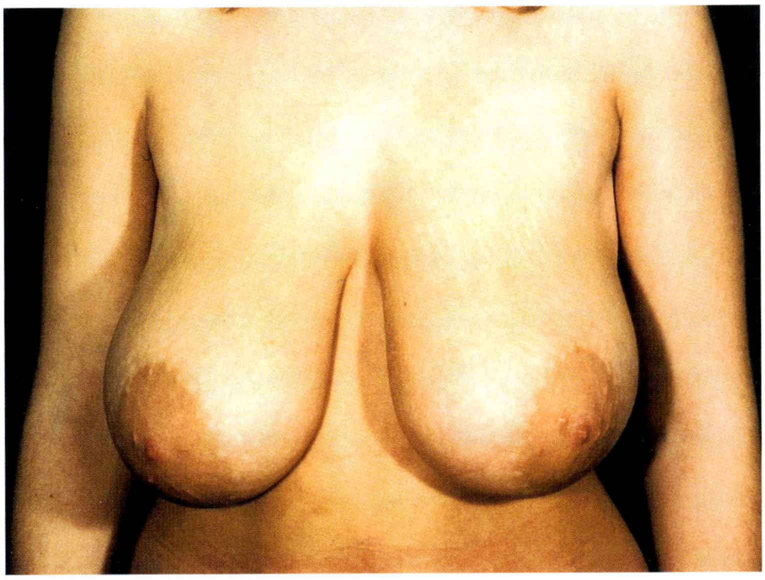

Figure 4.97a Breast hypertrophy and ptosis. Standard reduction (690 g per breast)

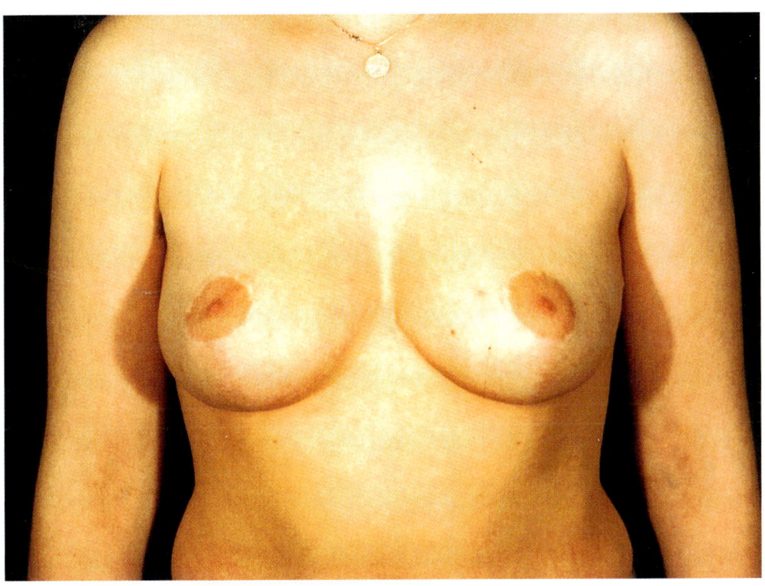

Figure 4.97b Late result – four years post-operatively. The long scars have faded. In this patient a vertical reduction would have been a good alternative.

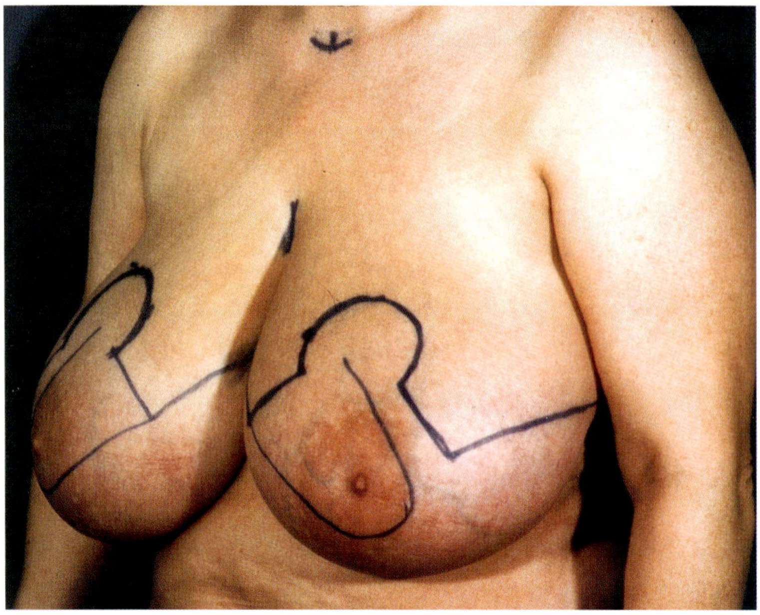

Figure 4.98a Standard reduction for gigantomastia. 1500 g were removed from each breast.

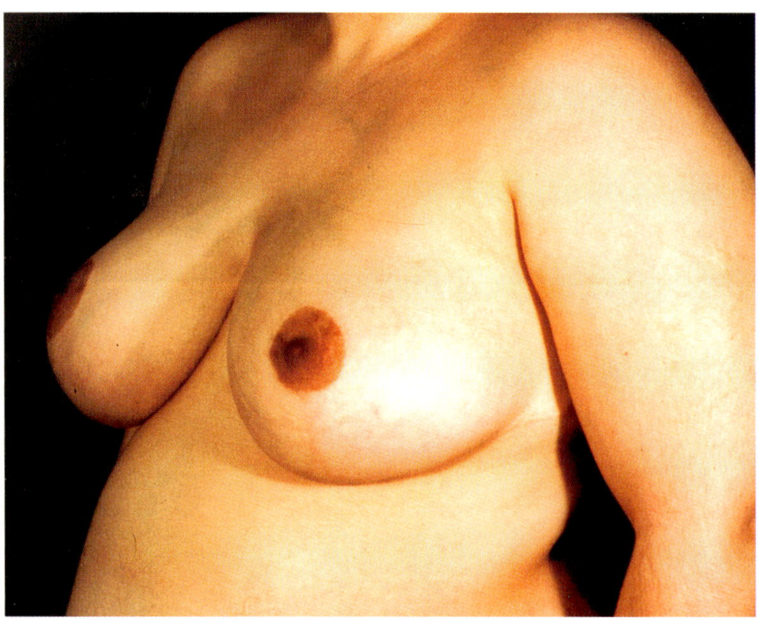

Figure 4.98b Late result – nine years post-operatively. Already two to three years following standard breast reduction scars have usually faded and thus are almost invisible (not always).

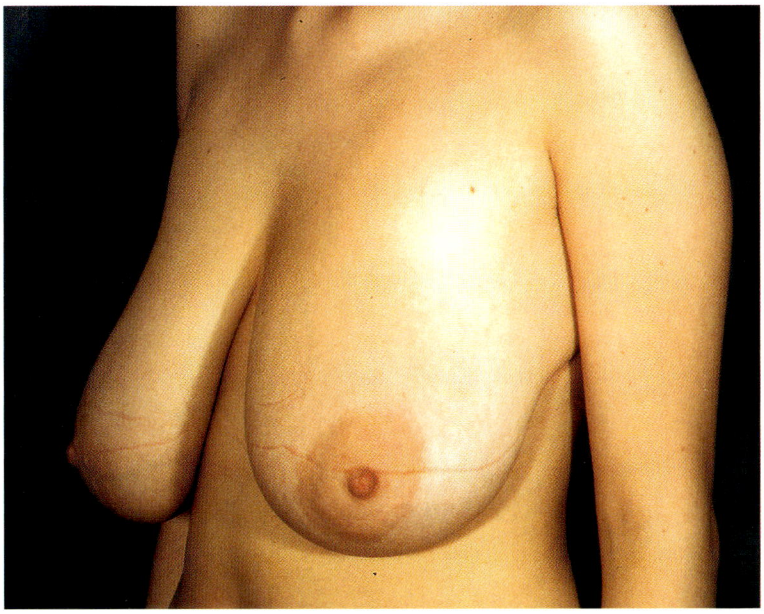

Figure 4.99a Juvenile hypertrophy with ptosis. A reduction was performed bilaterally with excision of 1100 g per breast.

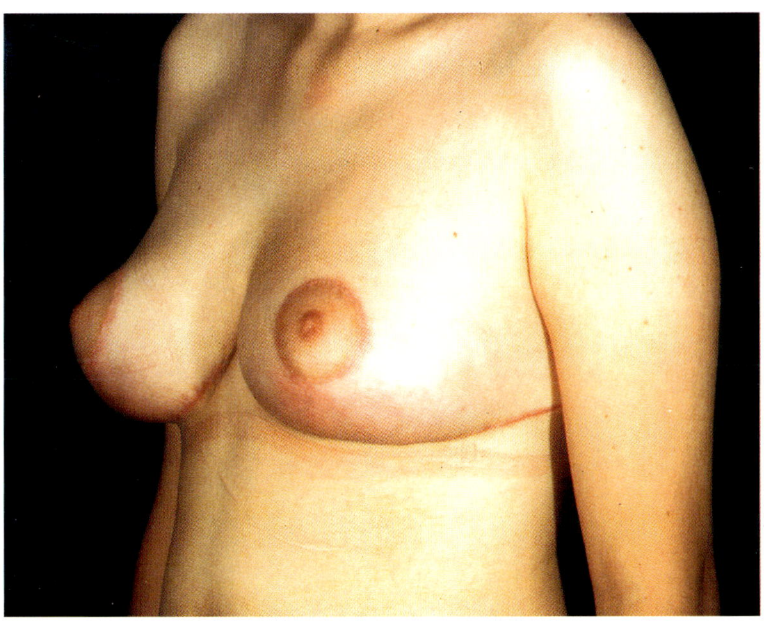

Figure 4.99b Six months postoperatively: Typically long transverse scar

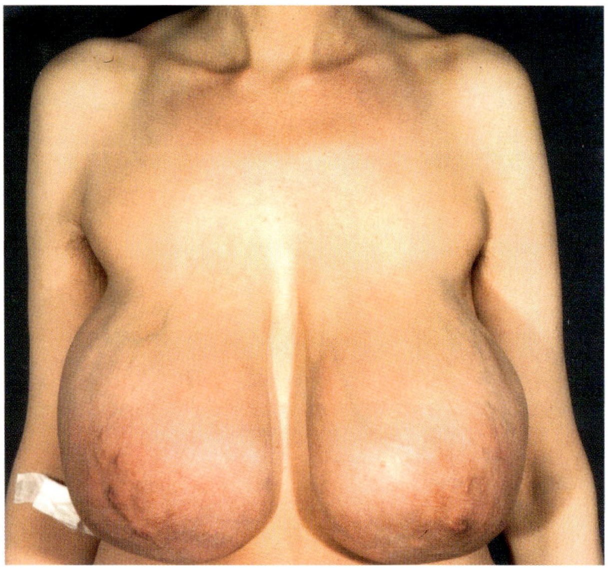

Figure 4.100a Painful glandular gigantomastia. This slender patient suffered extremely due to the breast weight. Almost the entire glandular breast was removed (2300 g per breast).

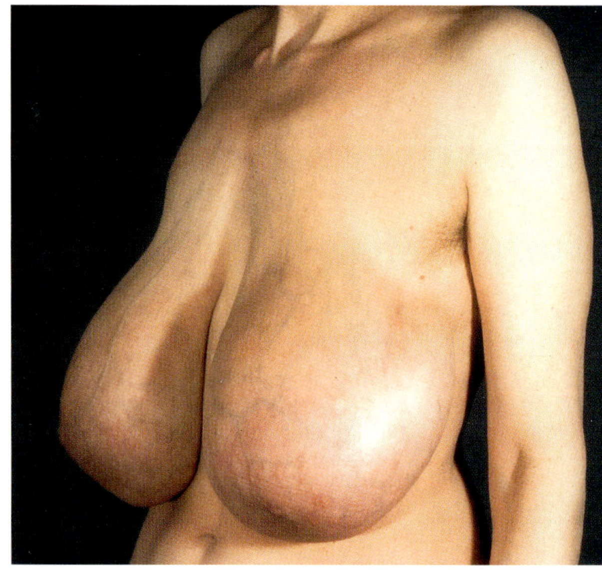

Figure 4.100b The nipple is located at the level of the umbilicus.

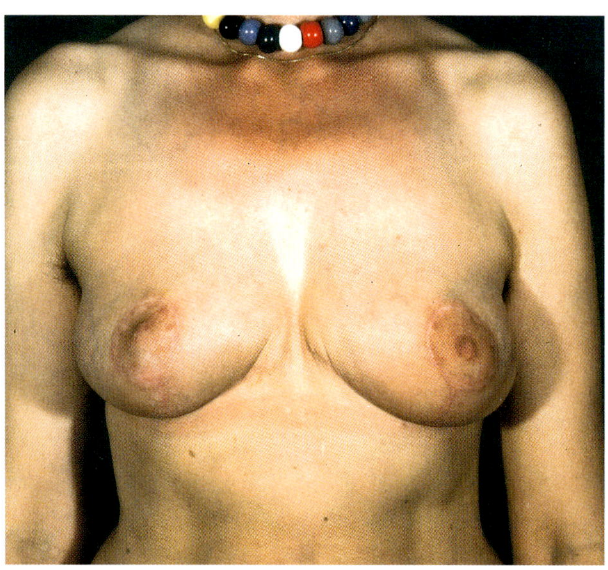

Figure 4.100c Fourteen months following a modified Strömbeck reduction

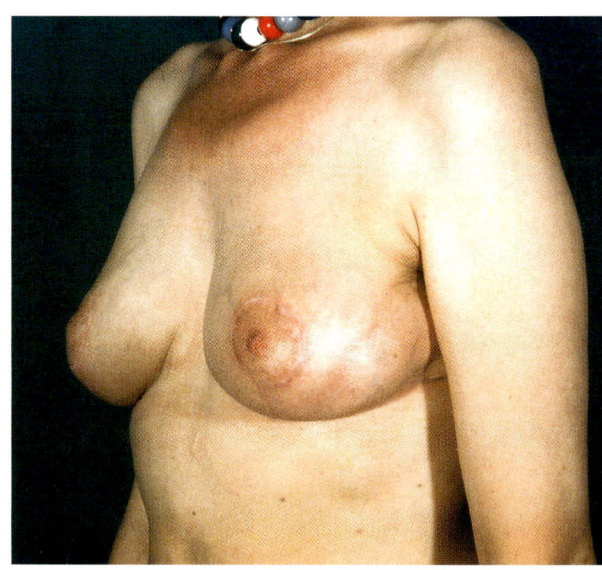

Figure 4.100d Oblique view fourteen months postoperatively

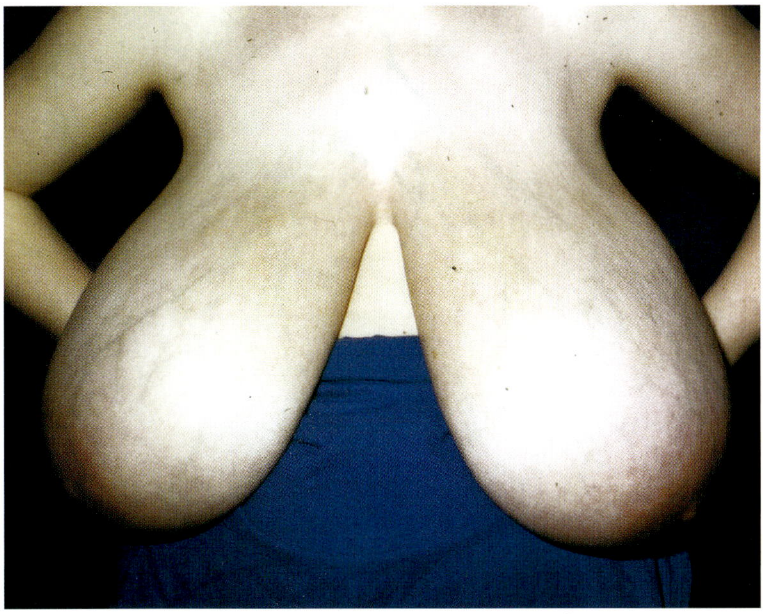

Figure 4.101a Gigantomastia with extreme breast weight related complaints – standard reduction. Six kilograms were removed from each breast.

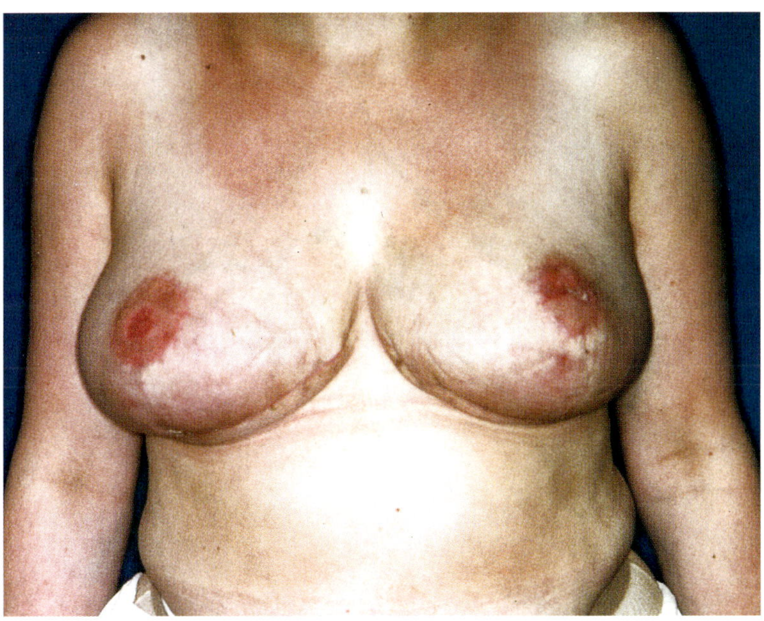

Figure 4.101b Three months postoperatively

b) Gigantomastia With Free NAC-Transplantation

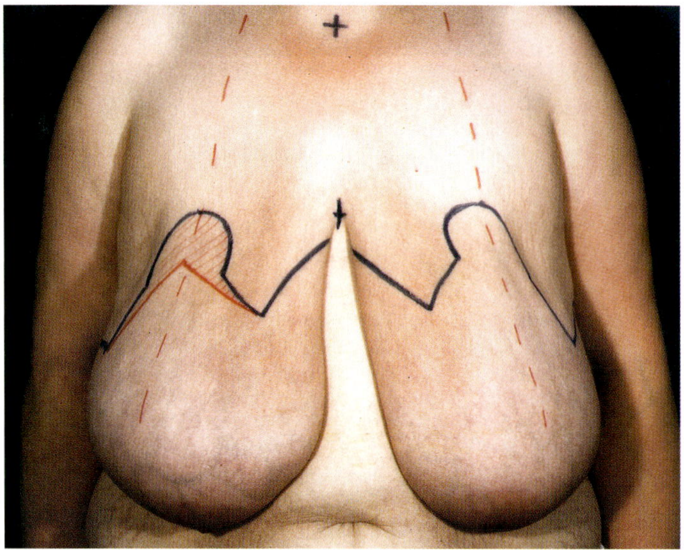

Figure 4.102a Gigantomastia: During preoperative marking the sternal notch-to-upper areolar border distance was defined to be 21 cm. Too little! The skin of a heavy breast stretches. It is better to choose a distance of 23 to 24 cm.

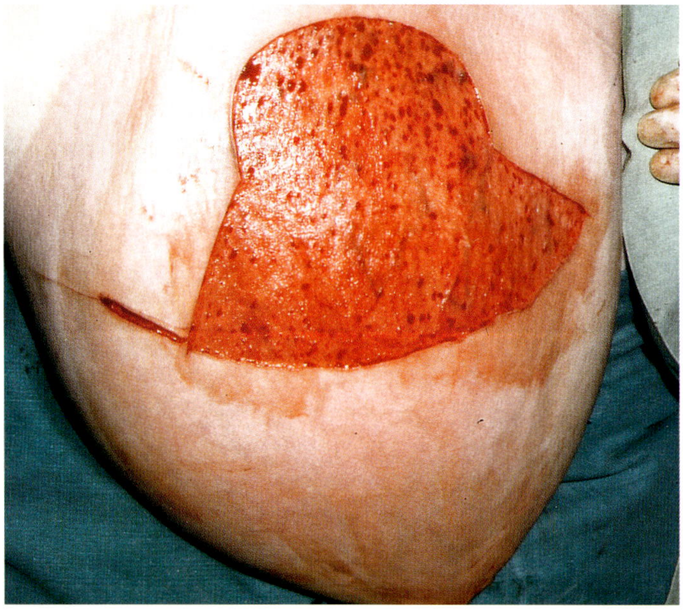

Figure 4.102b Reduction is performed without a pedicled nipple areola complex (NAC) but rather a free NAC transplant. Deepithelialization has to be performed with a scalpel. A dermatome should not be used in order to avoid epithelial cysts.

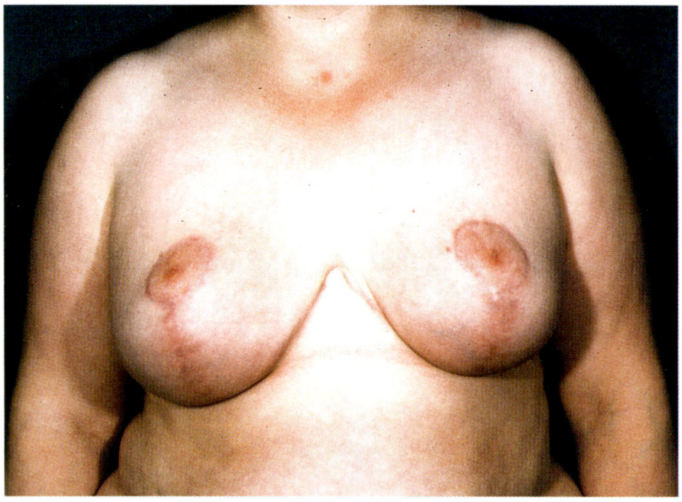

Figure 4.102c Six months following reduction and free NAC transplantation. 4200 g were removed from each breast. The superiorly located NAC results from a too little sternal notch-to-upper areolar border distance defined preoperatively. Correction is very difficult. On the contrary a low seated NAC can be corrected easily. NAC transplantation is rarely indicated.

c) Vertical Reduction (Lassus Technique)

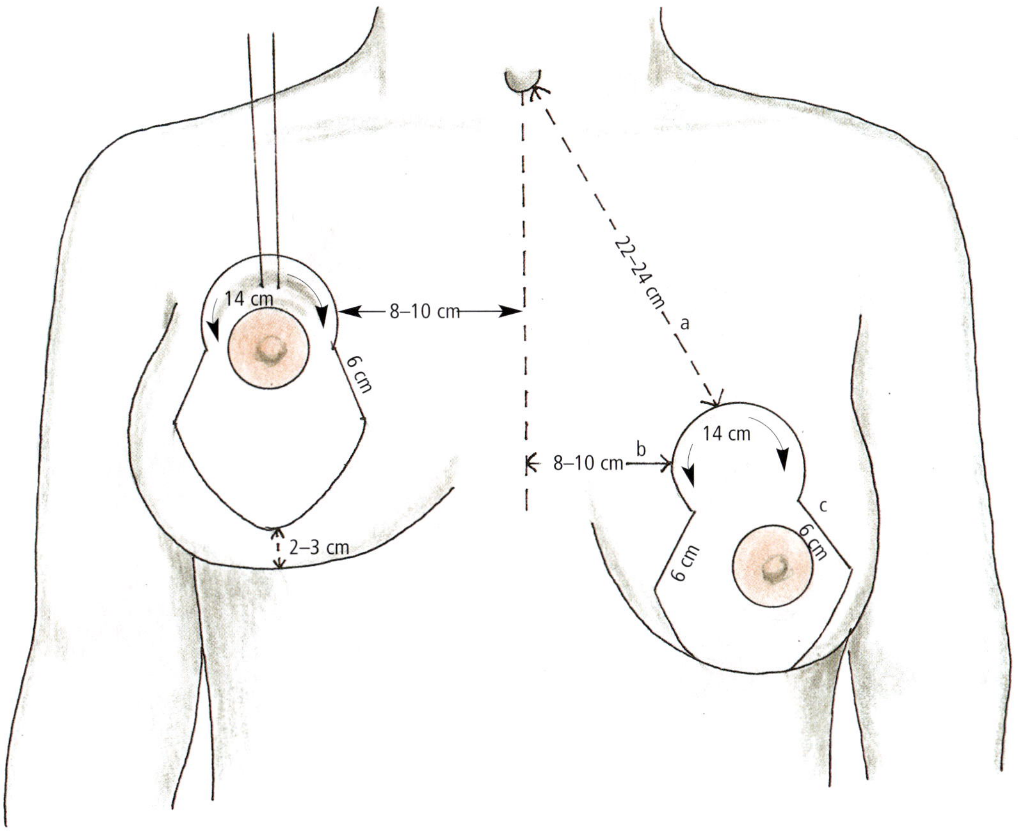

Figure 4.103 Vertical reduction (Lassus technique)

a) Sternal notch-to-postoperative upper areolar border distance: 22 to 24 cm (the larger the breast the longer the distance)
b) Median line-to-postoperative medial areolar border distance: 8 to 10 cm
c) The vertical incision should have a length of 6 cm
d) The areolar circumference has a length of 14 cm
e) Beginning from each vertical pillar (6 cm) the incision is continued inferiorly on both sides and connects with the contralateral incision 2 to 3 cm superior to the IMF forming an arc.

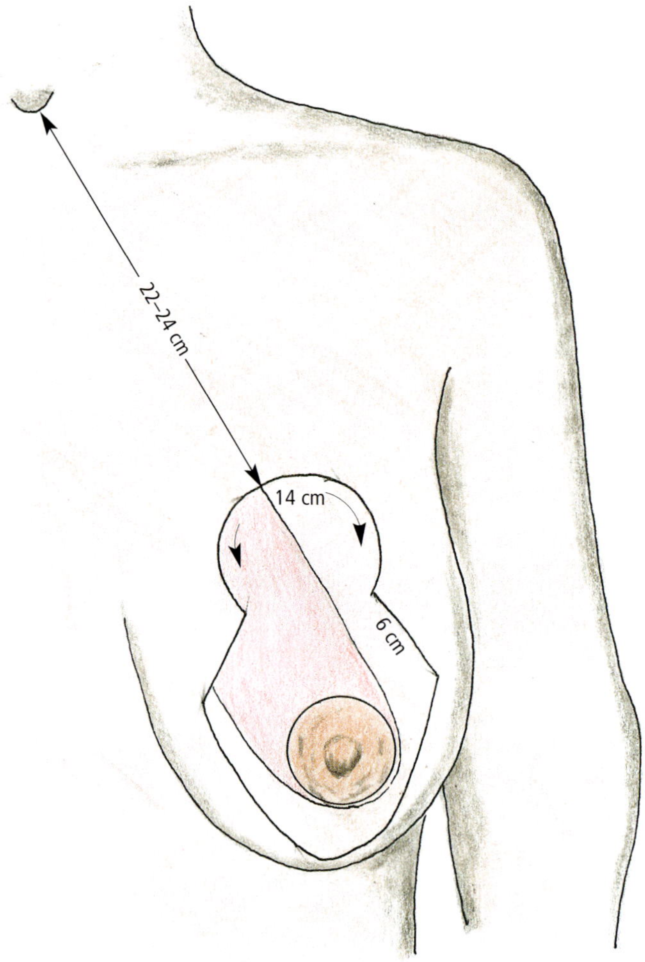

Figure 4.104 Vertical reduction (Lassus technique) – Modification. The areola does not have a large cranial pedicle but rather a medio-cranial. Thus the de-epithelialized flap displays an improved mobility. The areola is brought into its final position with less tension and kinking.

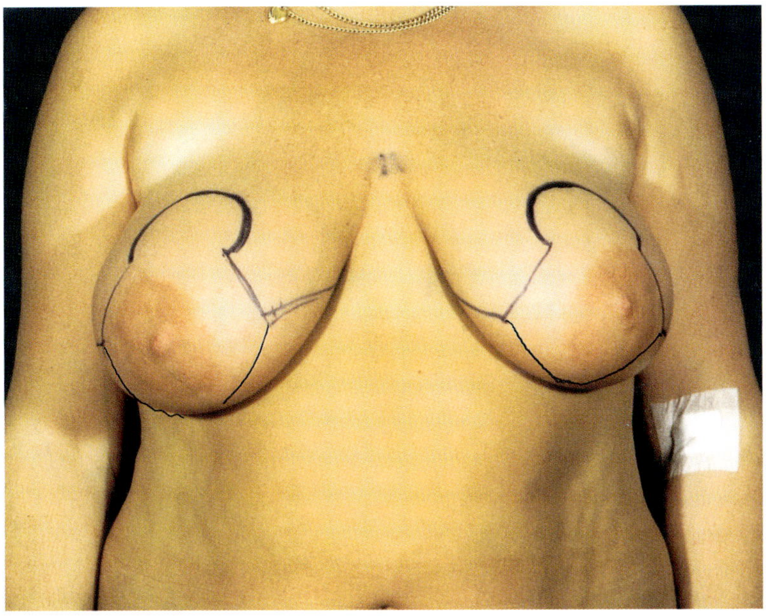

Figure 4.105a Asymmetric breast hypertrophy. Operative plan: For comparison only, markings according to standard reduction were conducted first with subsequent modification according to the vertical reduction technique (Lassus).

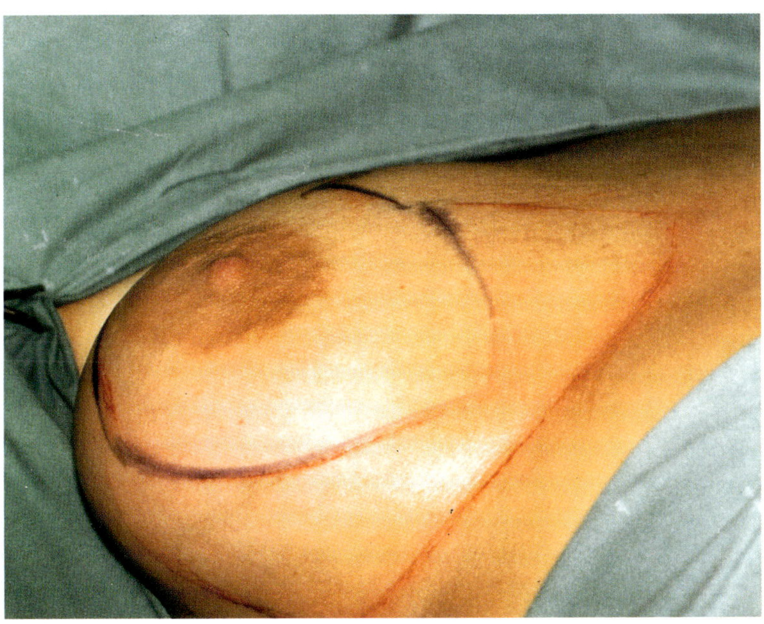

Figure 4.105b Note the clearly reduced length of the planned incisions. The vertical method results in considerably shorter scars.

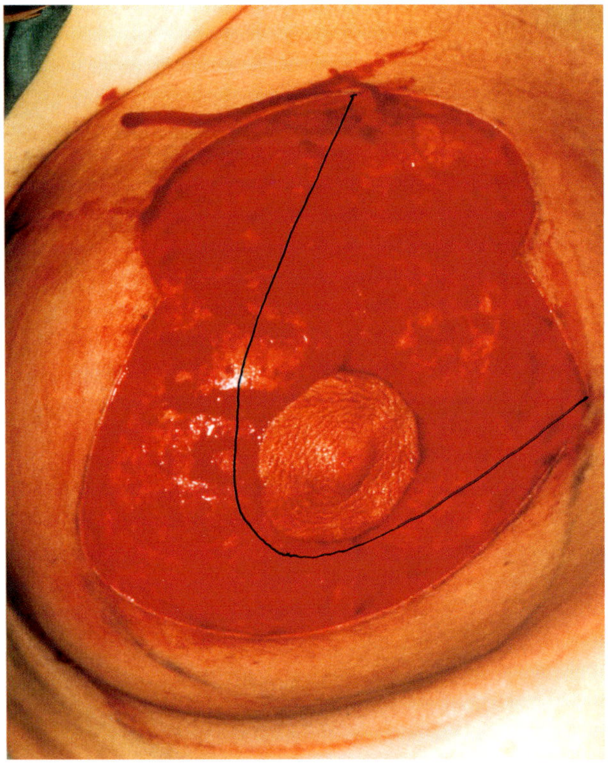

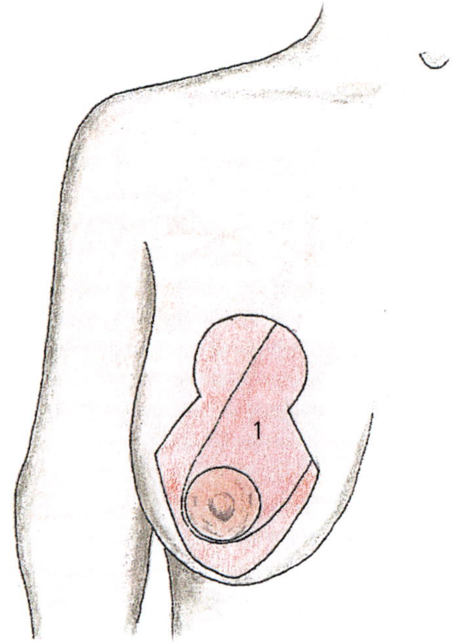

Figure 4.105c, d Deepithelialization

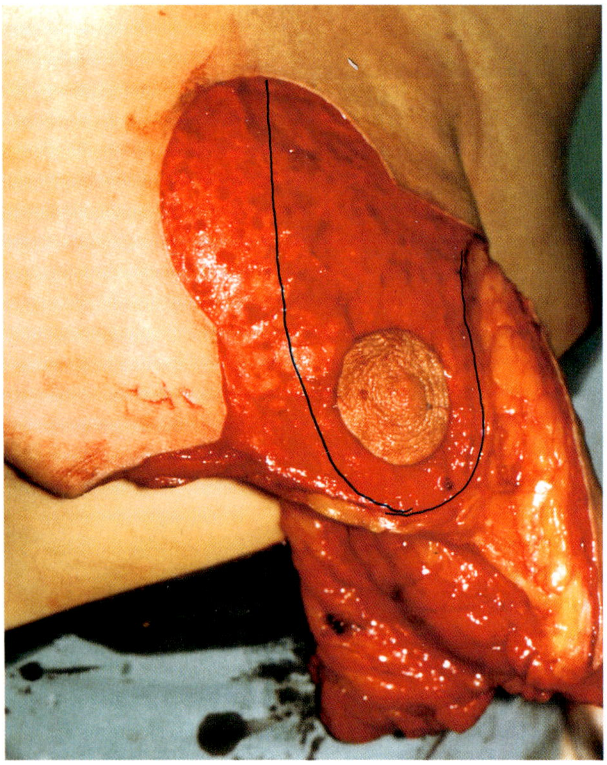

Figure 4.105e Excessive breast tissue is removed

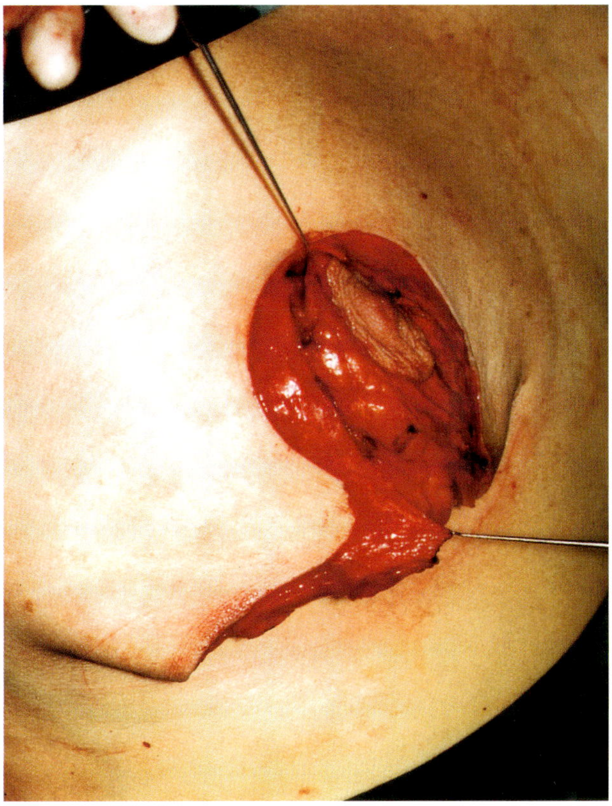

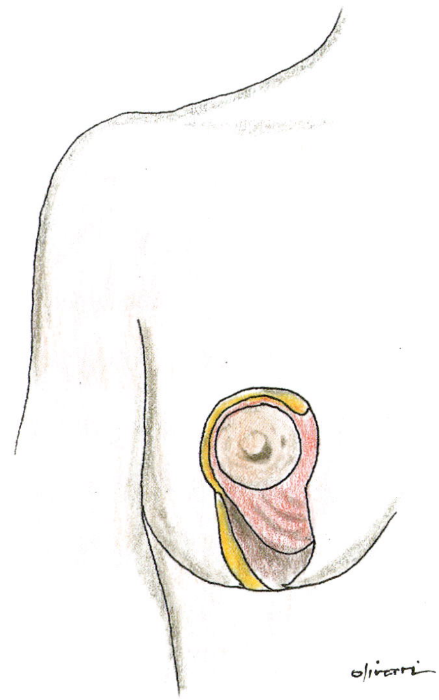

Figure 4.105f The medio-cranial pedicle allows a tension-free transfer of the areola into its final position; much easier than with a cranial pedicle.

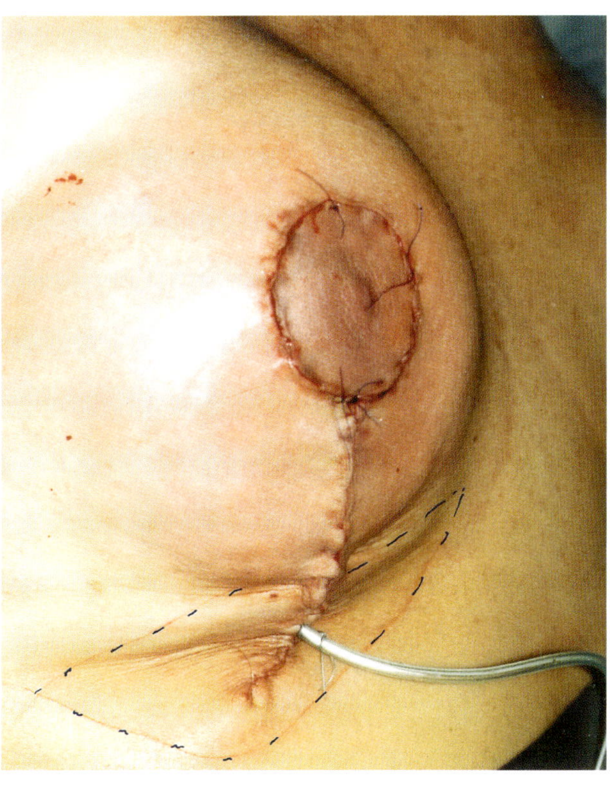

Figure 4.105g At the end of surgery. The dotted lines illustrate the additional incisions which would be done in standard breast reduction.

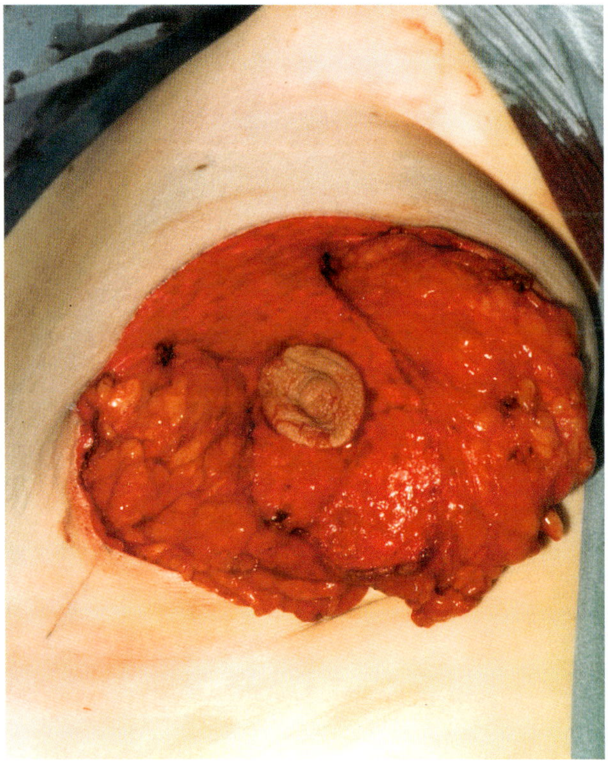

Figure 4.106a Appearance after resection

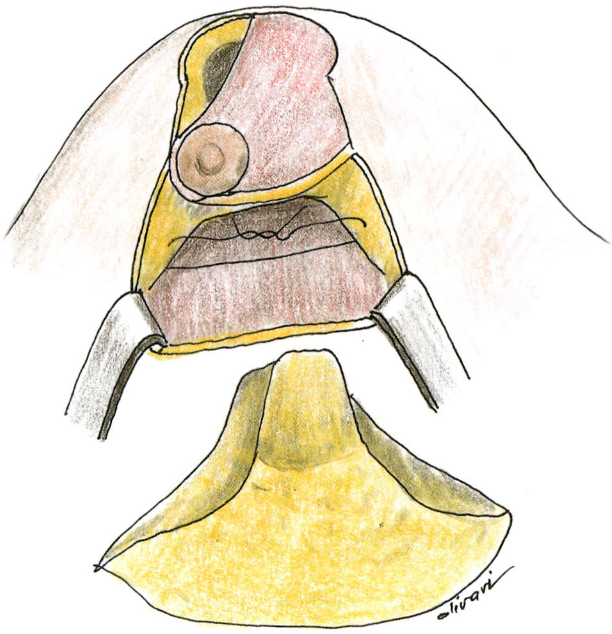

Figure 4.106b The excessive portion of the glandular breast has been removed and a medio-cranial NAC pedicle designed. The remaining glandular tissue is sutured together and fixed to the pectoral fascia.

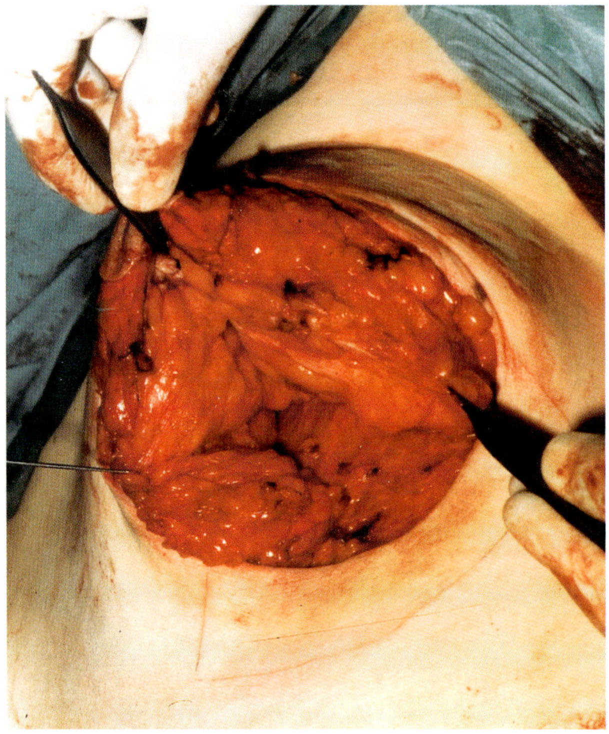

Figure 4.106c Plication of the remaining glandular breast tissue to the pectoral fascia

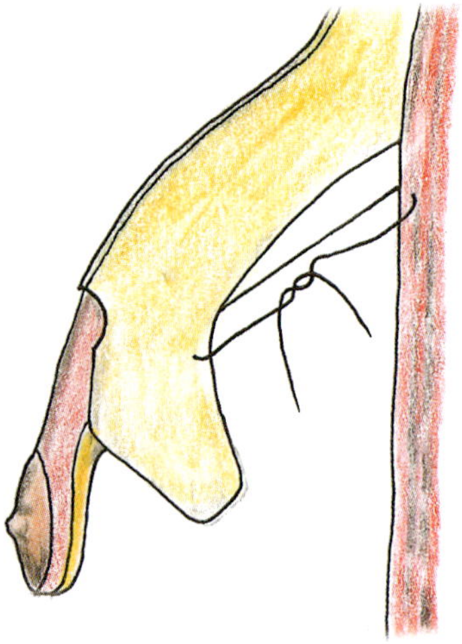

Figure 4.106d The remaining breast is fixated cranially to the pectoralis fascia with several stitches. Caudally, the remaining pillars of breast tissue are sutured to each other in order to create a nice breast mound.

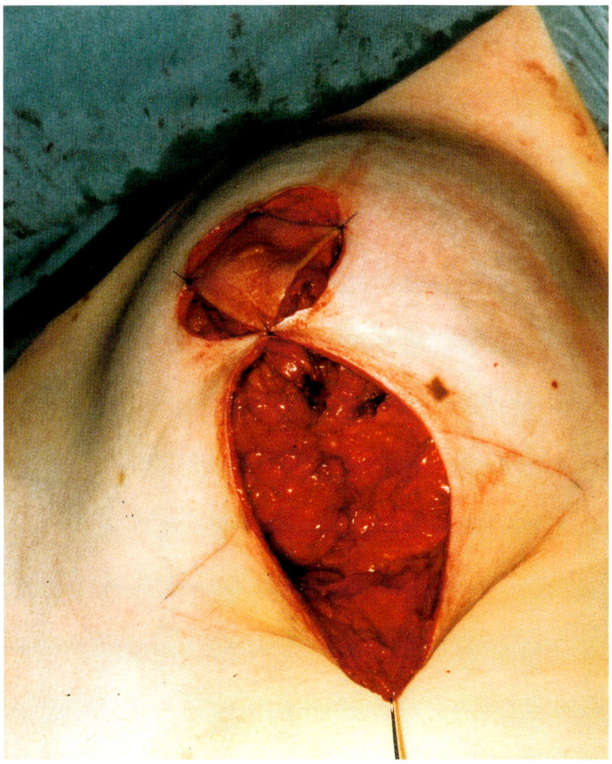

Figure 4.106e Compare: The marking displays the course of incisions in standard reduction. If at the end of surgery excessive wrinkling is observed in IMF one can immediately correct it by a short transverse incision.

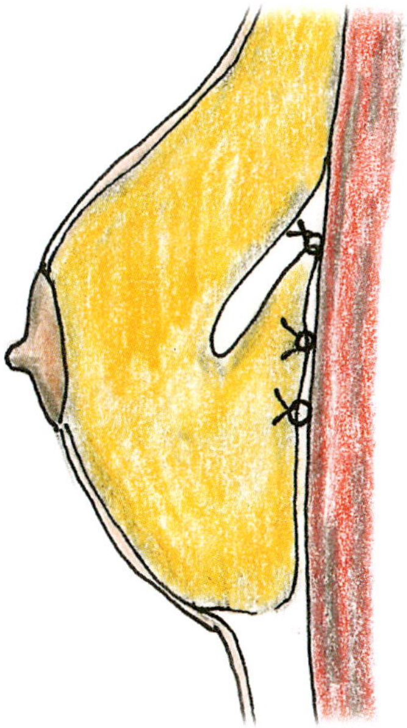

Figure 4.106f Fixation of the remaining breast to the pectoral fascia

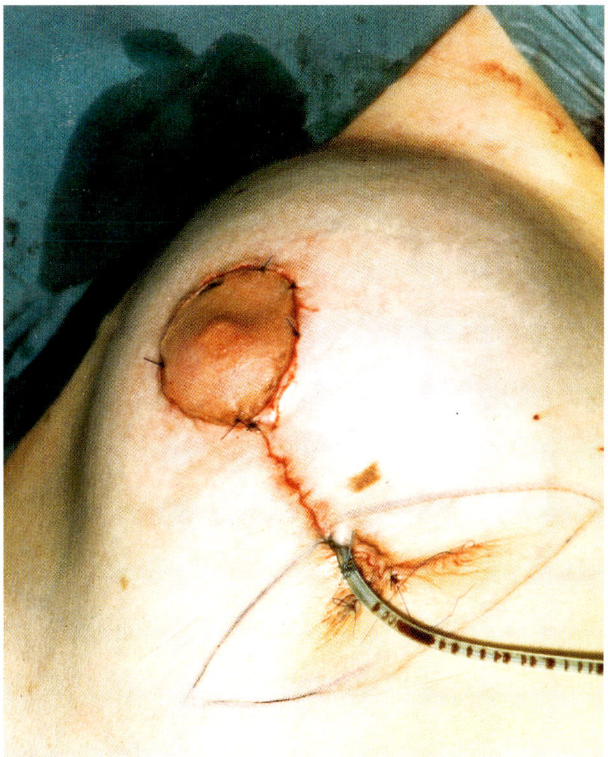

Figure 4.106g At the end of surgery: A short horizontal incision is barely visible and especially indicated if persistent wrinkling over the period of many months is suspected. The marking illustrates a horizontal incision which would be made in standard breast reduction.

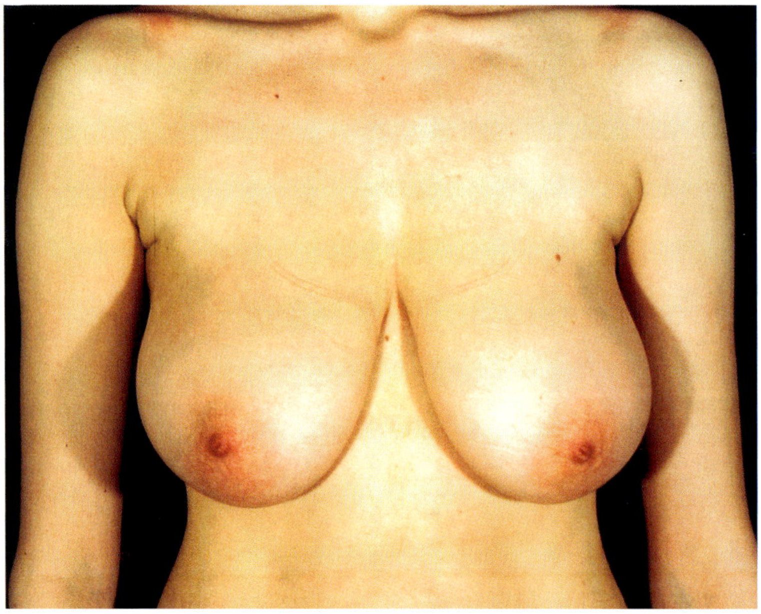

Figure 4.107a Breast hypertrophy. Vertical reduction: 750 g was resected from each breast.

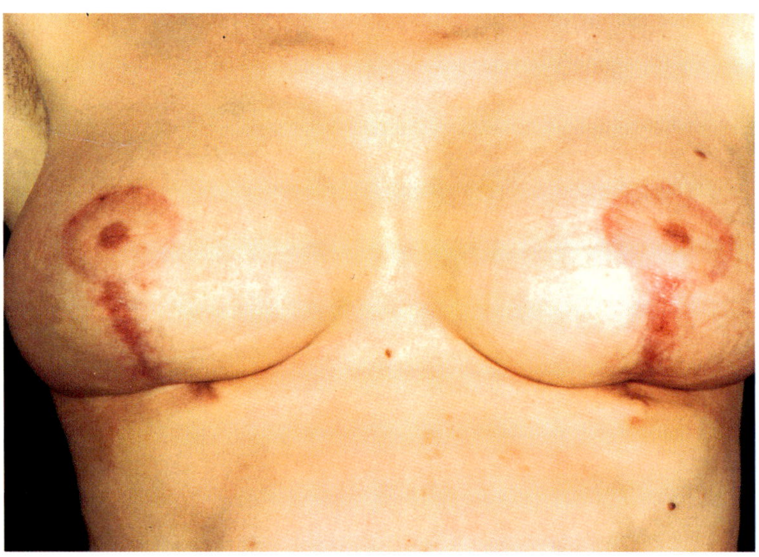

Figure 4.107b Status post breast reduction with the Lassus technique. Six weeks postoperatively scars as well as small skin folds in the inframammary region are still striking. This occurs commonly in the vertical technique and we warn the patient preoperatively regarding this.

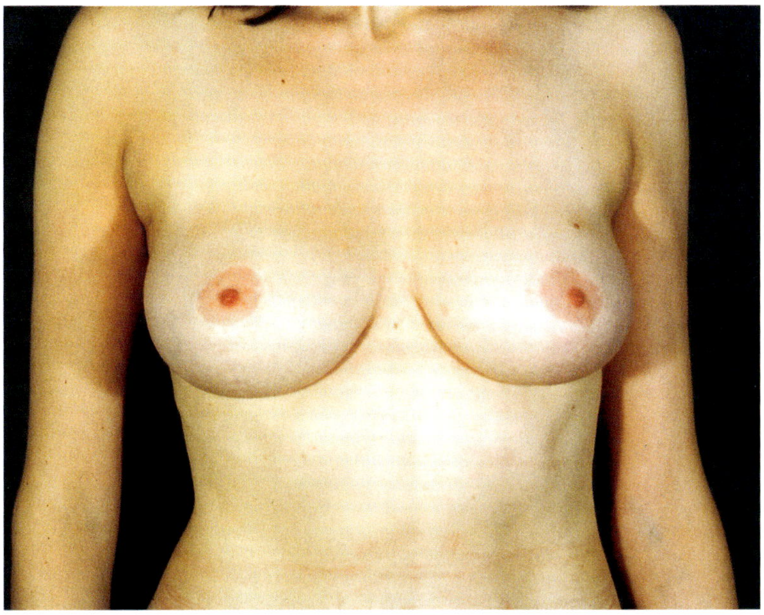

Figure 4.107c Two-and-a-half years postoperatively. Scars are barely visible. The breast has a very good shape.

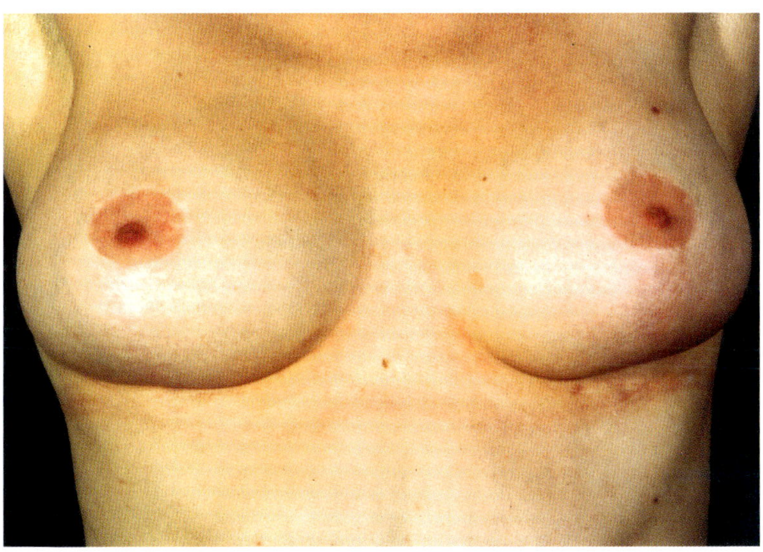

Figure 4.107d The IMF scar is well hidden

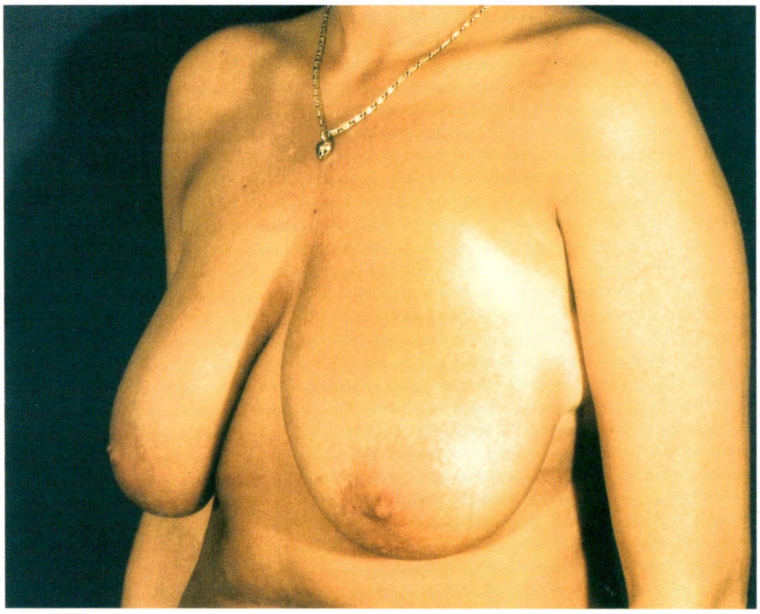

Figure 4.108a Breast hypertrophy and ptosis. A vertical breast reduction was performed with removal of 970 g from each breast.

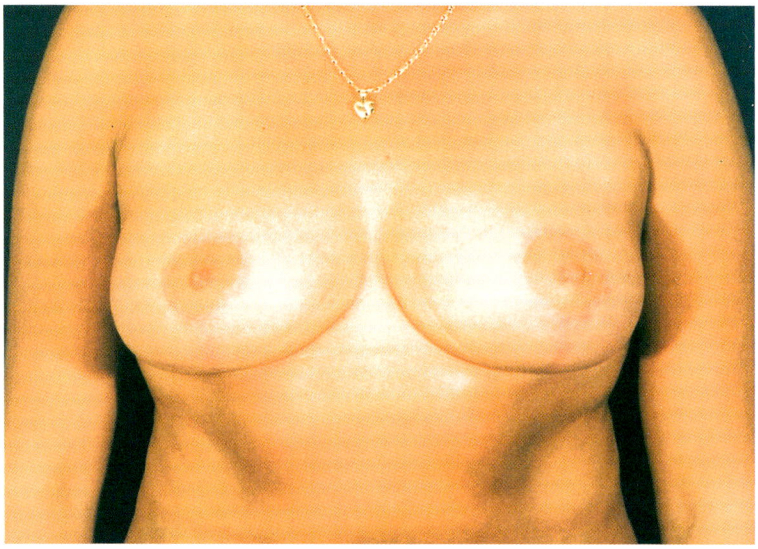

Figure 4.108b Six months postoperatively

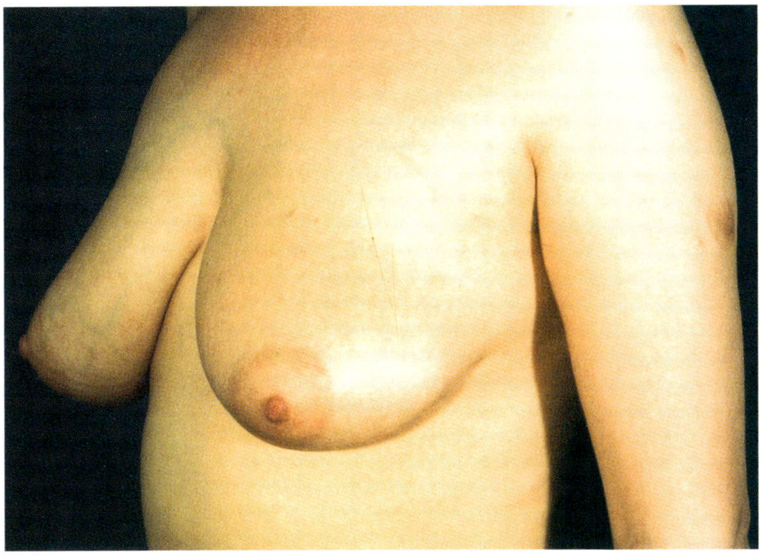

Figure 4.109a Breast hypertrophy with ptosis

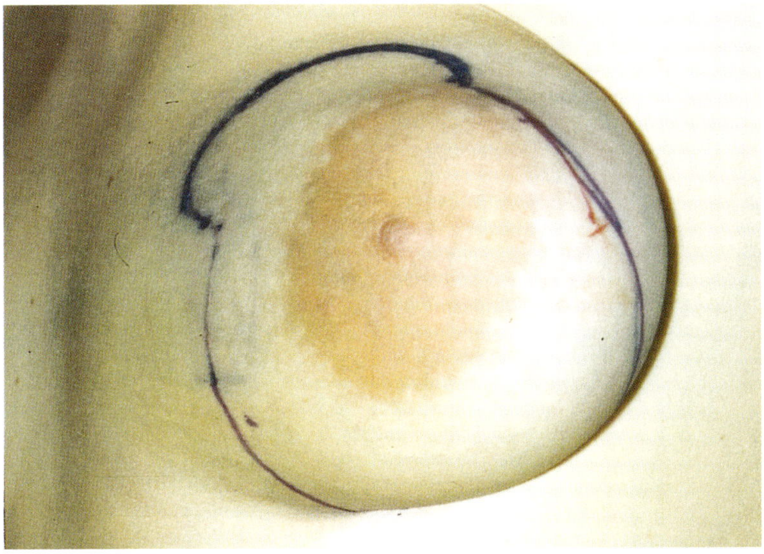

Figure 4.109b Typical preoperative marking with the patient in standing position. The upper part of the drawing is identical to the classic marking in standard reduction according to Strömbeck.

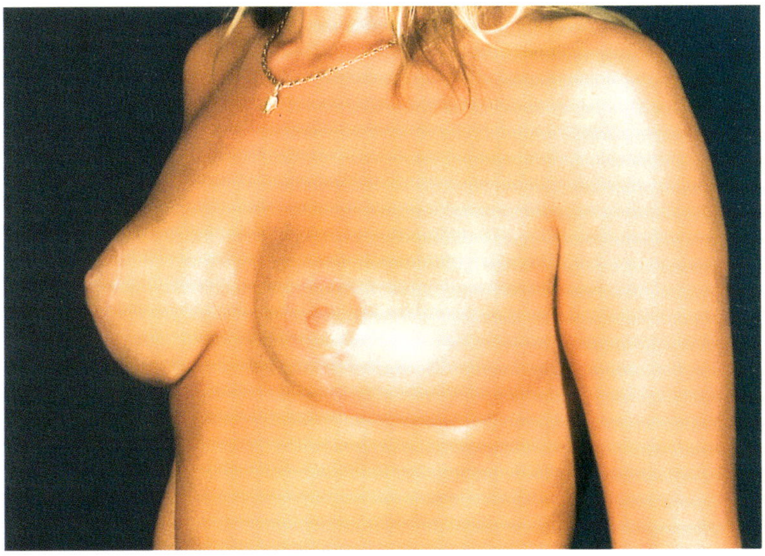

Figure 4.109c Two years postoperatively

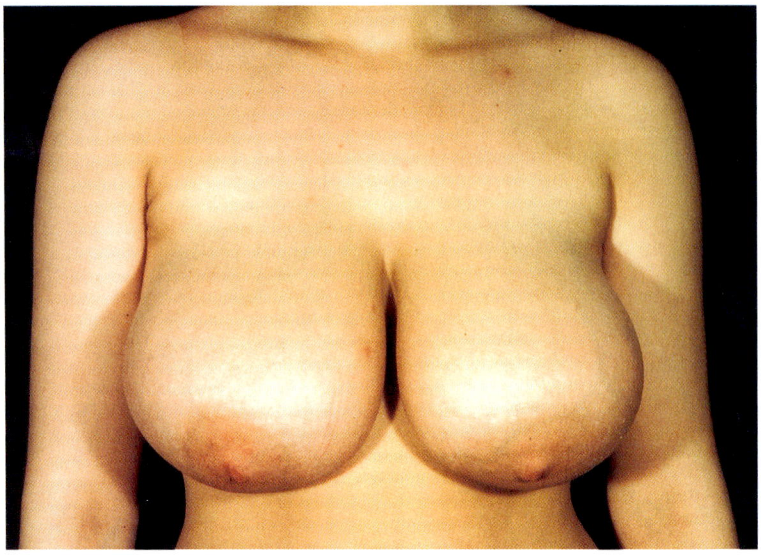

Figure 4.110a Juvenile macromastia. Preoperatively young patients must be clearly informed that ability to nurse a child postoperatively is almost never possible (Strömbeck 50 %)

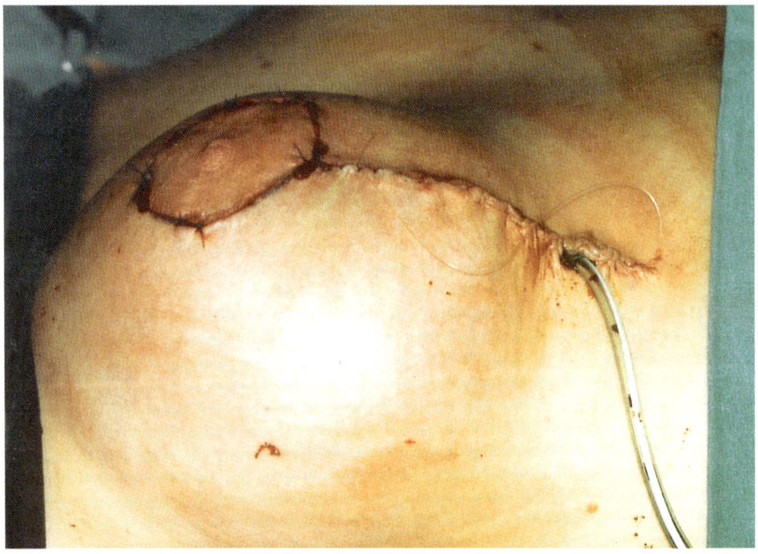

Figure 4.110b 1250 g were removed from each breast.

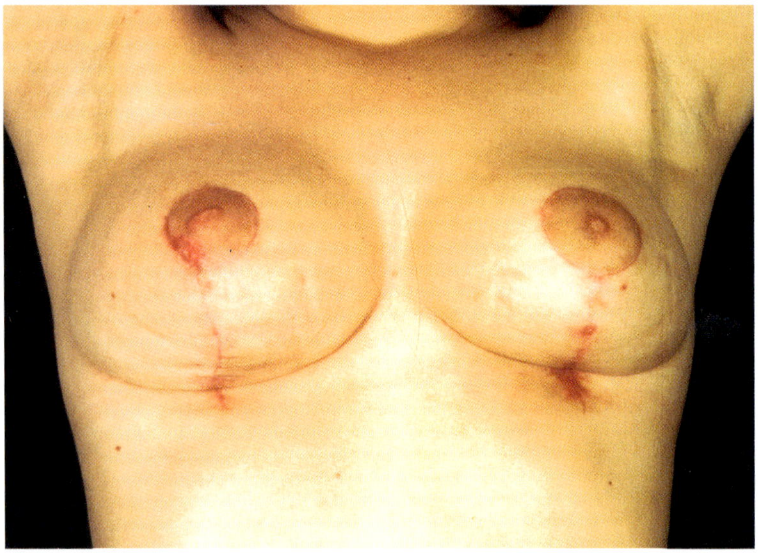

Figure 4.110c Four weeks postoperatively

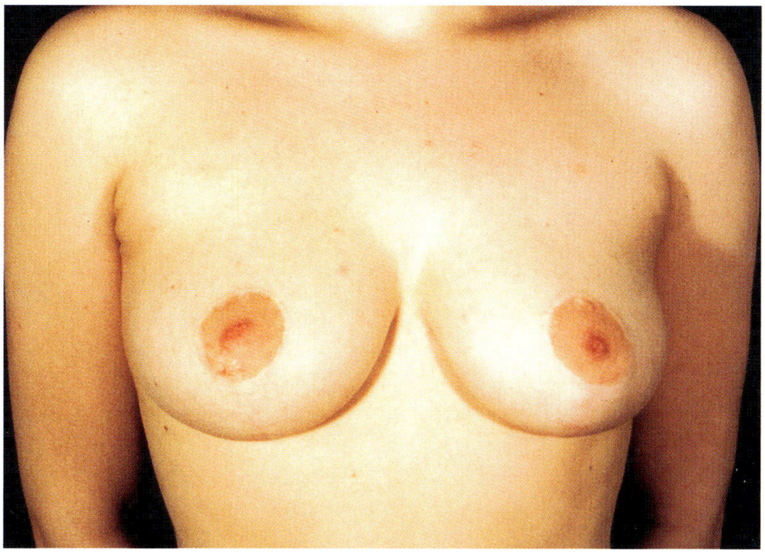

Figure 4.110d Two years postoperatively

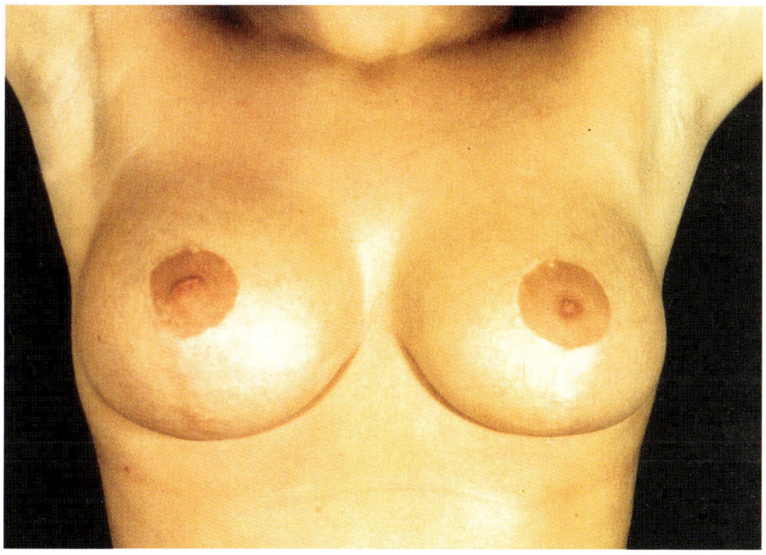

Figure 4.110e Two years postoperatively

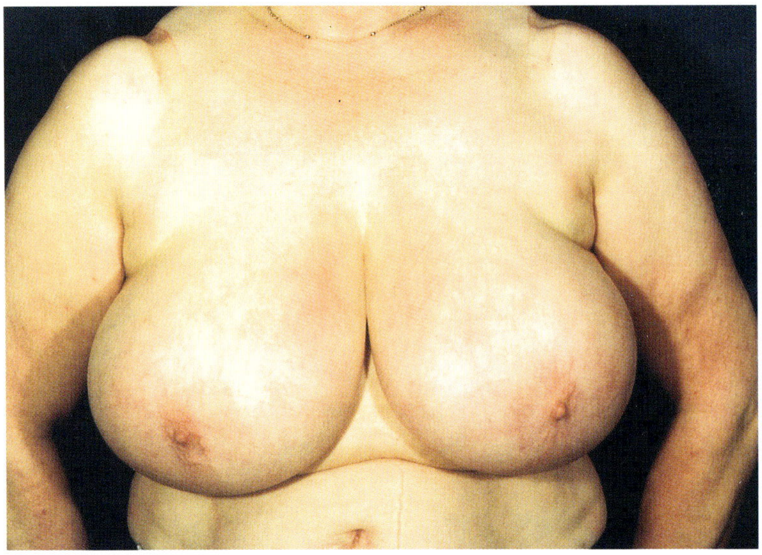

Figure 4.111a Macromastia in an obese patient

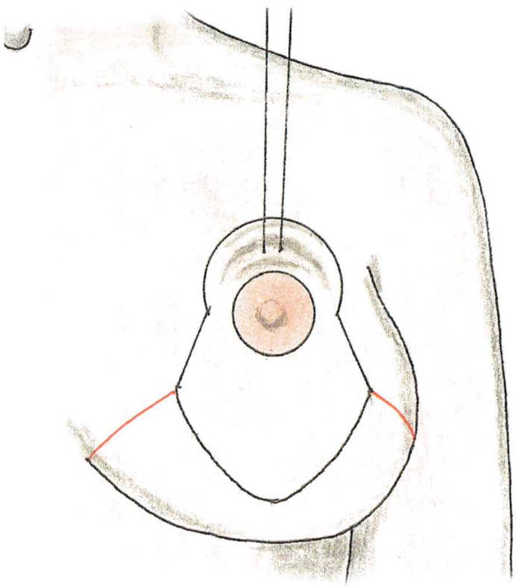

Figure 4.111b Preoperative surgical plan.
Marking: black – vertical technique;
red – standard technique. Just to see difference.

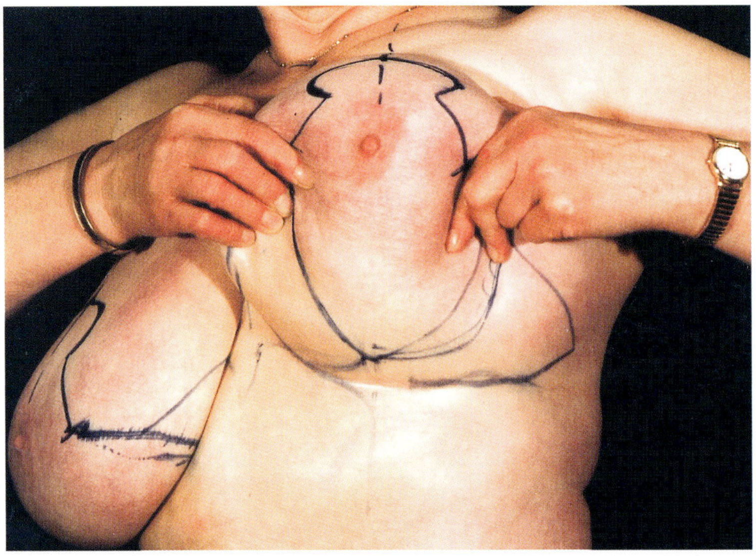

Figure 4.111c For comparison and delineation of existing differences markings are made for standard and vertical breast reduction.
1) The upper part displays identical markings.
2) Significant differences are noted in the lower part.
3) A vertical reduction was performed.

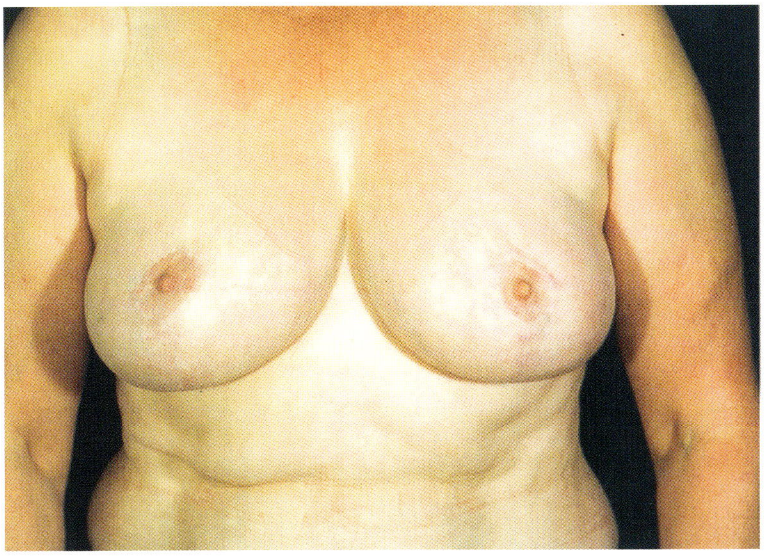

Figure 4.111d Two years postoperatively. 2100 g were removed from each breast.

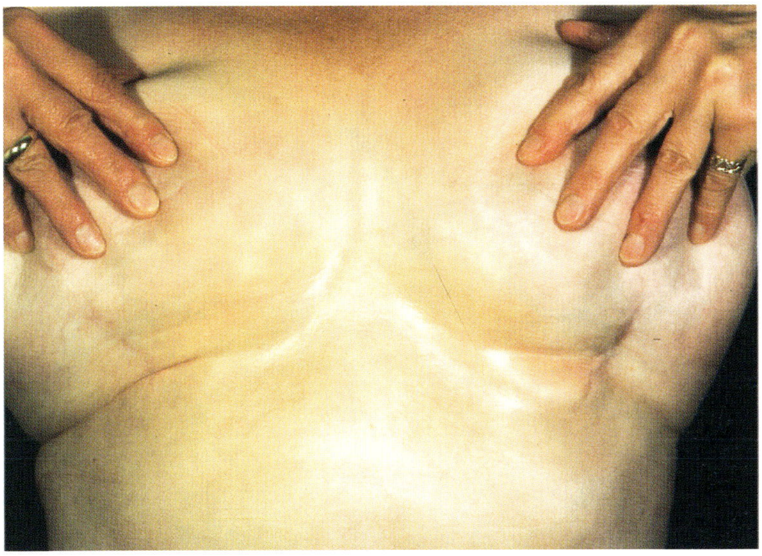

Figure 4.111e Relatively inconspicuous vertical scar two years postoperatively

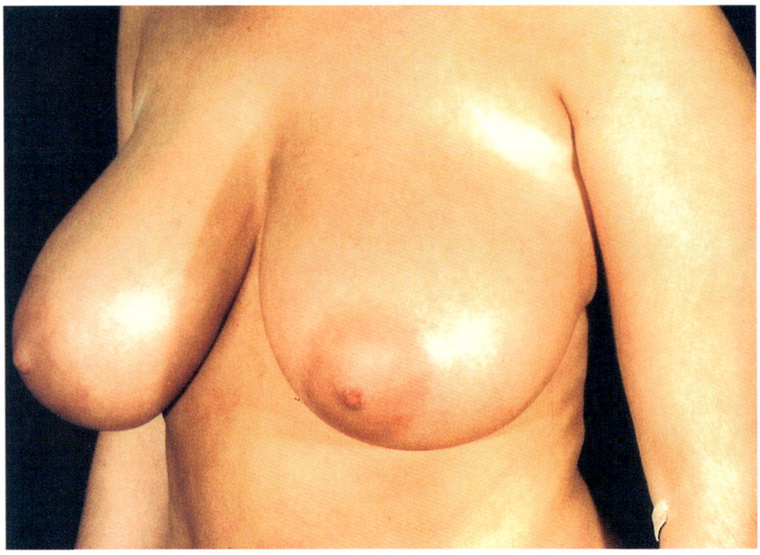

Figure 4.112a Macromastia. A vertical breast reduction (Lassus technique) was performed with removal of 1000 g per breast.

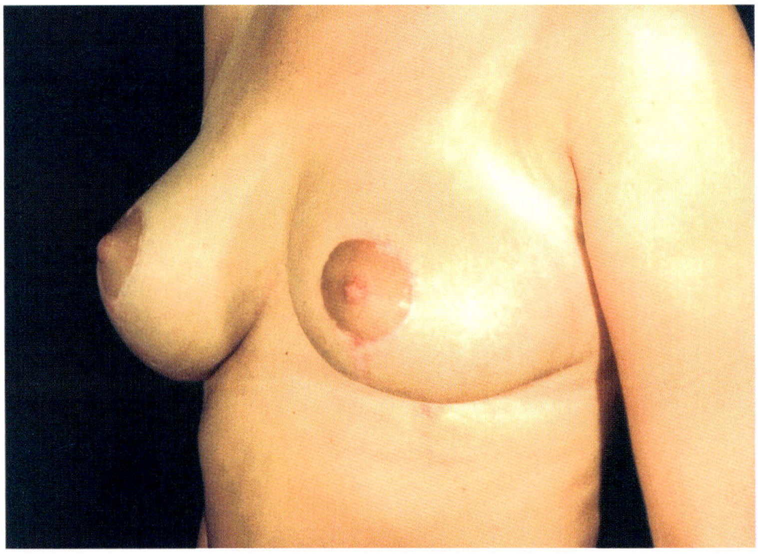

Figure 4.112b Three months postoperatively

d) Breast Ptosis and Asymmetry

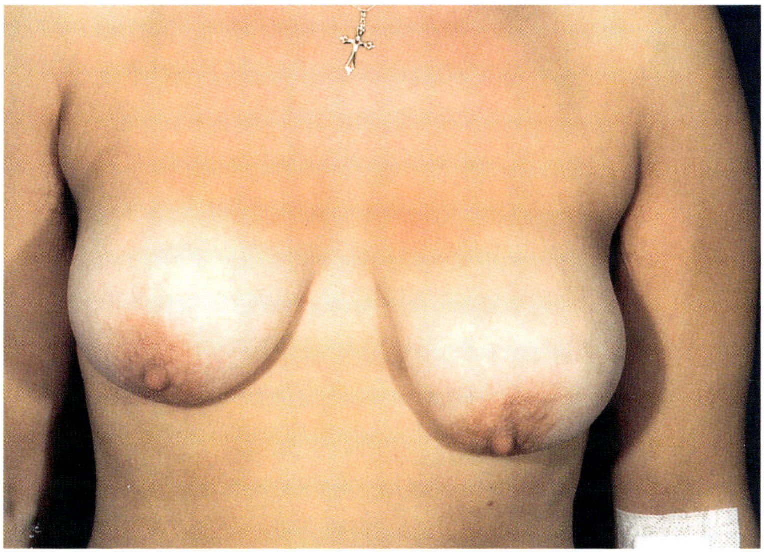

Figure 4.113a Breast asymmetry and ptosis. A vertical mastopexy was performed. 180 g were removed from the left breast with simple mastopexy of the right breast.

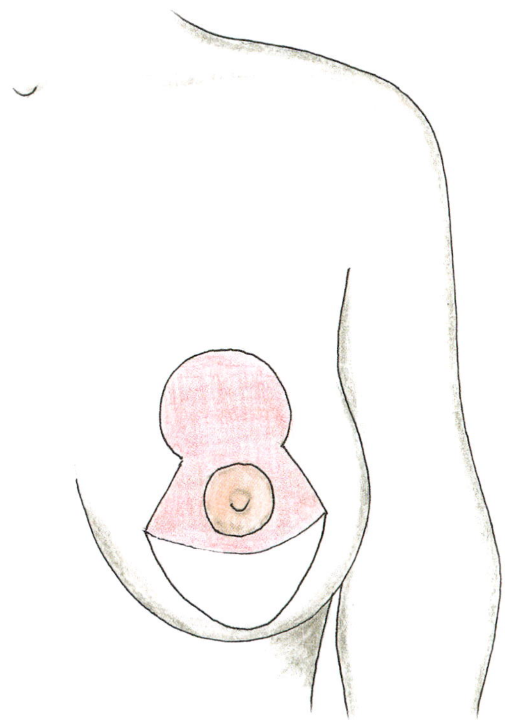

Figure 4.113b In ptotic breasts without persistent hypertrophy a cranially based areola is designed as recommended by Lassus and Lejour.

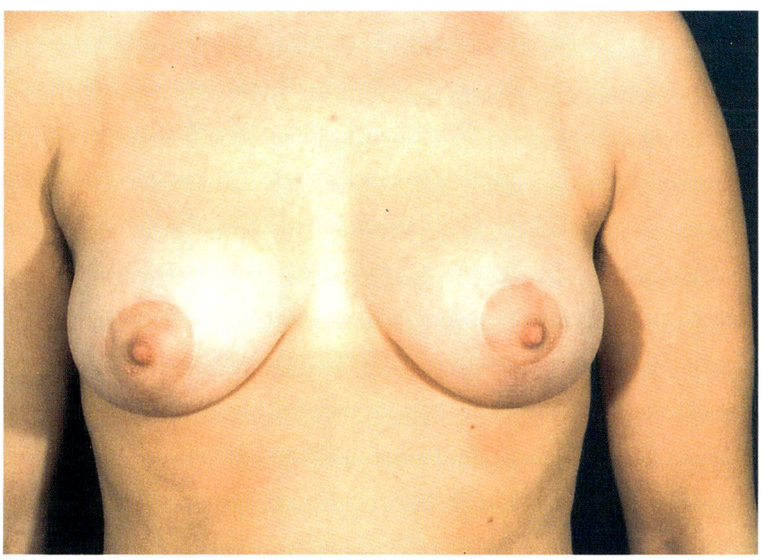

Figure 4.113c One year postoperatively

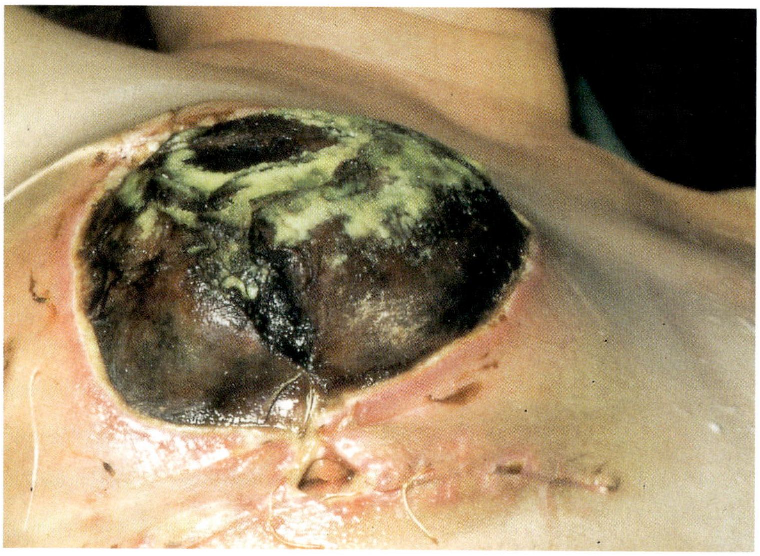

Figure 4.115a Status post reduction with extensive necrosis due to wrong operative technique. Treatment: Debridement and adaptation of remaining tissues in order to allow subsequent reconstruction.

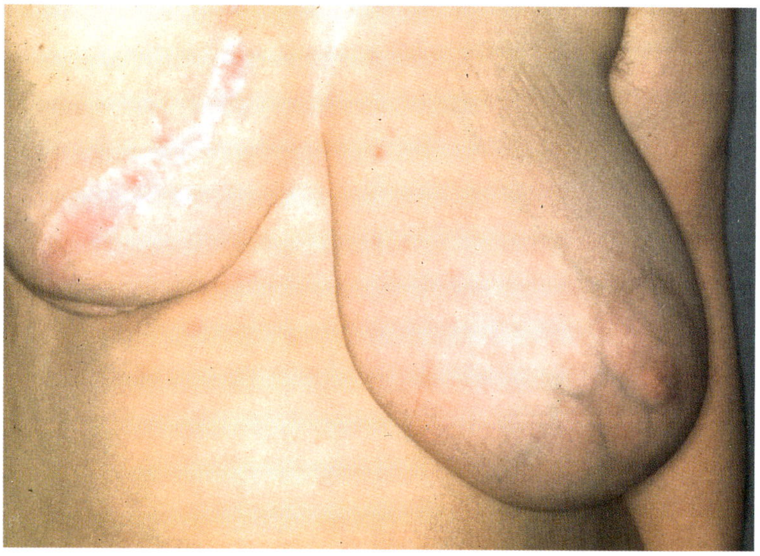

Figure 4.115b Four months later. No signs of infection. Hypertrophic scar. Treatment: Further improvement of breast shape, NAC reconstruction and left-sided breast reduction.

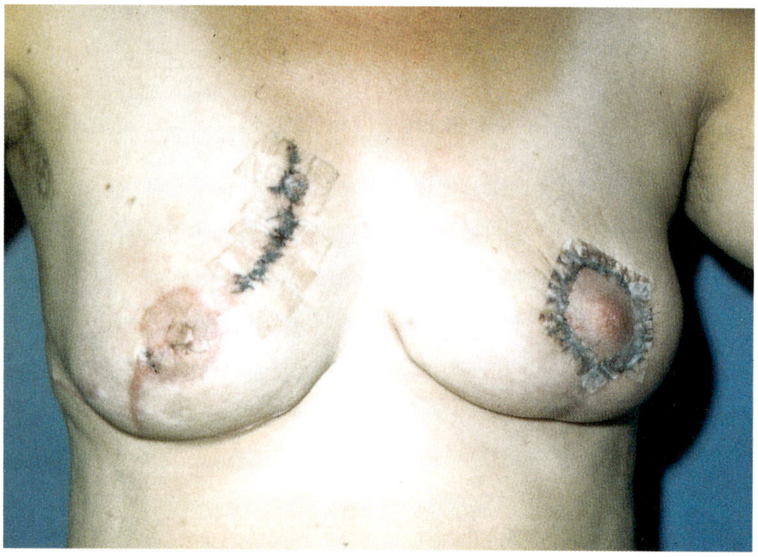

Figure 4.115c 1300 g were removed from the left breast. Areola reconstruction was performed using tissue from the periphery of very large areola of the left breast. Scar revision of the right breast.

Breast Reduction – Statistics

3346 breast reductions were performed in 1738 patients from 1982 to 1998.

Table 4.18 Frequency of standard vs. vertical reduction

Year	Standard reduction	Vertical reduction
1988	83 %	17 %
1998	27 %	73 %

Table 4.19 Volume removed

Technique	Mean weight
Standard reduction	760 g
Vertical reduction	440 g

In 78 % of all patients less than 1000 g was removed; more than 1000 g was resected in the remaining 22 %.

Table 4.20 Complications

Complications	Standard reduction	Vertical reduction
Hematoma	1.2 %	1.5 %
Infection	1.2 %	1.4 %
Fat necrosis	2.3 %	3.1 %
Partial areolar necrosis	0.9 %	1.5 %
Secondary healing	2.3 %	1.3 %

Table 4.21 Secondary surgery

Procedure	%
Dog ear excision	4.0 %
Scar revision	2.9 %
Necrectomy (fat)	2.1 %
Augmentation	0.5 %
NAC-correction	2.0 %

The development of breast reduction demonstrates the increasing frequency of the use of the vertical technique. It displays a slightly higher rate of complication, however, which may be reduced with increasing experience. The rate of secondary corrections around point G is reported in literature to be as high as 25 %. In our patients was 4 %.
Nonetheless, in special patients (gigantomastia, etc.) standard breast reduction (Strömbeck modification) remains the gold standard.

Patients

Seventy-two patients were operated on from 1983 to 1994 using the method described above (40 bilateral, 32 unilateral). Mean age was 34 years. In 1997 44 patients (76 nipples) presented for follow-up.

Results

1) In none of the nipples examined was a recurrence of inversion noted. All nipples had remained in their correct position.
2) Scars were not visible except in those nipples which had been treated by other techniques previously.
3) Surprisingly, four patients reported that they had been able to nurse. It is difficult to comment on this phenomenon. It could be assumed that a spontaneous re-approximation of the milk ducts had occurred in these patients. However, this is only an assumption.
   All patients had been informed that nursing would not be possible postoperatively.
4) After a mean follow-up of 23 months
   - 41 patients were very satisfied with nipple size and shape
   - 2 patients complained of nipples too small
   - 1 patient complained of a nipple too large

Conclusion

An inverted nipple causes functional and aesthetic problems.

Surgical techniques suggested for correction of this deformity as well as preservation of nursing ability are afflicted with a high rate of recurrence, unpleasing shape of the NAC as well as visible scars.

The technique presented in which all milk ducts, as well as fibrous bands reaching from the nipple to the deeper layers are transected, is characterized by:

- a simple surgical procedure performed under local anesthesia
- lack of scar visibility
- no recurrence of nipple inversion
- loss of nursing ability postoperatively; however, four patients reported on being able to nurse postoperatively
- nipple sensitivity returned to normal levels at three months postoperatively

Breast Reduction – Statistics

3346 breast reductions were performed in 1738 patients from 1982 to 1998.

Table 4.18 Frequency of standard vs. vertical reduction

Year	Standard reduction	Vertical reduction
1988	83 %	17 %
1998	27 %	73 %

Table 4.19 Volume removed

Technique	Mean weight
Standard reduction	760 g
Vertical reduction	440 g

In 78 % of all patients less than 1000 g was removed; more than 1000 g was resected in the remaining 22 %.

Table 4.20 Complications

Complications	Standard reduction	Vertical reduction
Hematoma	1.2 %	1.5 %
Infection	1.2 %	1.4 %
Fat necrosis	2.3 %	3.1 %
Partial areolar necrosis	0.9 %	1.5 %
Secondary healing	2.3 %	1.3 %

Table 4.21 Secondary surgery

Procedure	%
Dog ear excision	4.0 %
Scar revision	2.9 %
Necrectomy (fat)	2.1 %
Augmentation	0.5 %
NAC-correction	2.0 %

The development of breast reduction demonstrates the increasing frequency of the use of the vertical technique. It displays a slightly higher rate of complication, however, which may be reduced with increasing experience. The rate of secondary corrections around point G is reported in literature to be as high as 25 %. In our patients was 4 %.
Nonetheless, in special patients (gigantomastia, etc.) standard breast reduction (Strömbeck modification) remains the gold standard.

Inverted Nipple (Olivari Technique)

Inverted nipple is a congenital malformation. Instead of a normal nipple a more or less pronounced dimple may be observed. This inverted region is surrounded by contractile tissue reaching to the areola margin. The cylinder of musculo-fibrocollagenous elements which forms the nipple is thinner than normal. Fibrous bands cause its deep fixation in the glandular tissue [Schwager 1974].

Glandular ducts are short and underdeveloped [Broadbent, Woolf 1976]. The hereditary origin of this, either unilateral or bilateral, occurring malformation is evident [Skoog 1952]. Women with very large and ptotic breasts are affected more often. The incidence has been reported to be 0.5 % in the female population [Schwager 1974].

Symptoms

Inverted nipples cause three major problems:

1) Nursing. The infant is not able to suckle from the inverted nipple. Rarely, it is possible to temporarily correct this condition using a pump. The infant is, however, not able to overcome the elastic forces on a continuing basis. Therefore, affected women are frequent not able to nurse.
2) Infection. Adequate hygiene is not always possible due to the deep location of the milk ducts. Thus, local infections occur frequently.
3) Aesthetic problems. An inverted nipple poses a psychological burden for many females which may influence their sexual activity.

Treatment

Conservative treatment using vacuum cups over a period of six weeks is not very successful.

A great number of surgical techniques have been suggested for correction of the deformity, however, with the attempt to preserve the ability to nurse [Sellheim, Skoog and others]. Although preservation of nursing abilities was partially possible, however, aesthetic complaints remained due to excessive scar formation.

Our Approach

Surveys among affected females clearly revealed that the cosmetic aspect was much more important than the ability to nurse.

As a result, in 1983 we began to use a new method which

- does not aim to preserve nursing ability
- produces safe and pleasing aesthetic results
- is applicable to all forms of inverted nipples
- does not result in visible scar formation

Surgical Technique

1. A 3 mm incision is placed 5 mm lateral to the margin of the inverted nipple.
2. With a Gillies hook the centre of the nipple is pulled upwards.
3. All milk ducts as well as fibrous bands are transected with a scalpel and fine scissors (Aesculap BC 131). Complete transection may be tested by removing the Gillies hook. The nipple should not retract if all bands and ducts have been transected.
4. A purse-string suture is placed along the inner margin of the nipple with 4 × 0 Vicryl. However, this needs some practice. At least five to six stitches (inside) are necessary beginning at the superior margin of the incision and ending at the inferior margin. The knot is not pulled too tight and is subsequently buried.
5. Suturing the skin is not necessary. A simple dressing with antibiotic ointment (Neomycin) is used for two days.
6. The procedure is done under local anesthesia and takes 15 minutes per side.
7. This procedure is safe and applicable to all forms of inverted nipple.

Patients

Seventy-two patients were operated on from 1983 to 1994 using the method described above (40 bilateral, 32 unilateral). Mean age was 34 years. In 1997 44 patients (76 nipples) presented for follow-up.

Results

1) In none of the nipples examined was a recurrence of inversion noted. All nipples had remained in their correct position.
2) Scars were not visible except in those nipples which had been treated by other techniques previously.
3) Surprisingly, four patients reported that they had been able to nurse. It is difficult to comment on this phenomenon. It could be assumed that a spontaneous re-approximation of the milk ducts had occurred in these patients. However, this is only an assumption.
   All patients had been informed that nursing would not be possible postoperatively.
4) After a mean follow-up of 23 months
   - 41 patients were very satisfied with nipple size and shape
   - 2 patients complained of nipples too small
   - 1 patient complained of a nipple too large

Conclusion

An inverted nipple causes functional and aesthetic problems.

Surgical techniques suggested for correction of this deformity as well as preservation of nursing ability are afflicted with a high rate of recurrence, unpleasing shape of the NAC as well as visible scars.

The technique presented in which all milk ducts, as well as fibrous bands reaching from the nipple to the deeper layers are transected, is characterized by:

- a simple surgical procedure performed under local anesthesia
- lack of scar visibility
- no recurrence of nipple inversion
- loss of nursing ability postoperatively; however, four patients reported on being able to nurse postoperatively
- nipple sensitivity returned to normal levels at three months postoperatively

Inverted Nipple Olivari Technique

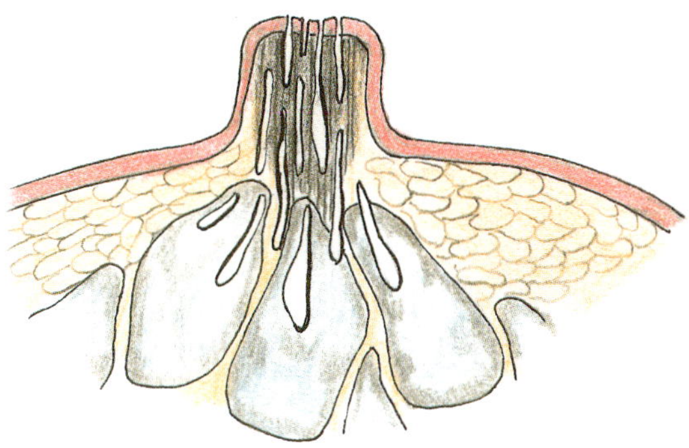

Figure 4.116a Normal nipple

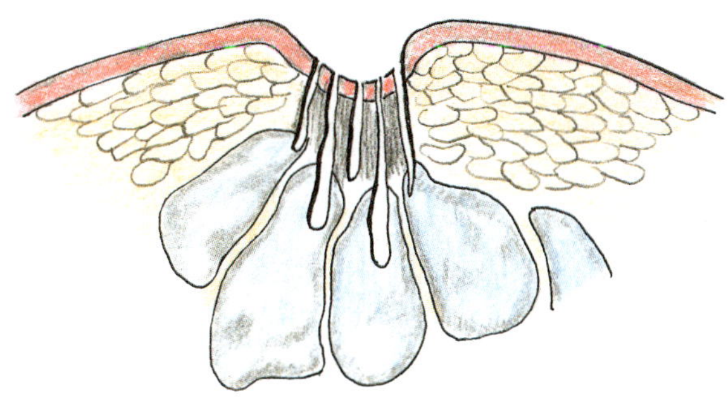

Figure 4.116b Inverted nipple

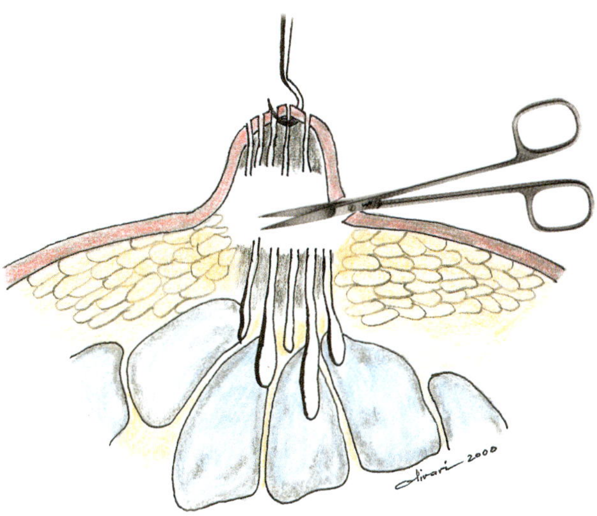

Figure 4.116b The nipple is pulled upward with a Gillies hook or with a suture. A 3 mm incision is placed along the lateral border of the nipple. Milk ducts and fibrous band are transected with scissors. When removing the hook the nipple should not revert to an inverted position. The procedure is possible under local anesthesia.

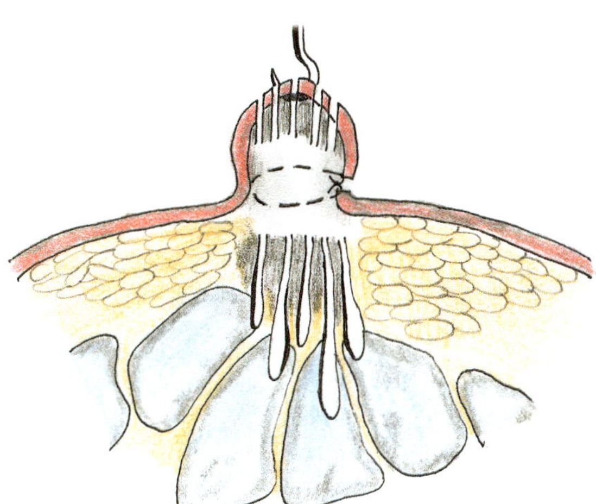

Figure 4.116c An internal "purse-string" suture with a buried knot is placed with 4×0 Vicryl with moderate tension. Suturing the skin is not necessary. Ointment dressing

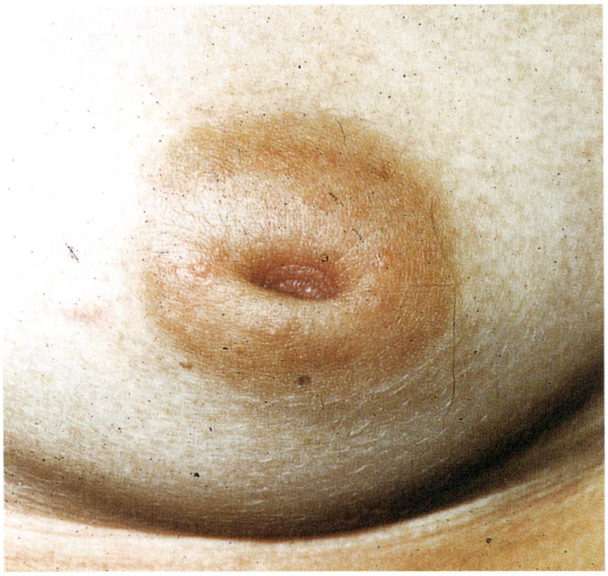

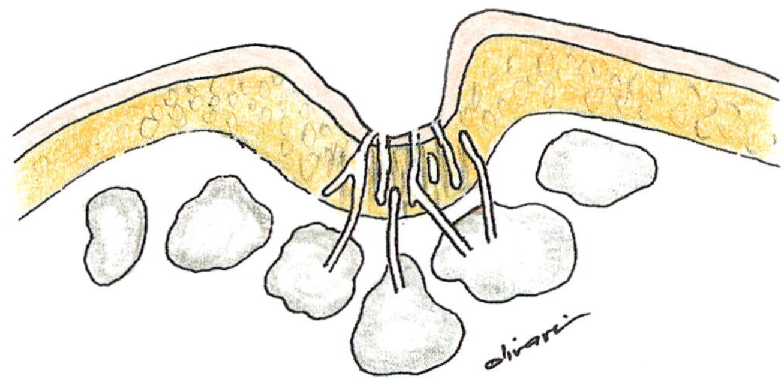

Figure 4.117a,b Typical inverted nipple

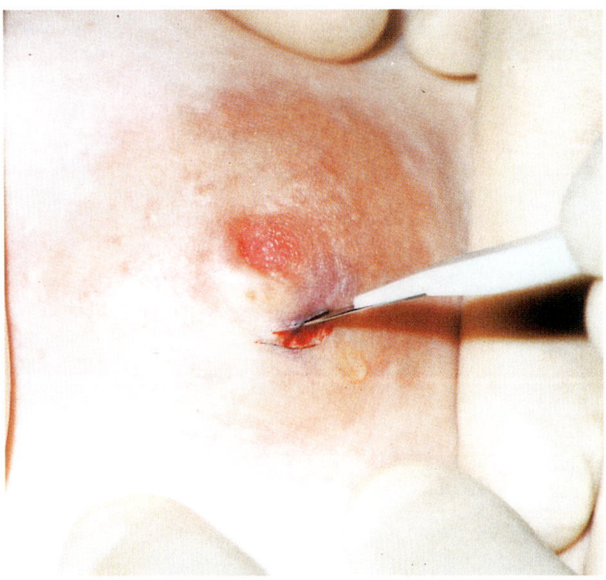

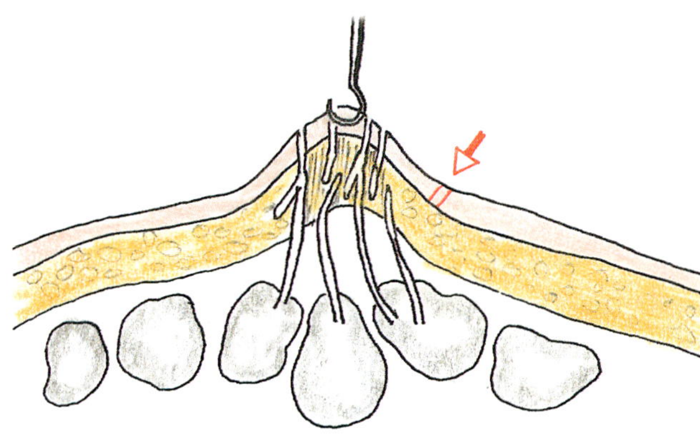

Figure 4.117c,d The incision lateral to the nipple has a length of only 3 mm.

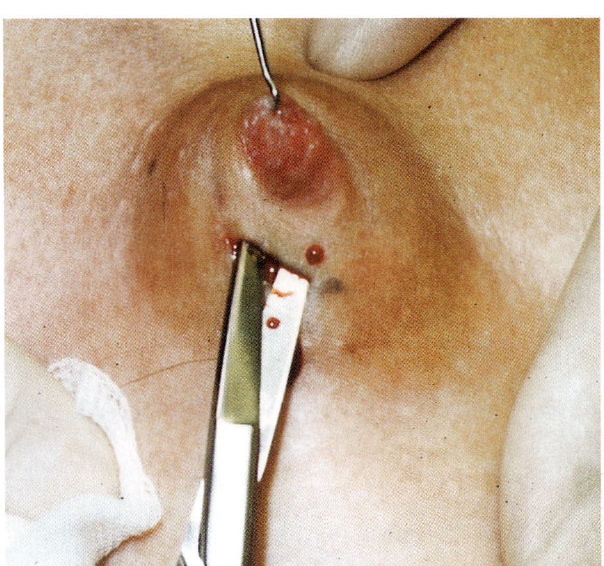

Figure 4.117e All milk ducts and fibrous bands are transected with pointed scissors.

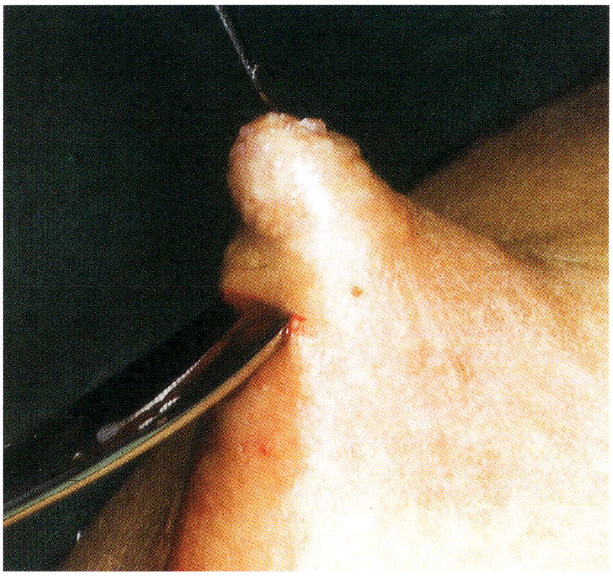

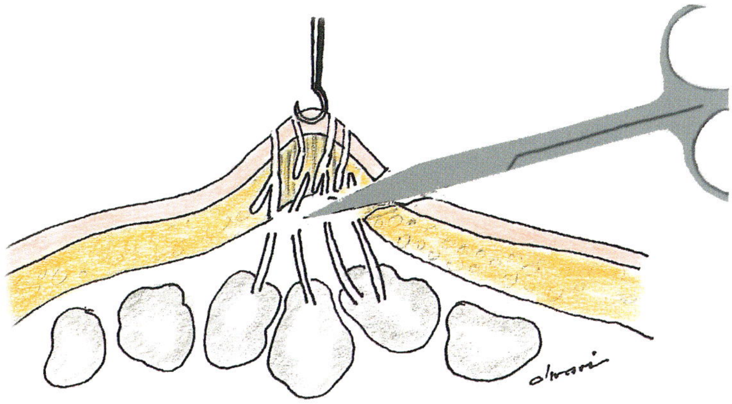

Figure 4.117f, g Following transection of milk ducts and fibrous bands the nipple takes up the right position.

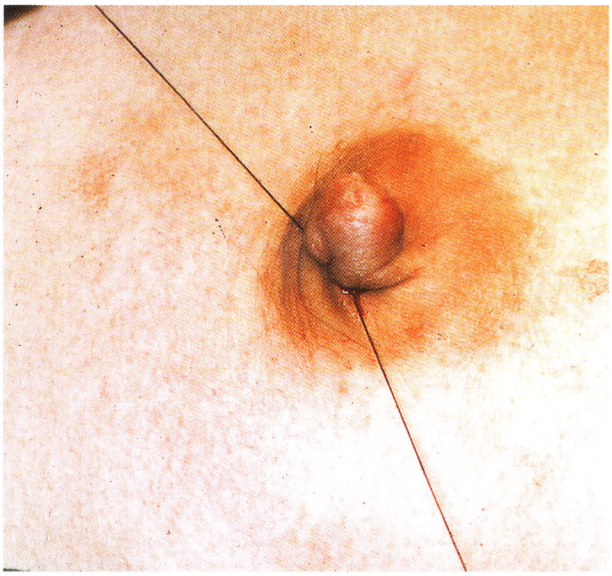

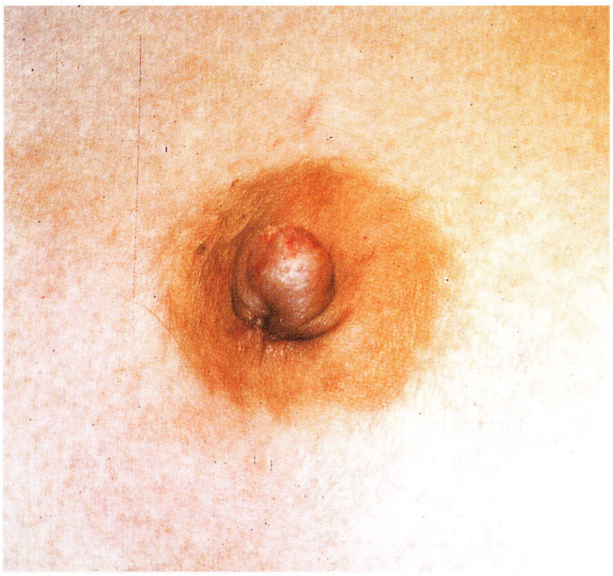

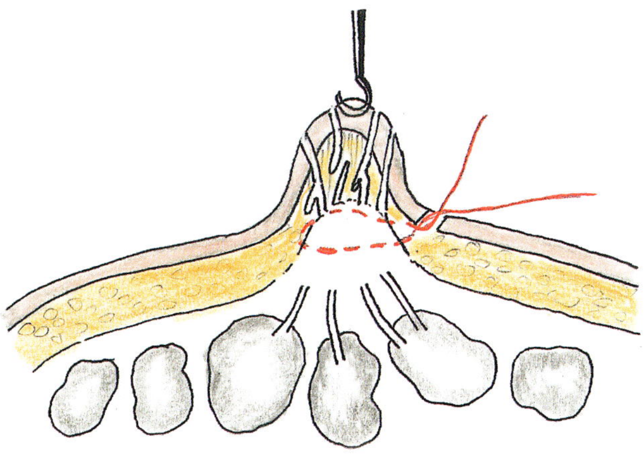

Figure 4.117h, j An internal suture with 4 × 0 Vicryl is placed. No skin closure!

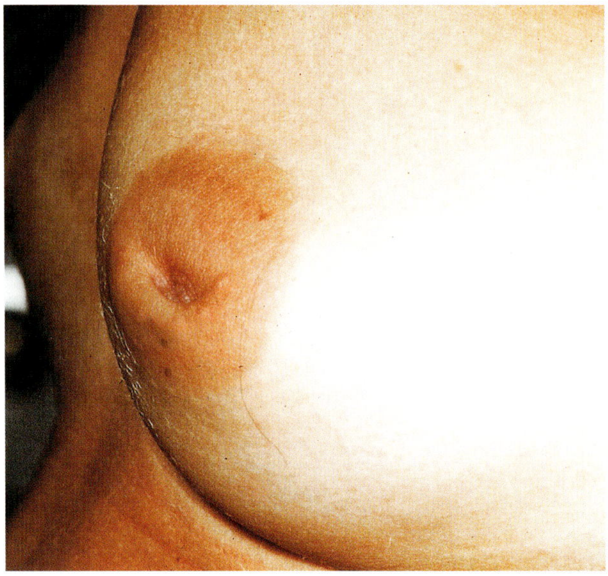

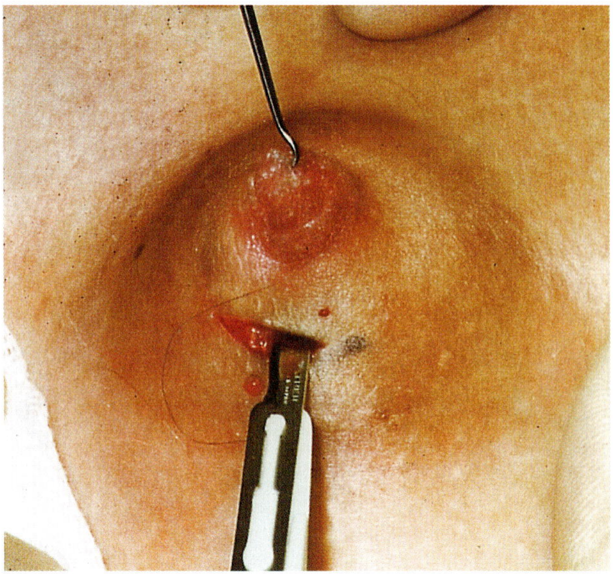

Figure 4.118a Marking the incision. An incision lateral to the nipple is made with a length of approximately 3 mm.

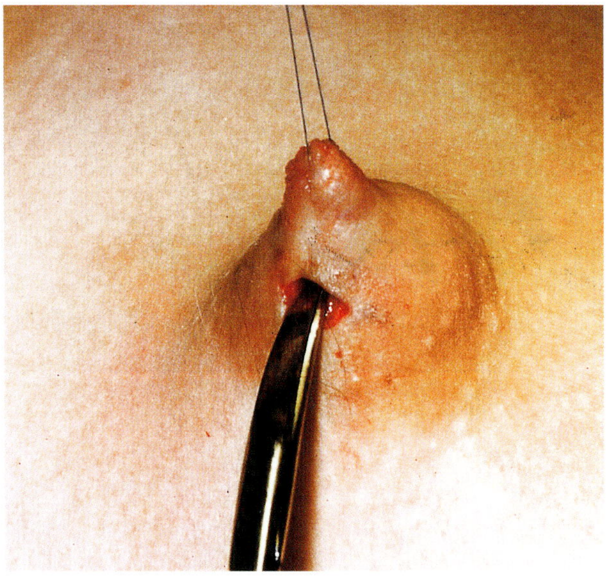

Figure 4.118b, c The nipple is pulled upward either with a Gillies hook or a stitch. All milk ducts and fibrous bands must be transected.

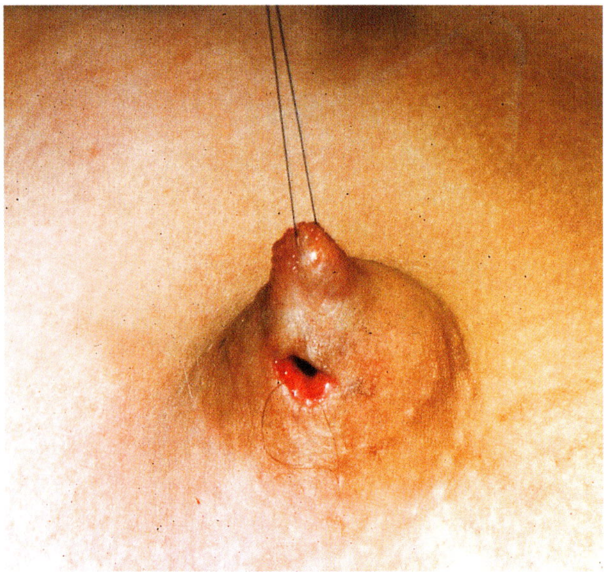

Figure 4.118d Following transection of milk ducts and fibrous bands the nipple displays no signs of retraction.

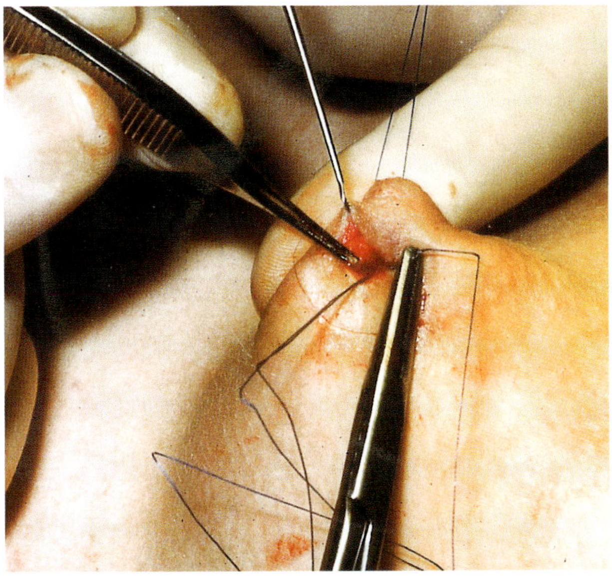

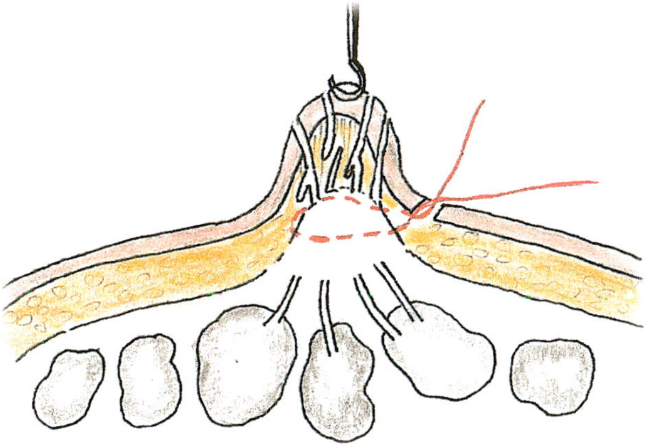

Figure 4.118e,f An internal purse-string suture is placed under moderate tension with 4 × 0 Vicryl. If a nipple is pale relieve tension.

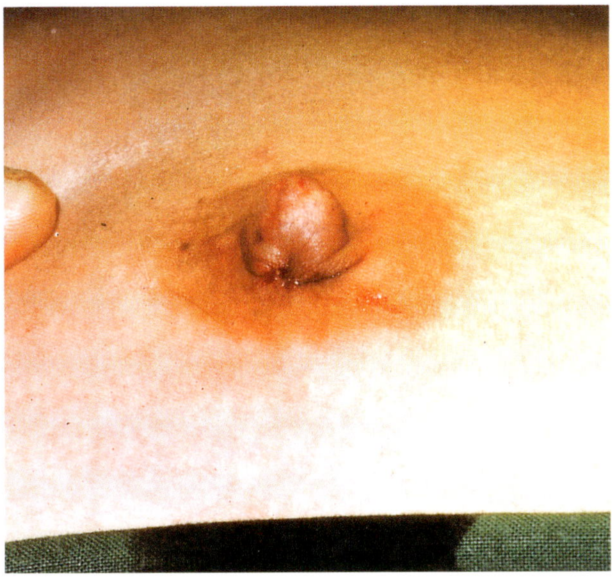

Figure 4.118g The knot is buried. Skin closure is not necessary. Ointment dressings for one week.

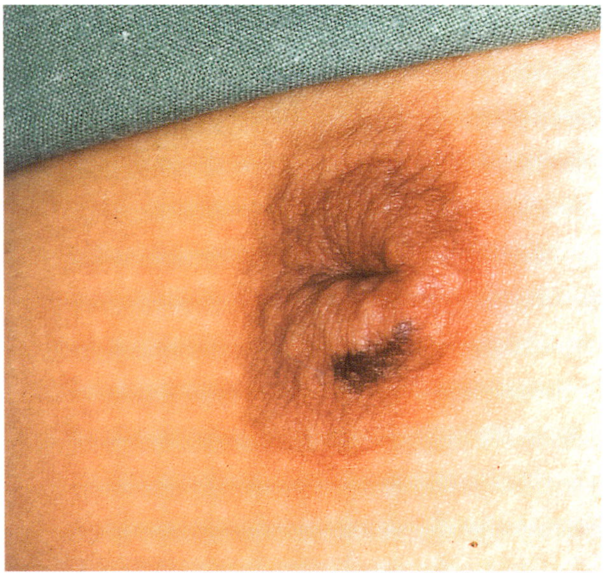

Figure 4.119a Inverted nipple

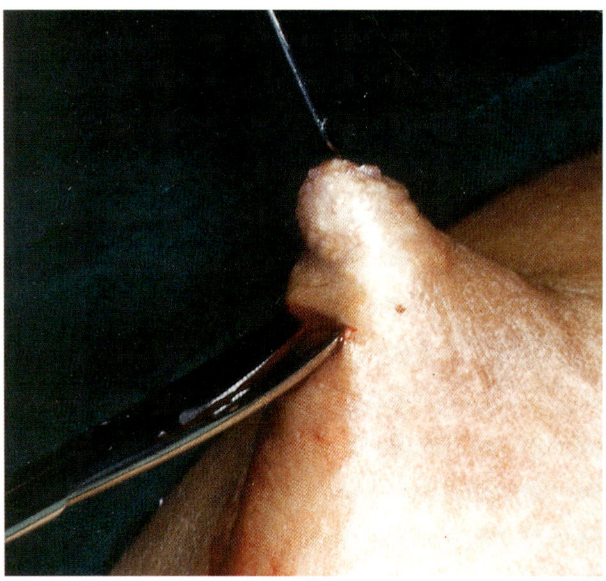

Figure 4.119b Surgery: Small incision is placed lateral to the nipple which is to be corrected. Milk ducts and fibrous bands are transected completely. Subsequently, an internal (inside) purse-string suture is placed with 4×0 Vicryl. No skin closure!

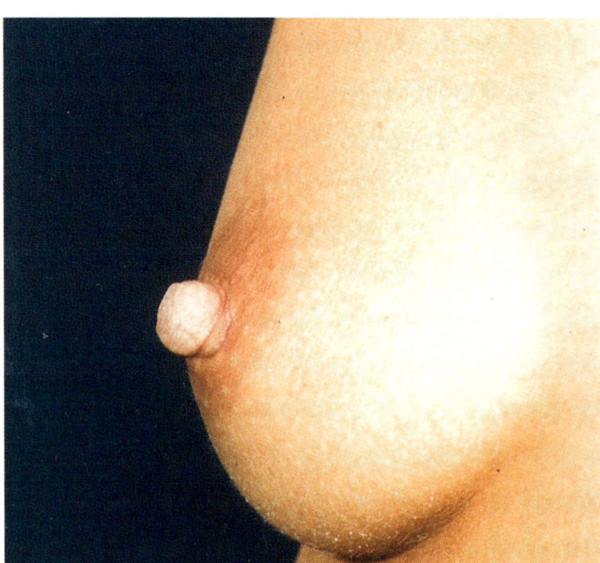

Figure 4.119c One year postoperatively: No scars

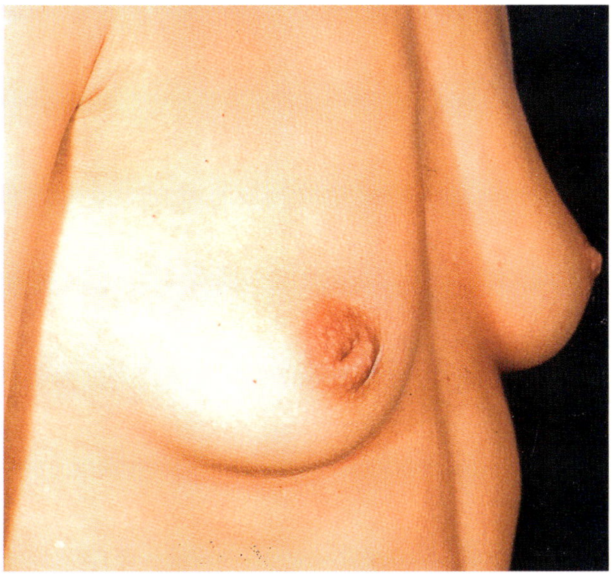

Figure 4.120a Status post unsuccessful procedures (×2) for correction of an inverted nipple

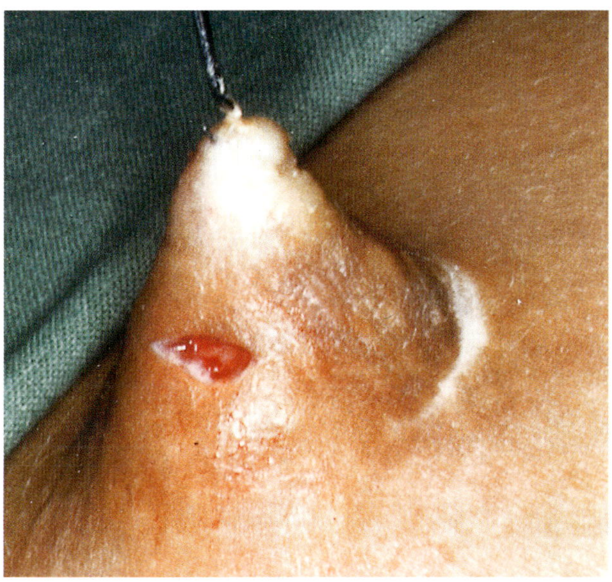

Figure 4.120b Milk ducts and fibrous bands are transected. The nipple demonstrates no signs of tension. One can see the scar from the previous procedure.

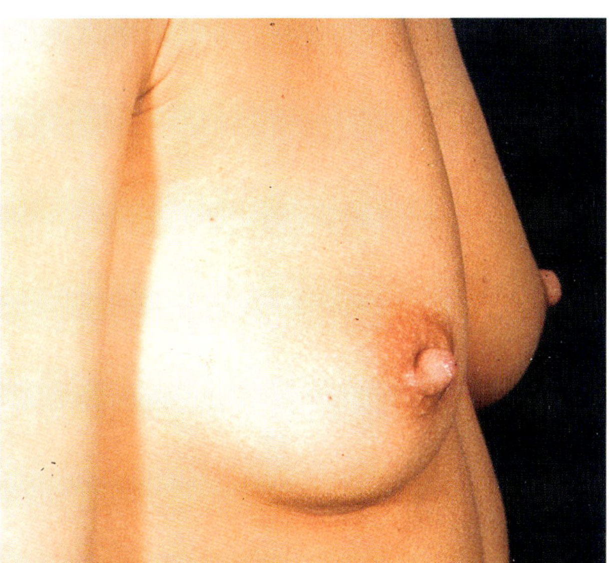

Figure 4.120c One year postoperatively

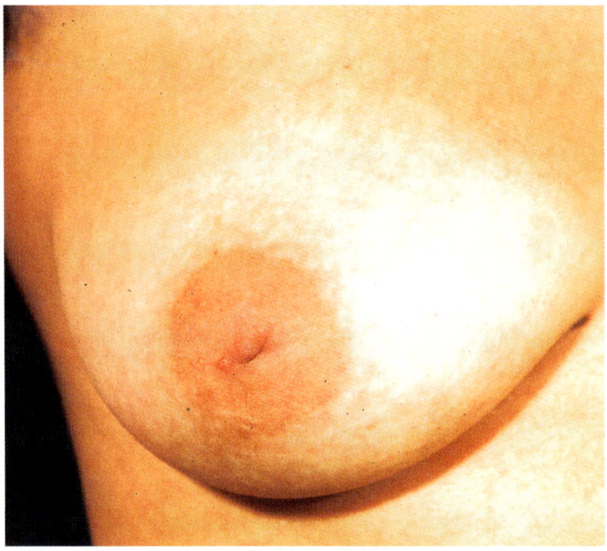

Figure 4.121a Inverted nipple

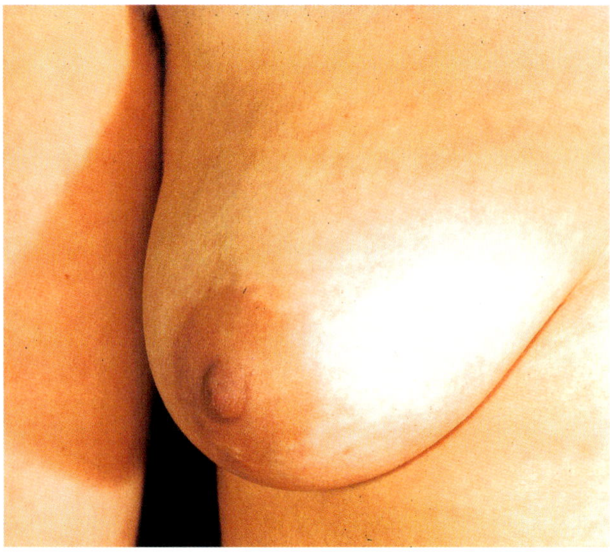

Figure 4.121b One year postoperatively.
The overcorrection noticed initially subsided. No scar!

Breast Hypertrophy With Inverted Nipple

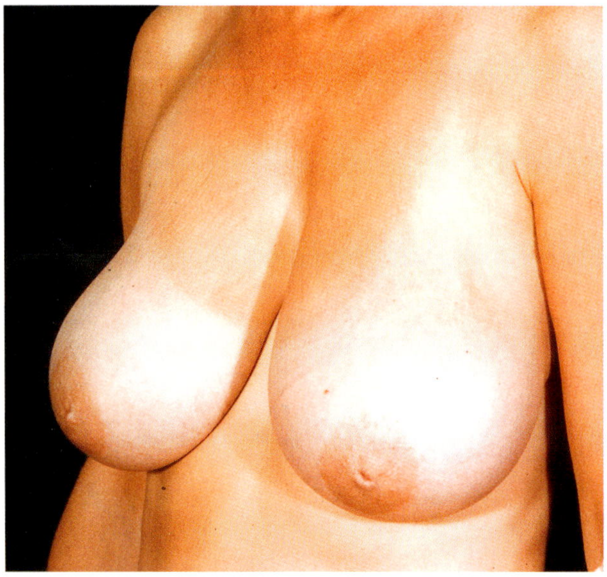

Figure 4.122a Breast hypertrophy with inverted nipples bilaterally

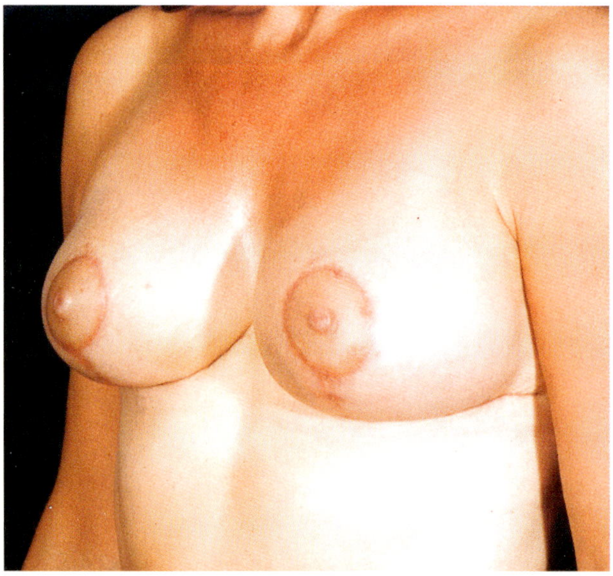

Figure 4.122b Six weeks postoperatively. Breast reduction (850 g per breast) and inverted nipple correction were performed simultaneously.

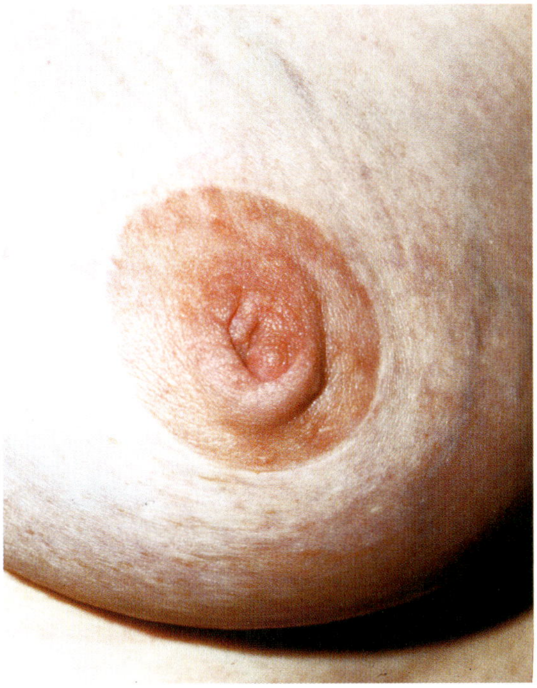

Figure 4.123a Status post breast reduction. Inverted nipples

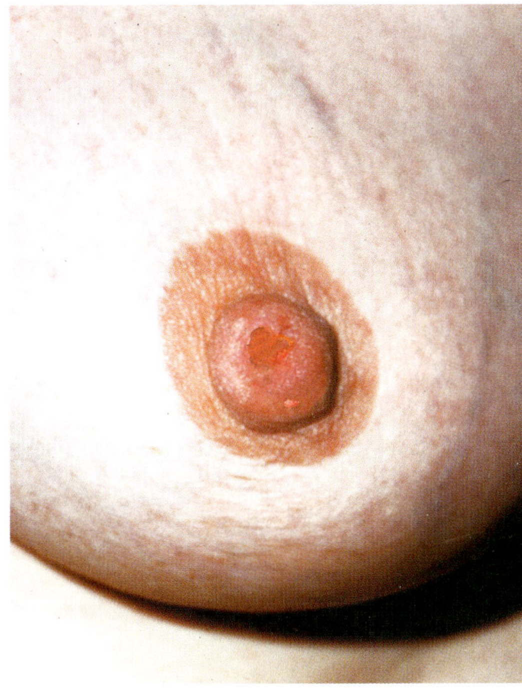

Figure 4.123b Six months postoperatively. The procedure was performed under local anesthesia.

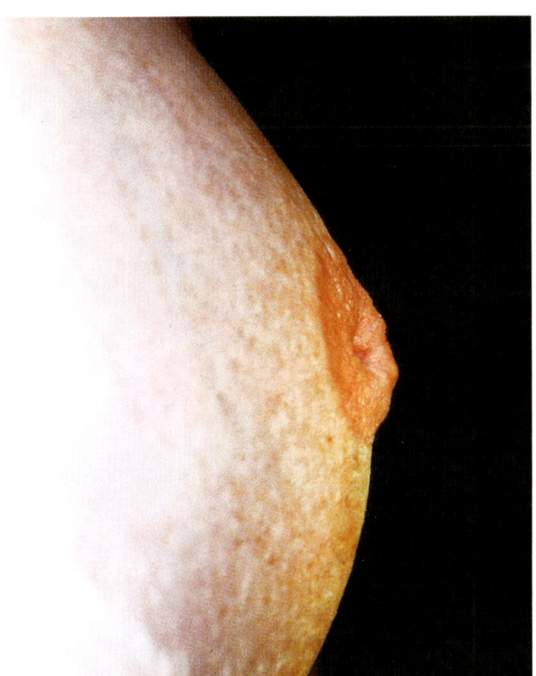

Figure 4.123c Lateral view preoperatively

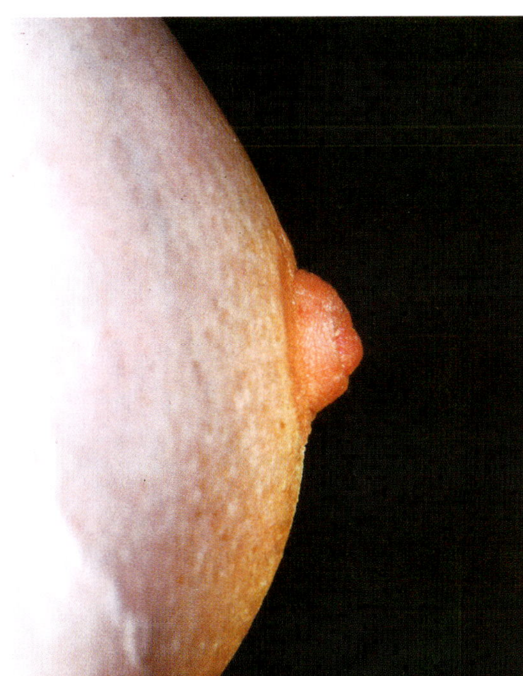

Figure 4.123d Six months postoperatively

Different Techniques of Nipple Reconstruction

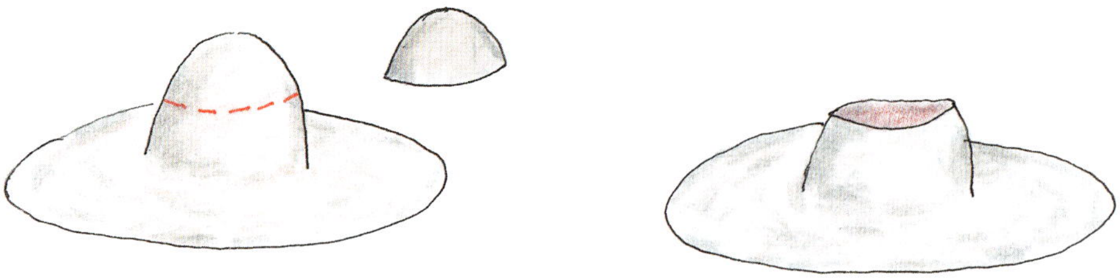

Nipple sharing using a tangential incision

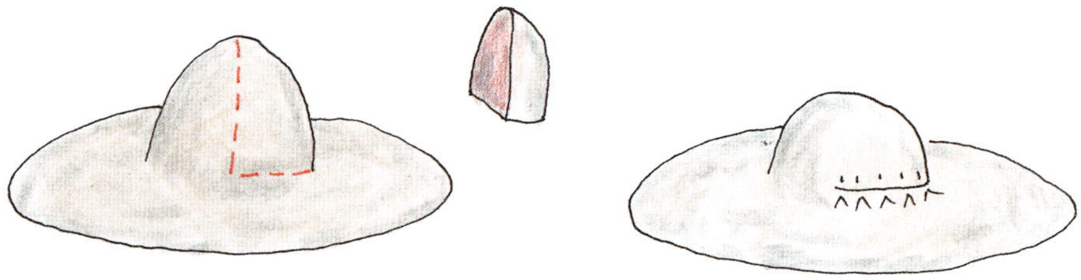

Nipple sharing using an L-shaped incision

These two methods are the ones most frequently performed!

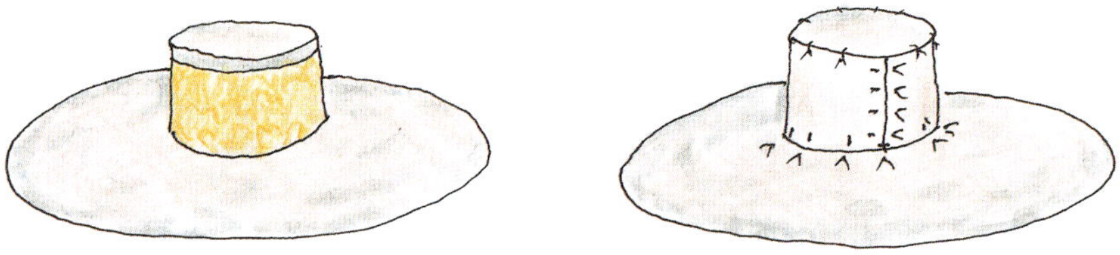

Circular incision of skin and subcutaneous tissues with subsequent lifting of a tissue cylinder and STS grafting of exposed tissues.

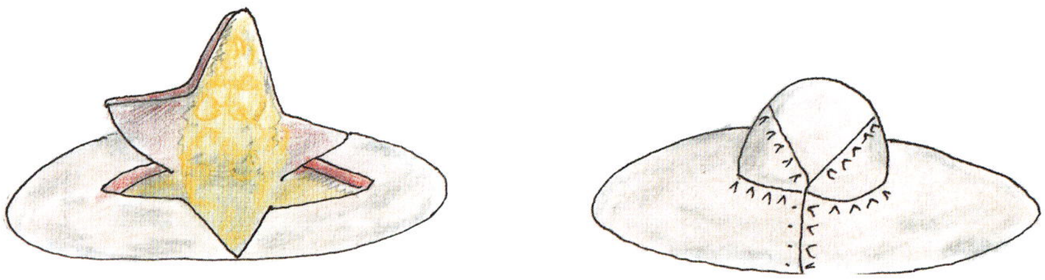

Reconstruction using star-like incisions

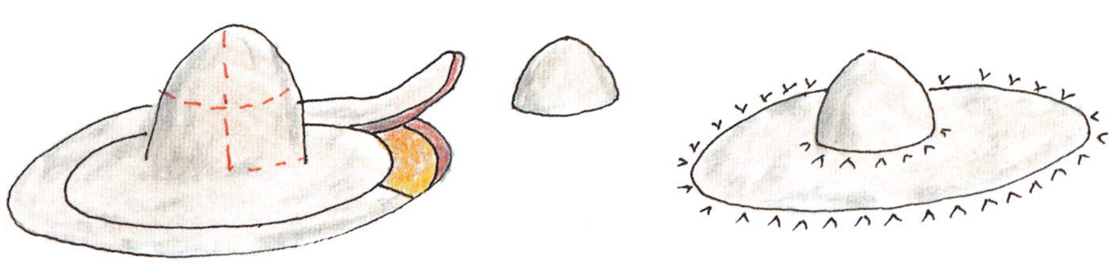

Reconstruction using a peripheral strip of the contralateral areola

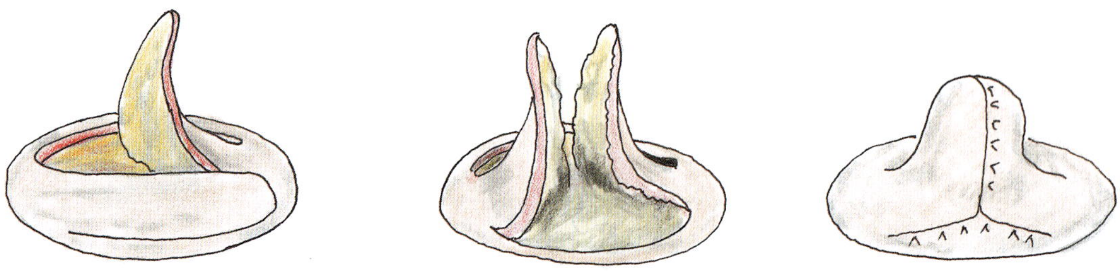

Reconstruction with two pedicled flaps

Breast Augmentation

Safety of Silicone Implants

a) Implants (cf. p. 459)

Although multiple types of implants are available the author recommends the use of implants displaying the following characteristics:

1) Double-shell implants, thus, minimizing silicone "bleed" as well as spontaneous perforation.
2) Viscous gel. Alternative: "cohesive gel", which even after implant disruption does not result in silicone leakage into adjacent tissues.
3) Textured surface. It is believed this indeed has reduced the rate of capsular contracture due to prevention of linear alignment of collagen fibres. It could be the truth.

Although several pathological features have been ascribed to silicone implants the following facts have turned out:

- A carcinogenic moiety has not been proven
- Damage to the immune system has not been demonstrated. Since capsular contracture occurs unilaterally even after bilateral placement an immunological process is unlikely.
- Mutagenic or teratogenic characteristics have never been proved.
- No increase in the incidence of rheumatic diseases.

Local reactions following leakage of silicone gel have been observed frequently, in particular in old implants with thinner shells and less viscous gels. Following introduction of double-shell implants and cohesive gels only microscopic particle grit has remained.

During the last 15 years several alternatives to silicone implants have been suggested:

1) Saline-filled implants: Even the best silicone shell is semipermeable. Saline crosses the shell at a mean rate 5 to 10 % per year. A reduction in breast volume ensues. Furthermore, many patients complain of audible "bubbles" in their breasts.
2) Hydrogel implants: These implants hardened by one year postoperatively requiring removal. Not to recommend.
3) Soya bean oil implants (Trilucent): The use of these implants is prohibited due to carcinogenic and mutagenic properties. Implants should be removed.

Aside from using textured implants the following recommendations should be adhered to for additional reduction in the occurrence of capsular contracture:

- Avoid hematomas. Hematomas promote fibrosis and facilitate infection.
- Consider irrigation of the implant pocket with antibiotics.
- After implantation, antibiotic coverage.

b) Capsular Contracture and Infection

During the last 35 years augmentation mammaplasty has gained widespread popularity. In the same time compatible silicone implants became available for placement. Furthermore, experience with this procedure has lowered the complication rate in a manner to ethically allow its performance in healthy individuals.

Unfortunately, complications may still occur which endanger a pleasing final outcome.

Postoperatively, a major problem is the occurrence of capsular contracture, which has an unknown etiology. A connection between capsular contracture and bacterial infections has been reported [Courtiss et al. 1979, Burkhardt et al. 1981, Burkhardt 1981].

In our clinic we tried to determine whether bacterial colonization could trigger the occurrence of capsular contractures. This was investigated in females with advanced capsular contracture requiring implant removal and capsulectomy.

Staphylococci, in particular S. aureus are suggested to be the causative organisms [Brandis, Pulverer 1988]. In recent years, however, scientific focus has shifted to coagulase-negative staphylococci (CNS). They belong to the regular flora of the human skin and mucous membranes and play an important role as an anti-infective barrier. In the past they were considered non-pathogenic (e.g. S. epidermidis).

They can be distinguished from S. aureus due to their lack of extracellular products such as plasma coagulase, clumping factor, and protein A.

They display a considerably lower virulence than S. aureus, however, they demonstrate a high degree of phenotypic variability. Furthermore, they are able to adapt rapidly to changing environmental factors.

Histological exams were conducted by Prof. Dr. P. Citoler (Cologne). We further thank Prof. Dr. Peters (Institute of Bacteriology, University of Münster) who performed the bacteriological exams.

Materials and Methods

In 88 patients with high-grade capsular contracture (Baker III) the following parameters were analyzed:

- 106 capsular excisions were analyzed histologically and bacteriologically
- 106 intracapsular swabs were sent for microbiological analyses
- 44 removed implant surfaces were sent for microbiological analyses

Histological Examination (Capsula)

Following histological analyses the specimens were classified [Baker et al. 1982, Smahel 1978]:

- Group 1: 0 patients

Fibrous/hyaline capsule without inflammation

- Group 2: 17 patients (16 %)

Fibrous/hyaline capsule with siliconomas

- Group 3: 71 patients (84 %)

Capsule with signs of subcutaneous/chronic inflammation

Table 4.22 Bacteriological analysis [N=88 patients]

Finding	N	%
Sterile	33	37.5 %
Positive	55	62.5 %

Table 4.23 Bacteriological colonization of the material

Material	N	Sterile		Colonized	
		(n)	(%)	(n)	(%)
Capsule (specimen)	106	70	66 %	36	34 %
Swabs	106	92	86.8 %	14	13.2 %
Implants	44	6	13.6 %	38	86.4 %

Table 4.24 Occurrence of single/mixed bacterial colonization in positive specimen

Material	N	Single		Mixed	
		(n)	(%)	(n)	(%)
Capsule (specimen)	36	31	86.1 %	5	13.9 %
Swabs	14	13	92.8 %	1	7.2 %
Implants	38	30	78.9 %	8	21.1 %

Table 4.25 Spectrum of germs (single colonization)

Germ	Capsule (specimen)		Swab		Implant	
	n	%	n	%	n	%
Grampositive bacteria						
CNS	21	67.7	9	69.2	25	83.3
S. aureus	2	6.5	2	15.4	2	6.7
Corynebacteria	1	3.2	1	7.7	–	–
Propioni bact.	4	12.9	–	–	1	3.3
Gramnegative bacteria						
Non-fermenting rods	1	3.2	1	7.7	–	–
Pseudomonas	–	–	–	–	1	3.3
Prot. mirabilis	–	–	–	–	1	3.3
E. coli	1	3.2	–	–	–	–
Fungi						
Aspergillus	1	3.2	–	–	–	–
Total (n)	31		13		30	

In all three specimen types CNS were the most frequently isolated germs: 65 to 85 %. The majority of isolated organisms were gram-positive.

Considering our results the following conclusions may be drawn:

Significant differences exist between the materials analyzed regarding the traceability of organisms. This is due to a significantly higher frequency of germ detection on polymerized synthetic material surfaces when compared to tissue specimen or swabs.

An explanation may be seen when considering the pathogenesis of polymer-associated infections caused by staphylococci [Peters et al. 1985]. This pattern of infection is due to the special feature of staphylococci to adhere irreversibly to polymer surfaces with subsequent proliferation [Peters et al 1982]. In the course of infection staphylococci produce an extracellular mucous substance. Finally, multiple layers of staphylococci exist within an amorphous matrix consisting of extracellular mucous substance and serum proteins such as fibrinogen and fibronectin [Herrmann et al. 1988]. This environment protects staphylococci against the host defense mechanisms such as opsonine-mediated phagocytosis as well as antibiotics [Peters et al. 1987].

Due to the course of capsular contracture and also the existence of CNS in the region of the areola and milk ducts [Rasjö 1985], attention focused on this population. Contamination during surgery, as well as a result of micro-lesions postoperatively is understandable.

The life-span of a silicone implant is estimated to be 8 to 12 years. Following this period removal is recommended.

Since CNS were not detected in only 2 cases of mixed germ colonization, the etiological impact of other germ species seems unlikely. In all three specimen types (capsule specimen, swab, and implant) CNS were demonstrated to exist in the majority of cases (65–85 %).

In conclusion, if bacteria cause the development of capsular contracture CNS are suggested to play the key role.

Clinical Impact

Application of strict aseptic techniques while performing augmentation mammaplasty is essential. The implant pocket should be irrigated with antibiotics (Neomycin). Furthermore, implants should be washed with an antibiotic solution prior to placement. Placement of a suction drain is recommended.

c) Positioning the Silicone Prosthesis

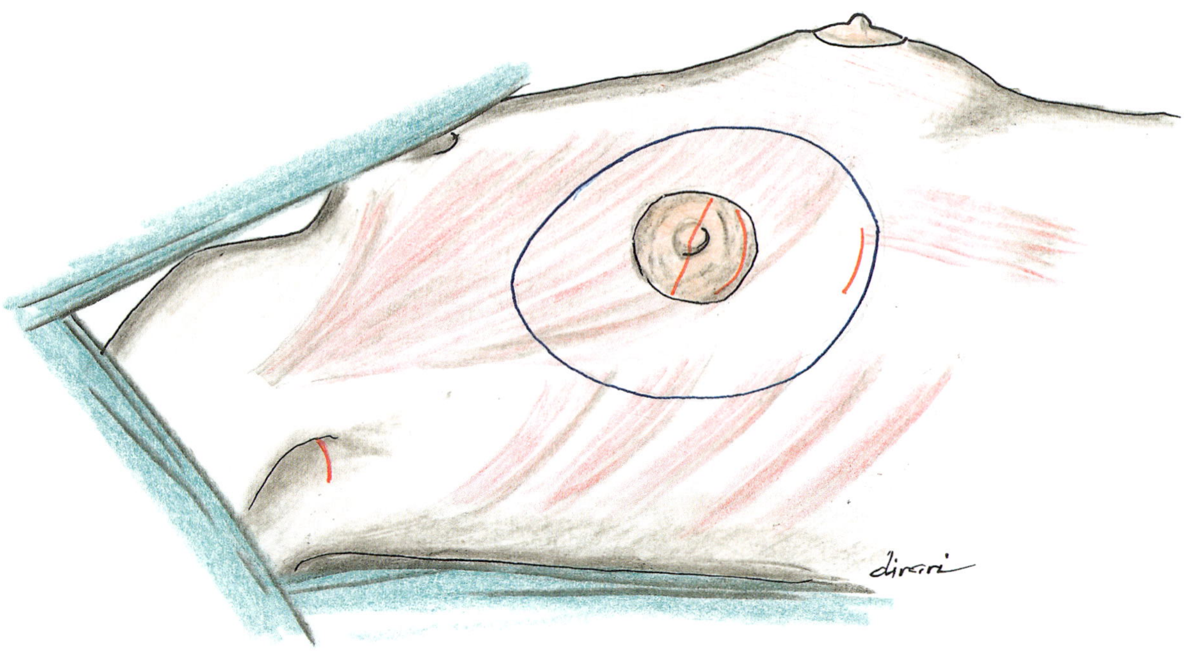

Figure 4.124 Incision sites and silicone implant position

Possible routes for implant placement are:

- Axilla
  Advantage: The scar is placed far-off the breast and is barely visible. With some practice, implant placement (epipectoral/subpectoral) becomes easy.
  Disadvantage: Due to a higher germ count in the axilla, higher rates of infection have been reported. If bleeding occurs caudally in the pocket problems may arise. In this case, endoscopy is helpful. In our patient population this was the preferred technique to implant inlays.

- Inframammary fold (IMF)
  An incision in the IMF allows good exposure with a long time visible scar.

- Areolar margin (caudally)
  Technically this method is more demanding. Caudal dissection should be performed subcutaneously. Either subpectoral or epipectoral implant placement is possible. The scar is barely visible if the incision is placed 2 mm within the areola.

- Transareolar incision
  The transareolar incision runs vertically through the areola and disrupts the milk ducts, which are frequently colonized by CNS. Hemostasis is rather difficult with this approach. Furthermore, pain and dysaesthesias of the areola may occur. The author does not recommend this technique.

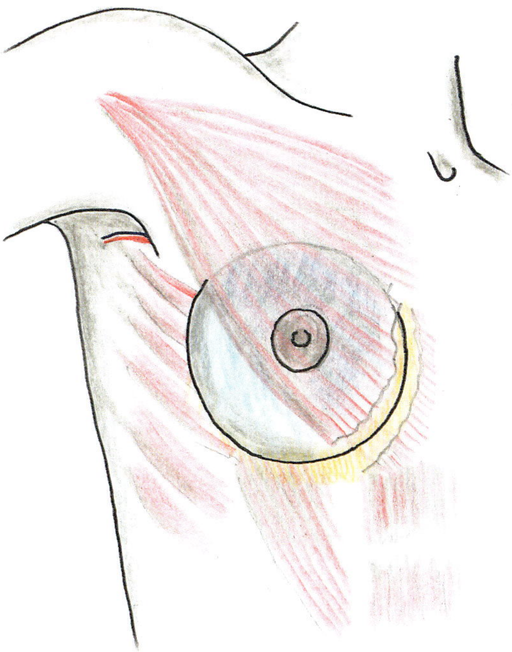

Figure 4.125a Retropectoral implant placement.
In fact, retropectoral implant positioning is not a correct term. Superiorly, the implant is positioned subpectorally. However, inferiorly and laterally the implant is covered by subcutaneous tissue only. For achievement of a nice breast shape the sternocostal insertions of the pectoralis muscle are transected. Here, the axillary technique of implant placement is illustrated. An endoscope is very helpful, however, not essential.

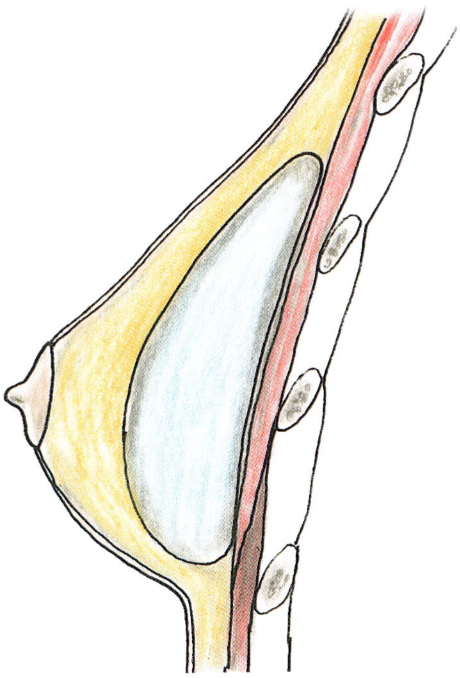

Figure 4.125b Subglandular implant placement. This position is indicated if sufficient subcutaneous as well as glandular tissue is present. One usually achieves a nice breast shape. In soft tissue coverage is not sufficient the edge of the implant may become palpable and visible.

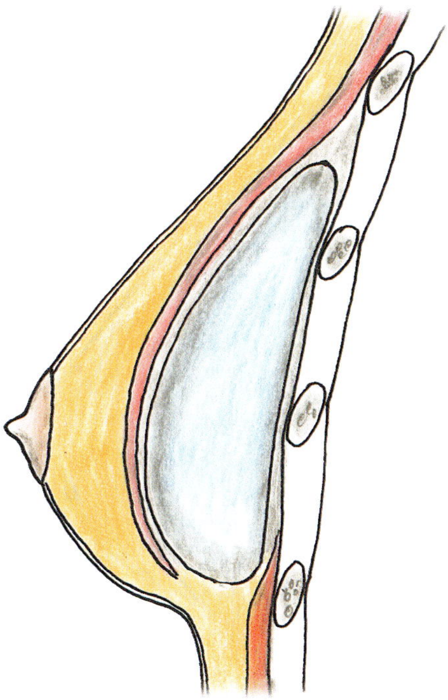

Figure 4.125c Subpectoral or rather partially subpectoral implant placement. Here, the inferior portion of the implant is covered by subcutaneous tissue. An advantage of subpectoral position is the fact that implant edges remain inconspicuous even in slim individuals. A drawback is frequent implant movement with arm movement.

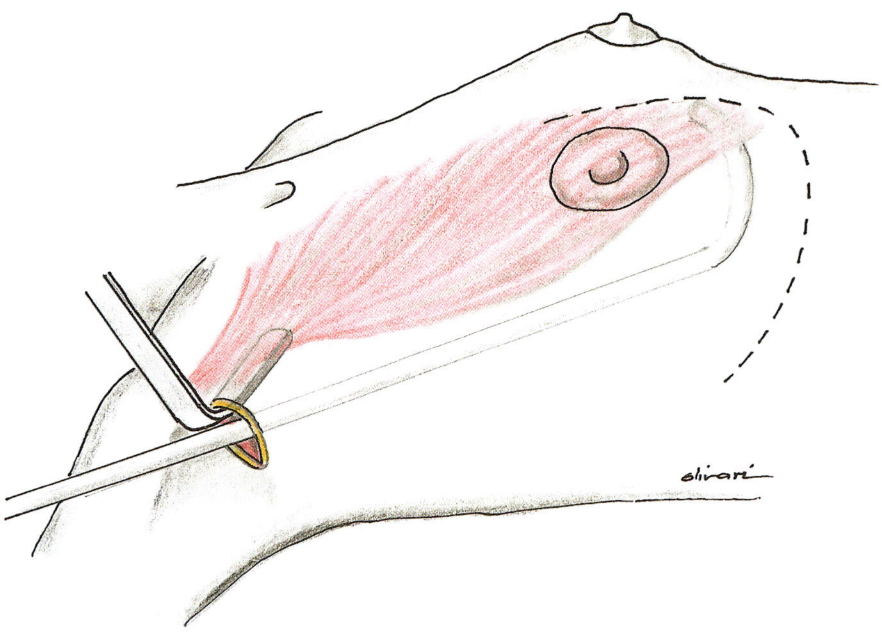

Figure 4.126 Subpectoral dissection of an implant pocket with a dissector. The sternocostal insertions of the pectoralis muscle are partly in lower part transected. The implant pocket borders extend beyond the pectoralis major muscle inferiorly and laterally, thus, the implant is not covered by muscle inferiorly. An endoscope facilitates dissection. Bleeding can be minimized if a diluted local anesthetic-epinephrine-solution is infiltrated. An endoscope is very helpful.

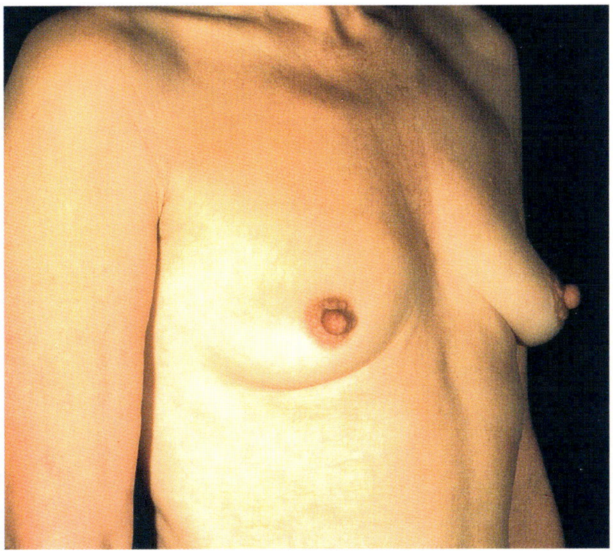

Figure 4.127a Hypoplastic breast following two pregnancies

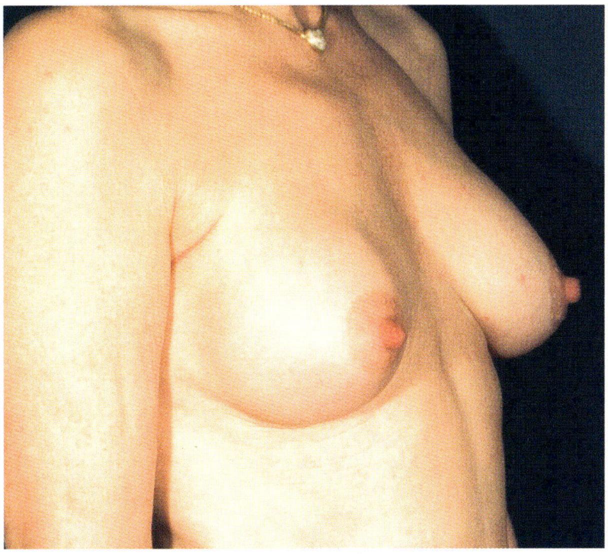

Figure 4.127b Six months postoperatively. Textured silicone-gel implants (270 ccm) were placed subglandularly via an axillary incision.

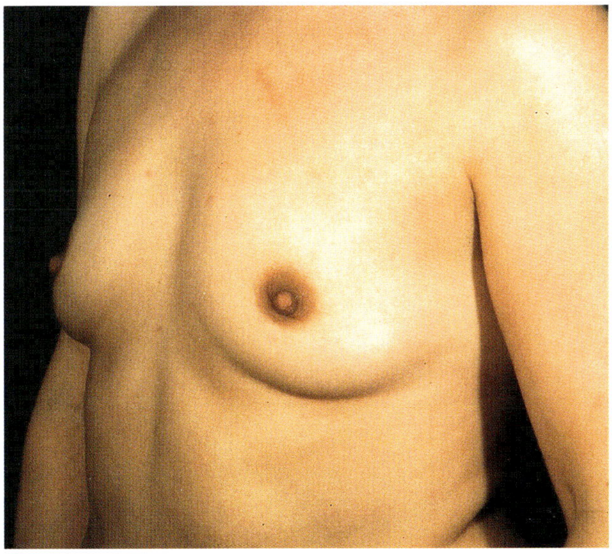

Figure 4.128a Hypoplastic breasts: Subglandular placement of textured McGhan implants (300 ccm) via an axillary incision

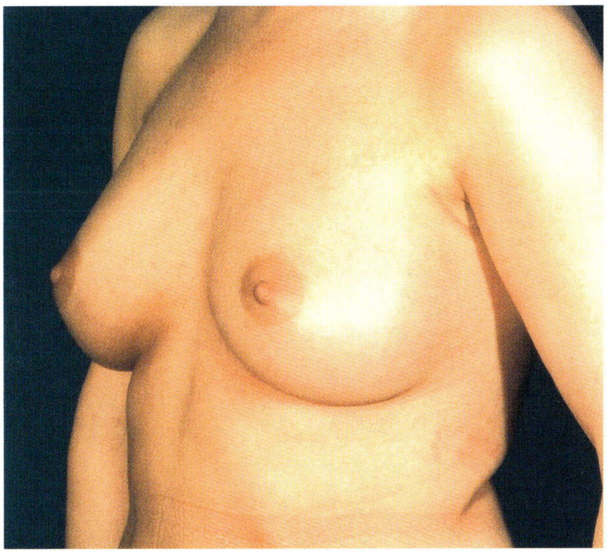

Figure 4.128b Seven months postoperatively

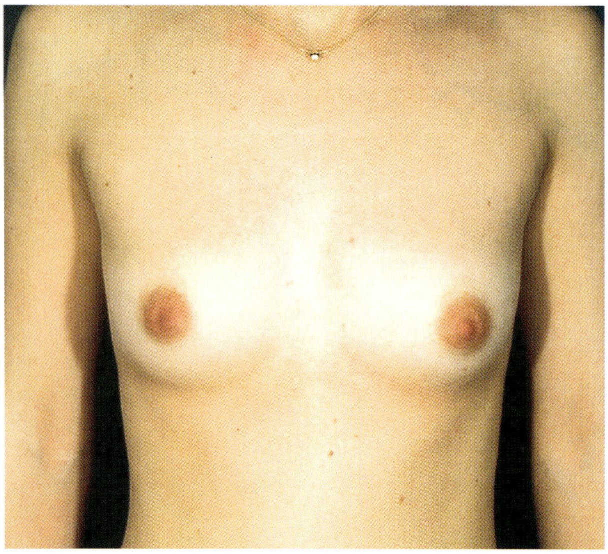

Figure 4.129a Juvenile breast hypoplasia: Subpectoral placement of 330 ccm McGhan CVI-implants via an axillary incision.

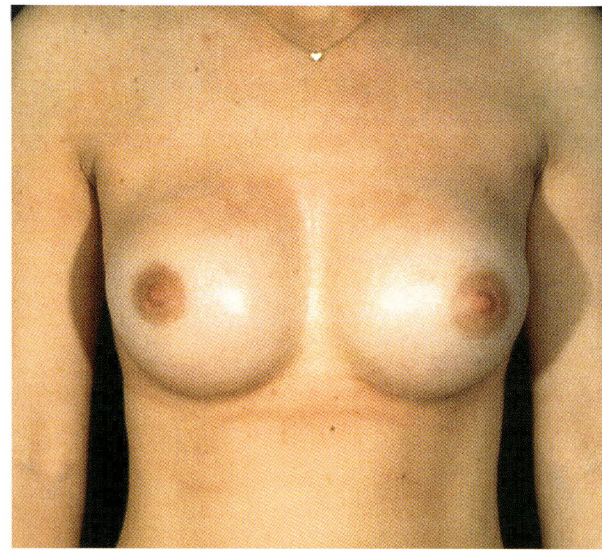

Figure 4.129b Three months postoperatively

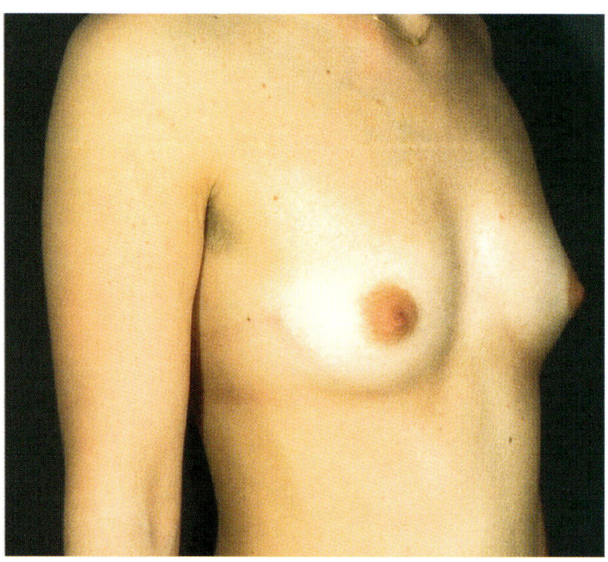

Figure 4.129c Preoperative oblique view

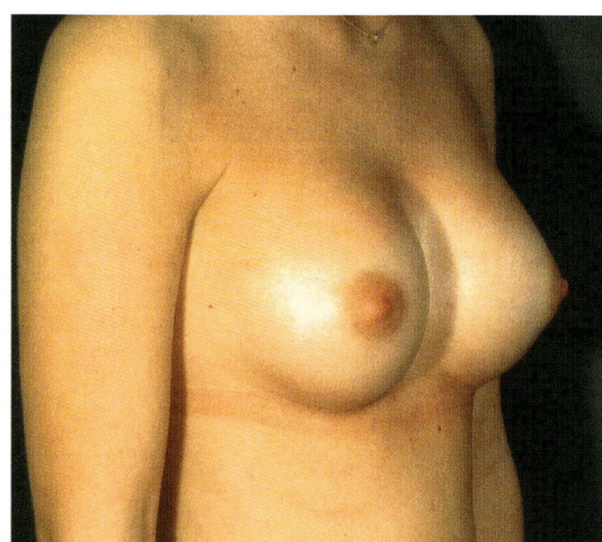

Figure 4.129d Three months postoperatively: No visible scars

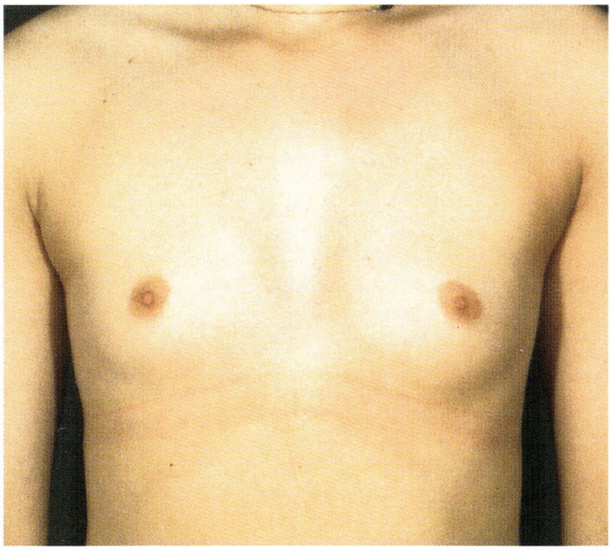

Figure 4.130a Juvenile breast hypoplasia

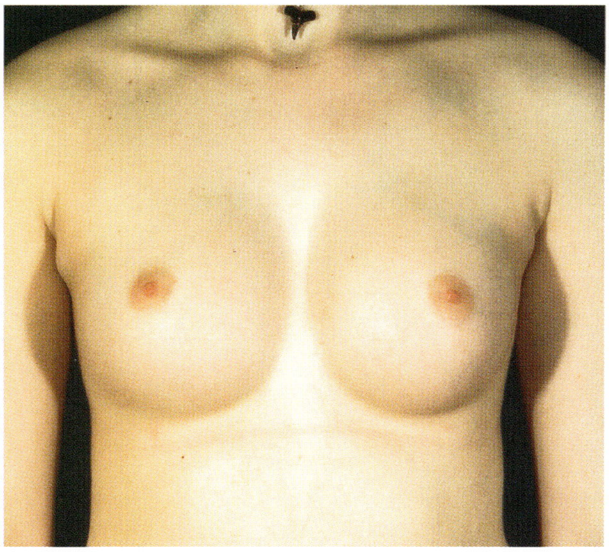

Figure 4.130b Subpectoral placement of 350 ccm implants (McGhan CVI) via an axillary incision. Nine months postoperatively.

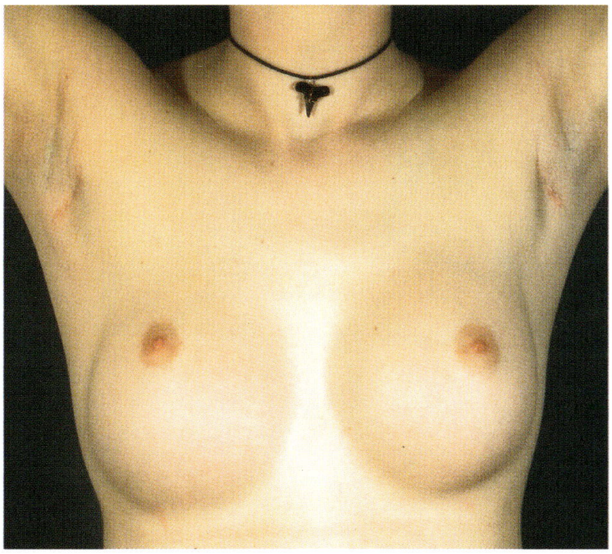

Figure 4.130c Nine months postoperatively. The scars in the axilla are still slightly visible.

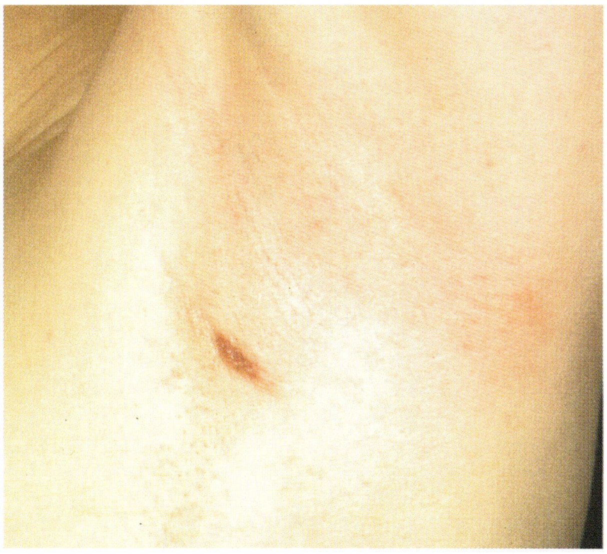

Figure 4.130d Complication: A minor skin infection can be treated easily.

Capsular Contracture

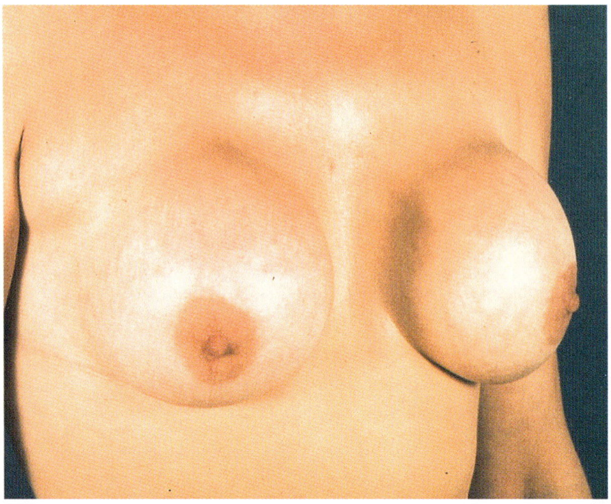

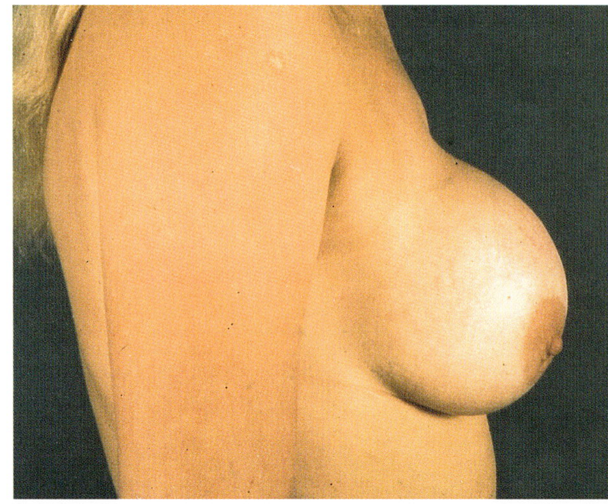

Figure 131a,b Four years following breast augmentation this patient suffered from a Baker III capsular contracture. The patient refused placement of new silicone implants.

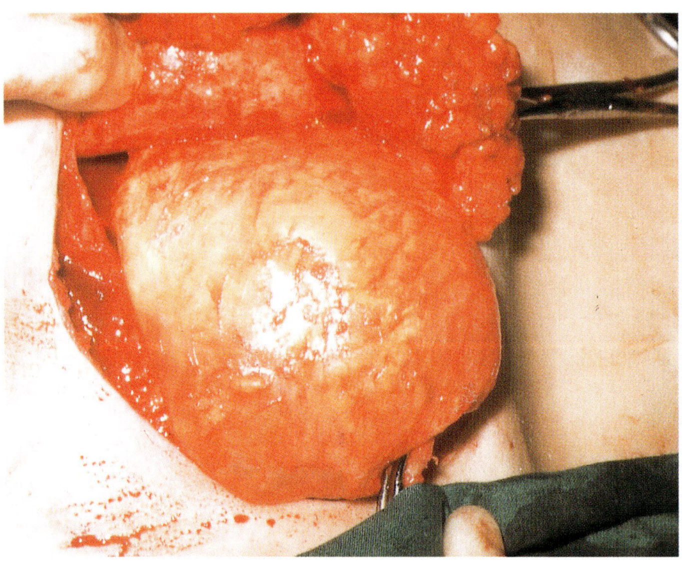

Figure 131c The implant is removed including the capsule (approx. 62 % of all severe capsular contractures are infected).

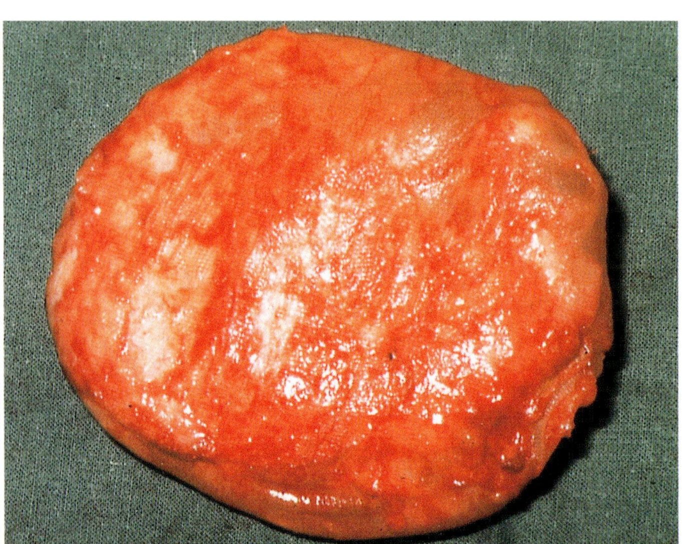

Figure 131d Excised implant with its fibrous capsule: Several advantages exist if an en-bloc removal of the implant with its capsule is accomplished:

1) Silicone particles in the capsule are removed by this means.
2) In case of implant perforation silicone leakage into the surgical field is prevented.
3) The infected content (cf. p. 645) does not reach the surgical field.

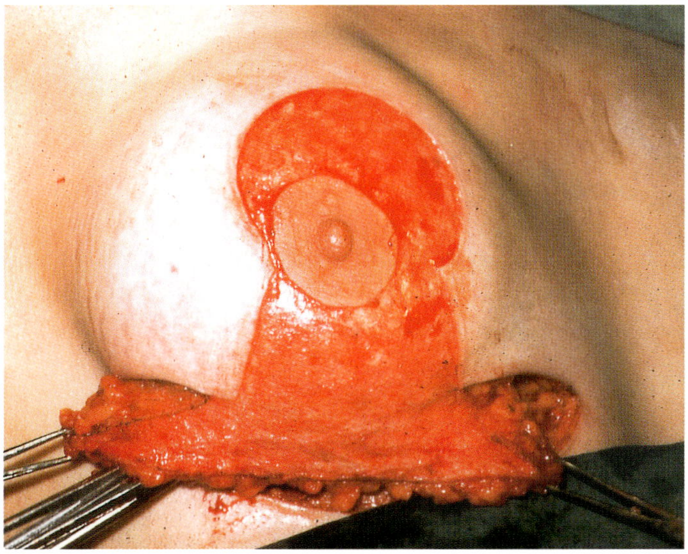

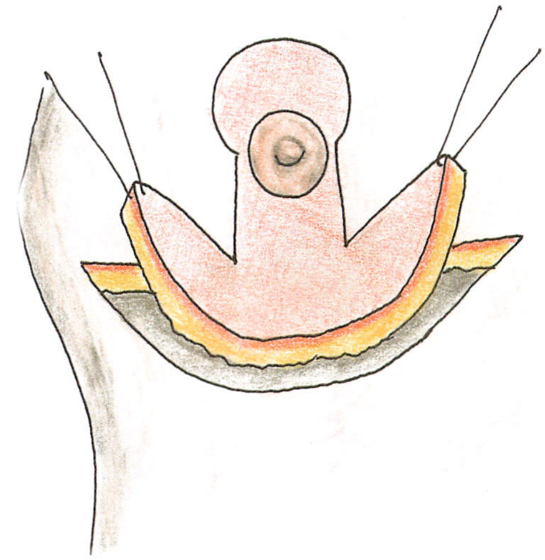

Figure 131e, f For breast volume preservation deepithelialization of an area, in particular inferiorly, is conducted. Medially and laterally a tip of deepithelialized small flaps and fixed to the pectoral fascia. Alternatives could be a TRAM flap or a deepithelialized latissimus flap.

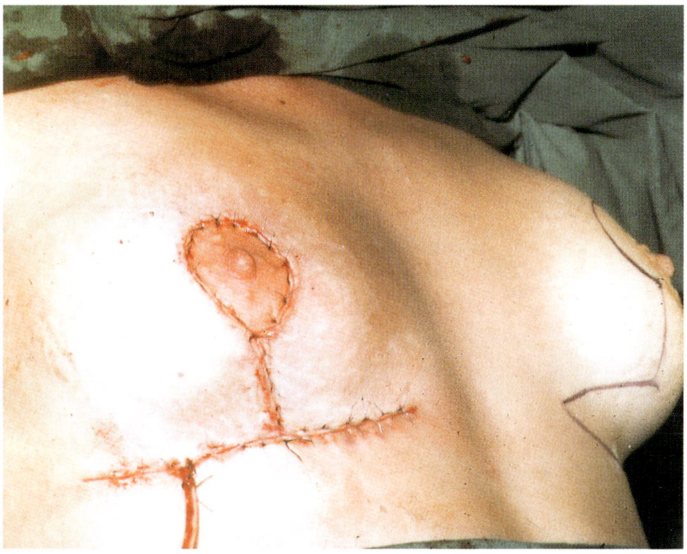

Figure 131g Status post shaping of the right breast, preoperative markings of the left breast

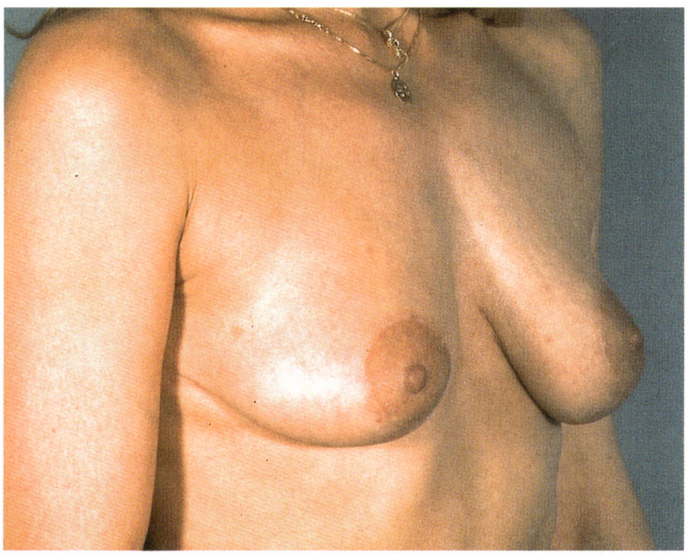

Figure 131h Three years postoperatively. Patient was happy with relatively small but trouble free breast.

Hidradenitis Suppurativa

This is a chronic, recurring, inflammatory and nodular disease of the apocrine glands.

The infection is predominantly caused by Staphylococci; rarely E. coli and Klebsiella are involved. Frequently, abscess formation is observed.

The human skin harbours sebaceous and sweat glands. Sweat glands are classified into eccrine and apocrine glands. Eccrine glands are small (20 μl) display a simple tubular structure and are innervated by cholinergic fibers of the sympathetic system. They produce odourless sweat and are distributed throughout the body.

Apocrine sweat glands are larger (200 μl) and are located deep within the dermis. They are innervated by adrenergic fibers of the sympathetic system and are localized in special areas only (axilla, perineum, groin, pubic hair). These glands secrete a viscous odourous fluid.

Only the apocrine glands are affected in hidradenitis suppurativa. It occurs following puberty and displays no sexual prevalence. In women the axillary region is affected more often, but in males this applies to the genital region.

The clinical course is characterized by multiple recurrences. Patients typically present with a long-standing history ranging from three to fifteen years (average: 4 years).

In addition to infection and pain, these patients also suffer psychologically.

The majority of patients have a history of multiple treatment trials (conservative and surgical). In recurring cases surgery is clearly indicated. Abscess incision generates temporary relief, but never cures the patient. Surgical treatment consists of wide excision, with an adequate safety margin as well, and defect coverage with a pedicled flap.

The excised area is irrigated with Neomycin. A suction drain is placed and antibiotic treatment commenced for five to seven days.

Some authors recommend letting the excised area heal by secondary intention, which of course takes several weeks, and generates painful scars or contractures. Thus, this method should be avoided.

The same procedure (excision and coverage with a local flap) was used for non-infected hidradenitis which primarily presented as excessive malodorous sweating. An alternative is subdermal liposuction.

a) Axillary Hidradenitis Suppurativa

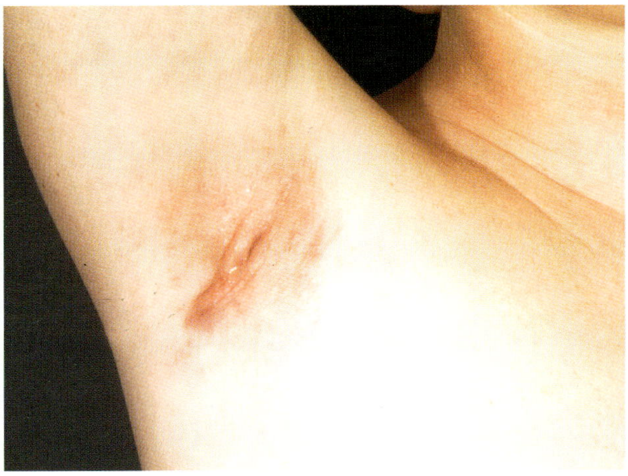

Figure 4.132a Hidradenitis suppurativa following multiple incisions. Remember: An incision never cures such a finding but rather results in a temporary relief.

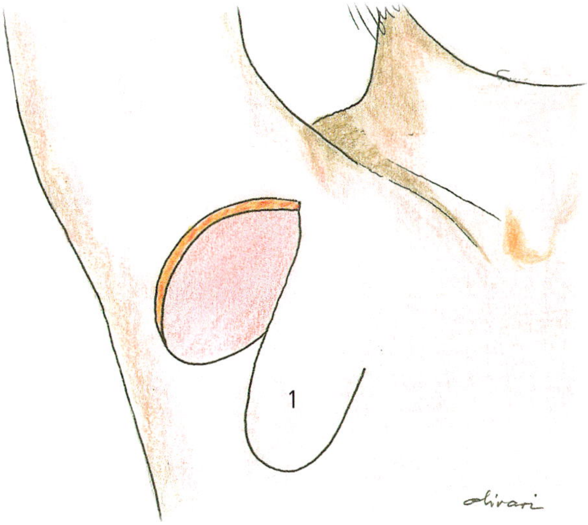

Figure 4.132b Surgery: The entire area needs to be excised including the subcutaneous extension of the process. En-bloc resection of eccrine and apocrine sweat glands is essential. A local flap is planned (1).

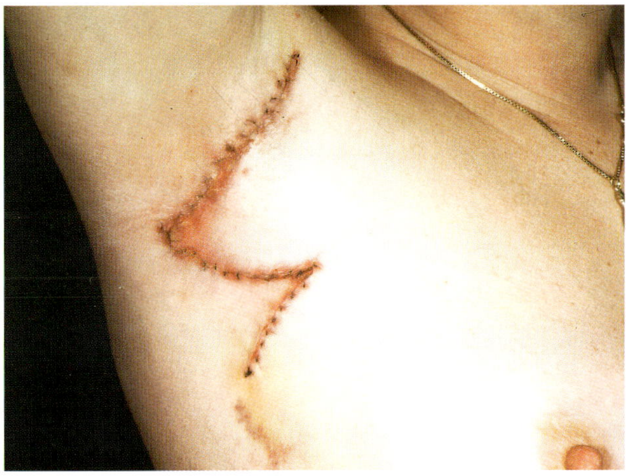

Figure 4.132c A local flap of unaffected skin is mobilized and transferred into the defect.

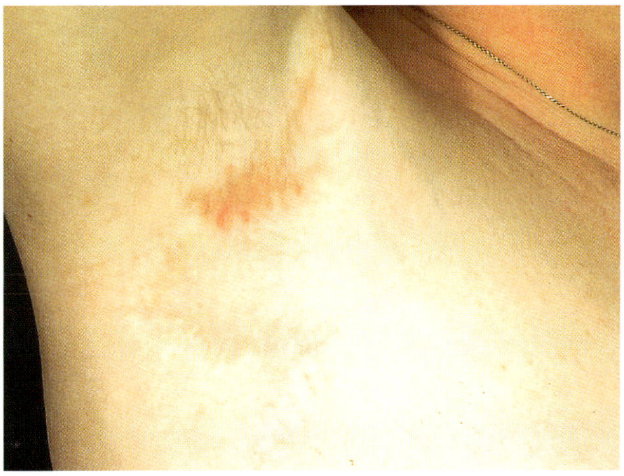

Figure 4.132d Three years postoperatively: No recurrence

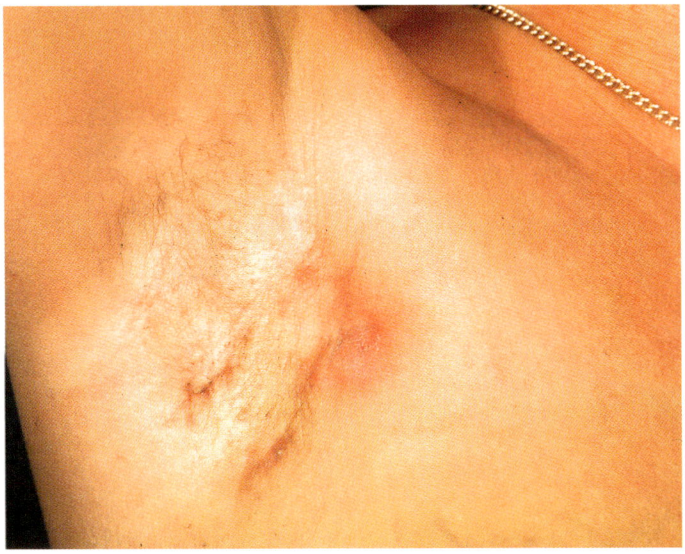

Figure 4.133a Hidradenitis suppurativa. Multiple incisions were done with a newly-formed abscess. Repeated incisions do not cure a hidradenitis suppurativa.

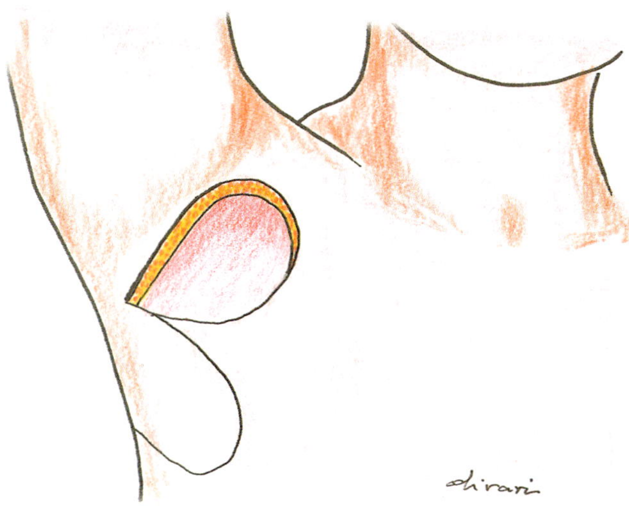

Figure 4.133b En-bloc resection of skin, eccrine and apocrine sweat glands. One should not wait until the infection has subsided. Moreover, the entire area should be excised en bloc.

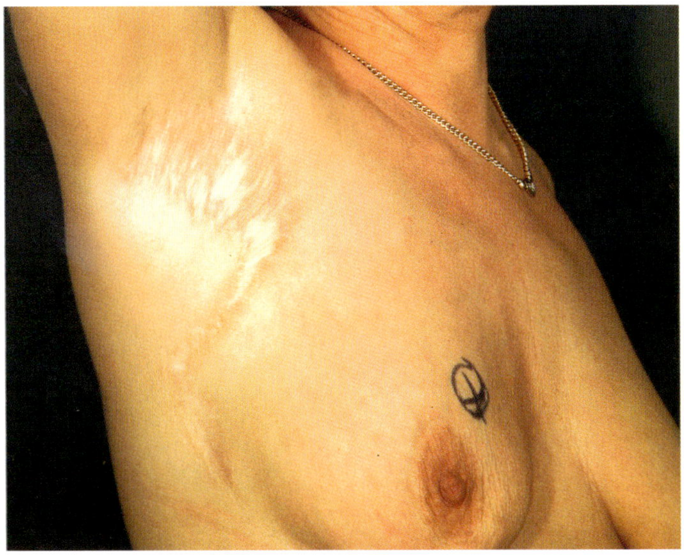

Figure 4.133c Three years postoperatively: No recurrence

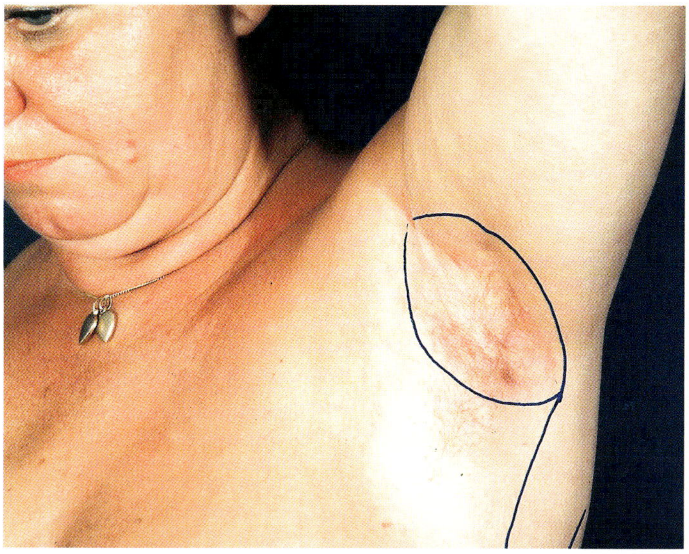

Figure 4.134a Status post multiple incisions (= 4), recurrent hidradenitis suppurativa. Operative plan: Excision of affected area with subcutaneous tissue and a local flap of unaffected skin is designed along the posterior axillary line.

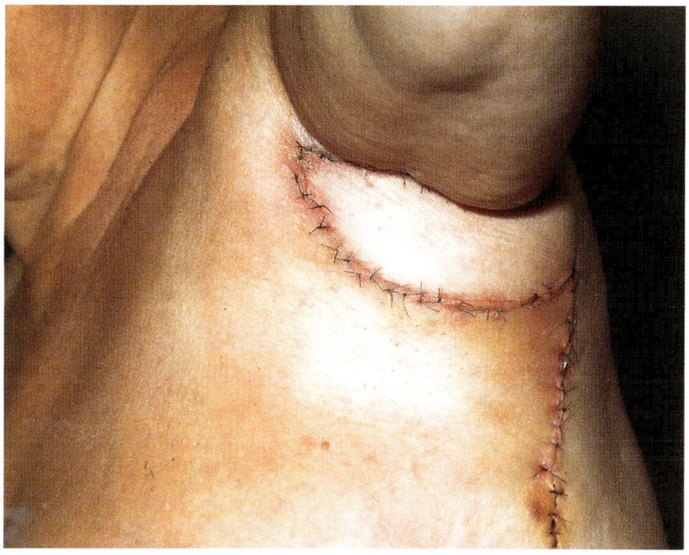

Figure 4.134b One week postoperatively. Postoperatively, the operative field is showered, cleaned, and treated with an antibiotic ointment daily beginning on postoperative day 1.

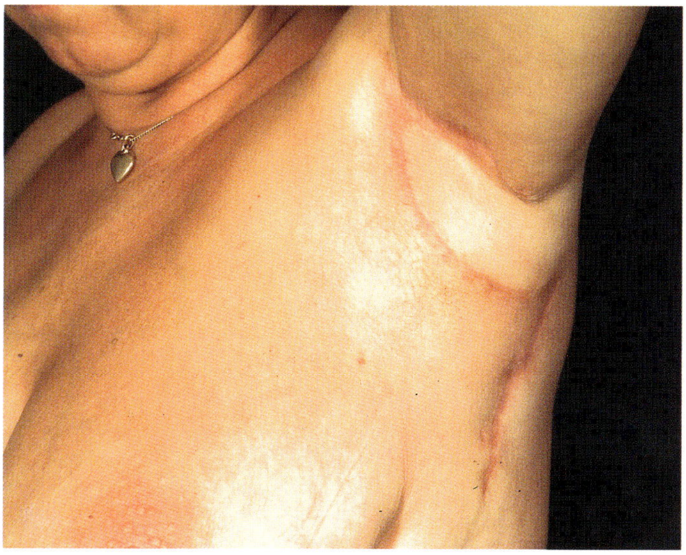

Figure 4.134c Six months postoperatively

b) Gluteal Hidradenitis Suppurativa

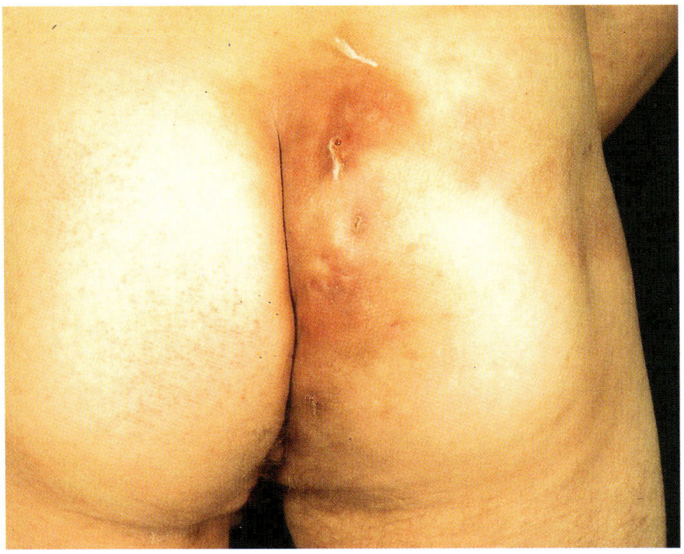

Figure 4.135a Hidradenitis suppurativa of the right gluteal and perianal region. The patient had to wear diapers for the past ten years. Eighteen incisions were performed over a period of eight years. The patient suffered from considerable social as well as occupational problems. Incision alone does not cure multifocal abscesses.

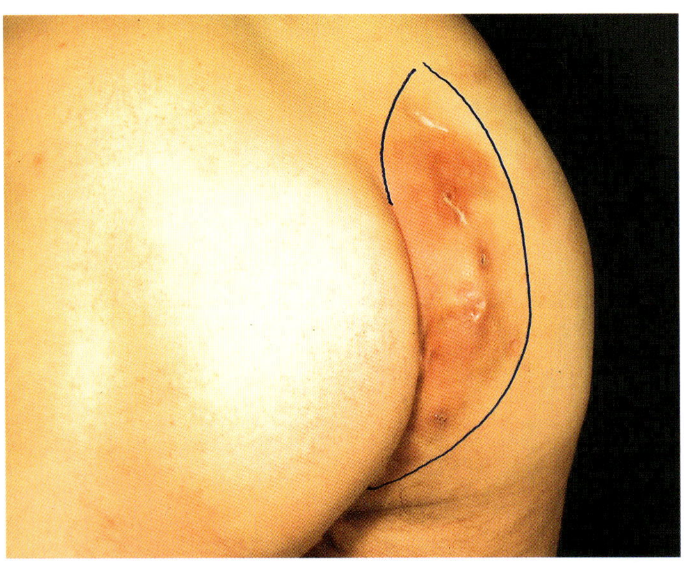

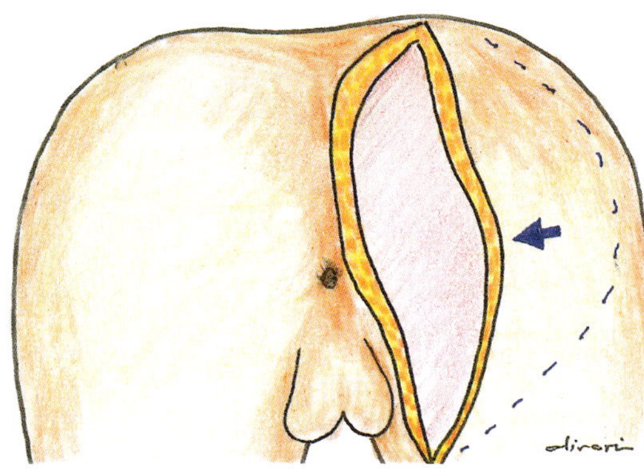

Figure 4.135c Excision (not incision) must include all affected tissues down to muscle fascia, with a safety margin of healthy tissue. Subsequently, extensive lateral mobilization and primary wound closure is performed. Three drains are placed and local as well as intravenous antibiotic treatment initiated.

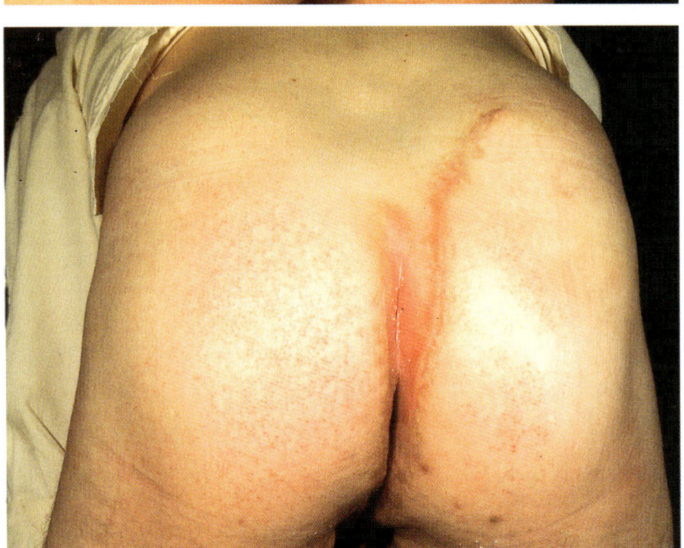

Figure 4.135d Fourteen months postoperatively

CHAPTER 5
Abdomen, Gluteal Region and Genitals

Abdomen

Extensive Abdominal Herniation

Etiology

- Following multiple laparotomies
- Traumatic abdominal wall hernia
- Rarely seen after multiple pregnancies
- Infections of the abdominal wall (secondary healing after laparotomy)
- Post TRAM procedure

In extensive abdominal wall hernias the defect cannot be adequately closed by direct suture of rectus muscle fascia. In the case of a smaller or medium-sized abdominal wall hernia, direct closure can be achieved using various techniques. These methods are usually performed by general surgeons and will not be discussed in this chapter. Extensive herniation of the abdominal wall requires specific operative techniques and frequently additional synthetic or biologic material is necessary to bridge larger-sized defects.

All this patient were admited to us by general surgeons.

We used the following procedures for the repair of larger abdominal wall herniation:

- Coverage of the defect using the tensor fascia lata muscle flap
- Full-thickness skin grafting
- Implantation of a non-resorbable mesh (Prolene® mesh)
- Biodegradable mesh implantation (Vicryl® mesh)
- The Ramirez procedure

Autologous Tissue Transfer

A versatile flap is the tensor fascia lata muscle flap which can be raised with a large part of the fascia. Tensor fascia lata muscle tissue is especially suitable for coverage of large defects of the lower abdominal wall. The challenging operative technique and the obvious upper thigh scar are considered as disadvantages of this method (Figure 5.1).

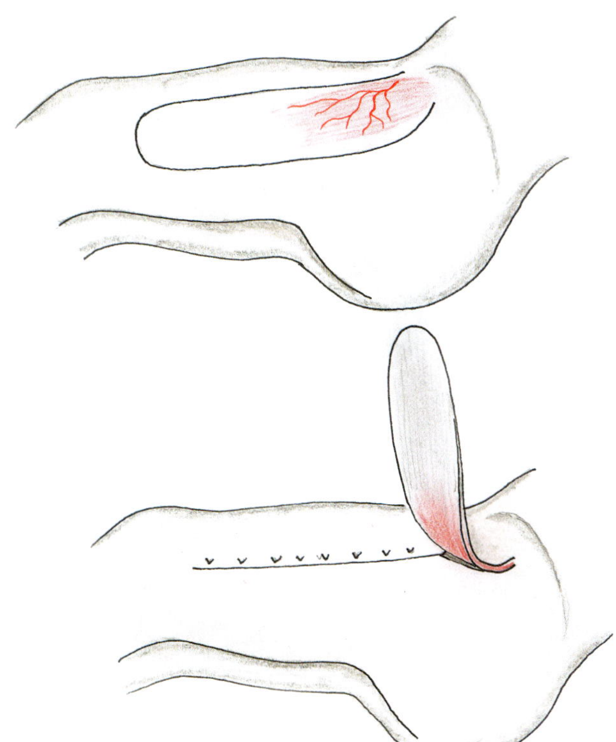

Figure 5.1 The tensor fascia lata muscle flap is an axial-pattern flap. Vascular supply is provided by a branch of the lateral femoral circumflex artery. The vascular supply enters the fascia through the muscle. The diameter of the artery measures about 2 mm and the pedicle length is approximately 7 to 9 cm. This can cover decubital defects in the trochanter region as well as the lower abdominal wall. The flap can be transferred as an island, pedicled or free tissue transfer.

a) Full-Thickness Skin Graft (Harvested from Spare Abdominal Skin)

Where there is excessive skin covering the hernia it can be used as a graft. Subtlety and patience are required to remove all the fat from the under surface of the skin. It is essential to fix the skin graft accurately and firmly using non-absorbable suture material to the dissected edge of the hernia. The epithelium is oriented ventrally and the corium is oriented dorsally. Fear of epithelial cyst formation is unsubstantiated: Grafted skin which is under tension does not lead to cyst formation.

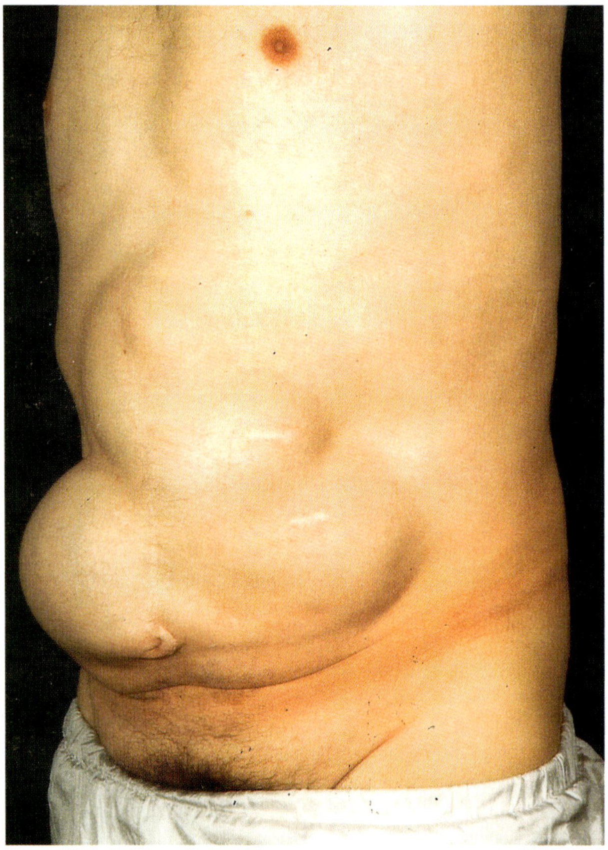

Figure 5.2a This patient presented with two large abdominal hernias. This was the situation following multiple laparotomies and attempts to close a hernia. The larger hernia, about 25 × 15 cm is located transversally around the umbilicus. The second hernia, 18 × 12 cm, is located sagittally in the epigastric region.

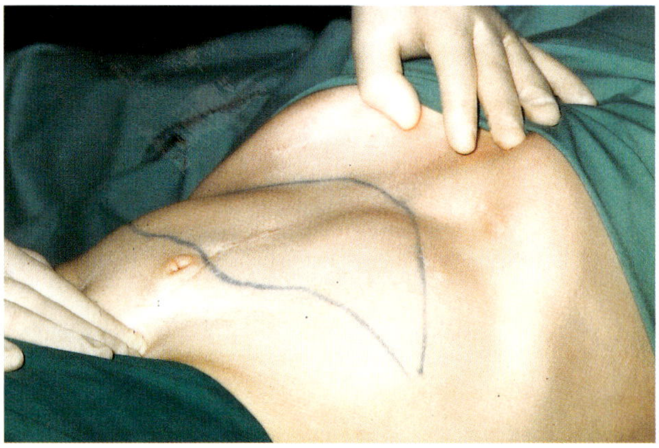

Figure 5.2b Planning of the procedure. A large full-thickness skin graft of about 30 × 18 cm is marked out supraumbilically then removed and carefully defatted.

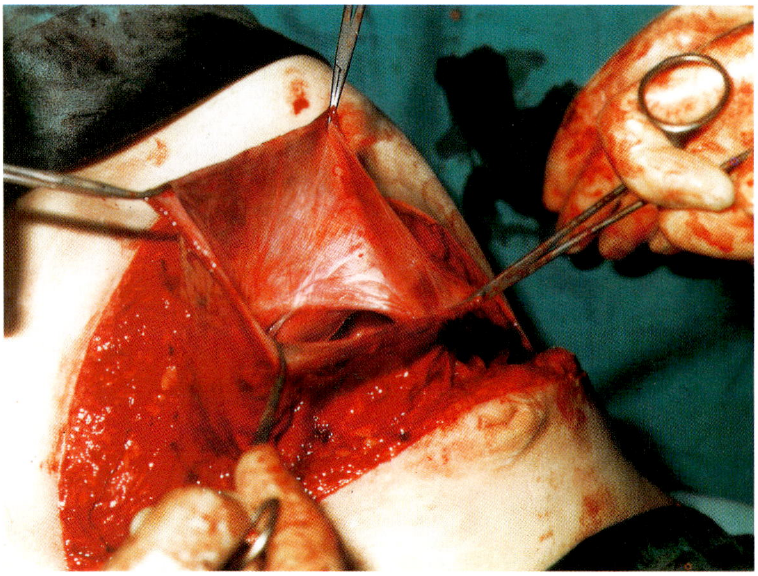

Figure 5.2c First, the larger caudal, hernia is repaired. The bowel is reposition and the peritoneal sac closed. The edge of the hernia is carefully prepared. No attempt was made to repair the cranial hernia at this session.

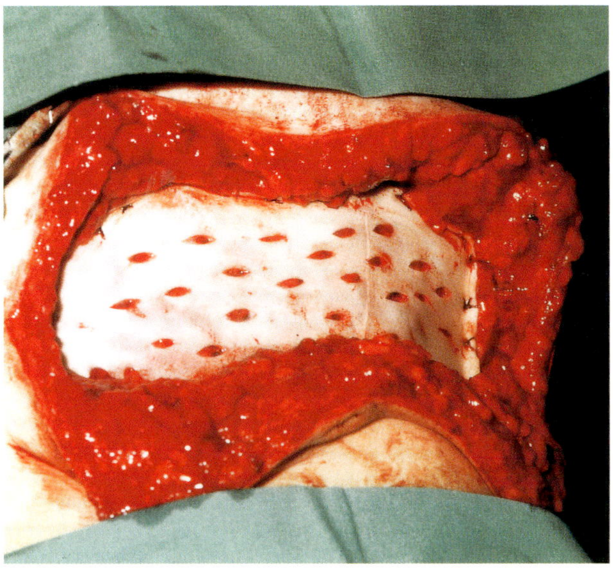

Figure 5.2d The full-thickness skin graft is sutured to the edge of the hernia using non-absorbable suture material. Multiple incisions are made to ensure adhesion of the underlying tissue to the graft. This prevents seroma formation. The epithelium is oriented ventrally.

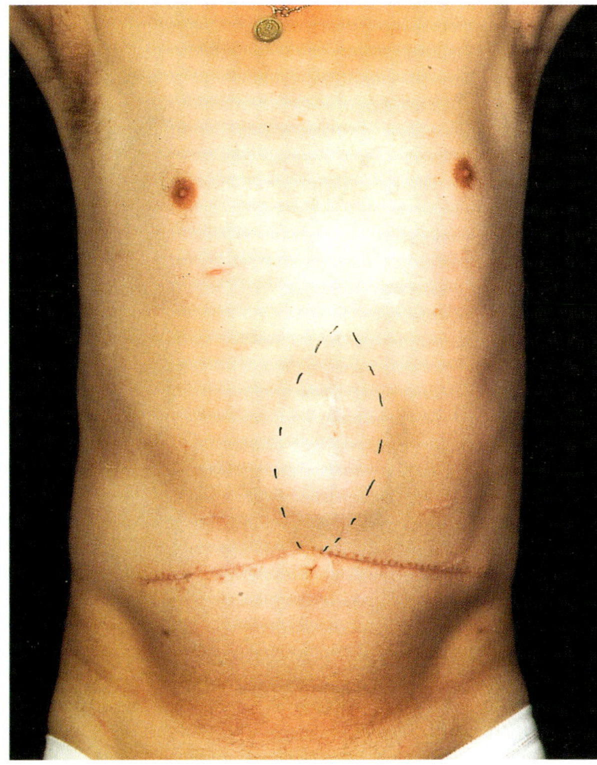

Figure 5.2e The cranial hernia is repaired six months later. Again, a full-thickness skin graft is harvested.

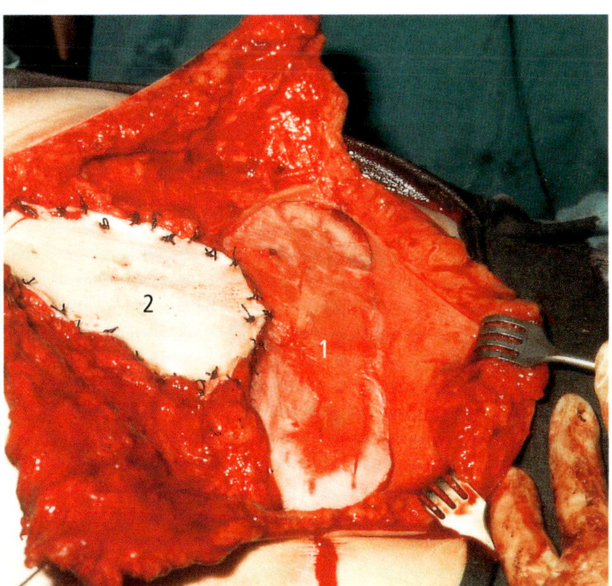

Figure 5.2f The full-thickness skin which was grafted six months earlier (1) is invaded by fibrous tissue and functions as fascia. Histological analysis revealed loss of almost all of the epithelium and massive fibrosis. The cranial hernia is now repaired using the full-thickness skin graft (2).

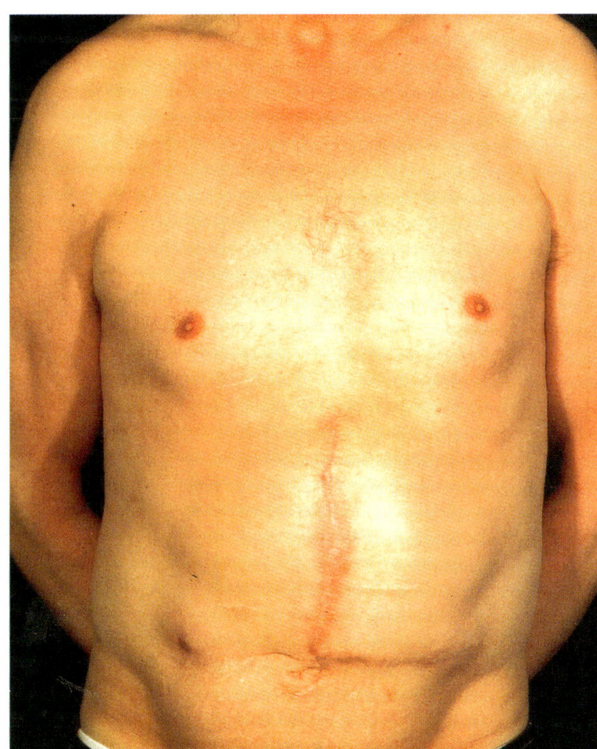

Figure 5.2g Situation three years after surgery

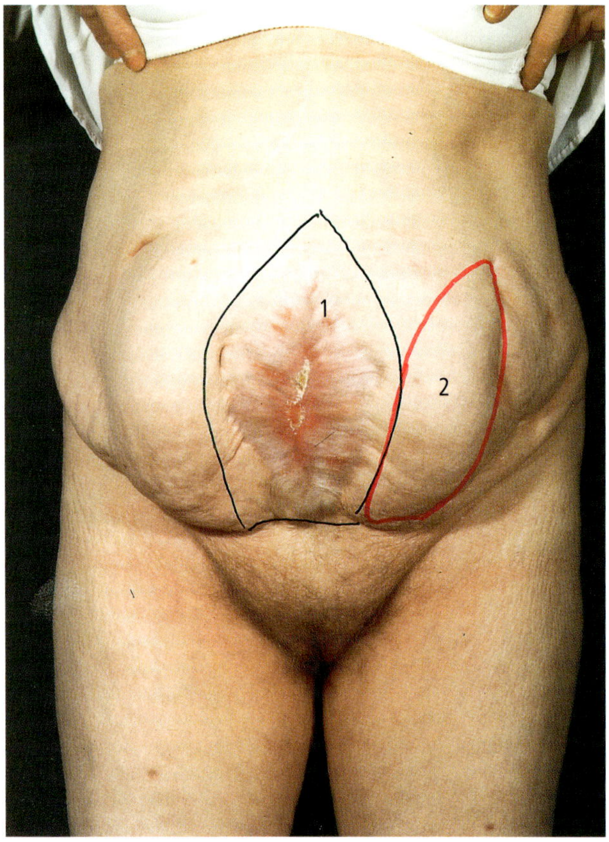

Figure 5.3a Abdominal wall hernia following multiple operations. The bowel is seen directly beneath the large, thin scar. *Planning of the procedure:* Black: Excision of scar tissue and preparation of the hernia edges. Closure of the peritoneum (1). Red: A full-thickness skin graft is harvested and used to close the defect (2).

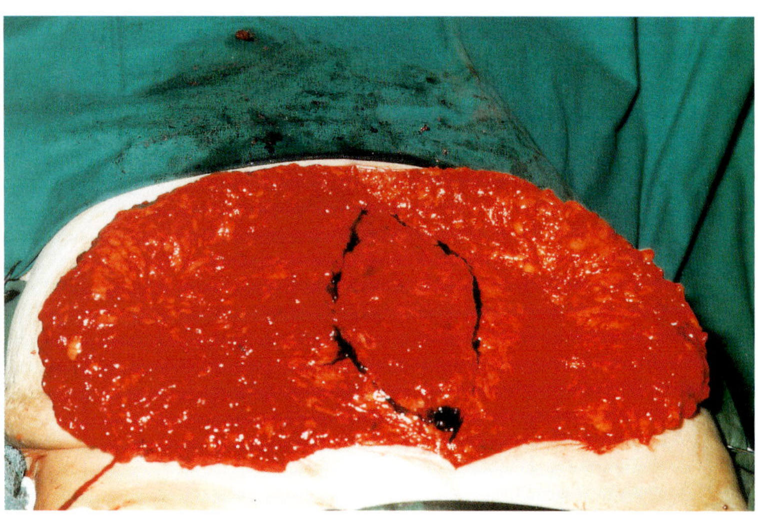

Figure 5.3b The edges of the hernia are prepared and the peritoneum is closed. Black marks: Abdominal wall hernia, will be repaired using the FTSG

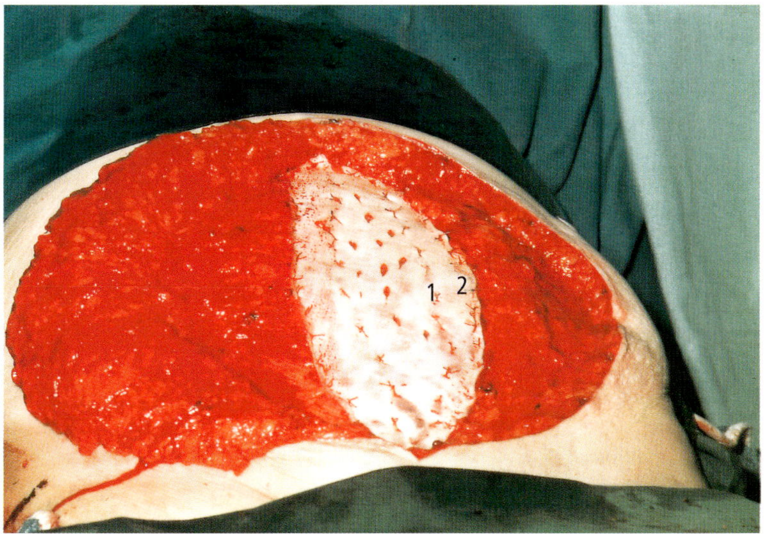

Figure 5.3c The full-thickness skin graft is sutured to the edges of the hernia using non-absorbable suture material (1). Subsequently, the FTSG is fixed using a second row of sutures 3–4 cm lateral to the edge of the hernia (2).

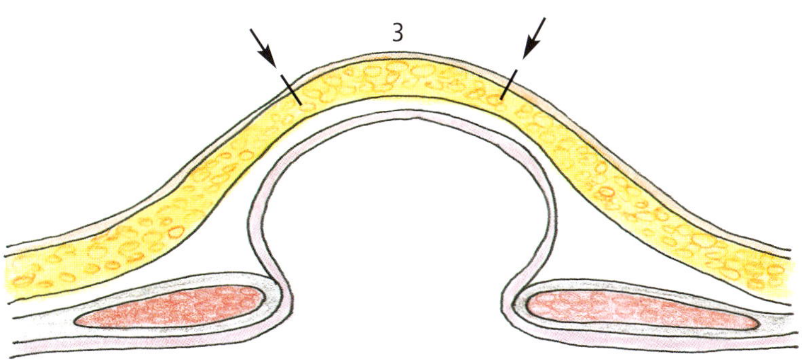

Figure 5.3d The full-thickness skin graft is harvested from the area between the arrows (3).

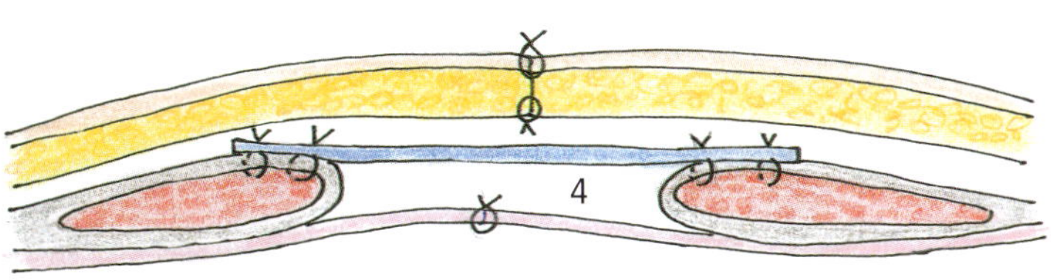

Figure 5.3e The FTSG is fixed to the rectus muscle and its fascia on both sides (two-rows) using non-absorbable suture material (4).

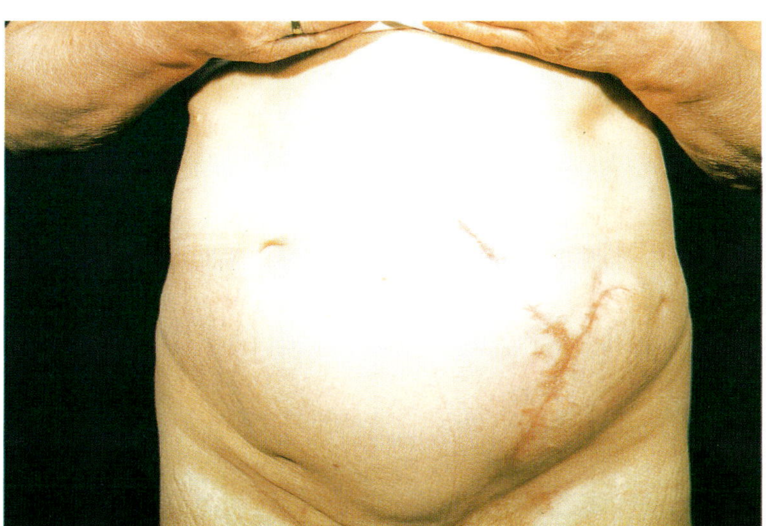

Figure 5.3f Situation six months after the operation: Stable abdominal wall

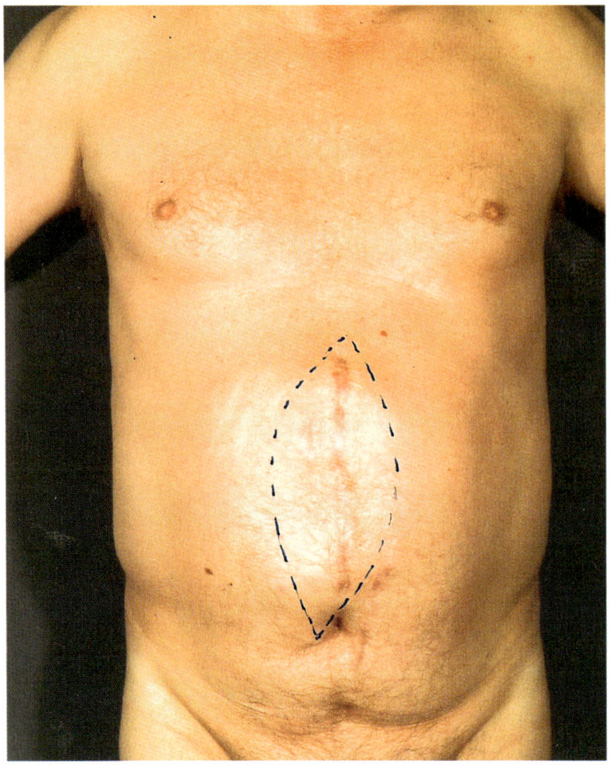

Figure 5.4a Large abdominal wall hernia following three attempts at surgical repair

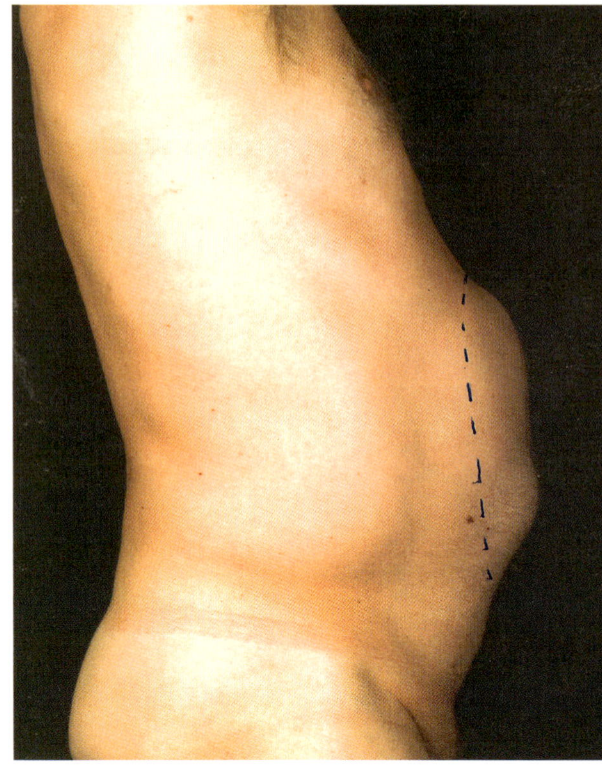

Figure 5.4b Fibrosis and retraction of the rectus muscle resulting from the multiple procedures made it impossible to achieve direct closure. The excess skin was taken as FTSG and used for closure of the large hernia.

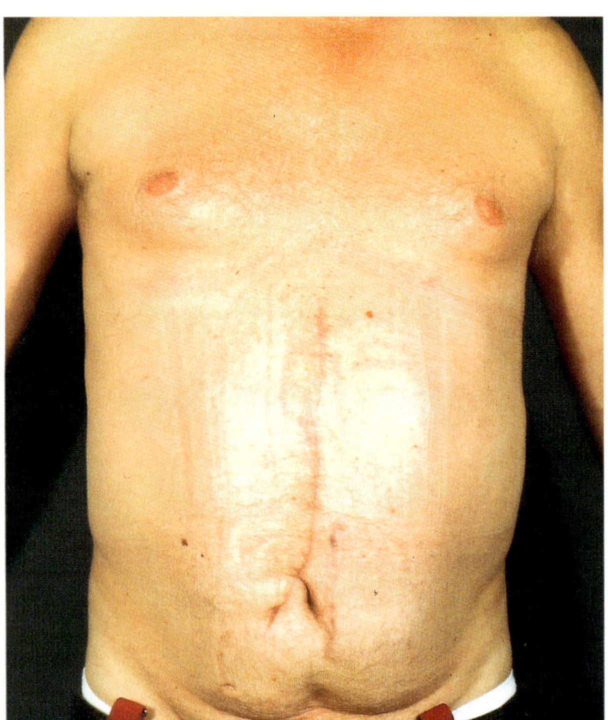

Figure 5.4c Postoperatively, the patient has to wear a supporting bandage for 12 months.

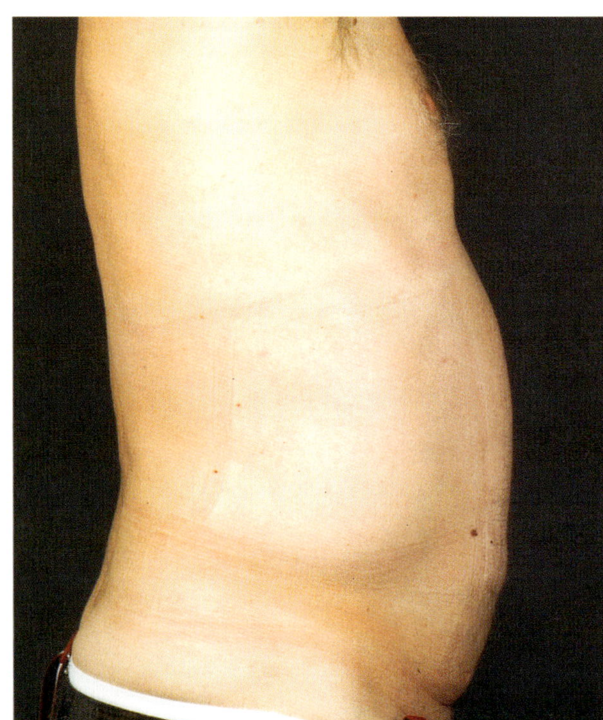

Figure 5.4d Postoperative situation after 12 months

b) Non-Absorbable Prolene® Mesh

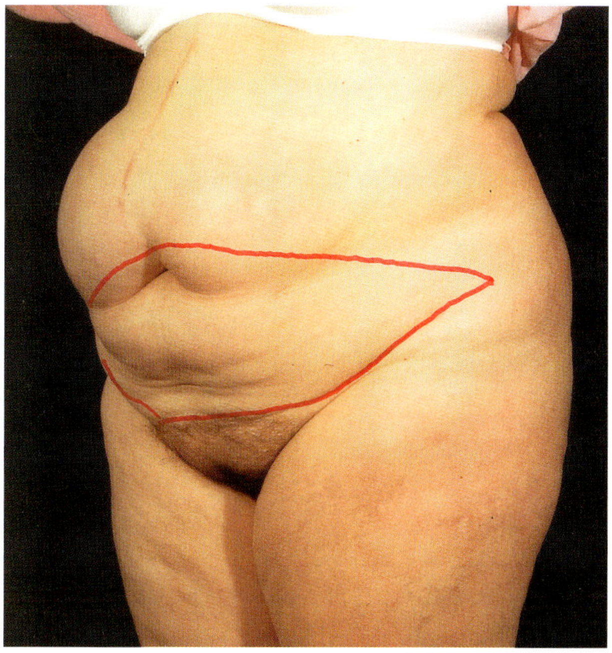

Figure 5.5a Large hernia of the abdominal wall following laparotomy.
Operative planning: The incisions are as for an abdominoplasty procedure. The area outlined by the red marks (1) is resected en bloc (skin and fat). The hernial contents are repositioned the peritoneum is closed. The edge of the hernia is dissected and a non-absorbable Prolene® mesh is fixed to support the abdominal wall.

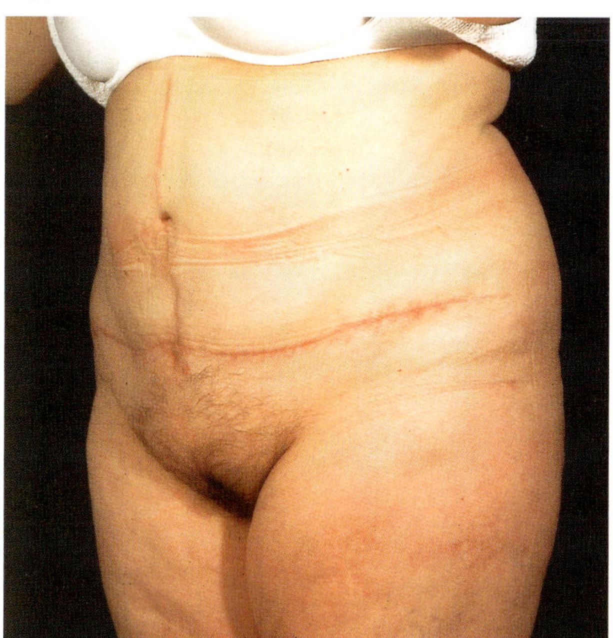

Figure 5.5b Postoperative situation seven months after the operation: Stable abdominal wall

There has been reluctance to use this material. However both plastic surgeons and general surgeons have been convinced by the evident successes of its use. The technique is easy, the procedures can be performed faster than methods using autologous tissue and there is no additional scar formation.

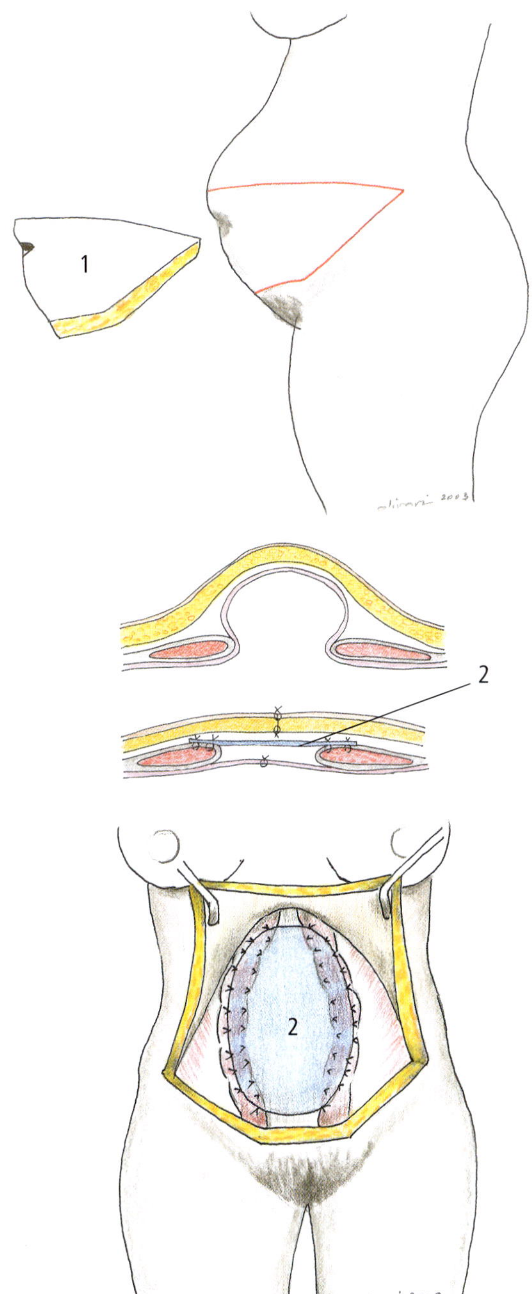

Figure 5.5c Position and fixation of the Prolene® mesh (two-rows of stitches, 2)

c) The Ramirez Procedure

This is a fascinating procedure which works well in slender patients. This technique is problematic in obese patients because of the high intra-abdominal pressure In future, non-absorbable material will probably be used more frequently for the repair of extensive abdominal wall herniation.

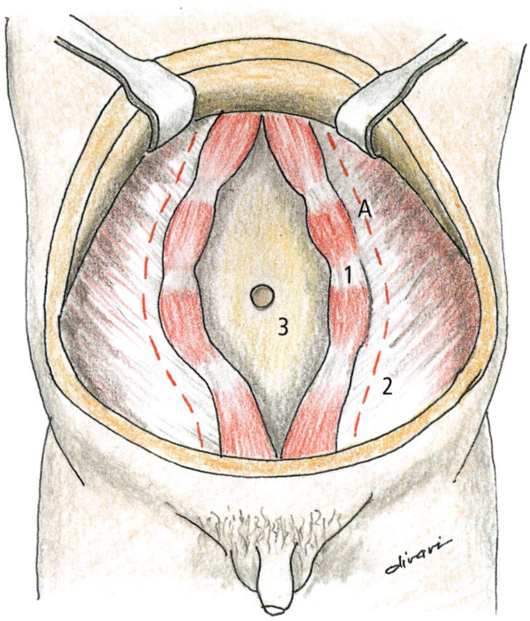

Figure 5.6a

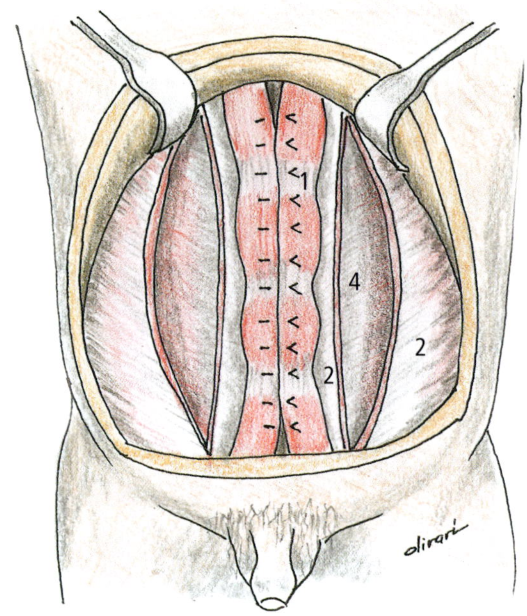

Figure 5.6b

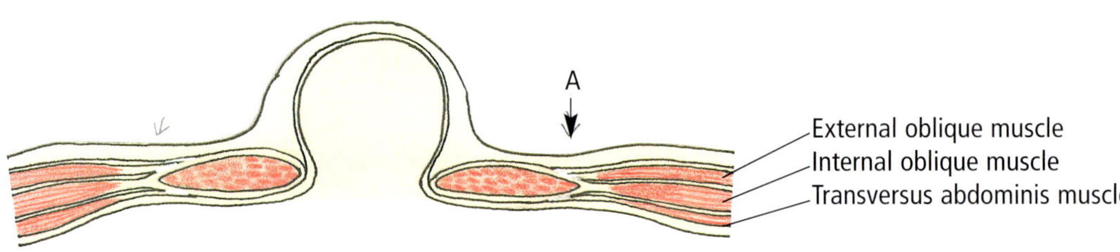

Figure 5.6c

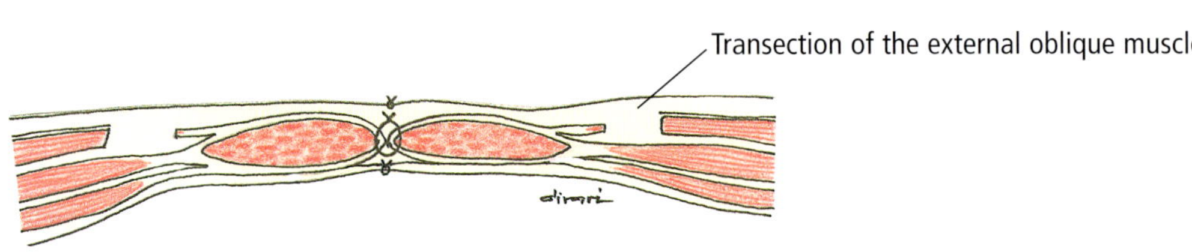

Figure 5.6d

Figure 5.6 a–d The Ramirez procedure: Sagittal transection of the external oblique muscle (red interrupted line – A). The internal oblique muscle and the transversus adominis muscle can be advanced medially by approximately 10 cm on each side. This cannot be done with the external oblique muscle. This method is considered a good choice for relatively slender patients. In very obese patients the use of a Prolene® mesh or a full-thickness skin graft is more suitable. 1) Rectus abdominis muscle, 2) External oblique muscle, 3) Hernia, 4) Internal oblique muscle

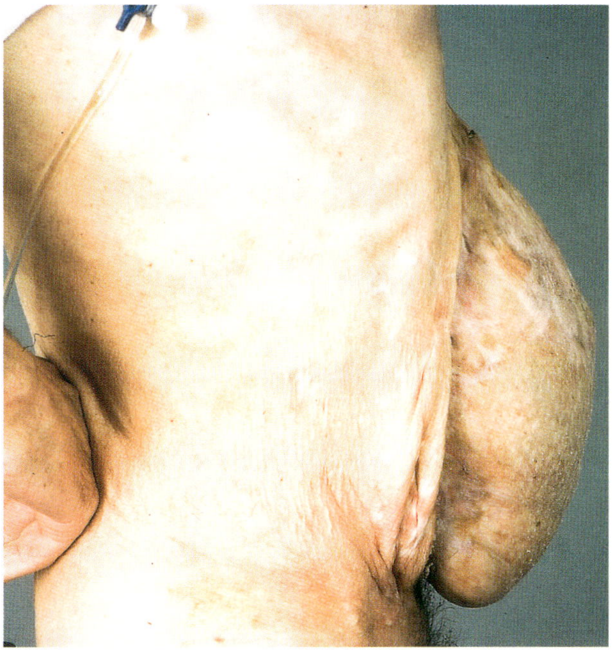

Figure 5.7a Abdominal sepsis and multiple laparotomies resulted in much of the abdominal contents lying outside the cavity. The prolapsed intestinal loops were covered with split-thickness skin grafts. Extensive abdominal wall hernia.

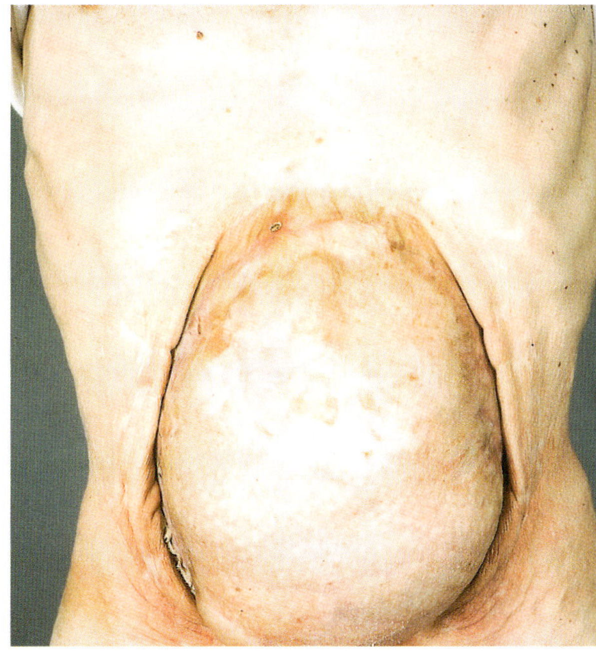

Figure 5.7b The rectus abdominis muscle on both sides was displaced far laterally.

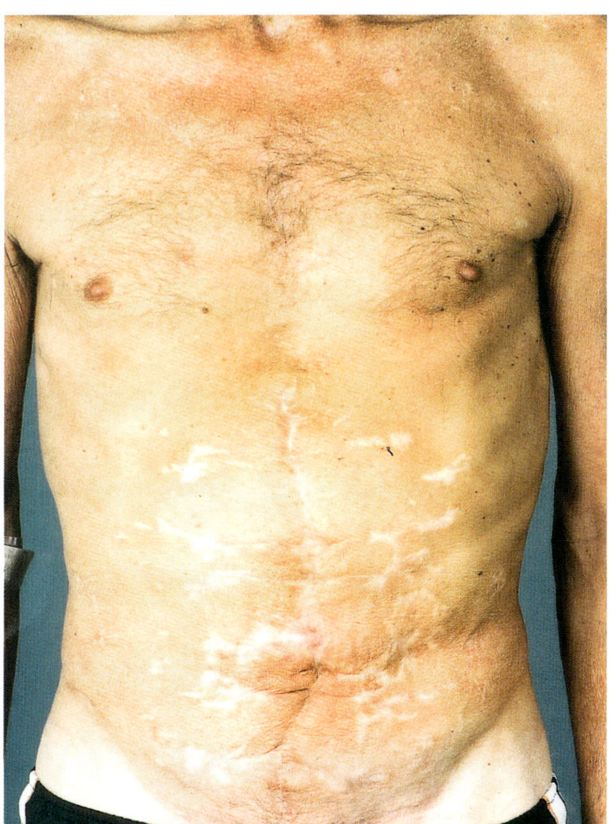

Figure 5.7c Situation one year after the Ramirez procedure

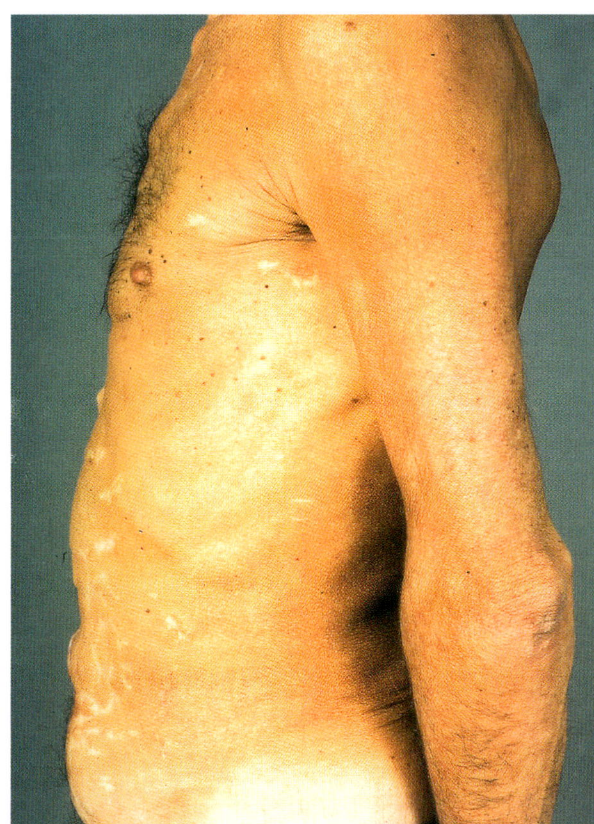

Figure 5.7d Follow-up of the patient one year after the operation

Tumor in the Flank Region

a) Epigastric Flap

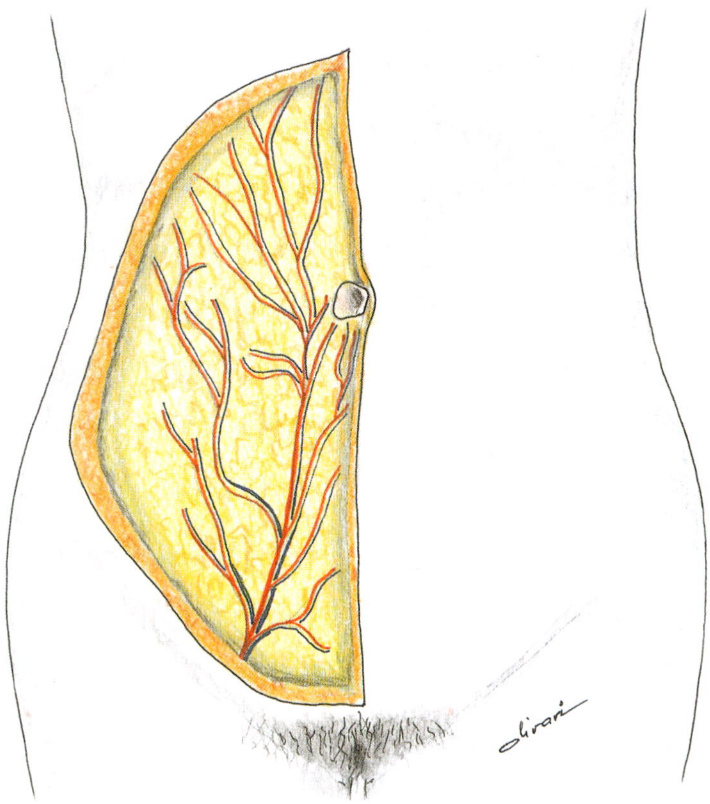

Figure 5.8 Anatomic course of the superficial inferior epigastric artery. It is the dominant vessel for the epigastric flap. The epigastric flap as an axial-pattern flap is well suited for coverage of local defects. Recently, this flap has also been used as a free flap.

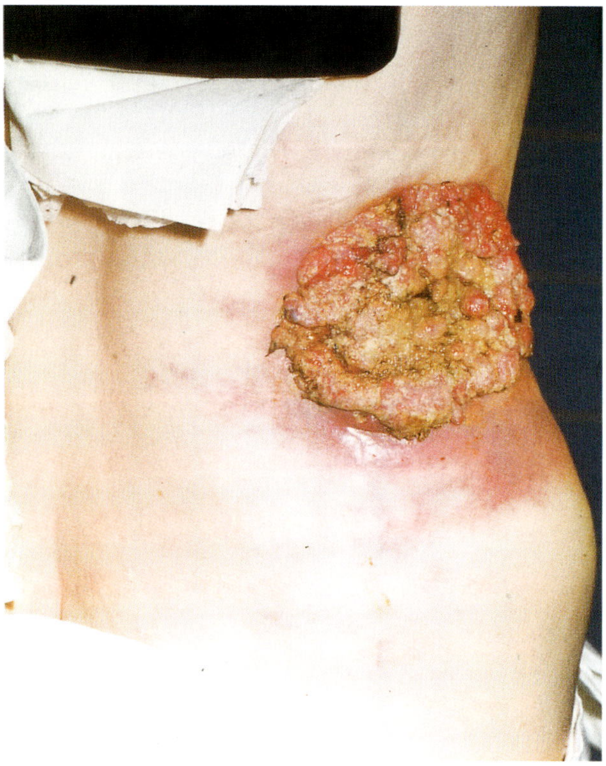

Figure 5.9a Squamous cell carcinoma of the right flank: Five years history.

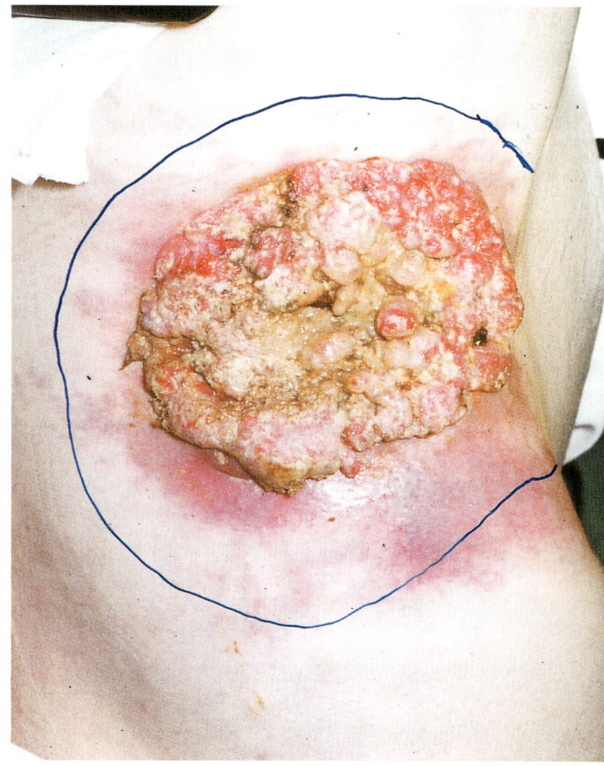

Figure 5.9b Extent of the excision

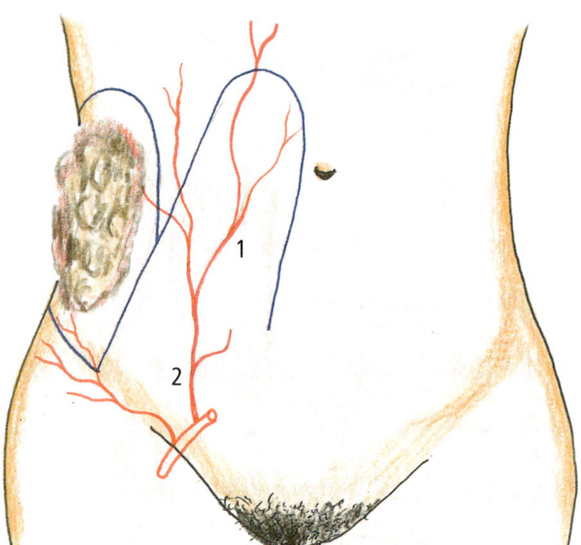

Figure 5.9c Operative planning: An epigastric flap (1) with the superficial inferior epigastric artery as the dominant vessel (2) is designed.

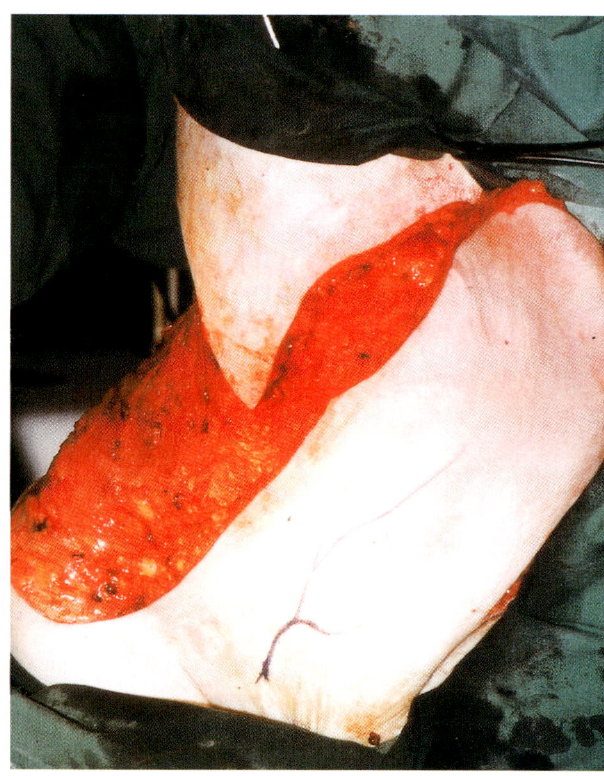

Figure 5.9d The large tumour is excised. The defect measures 20 × 18 cm. The flap size is 25 × 17 cm.

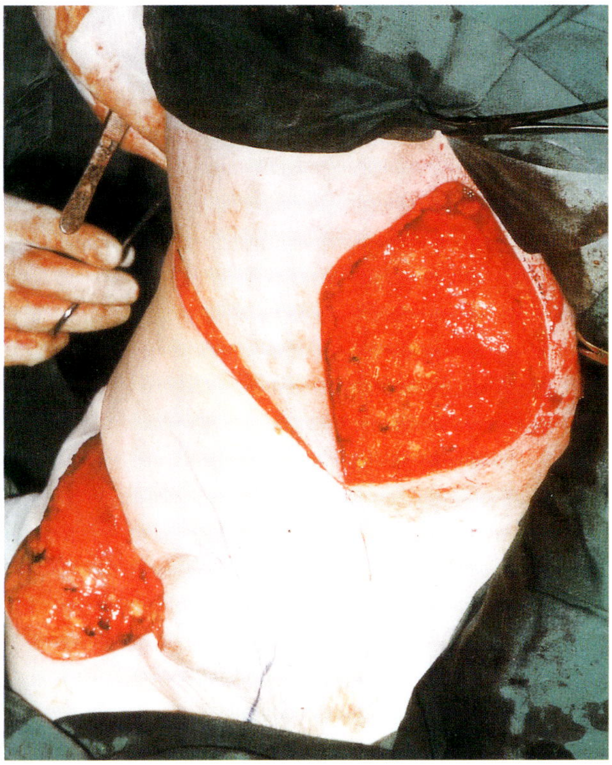

Figure 5.9e The epigastric flap is transposed into the defect after mobilisation. It is important to carry out extensive mobilisation of the skin on the contralateral side of abdominal skin and free the umbilicus.

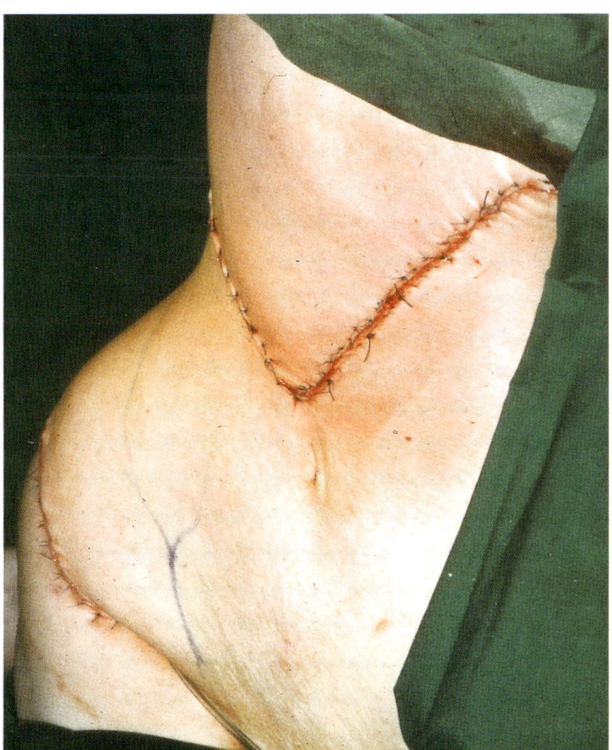

Figure 5.9f Situation at the end of the operation. Primary closure of the donor site defect was possible.

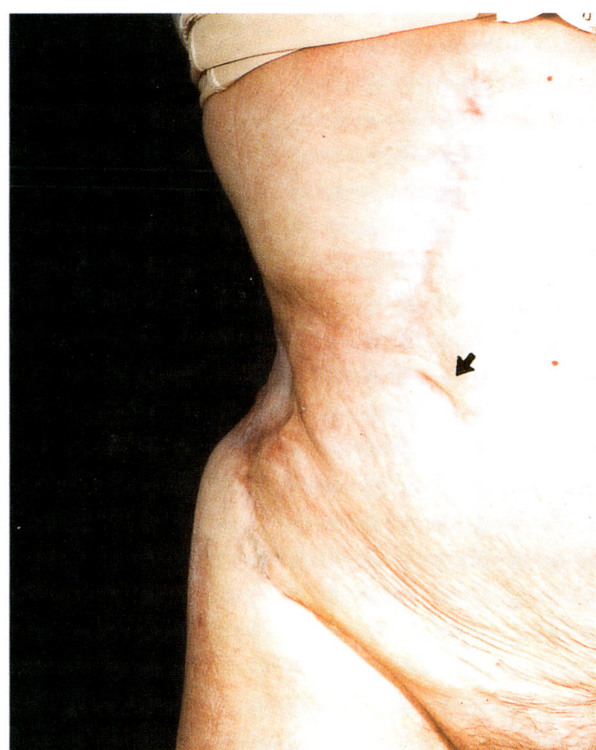

Figure 5.9g The patient six years after the operation. There is a significant displacement of the umbilicus (arrow) due to the necessary mobilisation.

Obesity

Obesity is a problem of modern times. Obesity is caused by

- more and more fast-food companies offering unappetizing fat and sugar-rich, cheap food.
- less and less physical activity
- TV and PC support this development

Obesity originates in the childhood. Children do less and play less out of doors. They sit in front of the PC playing stupid games that have been given to them by their parents or relatives instead of playing soccer. In addition, it is easier for many parents to send their children to McDonald's rather than cooking at home. The problem of obesity in children has on the increased greatly during the last 30 years (an increase of 25 % of the average body weight is estimated). Once obesity has occurred in childhood it is extremely difficult to correct. Success of treatment is about 20 % (in adults 15 %).

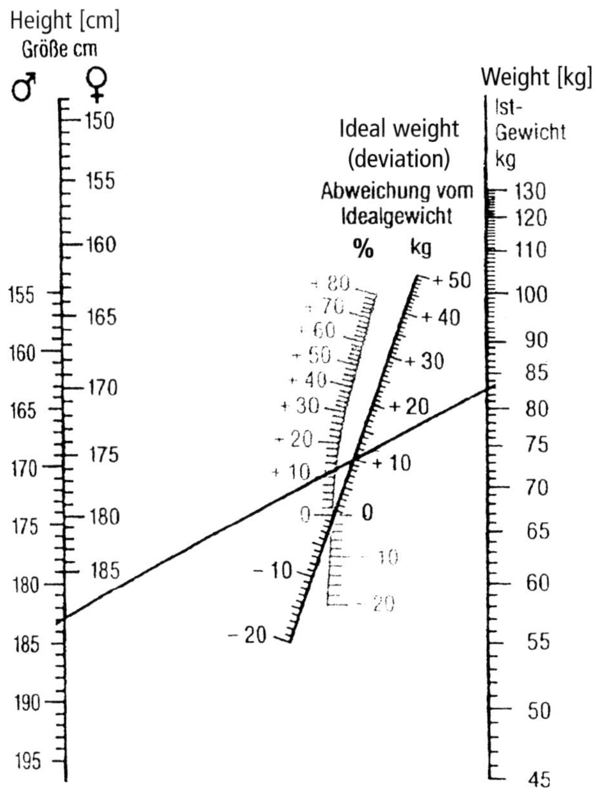

Figure 5.10 Nomogram (Broca's chart) for determining deviation from ideal weight (SD ± 5 %)

There are two ways of assessing if someone is overweight:

1. Broca's chart
The body weight and body height are measured and analyzed using a nomogram. Over and underweight can be assessed.

2. Body-mass index (BMI)
Recently, this method has become widely used; the body weight in kg is divided by the body height in meters, for example:

A woman who weighs 60 kg and is 1.65 m tall has BMI of 22

$$\frac{60}{1.65 \times 1.65} = \frac{60}{2.7} = \text{BMI } 22$$

or 90 kg body weight and 1.65 m height results in a BMI of 33

$$\frac{90}{2.7} = \text{BMI } 33$$

Table 5.1 Classification of body weight using the BMI

BMI	Body Weight
18–25	acceptable
26–30	marginal
31–35	overweight
36–40	severely overweight
40 and over	morbid obesity

Morbid obesity needs urgent treatment. The BMI has to be evaluated for each individual. A muscular, fit man is not overweight if he has a BMI of 30 whereas a little girl with a BMI of 25 is overweight. Severe overweight and morbid obesity are resistant to therapy. The success rate of conservative treatment is disappointingly low (15 %).

Morbid Obesity

Obesity with a BMI over 40 is considered a disease and requires specific treatment in an obesity centre. If dietary measures are not successful, surgical options such as gastric balloon, gastric bypass and gastric banding must be considered. Unfortunately the success of dietary measures in morbid obesity is low.

Sometimes, surgical fat removal is indicated if the anticipated weight of the resected tissue is 20 kg or more, even if dietary measures were ineffective. The thorax can be affected by a weight of 20 kg and more of abdominal fat with well known consequences. This is not an easy decision and the pros and cons have to be balanced carefully. However, the plastic surgeon cannot shirk his responsibility. In these cases, morbid obesity is "viewed as a huge lipoma, which compresses important organs" (Olivari).

Cooperation between dieticians, general surgeons and plastic surgeons is essential. Also, these patients represent a big challenge for the anesthesiologist.

Therapy
a) Liposuction

"Liposuction, the most popular of all aesthetic surgical procedures, has now come of age as a refined aesthetic tool. Technology and artistry have combined to enable the surgeon to sculpt the human form with accuracy, consistency, and safety." This quotation from a book about liposuction is very far from reality. Of all the aesthetic surgery procedures it has the highest complication rate at 9 % [Olbrisch 2004].

The idea of liposuction originally stems from Schrudde (1973), who removed undesirable accumulations of adipose tissue through a small incision using a curette.

The current method of liposuction was invented and developed by Kesselring (1976), who connected a large-bore cannula to a vacuum pump.

Everybody who has become famous for liposuction since has either used variations in the size of the cannula or administered additional fluids into the affected area or modified the original idea by the use of ultrasound.

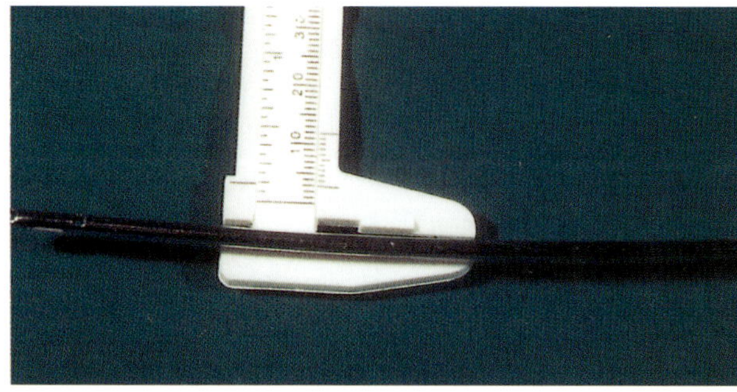

Figure 5.11 Liposuction cannula

Principles of liposuction.

1) Fine cannula 2–4 mm diameter.
2) Wet or super-wet technique. The tissue is infiltrated with either the exact or double the volume of fluid that one wishes to aspirate (Klein's tumescence technique). Standard fluid contains isotonic saline solution, epinephrine, bicarbonate and a local anesthetic. Postoperative swelling can be reduced by the addition of corticosteroid in this solution.
3) Light vacuum, depending on the site 0.2 to 0.5 bar.
4) Deep and superficial liposuction technique.
5) Combination of various instruments:
   - Ultrasound-assisted liposuction

   This can work well for the gentle aspiration of deeper fat. However, the ultrasound technique is not suitable for superficial liposuction because of the heat generation (skin necrosis)
   - Vibrating cannulae

   This is a precise technique especially useful in fibrotic or scarred tissue. A mechanical stroke-and-rotate motion is used (driven by electricity or compressed-air). Also, they spare the surgeon's arm. A good indication is the treatment of gynecomasty.

It must not be forgotten that liposuction induces a considerable inner wound area, which equals a significant trauma.

Even though some colleagues report aspirated volumes of 10 litres in one liposuction session, we strongly advise against these extremes.

Literature shows that currently about 500,000 patients in the United States and approximately 200,000 patients per year in Germany undergo liposuction.

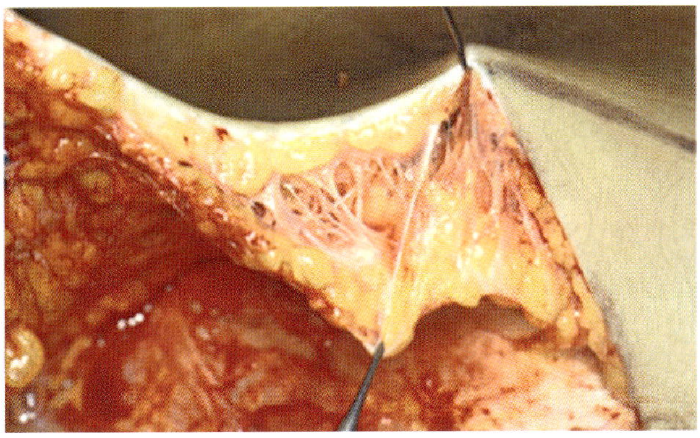

Figure 5.12 Note the absent fatty tissue and the spared septa containing the vessels and nerves after liposuction.

Complications of liposuction:

1)	Bleeding	approx. 1.0 %
2)	Local infection	1.0 %
3)	Lymphatic fistulae, seroma	1.5 %
4)	Superficial irregularities of the skin as a result of uneven liposuction (contour deformity)	10–20 %

5) Lethal DVT and PE (rare)
6) Rarely death results from toxic doses of local anesthetics
7) Local dysesthesia is common, but temporary in most cases
8) Deaths resulting from septicemia and fasciitis
9) Perforation of intestine

In 1999, 95 deaths were reported in the United States following liposuction; this is one fatality in 5000 procedures. In Germany, 12 deaths and 53 severe complications such as sepsis, bowel perforation, necrotizing fasciitis, skin necrosis, abdominal wall hernias, emboli and pulmonary edema have been reported in the period from 1998–2000 [Lehnhardt et al. 2004]. Of these 53 severe complications, 47 were operated as outpatients and six patients underwent liposuction as inpatients.

If one counts the frequent deformities after liposuction as well as the severe complications, the overall rate is 9 %, which is the highest of the aesthetic surgery procedures [Olbrisch 2004]. The deformities that occur after liposuction are rarely correctable.

Liposuction is being performed by dermatologists, gynecologists, ENT surgeons and even GP's. Quality control is non-existent, and there is no certification of adequate training.

Lehnhardt has reported aspirate volumes of up to 25 litres in one session. The indications are uncritical. Every patient is accepted. The author, an "old-fashioned" surgeon, has accepted less than 20 % of the patients desiring a liposuction.

The risk of a complication increases:

a) if more than three litres of fat tissue are aspirated in one session
b) if abdominoplasty and extensive liposuction are performed at the same time
c) if very large areas are operated on under local anesthesia
d) if the patient is older than 50 years
e) if there is a history of thrombosis

The indication for liposuction is the treatment of localised problem areas. Severe obesity must not be treated with liposuction!

Extensive liposuctions should be performed under general anesthesia. Some surgeons recommend this in all cases, because the production of dangerous methemoglobin increases when large amounts of local anesthetic is used. The amount of local anesthetic necessary is less under general anesthesia because of the modern postoperative pain control.

In some regions of the body (e.g. the abdomen), fat is divided into deep and superficial (1) layers by a fat fascia (Figure 5.13). For deep fat, a 4 mm cannula is used, superficial fat is treated with 2 mm cannula. Superficial wrinkle formation results when only the deep layers are liposuctioned.

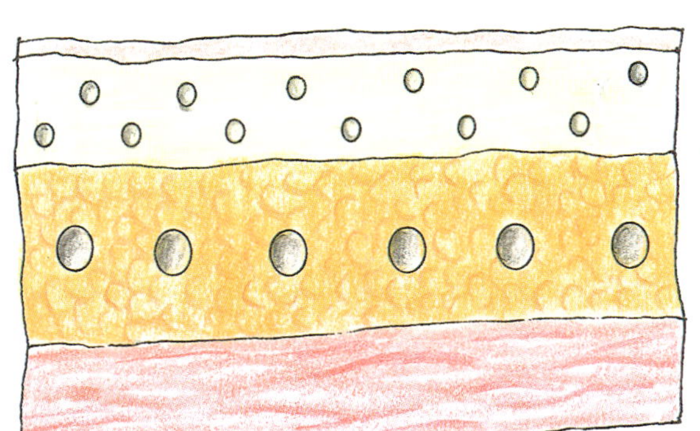

Figure 5.13 Layers of adipose tissue

Schematic Depiction of Liposuction (Idealized)

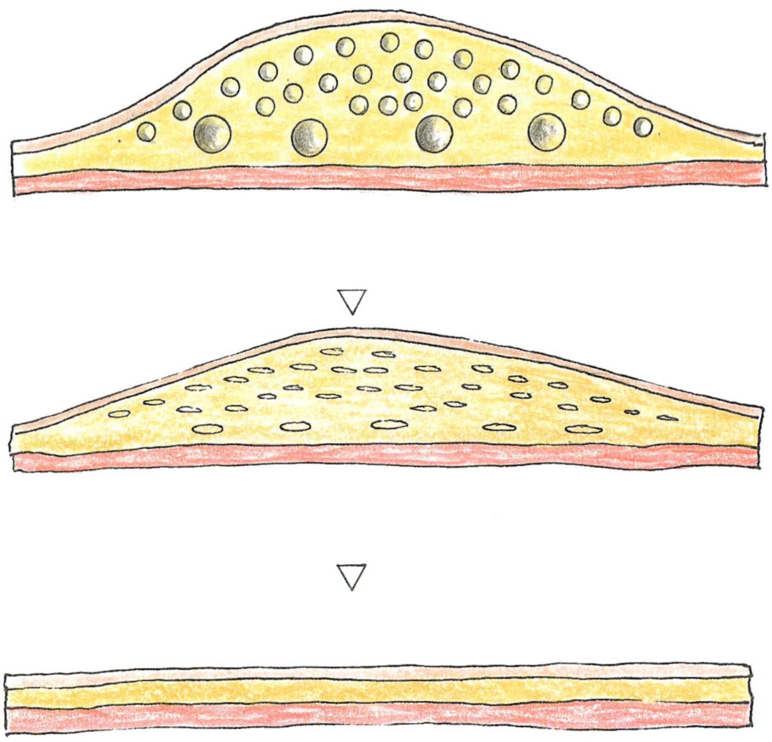

a

b

c

Figure 5.14
a) Deep fat is suctioned using 4 mm cannula, superficial fat is suctioned using 2 mm cannula.

b) Sometimes the skin is sufficiently elastic and shrinks without the formation of wrinkles or superficial irregularities.

c) The fat is suctioned, the oedema is gone and the elastic skin has adapted to the new form.

This idealized schema only applies to selective patients; be careful. If the skin is wrinkled before the procedure, the combination of lipectomy and liposuction is the better choice.

Infiltration in Liposuction

The technique of the traditional "dry" liposuction resulted in high blood loss 15 to 20 % of the aspirated volume, therefore only smaller areas could be dry liposucked.

Since Fodor (1986) and Klein (1987) developed the so-called "tumescent" technique, the blood loss has been drastically reduced (1 to 5 % of the aspirated volume). Tumescence solution is injected into the aspiration region in a 1:1 ratio, which means that if one litre of adipose tissue is to be aspirated, the area is infiltrated with one litre of tumescence solution. A solution-to-aspirate ratio of higher than 1:1 can be toxic, especially in the case of larger liposuction amounts (>4 litres).

The Klein formula for infiltration:

1000 ml	Saline (isotonic)
50 ml	Lidocaine 1 %
1 ml	Epinephrine 1:1000
12.5 ml	Sodium bicarbonate 8.4 %

Fodor's formula for infiltration

Ringer's lactate solution	1000 ml
1 ml epinephrine	1/500 (liposuction <2000 ml)
1 ml epinephrine	1/1000 (liposuction 2000–4000 ml)

Recipes for infiltration solutions vary from one author to another and by the time this book is published there are bound to be other recommendations which may be preferable. In extensive liposuction (>4 litres), thorough volume replacement and postoperative monitoring in hospital is essential.

The use of halothane for general anesthesia is not recommended because it can cause cardiac arrhythmia in combination with epinephrine.

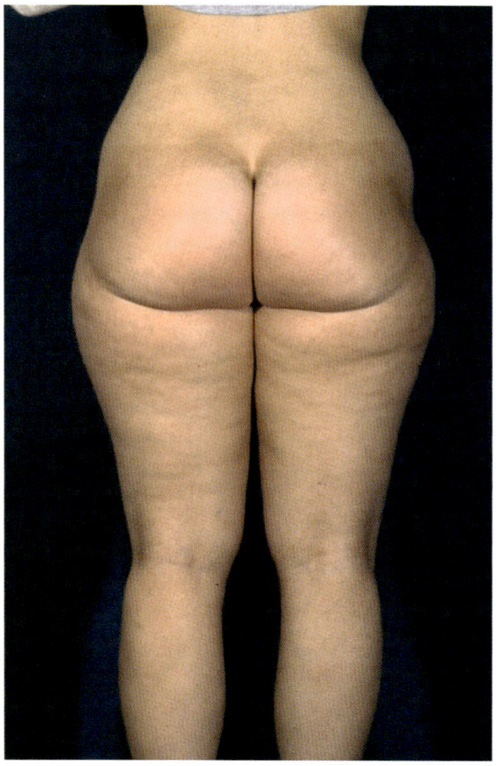

Figure 5.15a Local "saddle-bag" deformity, genetic etiology. This is a good indication for liposuction.

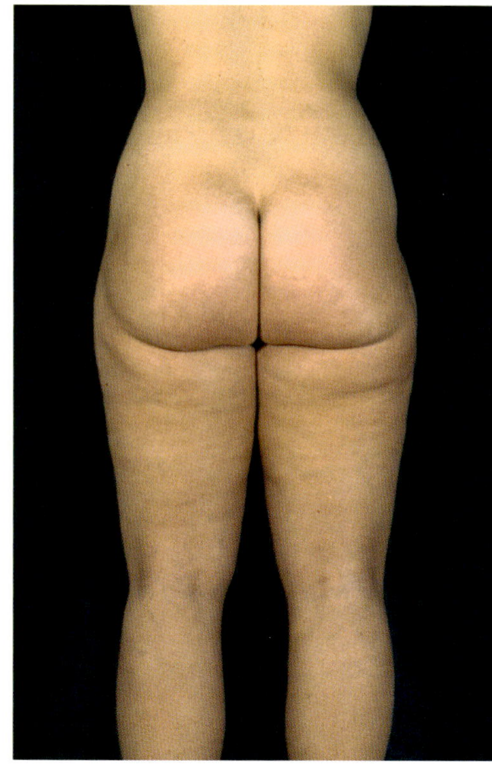

Figure 5.15b Situation after liposuction

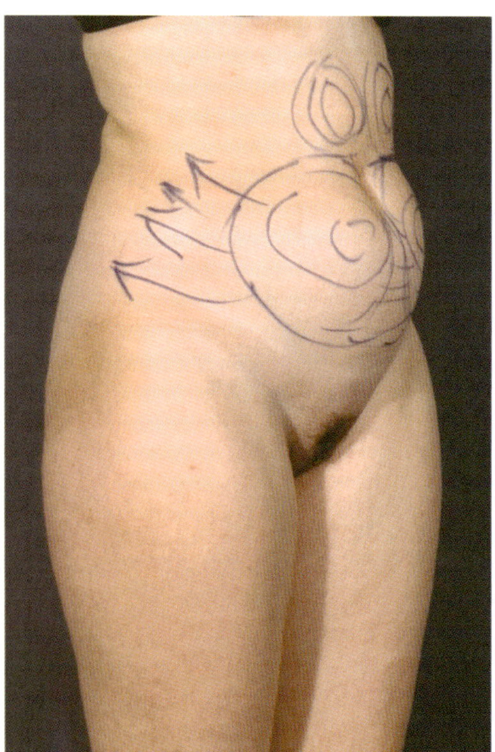

Figure 5.16a Isolated adiposity in the lower abdominal area. Ideal indication for liposuction. No distasis of the rectus muscle, elastic skin, young patient.

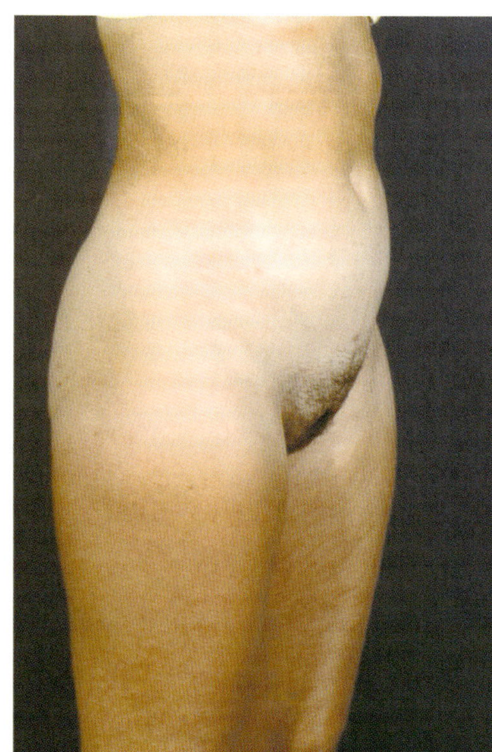

Figure 5.16b Situation post liposuction

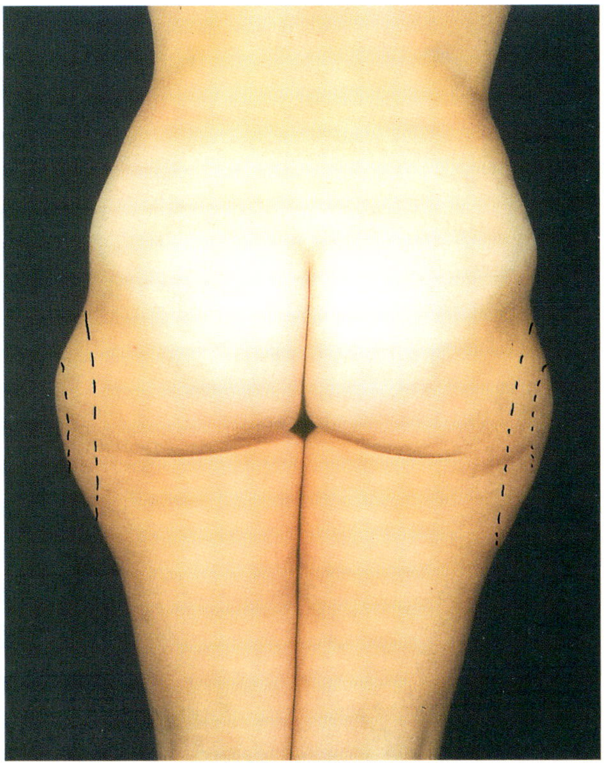

Figure 5.17a Genetically determined local lipodystrophy. This deformity cannot be corrected by dietetic measures. It is an ideal indication for liposuction. Great advantage is elastic skin in young female patients.

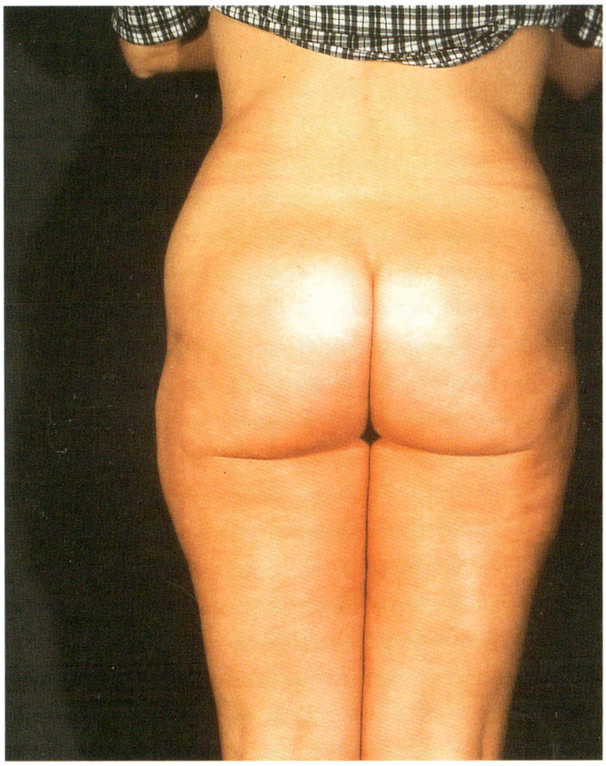

Figure 5.17b Situation one year after liposuction: Clear improvement of the body contour.

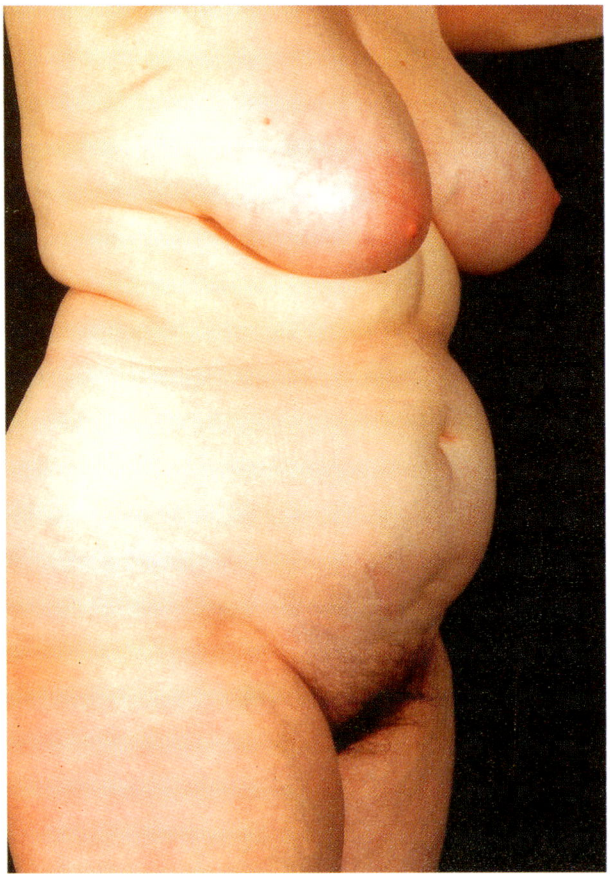

Figure 5.18a Liposuction of abdominal area and breast reduction.
Relative indication for liposuction in adipose abdomen. Here should be liposucted deep and superficial fat tissue. In case of rectus diastasis there is no indication for liposuction.

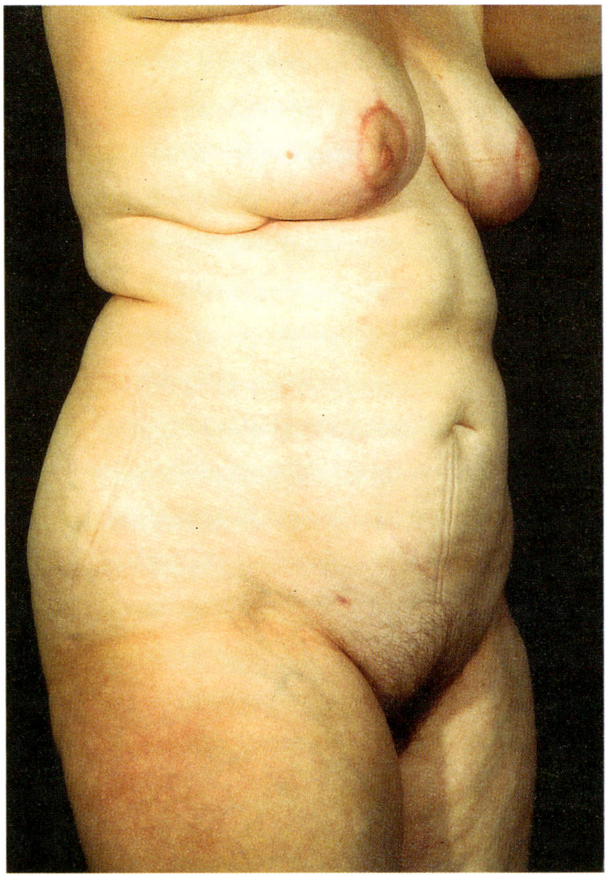

Figure 5.18b Situation six months after liposuction of abdominal area and simultaneously breast reduction.

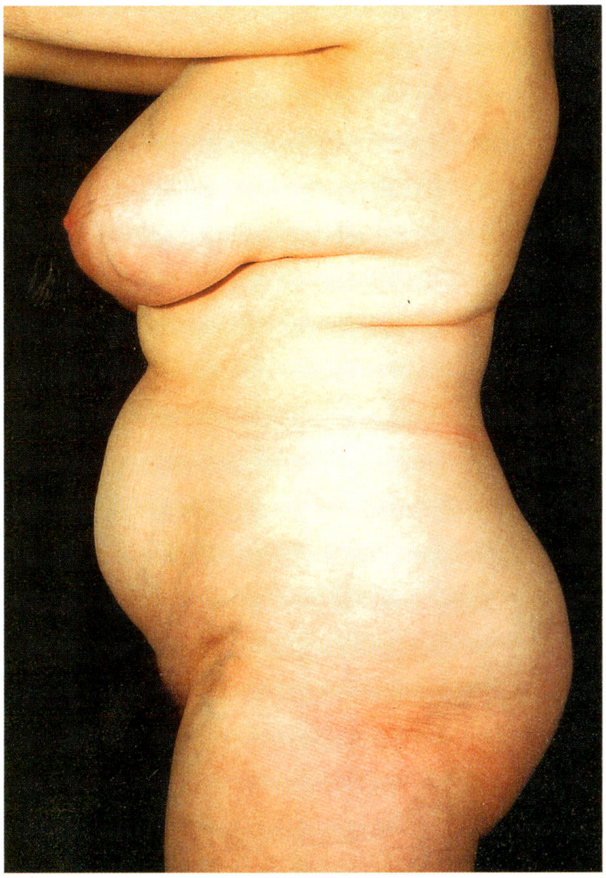

Figure 5.18c The same patient preoperative in profile

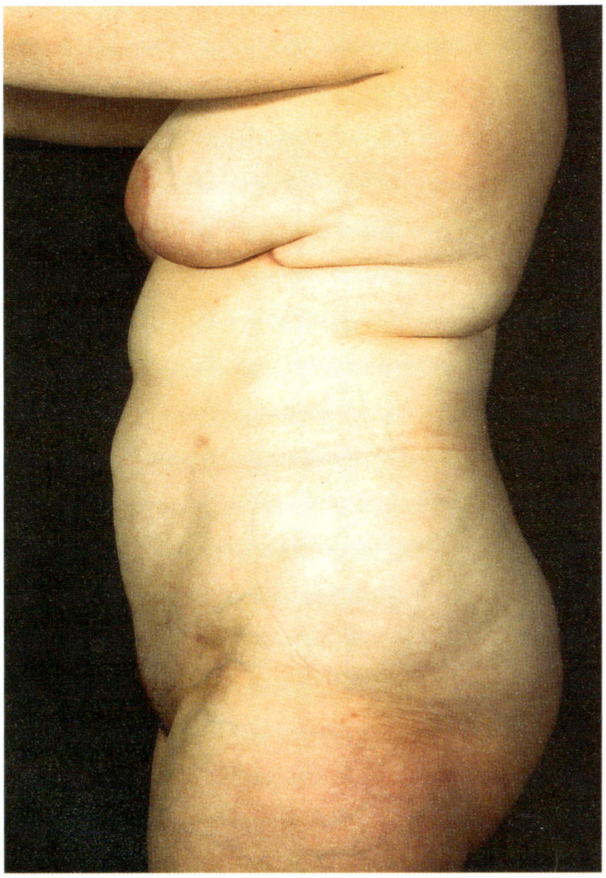

Figure 5.18d Postoperative in profile. Liposuction from abdomen (approximately 2.7 litres). Breast reduction 900 gram per site. Result: Almost good.

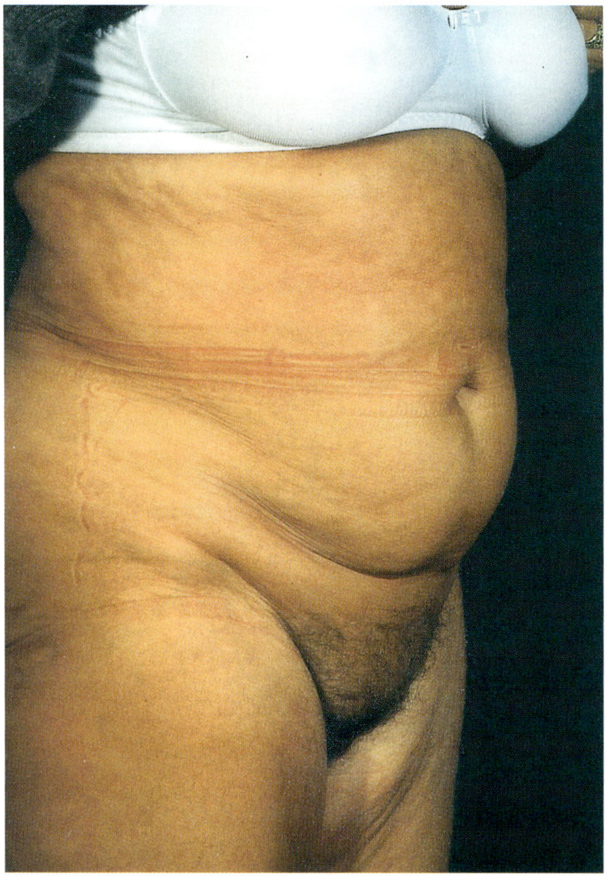

Figure 5.19a Alimentary local accumulation of fat in the abdominal and flank region

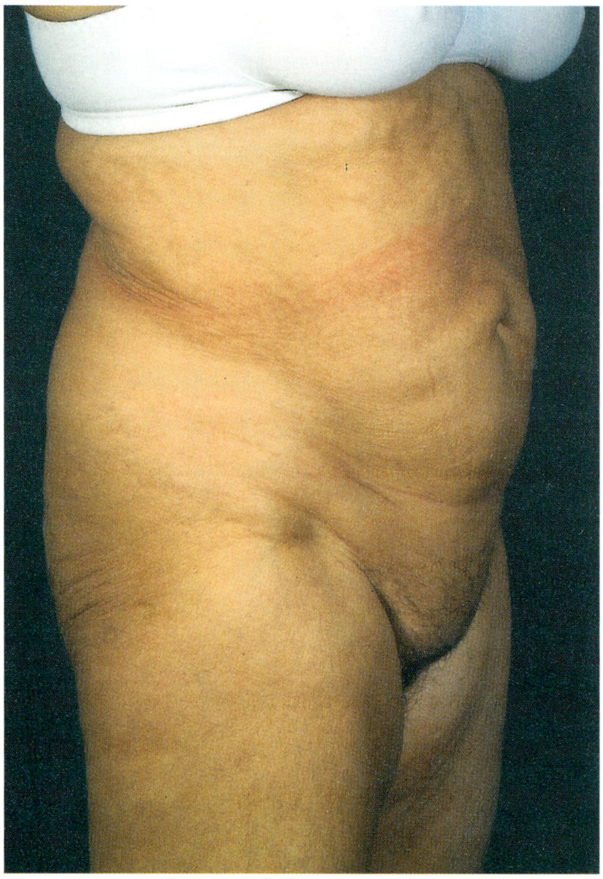

Figure 5.19b Deep and superficial liposuction can induce contraction of the skin (not always) which can improve skin contour.

b) Abdominolipectomy

Indication

Usually, abdominolipectomy is done for aesthetic reasons. Frequently there is an adjacent medical indication:

a) Recurrent intertrigo in the abdominal fold area
b) Status post marked reduction of body weight with extensive "apron-like" excessive abdominal fat and skin, inhibition of motion and rubbing of the excessive skin leading to superficial skin arosions
c) The indication is limited in adipose patients with extreme excess abdominal fat and/or hernia who do not lose weight despite multiple diet attempts

It is known that only 15 % of the patients suffering from obesity can durably reduce their body weight.

Aesthetic deformities of the abdominal wall, which can be improved by a surgical procedure:

1) Lax abdominal skin with marked formation of an abdominal fold and striae without accumulation of fat and without rectus muscle diastasis, most frequently after multiple pregnancies. For the surgeon, this patient collective is very thankful. The procedure is technically easy and the results are good.
2) Lax abdominal skin with rectus muscle diastasis. Besides the resection of the skin fat layer a rectus fascia suture is necessary.
3) Local accumulation of fat in the lower abdominal region with tight-elastic skin, without rectus rectus diastasis. In this case, a liposuction or a smaller resection in the caudal area combined with liposuction is indicated.
4) Marked excessive skin fat with "hanging tummy" and rectus muscle diastasis. In these cases, abdominolipectomy, frequently in combination with regional liposuction is indicated; also, suture of rectus fascia is indicated.

Preoperative Treatment

1) Heavily obese patients are escorted through a weight-loss program, which is best done with the help of dieticians, who also take the psychological treatment of the patients into account (Obesity Centres).
   If necessary, weight loss should be induced by the use of gastric balloon implantation or a gastric-bypass operation by visceral surgeon.
2) The timely referral to the anesthesiology service to check the operability is absolutely necessary.
3) The day before the procedure, the intestine has to be thoroughly cleaned (just like before a colonic procedure). A raise in the intra abdominal pressure results mainly from the suturing of rectus diastasis, which can favour venous thrombosis and pulmonary embolism (rare, but dramatic complication). The postoperative phase is easier without a filled abdomen.

Surgical Technique

The surgical technique depends on the deformity. Resection of the skin fat layer from the pubic hair line up to the region superior to the umbilicus is a standard method. The incisions vary due to the local specifities, but the concave upward-oriented arc-like incision is most of the times a good decision. However, fashion is playing a role in these circumstances (bathing suit!).

Abdominolipectomy Without Transposition of the Umbilicus, Without Suture of Rectus Fascia With Additional Selective Regional Liposuction

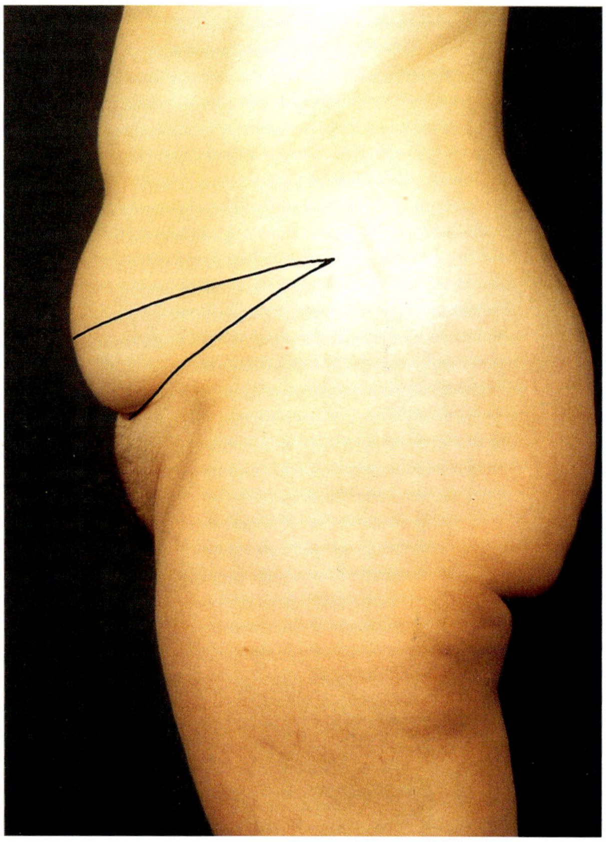

Figure 5.20a Lax, fairly adipose abdominal wall, no rectus muscle diastasis. Problem zone: Lower abdomen.

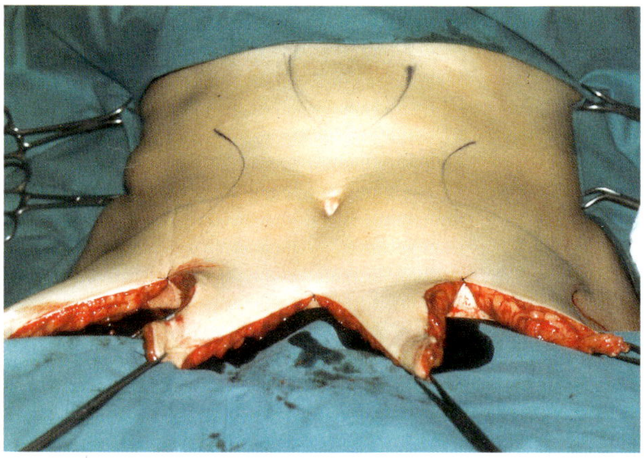

Figure 5.20b Mobilisation of the abdominal wall up to the umbilical height. The regions of the upper abdomen are marked for liposuction. No extensive mobilization of the tissue!

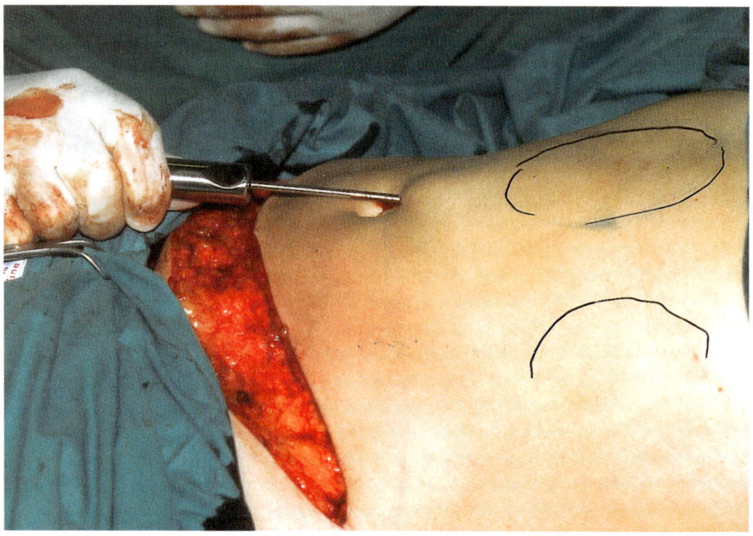

Figure 5.20c Liposuction in the middle upper abdominal region and in both lateral abdominal wall areas after resection of the excessive skin fat layer. The liposuction is done through a small umbilical incision.

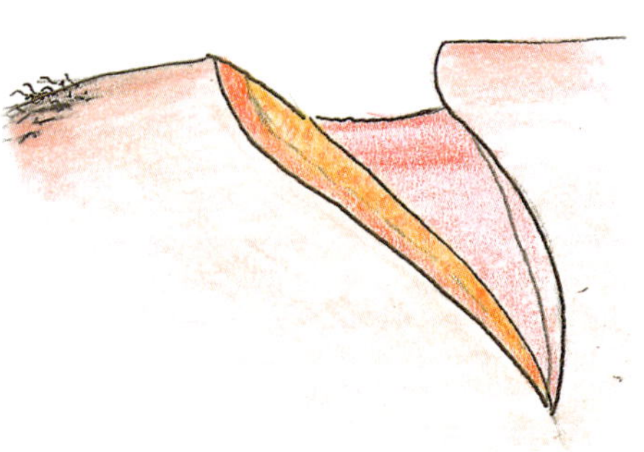

Figure 5.20d The caudal area is cut oblique to avoid retraction of the scar.

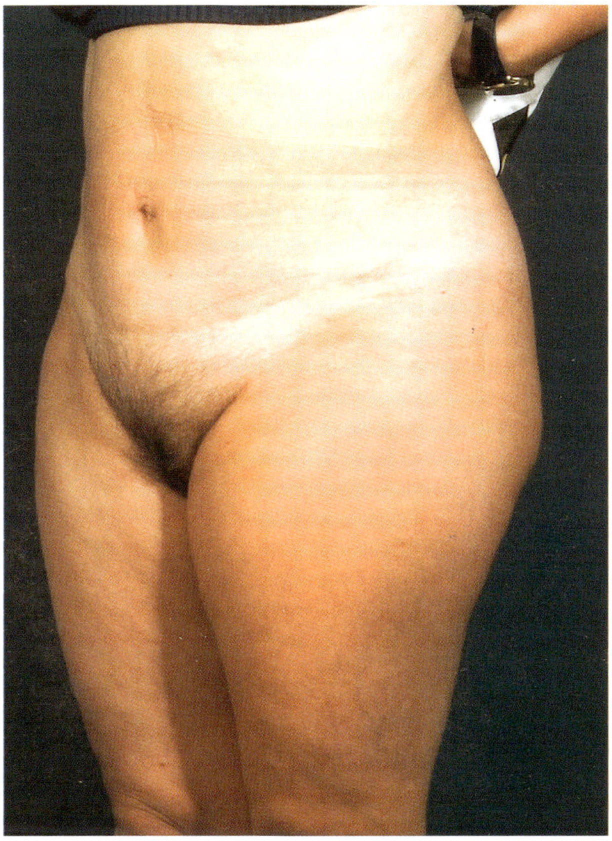

Figure 5.20e Status two years after the procedure. No retraction of the scar. Good result combining a smaller resection of the skin-fat layer and selective liposuction of the upper abdomen.

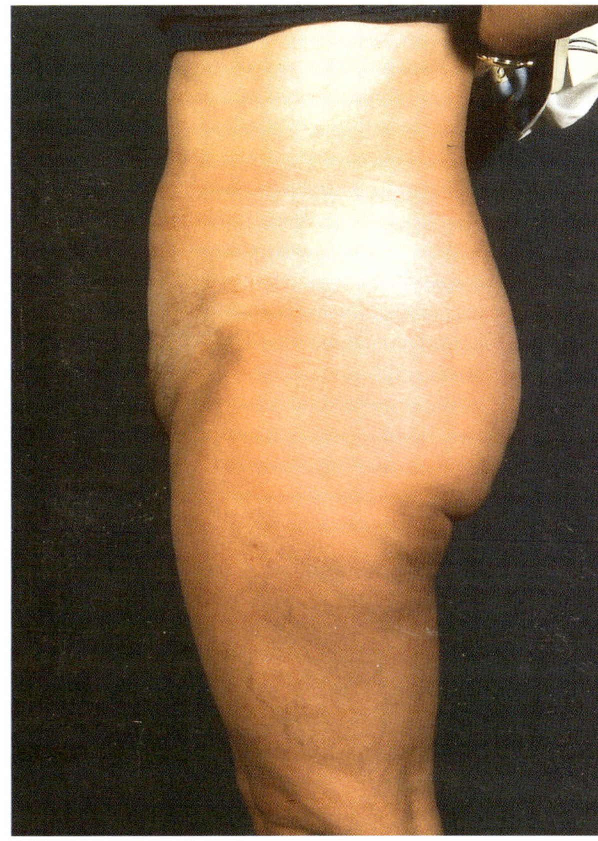

Figure 5.20f Lateral aspect

Abdominolipectomy With Transposition of the Umbilicus, Suture of Rectus Fascia and Selective Liposuction

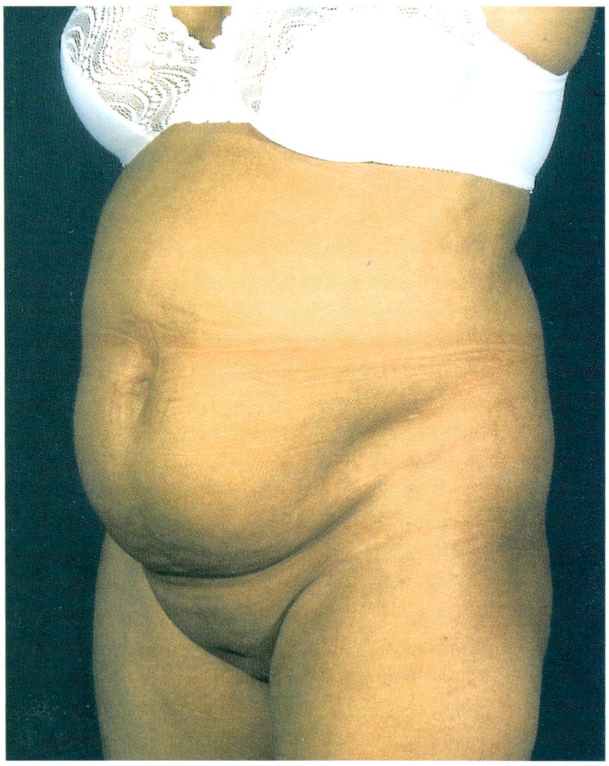

Figure 5.21a Lax adipose abdominal wall. Marked rectus muscle diastasis.

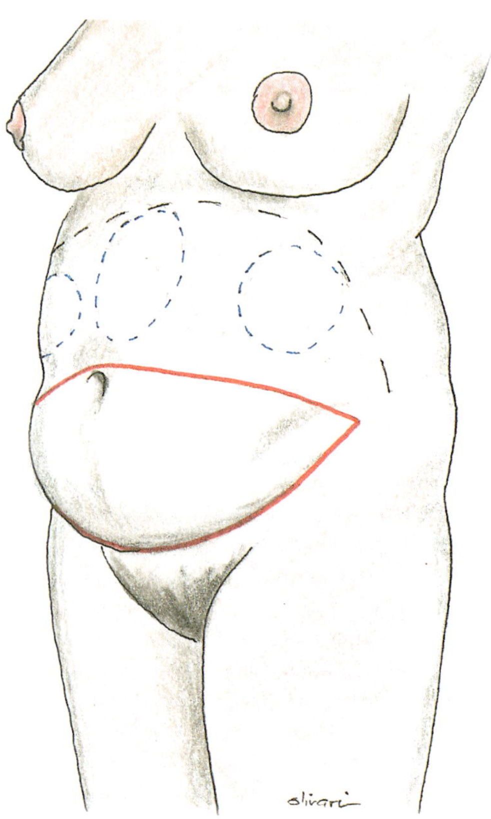

Figure 5.21b Surgical planning:

Red line: Resection of skin and fat down to the fascia.

Black line: Approximate extension of mobilization. In the case of tension, mobilisation should be performed up to the xiphoid and the rib bow.

Blue line: In these areas fatty tissue is removed by liposuction.

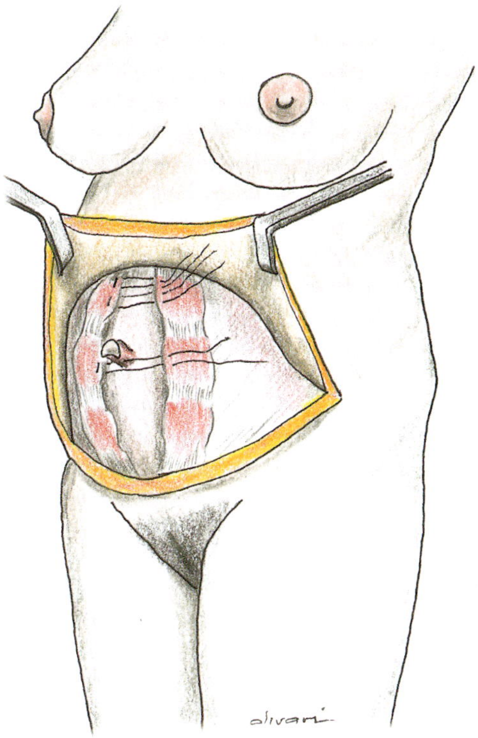

Figure 5.21c After the resection of the skin and fat layer, the remaining parts of the abdominal wall are mobilized up to the rib bow and the xiphoid, the rectus muscle diastasis is closed by suturing with non resorbable suture. This suture is done using 2×0 non-resorbable stitches (Ethibond). The umbilicus is fixated to its original position. The liposuction at the upper abdomen and the lateral abdomen is done.

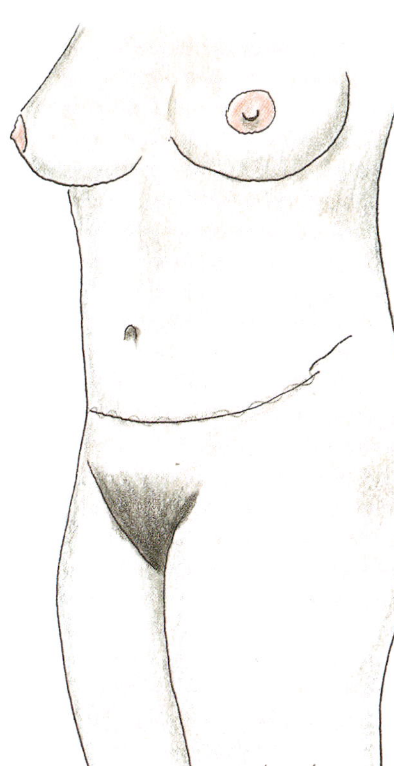

Figure 5.21d The subcutaneous suture is done using 3×0 Vicryl and the intracutaneous skin suture is performed using 3×0 Trofilene. 2 Redon-Drains.

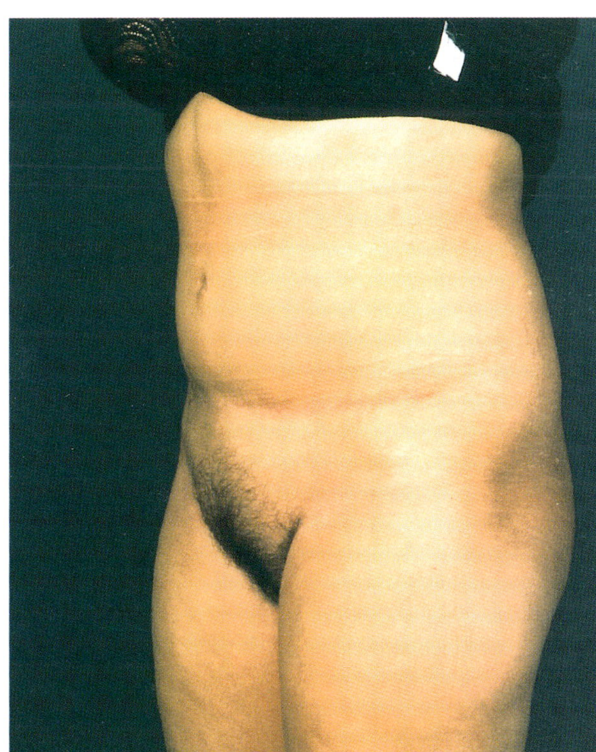

Figure 5.21e Status one year after surgery

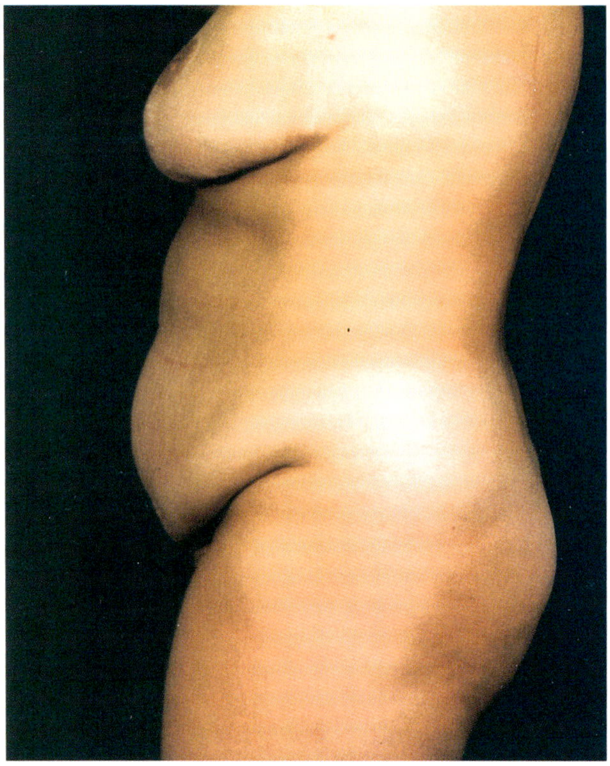

Figure 5.22a Apron-like abdominal fold, rectus muscle diastasis.

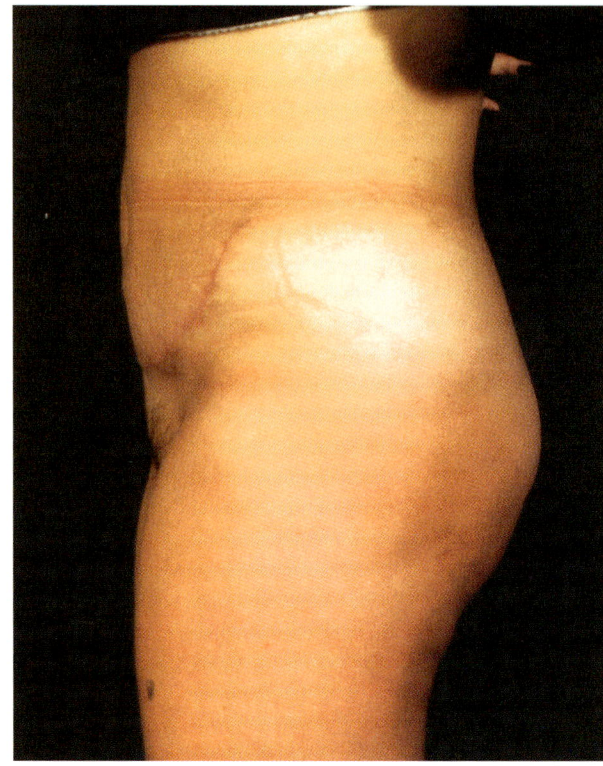

Figure 5.22b Status five weeks after abdominolipectomy, suture of rectus fascia and selective liposuction.

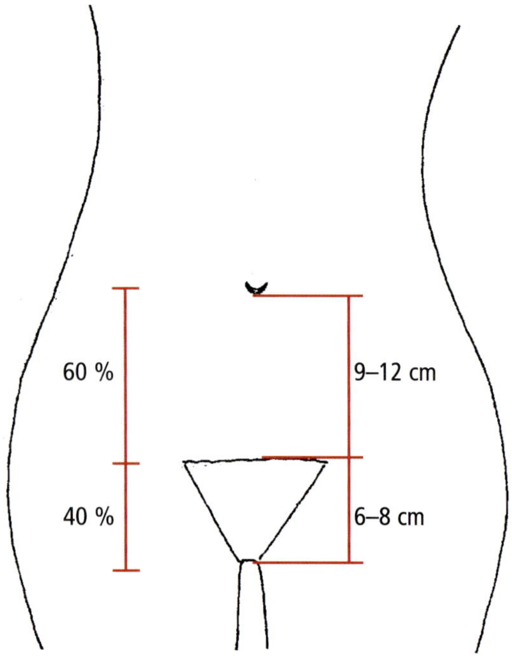

Figure 5.22c Measurements that should be respected in abdominolipectomy.

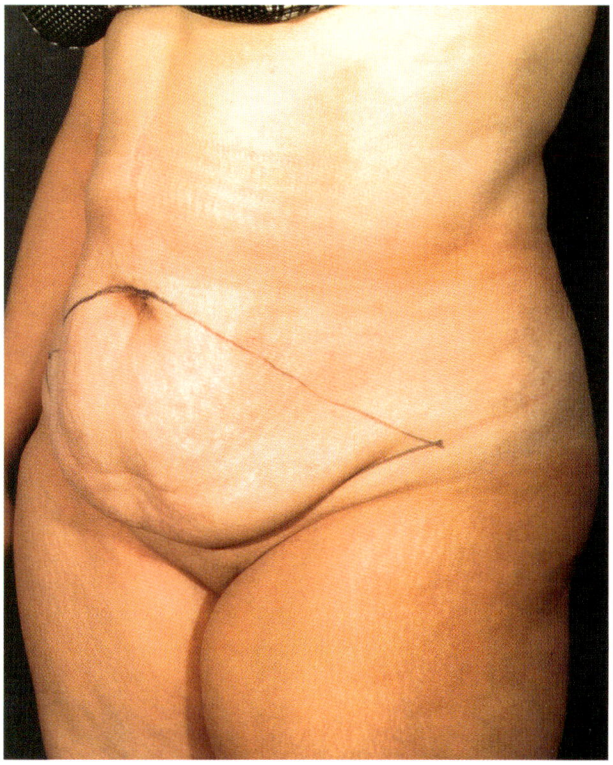

Figure 5.23a Lax abdominal wall with "apron" and rectus muscle diastasis in an adipose patient.

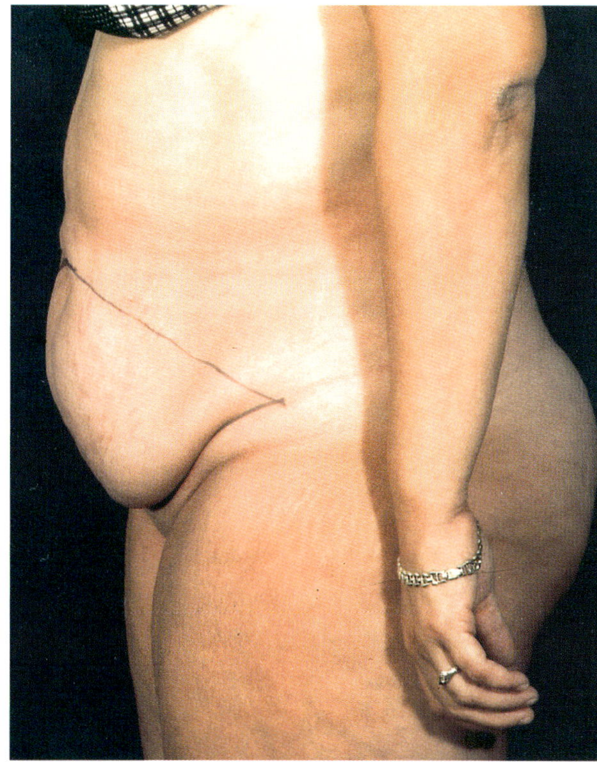

Figure 5.23b Marked "apron-like" abdominal fat-skin fold (always in standing position).

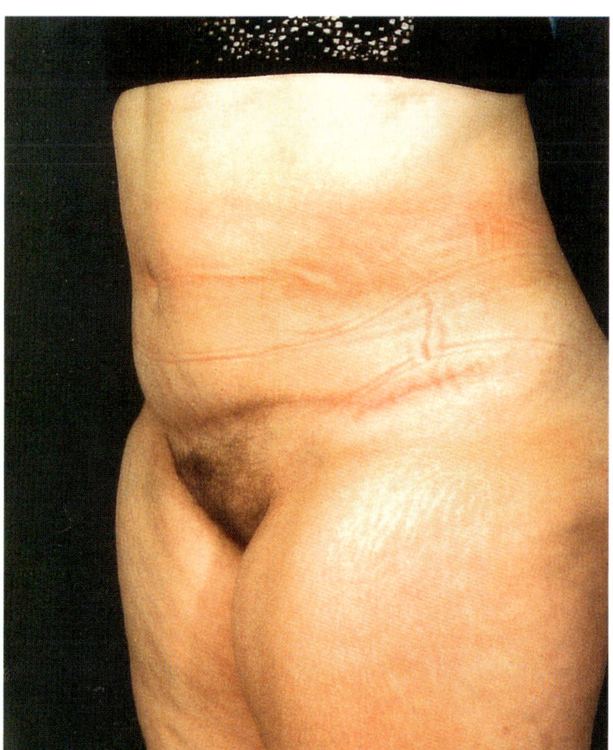

Figure 5.23c Status one year after the procedure

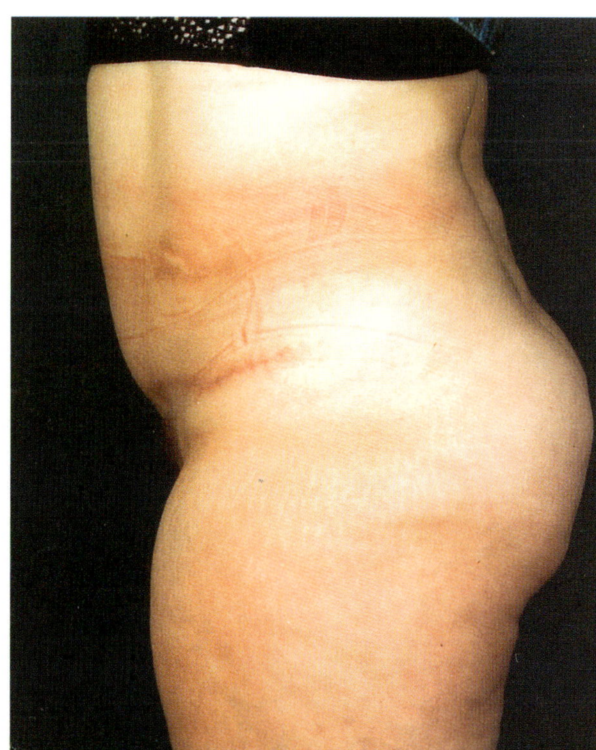

Figure 5.23d Lateral aspect

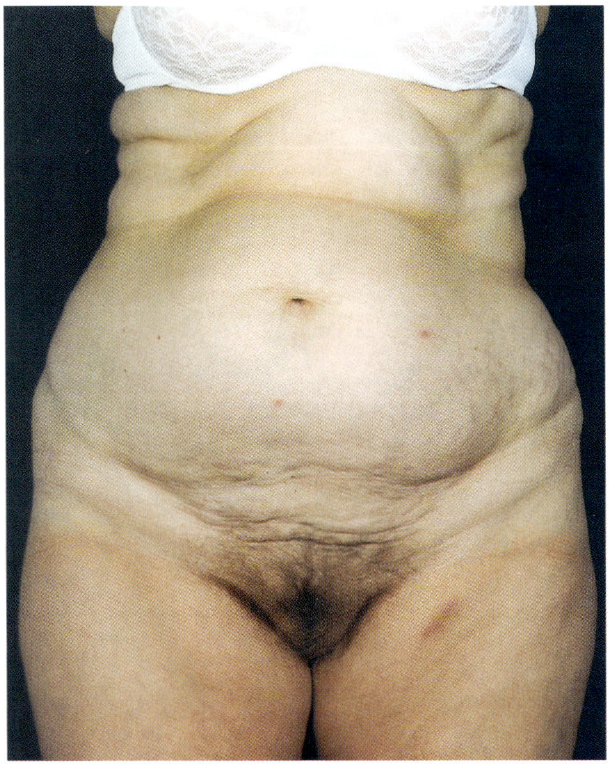

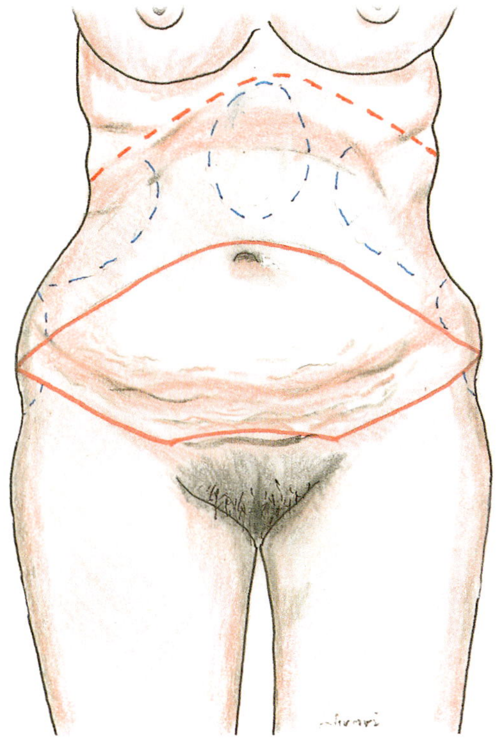

Figure 5.24a Rectus muscle diastasis in the upper and lower abdominal region, striae and irregular local adiposity

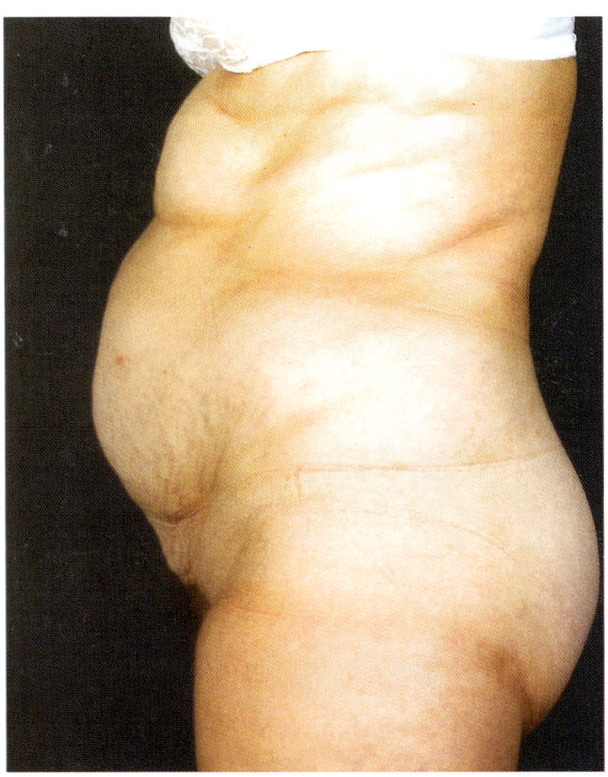

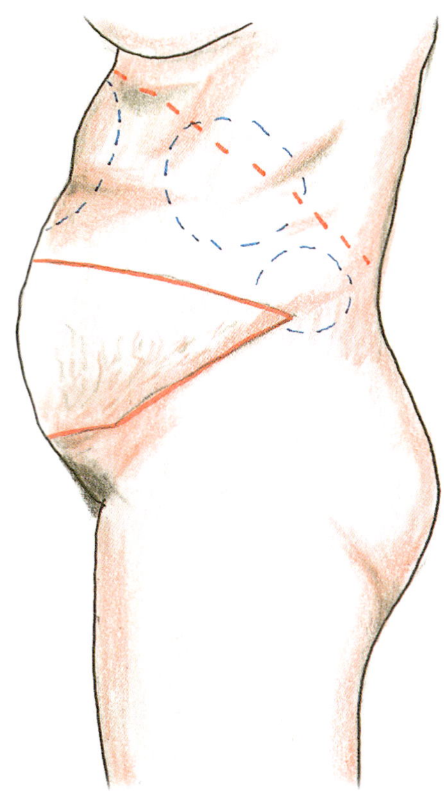

Figure 5.24b Preoperative status

Figure 5.24c Red = planned excision, red interrupted line = border of mobilization, blue = planned area for liposuction

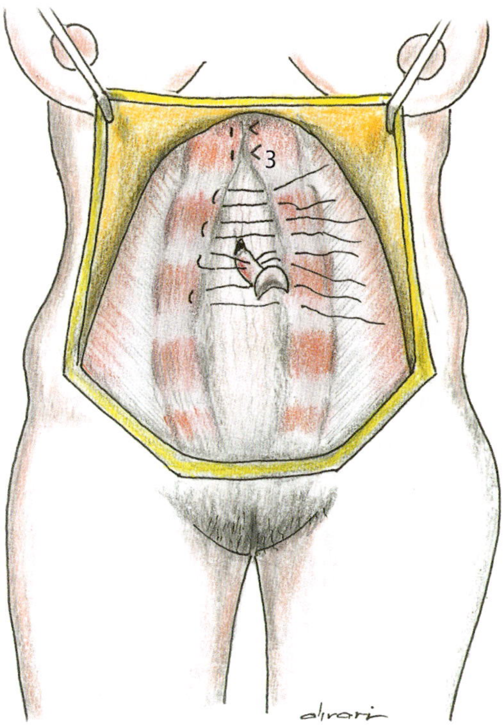

Figure 5.24d After resection of the excessive skin and fat, the mobilization up to the rib border is done, if needed even higher. Suture of rectus fascia (3)

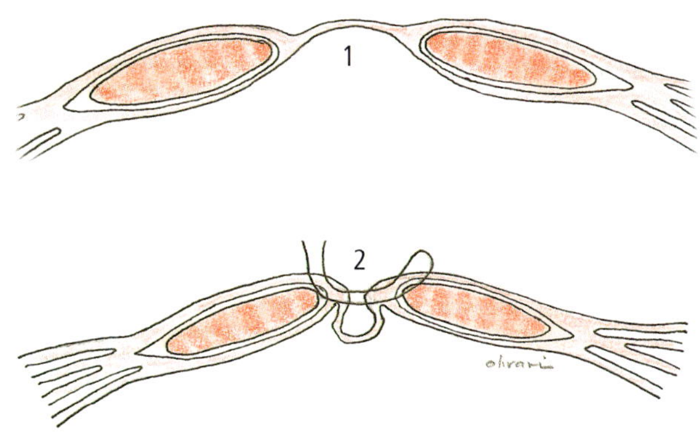

Figure 5.24e Rectus muscle diastasis (1), "doubling" of the fascia (2)

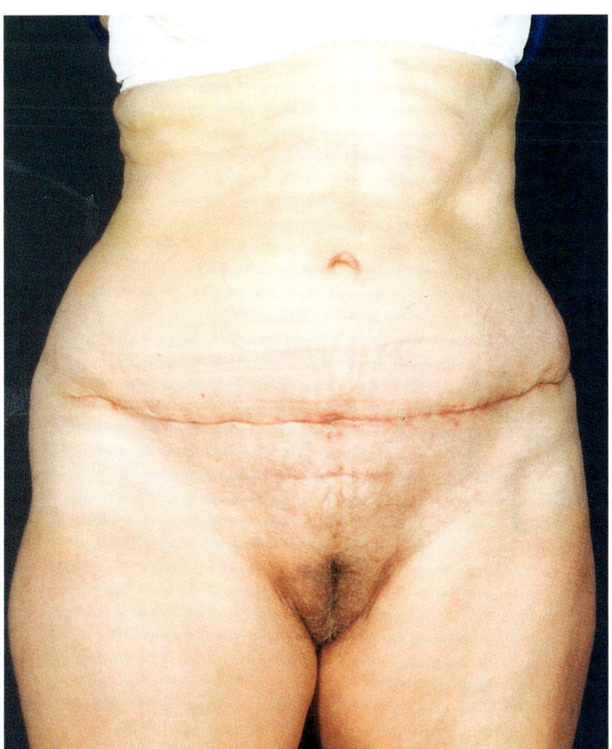

Figure 5.24f Status six weeks after the procedure. Note the form of the umbilicus!

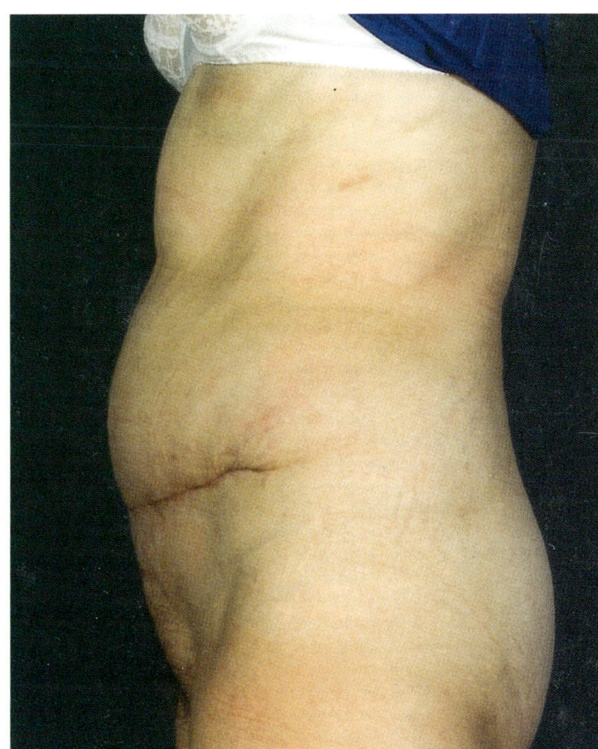

Figure 5.24g Lateral aspect

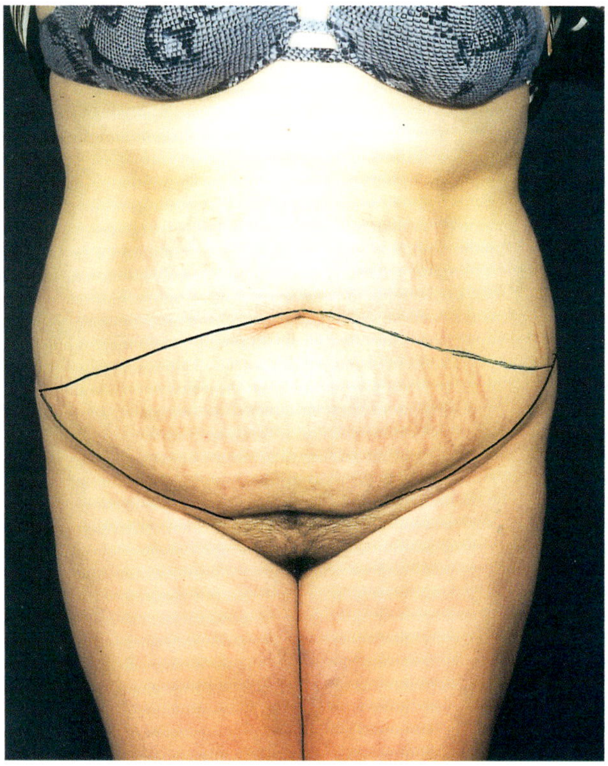

Figure 5.25a Apron-like abdominal skin-fat fold, rectus muscle diastasis.

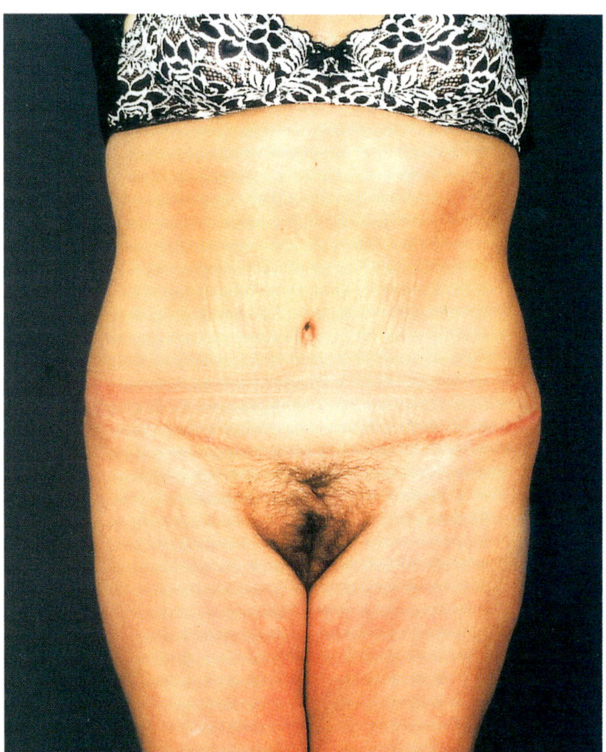

Figure 5.25b Status six months after the procedure. A skin-fat resection (abdominolipectomy) with "doubling" of the rectus fascia and partial liposuction has been done.

Modified Incision in Abdominoplasty

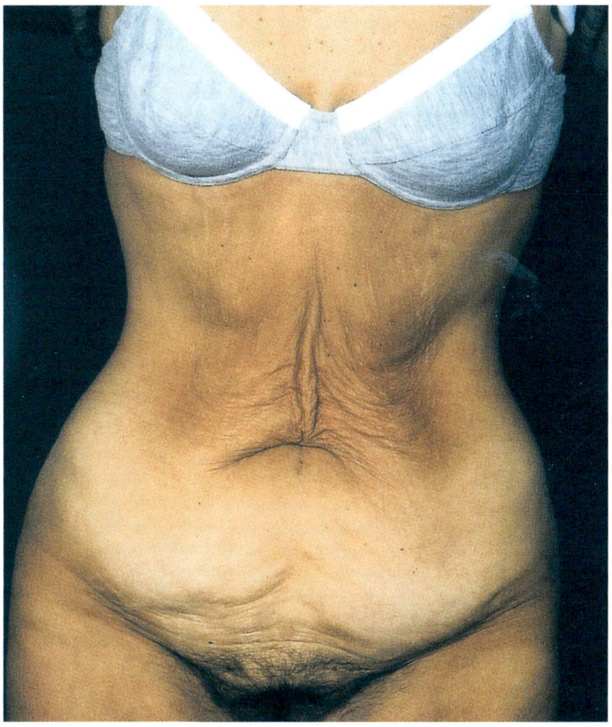

Figure 5.26a Lax abdominal wall after multiple pregnancies, otherwise slender patient.

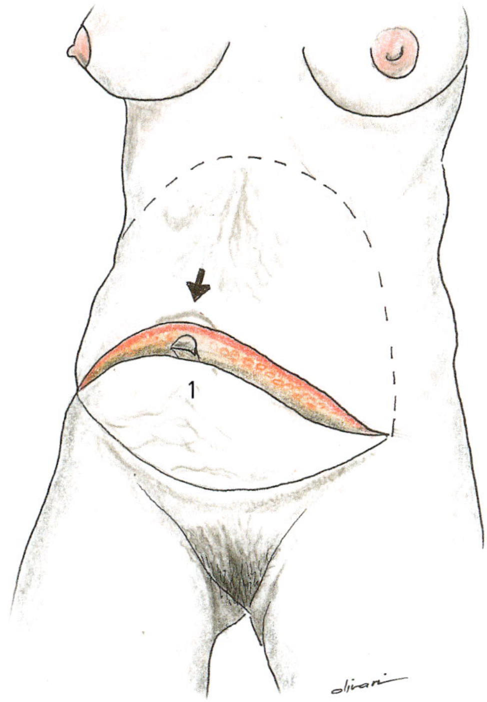

Figure 5.26b Here, modified incisions. These incisions facilitate the mobilization, require a certain experience. One has to be sure that the defect can be closed easily. Area of the resection (1).

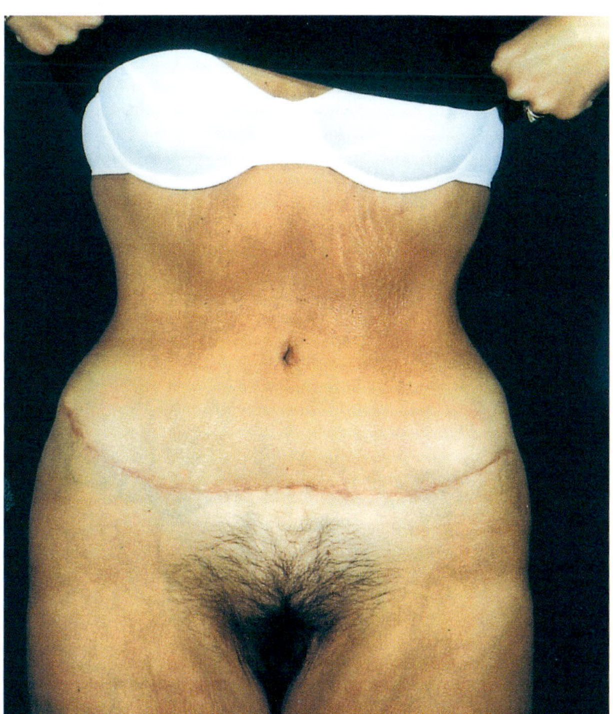

Figure 5.26c Situation ten months after the procedure

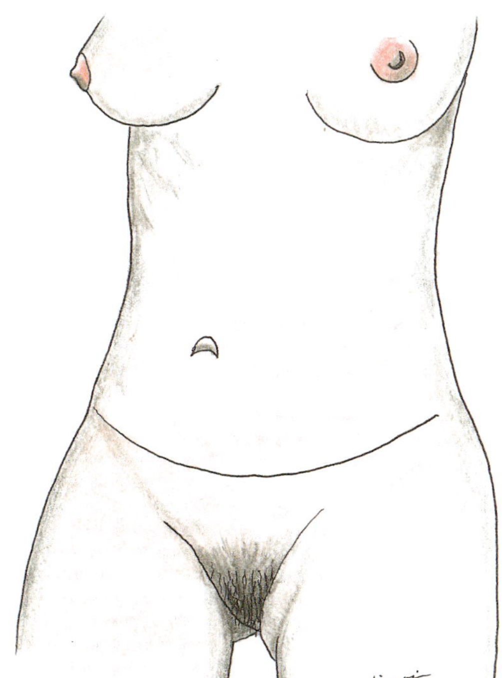

Figure 5.26d Subctaneous sutures are done using 3×0 Vicryl. The intracutaneous skin suture is done using 3×0 Trofilene. Two Redon drains.

Abdominolipectomy and Simultaneously Breast Reduction

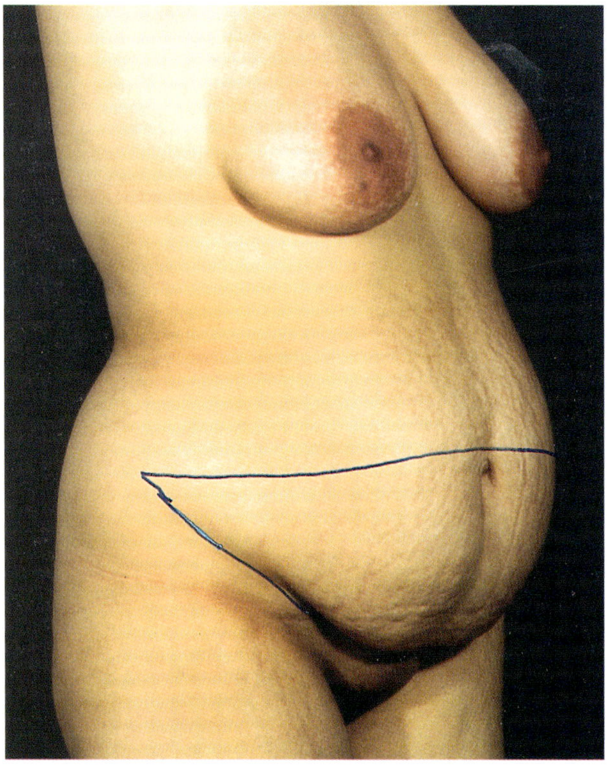

Figure 5.27a Breast ptosis and hypertrophy: Lax abdominal wall, rectus muscle diastasis

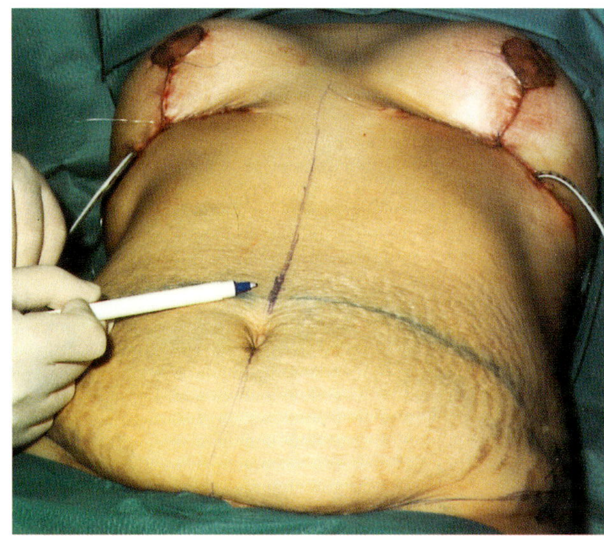

Figure 5.27b The breast reduction has been performed first. Planning of the abdominal resection.

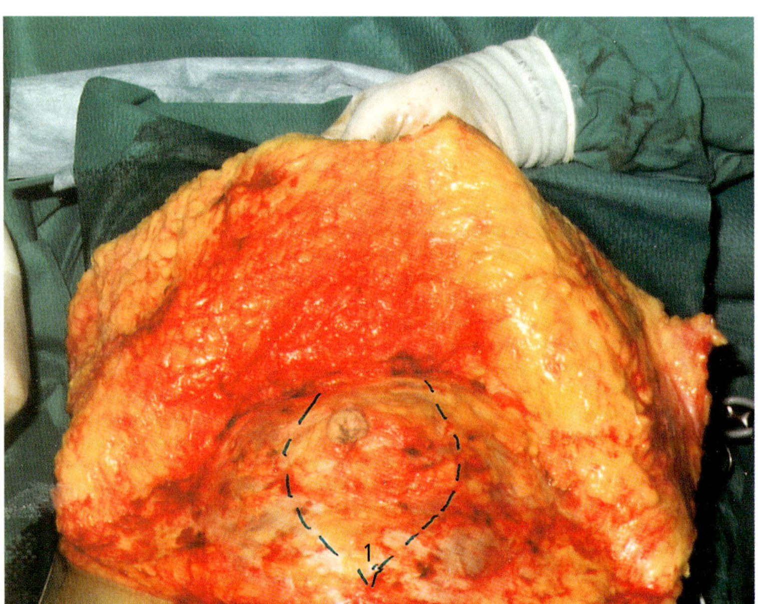

Figure 5.27c Mobilization of the skin-fat layer up to the xiphoid and the rib bow. Note the rectus muscle diastasis (1)!

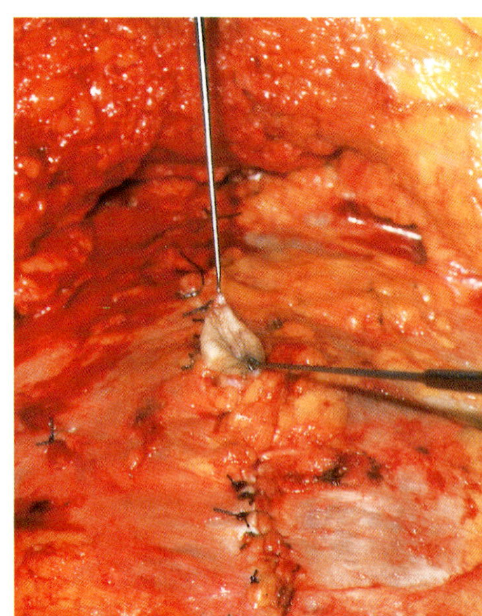

Figure 5.27d Status post "doubling" of the rectus fascia and fixation of the umbilicus to the fascia.

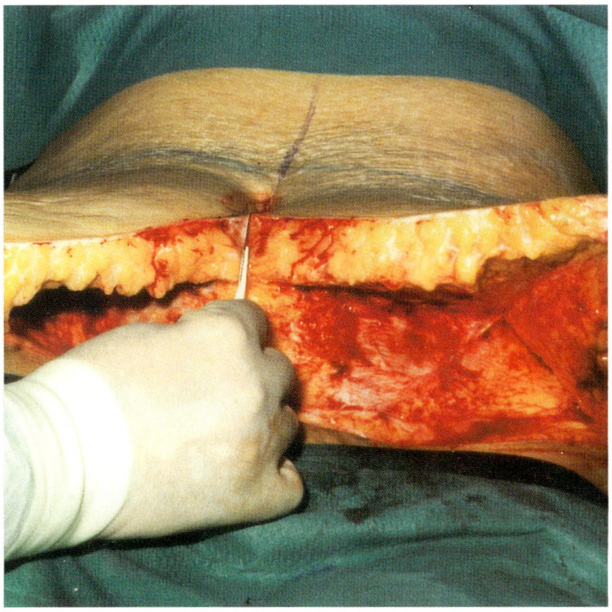

Figure 5.27e Resection of the skin-fat layer between the pubic hair line and above the umbilicus.

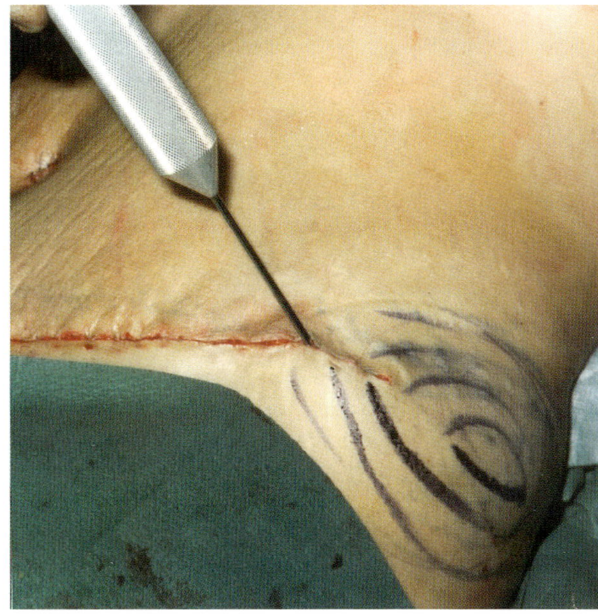

Figure 5.27f At the end of the operation a liposuction is done to avoid "dog ear" formation

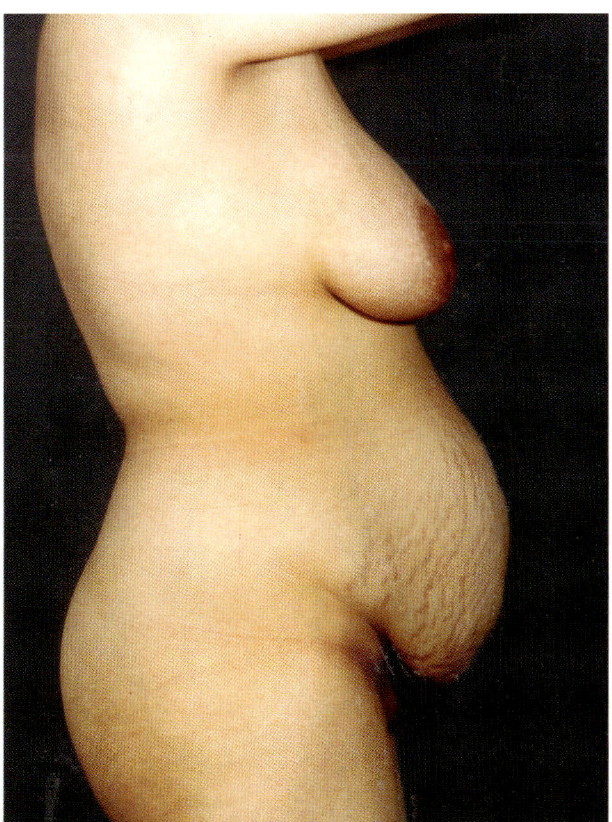

Figure 5.27g Preoperative status

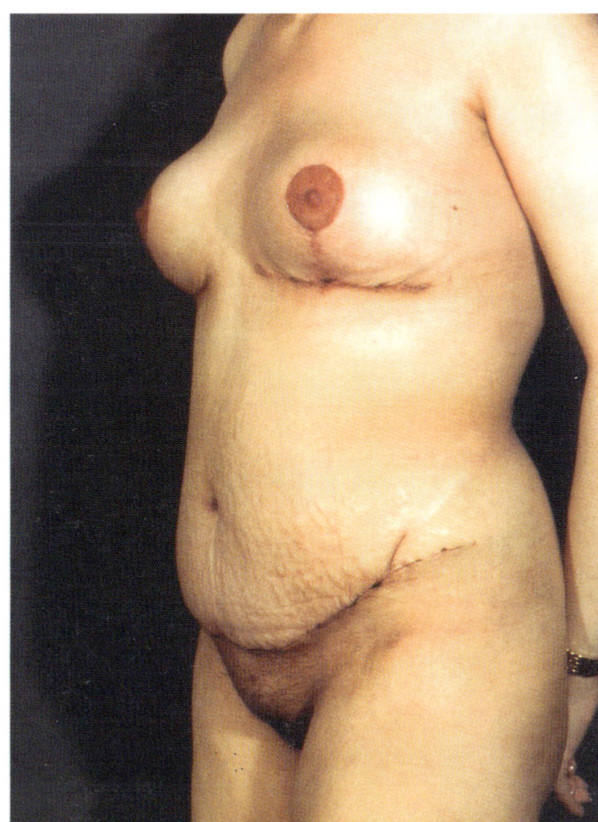

Figure 5.27h Status four weeks after surgery

How to Solve Umbilicus Problems

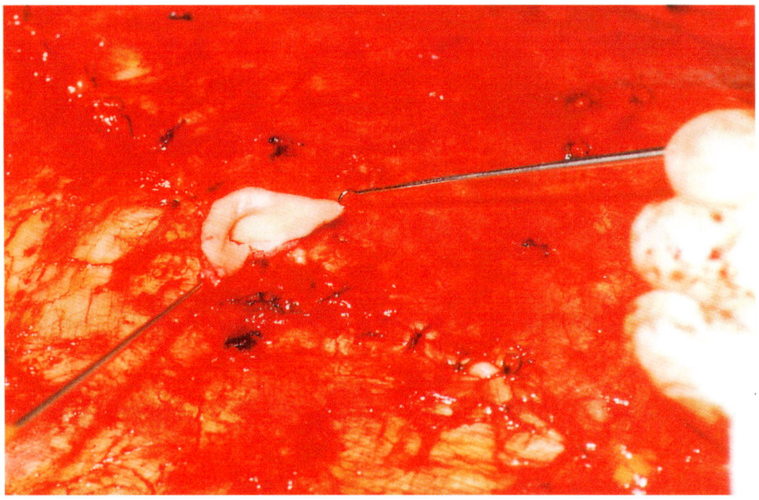

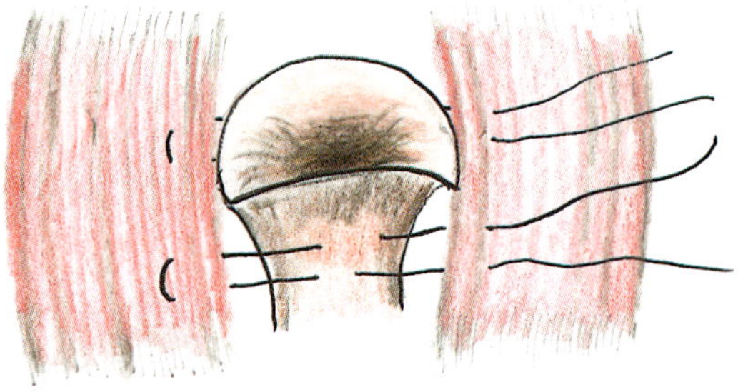

Figure 5.28a The umbilicus is incised out of the abdominal wall in a half-moon shape (cranially convex), not in a round fashion. The fixation to the rectus muscle is done.

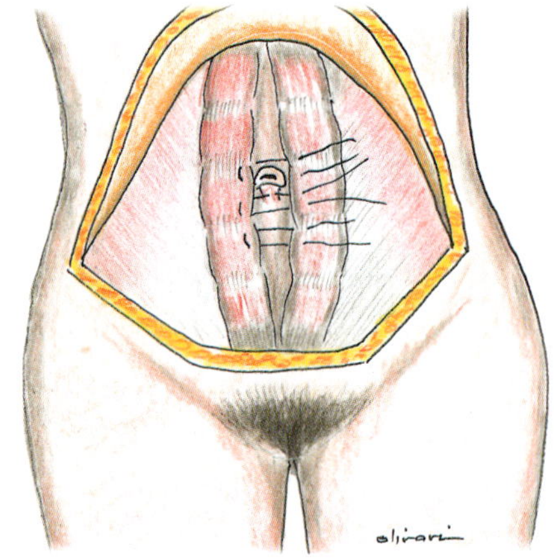

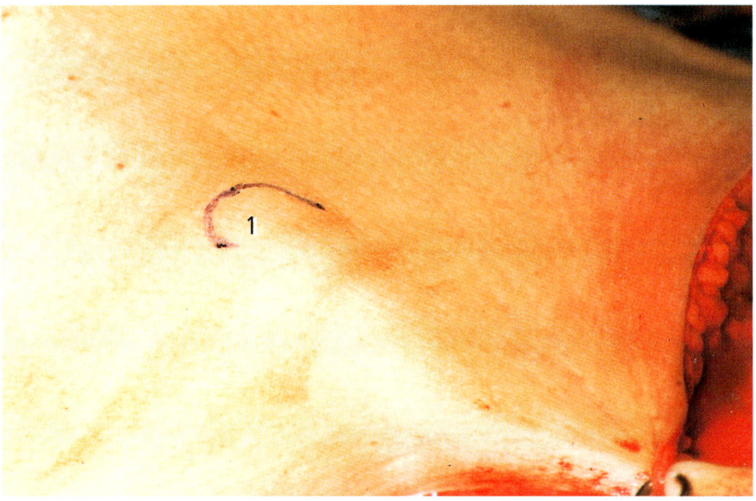

Figure 5.28b,c After doubling of the fascia and fixation of the umbilicus to the border of the rectus fascia, the skin opening for the umbilicus is incised, not excised, in a bow-like pattern (1).

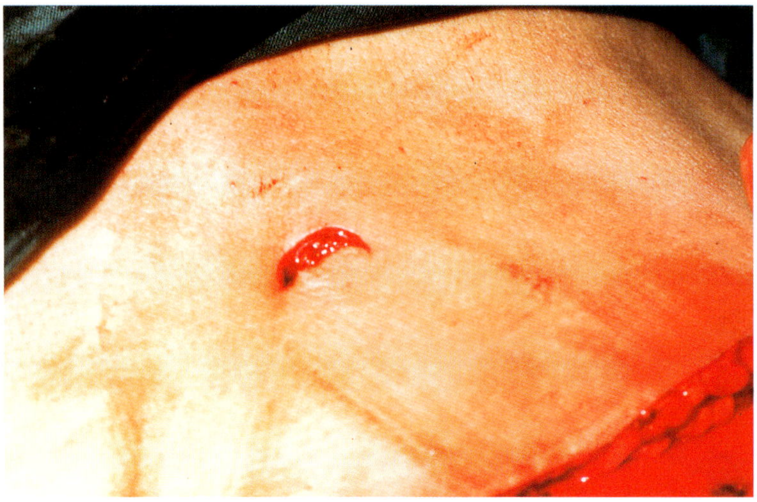

Figure 5.28d The bow-shaped incision (no excision) is cranially convex and should be located approx. one to two centimetres superior to the umbilicus, which is fixated to the fascia.

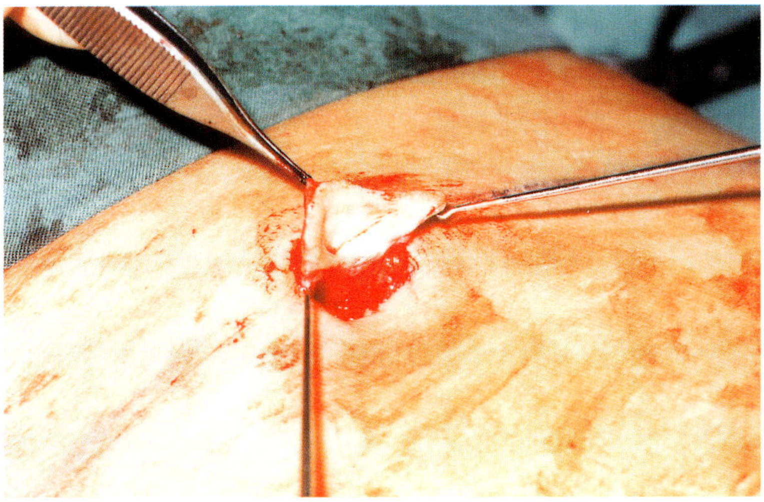

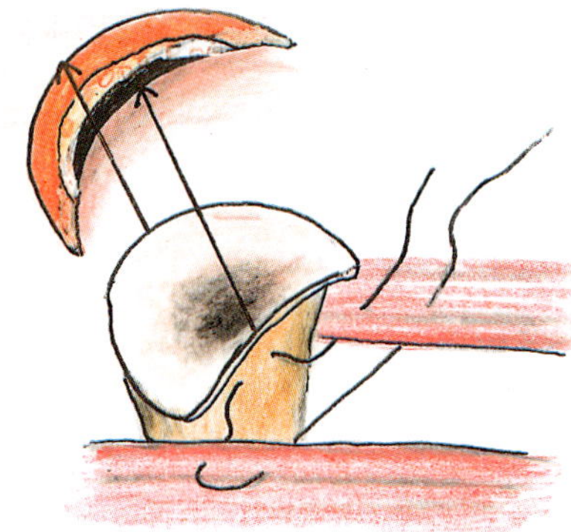

Figure 5.28e The umbilicus is pulled through the incision

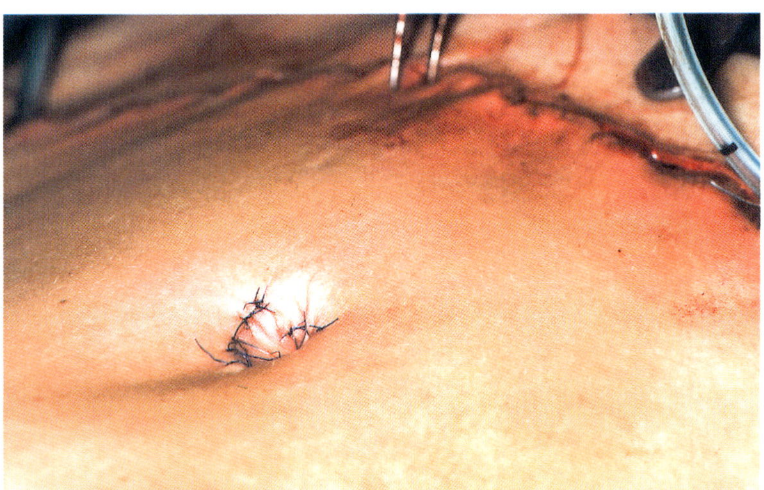

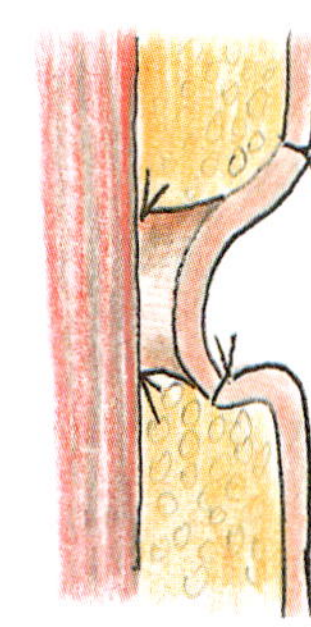

Figure 5.28f The umbilicus is fixated. Stitches at the lower border are not visible, so there are no scars later on. The new umbilicus has a more natural appearance by the slight caudal traction.

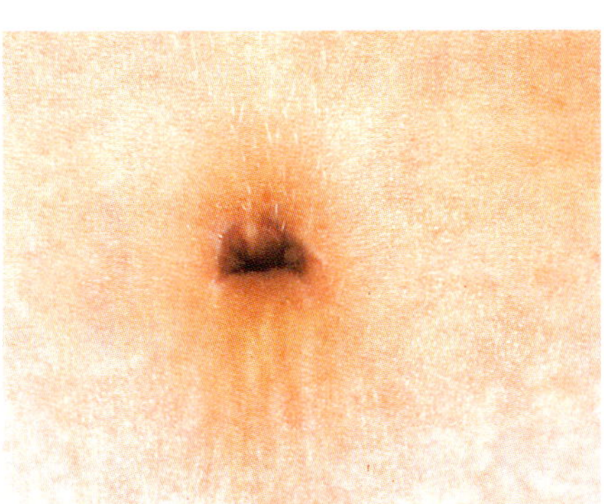

Figure 5.28g Six months postoperatively

Morbid Obesity (Indication for Operation)

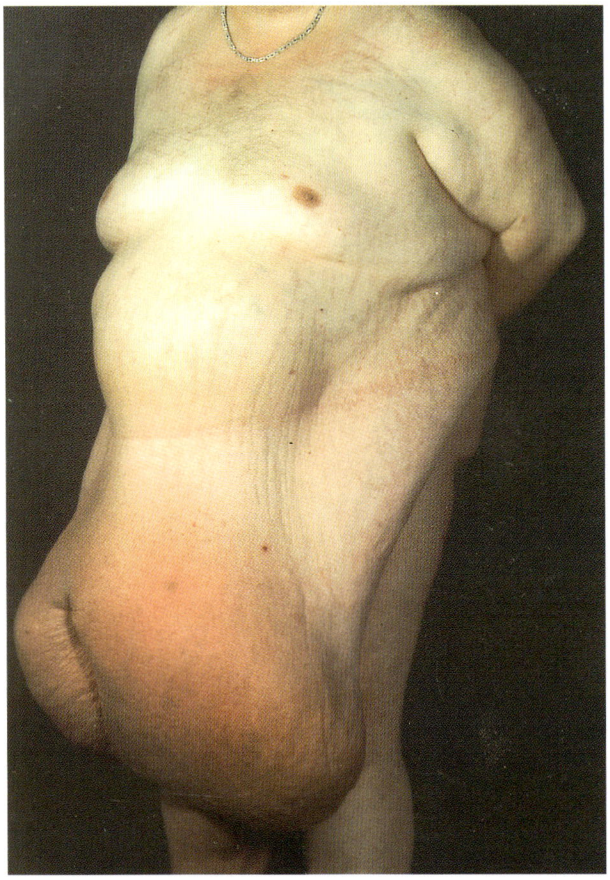

Figure 5.29a A patient weighing 210 kg. Status post multiple diet attempts without success. Marked problems in the laying position by compression of the abdomen and thorax with all known problems.

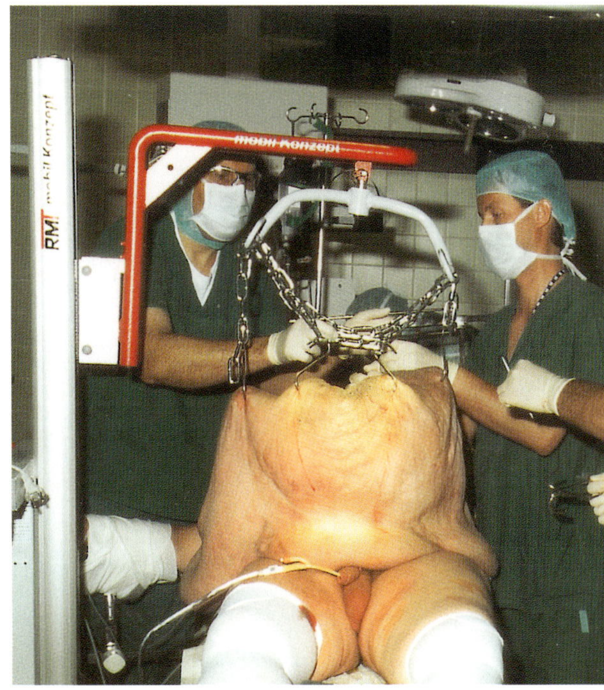

Figure 5.29b To make the operation possible, the abdominal wall is hooked up and lifted using a crane. First of all this has assistance function and secondly the blood is flowing from the very large fat area into the systemic circulation.

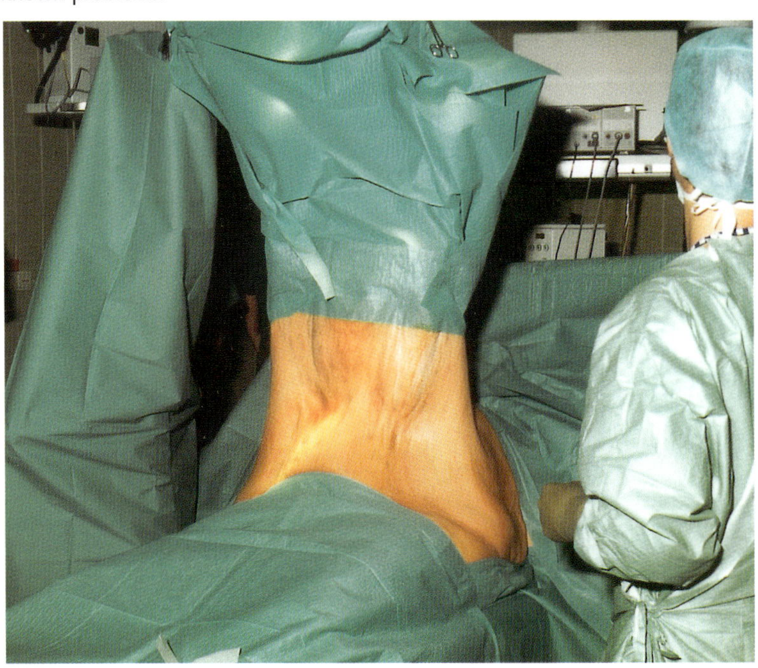

Figure 5.29c The blood that has flown back from the huge abdomen has an auto transfusion-like effect. Here, the situation before the procedure done by Dr. Dirk Richter (Wesseling) is shown.

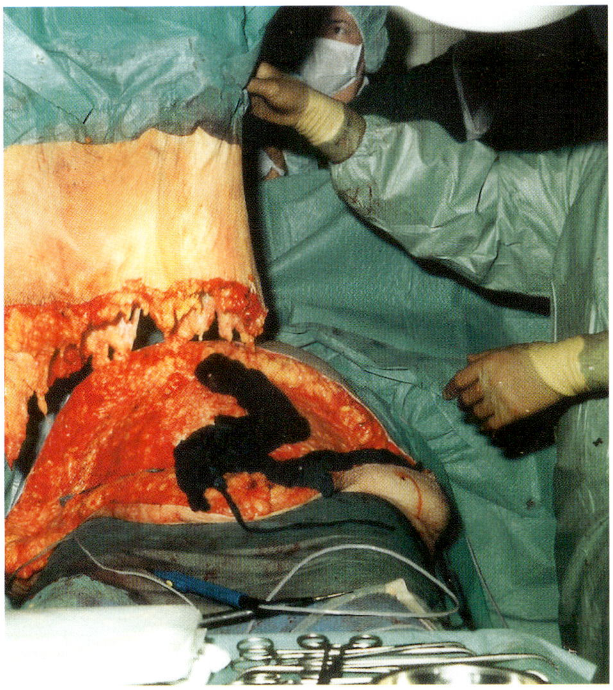

Figure 5.29d Status at the end of the resection. Note: No extensive mobilization!

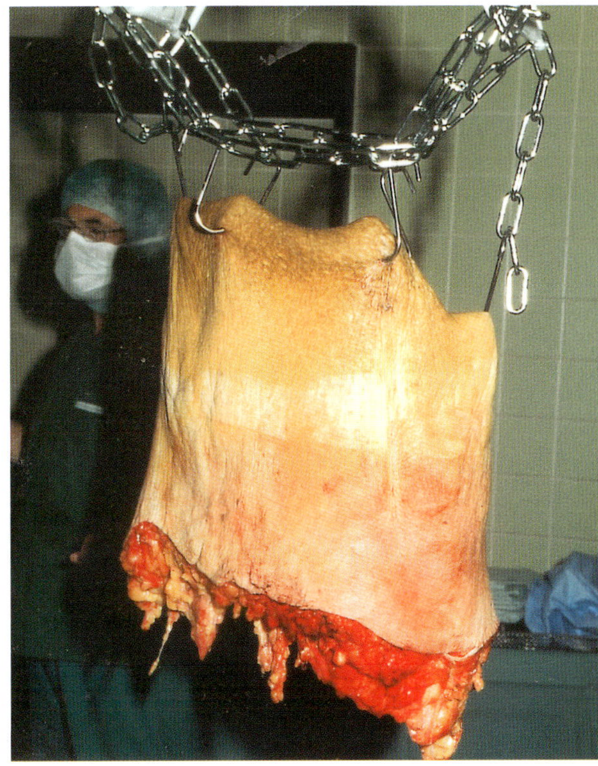

Figure 5.29e The resected tissue weighs 54 kg. An estimated three litres of blood have flown back from the abdominal fat into the systemic circulation.

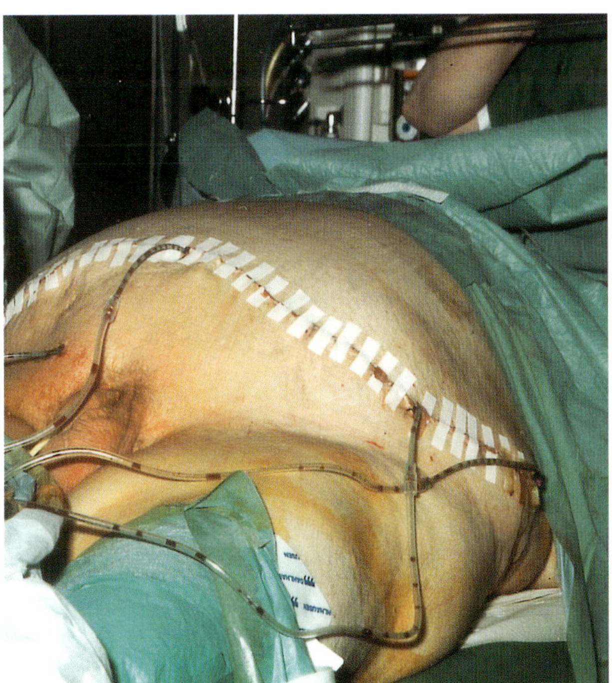

Figure 5.29f Status at the end of the procedure. No blood transfusion was necessary. The postoperative Hb-level was 13.2 despite the presence of a very large wound.

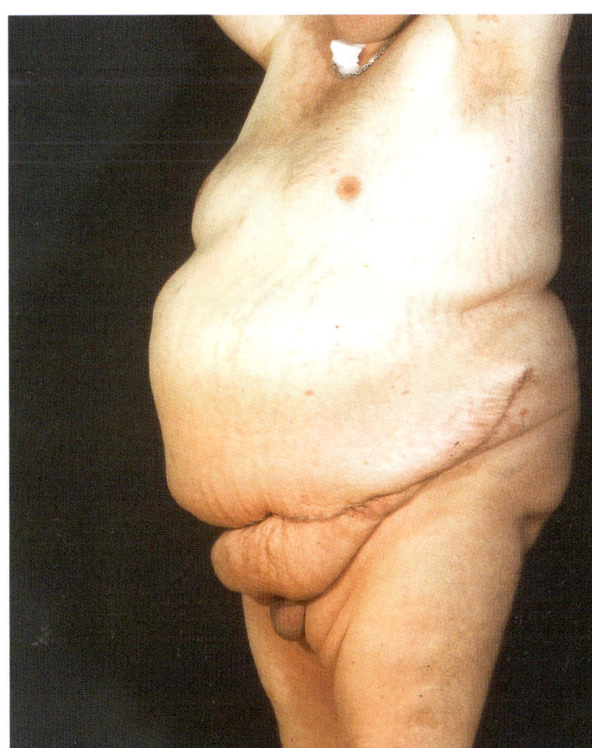

Figure 5.29g Status three weeks after the procedure: The patient now weighs 152 kg.

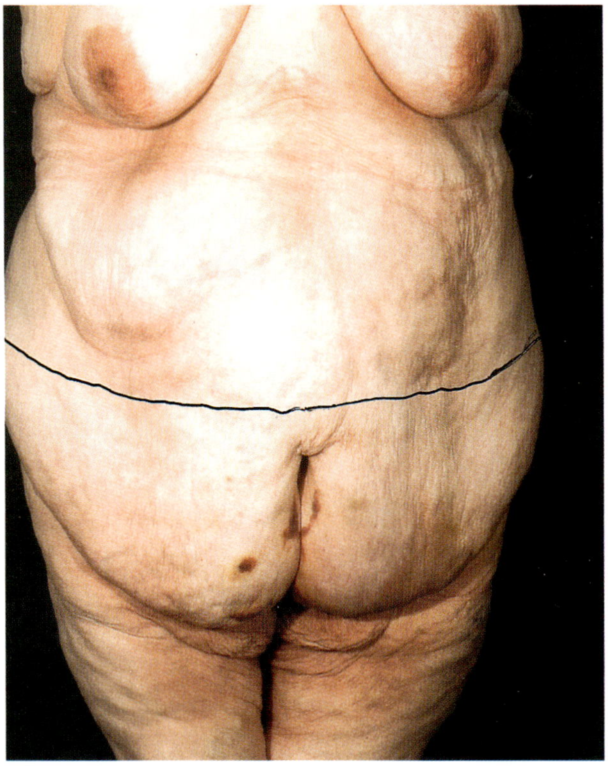

Figure 5.30a 67-year old obese patient with extreme apron-like abdominal skin-fat fold. Chronic intertrigo

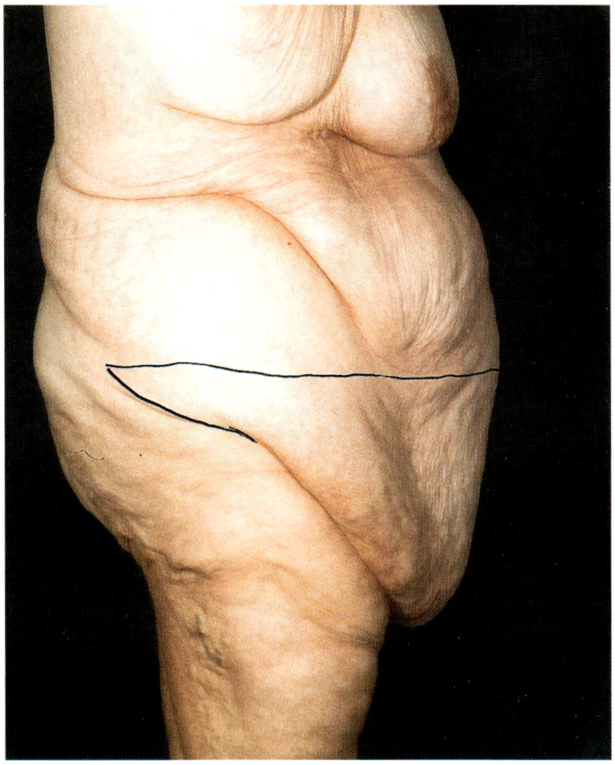

Figure 5.30b Marked functional problems are obvious.

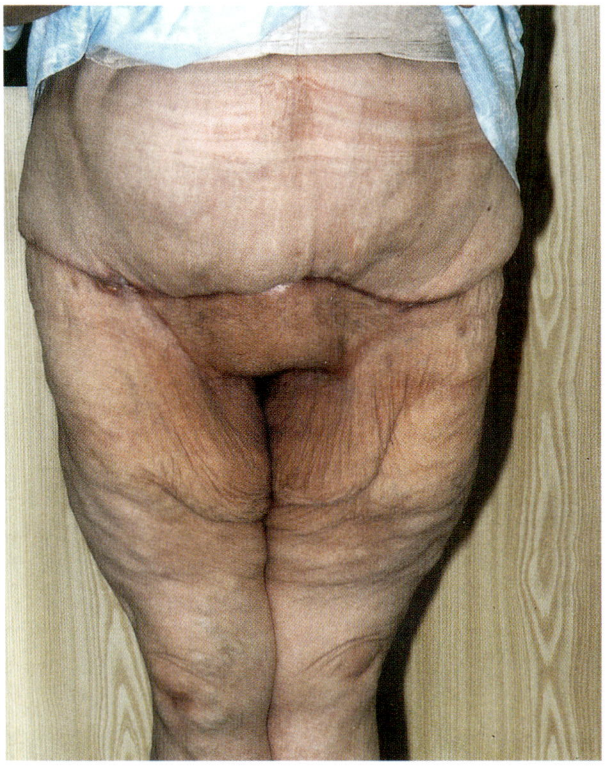

Figure 5.30c Status three months after the procedure: 17 kg have been resected.

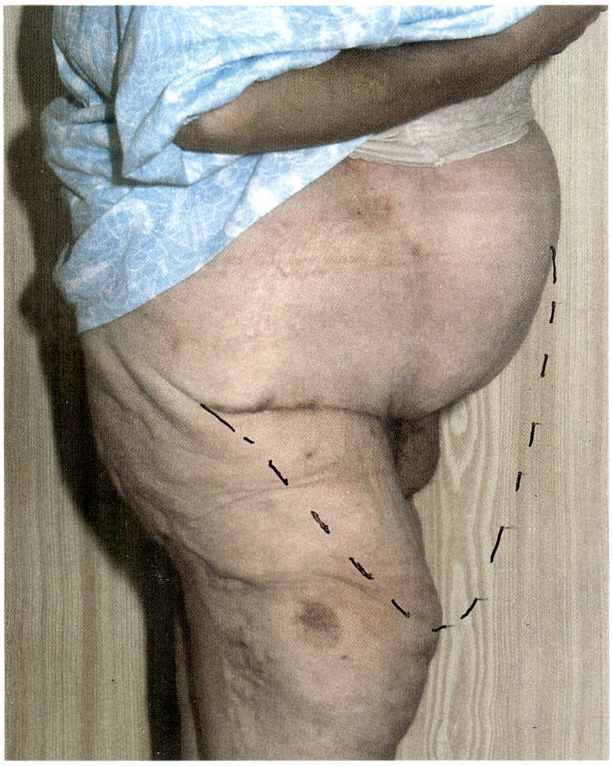

Figure 5.30d Marked functional improvement

Complication

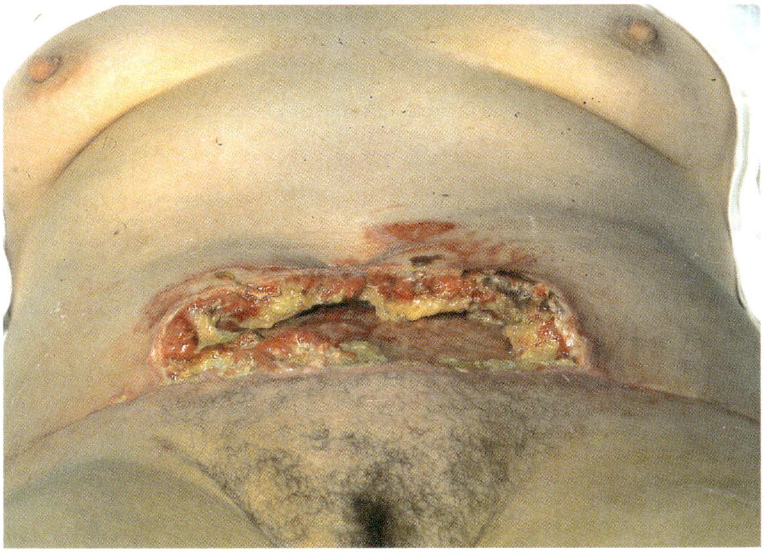

Figure 5.31a Abdominoplasty with complication. Necrosis of the skin and the fatty tissue between the pubic area and the umbilicus. Staphylococcus aureus infection. Reasons: Mobilization was not sufficient, suturing under too much tension. After wound closure, the midline area is the "last meadow" (e.g. the area most remote from the supplying vessel origin and therefore the area most prone to wound complications).

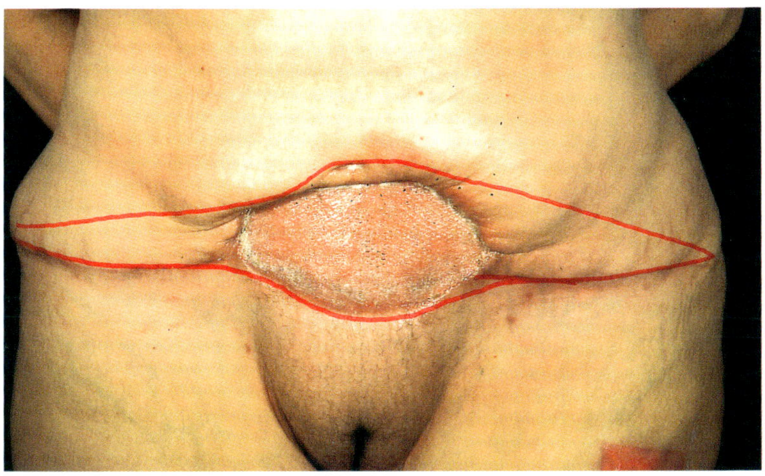

Figure 5.31b To close the defect, a mesh graft is applied after wound debridement and antibiotic therapy. Three months later, a modified abdominoplasty could be performed to close the remaining defect. At the same time, the umbilicus was reconstructed.

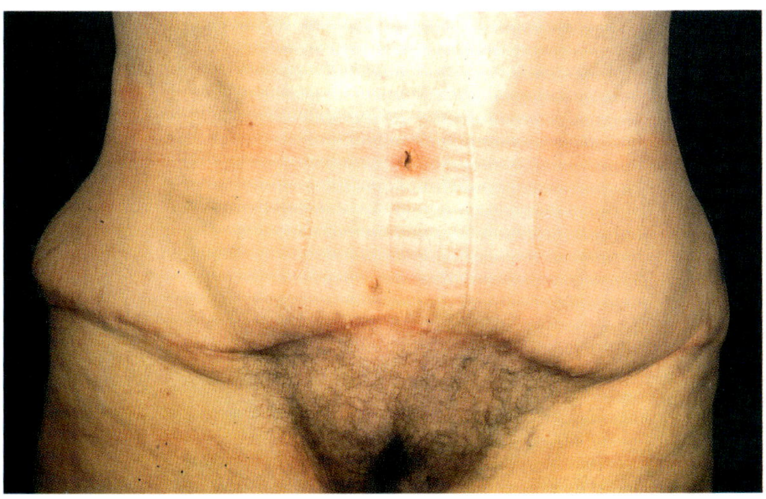

Figure 5.31c Status two years after the procedure. A marked dog ear is seen on the right side, which did not disturb the patient.

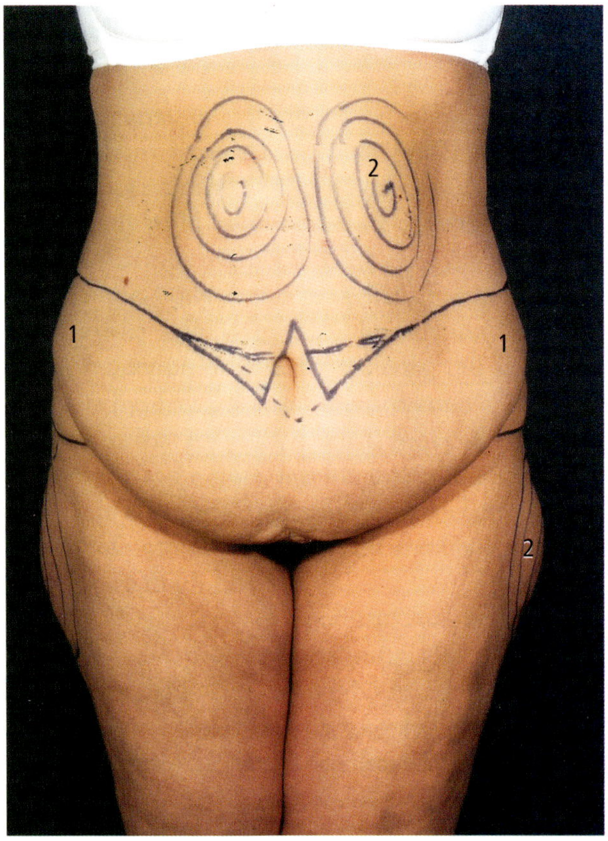

Figure 5.33a High-lateral-tension abdominoplasty (modification by Richter). Adipose, "hanging" tummy, which forms lateral tissue masses in both flank regions. Here, the incision is modified such that the incision is widely extended laterodorsally and markedly wider laterally than in the standard abdominolipectomy. The circles in the epigastric area and in the lateral thigh area indicate the planned regions for liposuction (2). With this method, the thighs are simultaneously lifted.

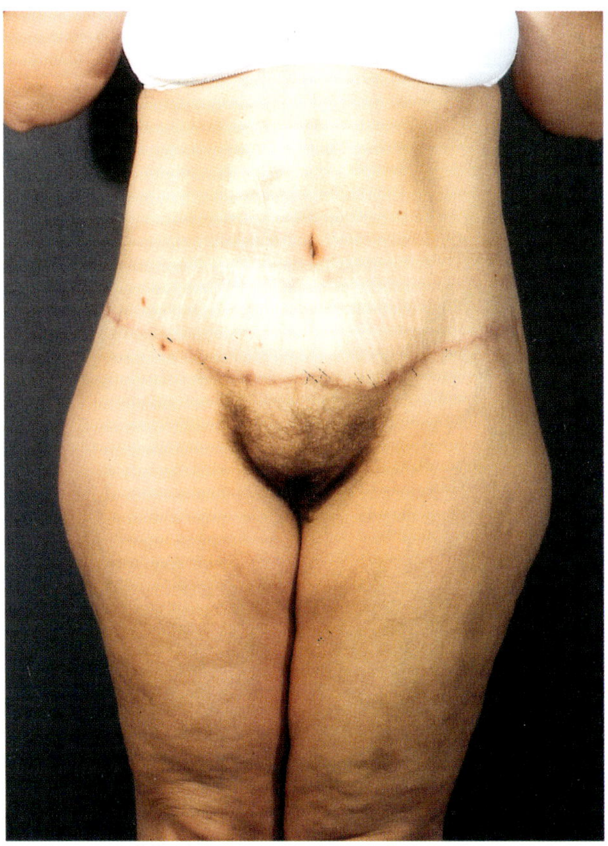

Figure 5.33b Status six months after the procedure. Very firm abdominal wall, but also lifting of the skin in the thigh area.

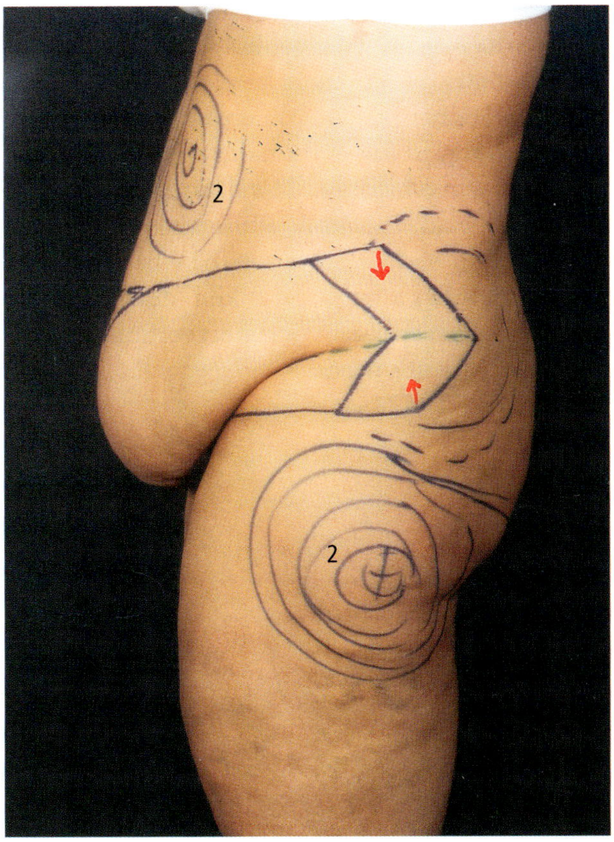

Figure 5.33c The laterally and dorsally extended incisions are clearly visible. This wide excision makes both an abdominal lift and a lift of the gluteal and lateral thigh region possible. Note the planned areas for liposuction (2). By raising the lower incisional margin and mobilization of the lateral thigh, the lateral thigh area is lifted.

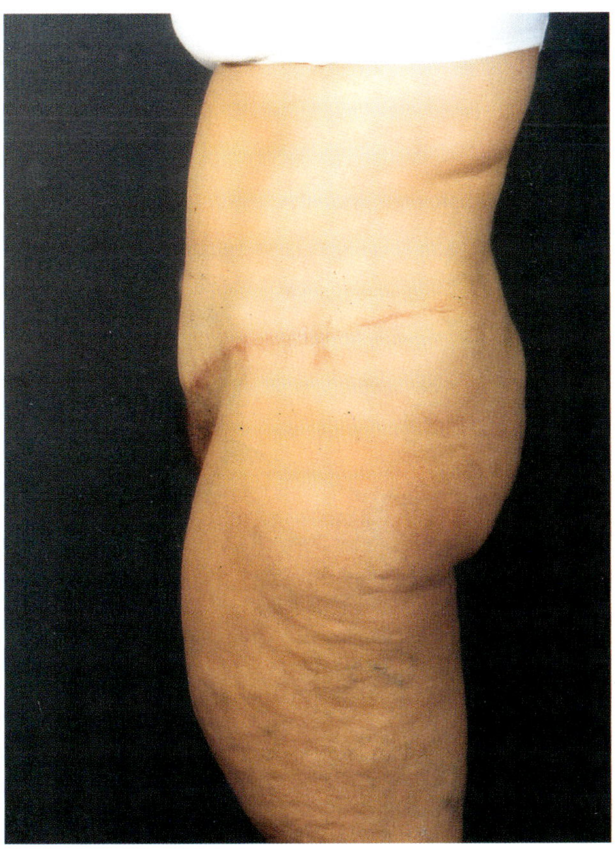

Figure 5.33d Status six months after the operation: The scar is very long. Marked lifting of the gluteal region and the thighs.

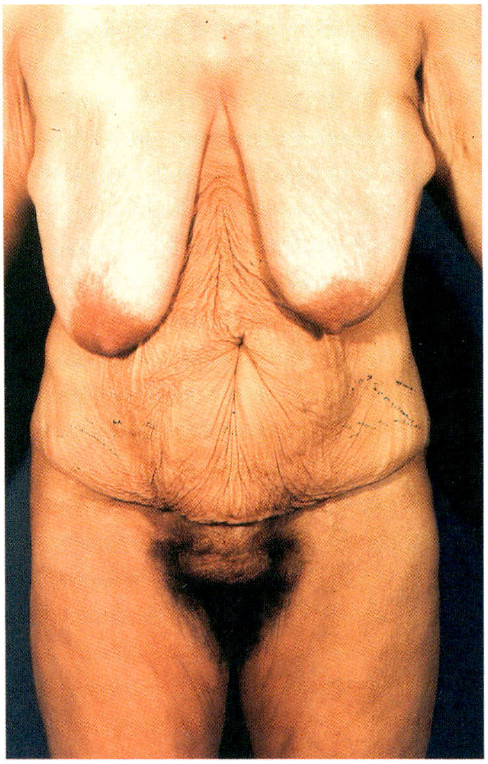

Figure 5.36a Problem case. Status post weight loss of 73 kg. Lax breast, abdomen and thigh skin.

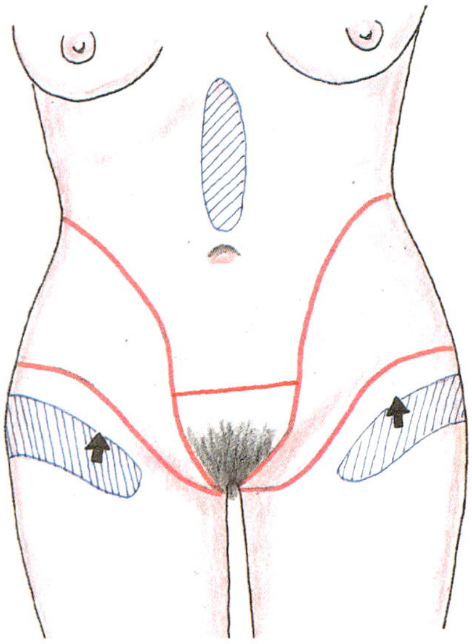

Figure 5.36b Planning of the Lockwood operation. At the same time, the abdomen, buttock and thighs are lifted. The skin of the thigh area is mobilized.

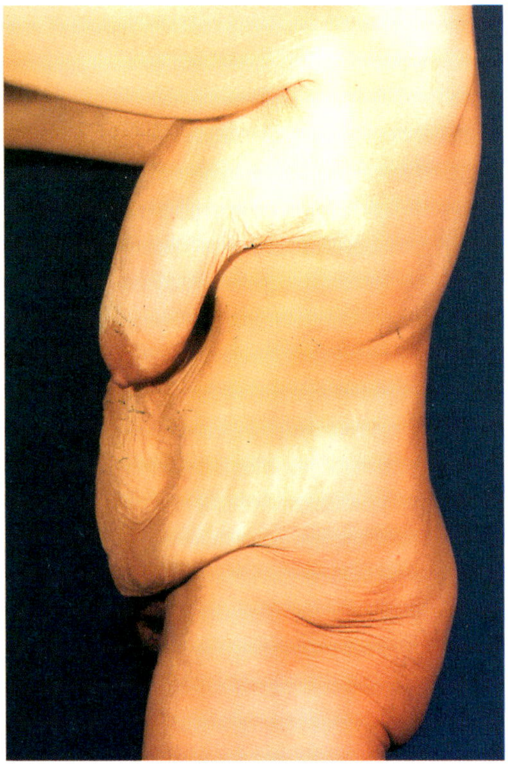

Figure 5.36c Preoperative situation, lateral aspect

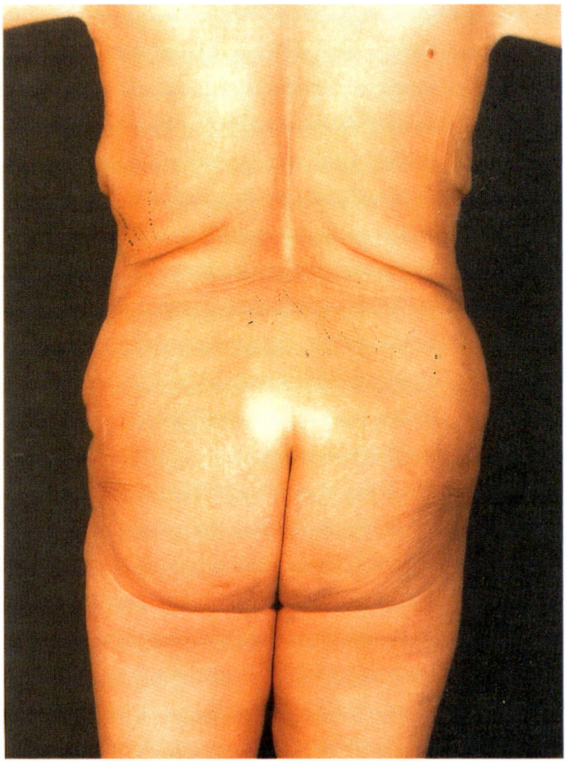

Figure 5.36d Preoperative situation, dorsal aspect

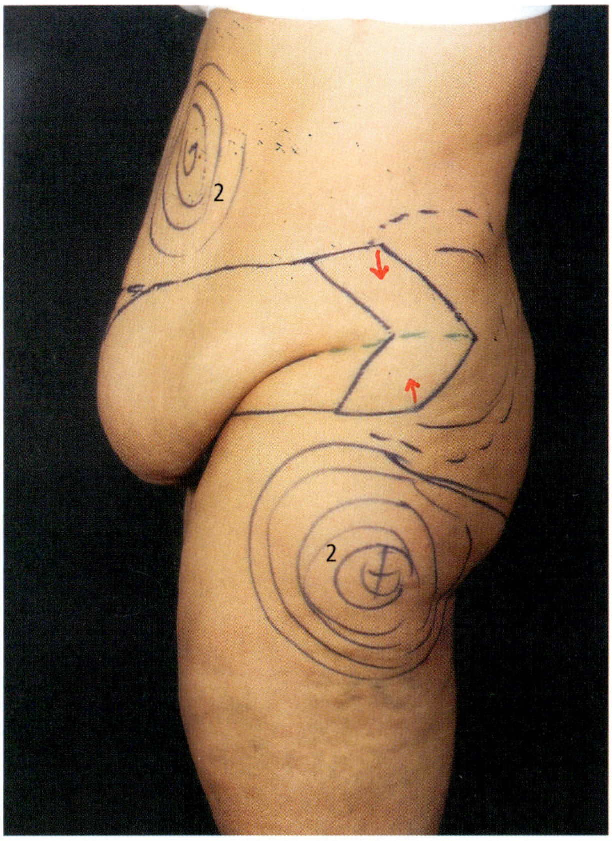

Figure 5.33c The laterally and dorsally extended incisions are clearly visible. This wide excision makes both an abdominal lift and a lift of the gluteal and lateral thigh region possible. Note the planned areas for liposuction (2). By raising the lower incisional margin and mobilization of the lateral thigh, the lateral thigh area is lifted.

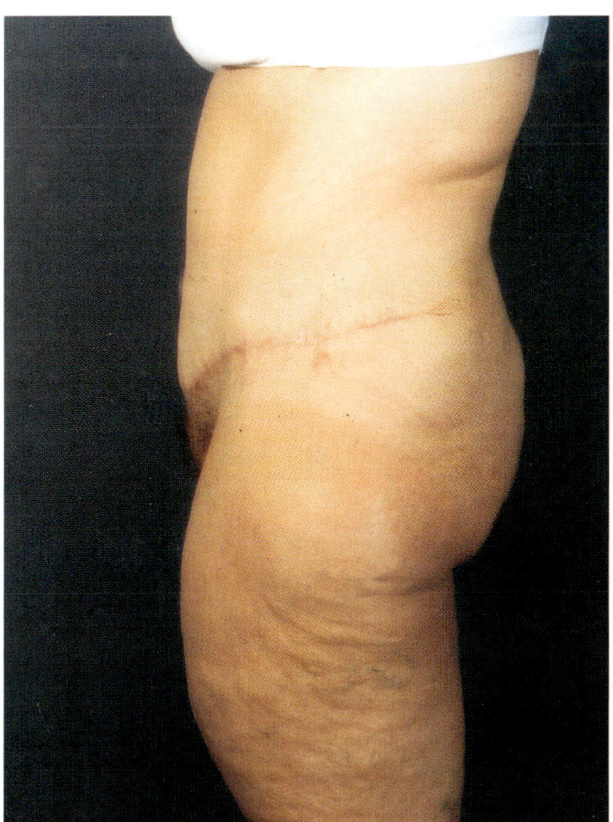

Figure 5.33d Status six months after the operation: The scar is very long. Marked lifting of the gluteal region and the thighs.

Body Lifting (Original Method by Tom Lockwood)

We discriminate two methods of lower body lifts. The original method was described by Lockwood (1993) and includes a steep bow-like incision from the medial aspect of the thigh following the pelvic area and then down to the rima ani. This method is particularly suitable if the laxity of the skin is mainly located in the medial and lateral thigh region and only moderately in the abdominal area. An umbilical transposition is not performed in this method, because the upper epigastrium is pulled tight by lateral tension and not only by vertical pull as in conventional abdominoplasty. Successful reposition of the frequently lax skin in the mons pubis area is done by a connective incision. The line umbilicus-symphysis can be taken as a rule of thumb for the degree of lifting: 60 % hairless, 40 % hair-bearing. The resulting scar has a "high-cut Bikini" design and can be modified (steep ascent or almost vertical) according to the patient's needs.

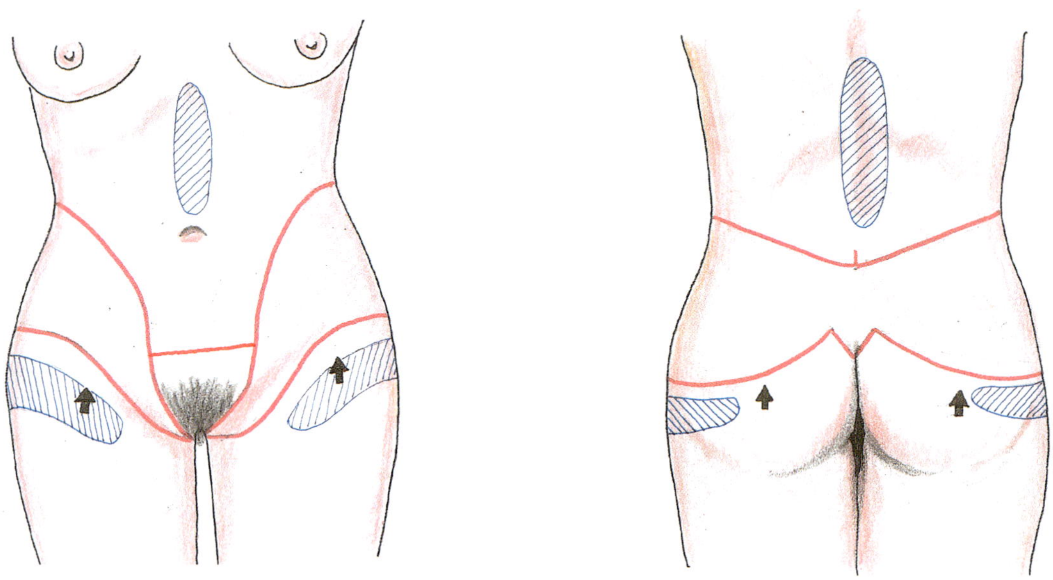

Figure 5.34a,b Design of the original method. The lower resection line is set by approximation under tension to the upper resection line. The blue areas are tightly adherent to the fascia, so that they have to be mobilized. The mobilization is only done in a caudal direction.

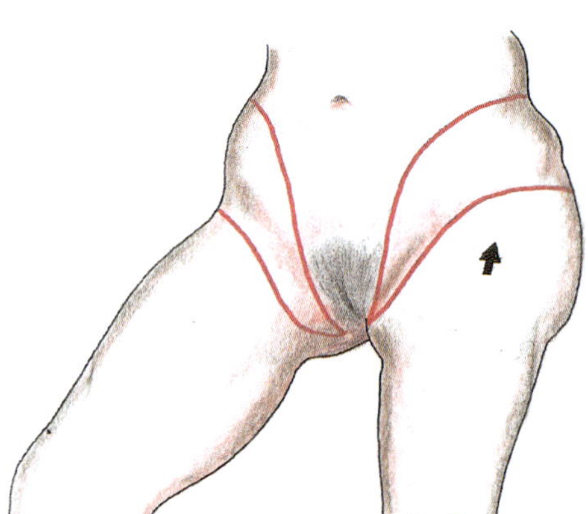

Figure 5.34c Incisional design of the lateral and medial part.

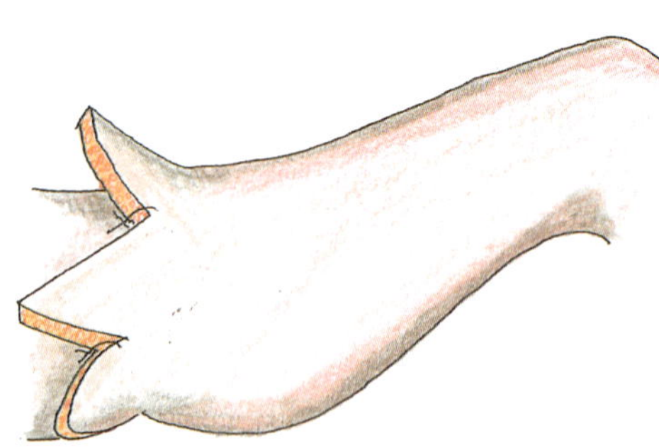

Figure 5.34d Lateral resection, by which particularly the thighs and the gluteal region is lifted.

Body Lifting (Modified by Tom Lockwood)

Is the laxity of the abdominal wall of a higher degree, the modified technique (1995) is recommended. In principle, it is a high-lateral-tension abdominoplasty with a continued thigh and buttock lift. To achieve this, the caudal incision is marked ventrally just like in conventional abdominoplasty, but the lateral tips of the incision do not converge, but stay almost parallel in the chosen distance tat has to be resected. A transposition of the umbilicus is mandatory.

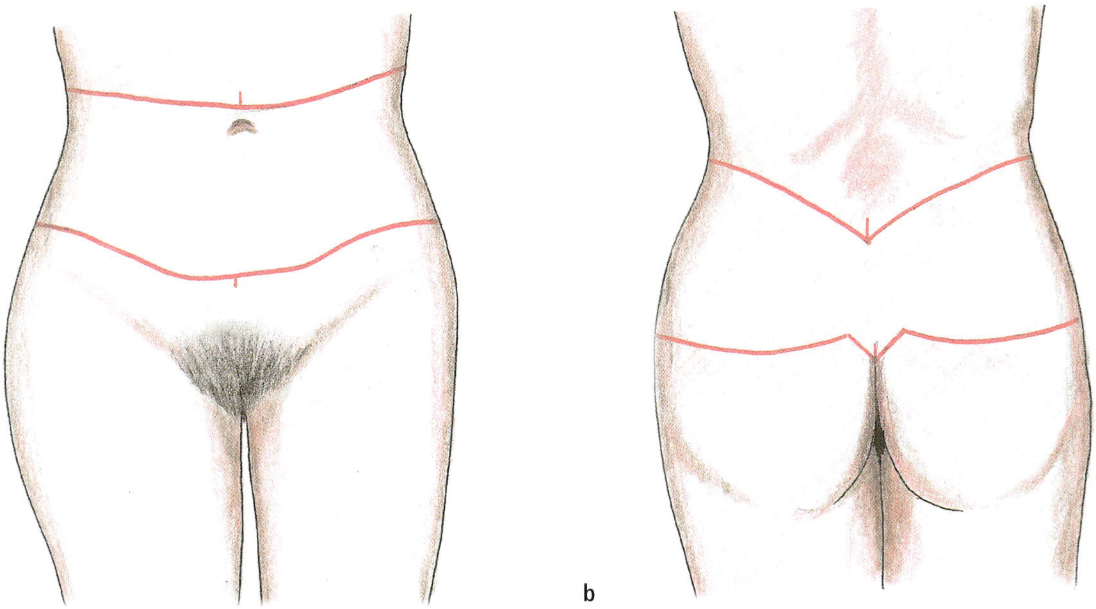

a b

Figure 5.35a, b Modified incisions by Lockwood: a) The ventral part is mobilized in a cranial direction up to the costal margin. b) Dorsally, mobilization is mainly done in a caudal direction. By doing so, the buttock and the thighs are lifted.

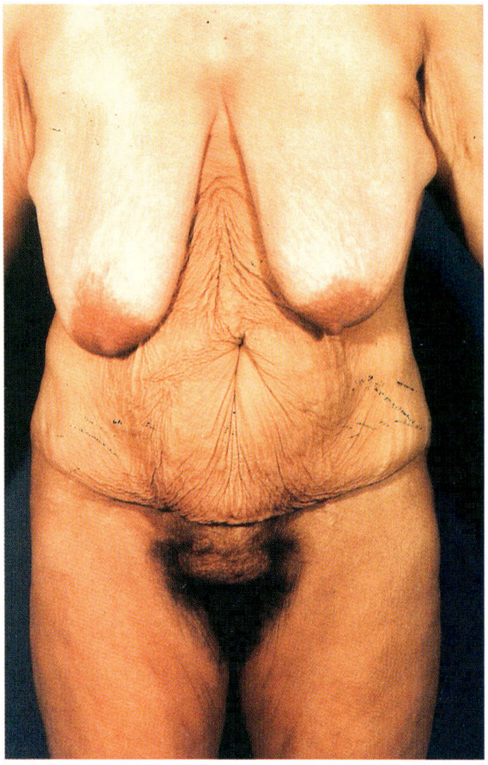

Figure 5.36a Problem case. Status post weight loss of 73 kg. Lax breast, abdomen and thigh skin.

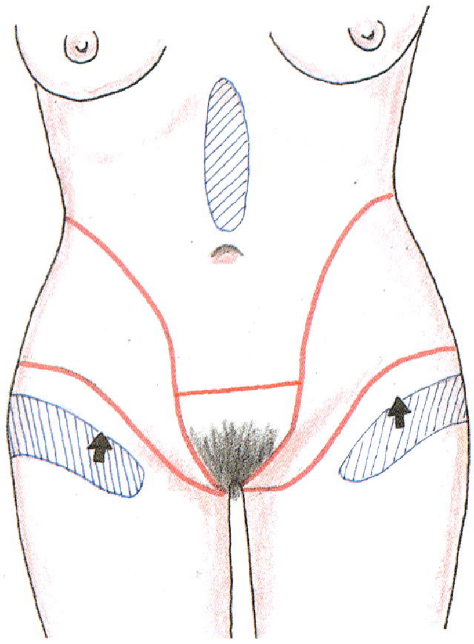

Figure 5.36b Planning of the Lockwood operation. At the same time, the abdomen, buttock and thighs are lifted. The skin of the thigh area is mobilized.

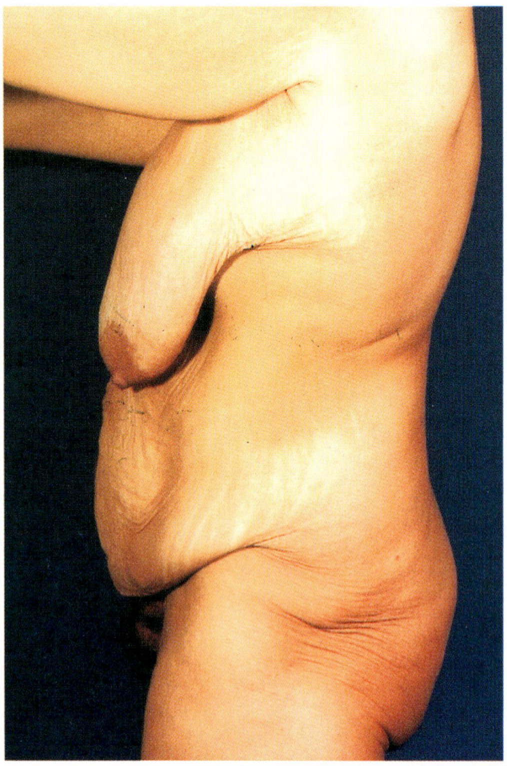

Figure 5.36c Preoperative situation, lateral aspect

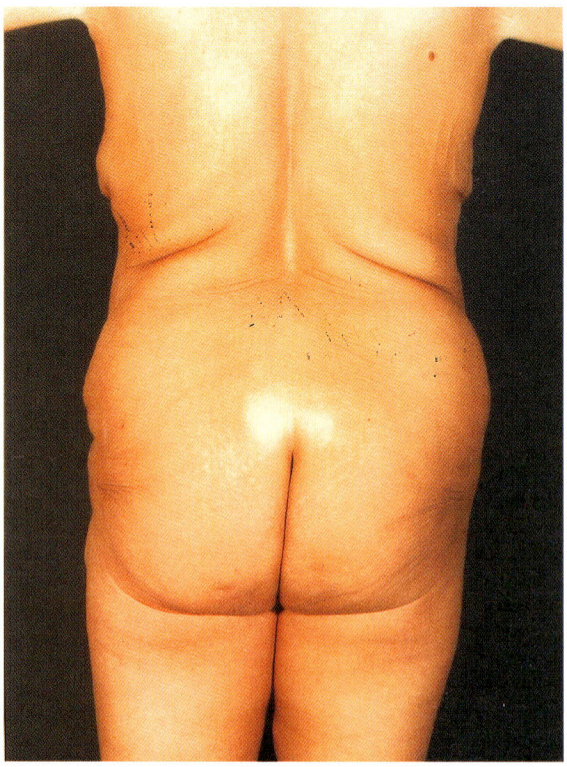

Figure 5.36d Preoperative situation, dorsal aspect

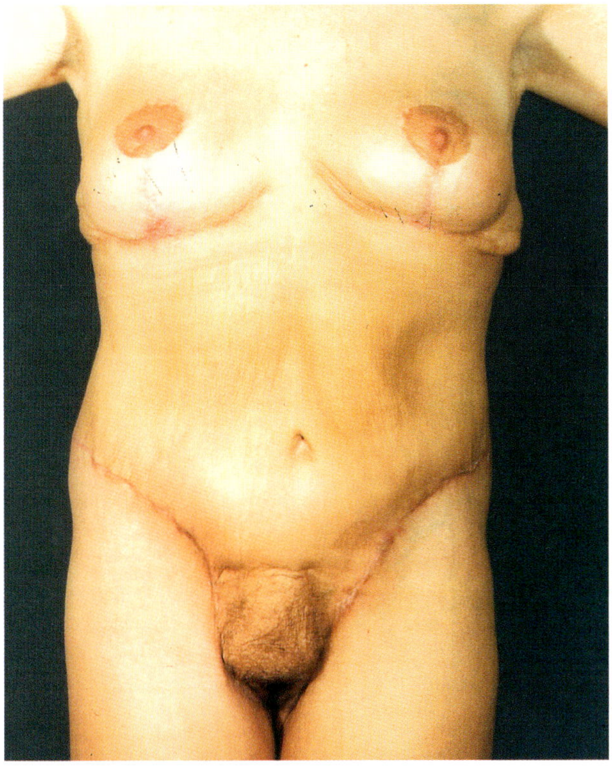

Figure 5.36e Status three months after the operation. Smaller corrections are planned.

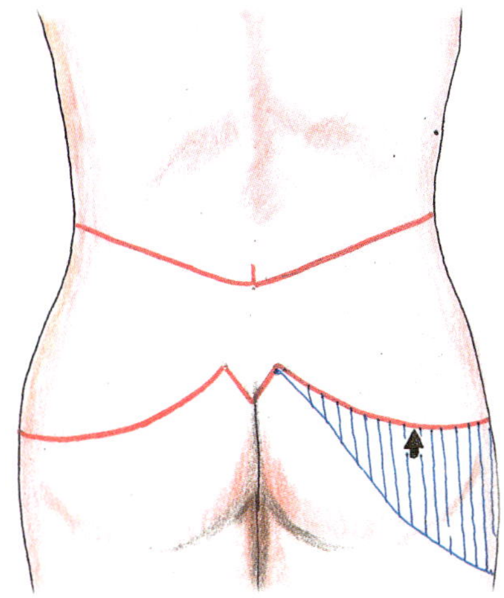

Figure 5.36f Dorsal incisions. Laterally, 28 cm dermofat have been resected, medially (dorsum) 17 cm. A mobilization in the caudal direction is sufficient.

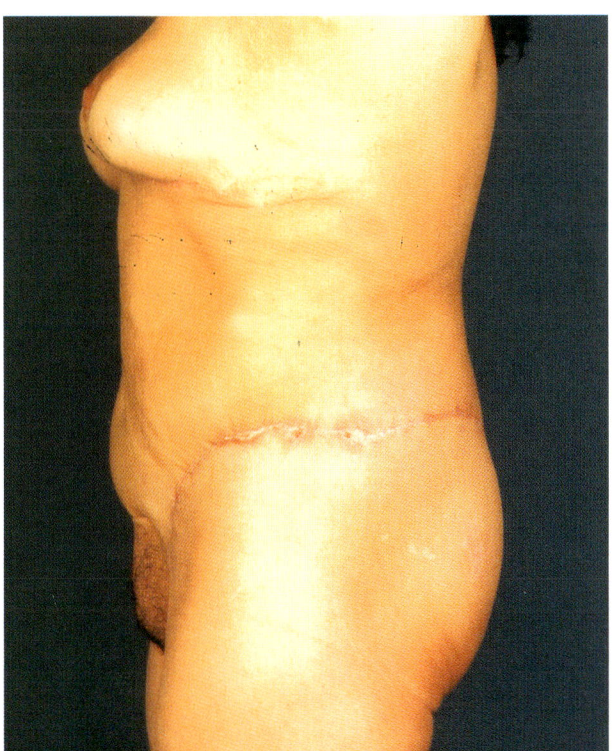

Figure 5.36g Postoperative result

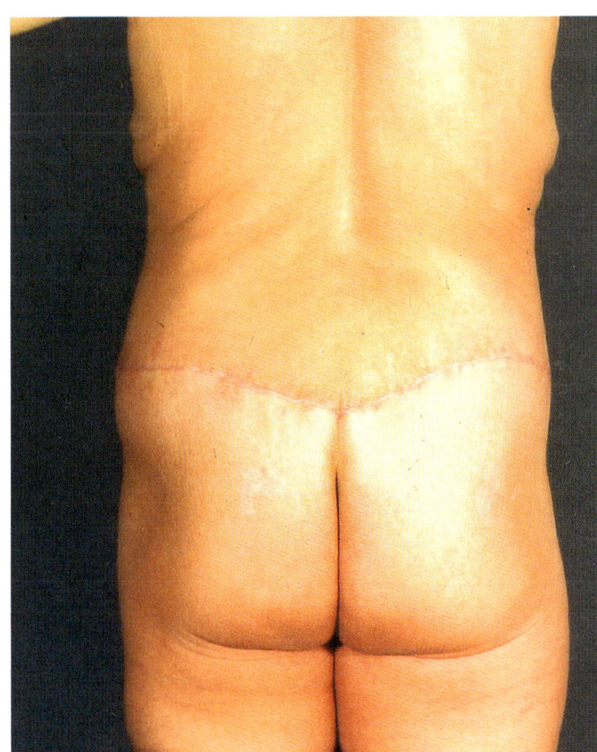

Figure 5.36h Marked improvement of the back contour and the gluteal region

Combination Method

Following the two published methods by Lockwood, we are using a "combination-method" since 1999 which is performed in the case of very lax abdominal and thigh skin, for example after excessive weight loss (>60 kg). Since the original method can be done very successfully in patients who already underwent abdominoplasty and particularly lifts the epigastric area by lateral tension, we had the idea to mobilize the central skin-soft-tissue strip of the original method so far downward that a transposition of the umbilicus is also needful. By doing so, an existing rectus muscle diastasis can be treated by doubling of the fascia. Also, one has the option perform a medial thigh lift – an area which is frequently also affected – at the same time. By the induced vertical pull in the central region of the abdomen in combination with lateral traction by the high lateral incision, an optimal lifting of the entire abdomen and particularly the epigastric area is the result. The resection between mons pubis and the umbilicus usually measures about 10 cm. It will be rarely more because of the tension distribution. This combination method is therefore solely indicated in cases with an extreme excess of skin in the central region.

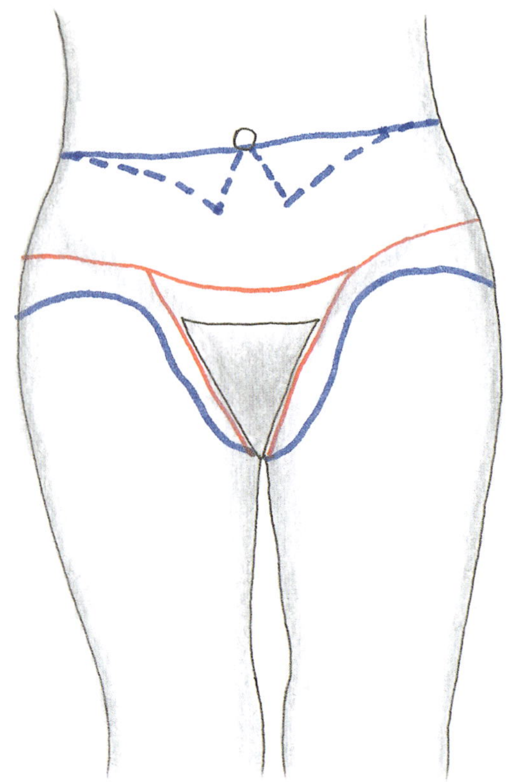

Figure 5.37 Incision marks of the combination method. First, the margins of the underwear (slip) have to be marked (red), where later on the scars will be located. Then the incision line is designed.

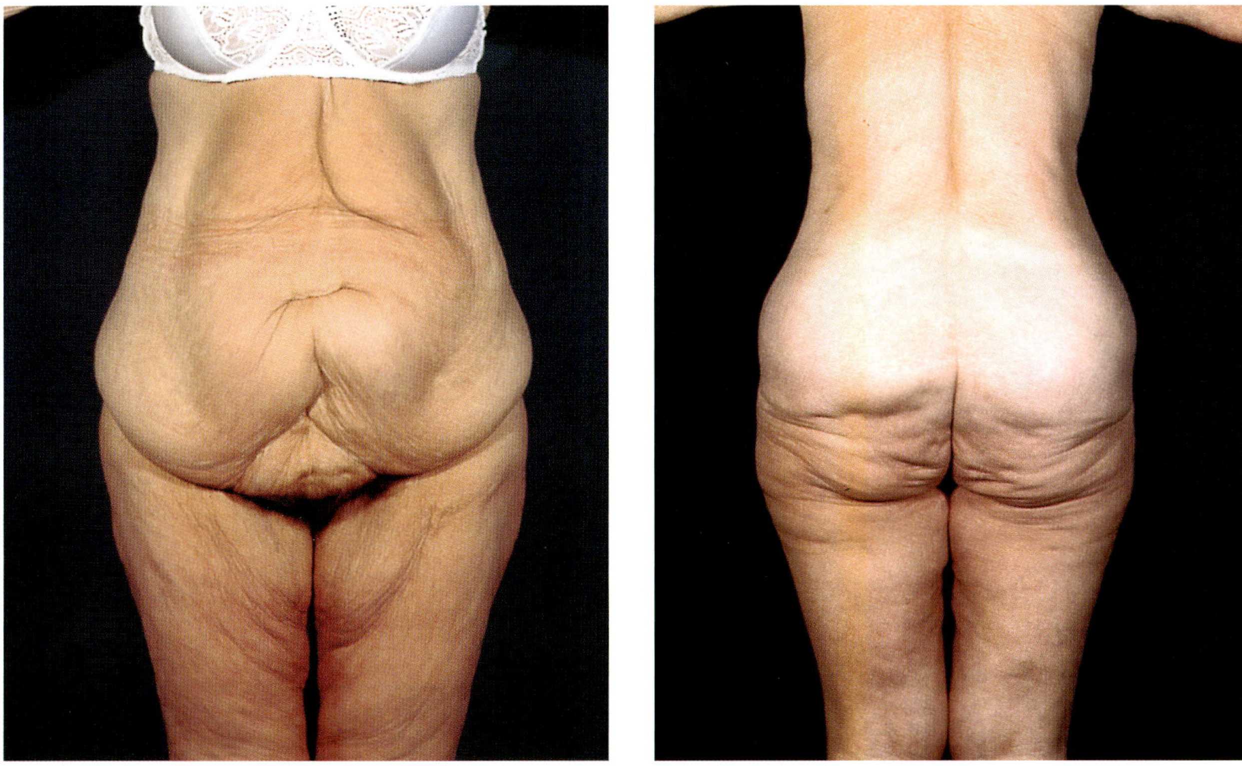

Figure 5.38a,b 63-year old patient: Status post weight reduction of 70 kg by gastric banding. Multiple recurrent scar herniations.

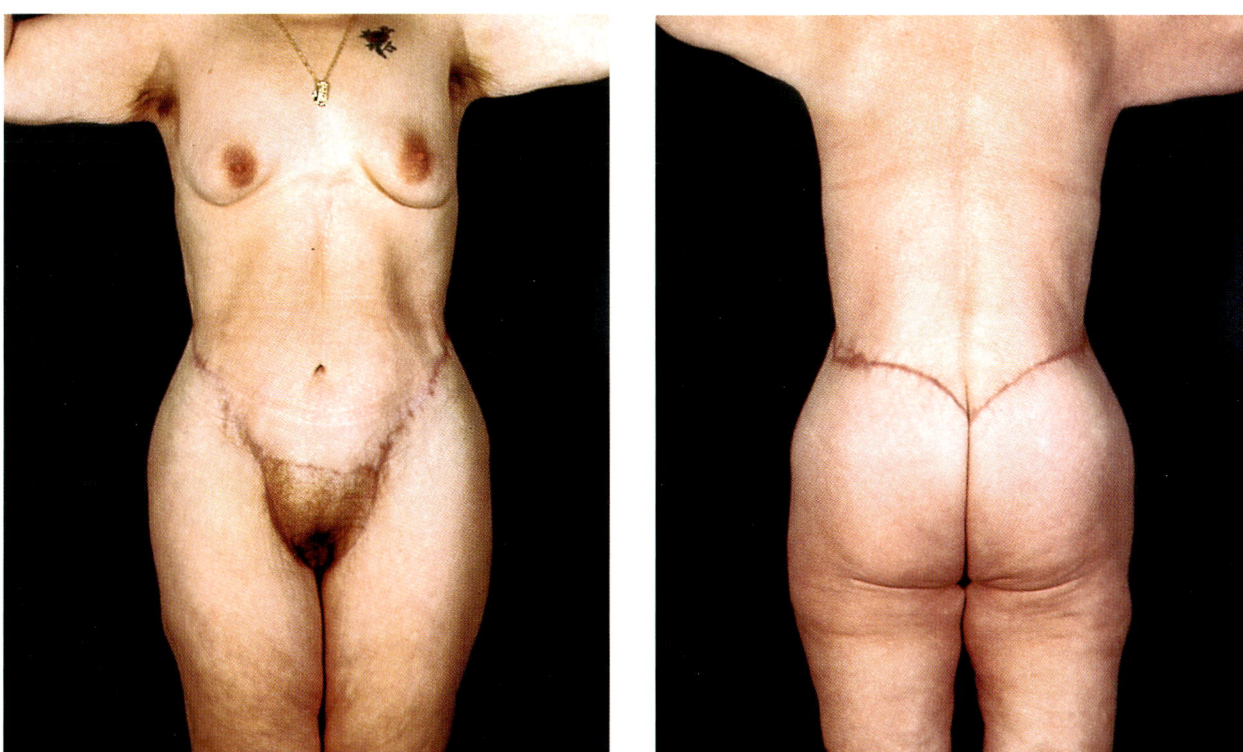

Figure 5.38c,d Status six months after lower body lift with umbilical transposition, herniotomy and Prolene®-mesh implantation over the entire abdominal wall.

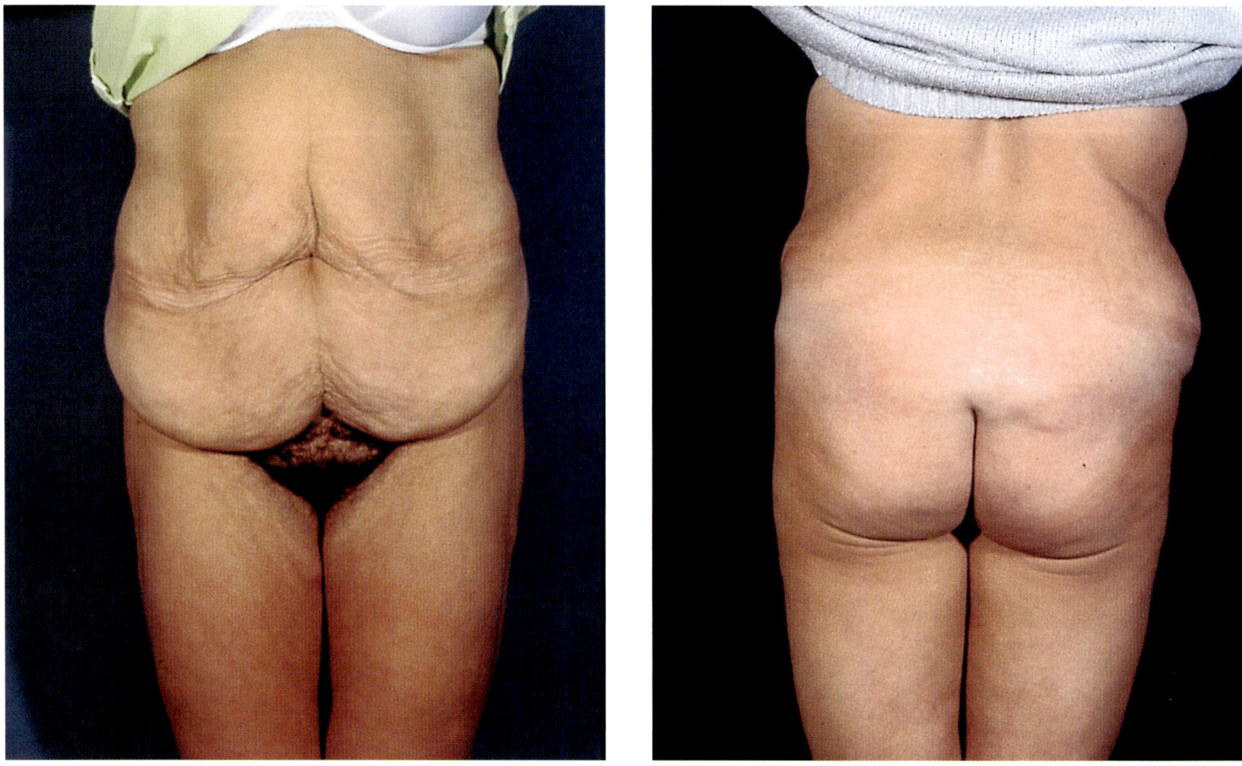

Figure 5.39a, b 36-year old patient with a weight loss of 70 kg

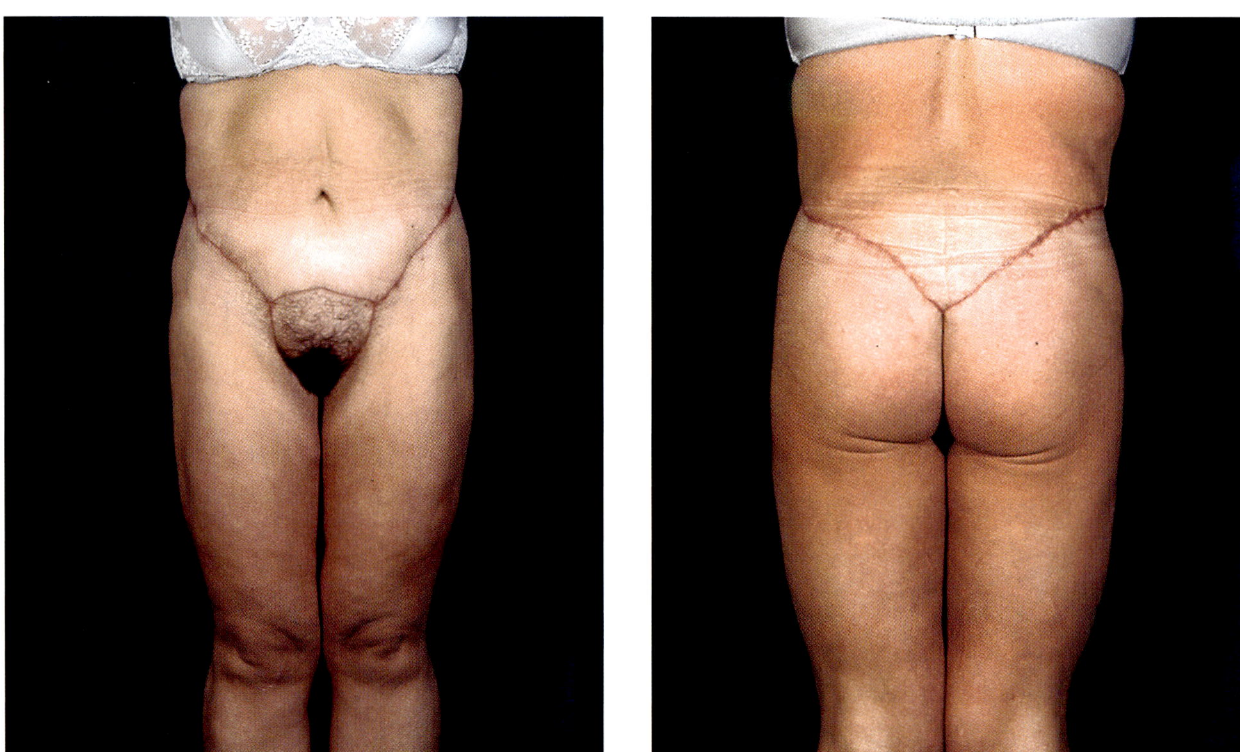

Figure 5.39c,d Status six months after lower body lift with doubling of the rectus fascia and umbilical transposition.

Results

Between January 1996 and June 2002, we have performed a total number of 91 body lifts with different indications. Only three patients were male. In 37 patients (96 %), weight reduction was the main indication and the resection volumes ranged from 10 to 150 kg. The resected dermo-fat flaps measured vertically (from the middle of the lateral thigh) between 13 and 37 cm. The average length of the procedure was 4.0 hours and the length of hospital stay 14 to 15 days. The objective and subjective improvement of skin quality, particularly in the lateral thigh region, was significant. The degree of satisfaction was in 96 % of the patients "good" to "very good". When asked, all patients would undergo the procedure again.

Summary

The methods described by Lockwood have revolutionized the range of lifting operations. In one single surgical stage, all problem zones such as abdomen, hip, thighs, buttock and back are durably addressed, with scars that can be easily covered with the clothing. Before, we only had one-step procedures for each of these problem zones, and the results were frequently disappointing without a significant improvement of skin quality. The contour transitions are fluent, and the improvement of the skin relief is significant even after liposuction with hump formation. The longer, more extensive operation with a larger wound area, which makes exact coagulation impossible, is a disadvantage of the method. Considerable efforts have to be made in the postoperative care and the feeling of tension can last for up to six months. The length of hospital stay is markedly shorter compared to the other, multiple single-step procedures. The long scar apparently loses significance by the improvement of skin quality and body contour.

The learning curve for this procedure is long. Before taking the decision to do this procedure, it is recommended to assist some of the operations with and experienced surgeon.

Complications

We have seen three (3.3 %) diffuse hematomas (which required blood transfusion), that could be managed by compression and also a regular decrease of the Hb-value of about 1.5 mg/dl because of the large wound area. Two (3.3 %) severe wound healing disturbances that could be managed by conservative treatment, healed with scarring. Two hypertrophic scars and an isolated keloid of the groin area could be improved by intensified scar and compression therapy. Longer lasting seroma formation (>14 days) were controlled by intralesional tetracycline injections in 14 patients (15.3 %). Circular dysesthesia around the scar were described as non-disturbing by almost all of the patients and the intensity decreased with time. Three patients (3.3 %) complained about a lasting dysesthetic area in the supply region of the lateral branch of the iliohypogastric nerve at the lateral border of the gluteus muscle.

We did not see complications that required surgical intervention, also, during follow-up, we did not see recurrent secondary laxity, lymphedema or infection.

In three patients, we performed circumscribed small liposuctions six months after the procedure to improve smaller contour differences. Widened scars were only corrected in two cases.

Gluteal Area

Pressure Ulcers

Pressure ulcers or pressure sores are seen in the following patient groups:
1) Paraplegic patients
2) Patients in the intensive care unit (longer LOC)
3) Geriatric patients
4) Drug addiction

These locations are most frequently affected:
a) Sacral area
b) Iliac area
c) Major trochanter

Pressure ulcers can also develop in the occipital region, the heels, the scapula, the elbow and the nasal vestibulum.

Pathogenesis

Pathogenetic mechanisms include external pressure exposure and the concomitant local ischemia which both lead to direct mechanical damage to the skin and subcutaneous fat tissue. Partial or total tissue necrosis results.

Pressure ulcers that have fully developed (break-up of the physical barrier skin) are always infected. In hemiplegic patients, one main pathogenetic factor is the decreased or absent sensibility, which favours the development of pressure ulcer formation. About 80 to 90 % of the patients, who present with pressure ulcers and need surgical interventions, are paraplegic. Despite that this chapter focuses on the surgical management of pressure ulcerations, pressure ulcer prophylaxis needs to be discussed. Effective prophylaxis is very time and resource-consuming in paraplegic patients. Pressure ulcer therapy though is way more time-consuming and expensive. A paraplegic patient must be admitted to a specialized rehabilitation centre. The patients get special beds equipped with pressure-changing mattresses and nursing is done by specially qualified personnel. Frequent position changes of the paraplegic patient and very diligent care of the vulnerable regions are of utmost importance. Periodical pressure relief and pressure-reducing garments are essential parts of the rehabilitation of wheelchair-bound patients.

There are many negative factors for paraplegic patients with pressure ulcers:
1) reduced immunity against urinary tract infections
2) worsening of bladder and bowel function
3) increased spasticity of the skeletal musculature
4) negative influence on protein metabolism and hemoglobin levels
5) psychological strain
6) Interruption of rehabilitative training
7) in severe cases risk of sepsis and osteomyelitis
8) need for multiple surgical interventions

The examination of pressure ulcers frequently reveals vast subcutaneous pocket formation. The surgeon frequently encounters a subcutaneous pocket that is about two to three-times bigger than the skin defect itself in pressure ulcers of the trochanteric region. In many cases, bones are exposed (os ischii, os sacrum, trochanter).

Surgical Therapy

The general condition of the patient should be maximally improved by admission to a rehabilitation centre prior to the surgical procedure. Laboratory parameters should of course be within the normal range (hemoglobin level, protein level etc.) and corrected if necessary. Infected ulcers are treated by at least two daily dressing changes and enzymatic wound cleaning. The iv administration of antibiotics is self-evident. Two to four PRBC should be supplied for the surgical intervention. The postoperative care of paraplegic patients must be done in specialized rehabilitation centres. On most surgical wards, the needed specialized care cannot be sufficiently provided for these patients. A close collaboration between the surgical team and the rehabilitation centre is absolutely necessary.

Surgical Procedure

Not only the ulcer, but also scar tissue should be excised. The subcutaneous pockets have to be debrided to the level of healthy tissue. Exposed bone (os ischii, trochanter etc.) should be osteotomized using a flat, wide chisel in a tangential fashion. The bone surface has to be smooth to avoid recurrencies. Defect coverage is done by myocutaneous flaps or – rarely – by fasciocutaneous flaps. The techniques are described in the following pages.

a) Gluteus Maximus Muscle Flap

Anatomic Situation

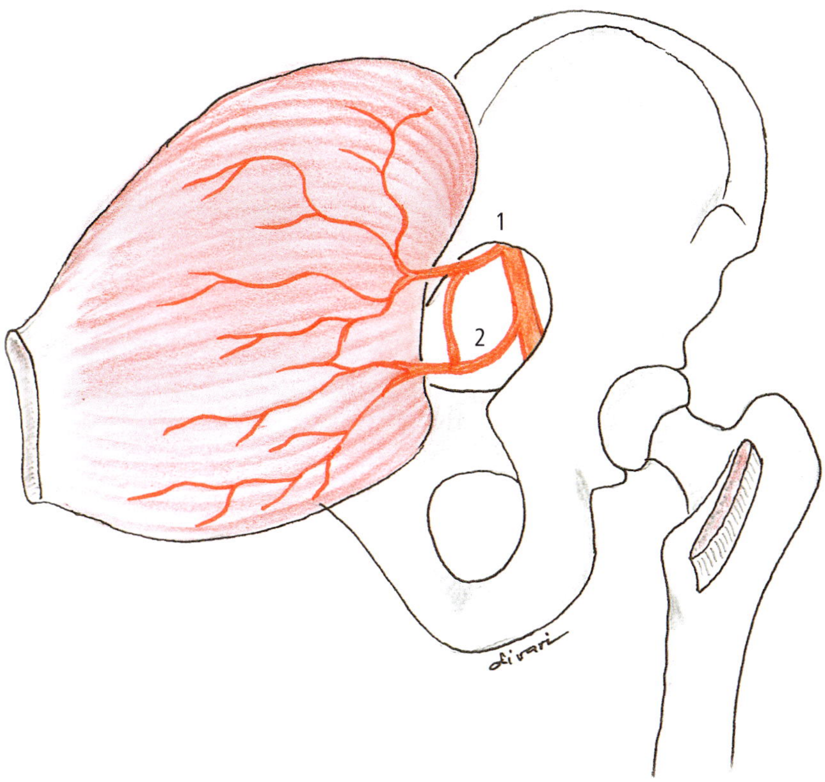

Figure 5.40 Blood supply of the gluteus maximus muscle: The gluteus maximus muscle has two dominant pedicles. Therefore, the whole muscle can be subdivided into two (vessel) parts either of which can be separately mobilized on his own pedicle (superior gluteal artery = 1, inferior gluteal artery = 2). Mobilization of the whole muscle on one pedicle is dangerous and extremely dependent on intramuscular anastomoses that may variably be present to a greater or lesser degree. In hemiplegic patients, both pedicles or the whole muscle must not be used to avoid functional impairment.

Myocutaneous Flaps

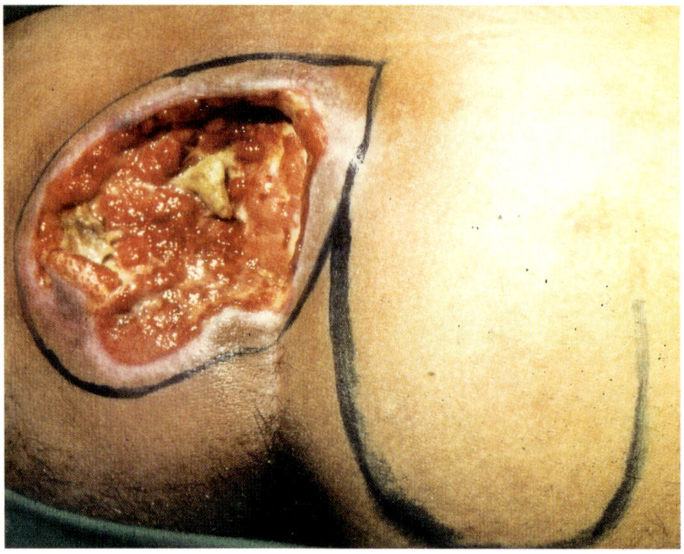

Figure 5.41a Pressure ulcer of the sacral region, mainly on the left side in paraplegic patients.

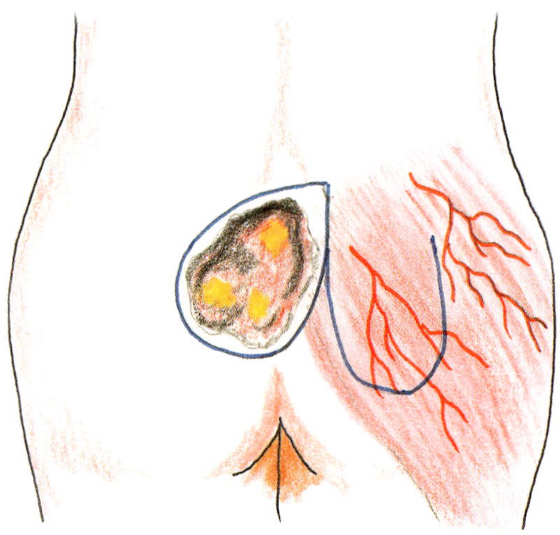

Figure 5.41b Preoperative planning. Excision of the ulcerated region and forming of a myocutaneous gluteus maximus muscle flap as a transposition flap.

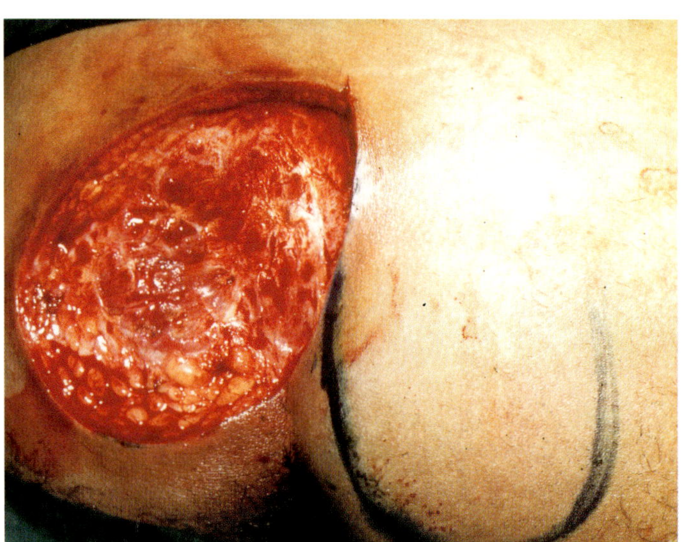

Figure 5.41c The central portion of the procedure is the radical debridement. Even a small piece of necrotic tissue will markedly impair wound healing.

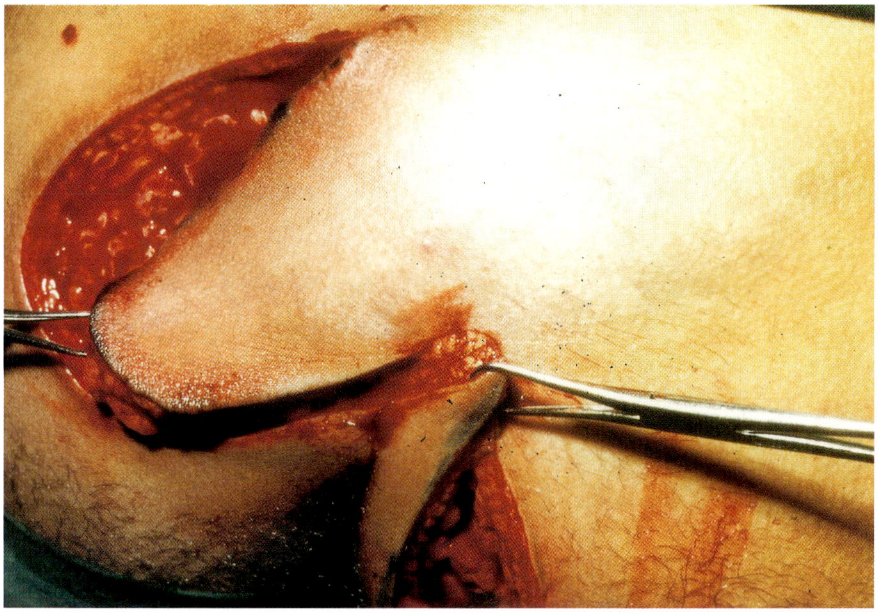

Figure 5.41d The gluteus maximus myocutaneous flap is mobilized and rotated into the defect. The secondary defect is closed after sufficient mobilization without tension.

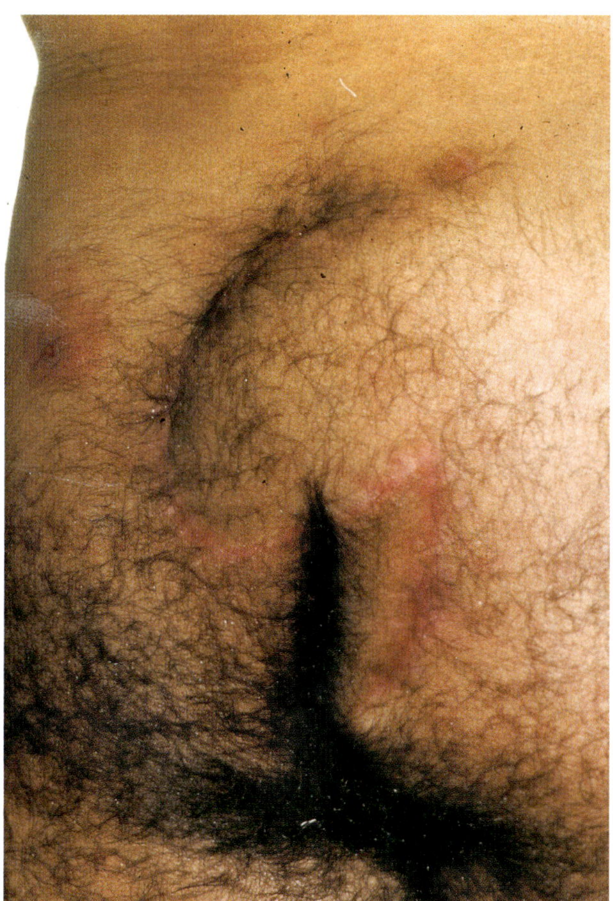

Figure 5.41e Status one year post surgery

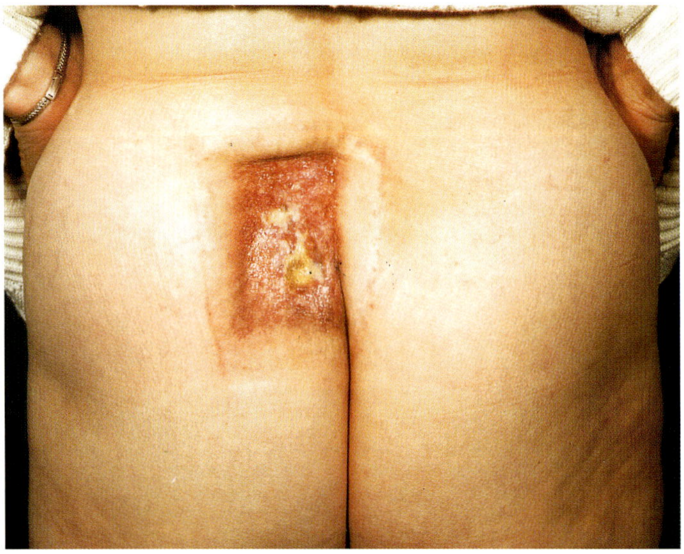

Figure 5.42a Sacral ulceration after radiotherapy. Pressure on the fragile, irradiated area led to the ulceration. Surgical strategy: A pedicled myocutaneous gluteal flap is raised and transposed into the defect after excision of the irradiated area.

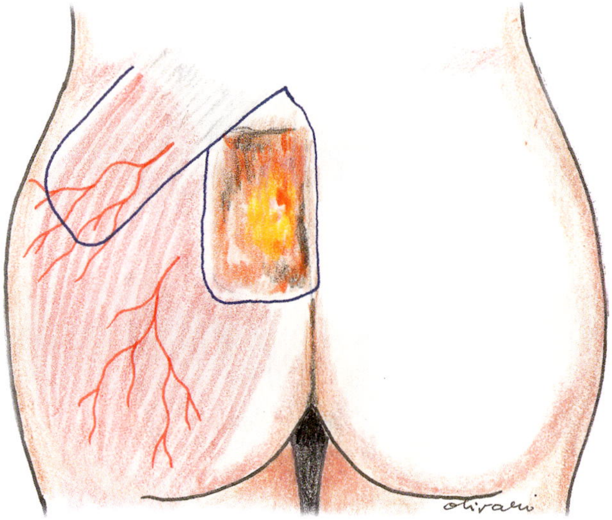

Figure 5.42b To allow for a better rotation, healthy skin is excised cranial from the defect.

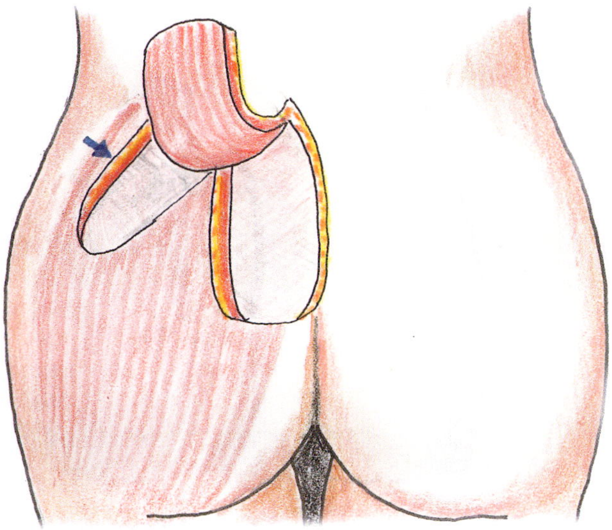

Figure 5.42c Tension-free secondary defect closure is done after lateral mobilization.

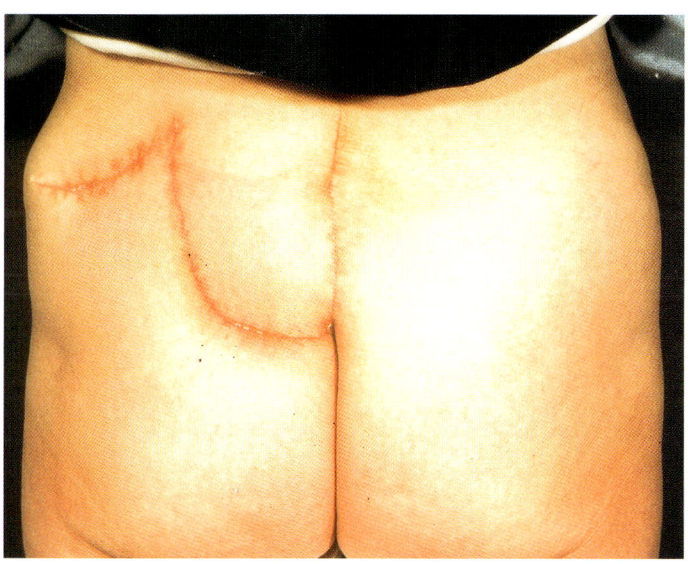

Figure 5.42d Status four months after surgery

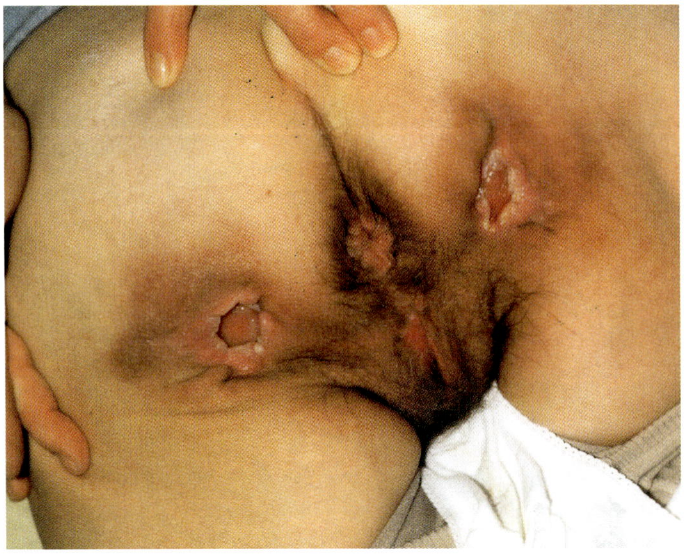

Figure 5.43a Two pressure ulcers of the sacral area (os ischii) in a hemiplegic patient. The ulcerations appear to be small in size, however, there is extensive subcutaneous pocket formation. There is exposed bone on both sides which is only covered with granulation tissue. The excision has to be extended to the healthy tissue. The subcutaneous pockets must be excised, also the heavily scarred skin regions. The surface of the os ischium is osteotomized using a flat chisel. By doing so, the bony surface is smoothened.

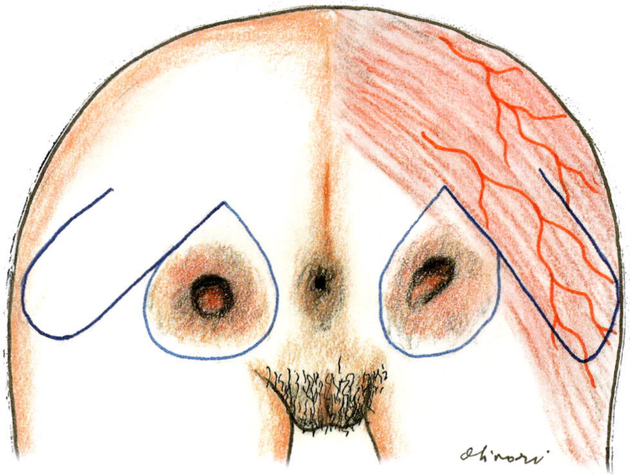

Figure 5.43b For coverage of the surgical defect a myocutaneous gluteal flap is raised on each side. The exposed bone is covered by the caudal portion of the gluteus maximus muscle with the inferior gluteal artery.

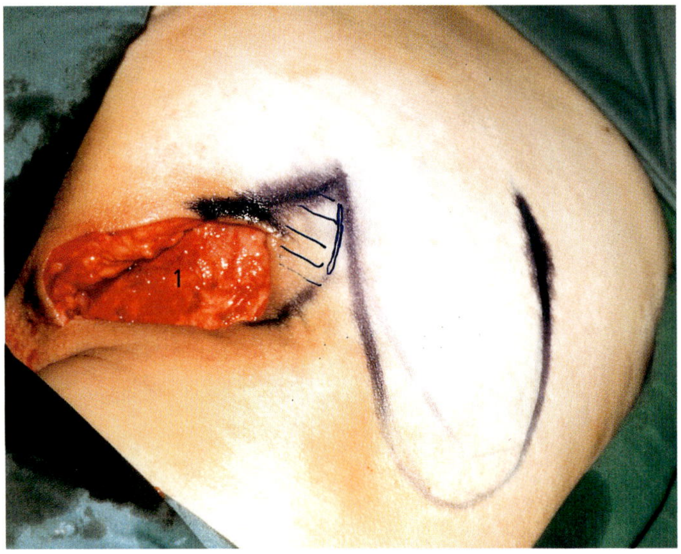

Figure 5.43c After the excision and chiselling of the superficial portion of the os ischium a part of surrounding healthy skin is excised (hatched) to allow for easier mobilization of the flap. Here, the smoothened os ischium is visible (1). The osteotomy also reduces relapse rates. The overlying muscle is well perfused and somewhat resistant to pressure force.

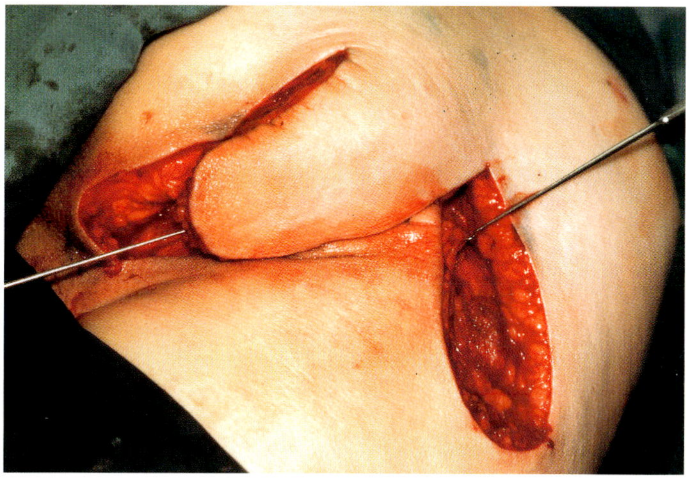

Figure 5.43d The myocutaneous gluteal flap is transposed into the defect.

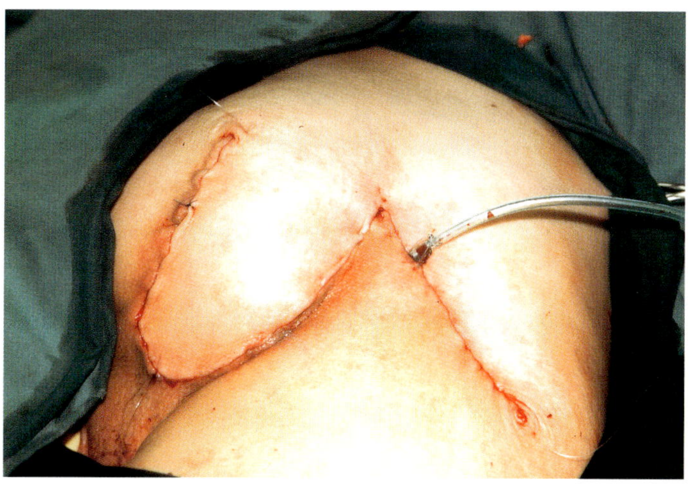

Figure 5.43e The donor site is primarily closed without tension on the suture. The left side is treated in the same fashion. Postoperatively, the patient must be admitted to a specialized rehabilitation centre with special focus on wound care and management of hemiplegic patients. There should be no pressure stress on the flap for at least four weeks.

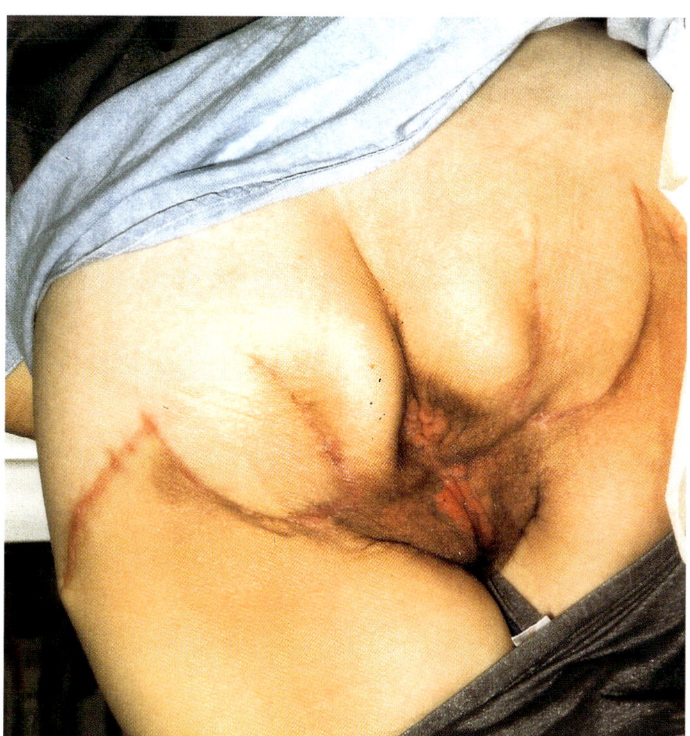

Figure 5.43f Status six months after surgery, full exposure to pressure stress.

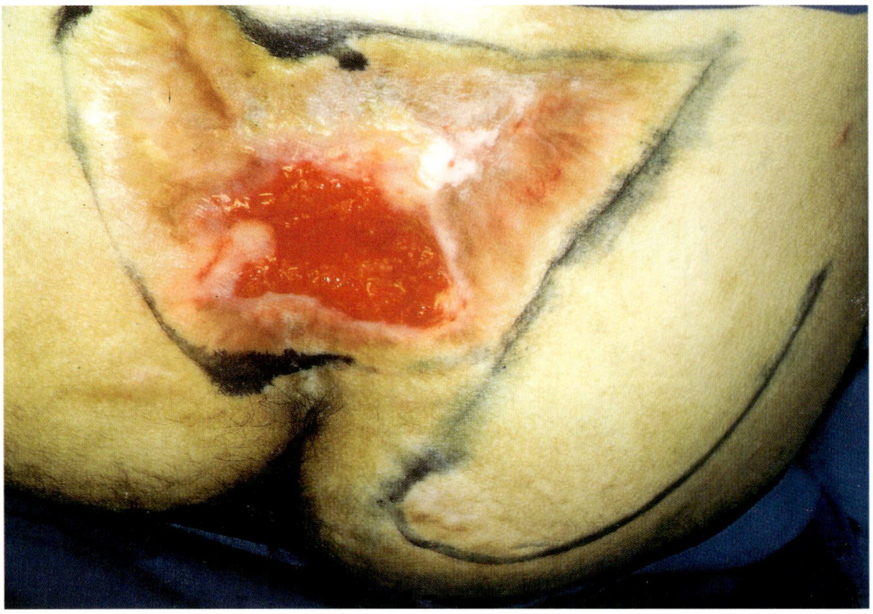

Figure 5.44a Sacral pressure ulcer in a hemiplegic patient. The patient has already been skin grafted twice.

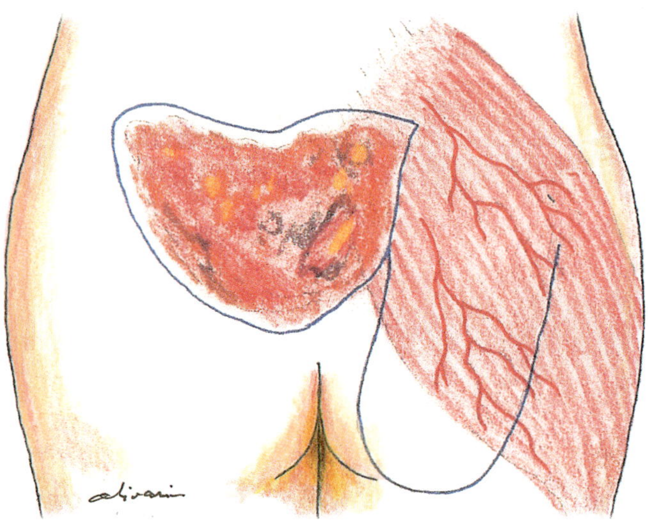

Figure 5.44b Surgical planning: A radical excision of the ulcer and the scar tissue is done. Raising of a myocutaneous gluteal flap, which is transposed into the defect. The tip of the flap is only a fasciocutaneous flap.

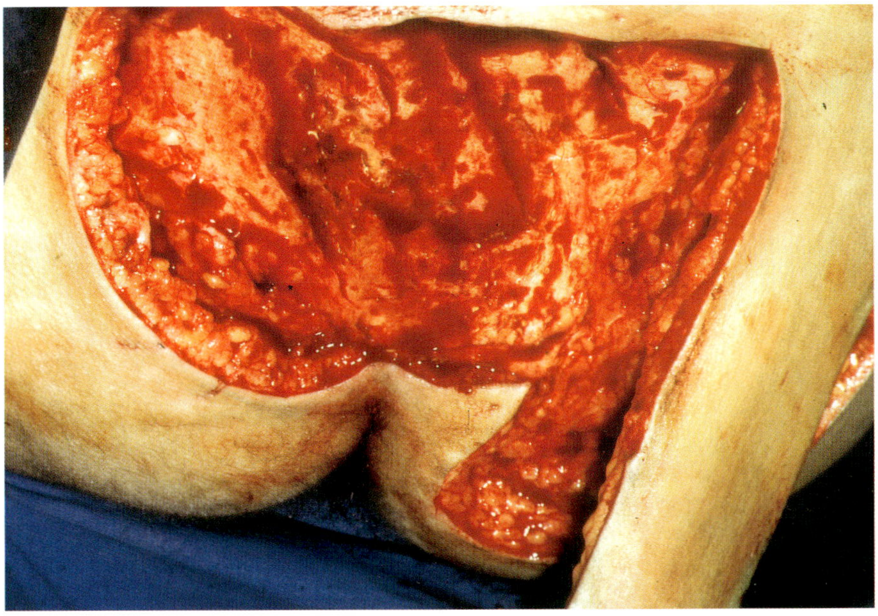

Figure 5.44c Status after radical excision, which is of utmost importance. The flap has been mobilized.

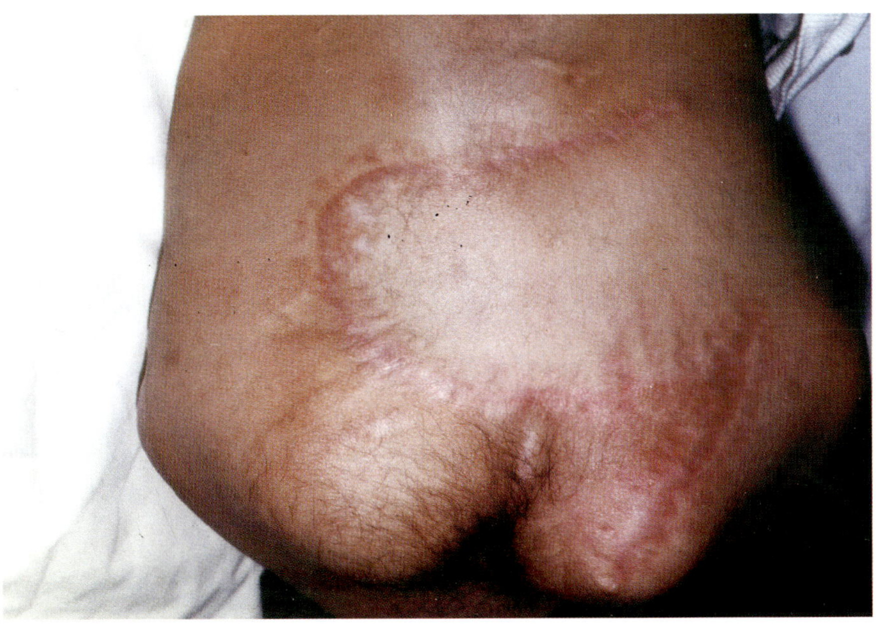

Figure 5.44d Status one year after surgery, full exposure to pressure stress.

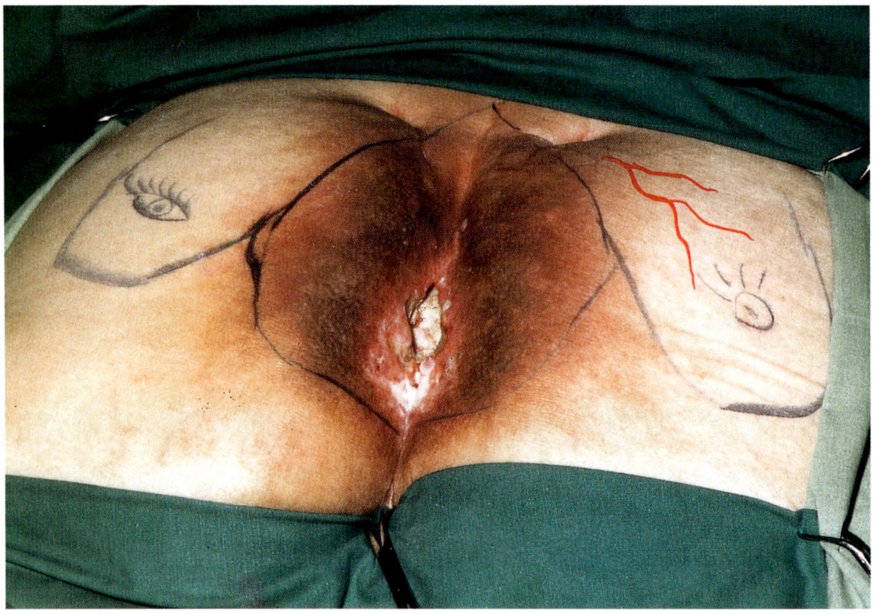

Figure 5.45a Ulcer induced by radiotherapy; radioderm of the sacral region.

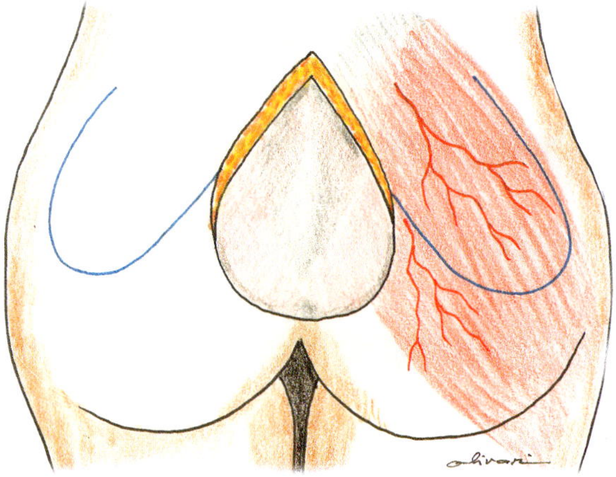

Figure 5.45b Surgical planning: First, all necrotic and fibrotic tissue is excised. The os coccygis is avitalized and resected. Two myocutaneous gluteal flaps are mobilized from both sides. The superior gluteal artery is located in the flap and maintains adequate perfusion of the flap. The donor site is closed primarily.

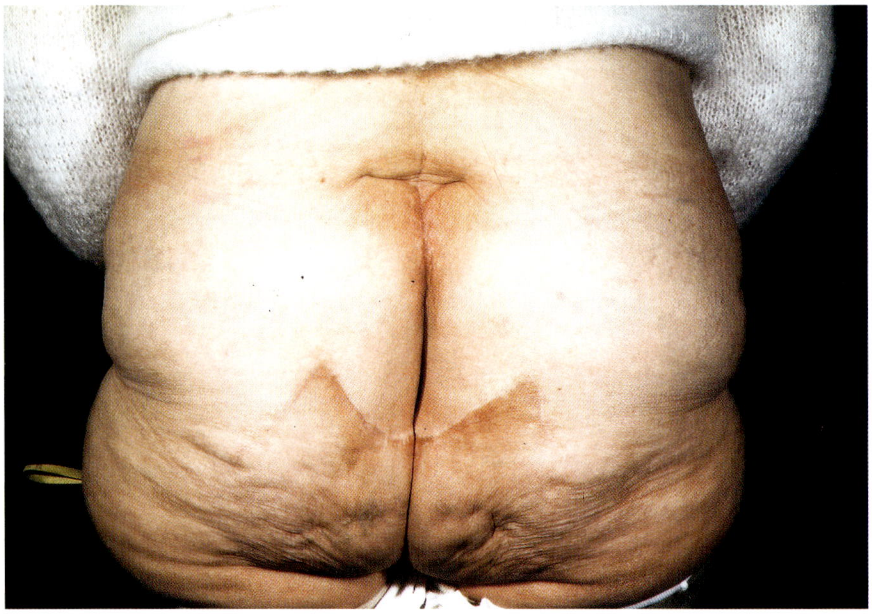

Figure 5.45c Status 18 months after surgery

VY-Myocutaneous Flaps

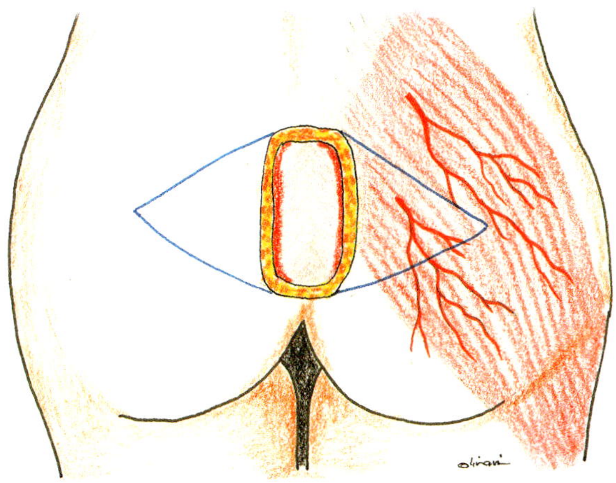

Figure 5.46a For defect coverage in the sacral region, a VY-plasty as a bilateral, myocutaneous flap is often utilized. In the cranial portion, the superior gluteal artery can be used. The caudal portion of the flap usually includes the inferior gluteal artery.

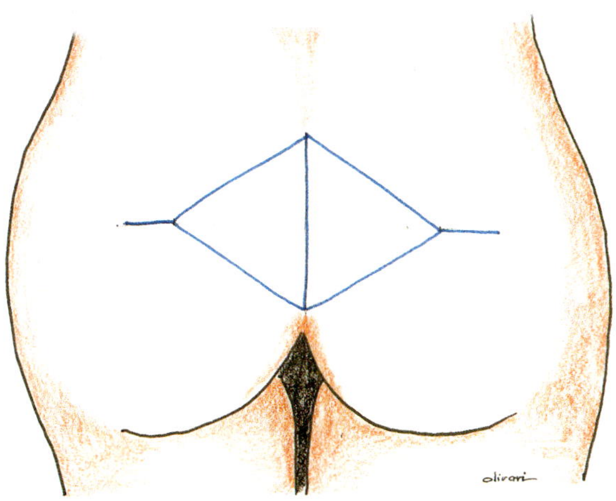

Figure 5.46b The flaps must be adapted medially without tension on the suture.

b) VY-Plasty and Tensior-Fascia-Lata Flap

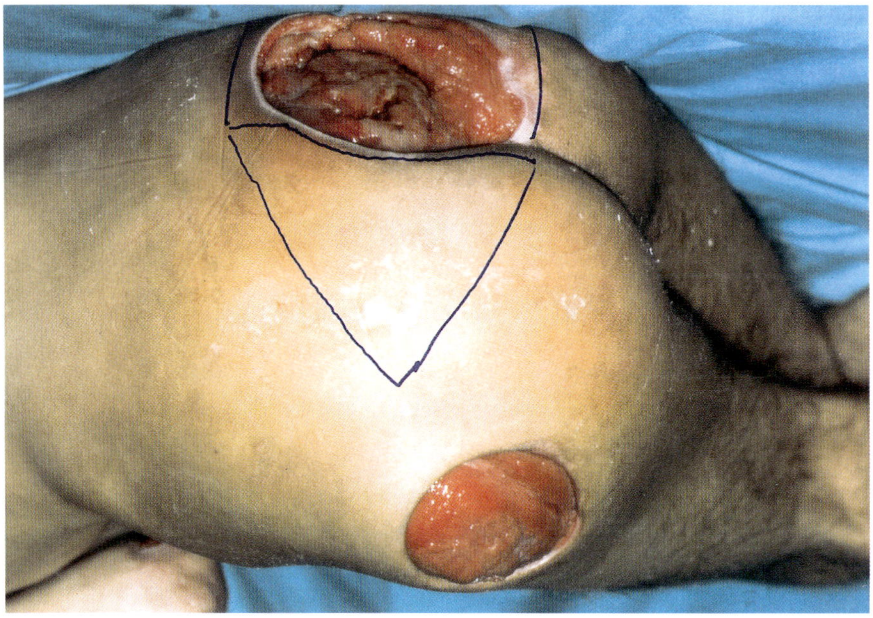

Figure 5.47a Paraplegia. Large ulceration in the sacral area and smaller ulceration in the left major trochanteric region.

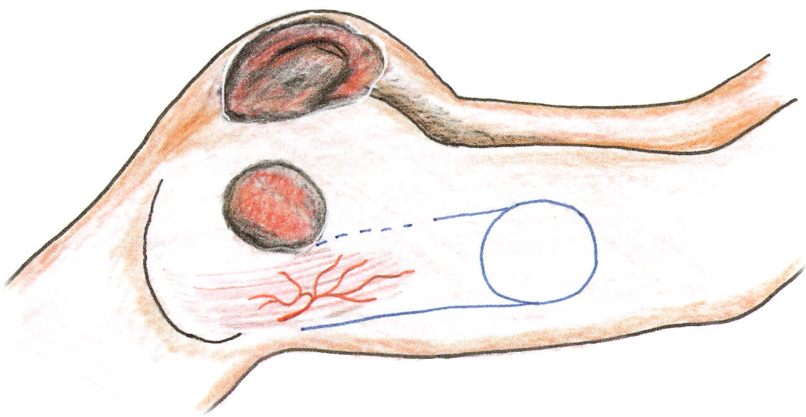

Figure 5.47b For the ulceration in the region of the major trochanter, a fascia-lata island flap is prepared.

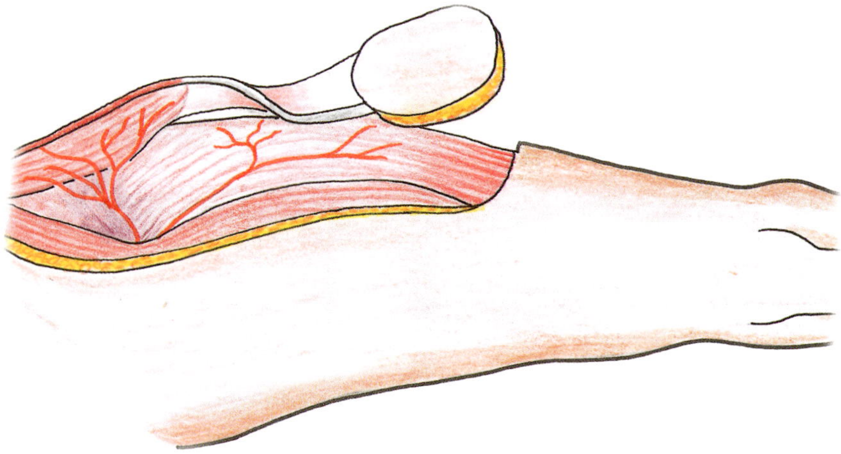

Figure 5.47c The tensor-fascia-lata flap is a musculocutaneous flap. Blood supply comes from a branch of the lateral circumflex femoral artery, which runs through the muscle and later surfaces and runs with the fascia. The diameter of the artery is 2 mm and the pedicle length is 7 to 9 cm. This allows for closure of defects in the major trochanter region and the lower abdominal wall (pedicled or island flap).

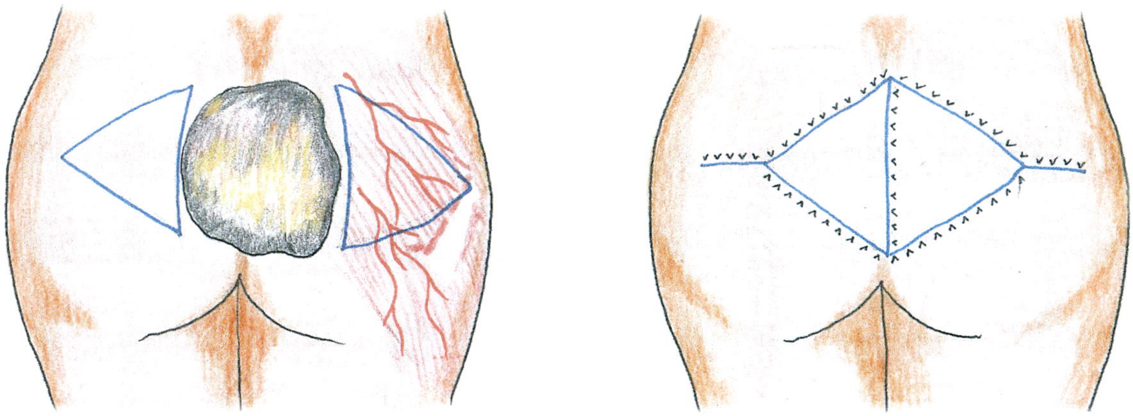

Figure 5.47d,e Two VY-myocutaneous gluteal flaps are bilaterally raised. To do so, the gluteus maximus muscle has to be latero-caudally transected. Care must be taken not to damage the superior and inferior gluteal arteries.

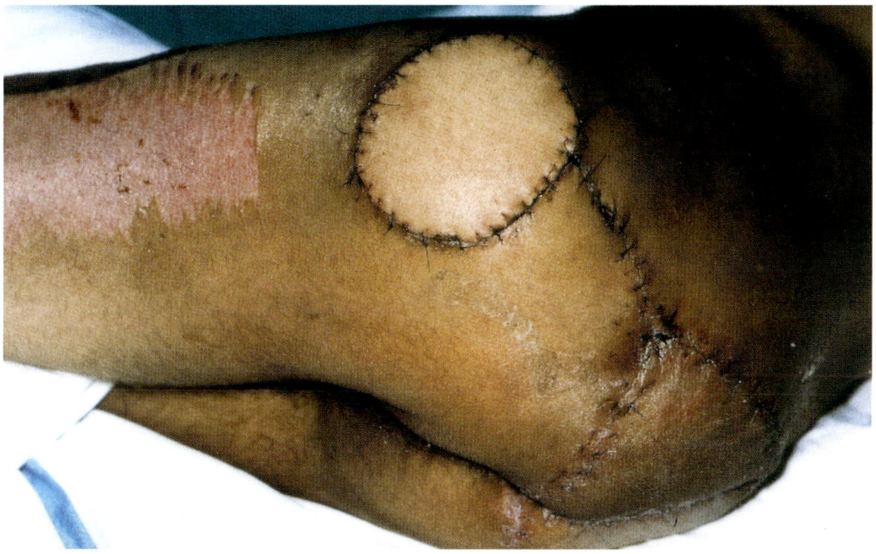

Figure 5.47f Status 16 days post surgery. The top portion of the picture shows the round tensor-fascia-lata flap. On the bottom of the picture, in the sacral region, the two VY-myocutaneous island flaps are seen.

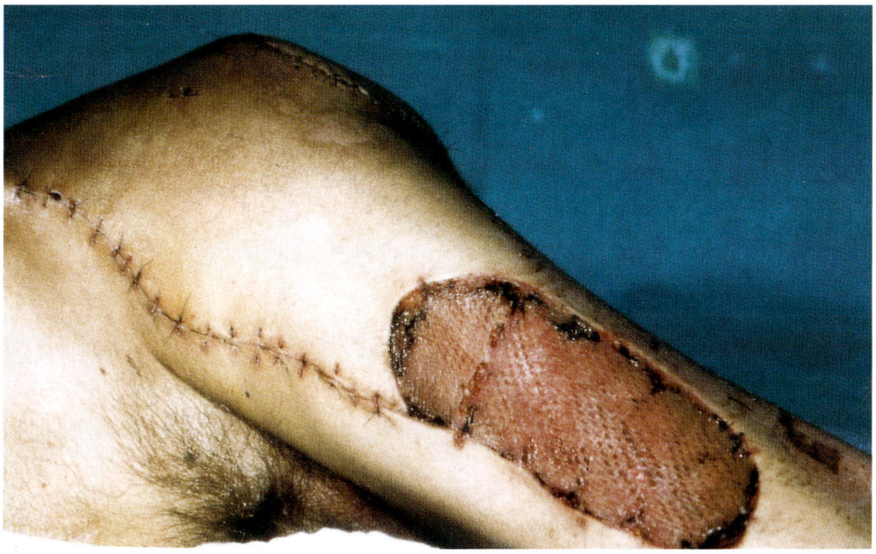

Figure 5.47g The donor site defect of the tensor-fascia-lata island flap is mesh-grafted.

c) Fasciocutaneous Flaps

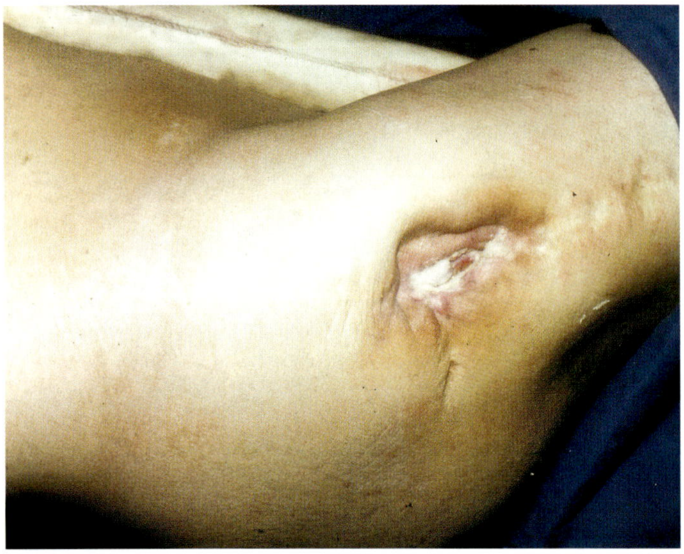

Figure 5.48a Pressure ulcer of the right major trochanteric region. Bone is exposed (paraplegia).

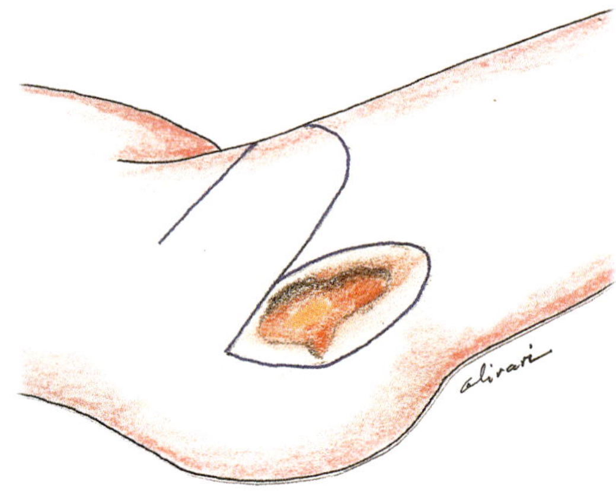

Figure 5.48b Excision of the necrotic tissue and superficial osteotomy of the major trochanter. A fasciocutaneous flap is raised from the ventral, not pressure-exposed part of the leg.

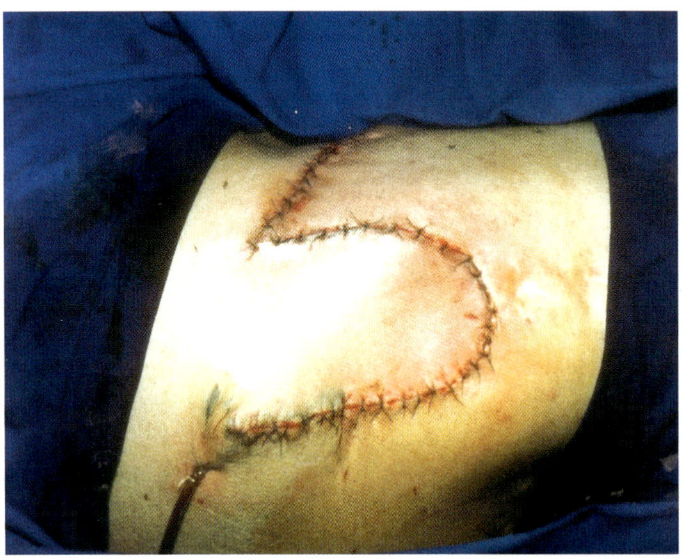

Figure 5.48c Status at the end of the procedure. The donor site defect is primarily closed without tension.

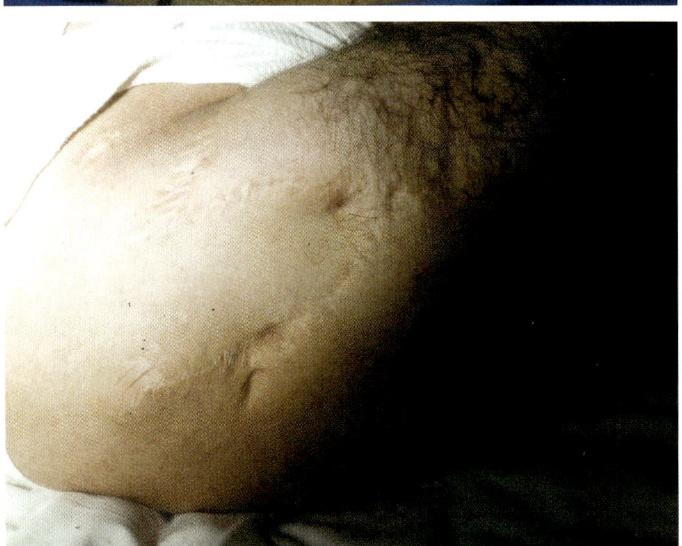

Figure 5.48d Status three years after the procedure

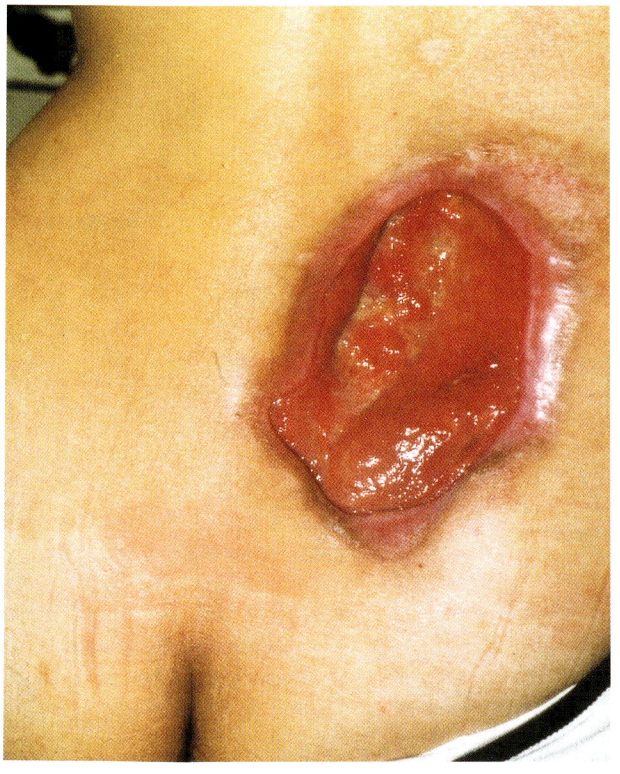

Figure 5.49a Pressure ulcer after longer coma

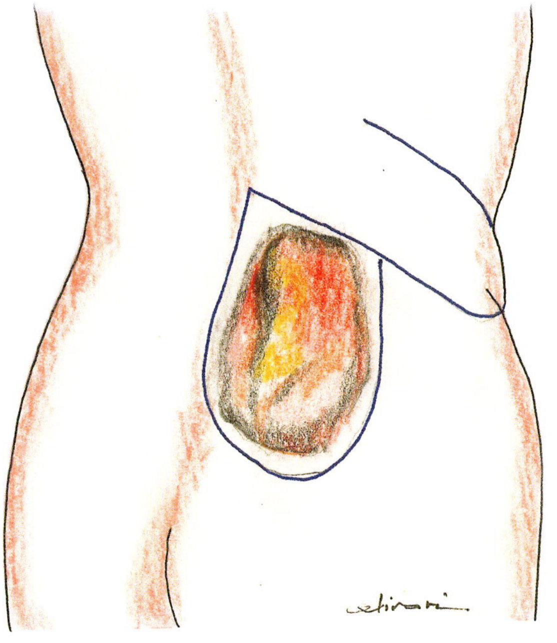

Figure 5.49b Surgical planning: Wide radical excision. A fasciocutaneous transposition flap is raised parallel to the intercostal vessels, mobilized and rotated into the defect. The donor site defect is closed primarily.

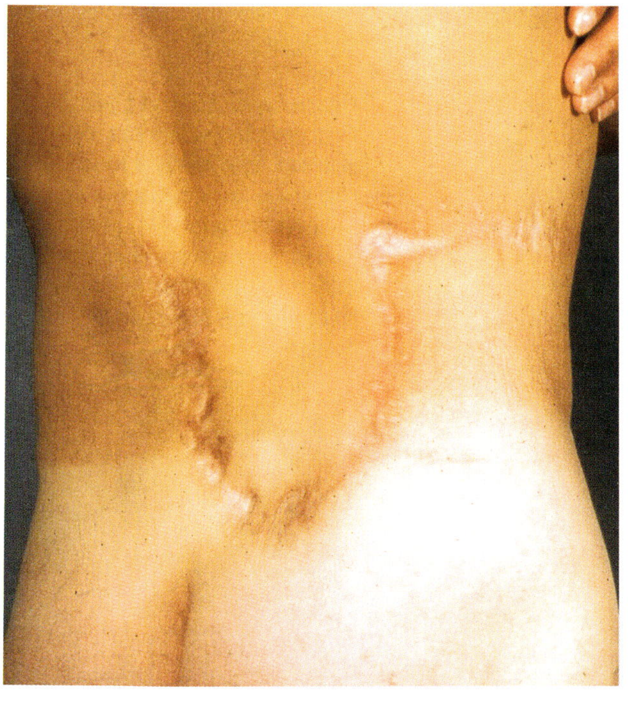

Figure 5.49c Status one year after the procedure

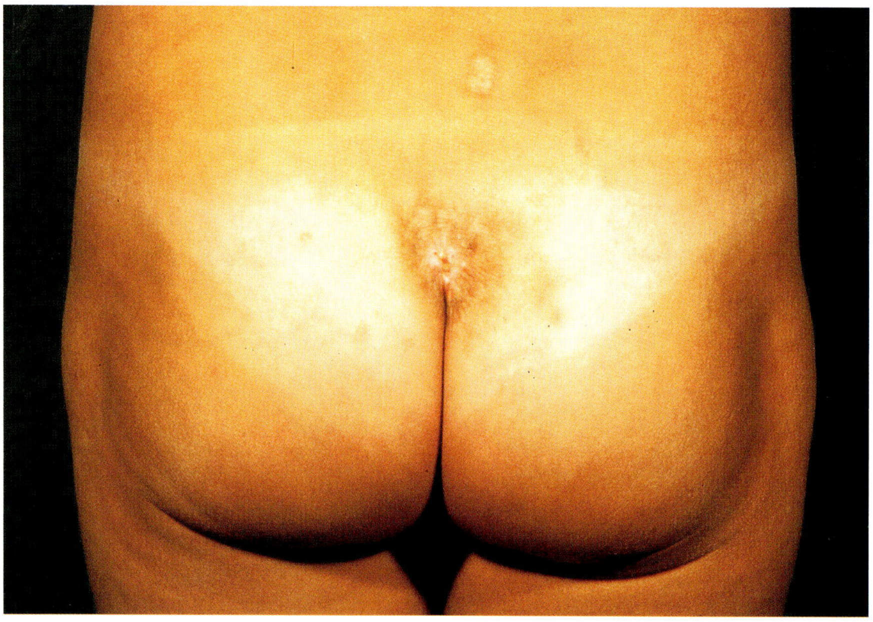

Figure 5.52a Pilonidal fistula after multiple infections

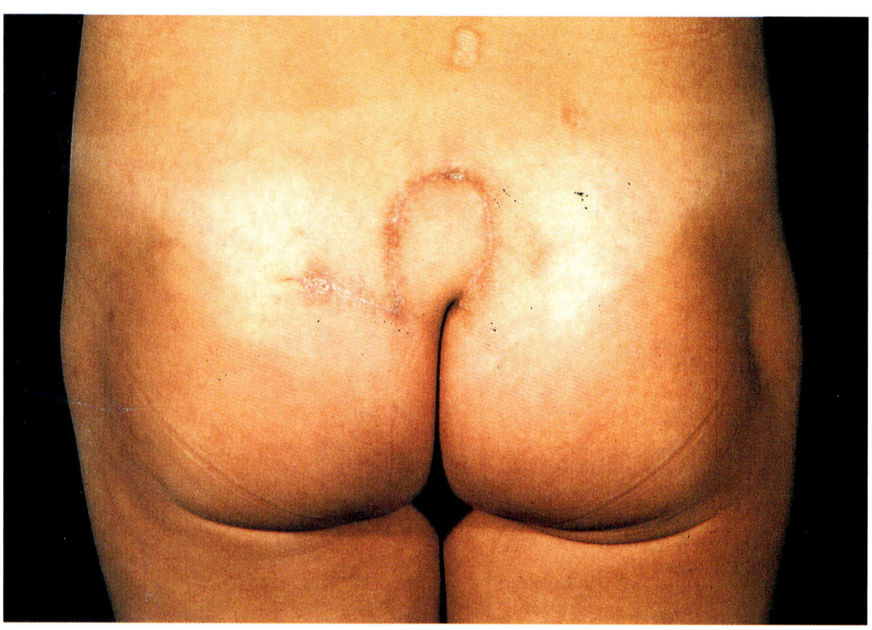

Figure 5.52b Status four weeks after the procedure

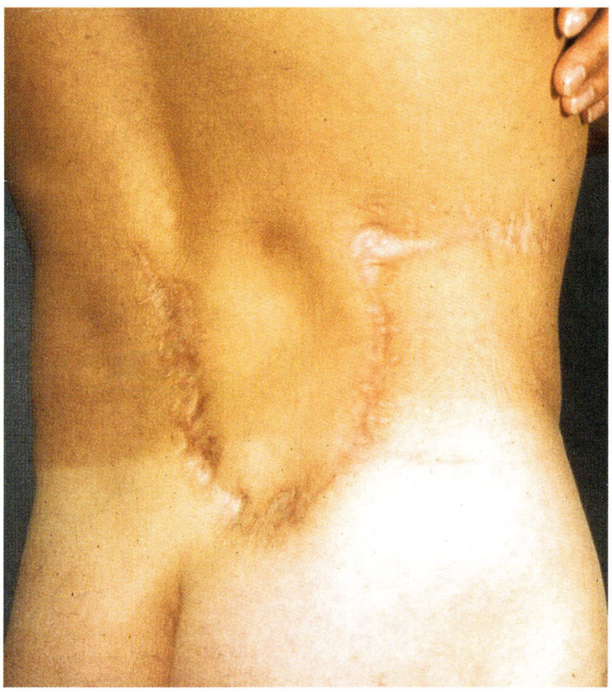

Rotation Flap

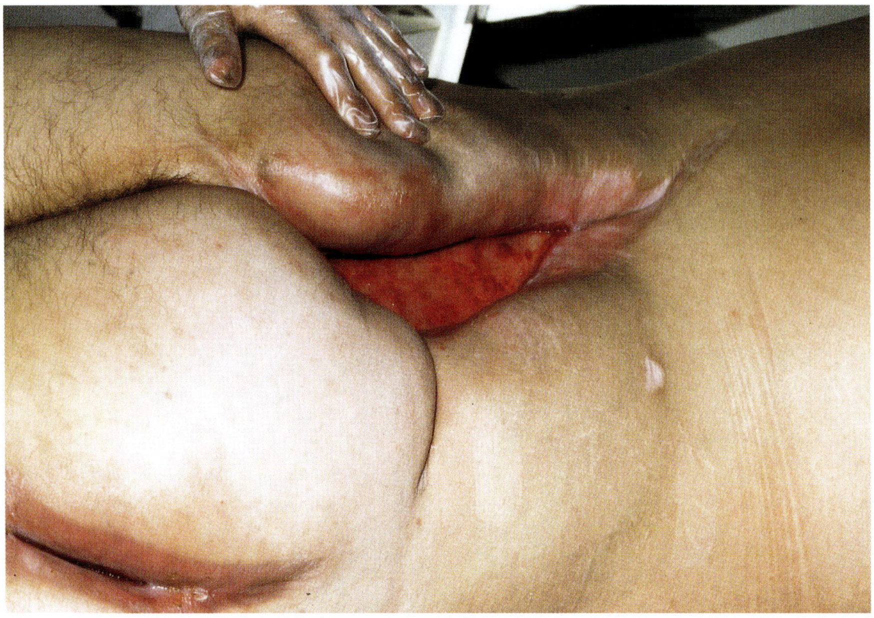

Figure 5.50a Ulceration in the lumbar spine region induced by irradiation of vertebral tumor metastases. Note the additional defect which developed after abscess incision in the lateral thigh region.

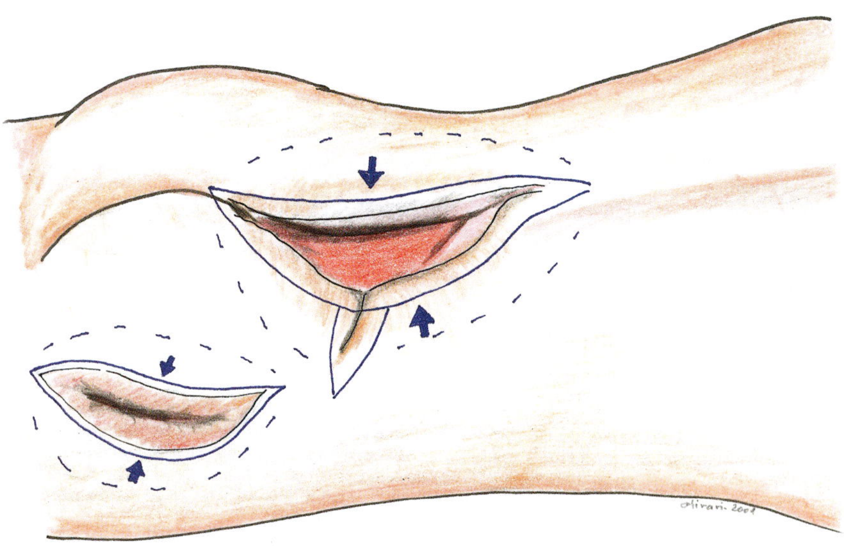

Figure 5.50b Surgical planning: First, granulation and scar tissue is resected. Then bilateral mobilization of the fasciocutaneous tissue layer is done until tension-free wound closure is possible.
Due of the wide base of the flap, its perfusion is expect to be excellent.

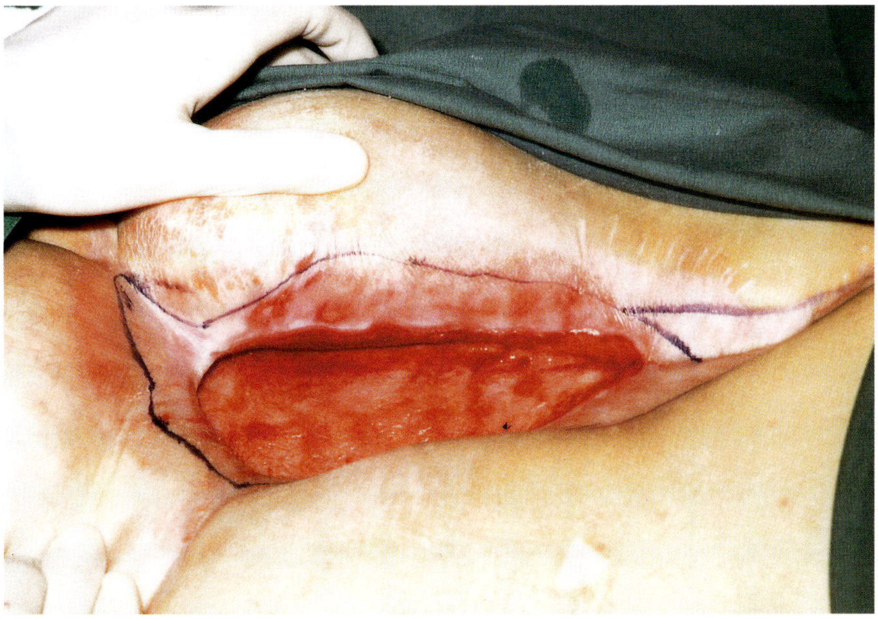

Figure 5.50c It is of utmost importance to excise the subcutaneous pockets entirely.

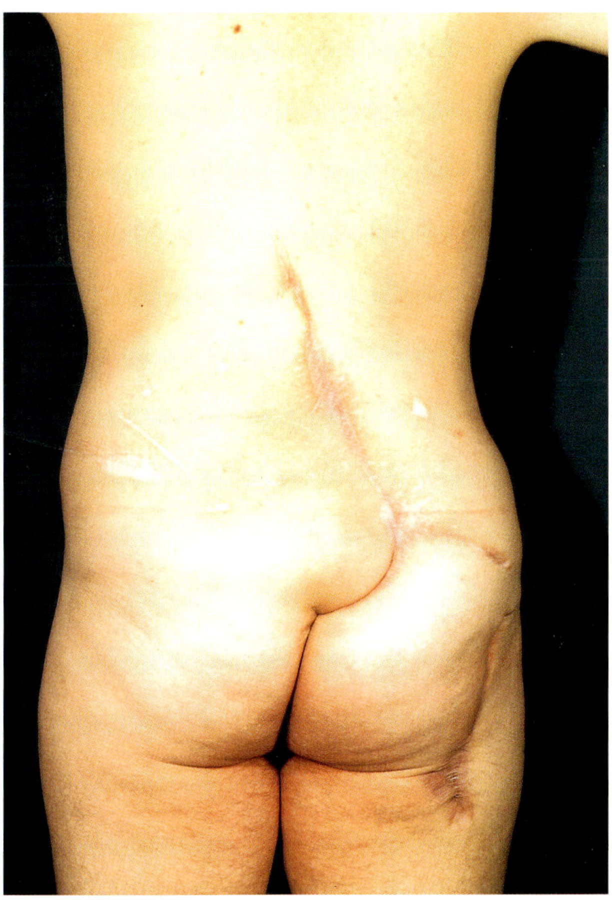

Figure 5.50d Status one year after the procedure. The surgical wounds have healed primarily.

Pilonidal Fistula (Sacrococcygeal Fistula)

Pathogenetic Aspects

The clinical picture of recurrent abscess and fistula formation in the sacral region is frequently being described in literature as sacraldermoid, pilonidal fistula or dermoid cyst.

The pathoanatomy includes an antrum in the sacral region or the caudal portion of the sacrum that is lined with a multilayer squamous epithelium. The depth of the antrum can reach down to the level of the presacral fascia, but it never reaches down to the bone. Usually, the fistula drains serous-putrid fluid through the skin of the rima ani. In moderate cases, the content of these cysts can contain conglomerates of bacteria-contaminated detritus, sebum and sudor. Skewered hairs can also be found in this material.

The original name pilonidal sinus stems from these morphologic and pathologic aspects. Since its introduction in 1880 by Hodges this name seems to be more and more accepted in literature.

Etiology

The exact etiology of pilonidal fistula formation is still debated. However, multiple facts count against the assumption of a congenital pathogenesis and for the (acquired) development of a pilonidal fistula most frequently between the second and third decade of life.

As described in literature, we did not see a "sacral dermoid" with its typical clinical appearance in children; all our patients presenting with a pilonidal fistula were between 16 and 39 years old.

Classically, almost all patients had noticeably intense hair-growth of the anal and perineal region, a hypertranspiratory predisposition and worked mainly in a seated position. It can be hypothesized that these factors in combination with mechanical stress lead to the retrograde skewering of hair, which is key to the development of a pilonidal sinus.

Capillary debris that is found in the "hair nest" also advocates the mechanial stress pathogenetic mechanism. The connatal pathogenesis based on dystopic ectoderm was confuted: Carstensen and Keichel microscopically and macroscopically examined histologic sections as well as excised pilonidal fistula specimen and did not find substantial support for the connatal theory of pilonidal fistula pathogenesis.

Diagnosis

The intermittent or continuous secretion from the opening of the fistula prompts only part of the patients suffering from pilonidal fistula to seek medical help. The majority of the patients note the process in the sacral region when inflammation and abscess formation is present.

Knowing the signs and symptoms of a pilonidal fistula, the diagnosis is not difficult to establish, especially when the patient presents with the typical sacral localization of the fistula opening and history.

False diagnoses such as furuncle, anal fistula or sacral osteomyelitis may be established in atypical cases when the surgeon faces atypical fistula localizations or the frequent relapses of a mistreated pilonidal fistula.

In our department, the standard diagnostic procedures do not include x-ray examination of the sacral bone anymore since our surgical experience over the years revealed that even large abscess formations or ramified fistulae never penetrate the presacral fascia.

Operation (The Olivari Sacral Dermoid Procedure)

The procedure is done even in the state of abscess formation without special preoperative preparation. We do not perform preoperative methylene blue injections into the fistula anymore since in our experience its extent is easy to determine even without the dye injection. The patient is prone positioned.

The opening of the fistula and the cyst or the duct should not be touched during the whole course of the operation. Rather, these structures should be tight-sealed in a sterile fashion against the operative field using sterile swabs, sutures or tape. The excision has to be done down to the level of the sacral fascia and must extend as far laterally as a margin of healthy tissue can also be resected (similar to the no-touch technique in oncologic surgery). This must be done in order to avoid the opening of the fistula in the operative field so that contamination and the associated risk of relapses is minimized. In order to achieve this, it is better to plan the operation so that a fairly generous "safety zone" of healthy tissue is resected rather than planning minimal tissue resection with the risk of inadvertent damage to the fistula in the operative field. In our experience, even large defects can later be easily closed by local flap. In this context, smaller flaps are also more prone to dehiscence and necrosis in our experience. According to the size of the defect, a flap is laterally marked and raised in a way that the flap completely contains the subcutaneous tissue, which extends in depth to the level of the fascia, and the blood vessels.

After hemostasis, an antibiotic solution is instilled into the wound area and a suction drainage is put in place via a separate incision. The flap should be sutured in place with fairly dense stitches using a bilayer technique. To avoid dislocation of the wound edges, the skin suture is done in a vertical mattress technique.

Supine position is not allowed until postoperative day 14, position changes between lateral recumbent position and prone position are possible. The suction drainage is removed on postoperative day 3, but no later than one week after the procedure. The suction drainage is of utmost importance, not only to remove potential hematoma or seroma, but also to achieve contact of the flap with the wound bed by the negative pressure. The first dressing change is done on postoperative day 1. During the whole postoperative phase, it is important to keep the surgical field maximally clean. Disinfection of the anal region after every defecation! The skin sutures can be removed 10 to 14 days after the procedure. Sitting can be allowed approximately three weeks after the procedure. Prophylactic broad-spectrum antibiotic treatment should be initiated at the time of surgery.

We have treated 36 patients with this method. The average hospitalisation was 10 days; at the time of discharge from the hospital, all surgical wounds healed completely. One patient developed postoperative surgical wound infection which was most probably caused by insufficient resection of the fistula. The average time of inability to work after the procedure was 22 days (compared to 45 days with the method of resection and secondary wound healing).

We are well aware of the fact that an infected wound must not be closed primarily. However, since it is possible to avoid any contact of the surrounding tissue with the fistula using the no-touch technique and wide excision, we think that our method is warranted mainly in cases with large abscess formation or branched fistulae. Conditions sine qua non are radical excision of the fistula and functional suction drainage. We have not seen any long-term relapses yet.

A main advantage of our technique is that there is no scar plate formation with thin epithelium, rather, functional skin – with altered hair growth direction – and subcutaneous tissue is conserved and transposed into the defect. Some authors criticized the procedure for its complexity, however, this is relative if we take into account the comparatively short duration of the procedure which was 27 minutes on the average (own patient collective).

Therefore, the author does not recommend a simple excision with secondary healing by wound bed granulation. Also, excision and primary closure of the defect is not recommended because of high tension on the surgical wound.

Our patient collective (n=36) consisted of:

- Male patients: n=29
- Female patients: n= 7

The mean history of the disease was between six months and 10 years, 34 months on the average. The length of hospital stay was six to 14 days with an average of ten days.

Treatment course (n=36):

- 31 patients revealed an uneventful pre- and postoperative course
- 4 patients developed seroma which were successfully treated within 2 to 3 weeks
- 1 patient with abscess formation and relapse needed re-excision

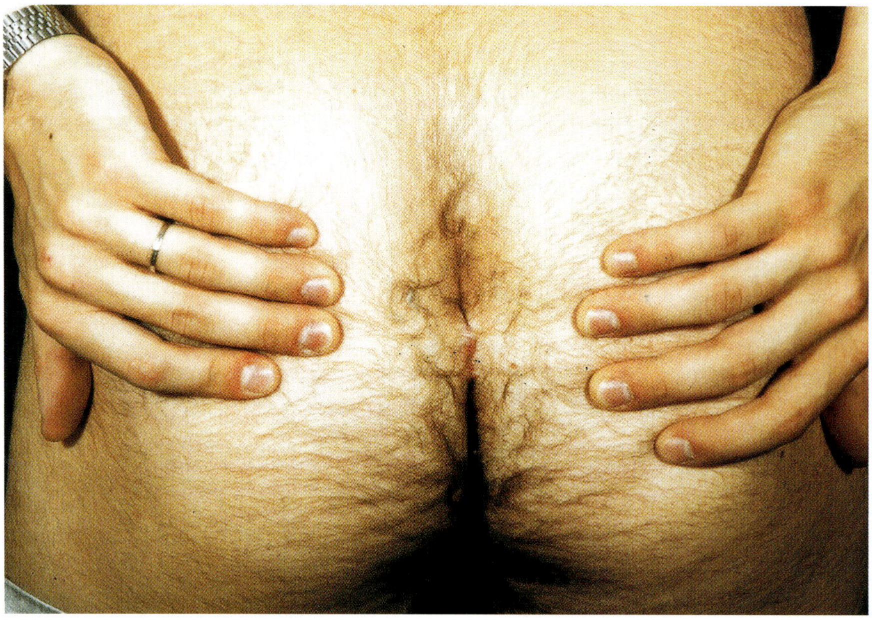

Figure 5.51a Recurrent infected pilonidal cyst (multiple recurrent infections)

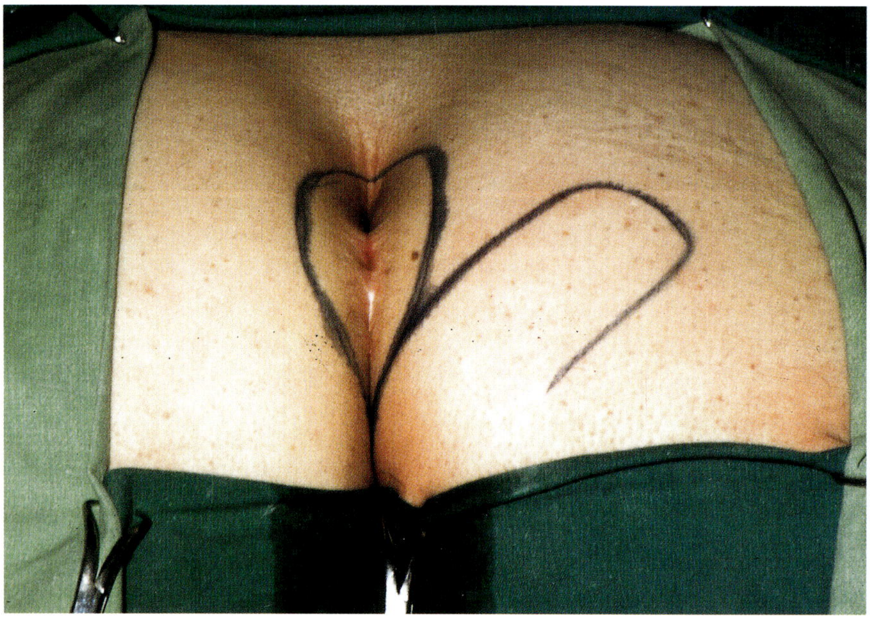

Figure 5.51b Excision of the pilonidal cyst down to the level of the sacral fascia.
Planning of a large flap.

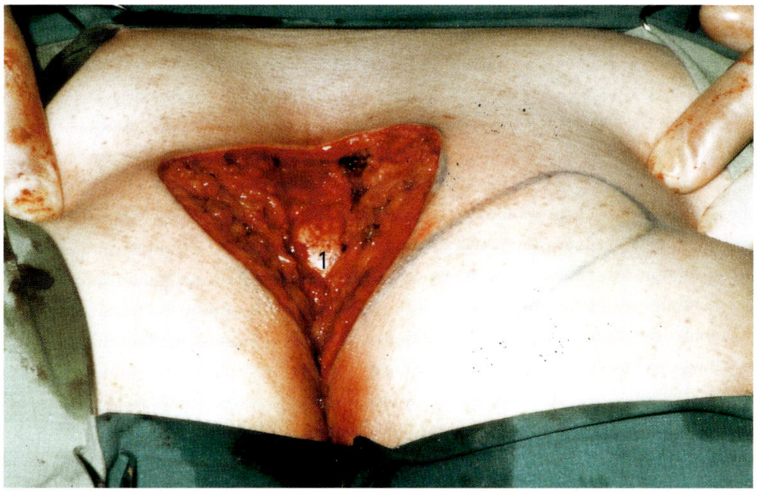

Figure 5.51c Wide in sano excision. The presacral fascia is visible (1). The excision must be done down to this fascia level. A caudally pedicled flap is planned for defect coverage.

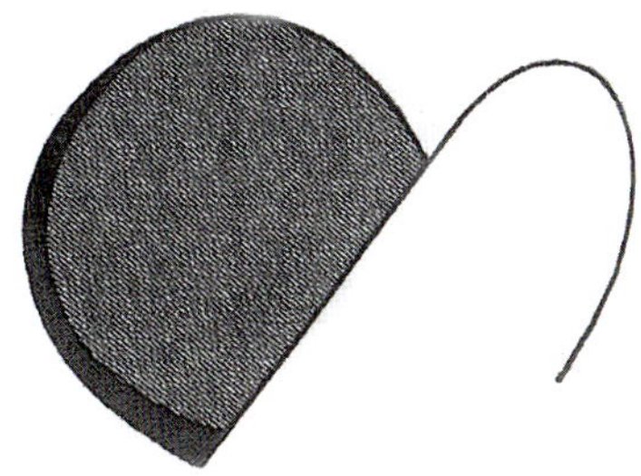

Figure 5.51d

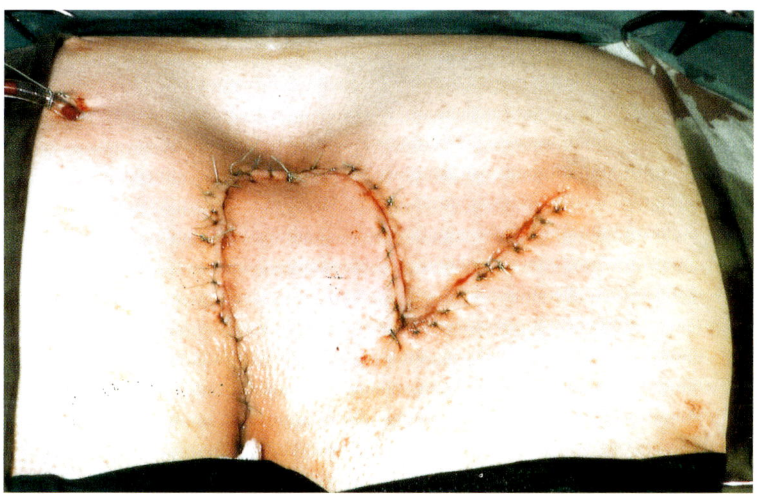

Figure 5.51e Status after the procedure

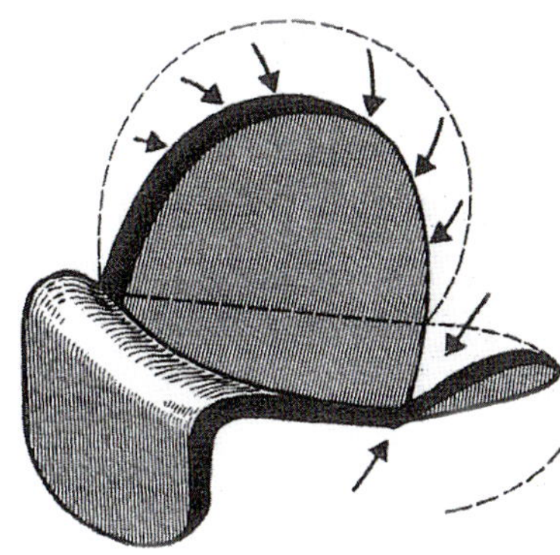

Figure 5.51f

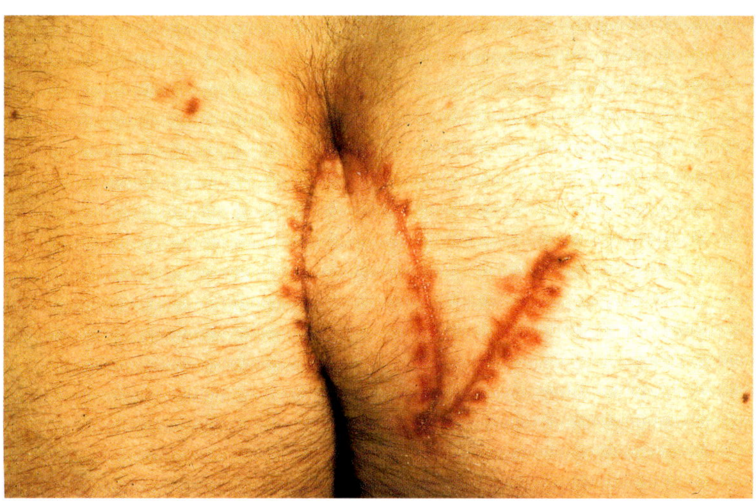

Figure 5.51g Status three weeks after the procedure

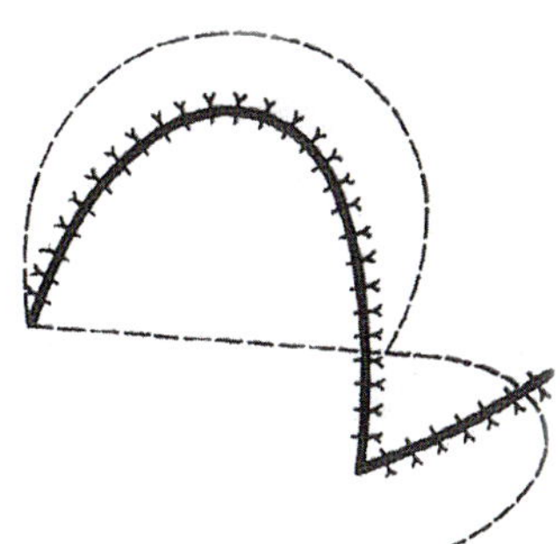

Figure 5.51d, f, h

Figure 5.51d, f, h Drawings from "Die operative Behandlung des infizierten Sakraldermoids" by N. Olivari et al. in Bruns Beitr Klin Chir 220 (1973) 306–312.

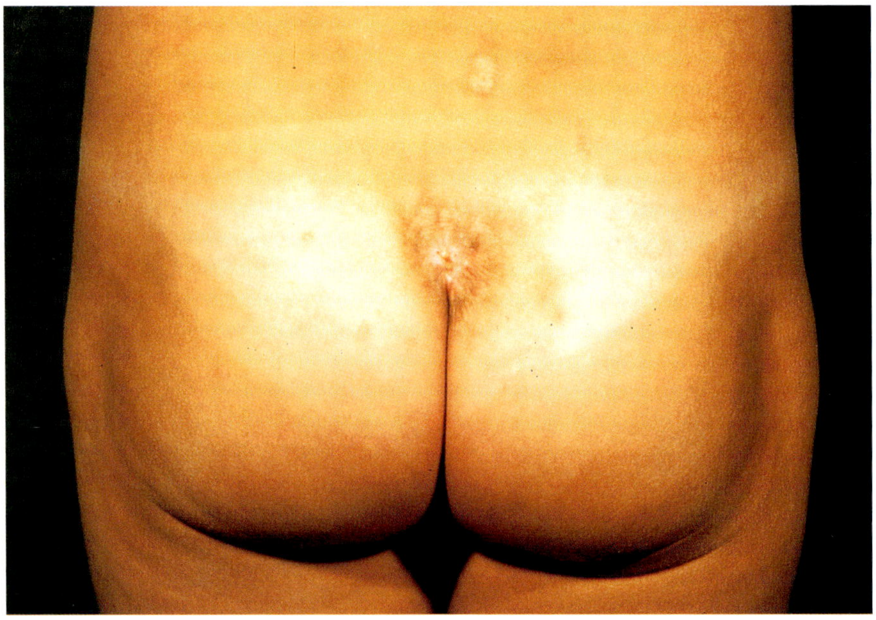

Figure 5.52a Pilonidal fistula after multiple infections

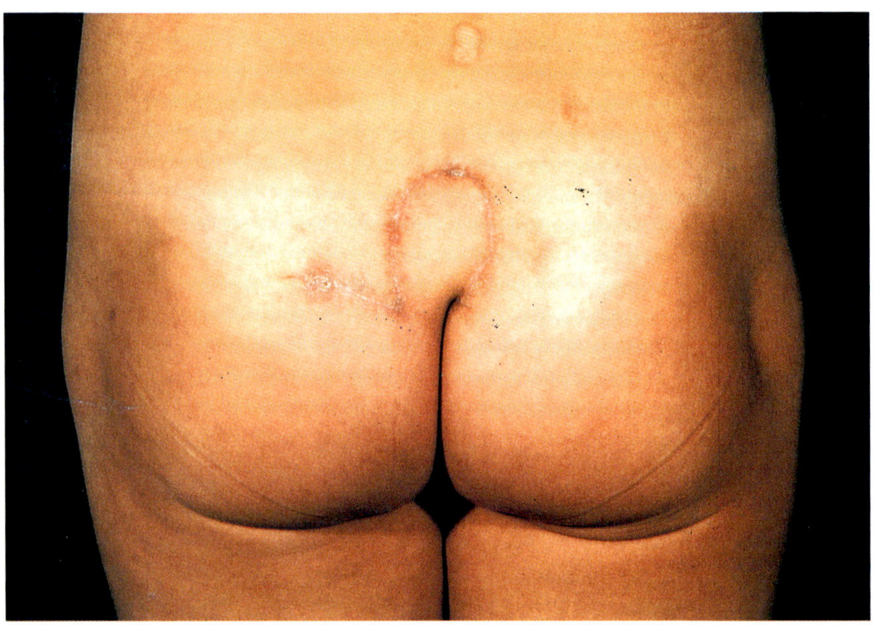

Figure 5.52b Status four weeks after the procedure

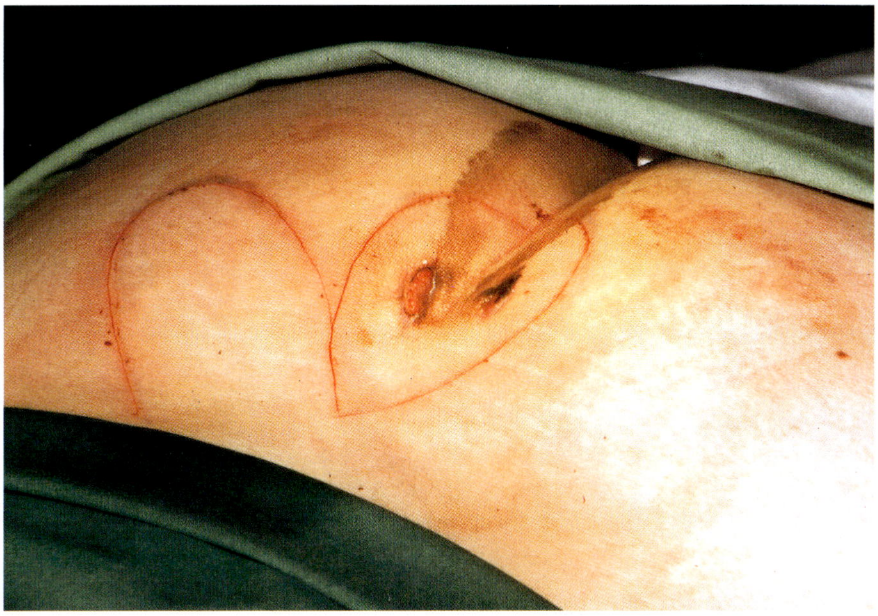

Figure 5.53a Pilonidal fistula after multiple infections. In this patient, the transposition flap is cranially pedicled because of extensive scarring of its caudal portion.

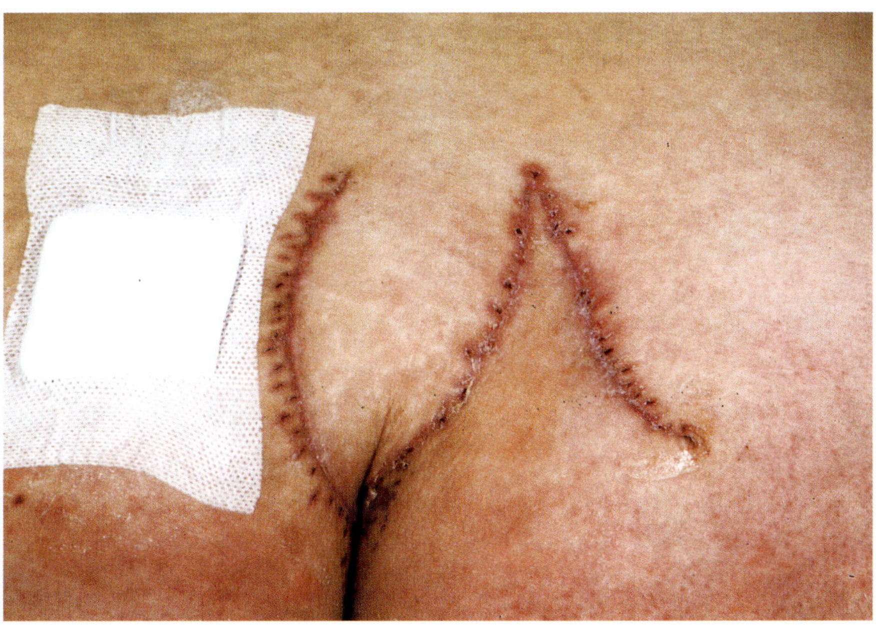

Figure 5.53b Primary healing. The caudally pedicled flap is superior to the cranially pedicled flap.

Hairy Nevus (Nevus Pilosus) – Expander Treatment

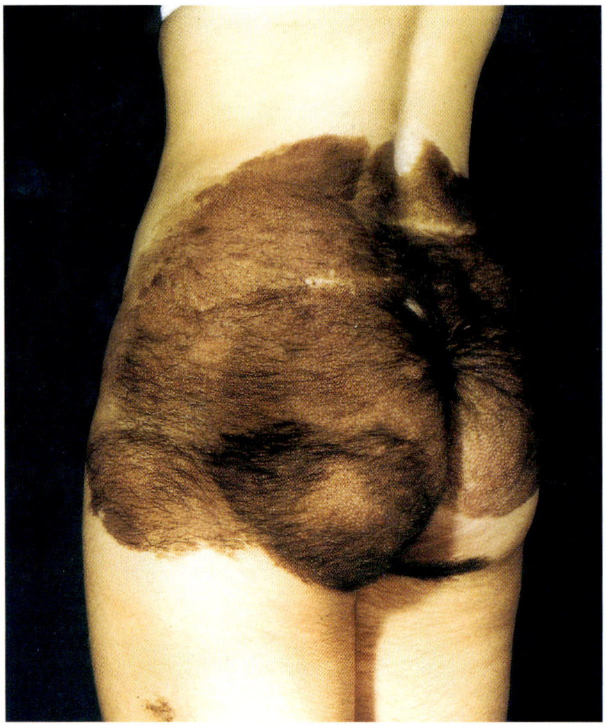

Figure 5.54a Hairy nevus of both gluteal regions

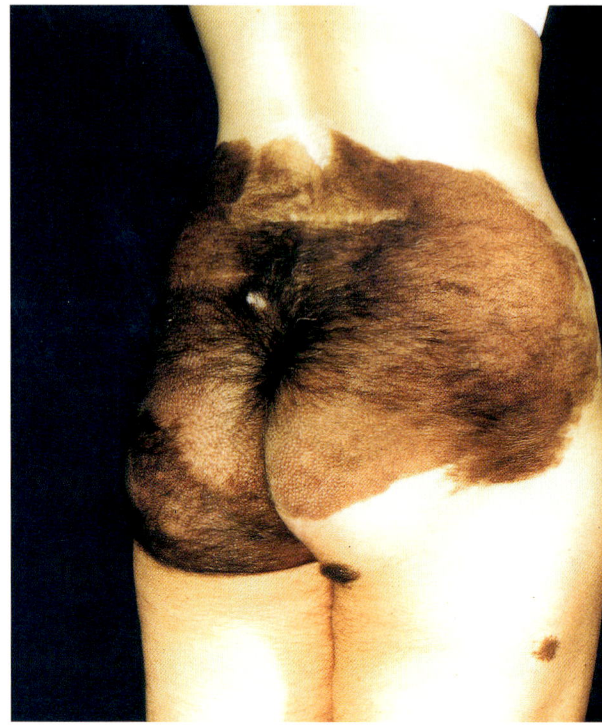

Figure 5.54b Oblique view. Note the affection of the lower dorsum and both flanks.

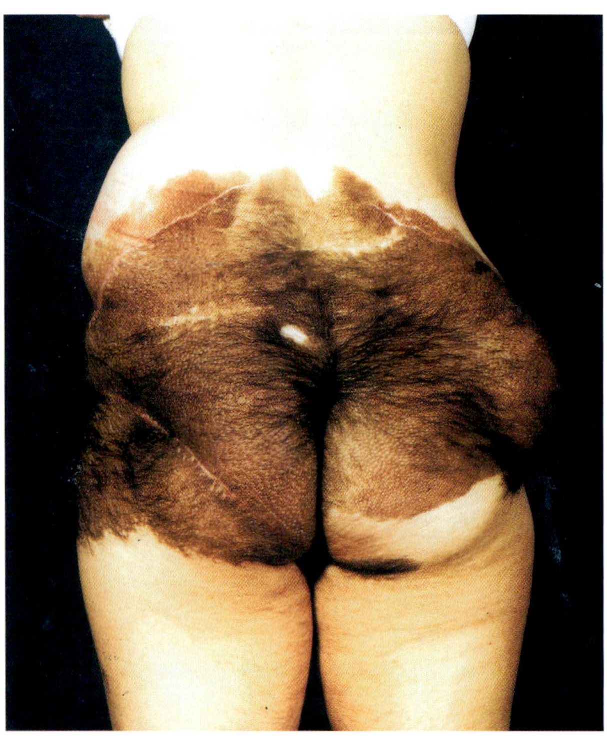

Figure 5.54c Three expanders are filled with up to 500 ccm and 1000 ccm of saline. After six weeks, parts of the tumor are excised.

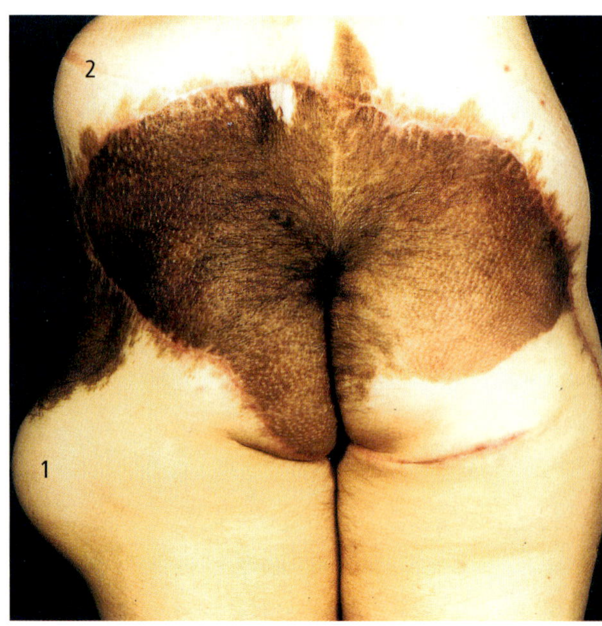

Figure 5.54d Four months after partial excision. New expanders are implanted, visible in the left thigh and hip region (1, 2).

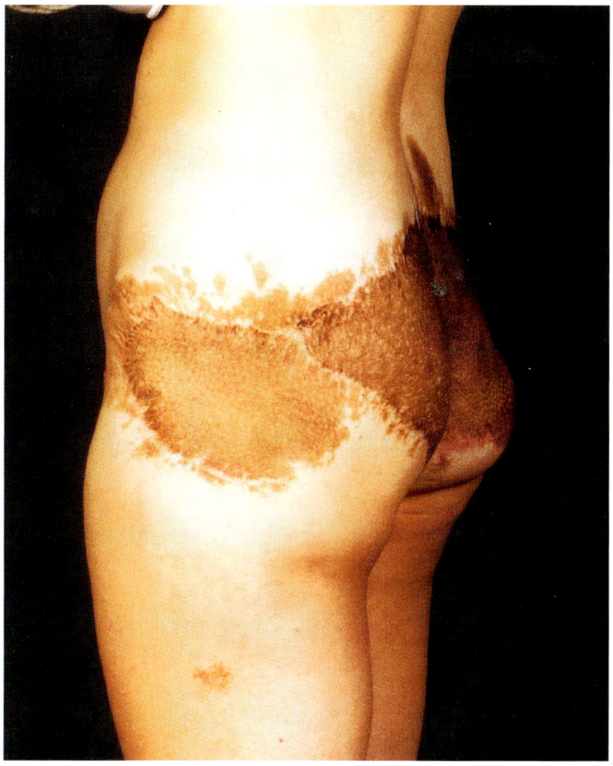

Figure 5.54e Stepwise excision on the right side and implantation of new expanders on the left side.

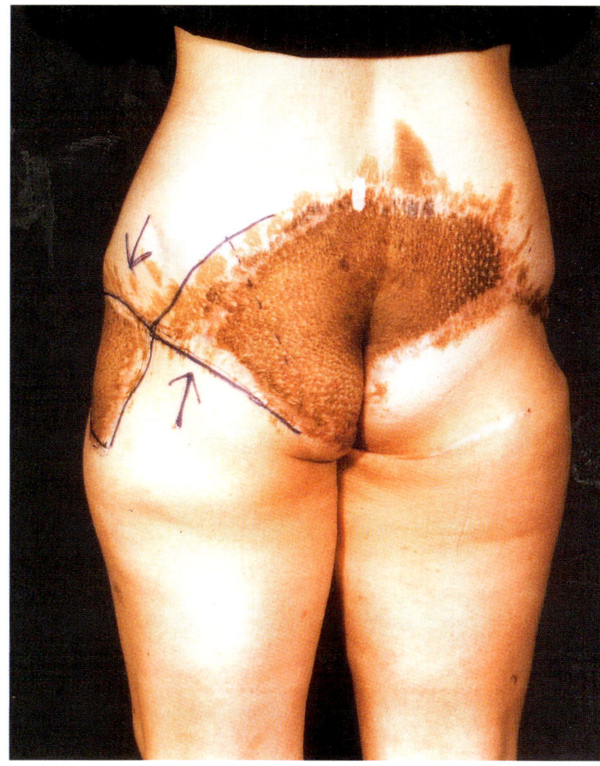

Figure 5.54f Surgical planning of further excisions: Defect coverage with rotational flap and implantation of new expanders.

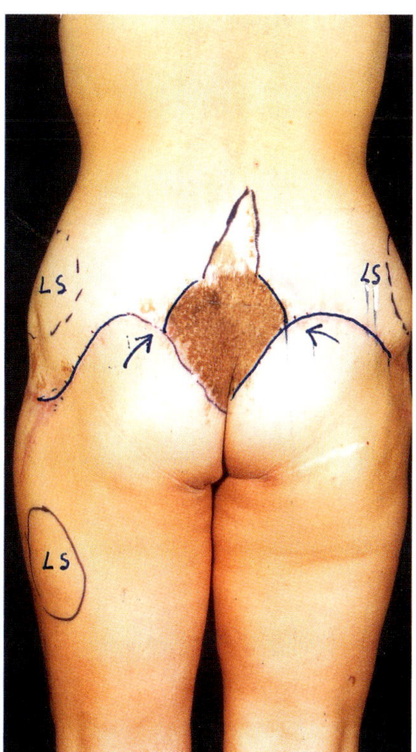

Figure 5.54g Last operation: Two rotational flaps are raised from both sides and combined with adjuvant liposuction (LS).

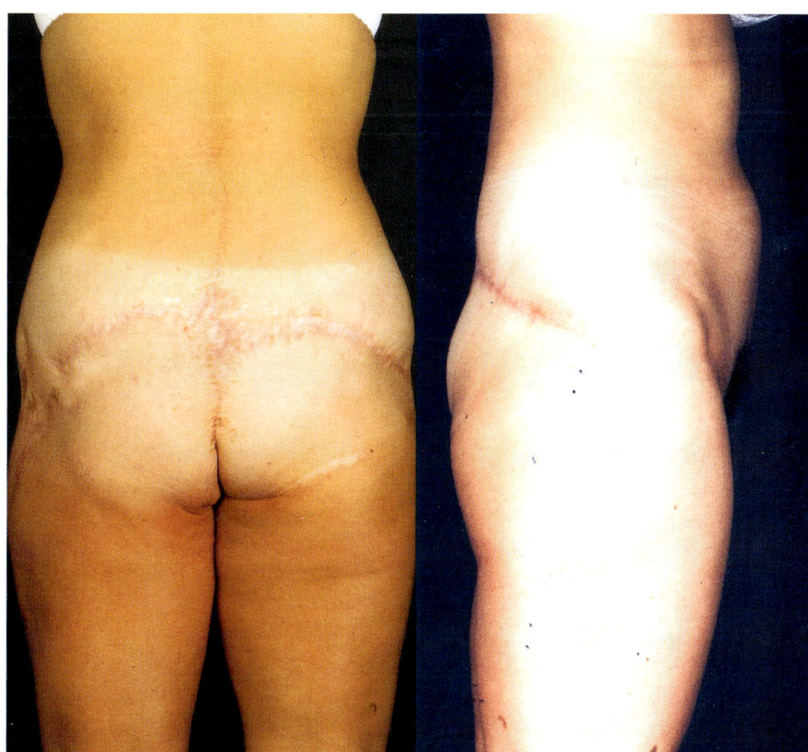

Figure 5.54h Status after seven surgical procedures within five years

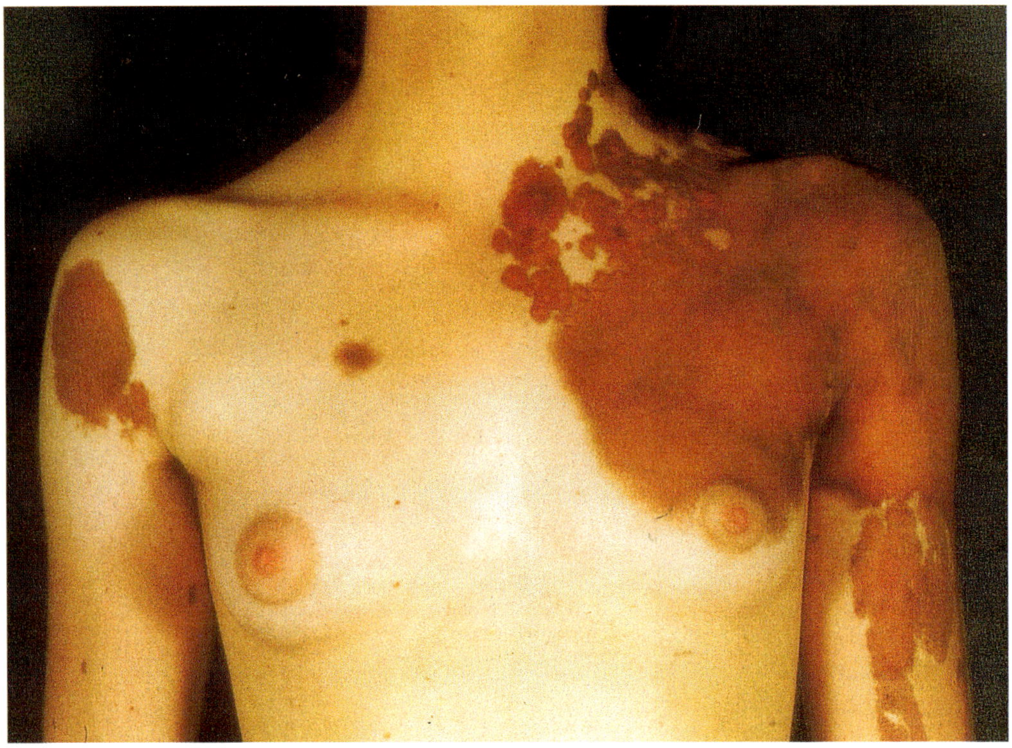

Figure 5.55a 16-year old female patient presenting with hairy nevus. Surgical planning: Tangential full-thickness excision. Defect coverage with split-thickness skin grafting (mesh grafts).

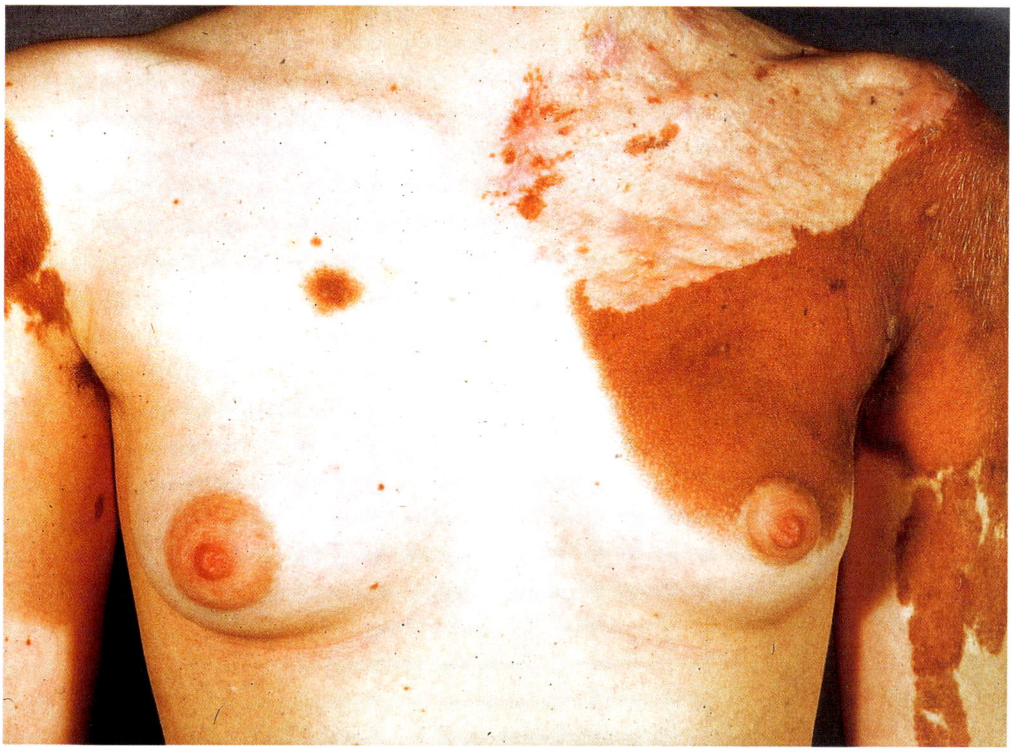

Figure 5.55b Status six months after the first excision. The result is acceptable, however, rests of the nevus infiltrate the skin graft. This demonstrates that full-thickness skin excision is essential.

Genitalia

Penile contracture

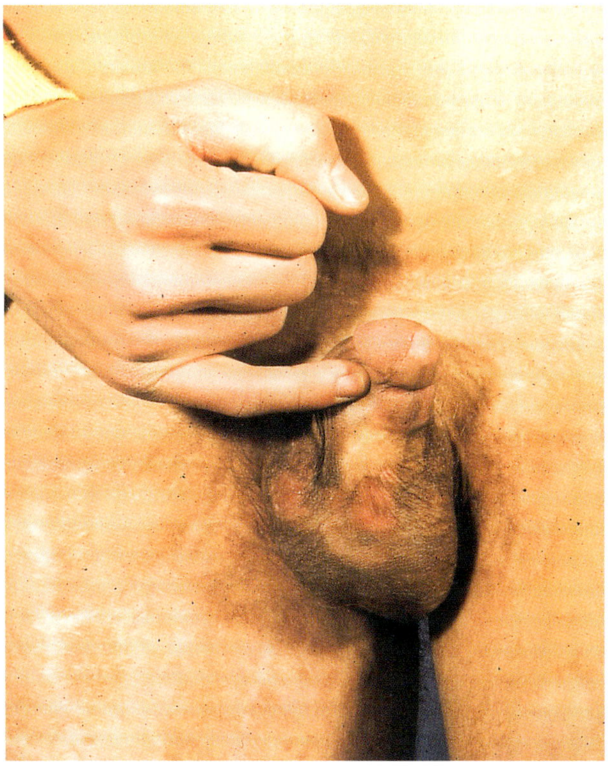

Figure 5.56a Extensive contracture of the penis induced by scar formation after full-thickness burn. An erection is impossible.

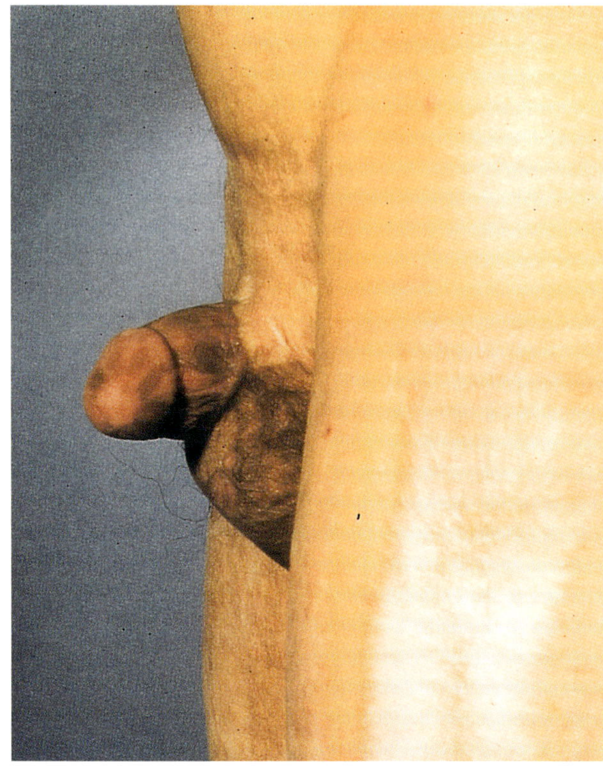

Figure 5.56b Initial aspect: Lateral view

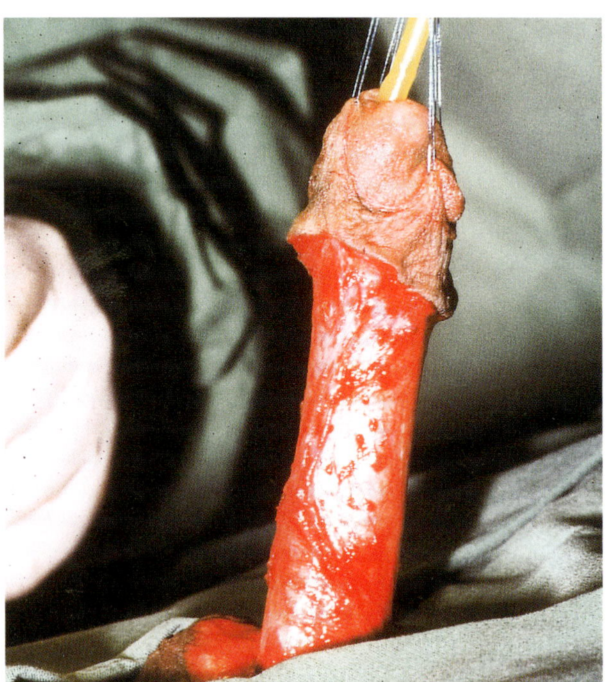

Figure 5.56c Intraoperative view. A circular incision of the scar is done down to the level of the tunica albuginea. *No excision of the scar.* This shows the extent to which the scar contracture has shortened the penis.

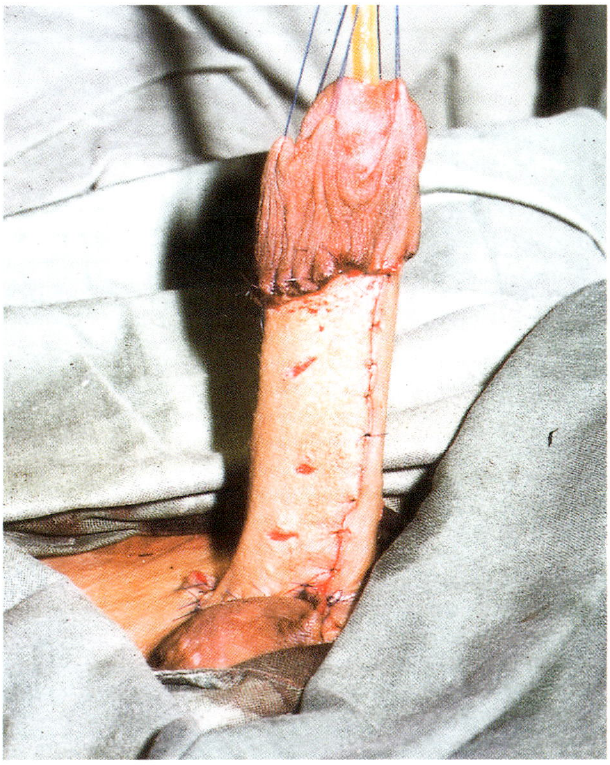

Figure 5.56d The resulting area (corpus cavernosus) is covered with a full-thickness skin graft. The graft has been sutured in place without tension. Some perforations in the graft drain potential seroma or hematoma formation. The full-thickness skin graft has been harvested from the groin region.

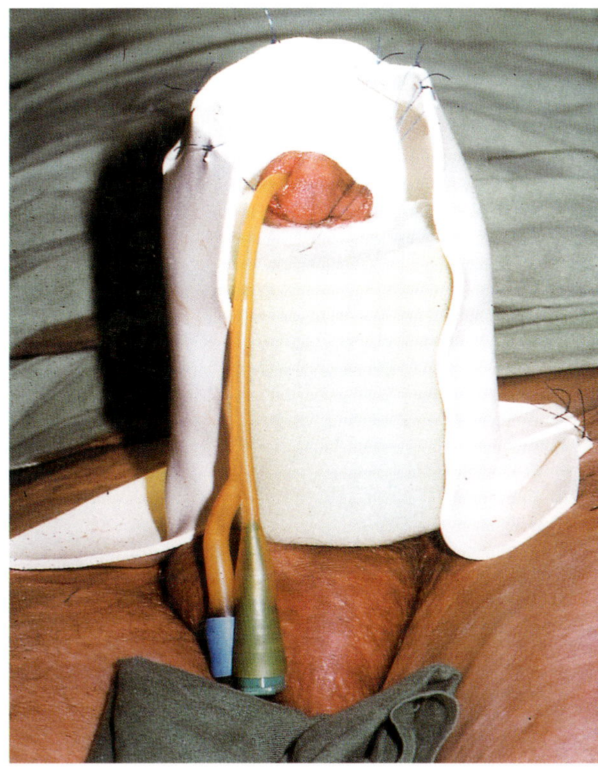

Figure 5.56e Important! The fixation of the penis using isoprene in erected position. The penis is fixated to the shaft of the isoprene roll and the base of the penis with sutures. Dressing: Gauze and elastic bandage. The patient was sedated for five days.

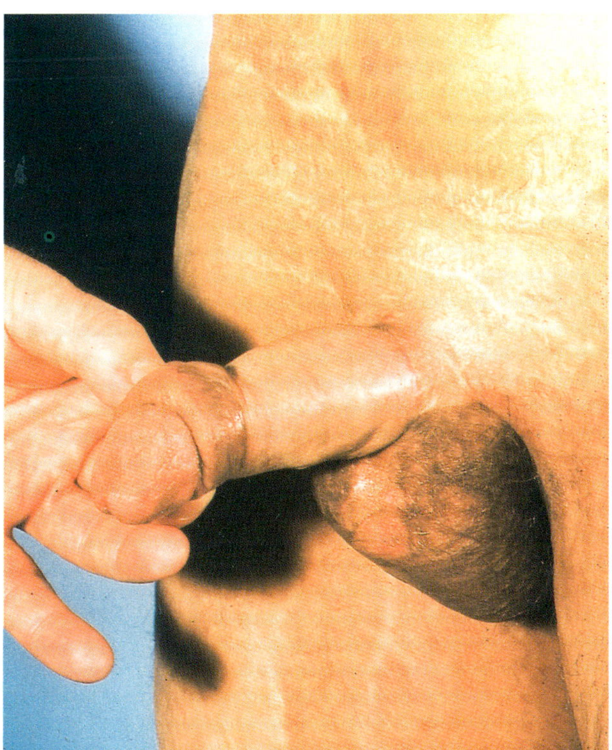

Figure 5.56f Status six months after the procedure. The erection is complete, which is made possible by the full-thickness skin graft. There is no indication for split-thickness skin grafting. Should the swelling in the sulcus persist, another excision and primary closure could be done.

Perineal Defect

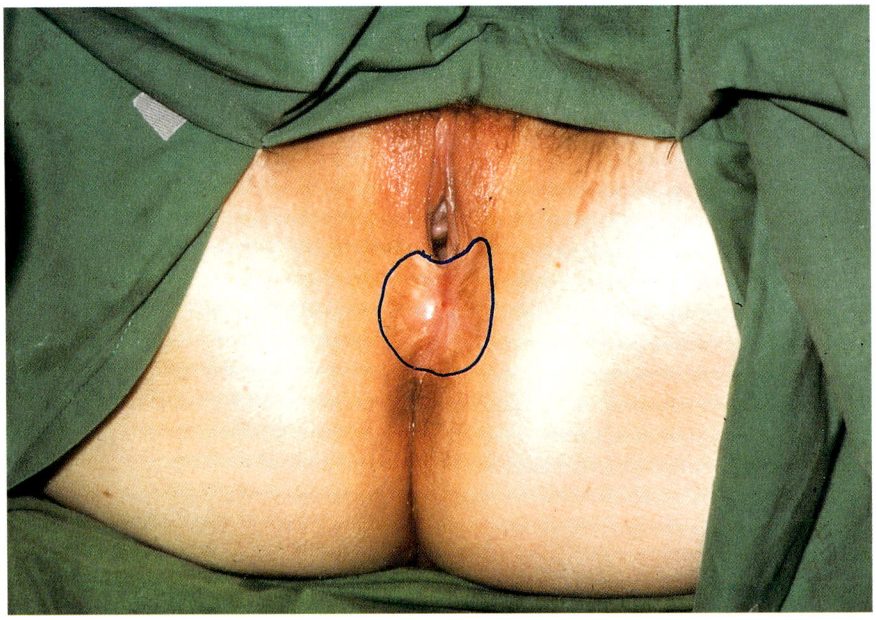

Figure 5.57a Perineal defect due to episiotomy. Status post secondary healing of a perineal rupture after labor. Excessive scarring and functional narrowing of the vaginal introitus, pain, sexual intercourse is impossible.

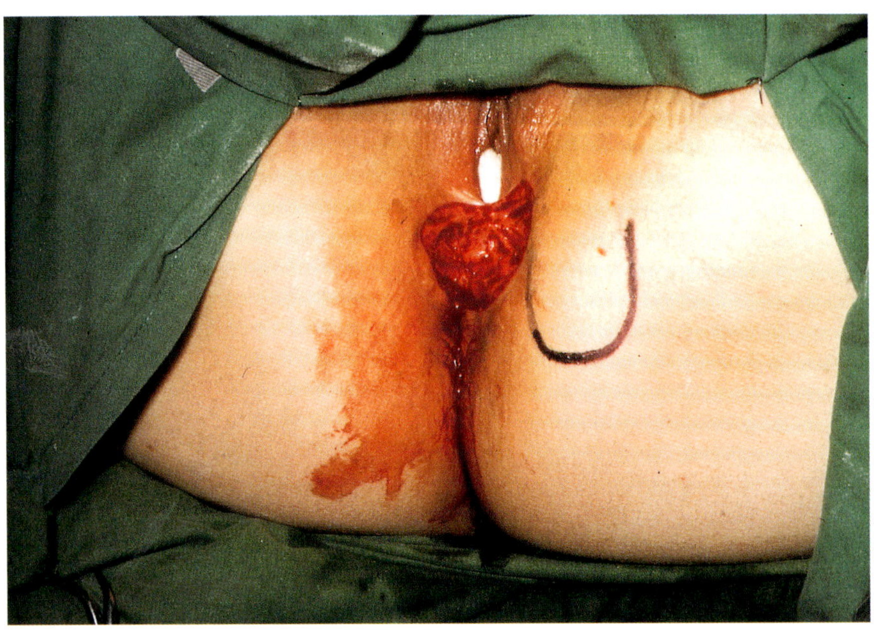

Figure 5.57b Important! The entire scar must be excised including the deeper portions of the scar. A ventrally pedicled local flap is raised. **Cave:** The sphincter muscle in females is very weak in the perineal portion!

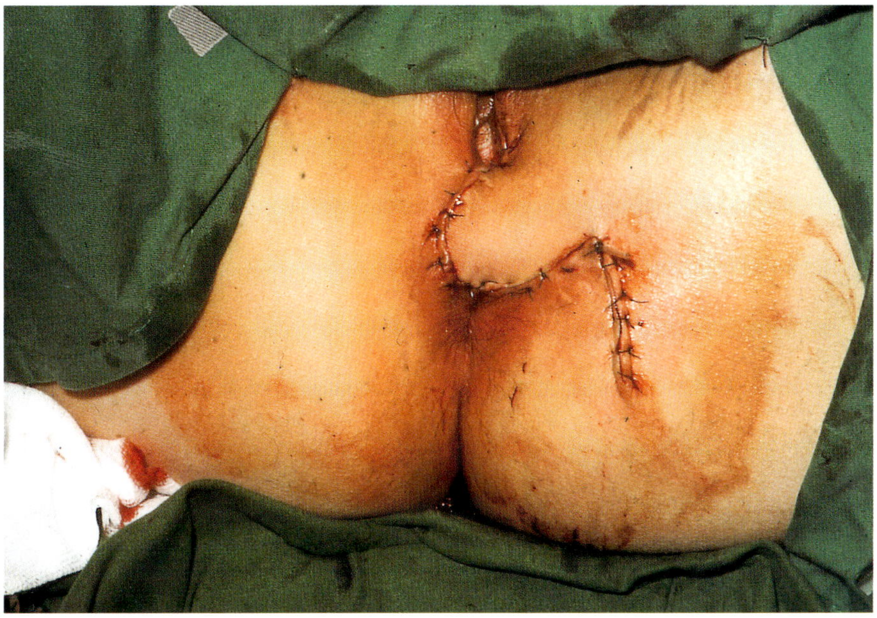

Figure 5.57c The donor site is closed primarily

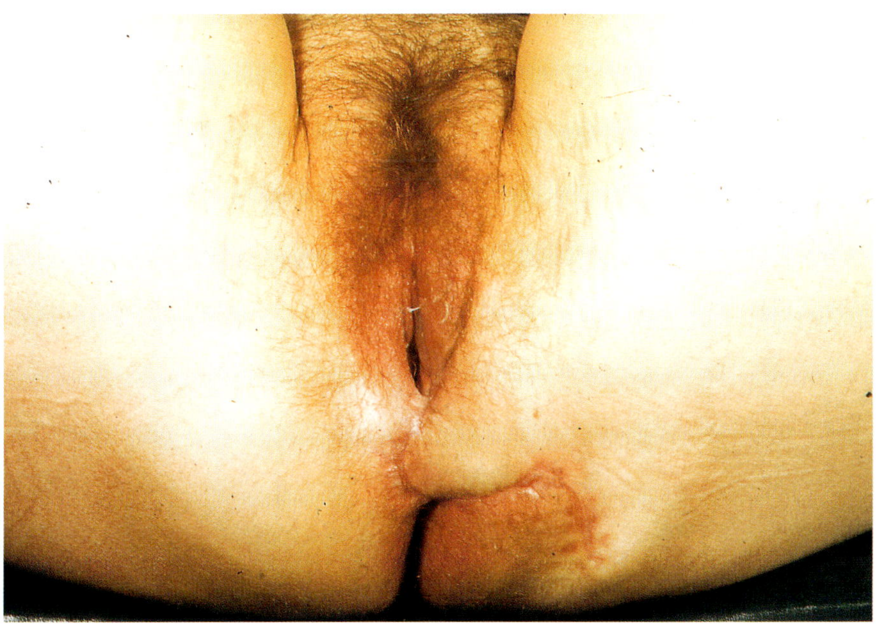

Figure 5.57d Status six weeks after the procedure. The vaginal introitus is open and elastic; the patient is pain-free.

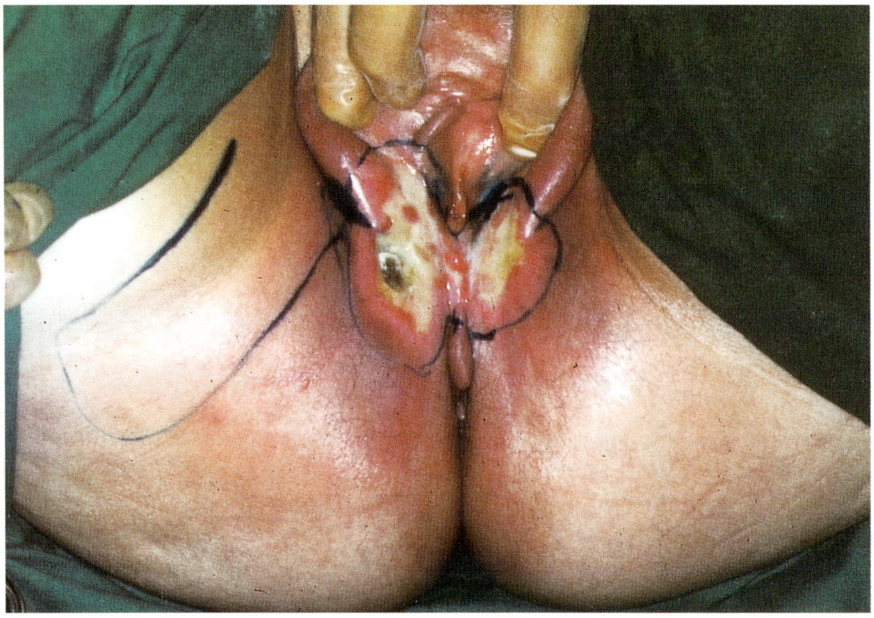

Figure 5.58a Bowen´s disease. Status after irradiation with subsequent ulceration, tissue necrosis and infection. Steady intensive pain.

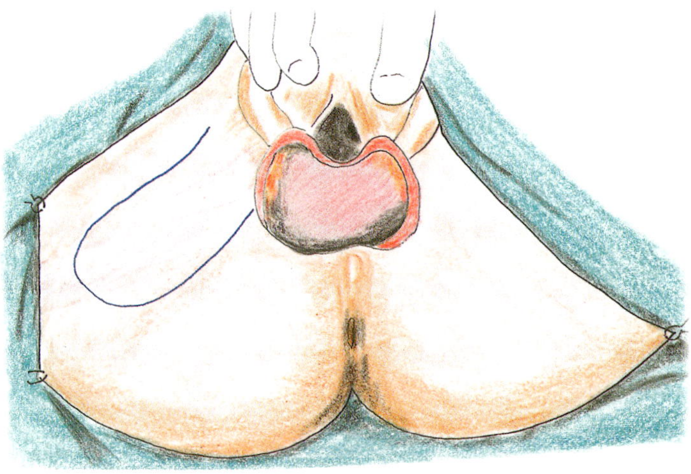

Figure 5.58b The damaged tissue is removed by radical excision. A medially pedicled transposition flap is raised and sutured into the defect. The donor site can be closed primarily.

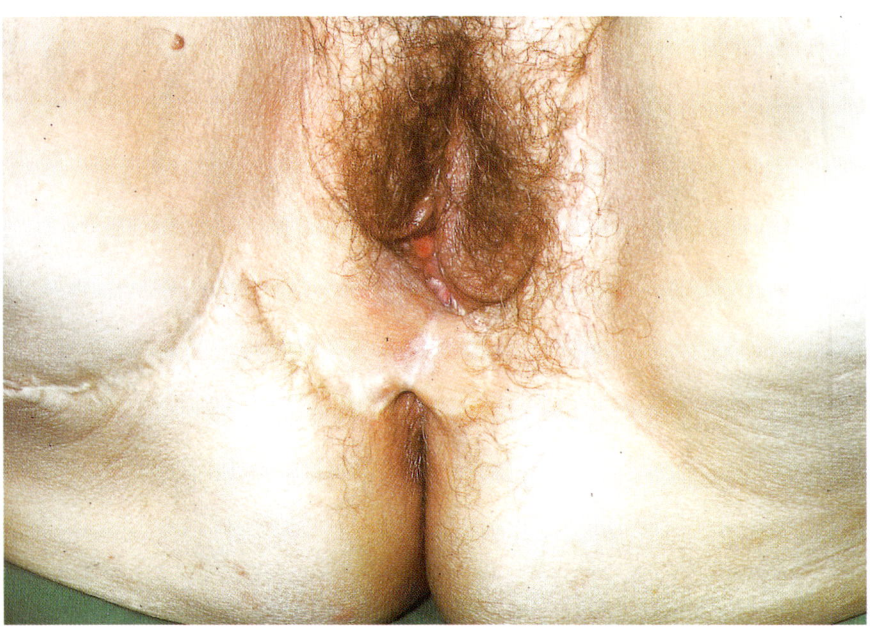

Figure 5.58c Status two years after the procedure. The patient does not complain about pain or functional problems.

Bladder Ectopy

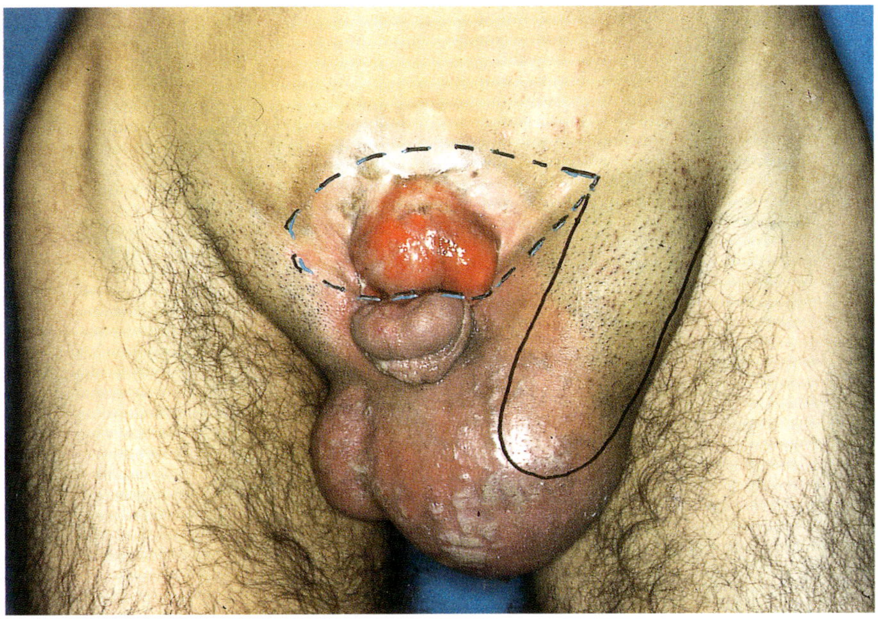

Figure 5.59a Bladder ectopy and epispadias with concomitant left inguinal herniation. Earlier, the patient underwent a Bricker procedure, the Bricker bladder was functional.
Surgical planning:
a) Resection of the secreting dorsal wall of the bladder
b) Reconstruction of the abdominal wall using fascia lata
c) Defect coverage using a transposition flap raised from the left groin and the scrotum
d) Hernia repair (single-stage procedure with c)

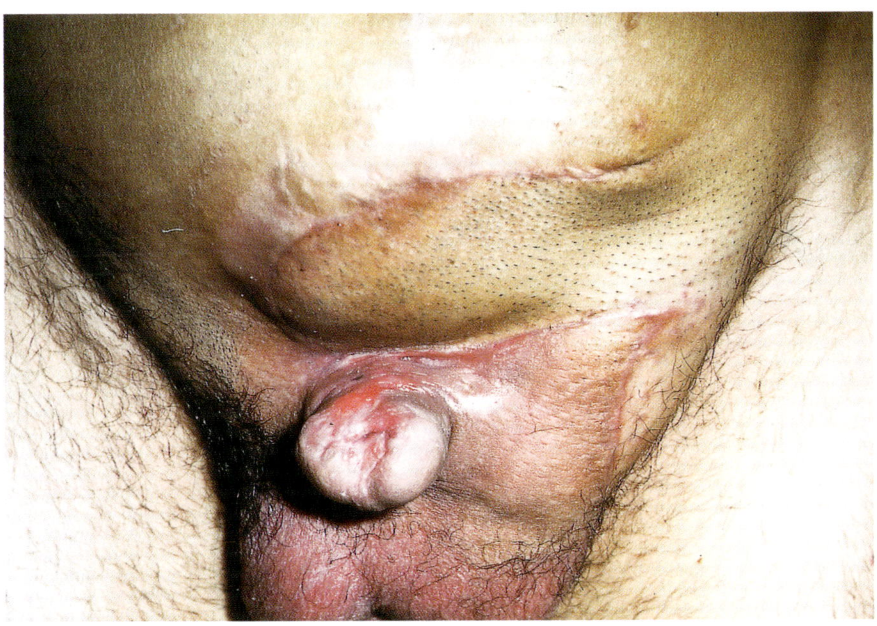

Figure 5.59b Status six months after the procedure. The abdominal wall is stable.

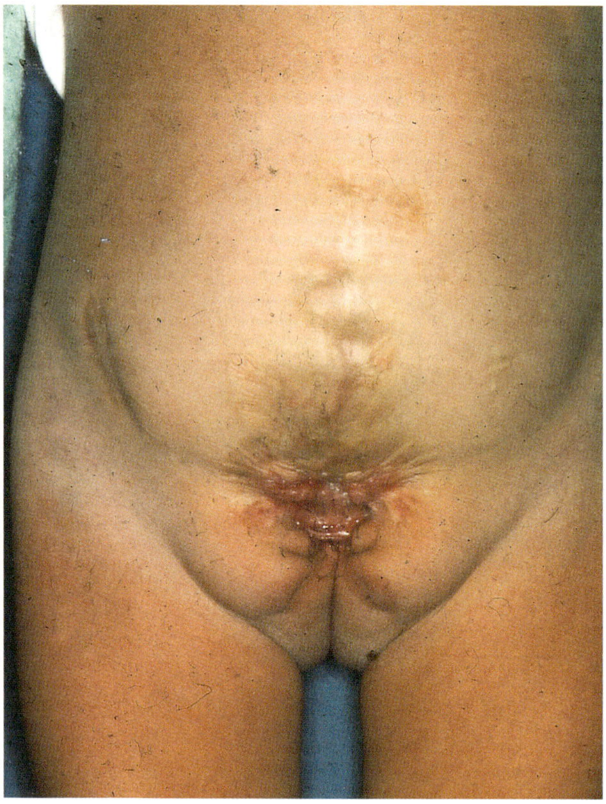

Figure 5.60a Bladder ectopy, excessive scarring. Status post Bricker procedure with good function

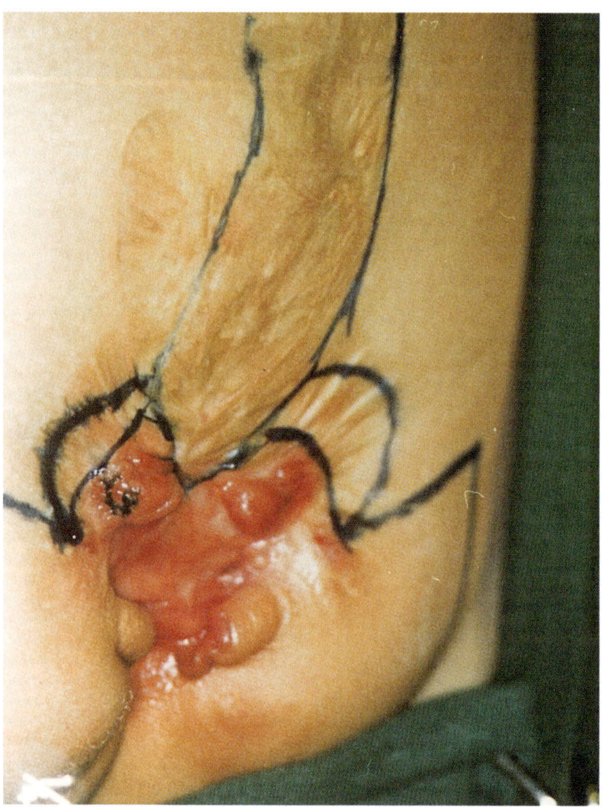

Figure 5.60b Surgical planning

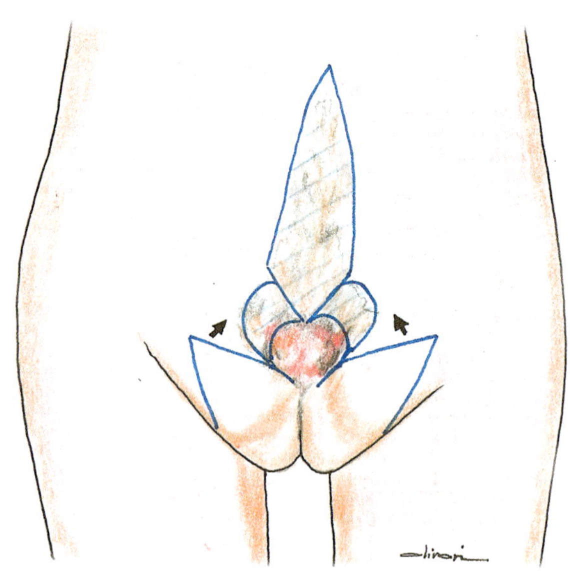

Figure 5.60c The hatched portion is excised. Two triangular flaps are raised and sutured in place with medial contact.

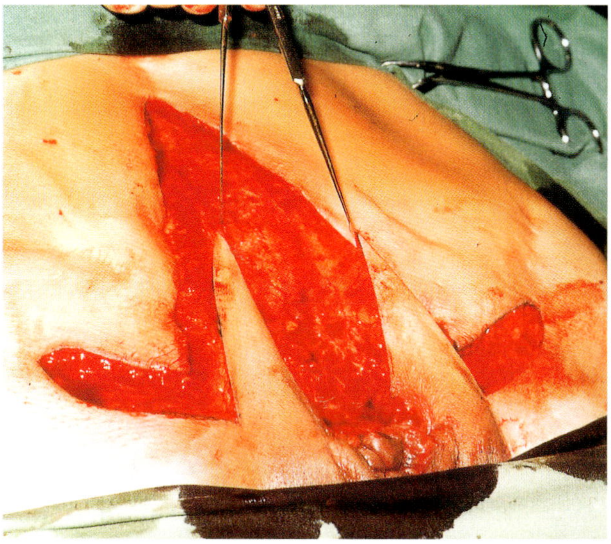

Figure 5.60d The triangular flaps are raised and transposed into the defect

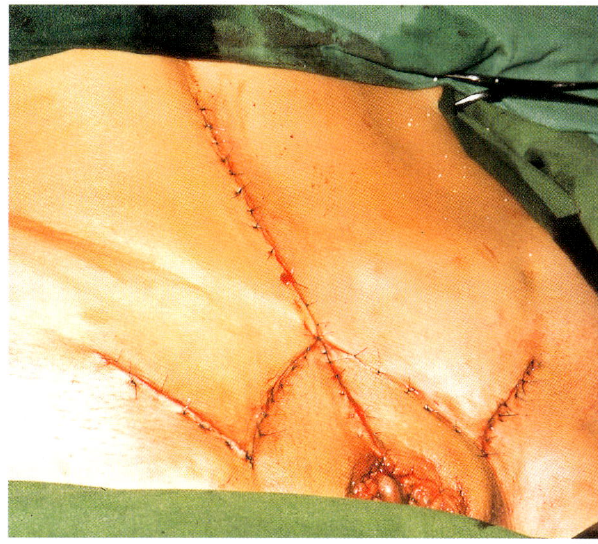

Figure 5.60e Status at the end of the procedure

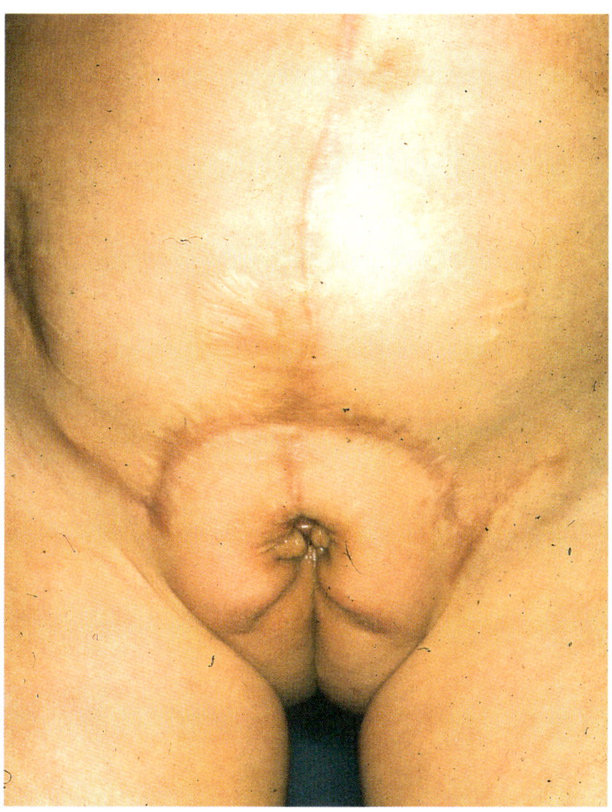

Figure 5.60f Status six months after the procedure

CHAPTER 6
Skin and Soft Tissue Defects in the Extremities

The Lower Extremities

Random Pattern Flap

The poor mobility of soft tissue of the lower limb limits the use of random pattern flaps. This contrasts with the situation of the chest, abdominal wall, head and neck, where they can be used to close large defects. The further distal on the limb the more risky they are and in the lower legs and feet they are rarely indicated, particularly as there are a variety of axial pattern fasciocutaneous flaps and free flaps available. When planning of random pattern flaps in the lower limb a ratio of 2 : 1 (length : width) is appropriate.
This kind of flap is most suitable in the upper thigh.

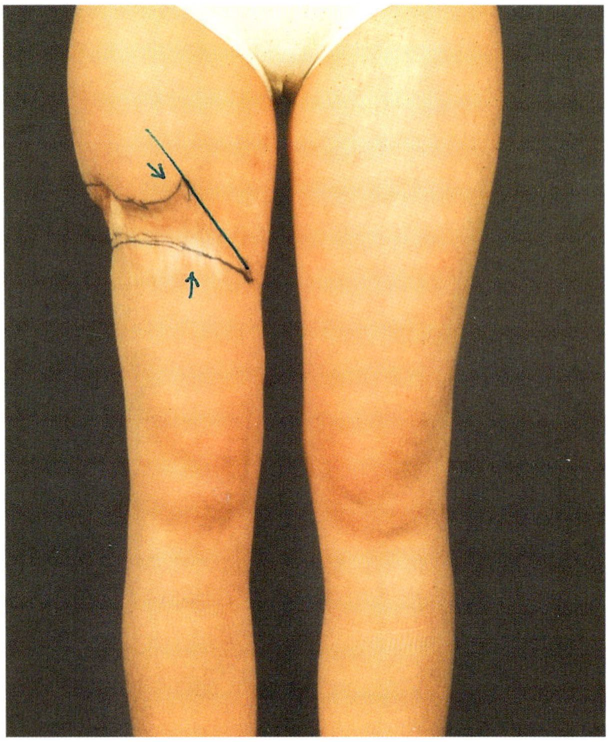

Figure 6.1a Post-traumatic defect of the right upper thigh. Two sliding flaps are planned one from above and another from below to cover the ventral defect.

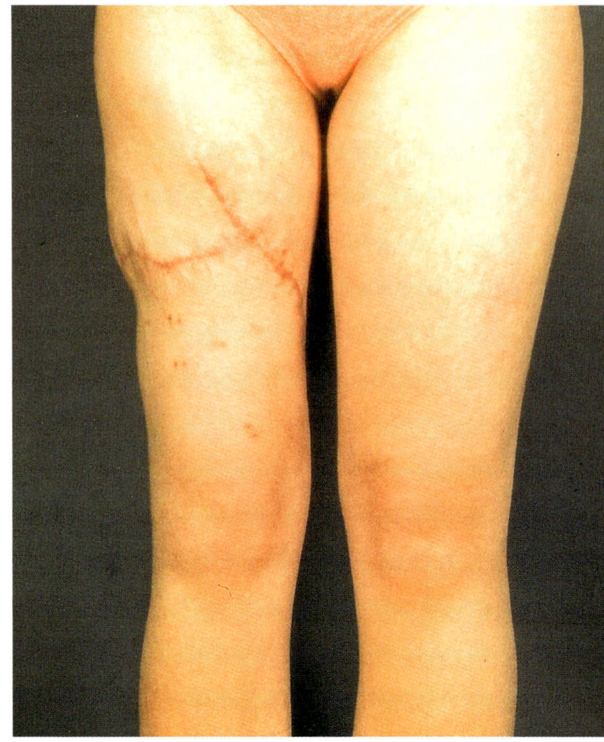

Figure 6.1b Result after six months

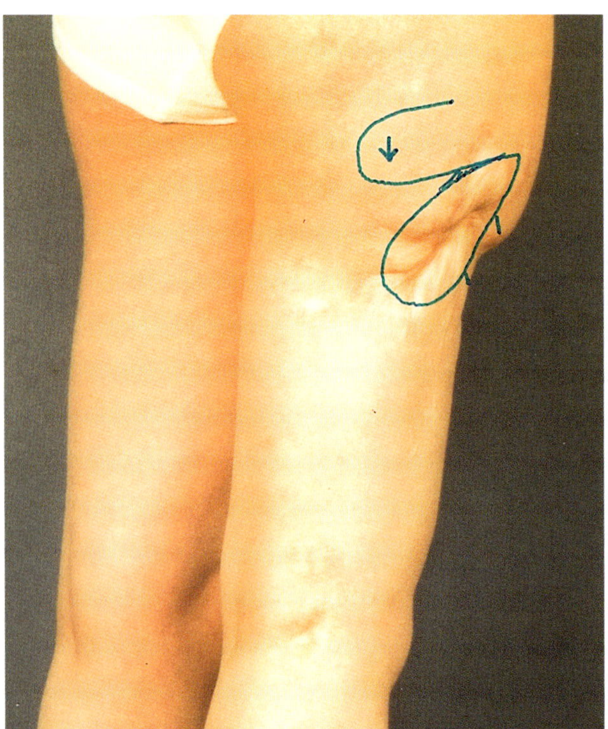

Figure 6.1c The lateral defect is covered with a transposition flap from above.

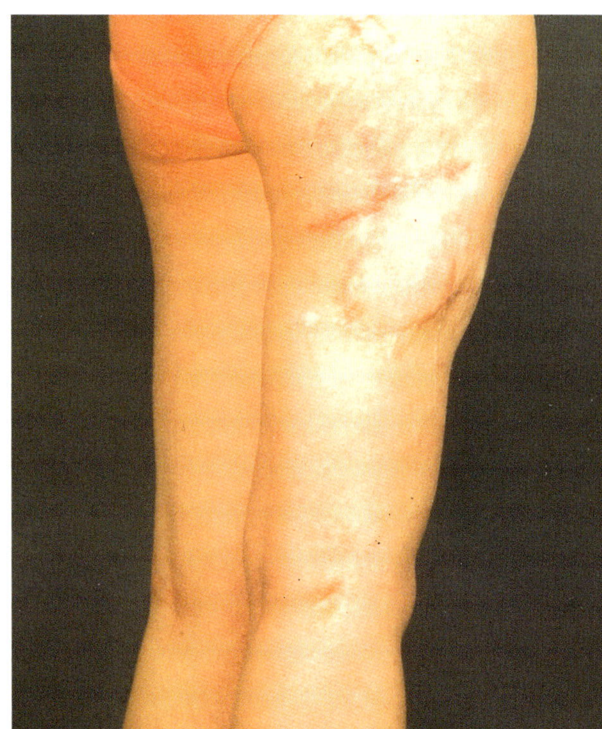

Figure 6.1d Result after six months

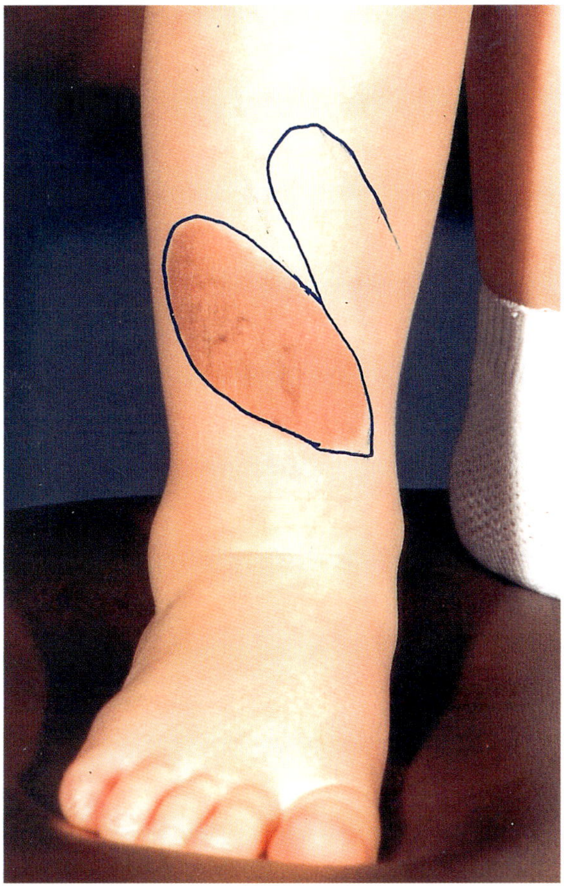

Figure 6.2a Nevus of the right lower leg of a 4-year old child.
Planning of the operation: Transposition flap. A defect of this size can be treated with local flaps in children. In adults this would be too risky; an alternative would be a split-thickness graft or a fasciocutaneous flap.

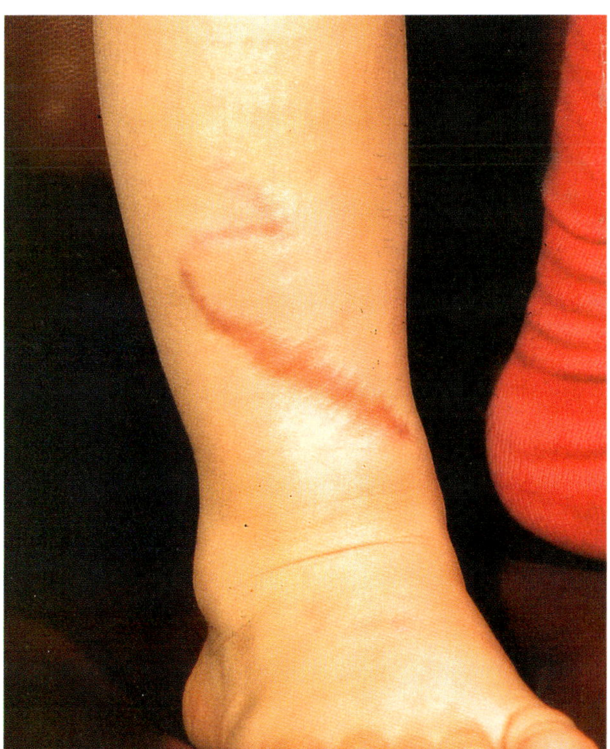

Figure 6.2b Result after four months

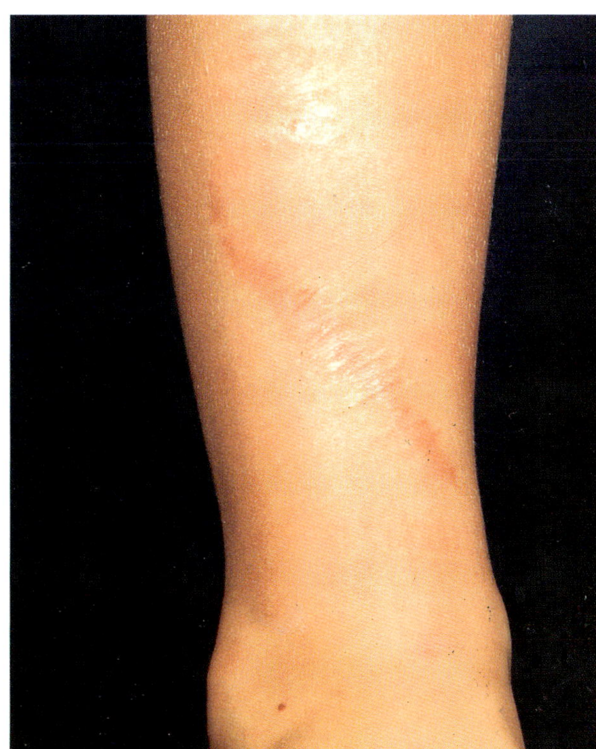

Figure 6.2c Result after four years:
The cosmetic result after local flap is better than after split-thickness-graft.

Fasciocutaneous Flaps

a) Medial Plantar Flap

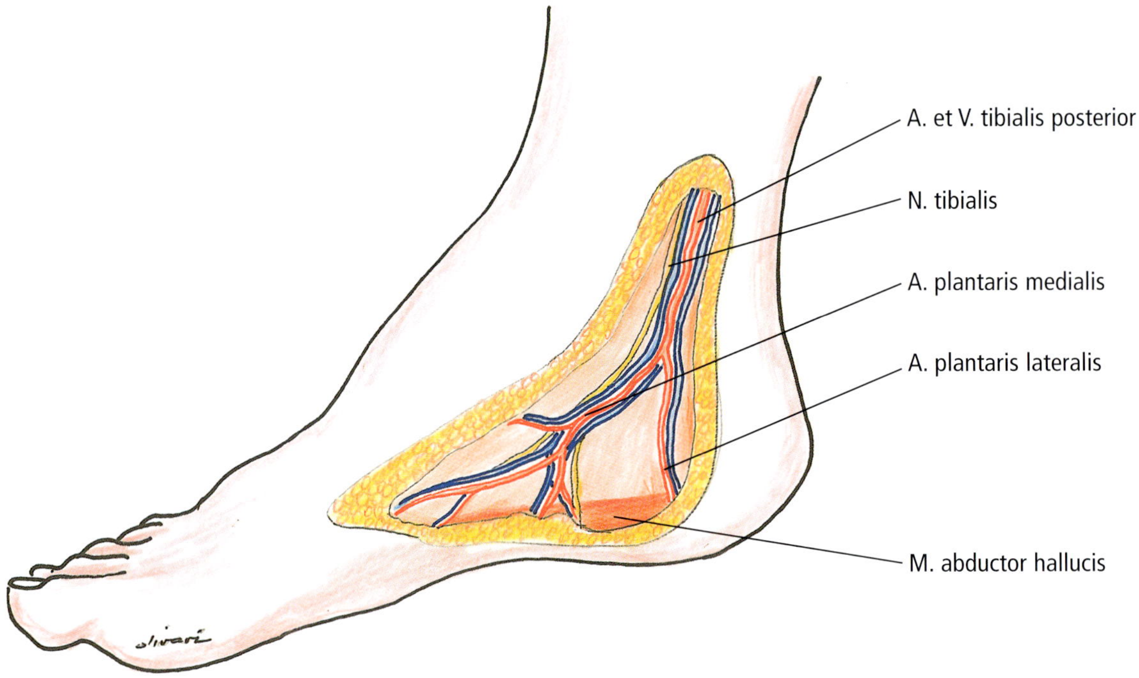

Figure 6.3a Anatomy of the medial plantar flap.
The vascular pedicle of this flap is the medial plantar artery and vein. This is a branch of posterior tibial artery and vein; the lateral plantar artery and vein are left intact. The medial plantar nerve is included and thus, the medial plantar flap has sensation. The competence of the vessels is checked preoperative with duplex ultrasound or angiography.

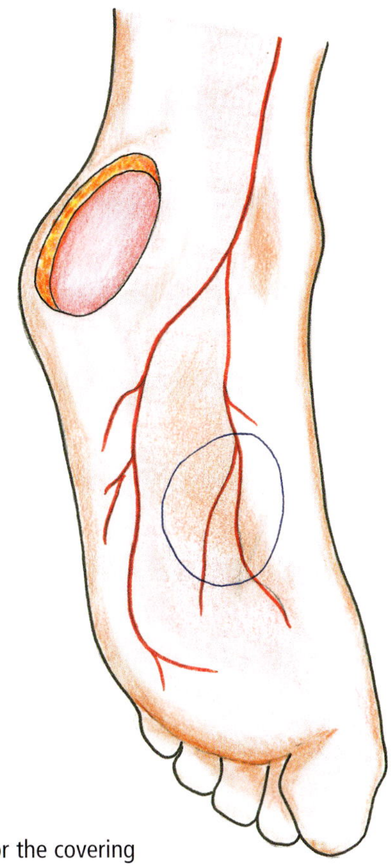

Figure 6.3b The medial plantar island flap is very suitable for the covering defects of the heel. The weight bearing quality of skin is of great advantage. This flap can be used also as a free flap.

Medial Plantar Island Flap

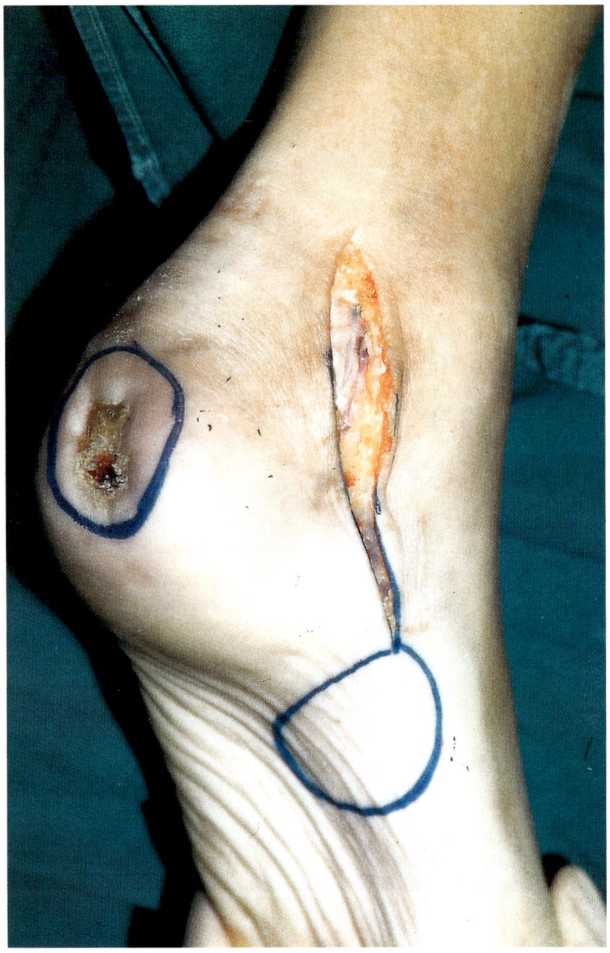

Figure 6.4a Defect of the heel.
A fasciocutaneous medial plantar island flap is planned to cover the defect. The posterior tibial artery is exposed and followed distally to its bifurcation.

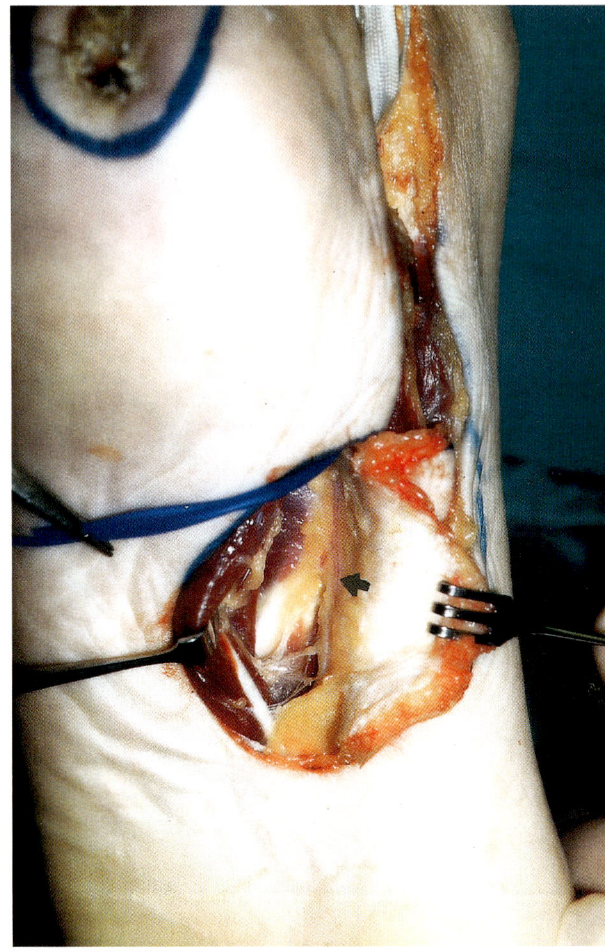

Figure 6.4b The posterior tibial artery divides into the lateral and medial plantar arteries below (distal) to the medial malleolus. A fasciocutaneous plantar island flap of appropriate size is prepared and freed with the medial plantar vessels (Arrow: The vascular and nerve bundle is clearly visible).
The flap contains the fascia of the abductor hallucis muscle. For mobilization of the island flap around the heel the abductor hallucis muscle is divided in the middle and afterwards repaired. The digitalis proprius nerve must be identified during the dissection. The flap has sensation by including the branch of the medial plantar nerve.

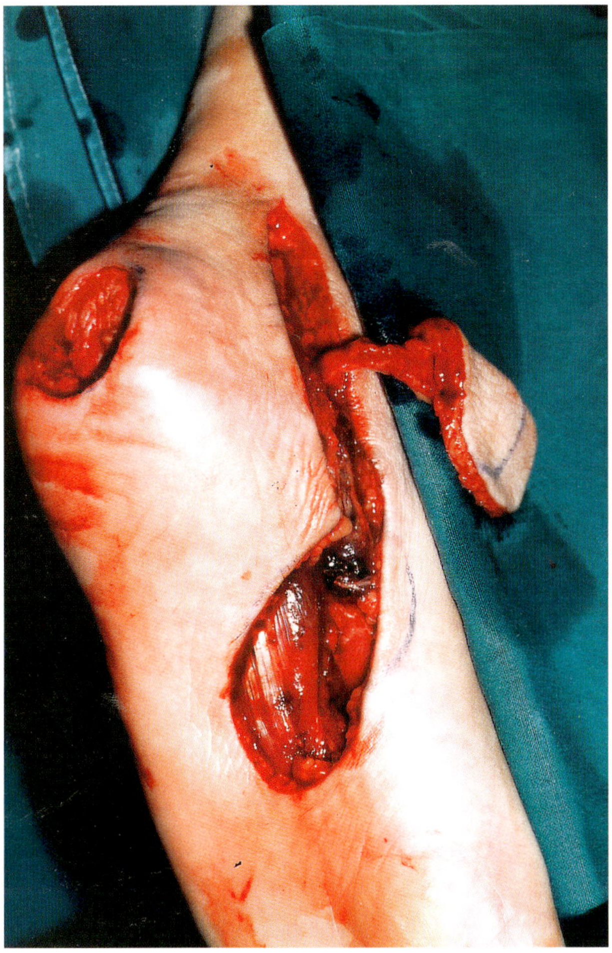

Figure 6.4c The medial plantar island flap is mobilized as a fasciocutaneous island flap and is moved through a subcutaneous tunnel to the defect.

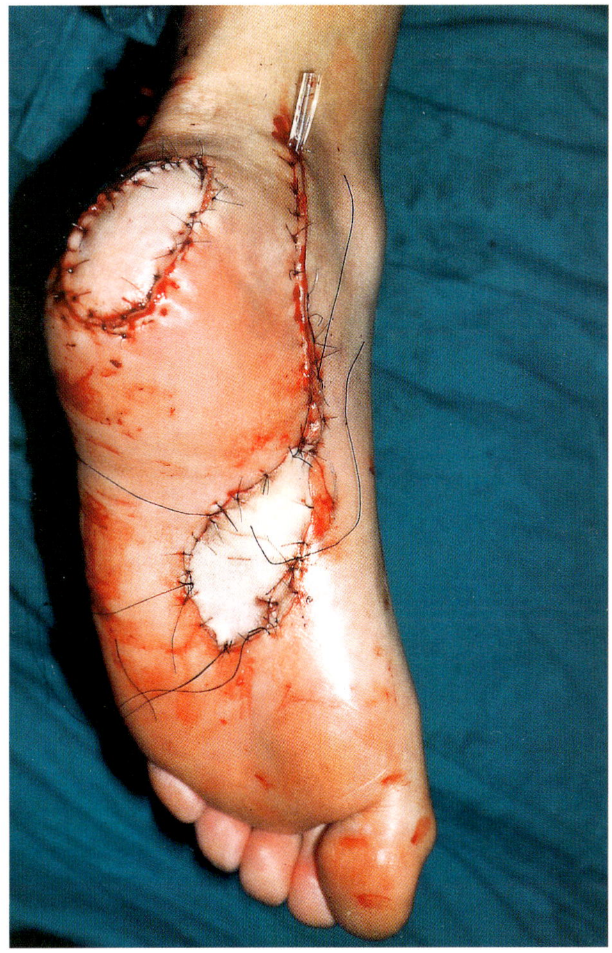

Figure 6.4d The donor site is covered with a skin graft. One can see the excellent blood supply of the flap.

b) Lateral Calcaneal Artery Island Flap

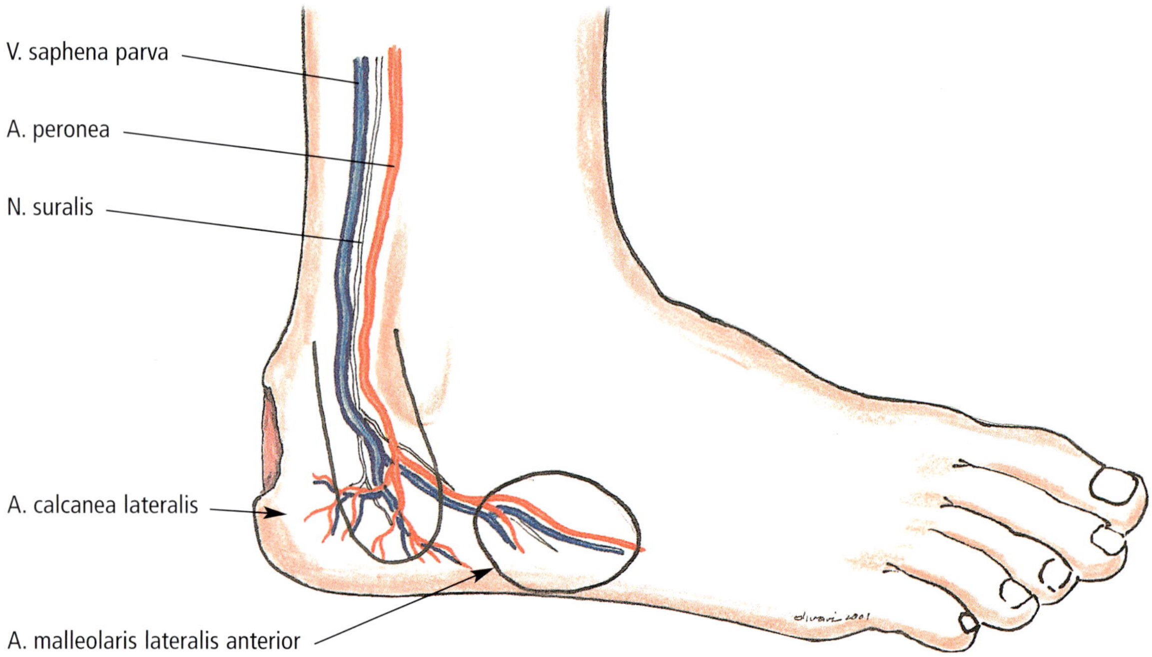

Figure 6.5 The fasciocutaneous lateral foot flap can be used as an axial pattern flap or as an island flap. It is suitable for covering defects over the lower part of the Achilles tendon, but not for the lower part of the heel, as the skin is not designed for weight bearing. For the heel the medial plantar flap is better. The blood supply is derived from the peroneal artery, anterior malleolar artery and lateral calcaneal artery. The venous outflow is guaranteed by the short saphenous vein. The flap is innervated by the sural nerve.

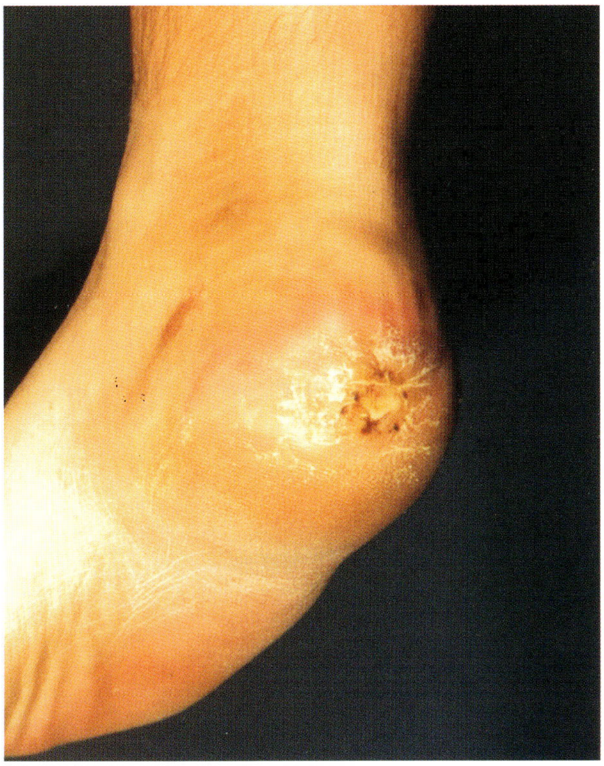

Figure 6.6a Defect of the heel

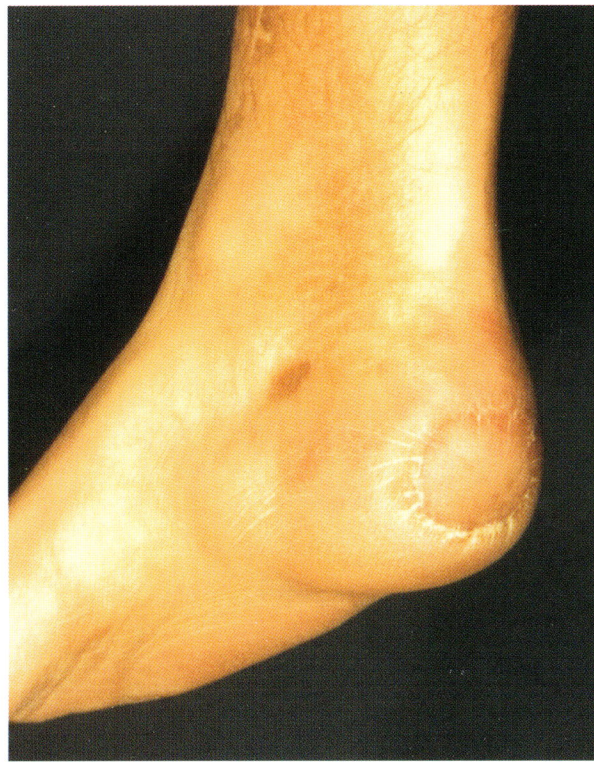

Figure 6.6d Result two years after operation

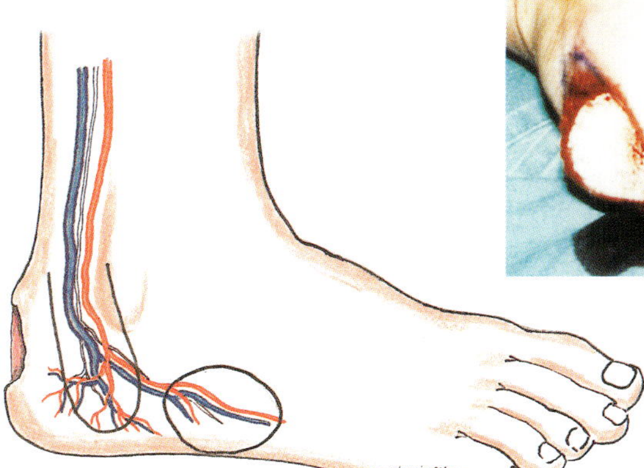

Figure 6.6b The lateral calcaneal artery skin flap is used to cover the defect. This fascio cutaneous island flap has a vascular pedicle consisting of the peroneal artery, the antero-lateral malleolar artery and short saphenous vein. It can also be utilized as a pedicled flap. In this case the blood supply is derived of the lateral calcaneal artery.

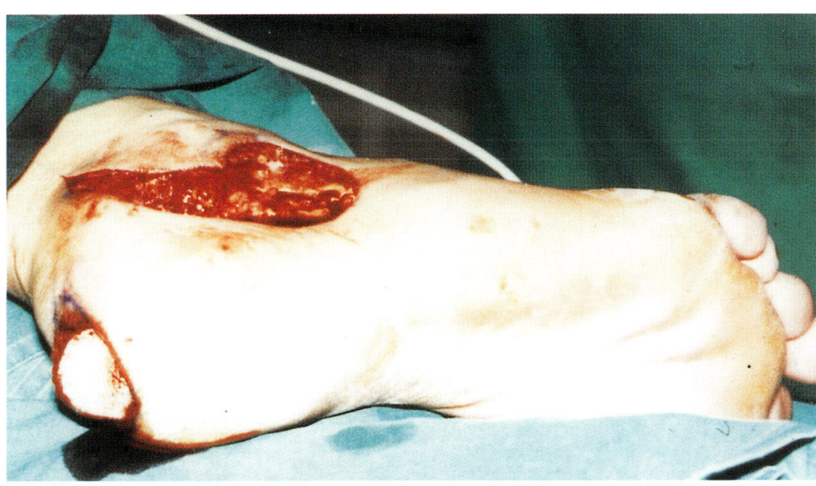

Figure 6.6c The island flap is mobilized and passed through a subcutaneous tunnel. Afterwards it is fixed in the defect and the donor site is closed by a mesh graft.

c) Distally Pedicled Fasciocutaneous, Sural Sensory Flap

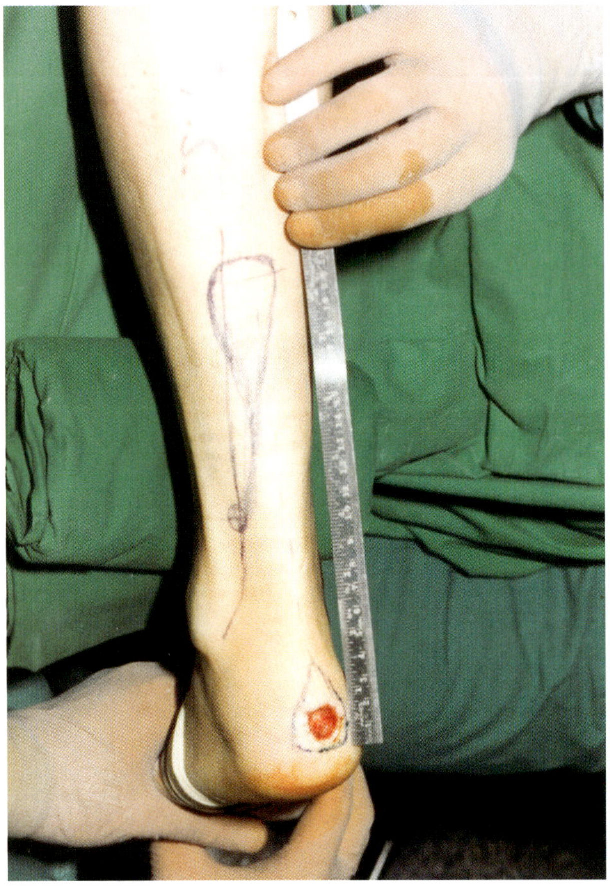

Figure 6.7a Defect at the heel below the Achilles tendon. A distally pedicled sural sensory fasciocutaneous flap is planned. The pathway of the sural nerve is marked. The upper edge of the island flap is marked about 22 cm above the margin of the calcaneum.

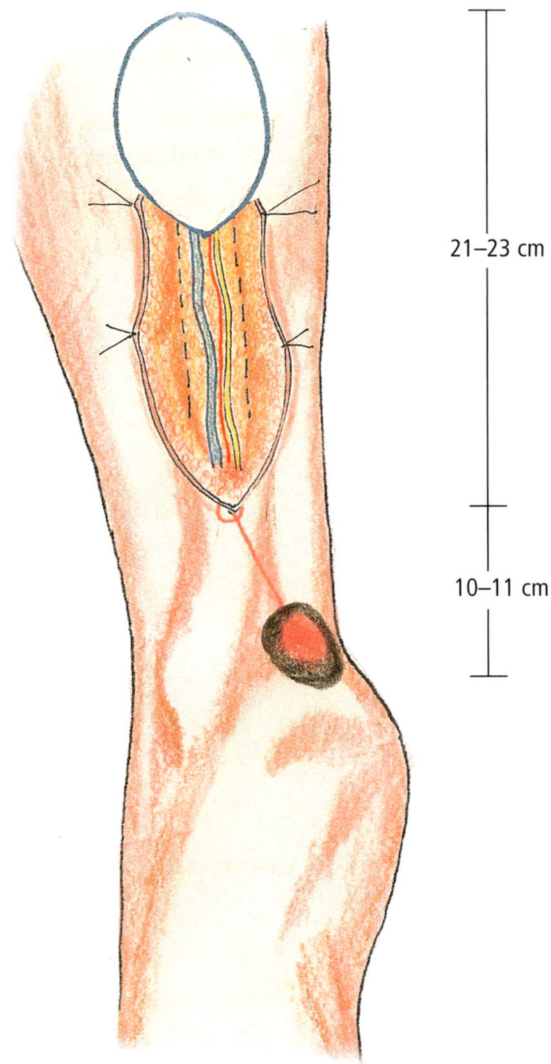

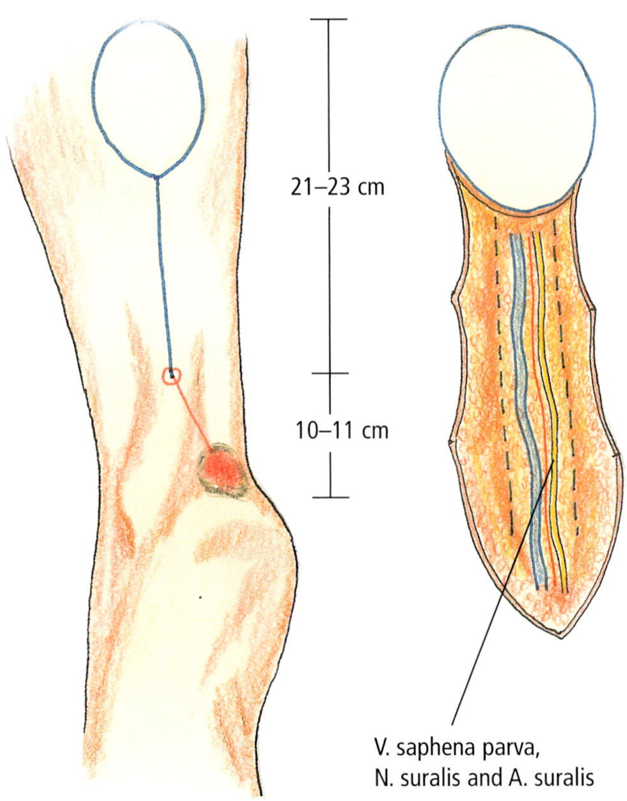

△ **Figure 6.7c**

◁ **Figure 6.7b** The flap and the pedicle are mobilized with the crural fascia. The commencement of the pedicle is located 5 cm proximal to the lateral malleolus (red circle). Distally the skin is incised to mobilize the pedicle (red line).

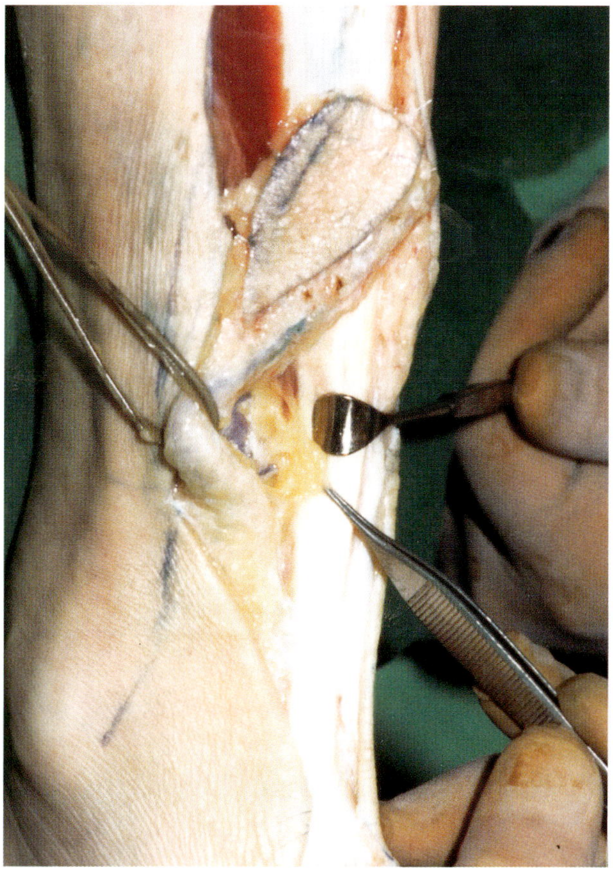

Figure 6.7d The sural flap is mobilized as an island flap. The pedicle consists of subcutaneous tissue, crural fascia and contains the sural nerve short saphenous vein.

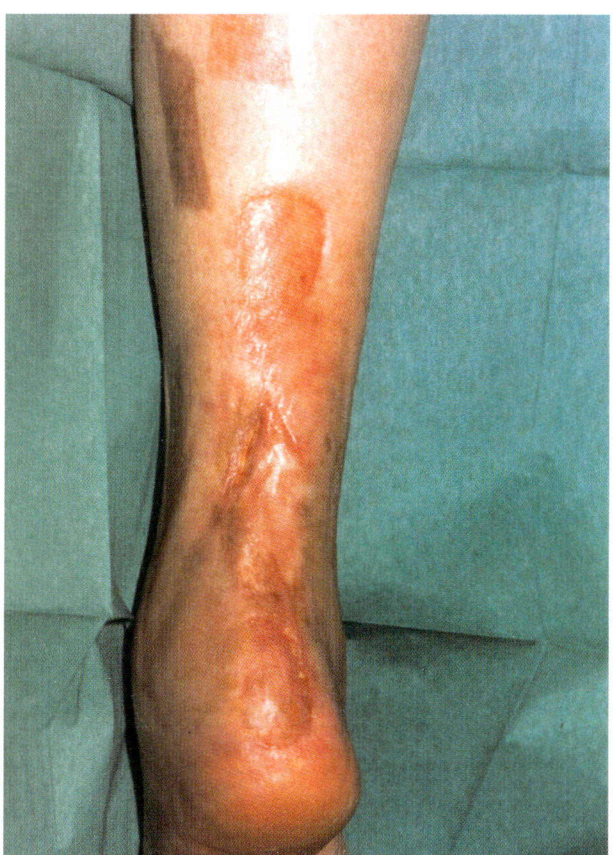

Figure 6.7e Result one year postoperatively. The donor site was closed with split-thickness graft.

Sural Flap (Distal Pedicle)

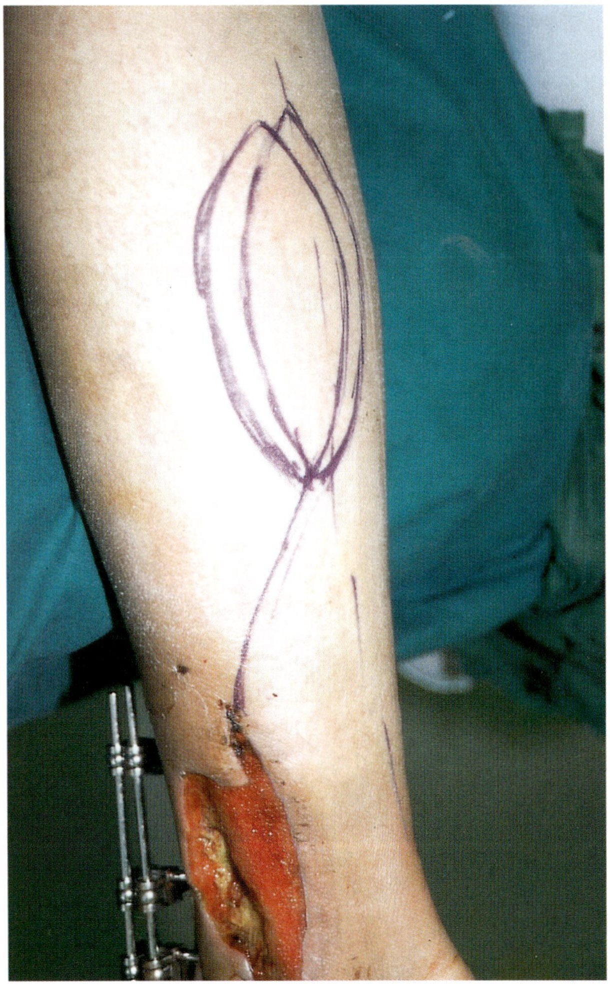

Figure 6.8a Traumatic defect on the left lower leg above the malleolus with external fixation of a fracture. A distally pedicled fasciocutaneous sural island flap is planned.

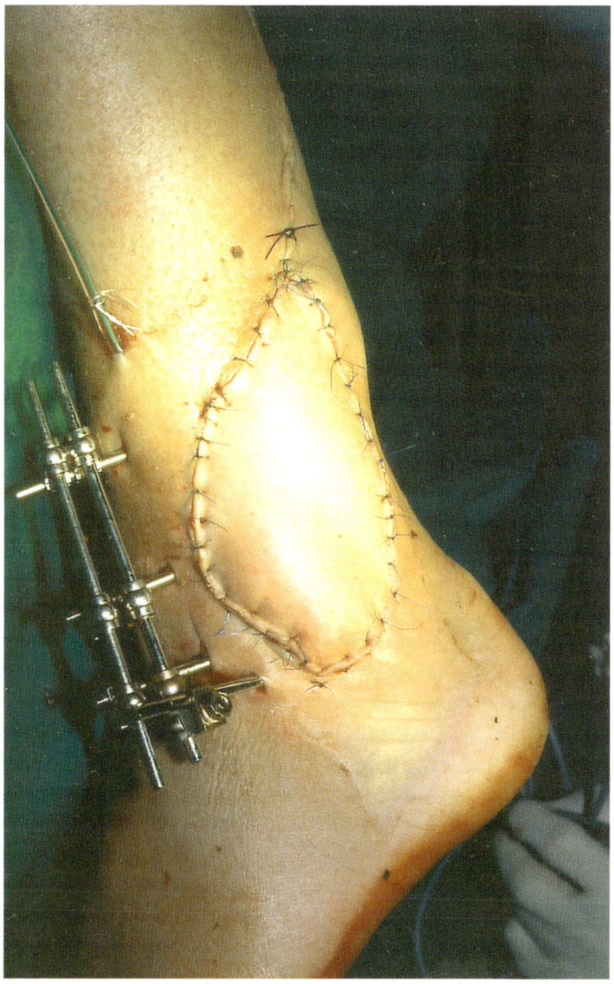

Figure 6.8b Result 24 hours after the operation

d) Fasciocutaneous Foreleg Flap (Ponten Flap)

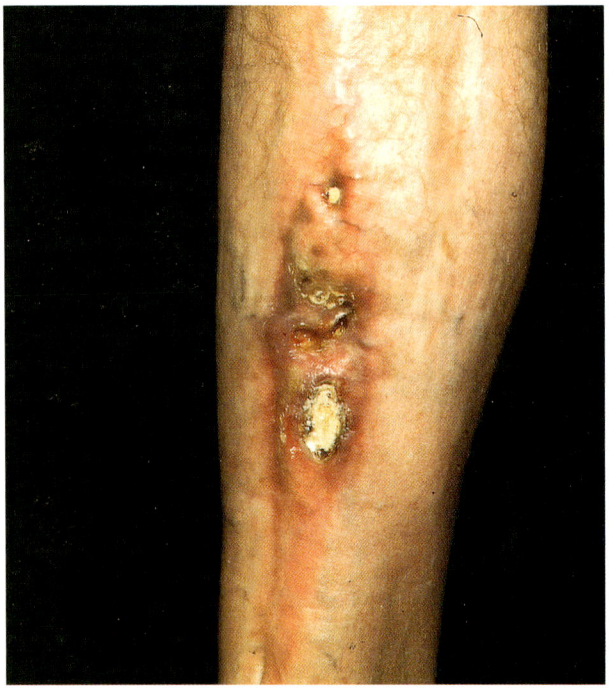

Figure 6.9a Osteomyelitis of the tibia (post trauma), unhealed for one year

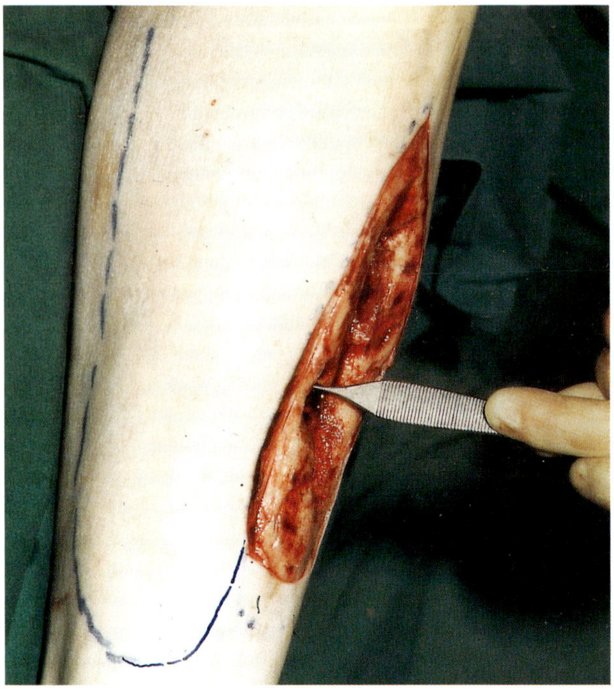

Figure 6.9b Result after debridement. It is very important, that the infected and necrotic parts of the bone are completely debrided with chisel. Healthy parts of the bone show punctate bleeding.

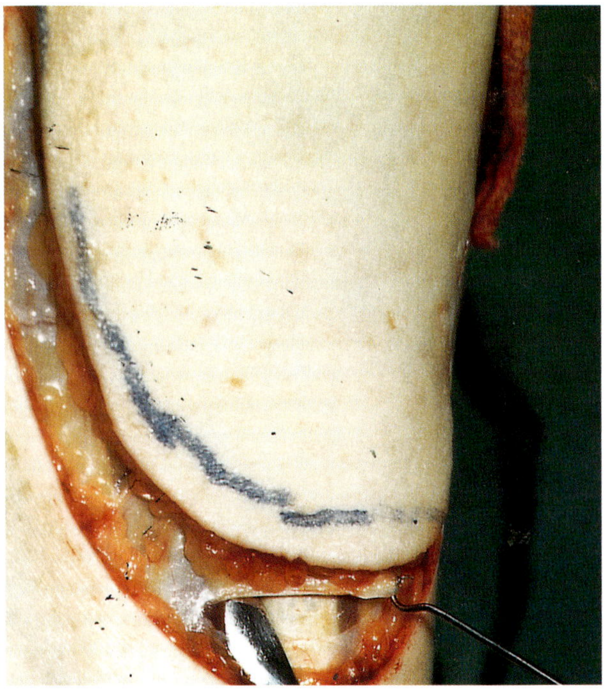

Figure 6.9c The fasciocutaneous flap is mobilized with blunt dissection from distally to proximally.

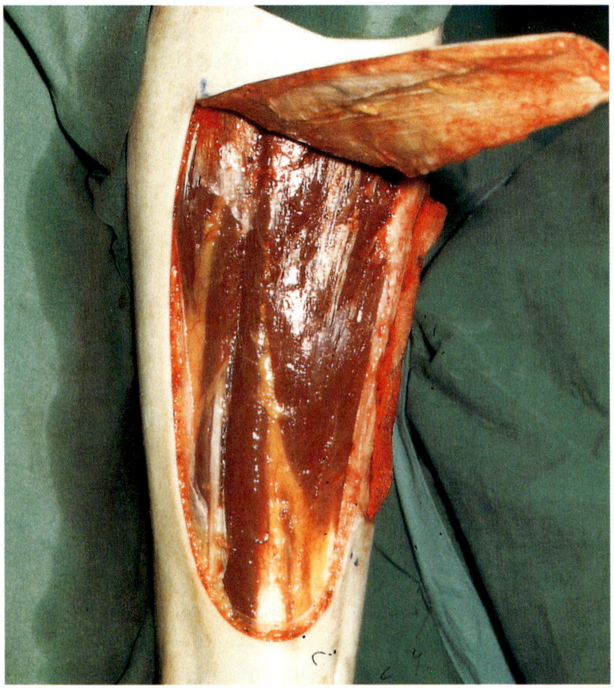

Figure 6.9d The fasciocutaneous flap after complete mobilization. **Notice** the large fascial (and skin) pedicle of the flap.

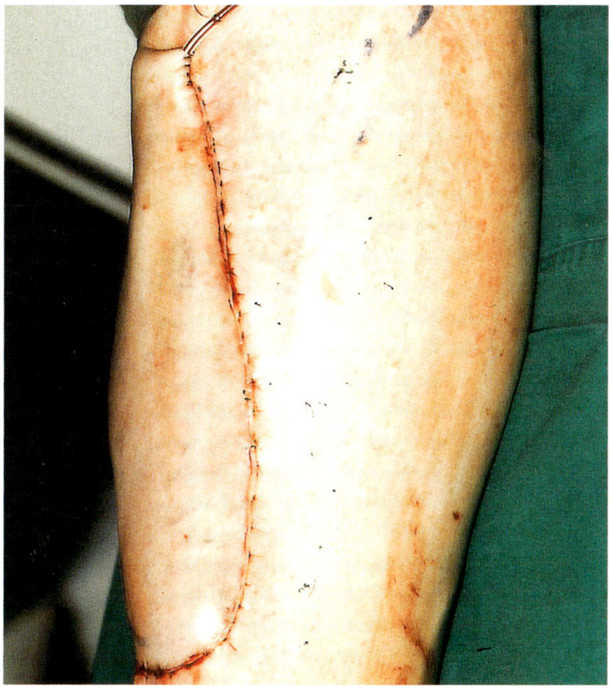

Figure 6.9e Result at the end of the operation. The blood supply of the flap is excellent. However there was a necrosis of the medial part of the tip of the flap due too tight a dressing but fortunately away from the tibia.

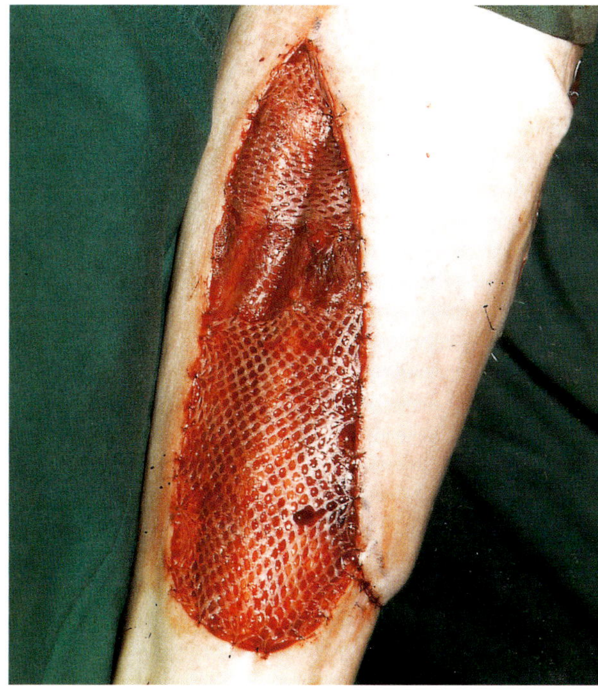

Figure 6.9f The donor site was closed with mesh graft

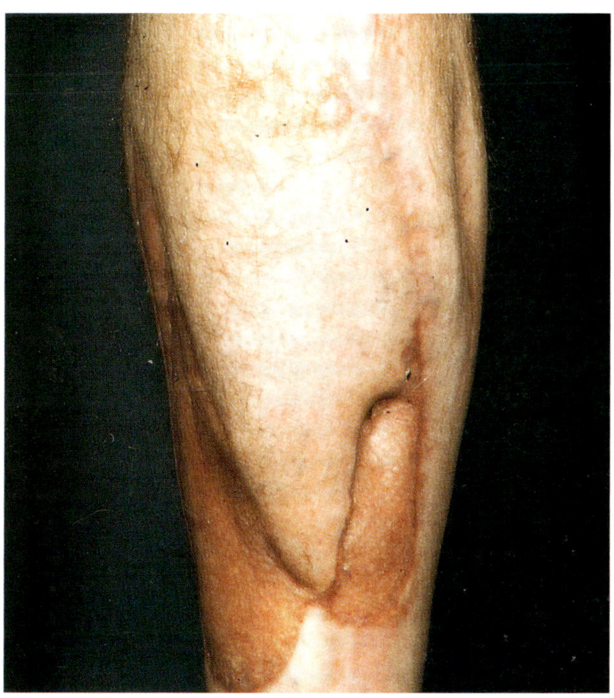

Figure 6.9g Result three months after operation. The defect of the bone is located beneath healthy part of the flap. This demonstrates that a surgeon needs some luck besides his good technique!

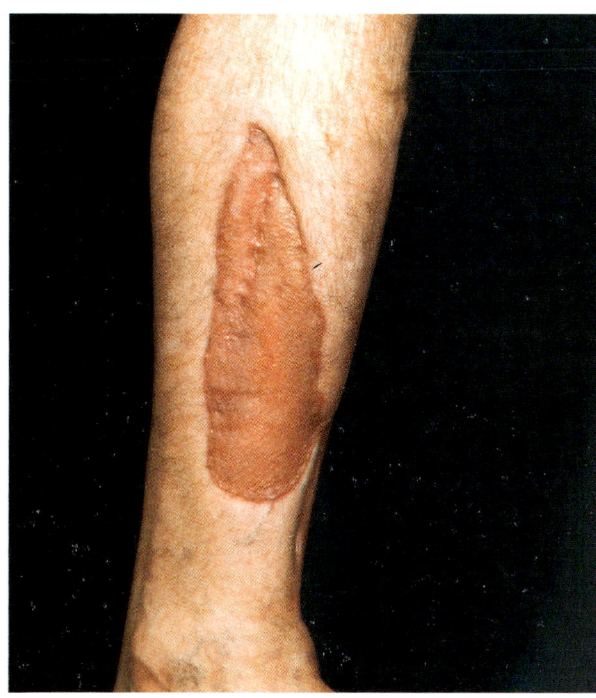

Figure 6.9h The defect in the flap apex of the flap was covered with a mesh graft

Bilateral Fasciocutaneous Bridge Flap

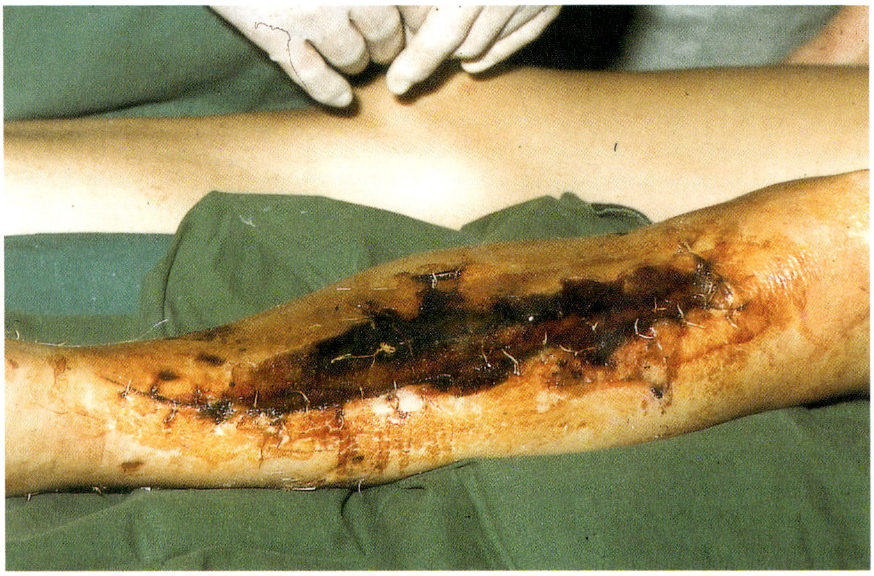

Figure 6.10a Internal fixation of a lower leg fracture. The primary wound closure was too tight and resulted in a large area of necrosis with infection.

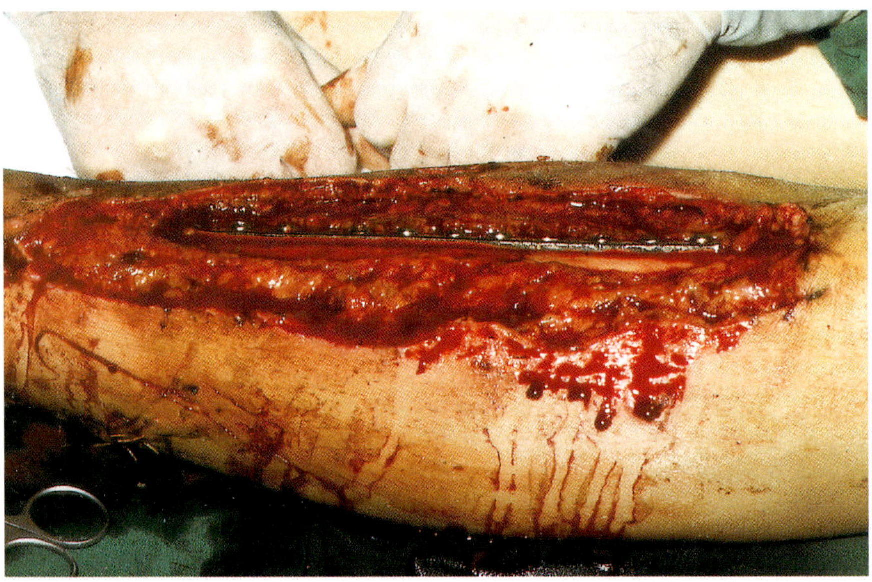

Figure 6.10b Radical debridement and irrigation of the wound with Betaisodona solution and Neomycin sol. (Nebacetin®). Intravenous infusion of antibiotics.

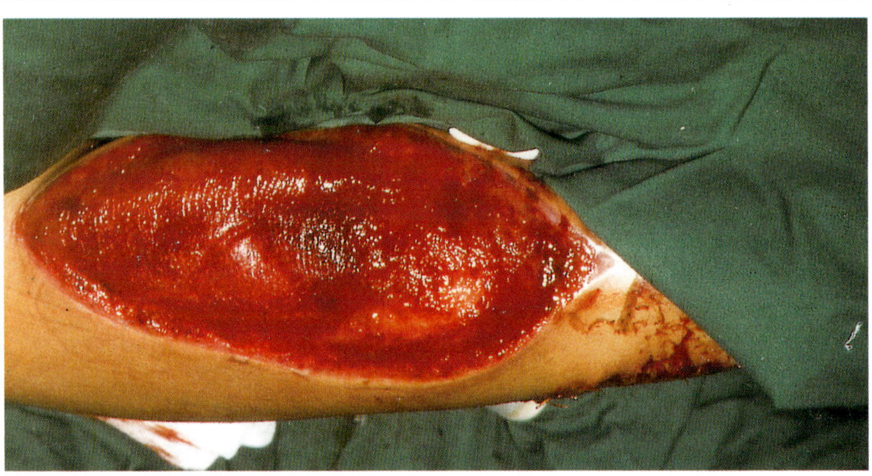

Figure 6.10c Sagittal midline incision of the calf down to the muscle layer. Then subfascial mobilization in medial and lateral direction, creating two fascio-cutaneous bridge flaps, each with a cranial and a caudal pedicle.

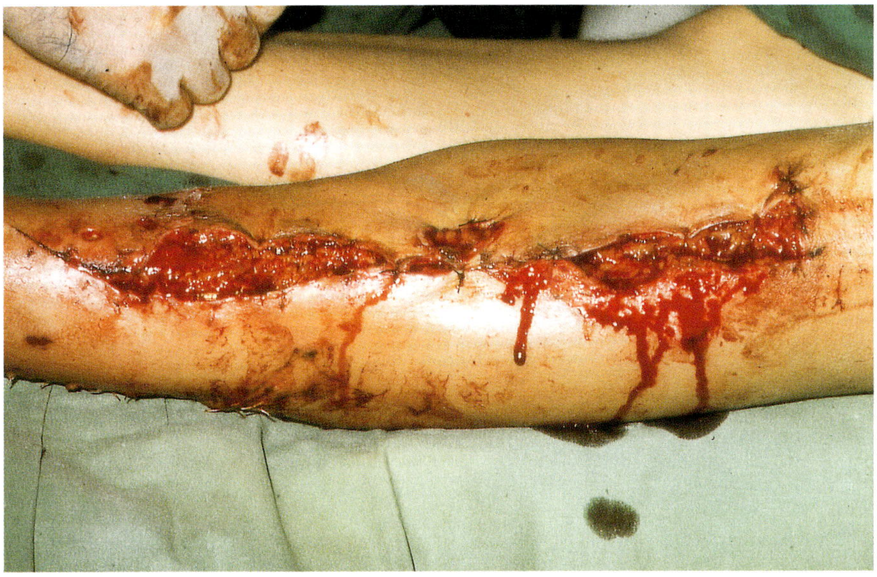

Figure 6.10d After mobilization of these two fasciocutaneous flaps the defect is closed without tension. The defect in the middle of the calf is closed by mesh graft.

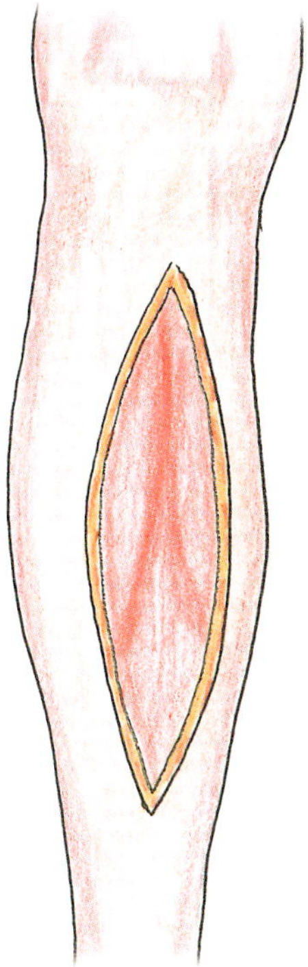

Figure 6.10e The donor site is covered with mesh graft

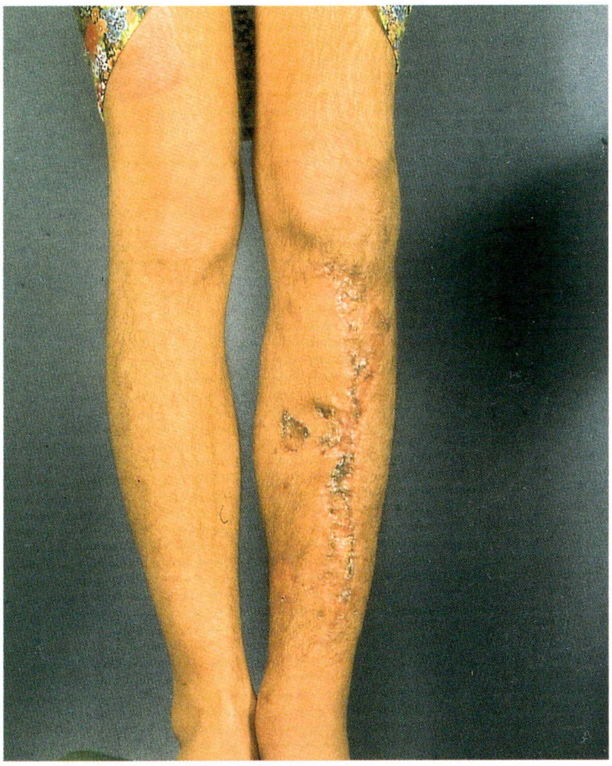

Figure 6.10f Result five months postoperatively.
Just for critics: Of course, the author knows that a free flap could be used in this case, but this was a good and simple alternative.

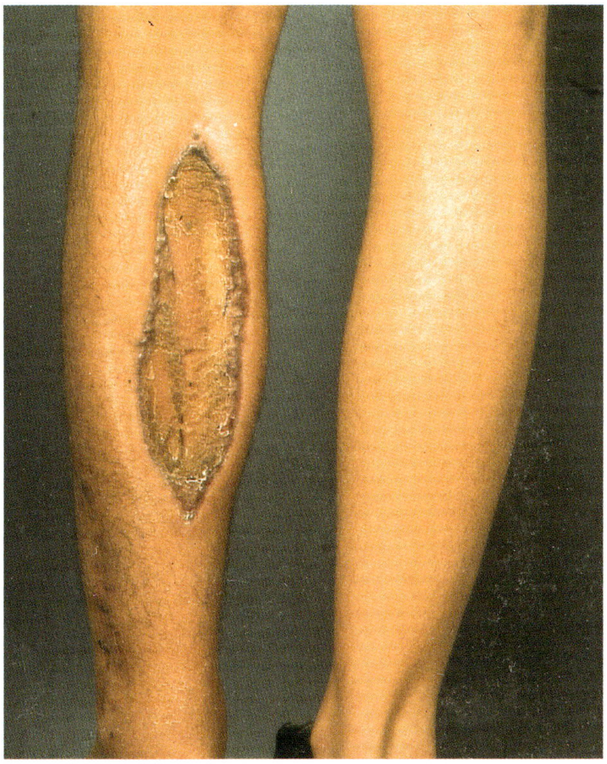

Figure 6.10g The mesh graft of the calf five months postoperatively

Myocutaneous Flaps

a) Gastrocnemius Flap

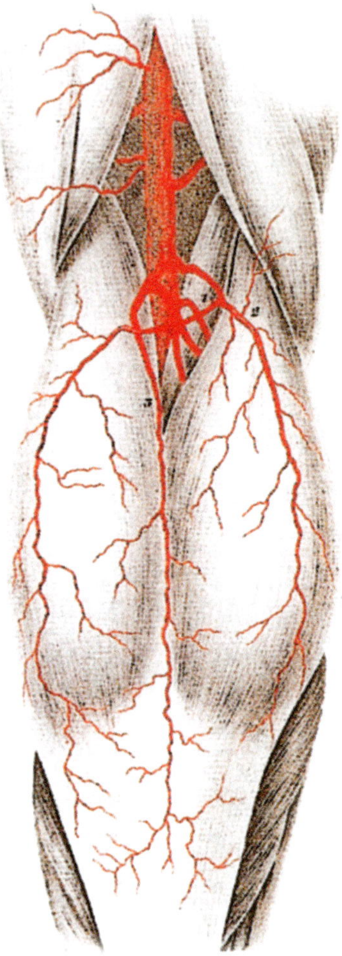

Figure 6.11a Carl Manchot (1889) in his work: "Die Hautarterien des menschlichen Körpers" (The skin arteries in the human body) gave a precise description of the blood supply in this region.

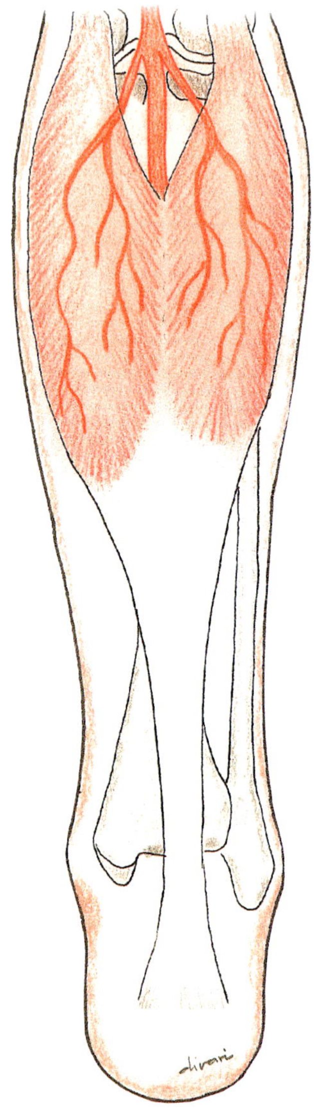

Figure 6.11b Blood supply of the gastrocnemius flap: The popliteal artery gives off a branch to the medial head and another to the lateral head of the gastrocnemius muscle. Each head of this muscle can be used as a pedicled muscle flap or myocutaneous flap. The medial head is large and is located in a better position for the covering defects in the knee area.

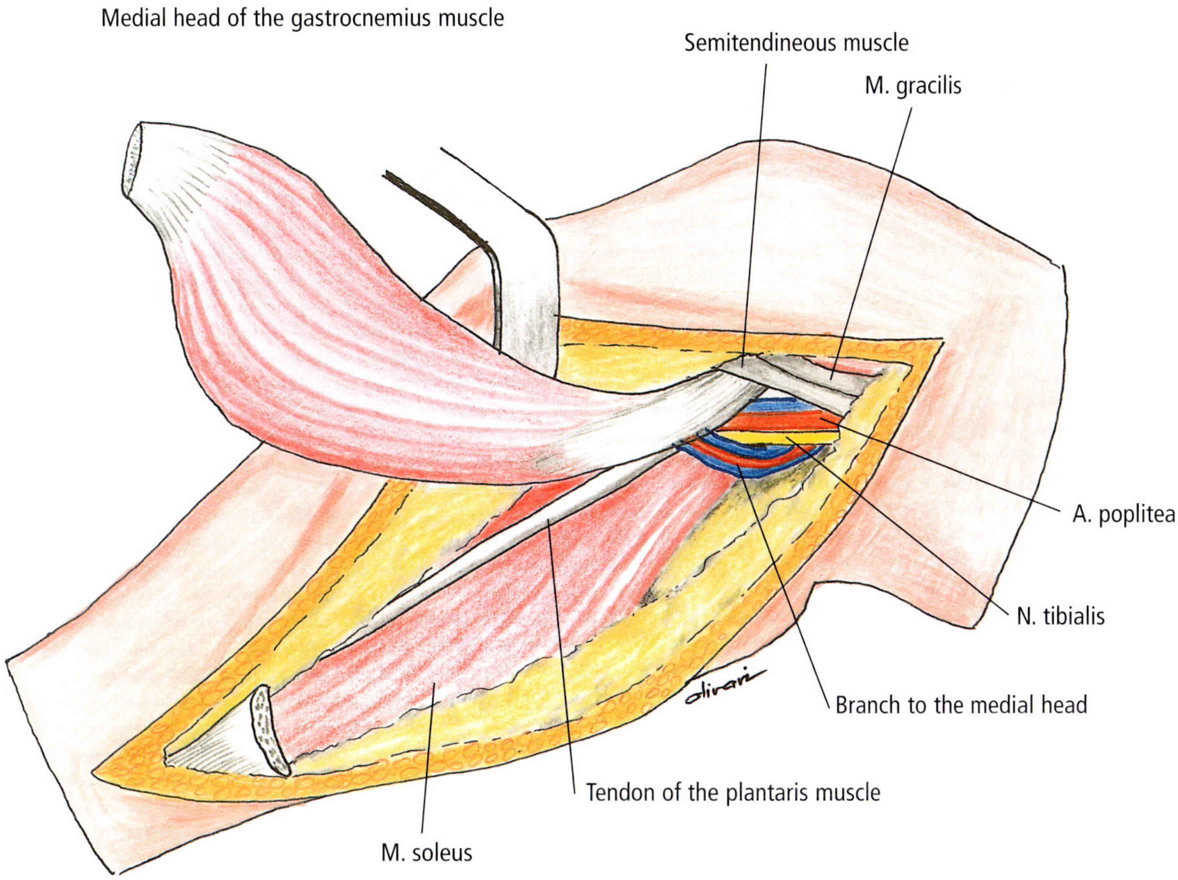

Figure 6.12 Anatomy for raising the medial head of the gastrocnemius muscle.

Medial Gastrocnemius Island Flap

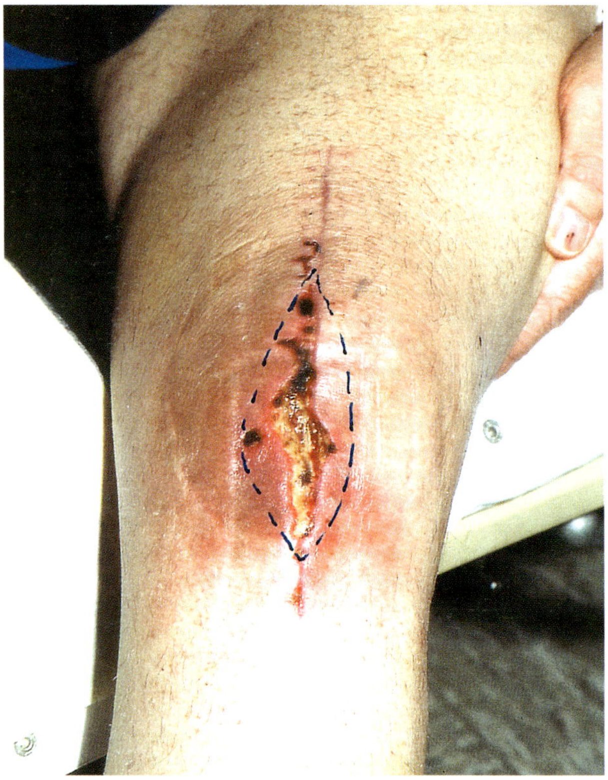

Figure 6.13a Situation after implantation of a knee prosthesis. Soft tissue necrosis and infection. All the necrotic and infected tissue is radically excised.

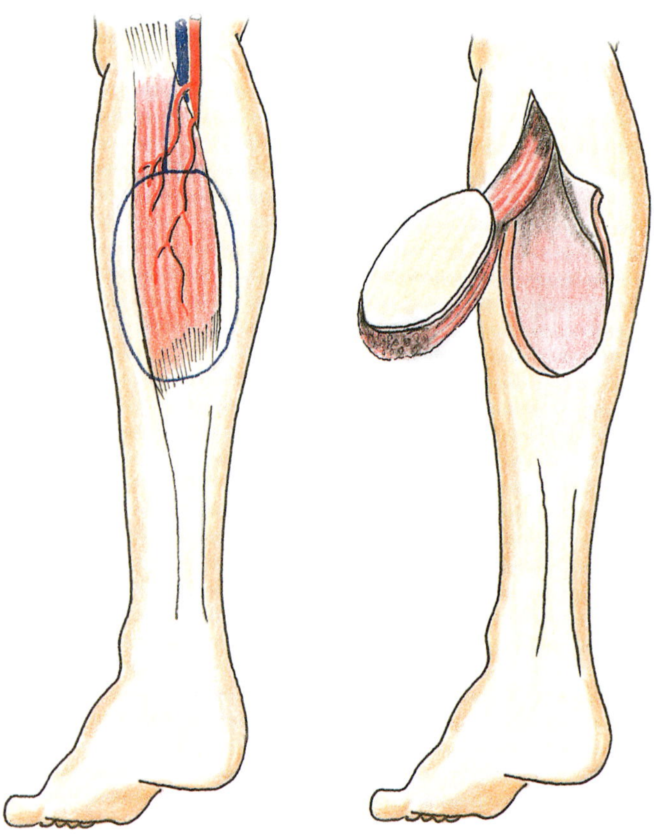

Figure 6.13b Planning of the operation:
Gastrocnemius island flap. The medial head of gastrocnemius muscle is dissected as myocutaneous flap working from distal to proximal. It is important to identify the supplying vessel and avoid any injury or distortion. The island flap is tunnelled to the defect.

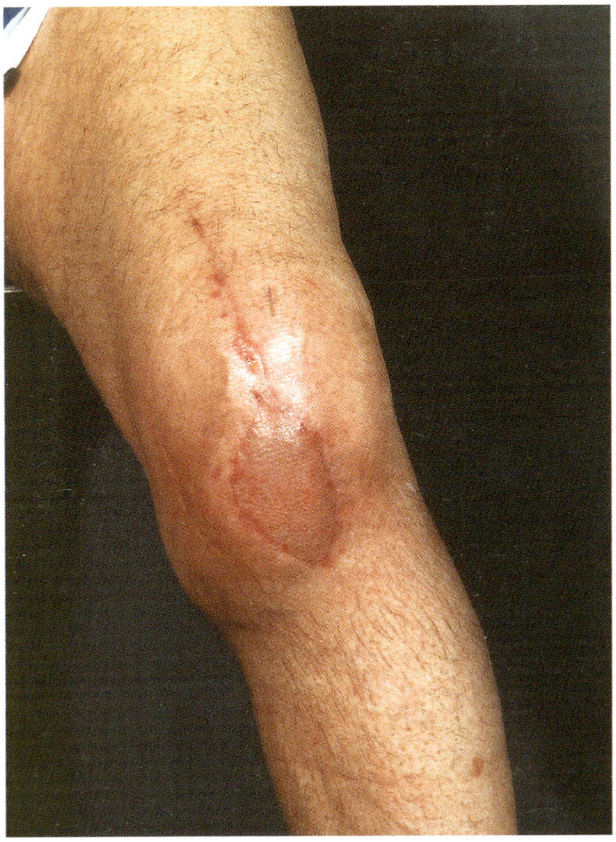

Figure 6.13c Result four months postoperatively. The gastrocnemius island flap has healed in without any problems. The knee prosthesis is functioning well.

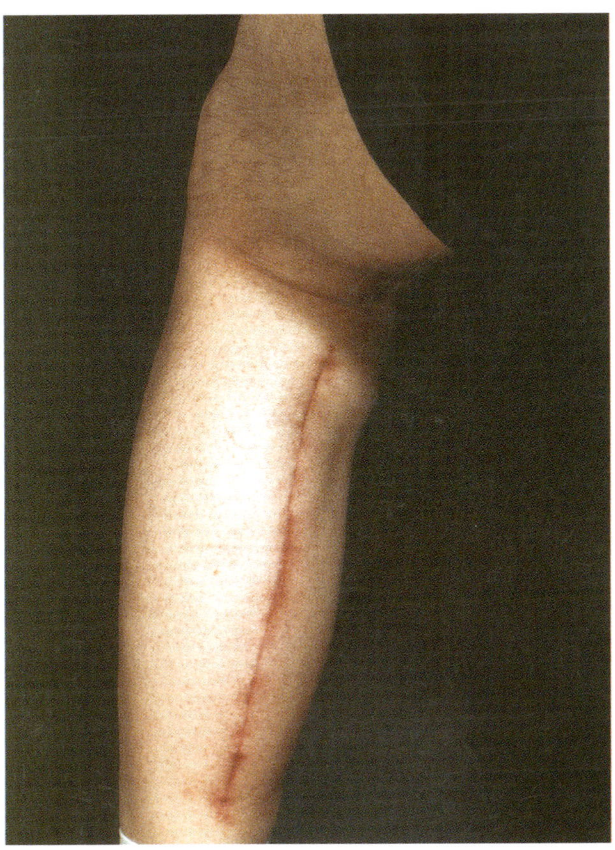

Figure 6.13d Skin part of gastrocnemius flap was small so it was possible to close the donor site primarily.

Medial Head of the Gastrocnemius Muscle as a Muscle Flap Alone

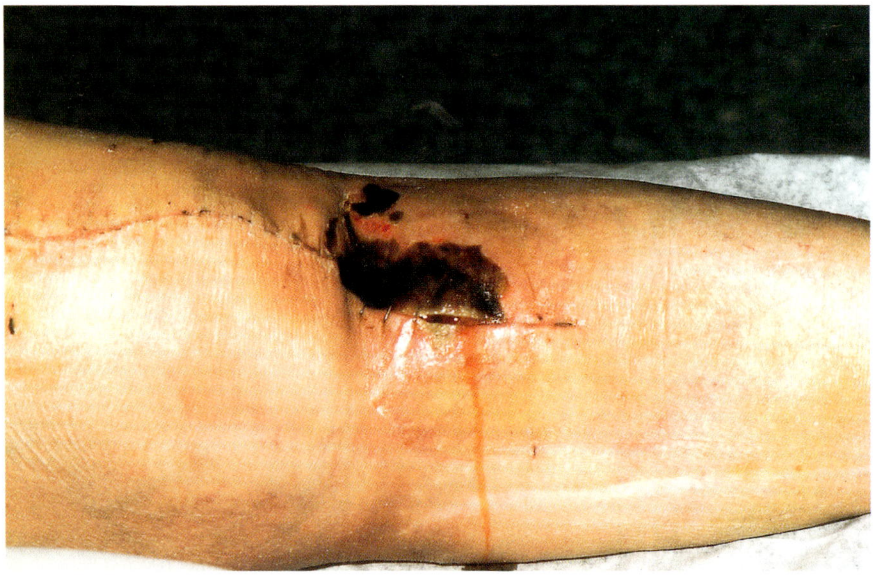

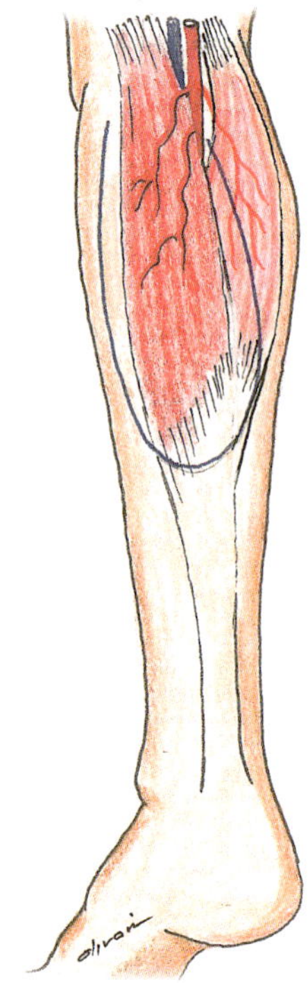

Figure 6.14a Prosthetic knee replacement. Necrosis of the skin and infection of the soft tissue. Aim of operation is to save prosthesis.

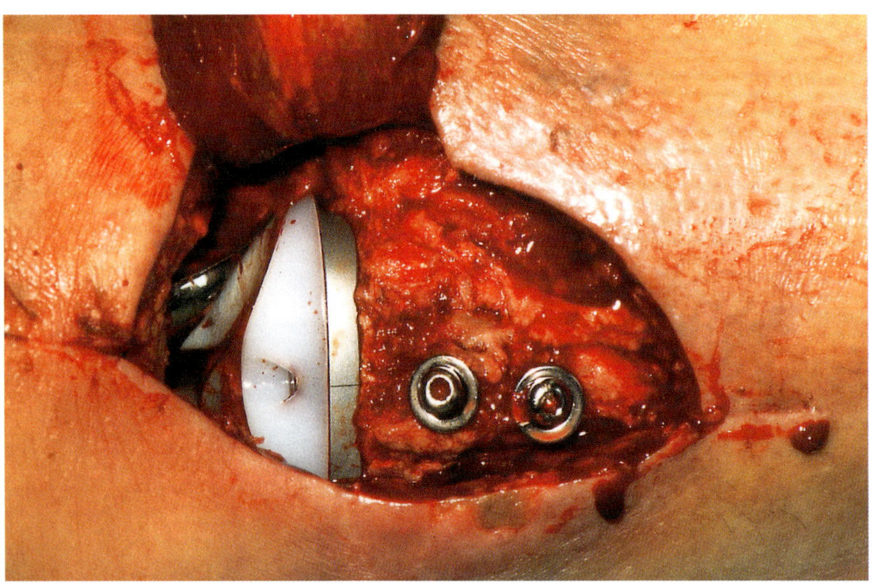

Figure 6.14b Radical resection of the necrotic material extending to the healthy tissue. Irrigation with medical soap, Betaisodona and Neomycin solution. High-dose antibiotics.

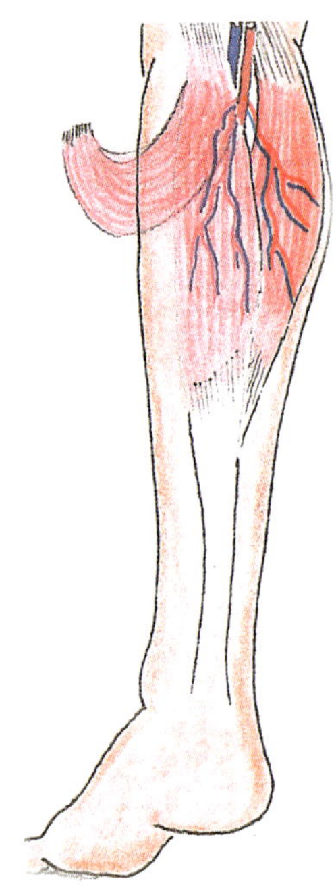

Figure 6.14c The medial part of the muscle is mobilized without skin and moved to the defect through a subcutaneous tunnel.

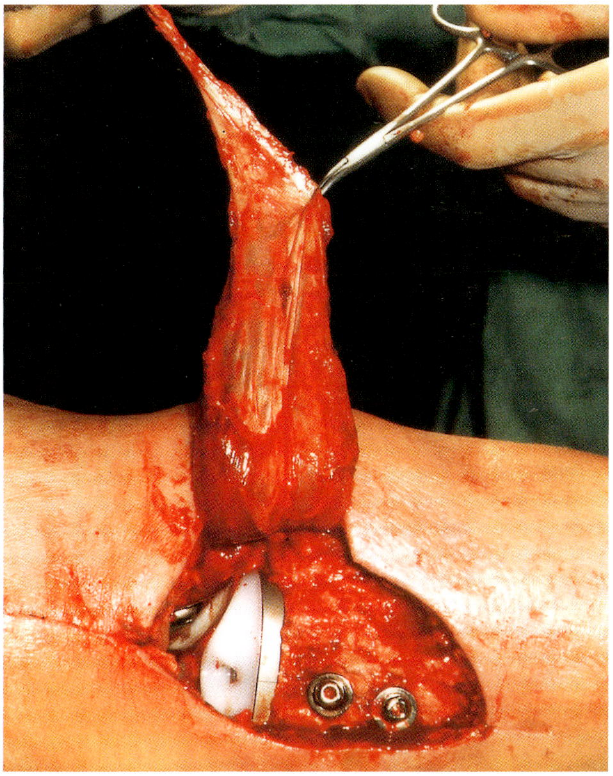

Figure 6.14e The medial head of the gastrocnemius muscle is dissected and moved to the defect.

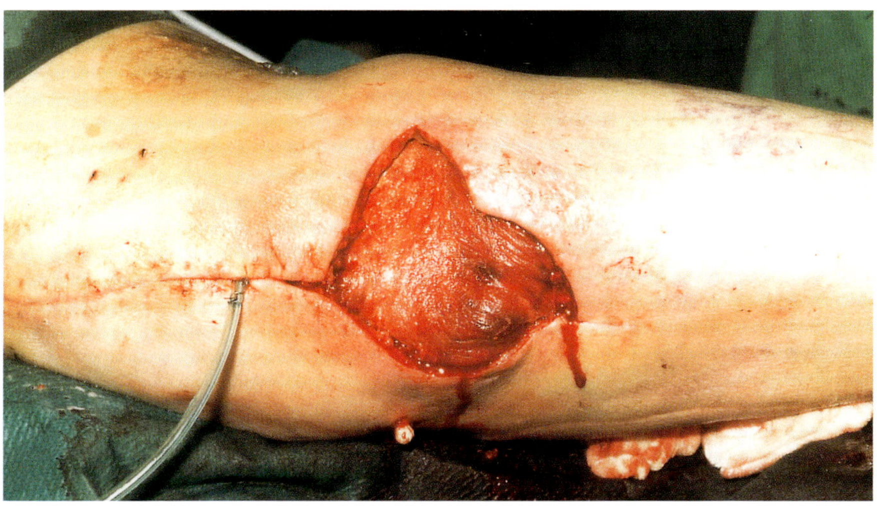

Figure 6.14f The defect and especially the prosthesis are covered with muscle. The muscle is covered with mesh graft.

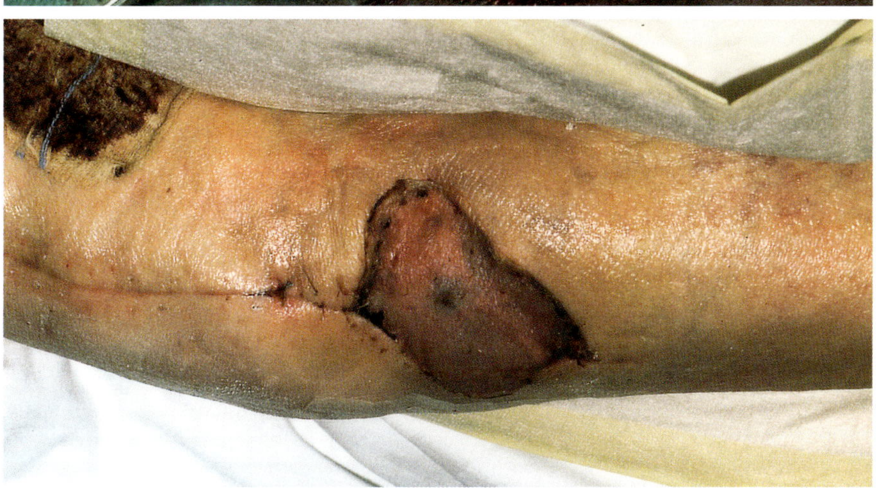

Figure 6.14g Result 16 days after the operation.
Cooperation between orthopaedic surgeon and plastic surgeon is very important. Such defect should be covered as early as possible; otherwise the prosthesis will need to be removed.

Medial Head of the Gastrocnemius Muscle and Tibialis Anterior Muscle

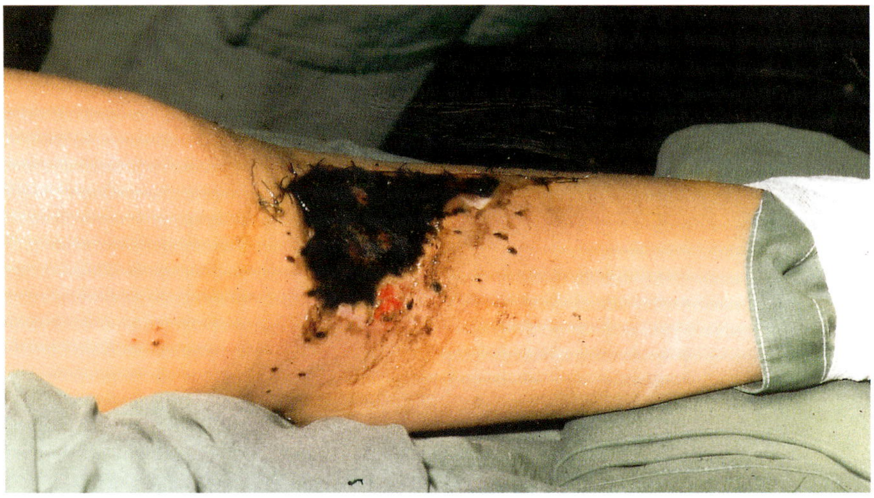

Figure 6.15a Condition after plating of a compound proximal tibial fracture. Wide necrosis of the skin.

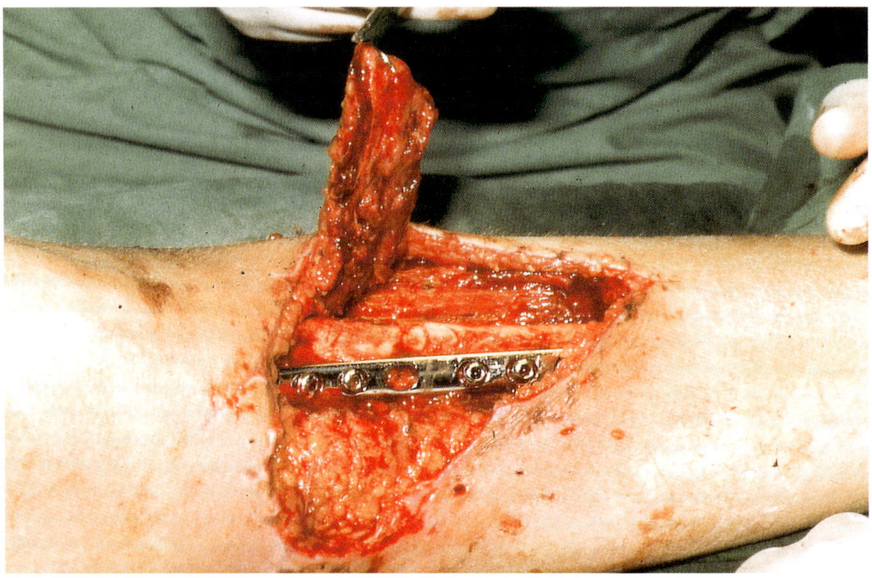

Figure 6.15b The necrotic tissue is completely excised. A part of the tibialis anterior muscle is mobilized. But only a part of the defect can be closed with this.

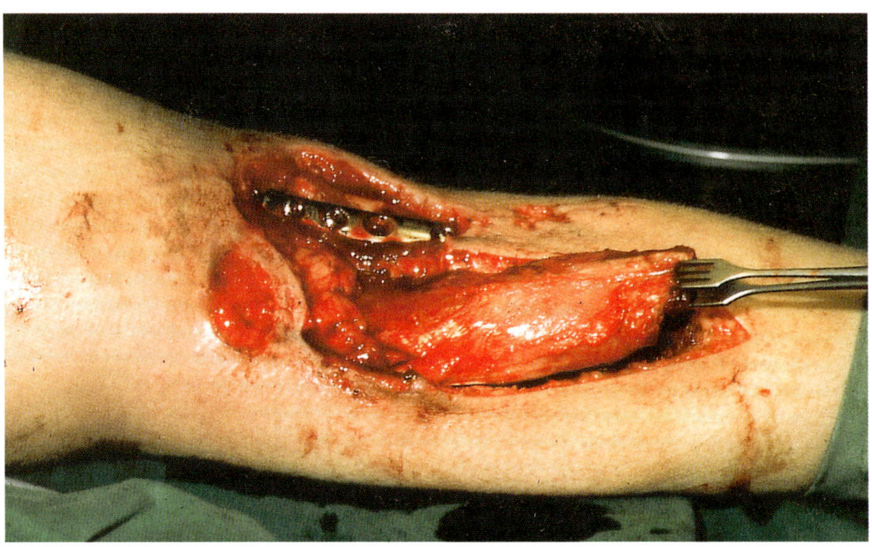

Figure 6.15c In order to close the whole of the defect the medial head of the gastrocnemius muscle was raised and transferred.

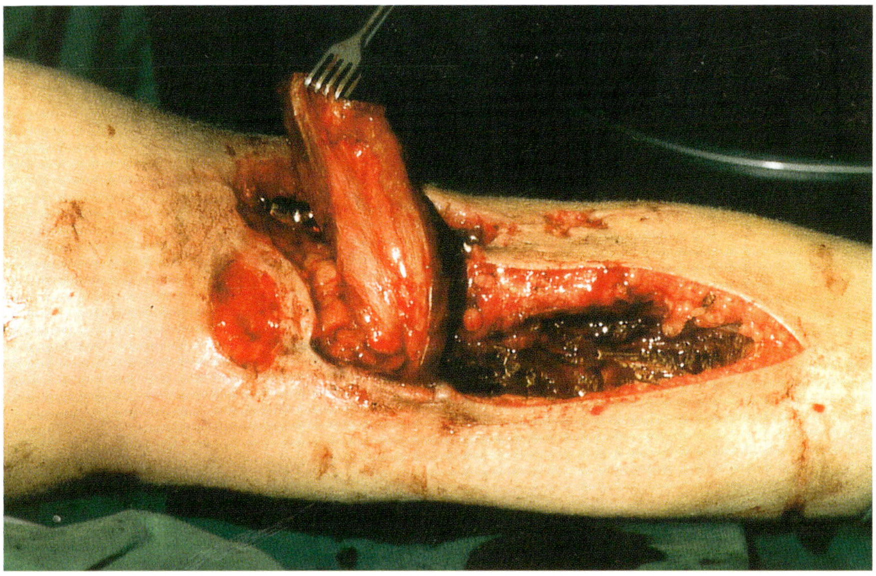

Figure 6.15d By transposing the medial head of the gastrocnemius muscle the remaining defect can be closed completely.

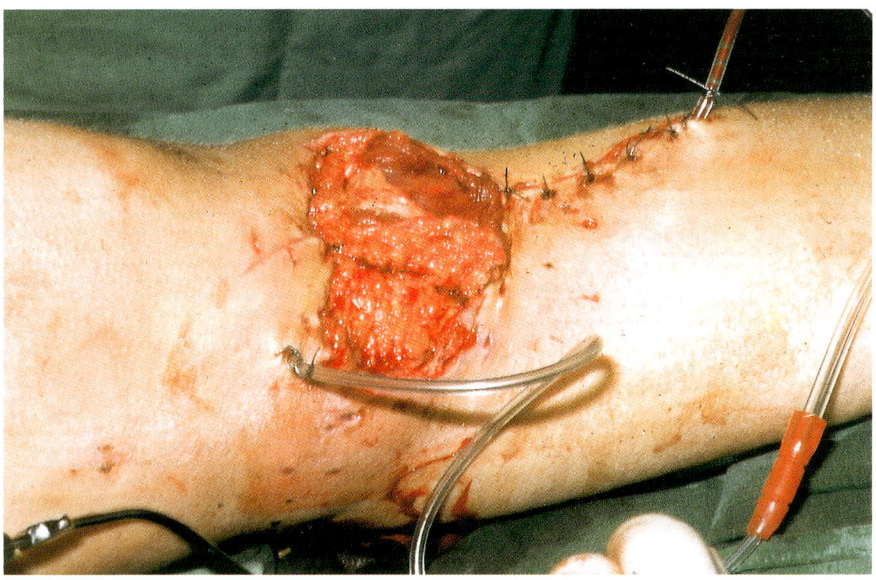

Figure 6.15e Result at the end of the operation, just before the muscle is covered by mesh graft.

Gastrocnemius Muscle Flap

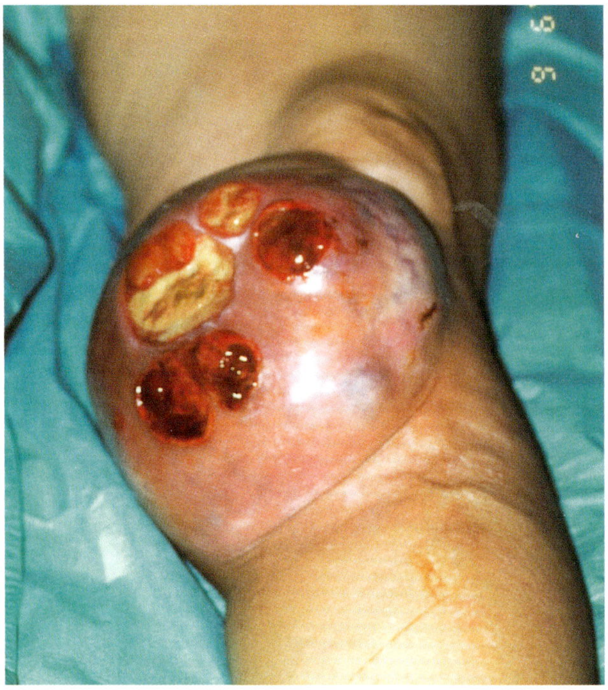

Figure 6.16a Myxoid liposarcoma in left the knee area. After excision of the tumor there was a large defect (22×20×10 cm). This was closed with the medial head of the gastrocnemius muscle and covered with split thickness skin graft.

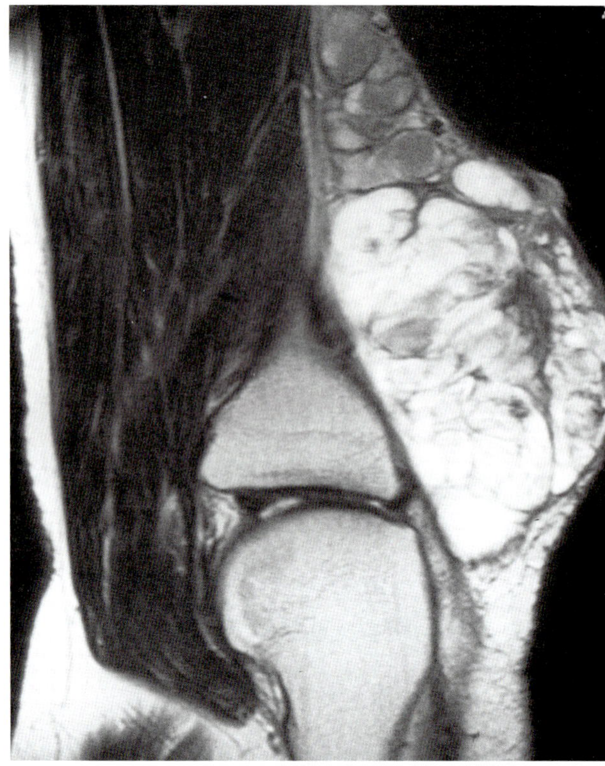

Figure 6.16b The MRI-scan shows the dimension of the tumour

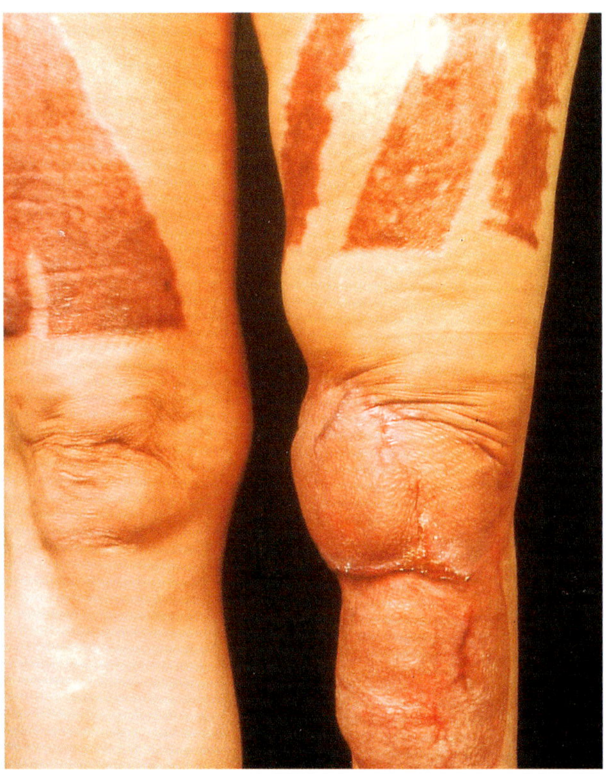

Figure 6.16c Result four months after operation

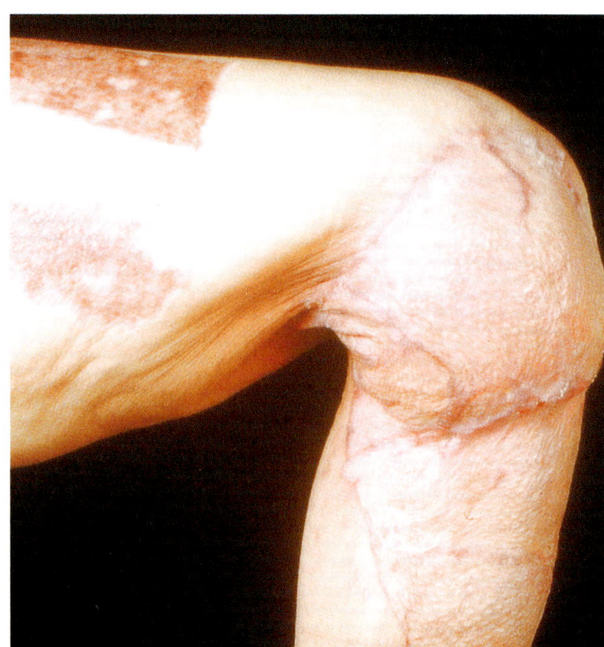

Figure 6.16d Functional result

Lateral Head of the Gastrocnemius Muscle

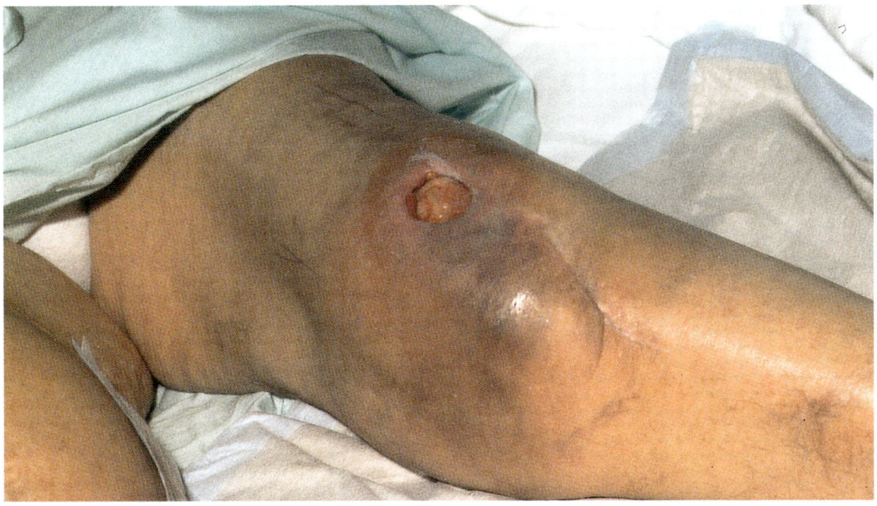

Figure 6.17a The insertion of a knee prosthesis was followed by an infected soft tissue defect on lateral side of the knee. Excision of the necrotic and inflammatory tissue and the repair planned. The preference is to use the lateral head of the gastrocnemius muscle and cover with a mesh graft because the defect is located in the lateral side of the knee.

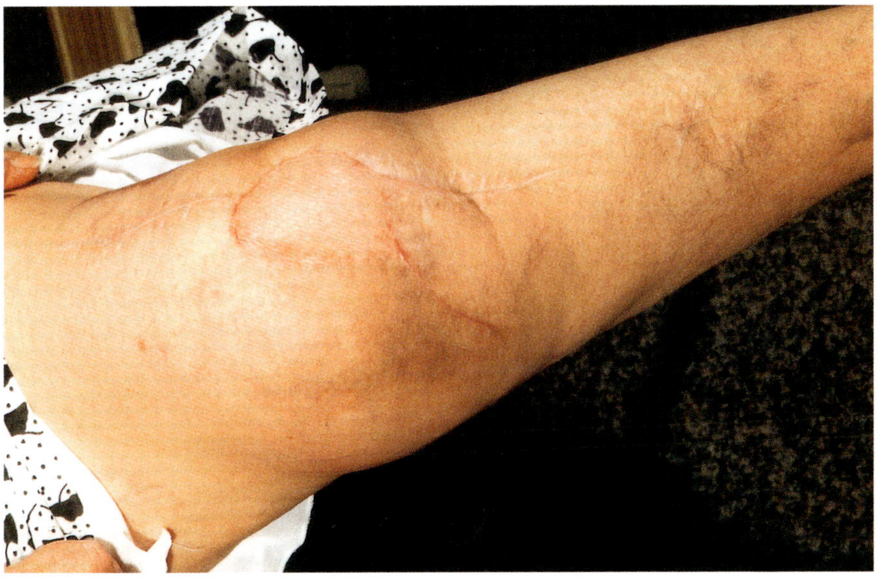

Figure 6.17b Result five months after operation. Good functional result

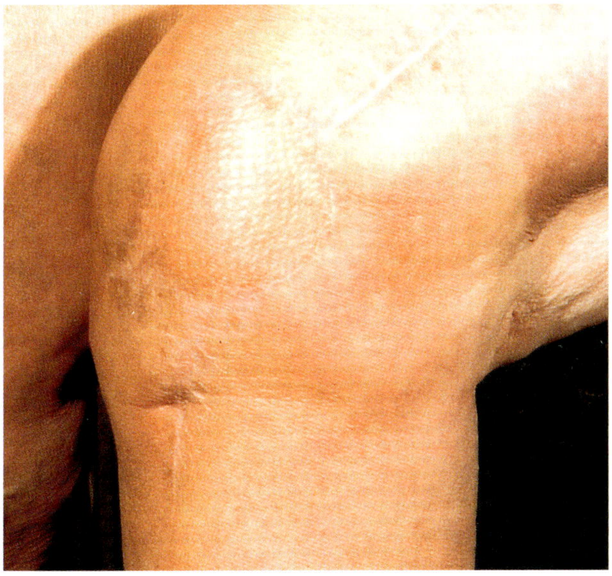

Figure 6.17c Result five months after operation

Lateral Upper Arm Flap

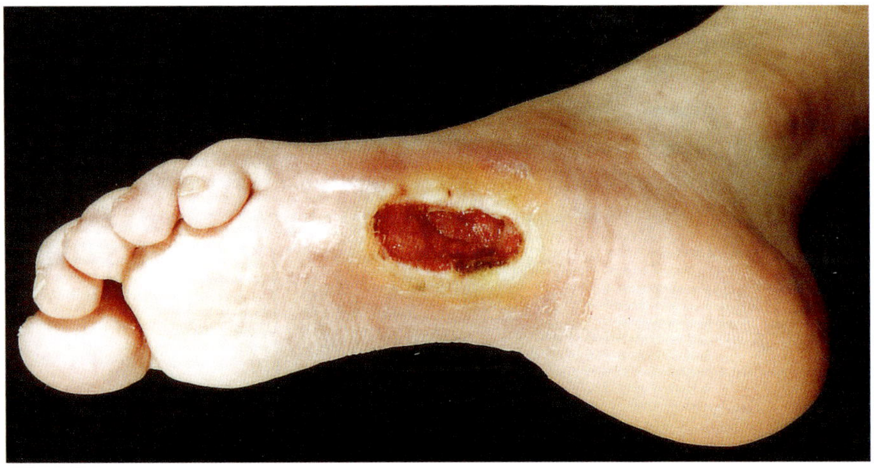

Figure 6.19a Defect in the lateral part of the left sole of the foot. The surrounding scar tissue is completely excised.

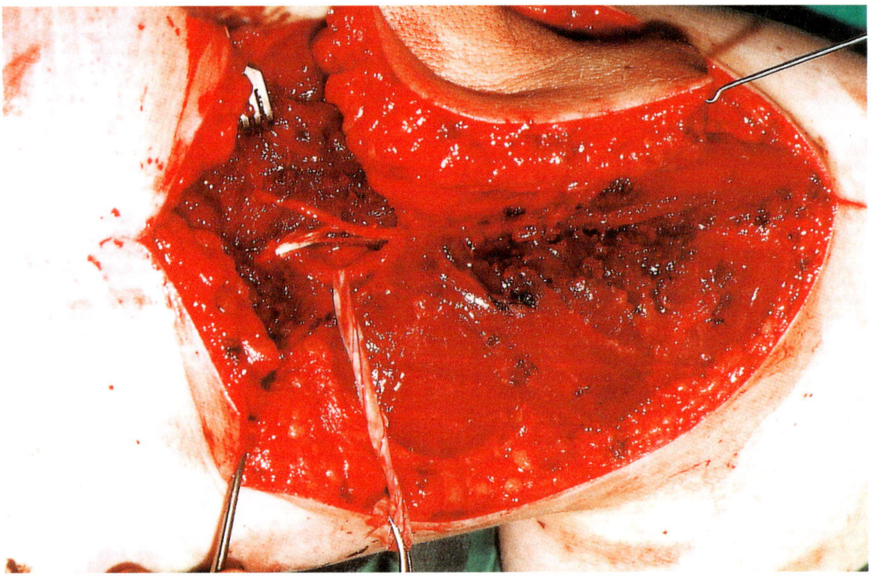

Figure 6.19b Preparation of the upper arm flap 15 × 7 cm. The flap is supplied with blood from the superior collateral artery.

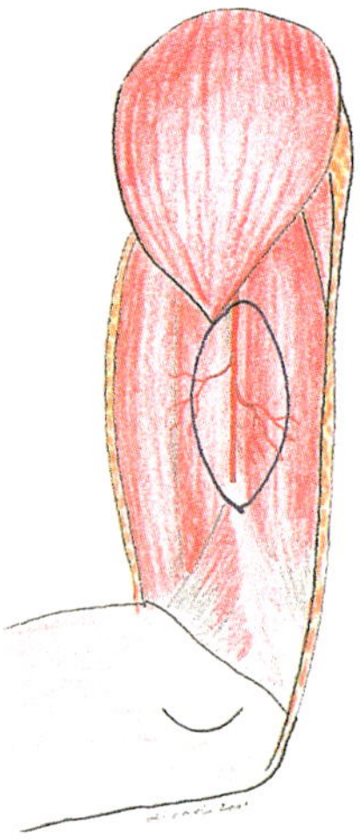

Figure 6.19c Diagram of the profunda brachii artery, which runs in the groove between the deltoid muscle and the lateral condyle.

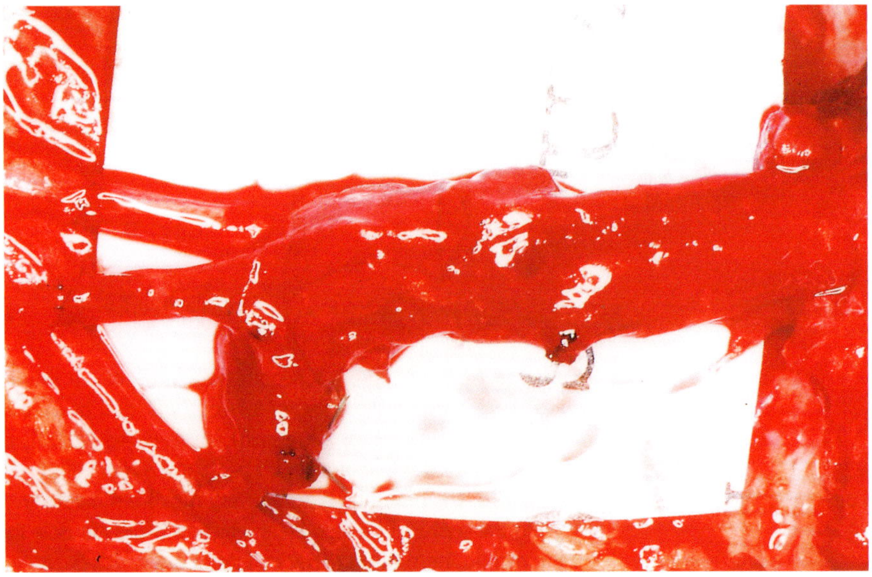

Figure 6.19d The anastomosis of dorsalis pedis artery and the superior radial collateral artery.

Lateral Head of the Gastrocnemius Muscle

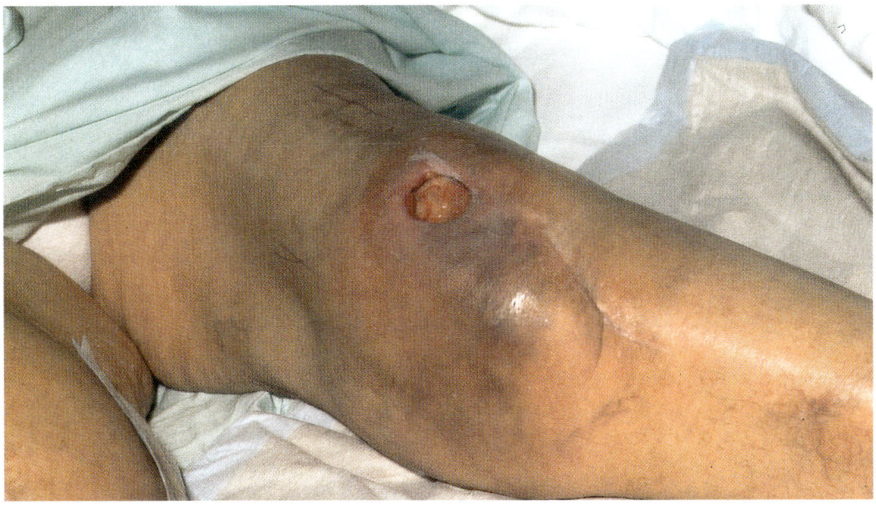

Figure 6.17a The insertion of a knee prosthesis was followed by an infected soft tissue defect on lateral side of the knee. Excision of the necrotic and inflammatory tissue and the repair planned. The preference is to use the lateral head of the gastrocnemius muscle and cover with a mesh graft because the defect is located in the lateral side of the knee.

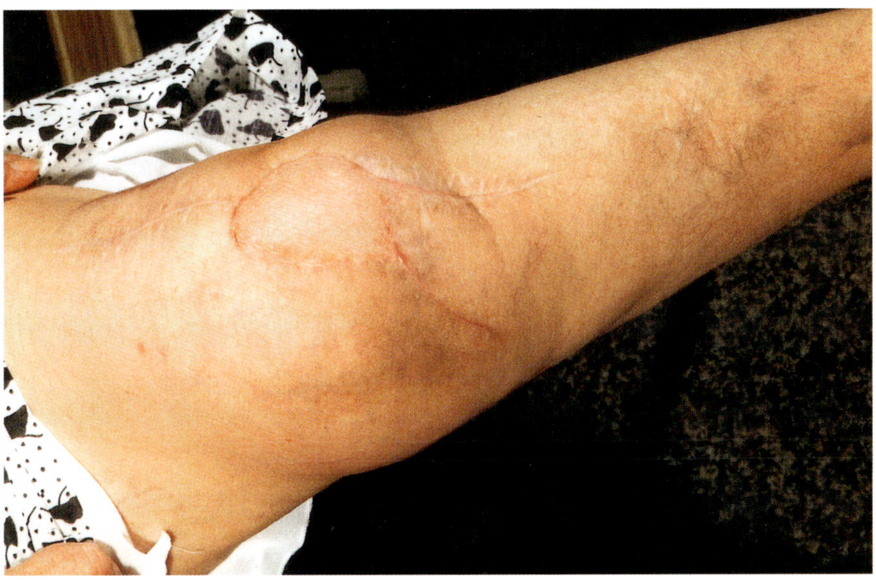

Figure 6.17b Result five months after operation. Good functional result

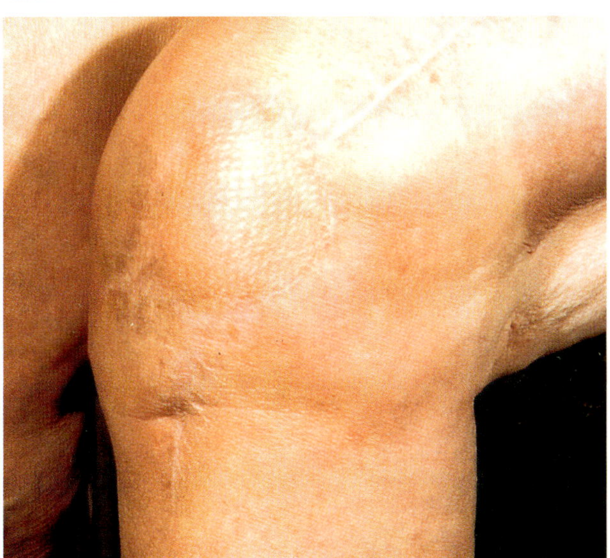

Figure 6.17c Result five months after operation

Free Flaps

a) Lateral Upper Arm Flap

The lateral upper arm flap is a fasciocutaneous free flap which is suitable for small to medium defects. Occasionally it can be used as a local flap to cover defects in the elbow and shoulder area.

Because of its proximal pedicle it can reach the axilla, but a scapula flap or a latissimus dorsi flap is preferable. The donor site of free upper arm flap is inconspicuous.

It is conventional to use the free upper arm flap to cover of defects of the hand, foot and lower leg. It is also suitable for the head region. The blood supply is derived from the collateral radial superior artery, which arises from the profunda brachii artery. The pedicle of the flap is dissected down to the profunda brachii artery. Care must be taken not to damage the radial nerve. The pedicle is about 7 to 8 cm long and the artery has a diameter of about 2 to 2.5 mm.

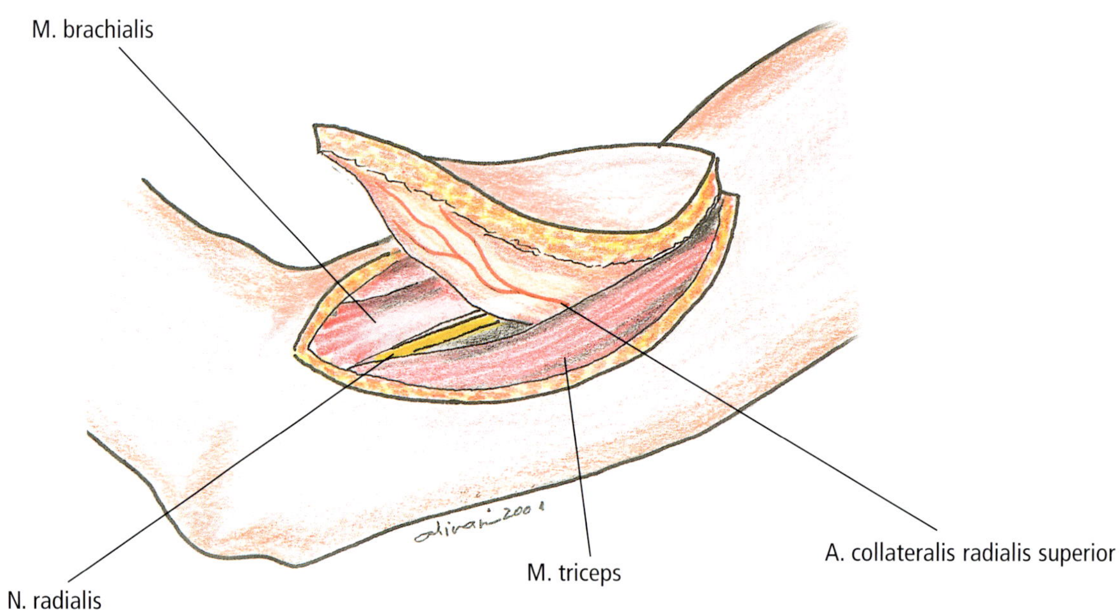

Figure 6.18a The blood supply of the lateral upper arm flap is derived from the superior radialis collateral artery, which is situated between the triceps and the brachialis muscles. The radial nerve is located directly underneath!

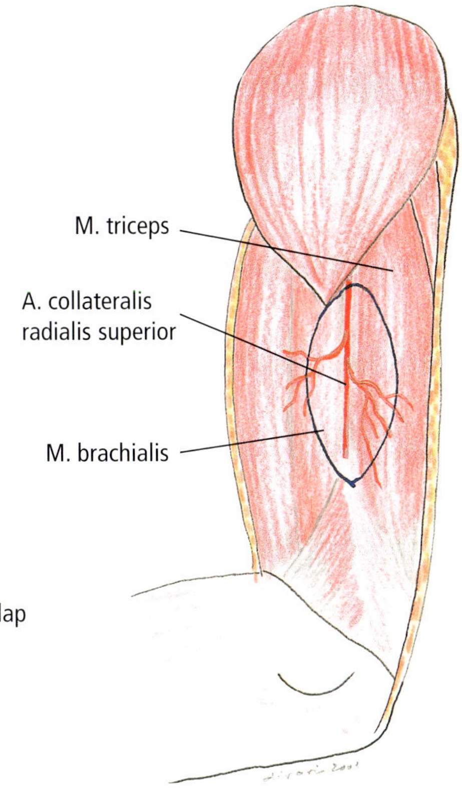

Figure 6.18b The blood supply of the lateral upper arm flap is derived from the superior radial collateral artery, which arises from the profunda brachii artery.

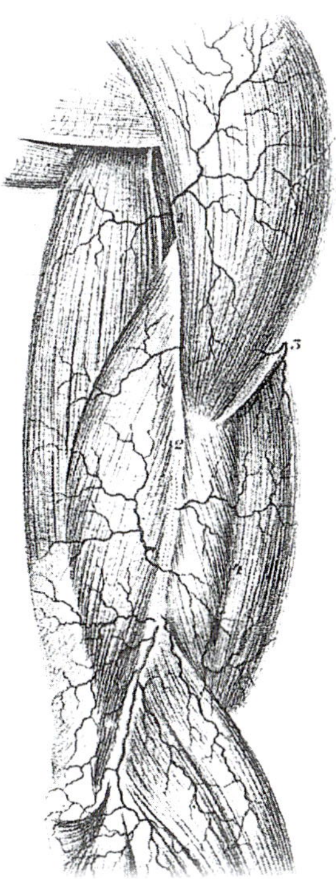

Figure 6.18c Carl Manchot from Leipzig described the arteries of the skin in 1889.

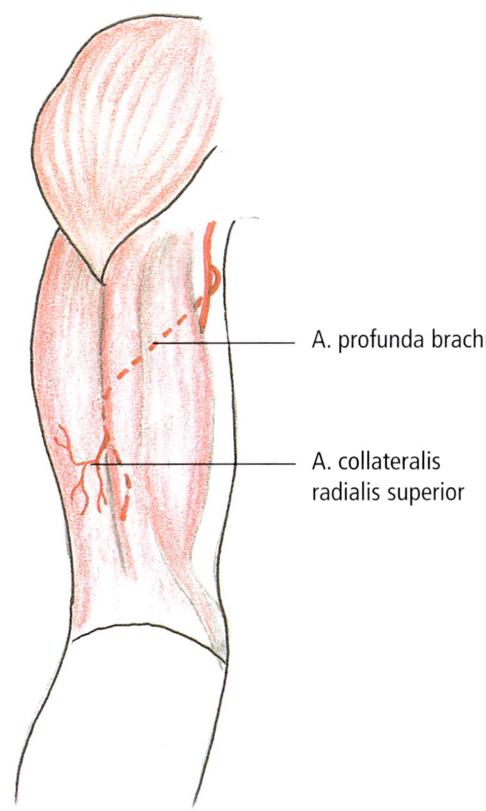

Figure 6.18d The profunda brachii artery runs from medially following the septum between brachialis and triceps muscle in distal direction. Here the superior collateral artery arises.

Lateral Upper Arm Flap

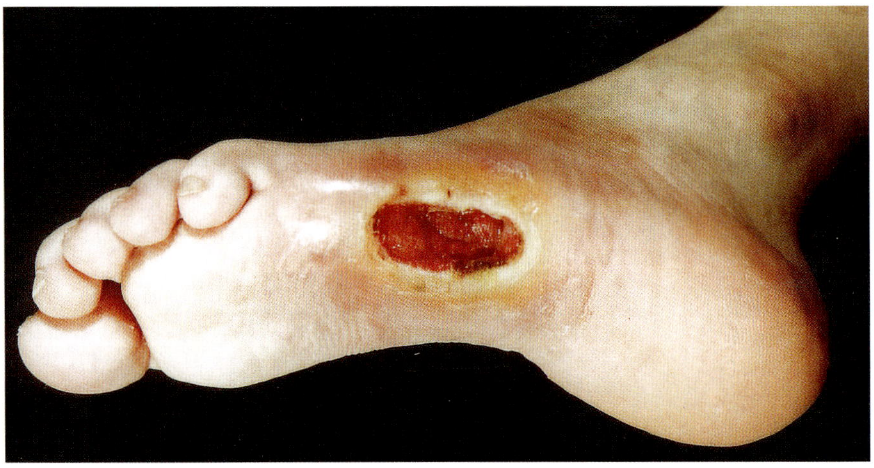

Figure 6.19a Defect in the lateral part of the left sole of the foot. The surrounding scar tissue is completely excised.

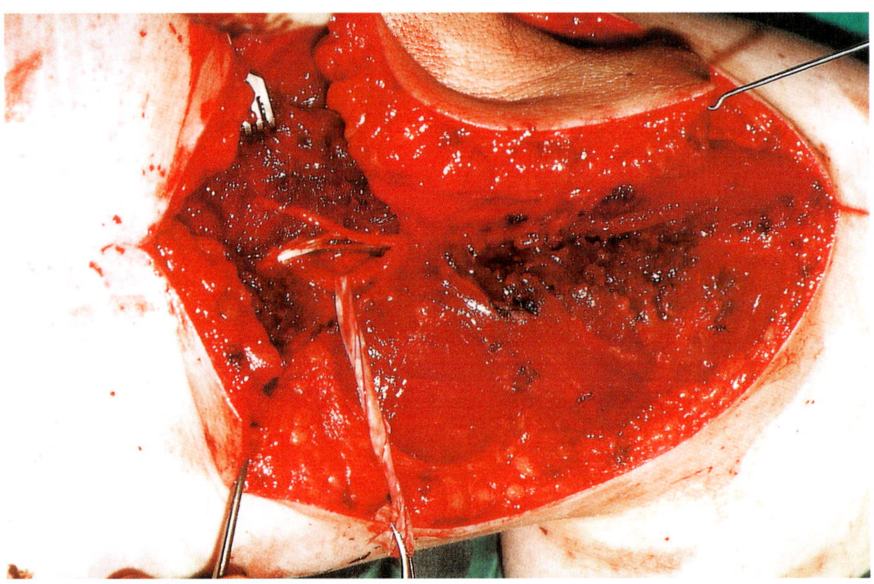

Figure 6.19b Preparation of the upper arm flap 15 × 7 cm. The flap is supplied with blood from the superior collateral artery.

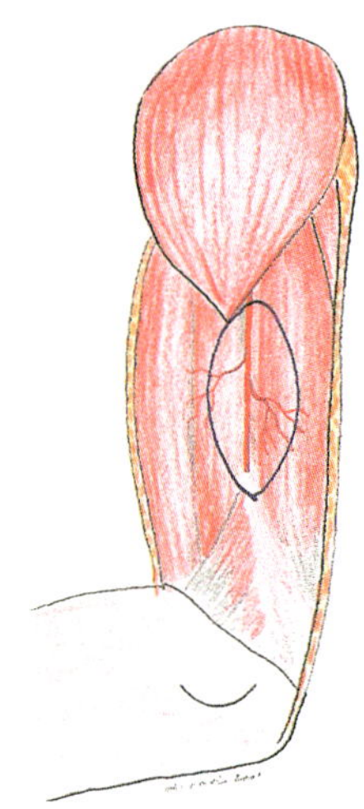

Figure 6.19c Diagram of the profunda brachii artery, which runs in the groove between the deltoid muscle and the lateral condyle.

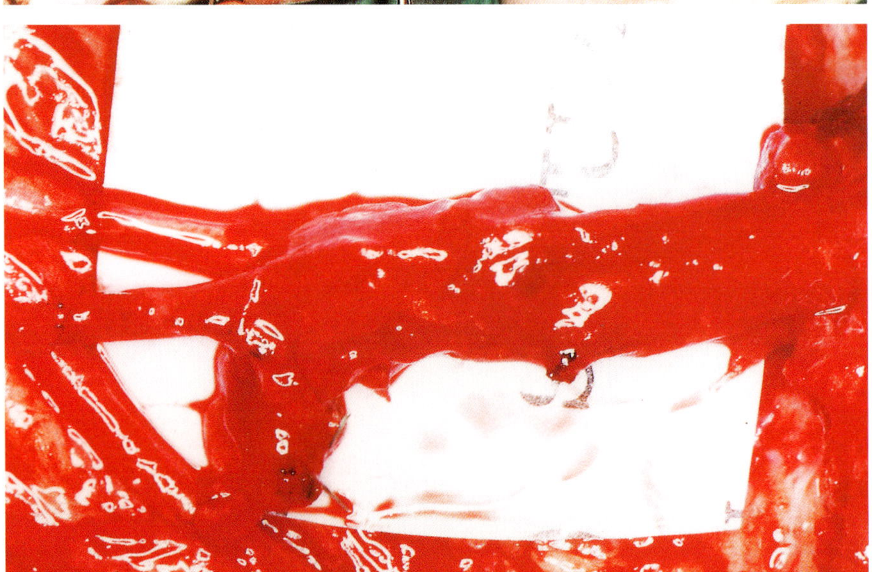

Figure 6.19d The anastomosis of dorsalis pedis artery and the superior radial collateral artery.

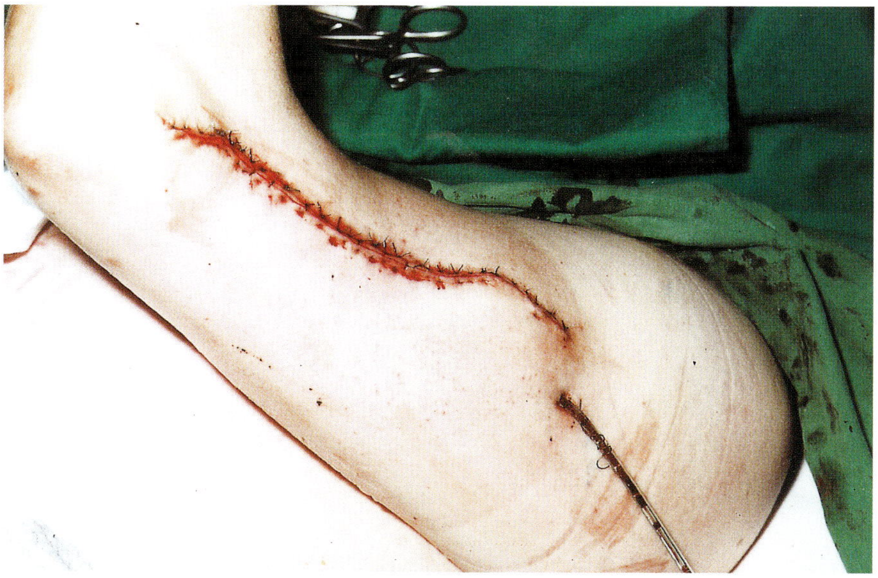

Figure 6.19e The donor site is closed primarily. The width of the flap depends on the diameter of the upper arm and averages 6 to 8 cm.

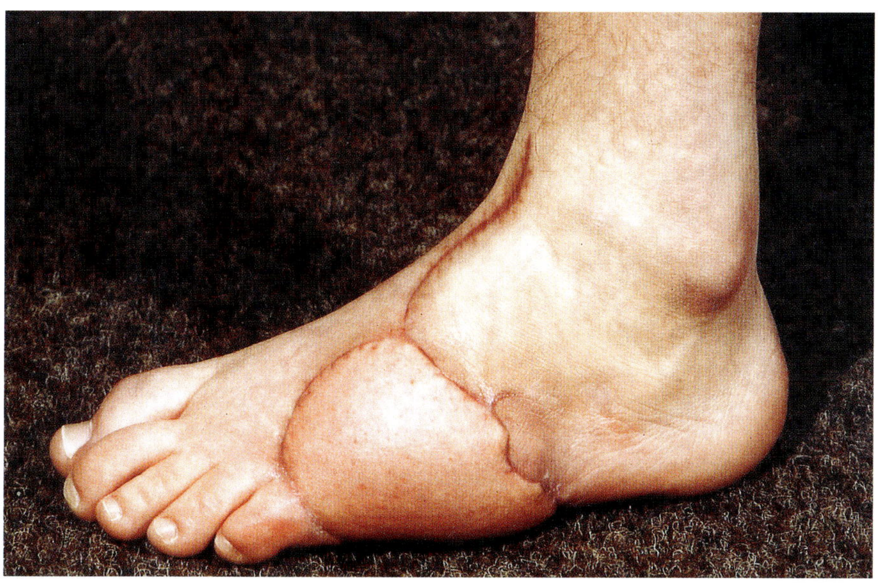

Figure 6.19f Result four months postoperatively: The foot can bear full weight

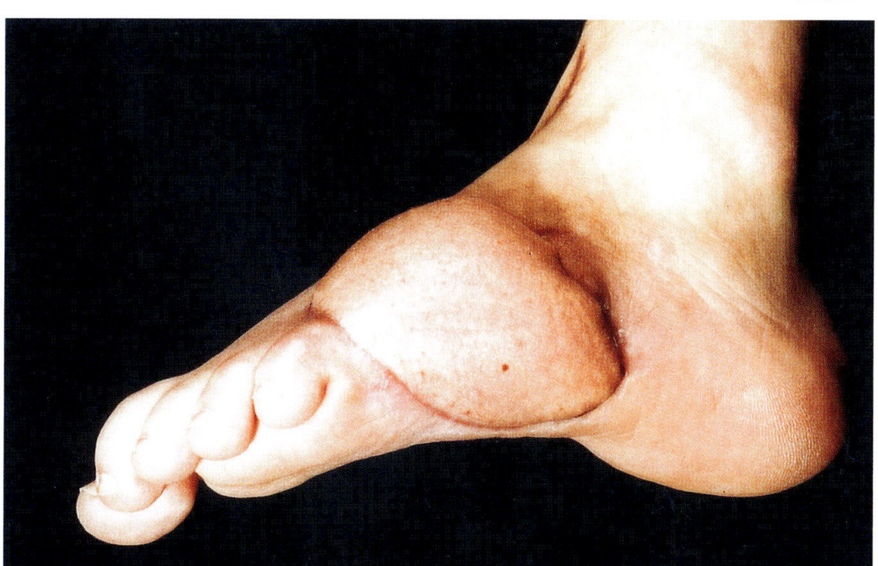

Figure 6.19g Result four months postoperatively

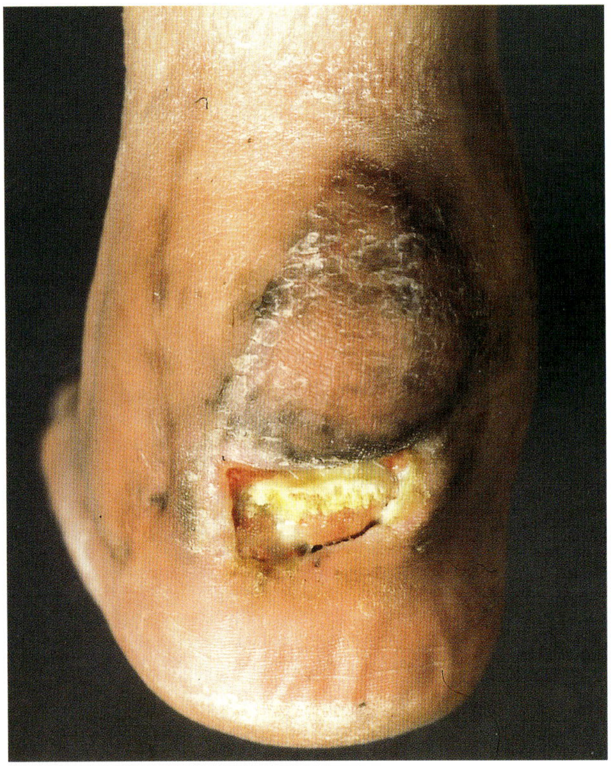

Figure 6.20a Post-traumatic chronic defect of the heel

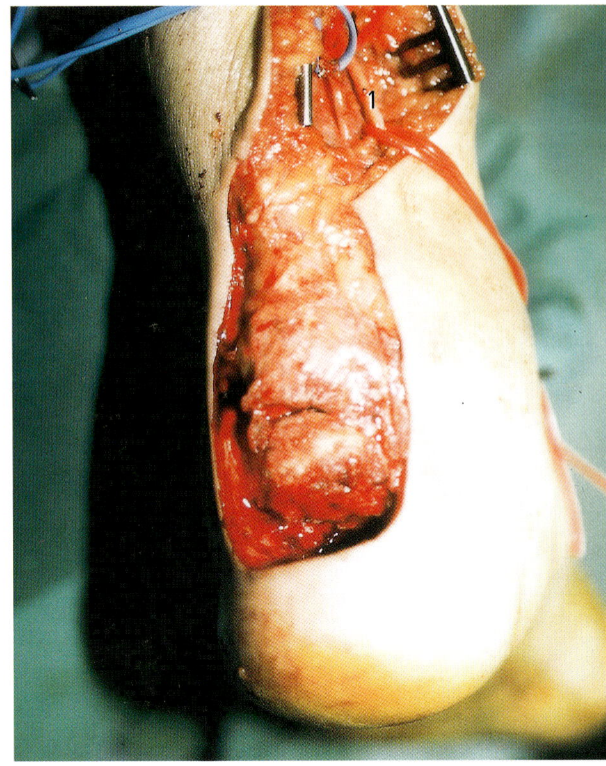

Figure 6.20b Radical debridement and preparation of the posterior tibial vessels (1)

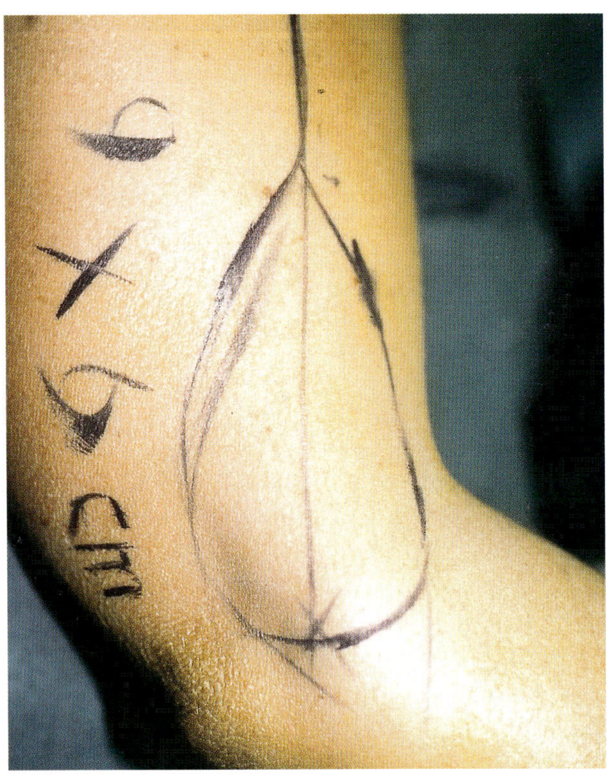

Figure 6.20c Planning of a lateral upper arm flap

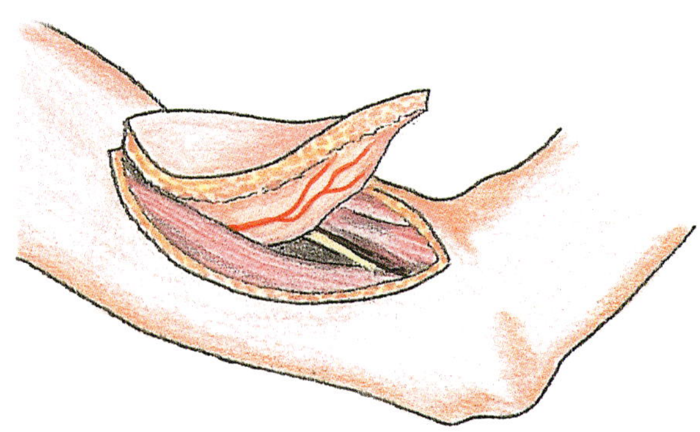

Figure 6.20d Raising of a lateral upper arm flap. **Mind:** Radial nerve. The pedicle of the flap and the radials nerve are located between the brachialis and the triceps muscles.

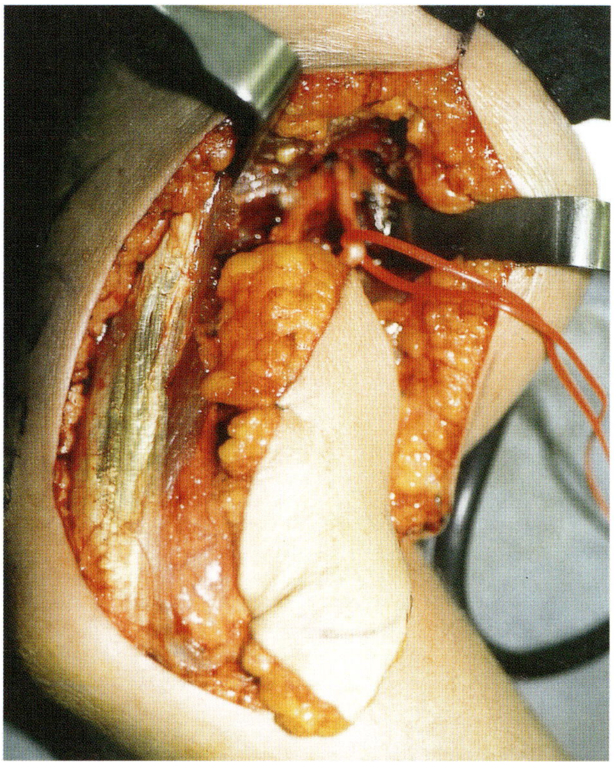

Figure 6.20e The lateral upper arm flap is mobilized and the pedicle (superior radial collateral) is prepared and anastomosed end to side with the posterior tibial artery and end-to-end with a comitant vein.

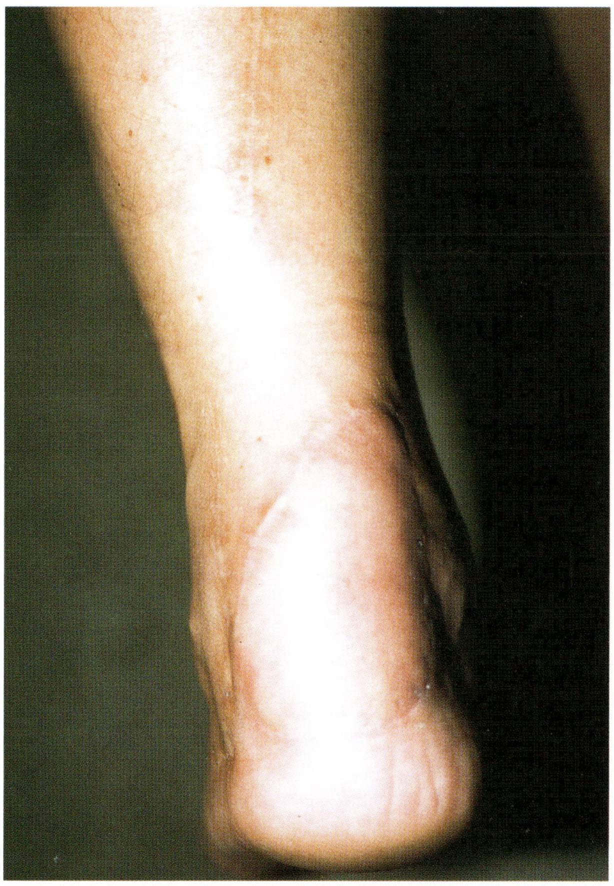

Figure 6.20f Result two years after the operation

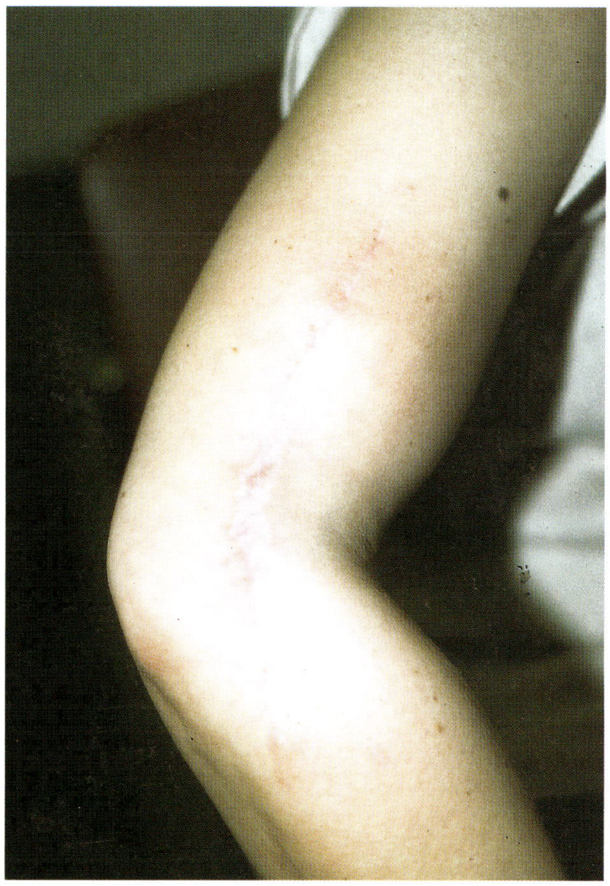

Figure 6.20g The donor site is tolerable

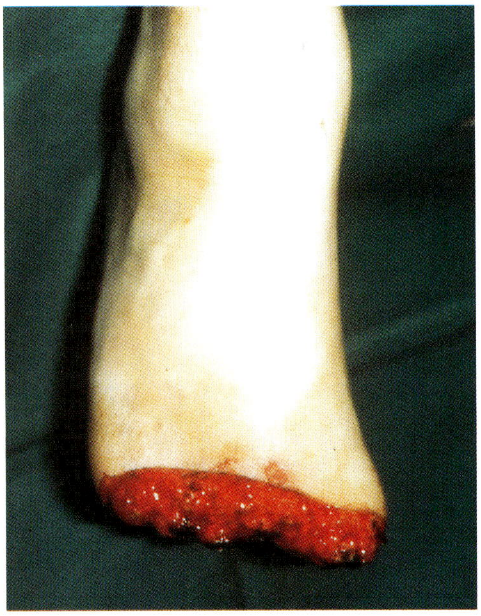

Figure 6.21a Traumatic forefoot amputation

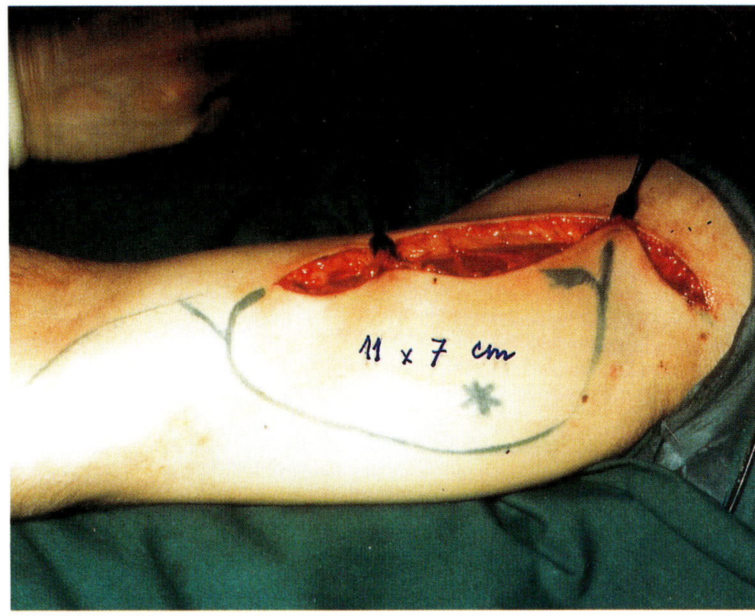

Figure 6.21b Preparation of the lateral upper arm flap with a size of 11 × 7 cm. This is about the maximum size which allows primary closure of the defect.

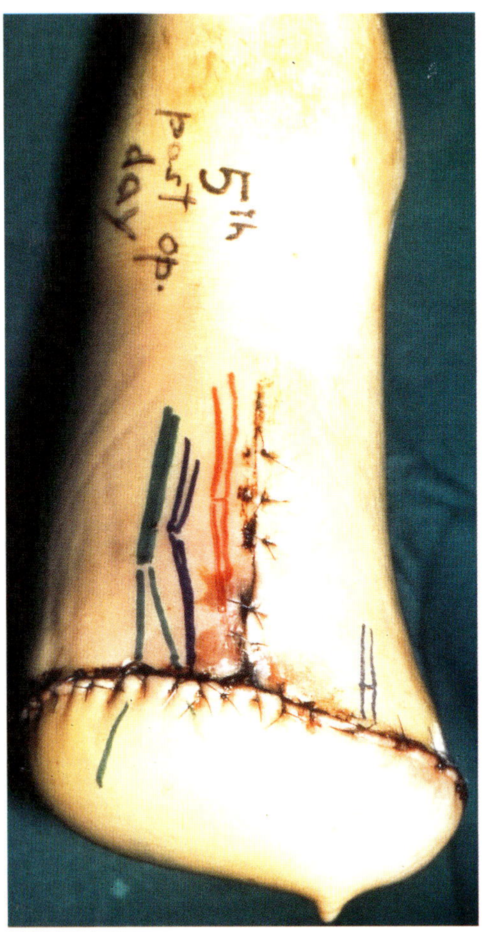

◁ **Figure 6.21c** Anastomosis of the superior radial collateral artery and vein with the dorsalis pedis artery and vein.

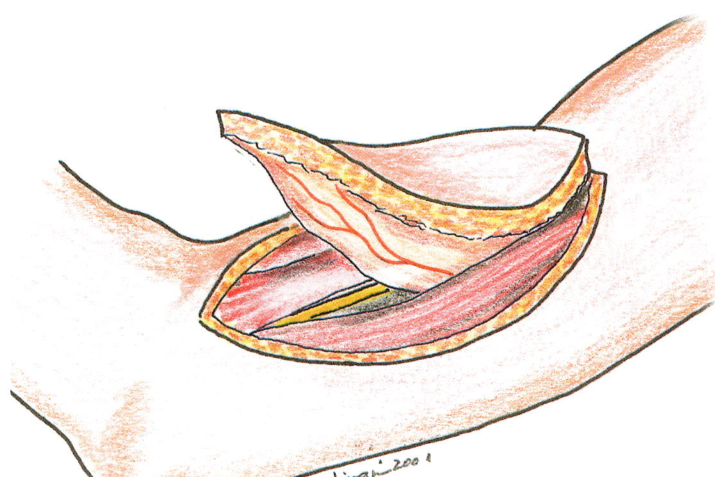

Figure 6.21d Situation five days after operation

b) Radial Forearm Flap

The radial forearm flap is a versatile and safe fasciocutaneous flap which is suitable as free flap but also as a distally pedicled flap for the covering defects in the hand. It is also convenient as proximal pedicled flap for the closure of defects in the elbow region.

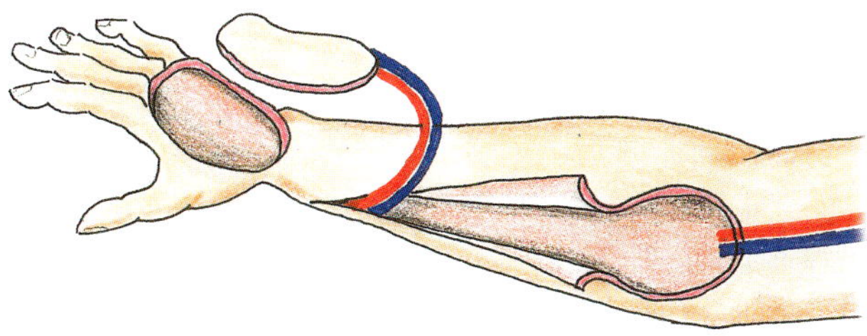

Figure 6.22a Distally pedicled radial flap

Anatomy

The flap is supplied by the radial artery, which has many small branches which perforate the antebrachial fascia and nourish the skin. In the distal third of the forearm there are more perforators than in the proximal third. The venous drainage is by the comitant veins and the subcutaneous veins.

The cutaneous antebrachial nerve supplies the rather moderate sensation.

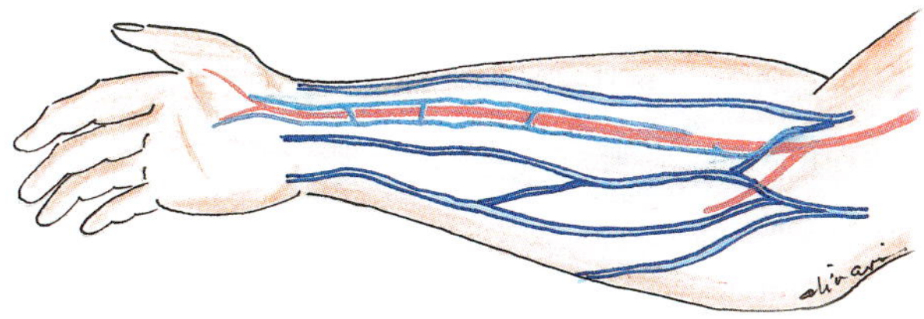

Figure 6.22b Blood supply of the radial flap

Indications

As a proximally pedicled flap it is suitable for wound closures in the elbow region. As a distally pedicled flap it is excellent for defects in the hand and fingers (CF. pages 46–47).
As a free flap commonly used in the following locations:

- Head and neck region
- Foreleg and foot region
- Genital region
- In combination with the radial bone as composite transfer or with adjacent tendons for reconstruction of the Achilles tendon.

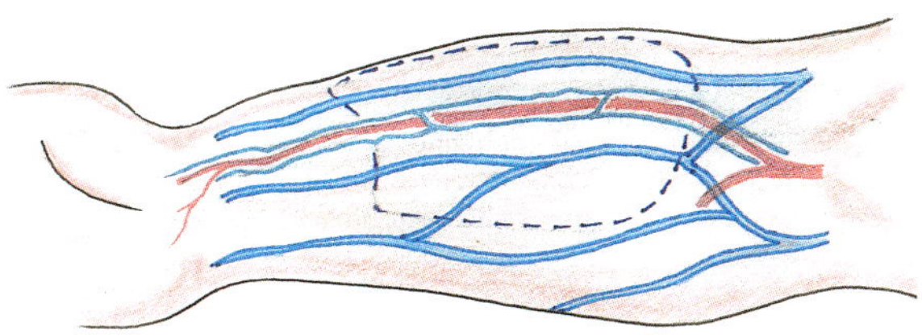

Figure 6.22c Planning of the free radial forearm flap

Disadvantage

Sacrification of the radial artery can lead to mild weakness of the forearm and hand muscles. Additionally patients with cold intolerance of the hand area are reported. Furthermore there can be poor appearance of the donor site.

Radial Flap With Vessel Interposition

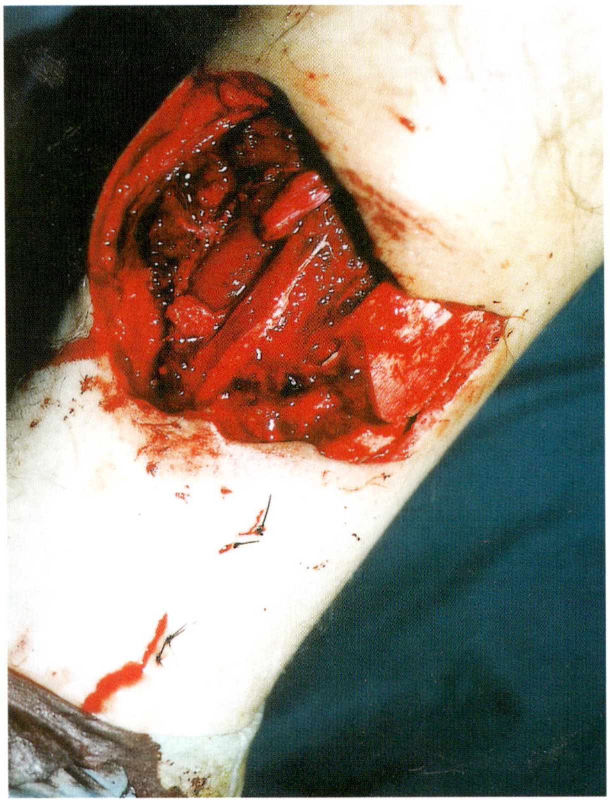

Figure 6.23a Traumatic defect of the left lower leg. Fracture of the tibia, defect of the posterior tibial artery of 12 cm length, defect of the tibialis posterior muscle and the flexor digitorum longus muscle.

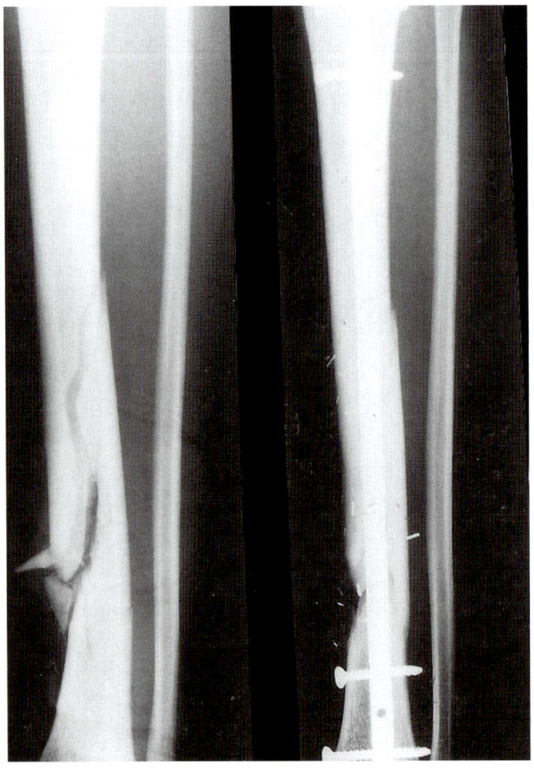

Figure 6.23b First the tibial fracture is stabilized by nail plate

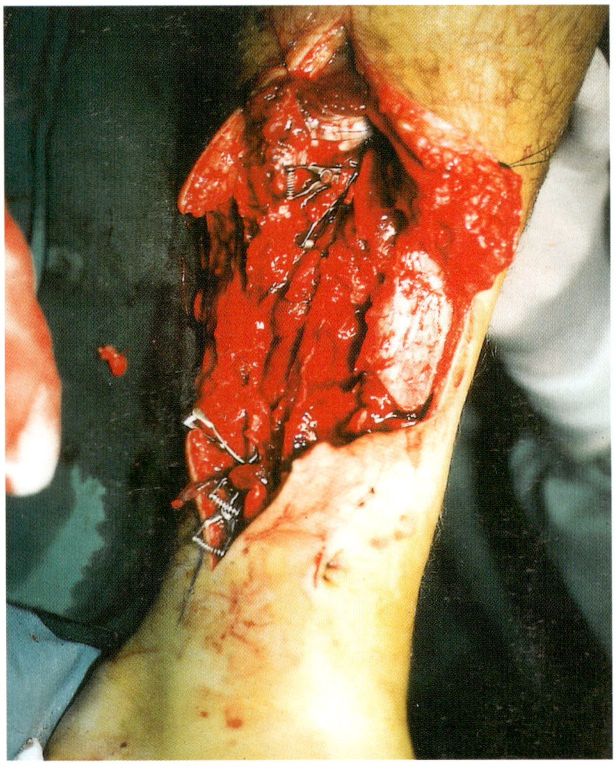

Figure 6.23c Debridement of the wound. Both ends posterior tibial artery are prepared for an artery interposition.

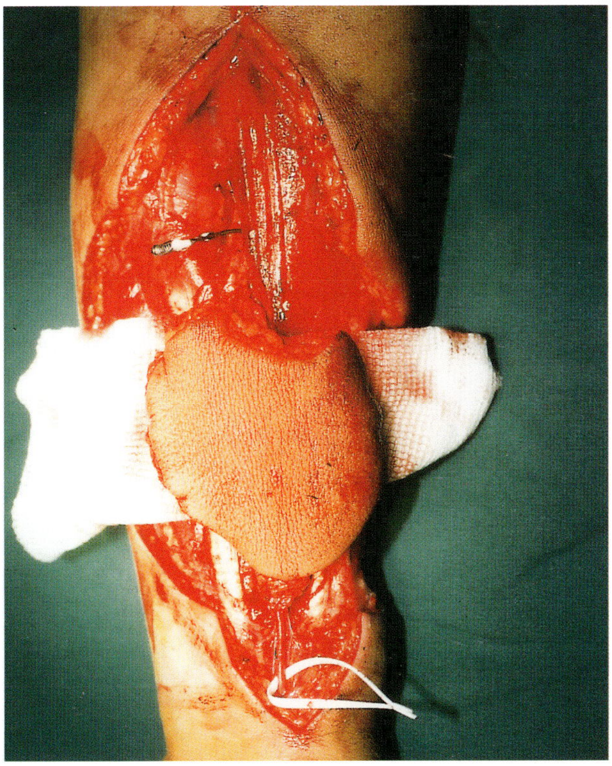

Figure 6.23d A radial forearm flap with two long pedicles, proximal and distal is mobilized.

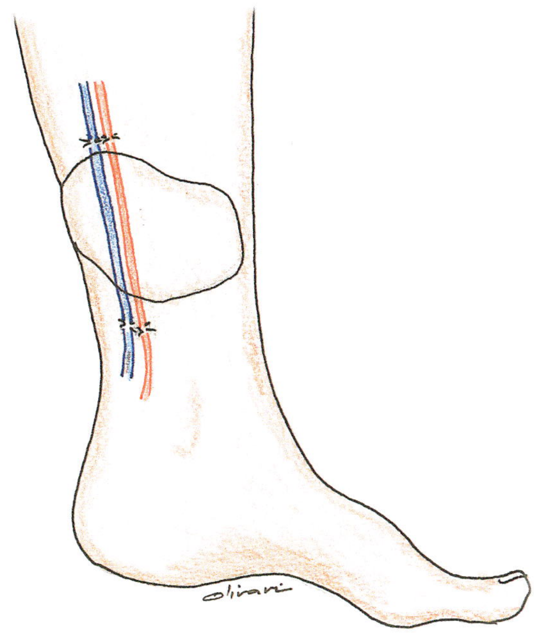

Figure 6.23e The radial forearm flap is used to cover the defect. The radial artery functions as vessel interposition, so that there is continuity of the posterior tibial artery.

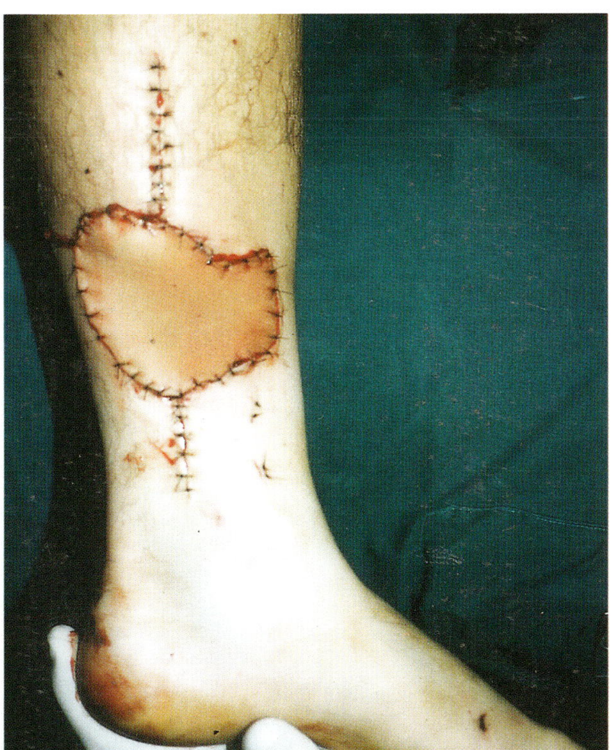

Figure 6.23f Result at the end of the operation

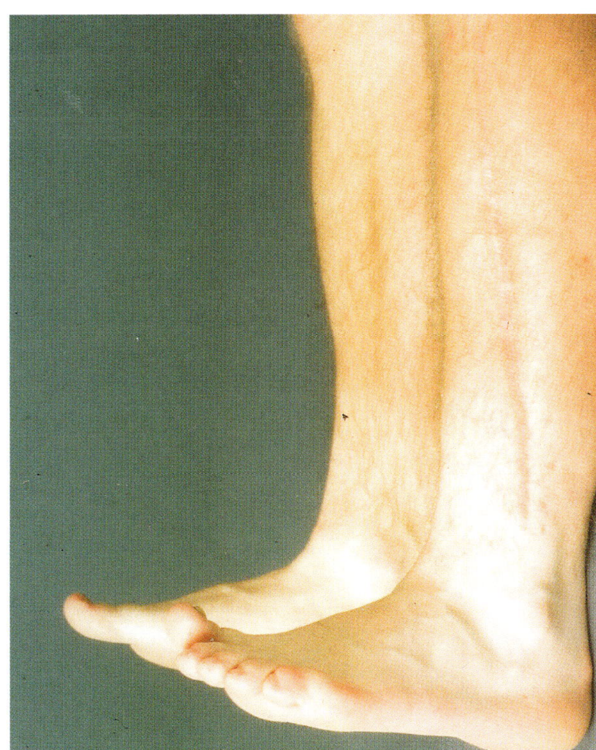

Figure 6.23g Functional result one year after the operation

Radial Forearm Flap

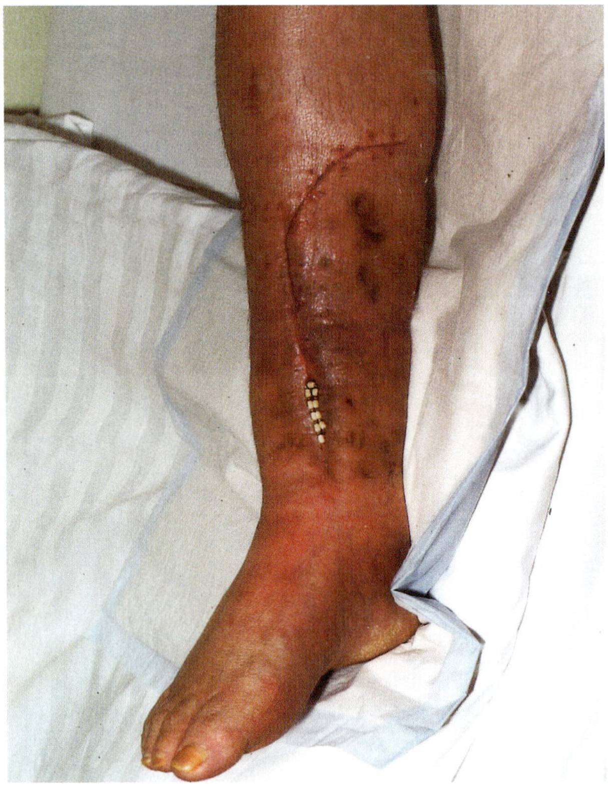

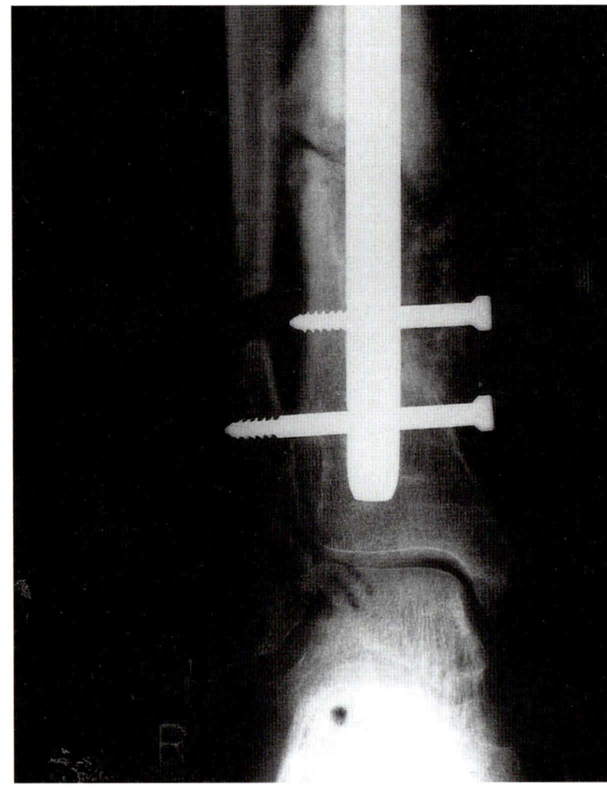

Figure 6.24a, b This was the situation following internal fixation of a complex right lower leg fracture. Infection has been present for three months. The metal is exposed and there is osteomyelitis of tibia.

Operation: Radical debridement of the soft tissue. The bone of the tibia is tangentially removed with a chisel until punctate bleeding is visible.

A radial forearm flap has been mobilized from the left forearm and attached end to side with the tibial artery. So the arterial supply of the foot is not affected.

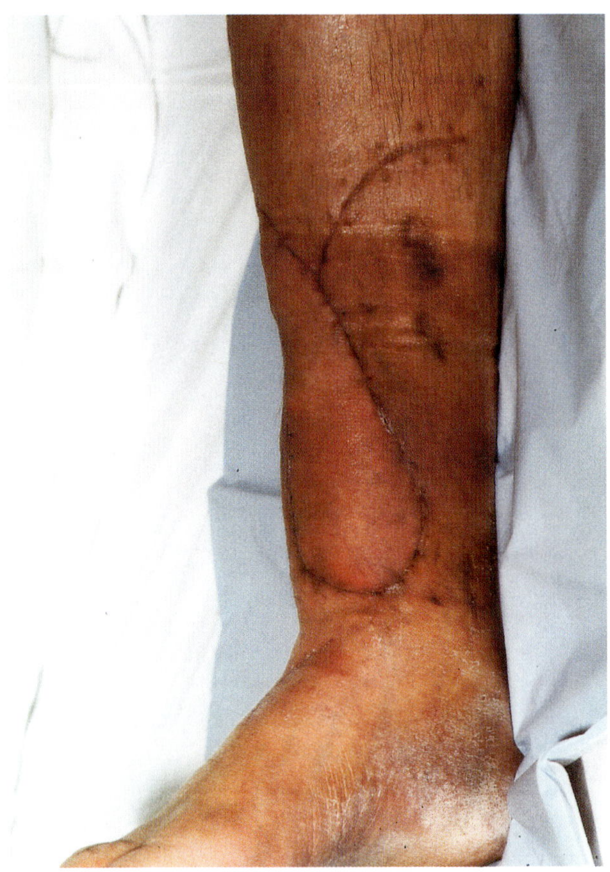

Figure 6.24c Result four weeks after the operation

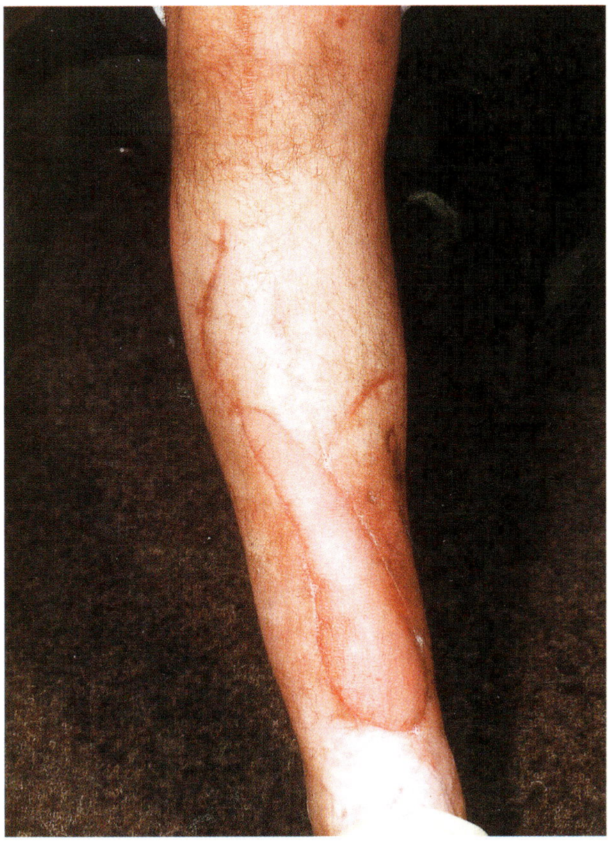

Figure 6.24d Result seven months after operation

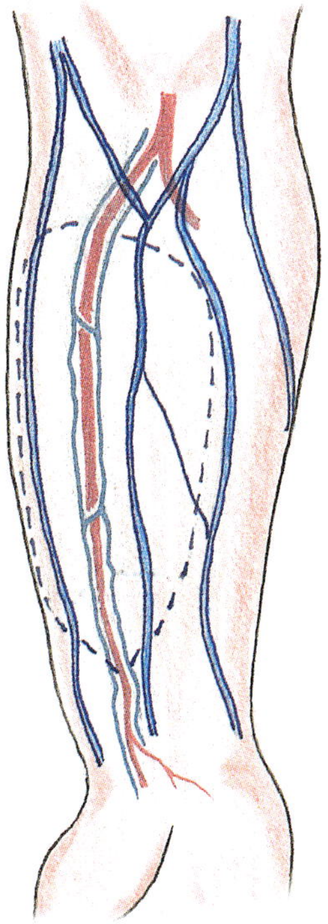

Figure 6.24e Radial forearm flap

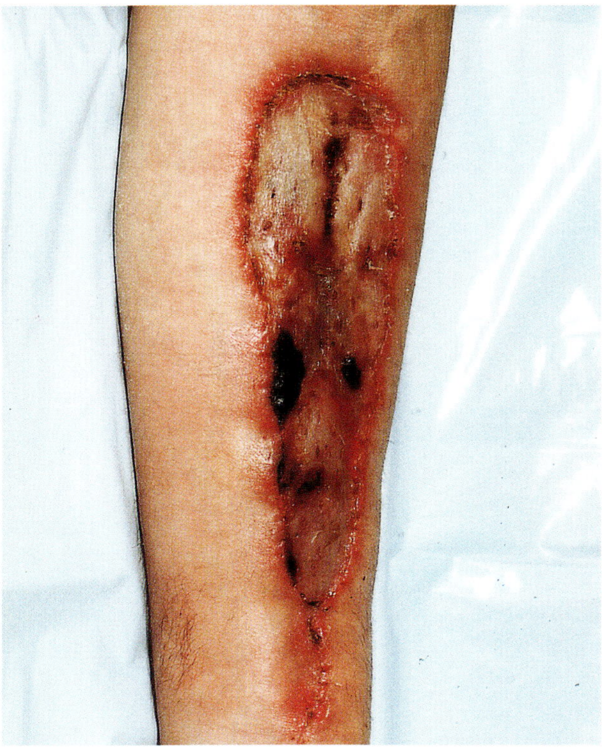

Figure 6.24f Donor site four weeks postoperatively with only partly healed split-thickness skin graft.

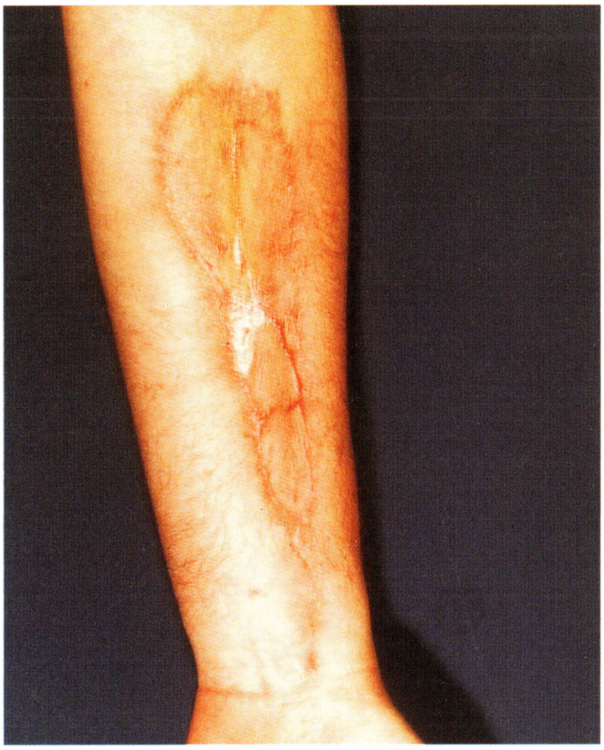

Figure 6.24g Donor site seven months postoperatively

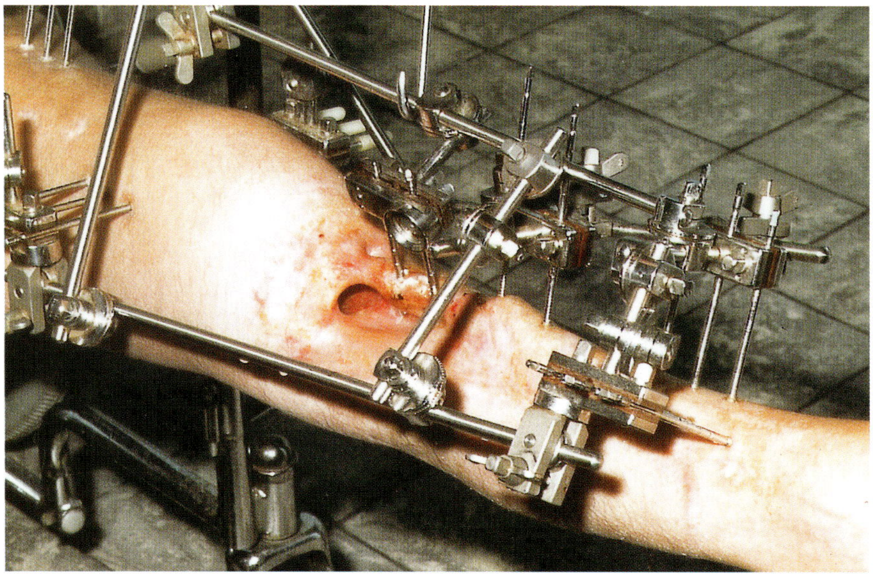

Figure 6.25a The situation at six months after a compound fracture of the lower leg and external fixation.

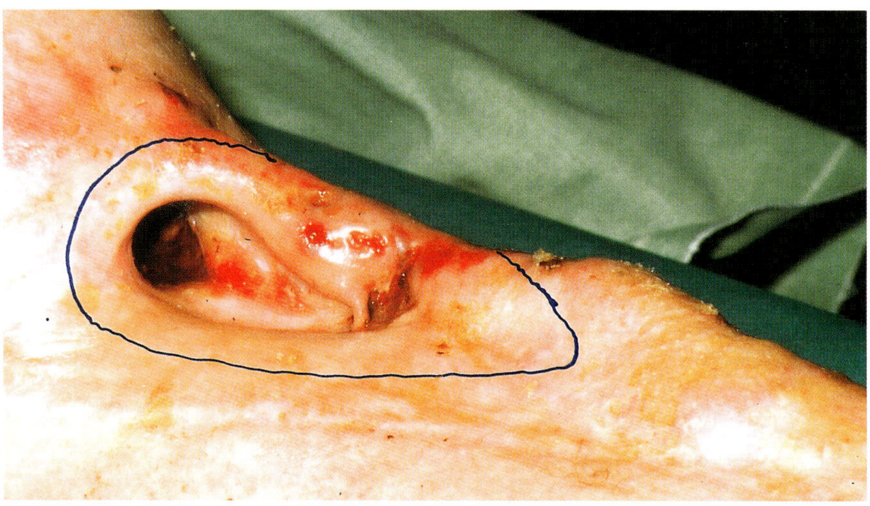

Figure 6.25b Osteomyelitis of the tibial head and loss of soft tissue. The infected and scared tissue is resected. The bone is debrided down to healthy tissue and all the osteomyelitis removed. Inlay of a gentamycin chain.

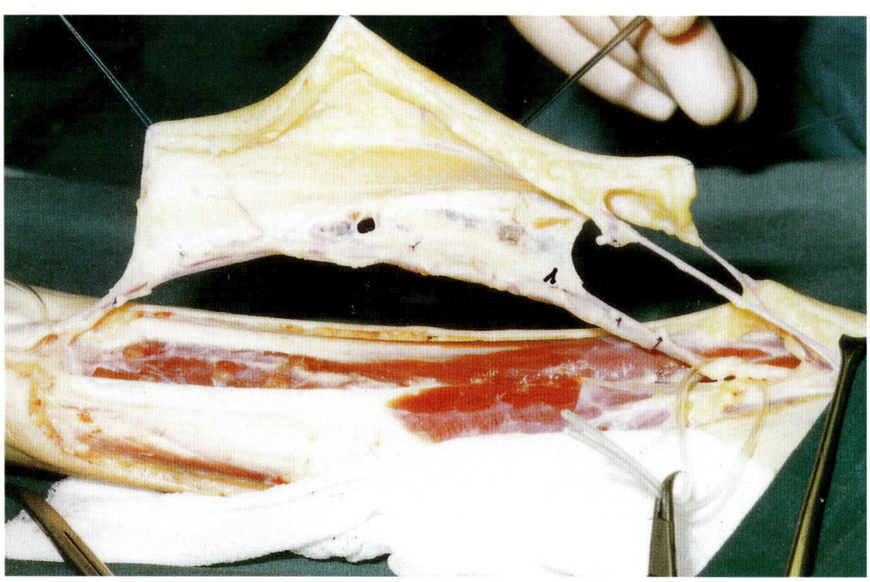

Figure 6.25c A fasciocutaneous radial flap is mobilized. The radial artery (1) is clearly visible.

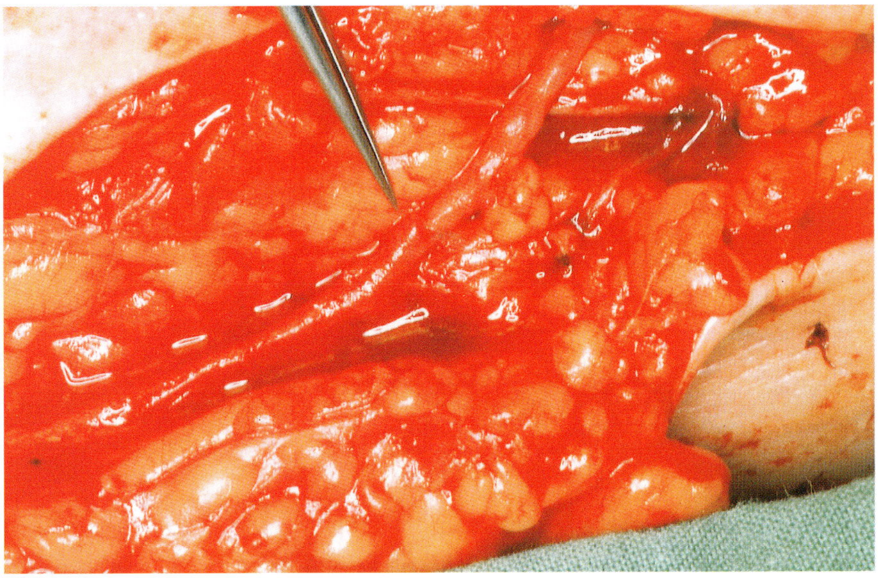

Figure 6.25d Anastomosis between radial artery and anterior tibial artery

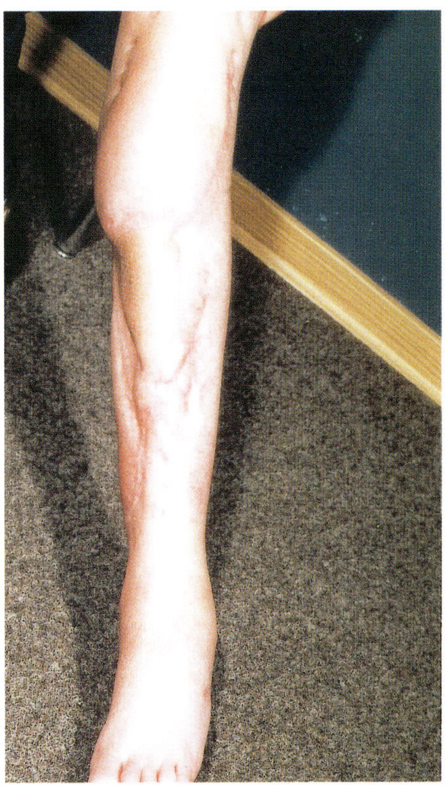

Figure 6.25e Result seven months after operation: The leg is fully weight bearing

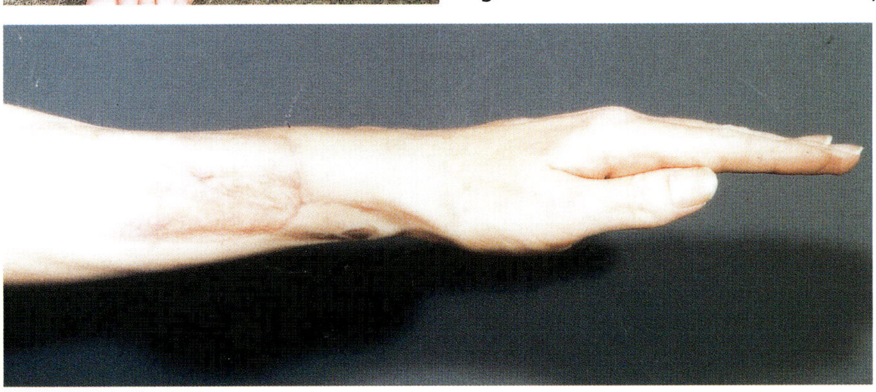

Figure 6.25f The donor site seven months postoperatively

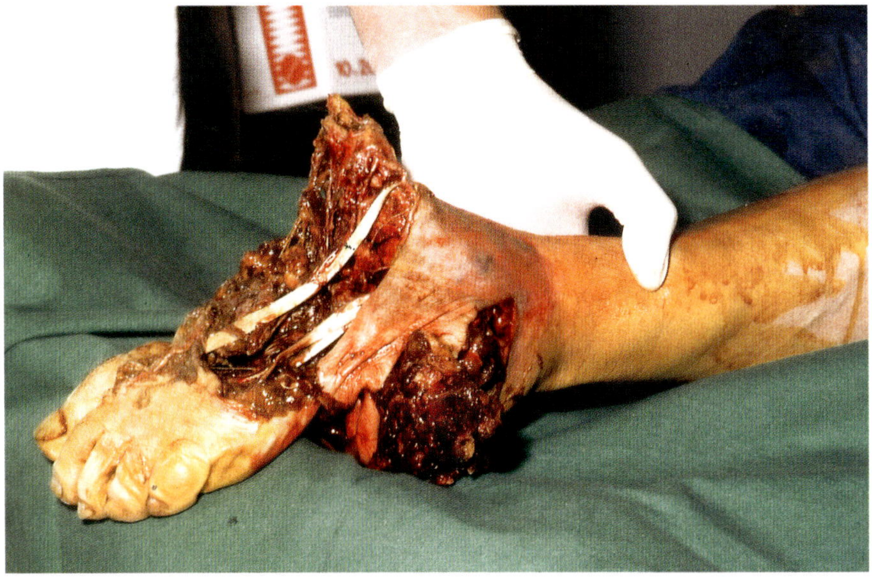

Figure 6.26a Crush injury of the left foot. There is so much damage to the foot structures that a replantation is impossible. The aim is to form a convenient stump.

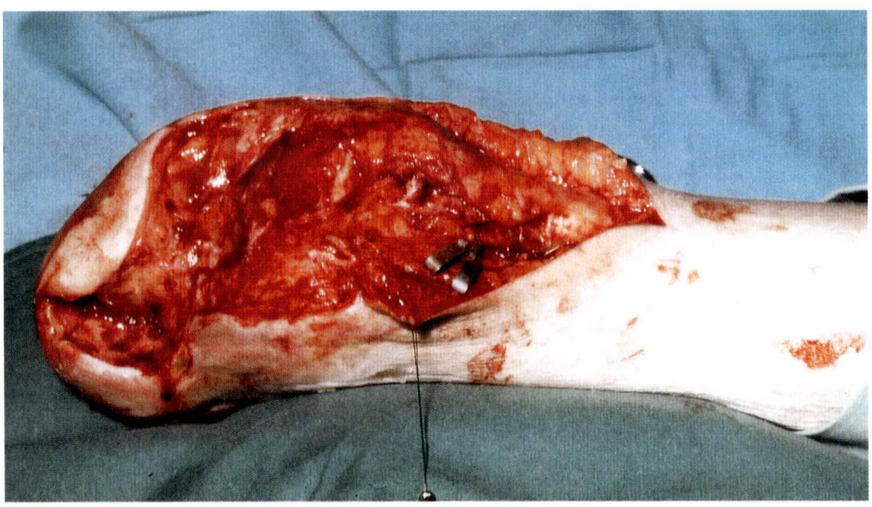

Figure 6.26b After excising the crushed necrotic tissue (which is not easy job) the calcaneum and proximal part of foot are successfully covered with the remaining well vascularized tissue. There remains a large defect on the ventral surface. The anterior tibial artery is prepared for the anastomosis.

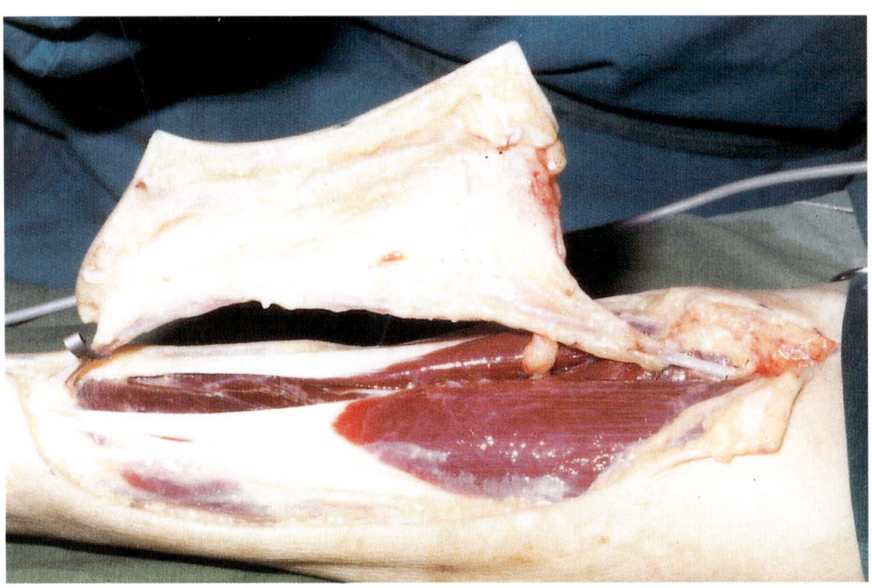

Figure 6.26c Mobilizing of a fasciocutaneous radial forearm flap

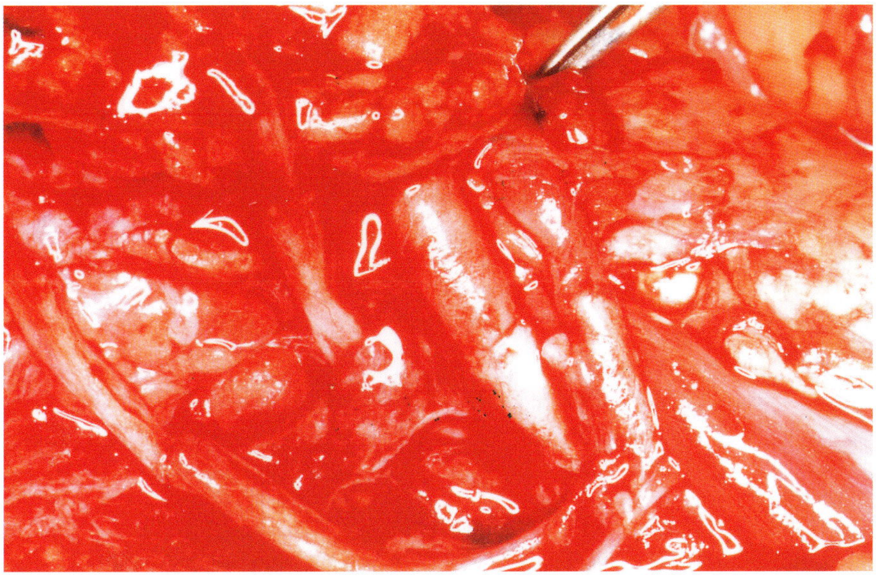

Figure 6.26d The radial vessels are anastomosed with anterior tibial artery and vein, end-to-end.

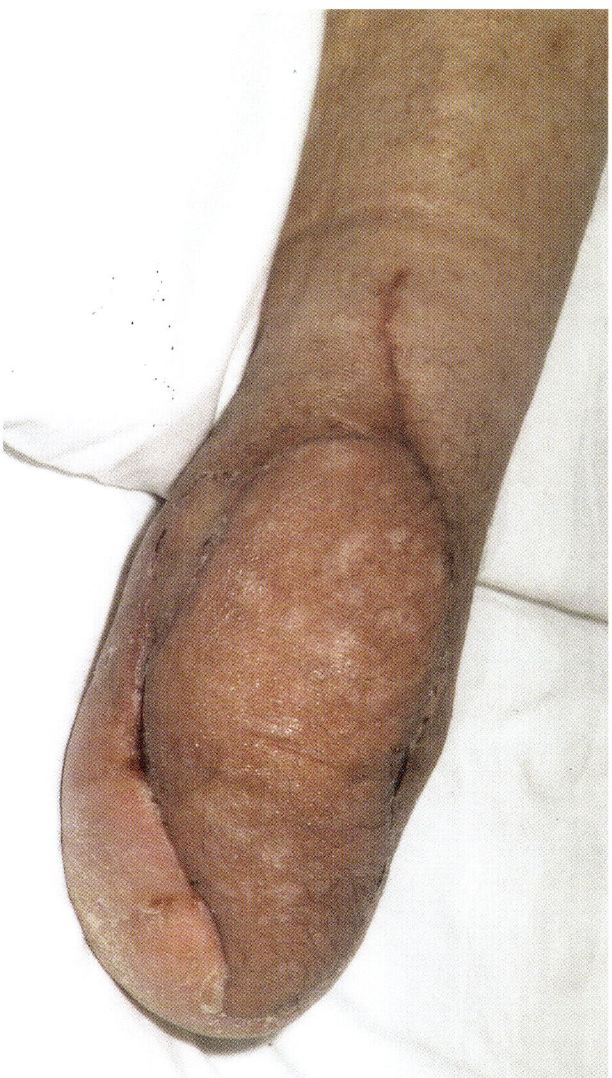

Figure 6.26e Result after three months post trauma. One can see the weight bearing stump. This case shows the importance of a definitive primarily therapy in such a severe injury.
The primarily transplantation shortened the period of healing and prevented secondary infection. In patients with multiple injuries transplantation should delayed to second operation, but whenever possible within one week.

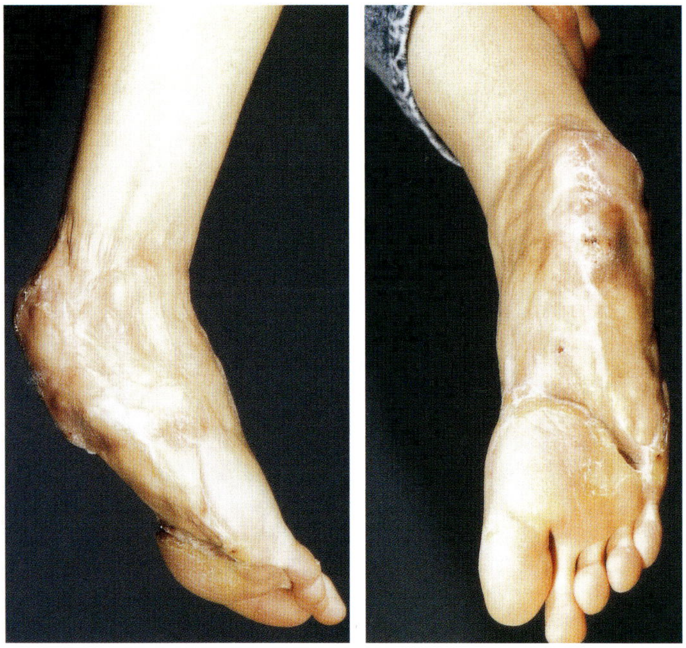

Figure 6.27a Extensive soft tissue defect of the right heel and sole of the foot (trauma one year ago). Initially the wound was covered with mesh graft but this did not provide a surface that could stand up to weight bearing.

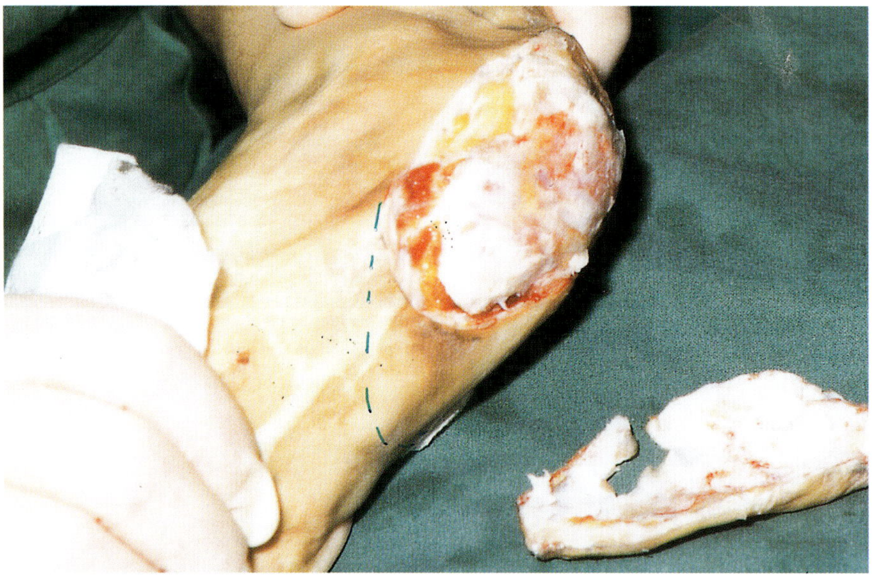

Figure 6.27b Excision of the scar area at the heel and sole of the foot

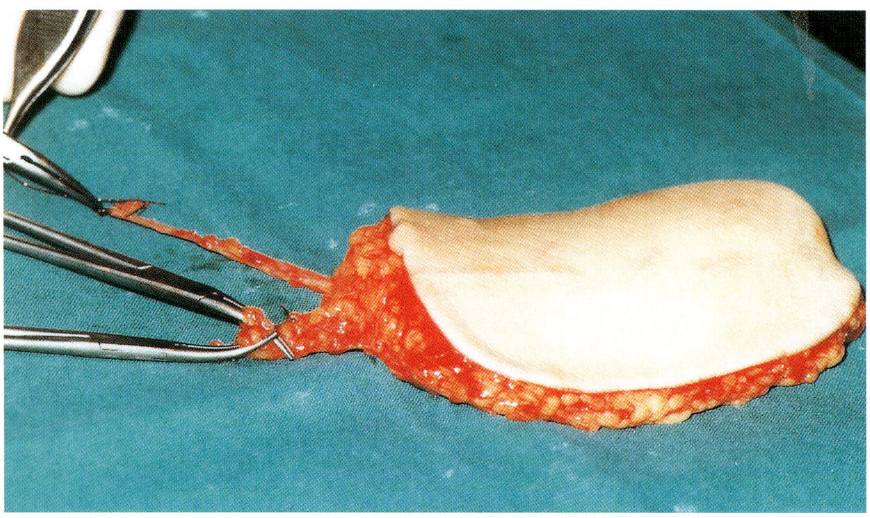

Figure 6.27c A fasciocutaneous radial forearm flap is prepared for transplantation

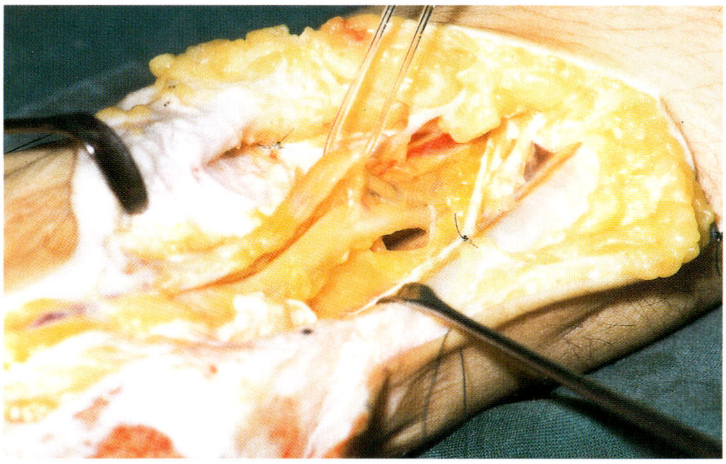

Figure 6.27d Posterior tibial artery and vein are prepared for the anastomosis

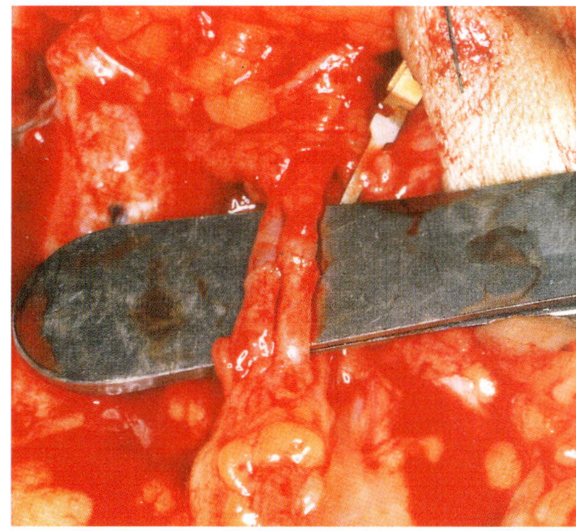

Figure 6.27e An end-to-end anastomosis is performed because the distal part of the posterior tibial artery was destroyed.

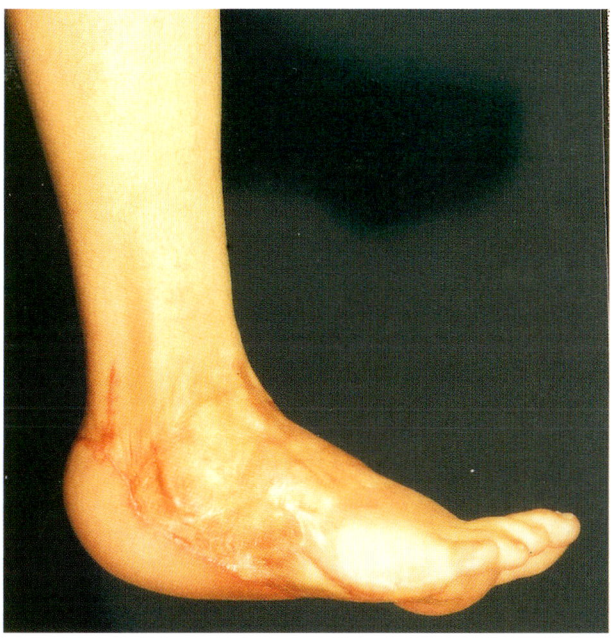

Figure 6.27f The foot is weight bearing seven months postoperatively

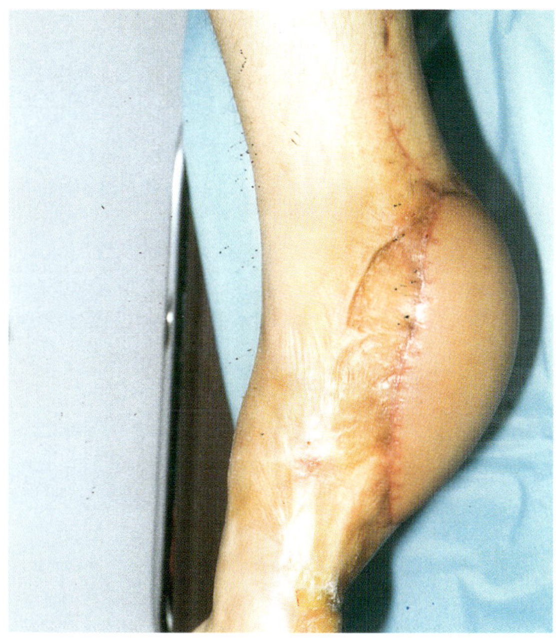

Figure 6.27g Good functional result

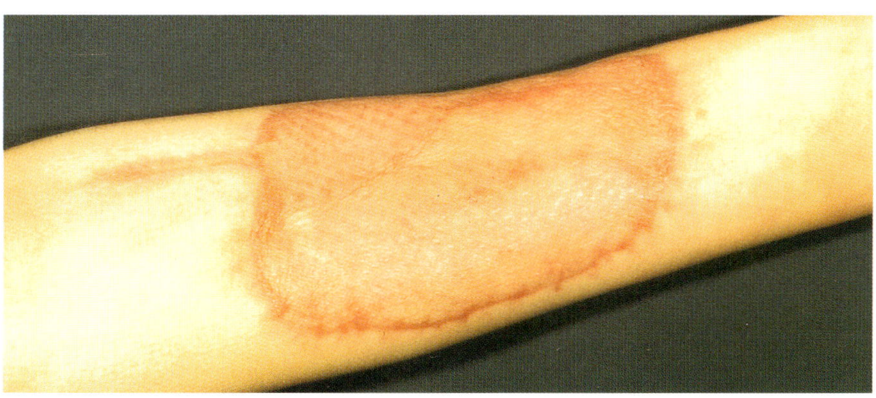

Figure 6.27h The secondary defect of the forearm seven months postoperatively

Radialis Flap With Tendon Interposition

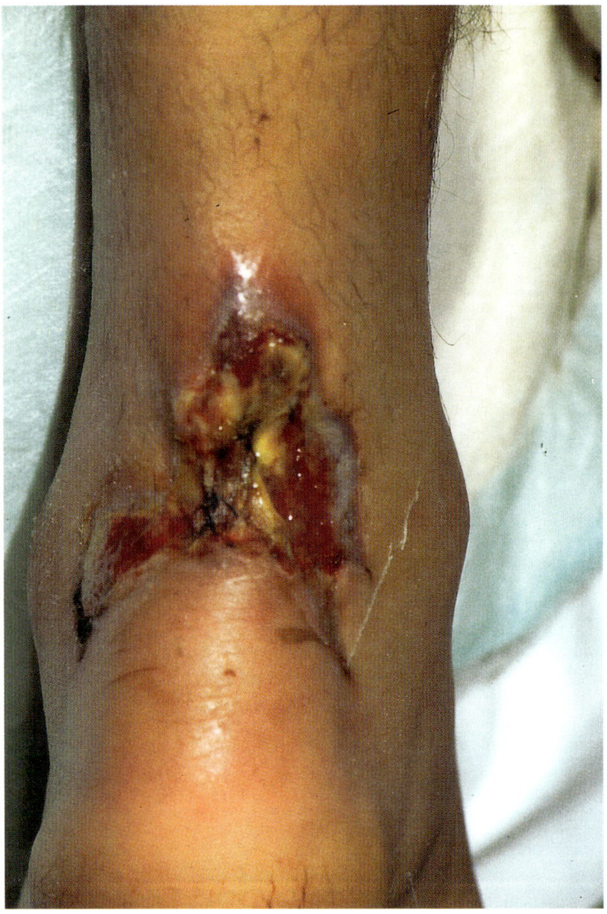

Figure 6.28a Injury of the left heel with defect of the Achilles tendon

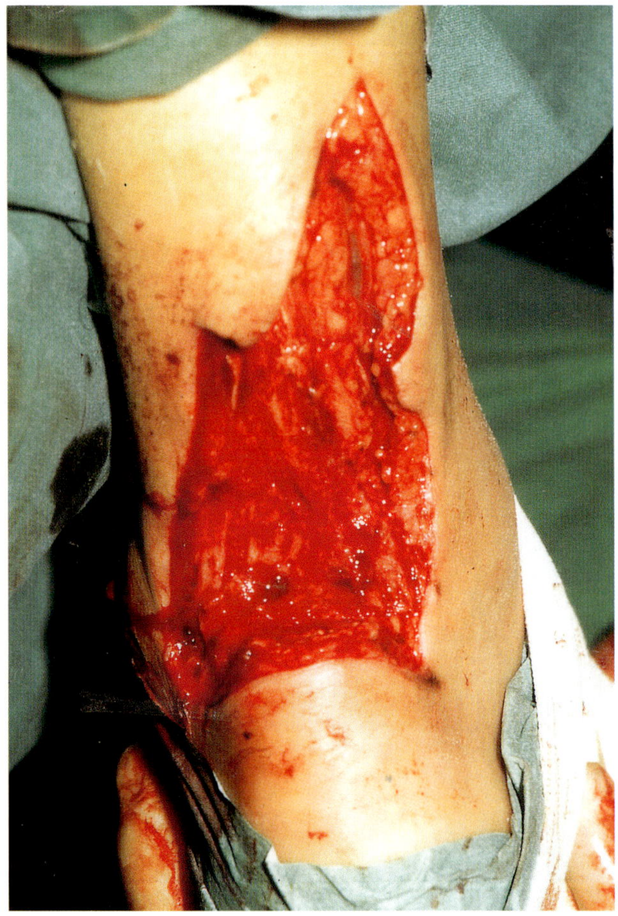

Figure 6.28b Result after debridement. The Achilles tendon shows a defect of 4 cm. The posterior tibial artery and vein are prepared for the anastomosis, end-to-side.

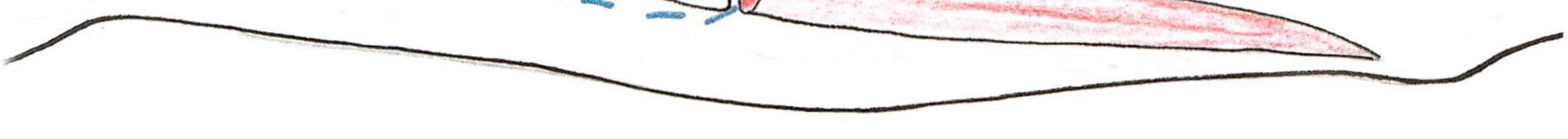

Figure 6.28c A radial forearm flap is prepared. The flap contains the tendons of palmaris longus muscle (1) and brachioradialis (2). They serve for reconstruction of the Achilles tendon.

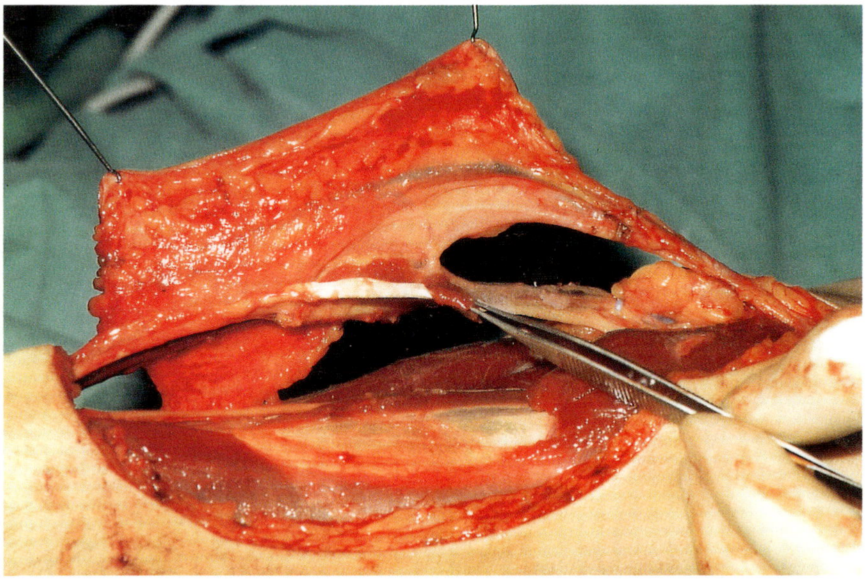

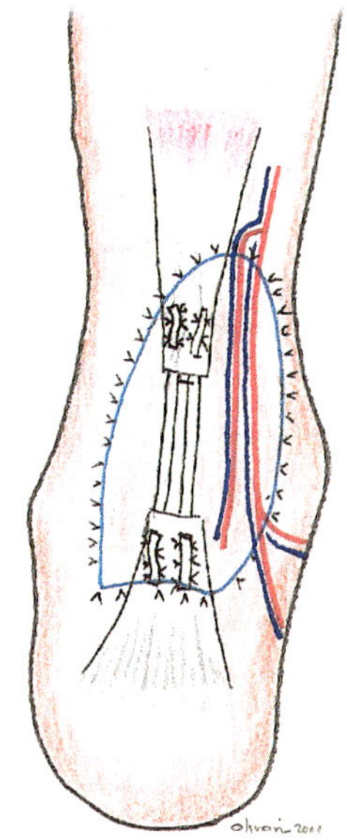

Figure 6.28d Mobilization of the radial flap together with the tendons of the palmaris longus and the brachioradialis muscles. Both tendons are used to interpose to reconstruct the Achilles tendon. The radial artery is anastomosed end-to-side to the posterior tibial artery.

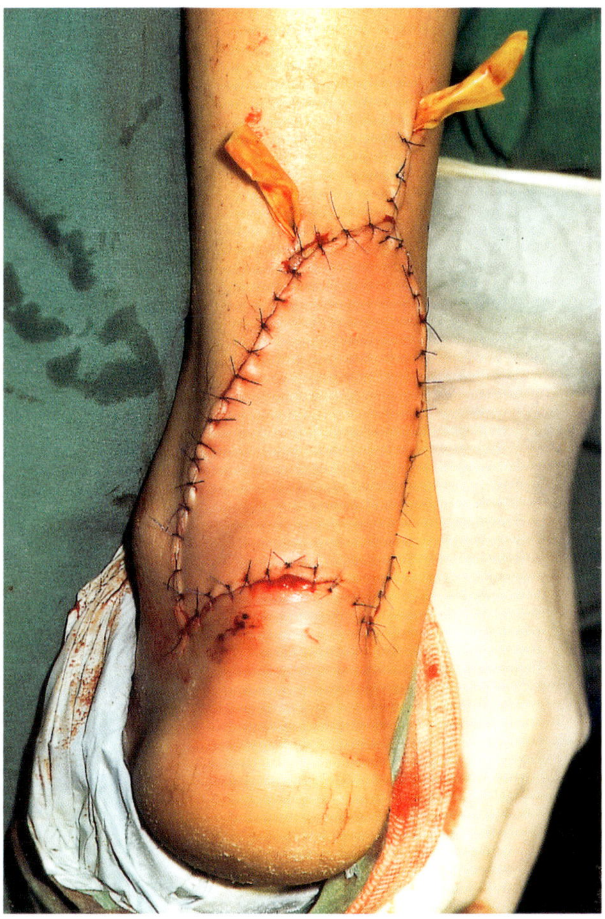

Figure 6.28e Result at the end of the operation

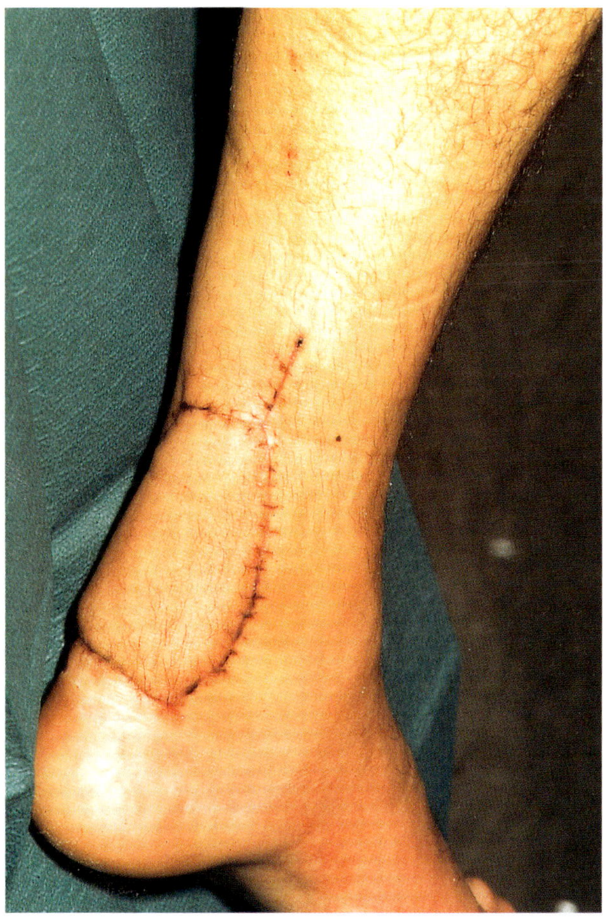

Figure 6.28f Result three weeks postoperatively

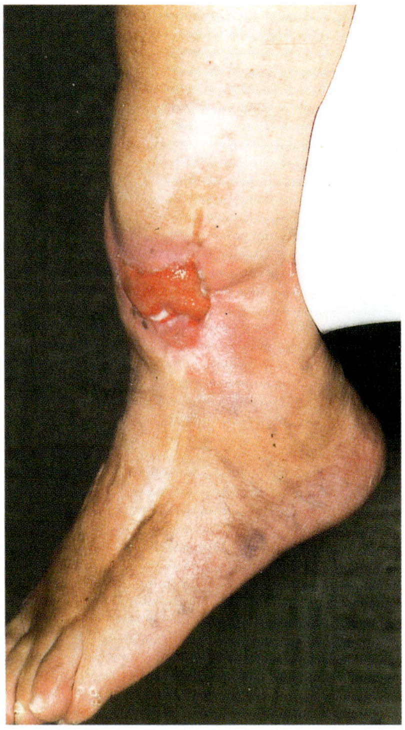

Figure 6.29a Post-traumatic defect, one year conservative therapy. Initially a radical debridement was necessary.

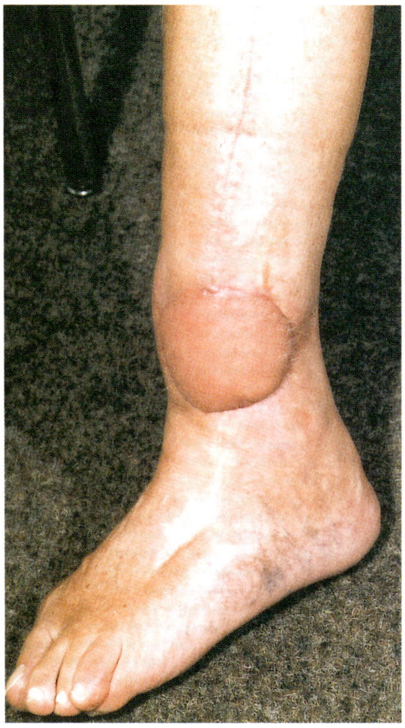

Figure 6.29b Result four months after operation

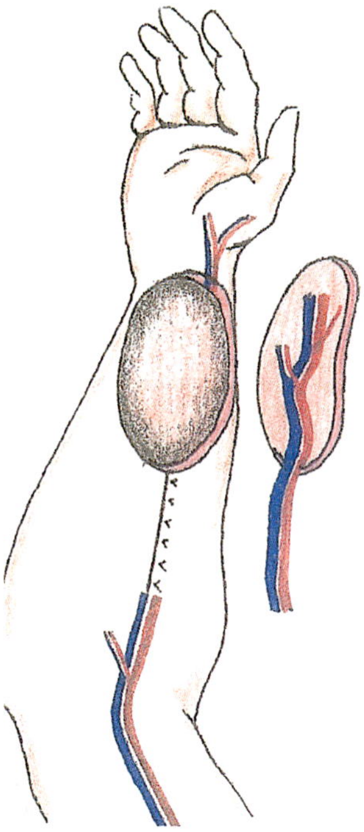

Figure 6.29c A radial flap with a very long pedicle is mobilized so that the anastomosis is far from the chronically infected area. An end-to-side anastomosis to the anterior tibial artery is performed.

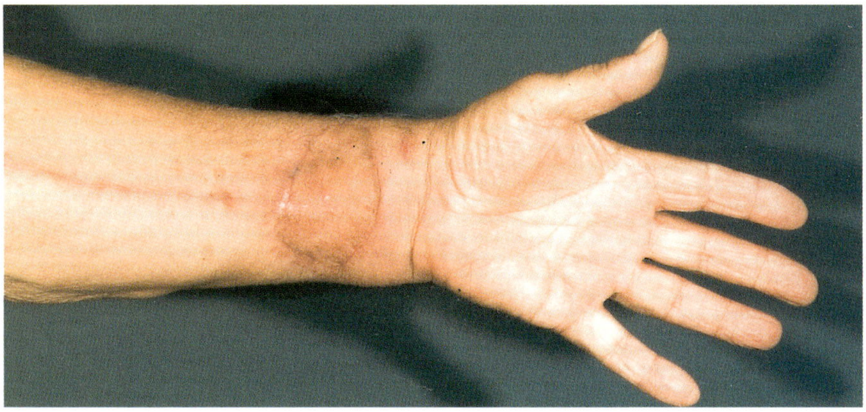

Figure 6.29d The donor site four months postoperatively

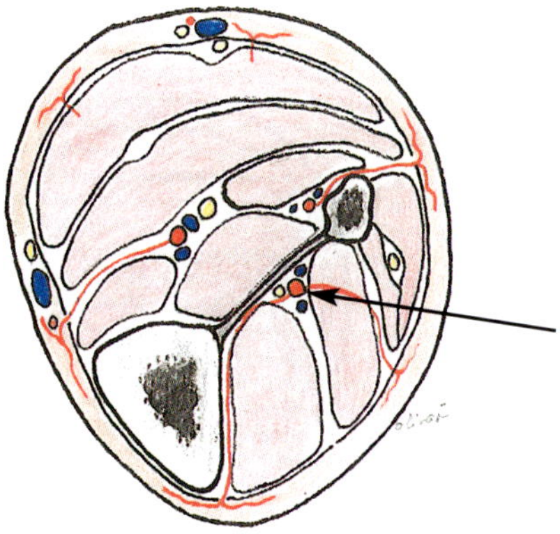

Figure 6.29e Cross section diagram of the left lower leg showing the position of the anterior tibial artery (arrow). It is located between tibialis anterior muscle and extensor digitorum longus muscle.

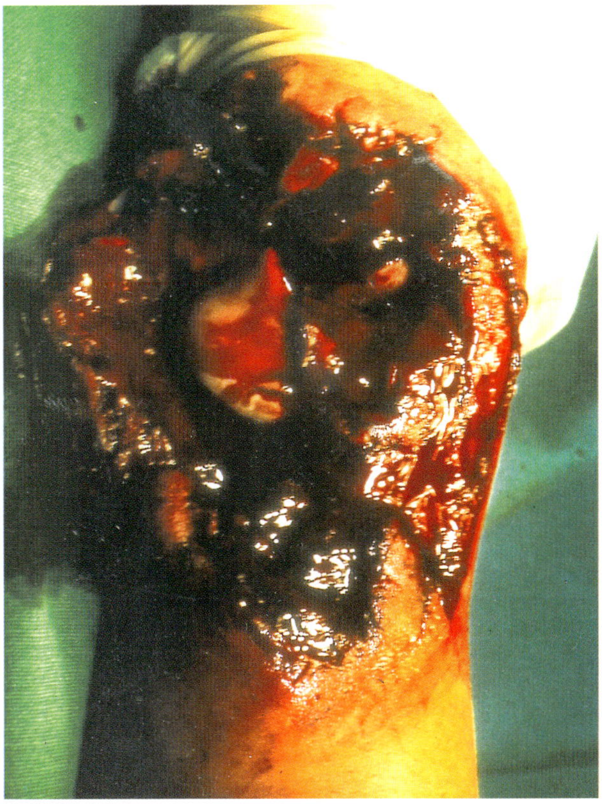

Figure 6.30a Severe fracture of the distal third of the lower leg with a soft tissue defect and loss of all extensor tendons. Avascular foot. Primary treatment: external fixation, reconstruction of extensor tendons using multiple strips of fascia lata (extensor hallucis longus, extensor digitorum longus, anterior tibial muscle), free radial forearm flap using the radial artery as an interpositional vessel to revascularize the foot.

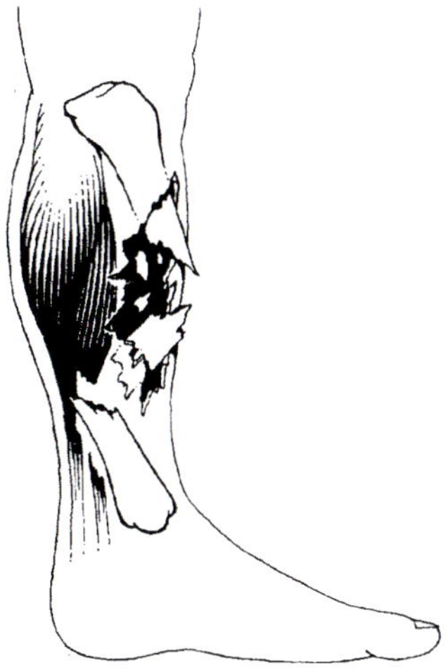

Figure 6.30b Fourth-degree open fracture of the lower leg after a high speed trauma. Soft tissue defect and ischemia of the foot following blood vessel rupture due to the crush injury. Primary reconstruction with free flap is essential to preserve the foot.

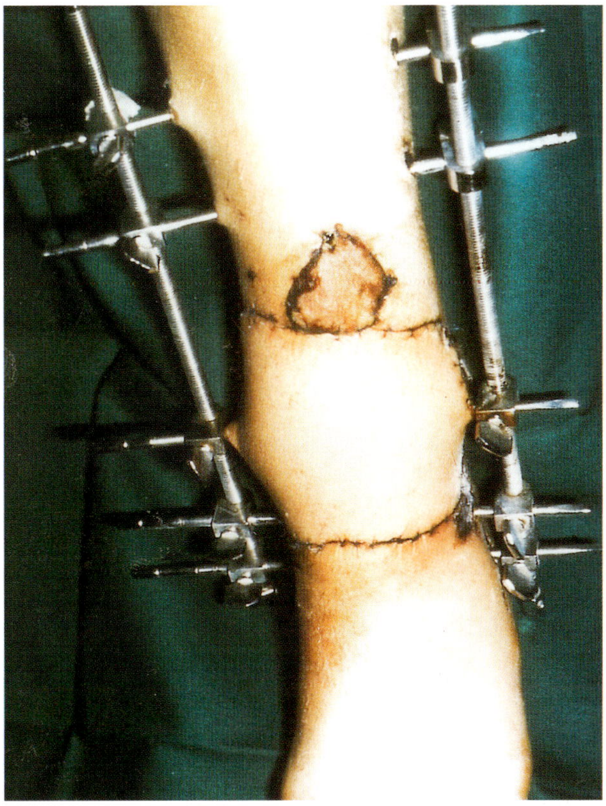

Figure 6.30c Result after two weeks

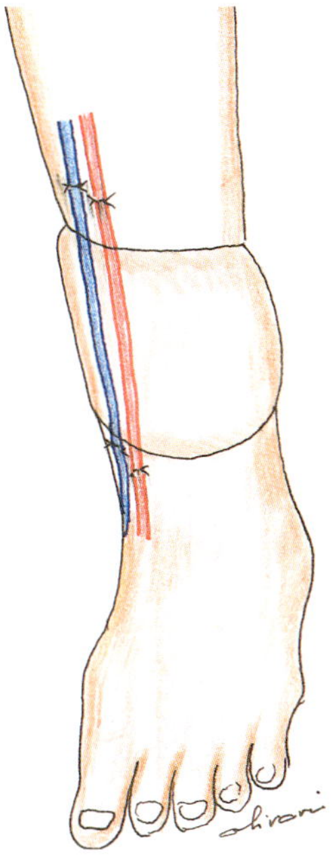

Figure 6.30d The radial artery is not only the nutrient vessel of the flap but is used to reconstruct the anterior tibial artery and revascularize the foot.

c) Latissimus Dorsi Free Flap

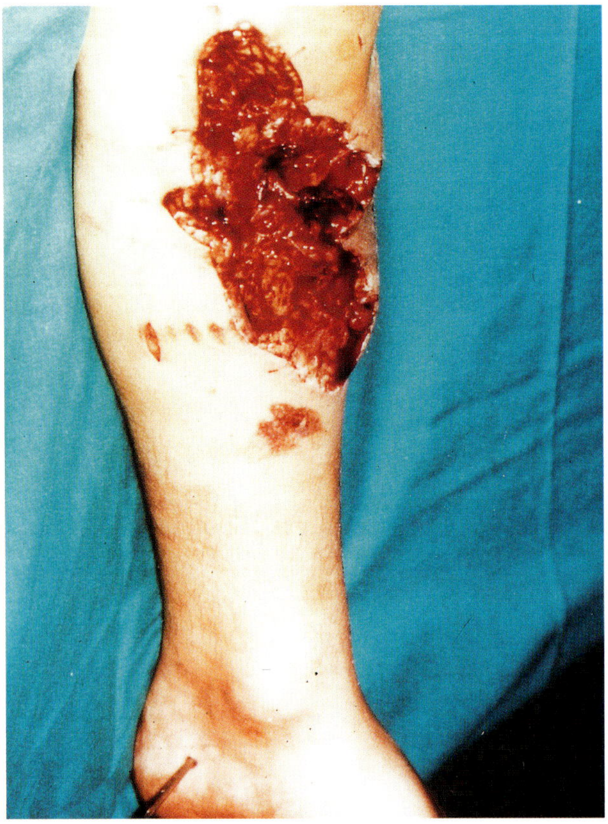

Figure 6.31a Open fracture of the tibia and fibula in the left lower leg due to a car accident. A large area of the skin was avulsed.

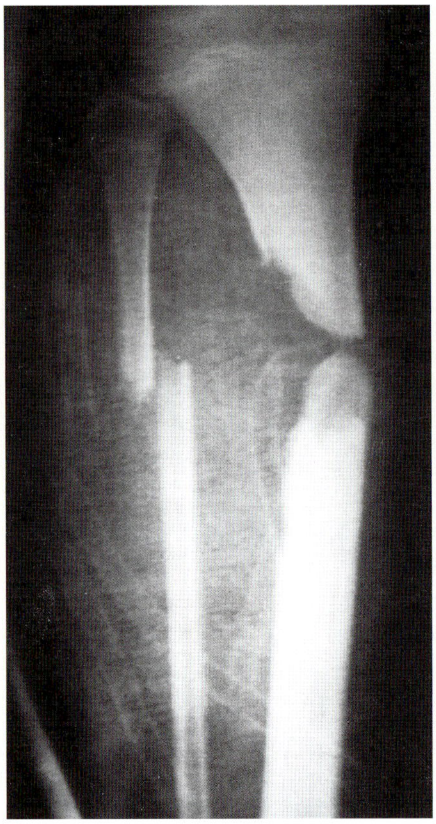

Figure 6.31b Treatment plan: a) external fixation, b) primary reconstruction of the soft tissue defect using a free latissimus dorsi flap.

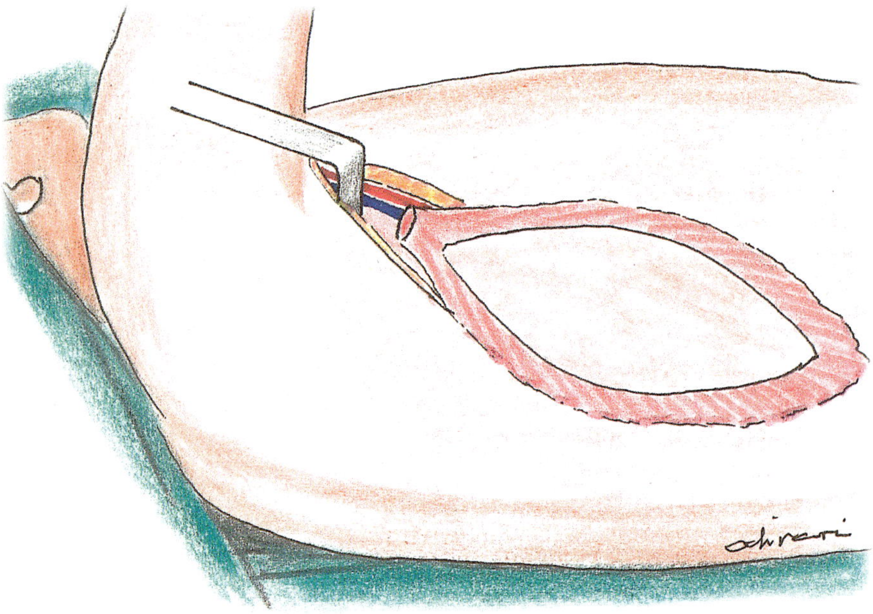

Figure 6.31c After external fixation the avascular tissue of the wound was removed and a latissimus dorsi flap was prepared for a microsurgical transfer.

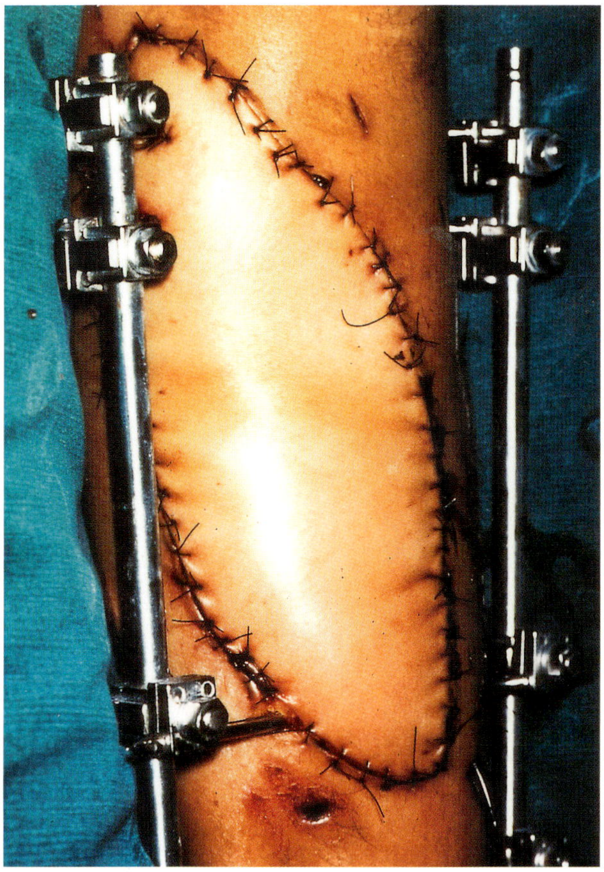

Figure 6.31d 24 hours after the flap procedure. End-to-side anastomosis of the thoracodorsal artery with the popliteal artery.

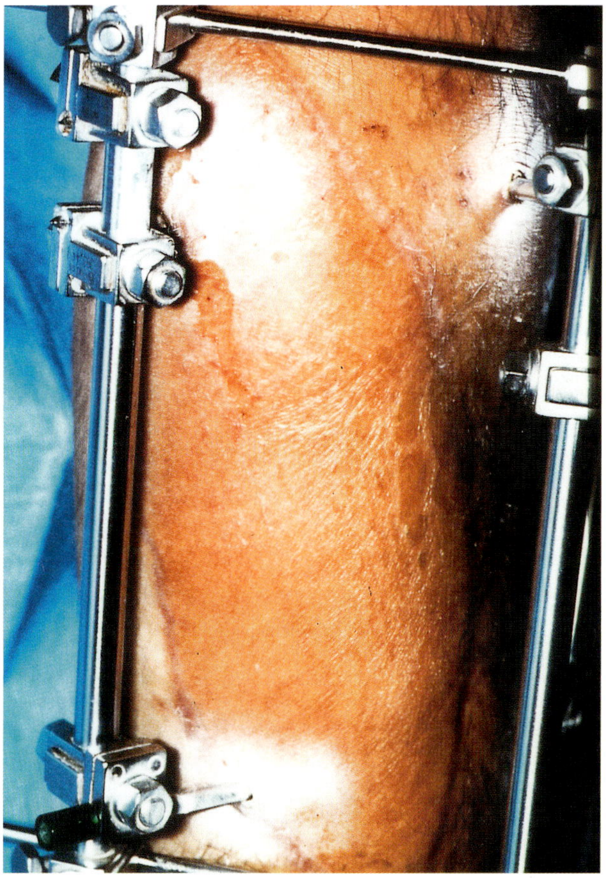

Figure 6.31f The external fixation remains until the tibial bone has healed completely.

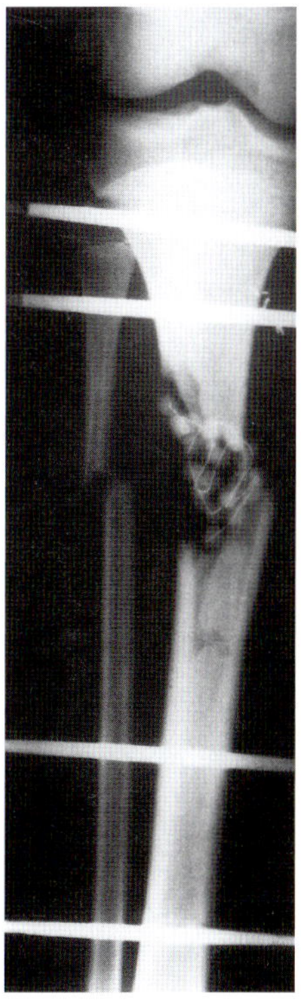

Figure 6.31e The condition five months after flap surgery. Note that an osteoplasty was performed to stabilize the fracture two months after the Latissimus dorsi flap surgery.

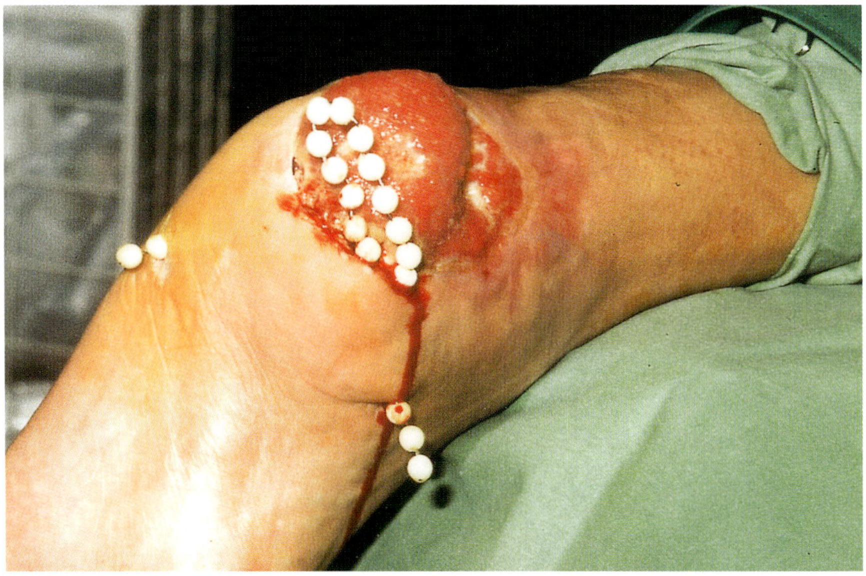

Figure 6.32a Avulsion injury of the left heel: Four months after conservative treatment.

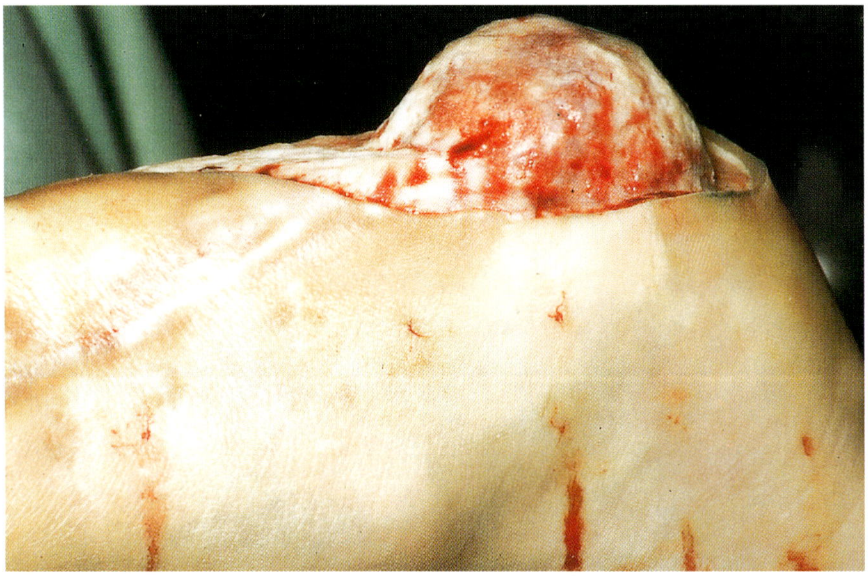

Figure 6.32b Radical debridement

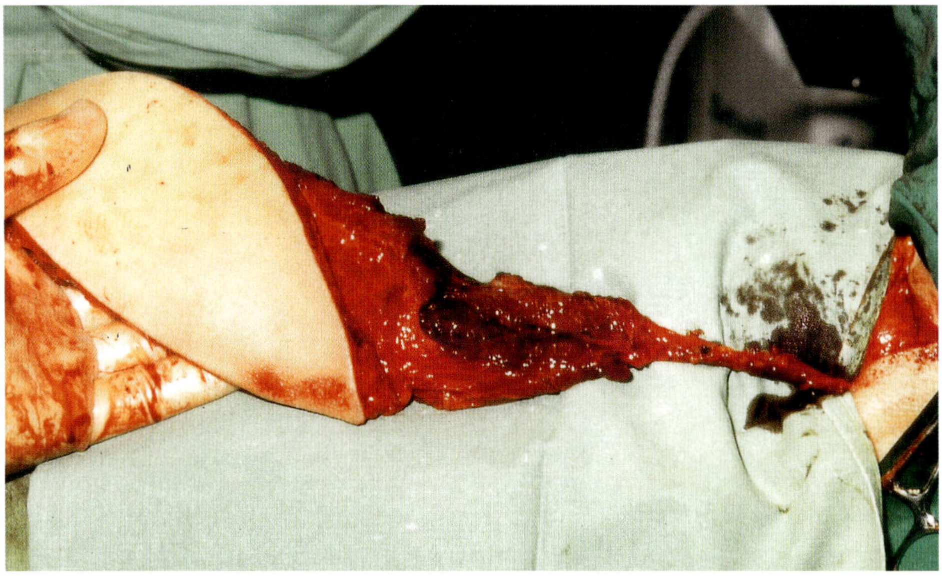

Figure 6.32c An ipsilateral latissimus dorsi flap is elevated

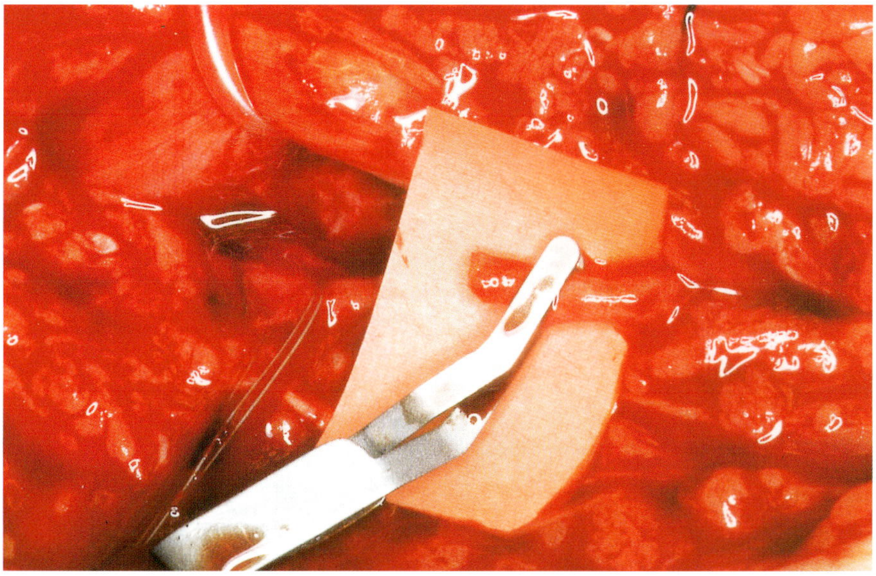

Figure 6.32d An end-to-side anastomosis of the thoracodorsal artery to the posterior tibial artery and an end-to-end anastomosis of the vein

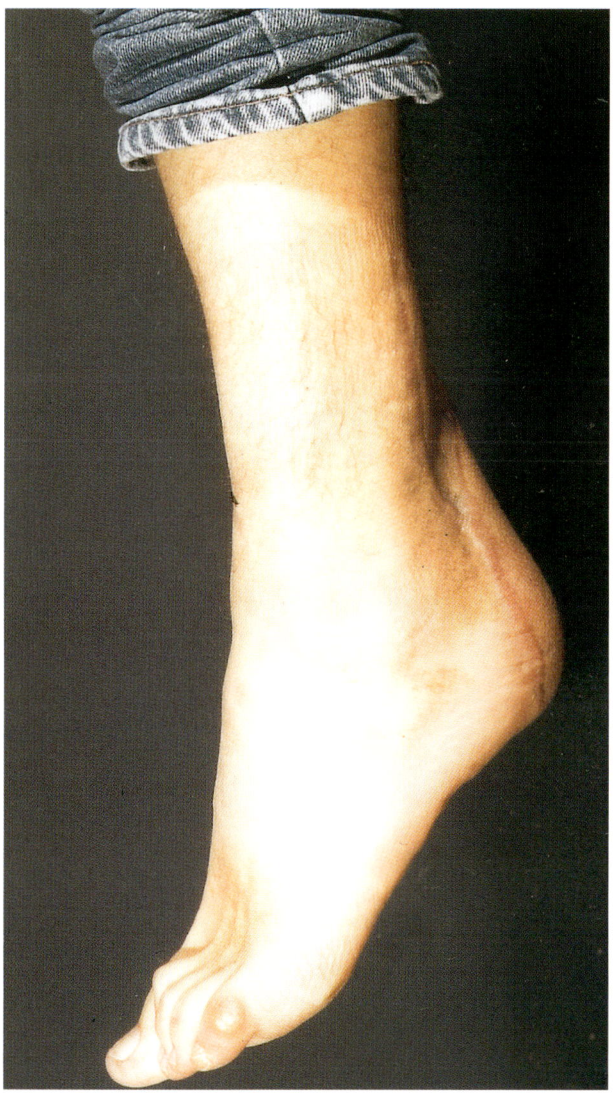

Figure 6.32e Three years after the operation. The patient is able to walk without any restriction.

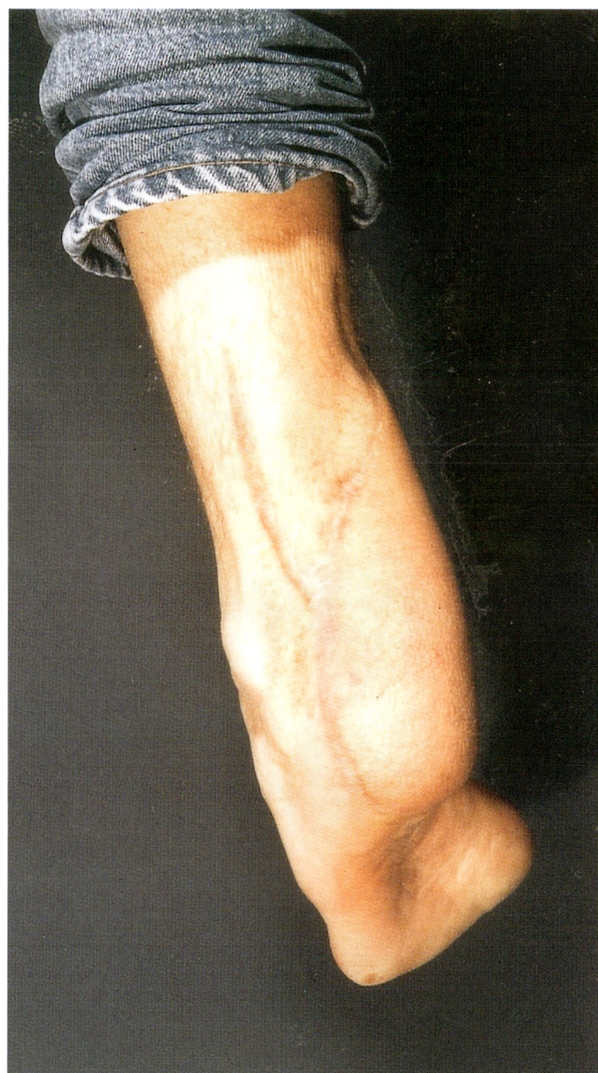

Figure 6.32f Good functional result

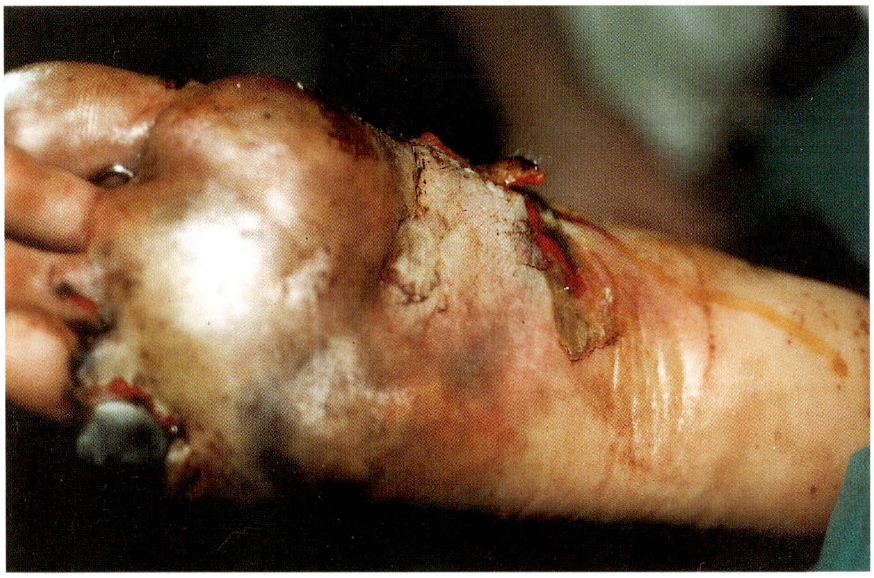

Figure 6.33a Severe crush injury of the foot (fourth degree). It was not possible to judge immediately level of debridement.

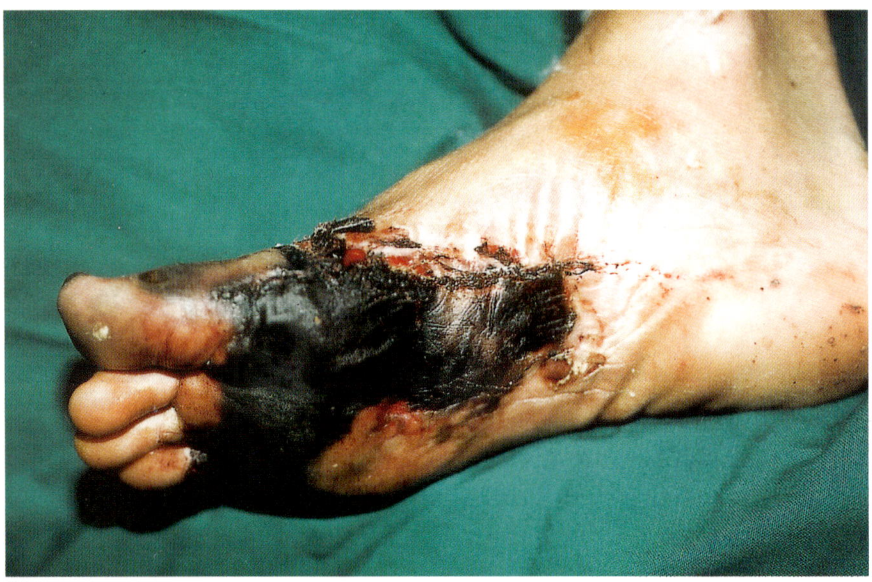

Figure 6.33b Five days after trauma demarcation of the necrotic tissue is quite clear.

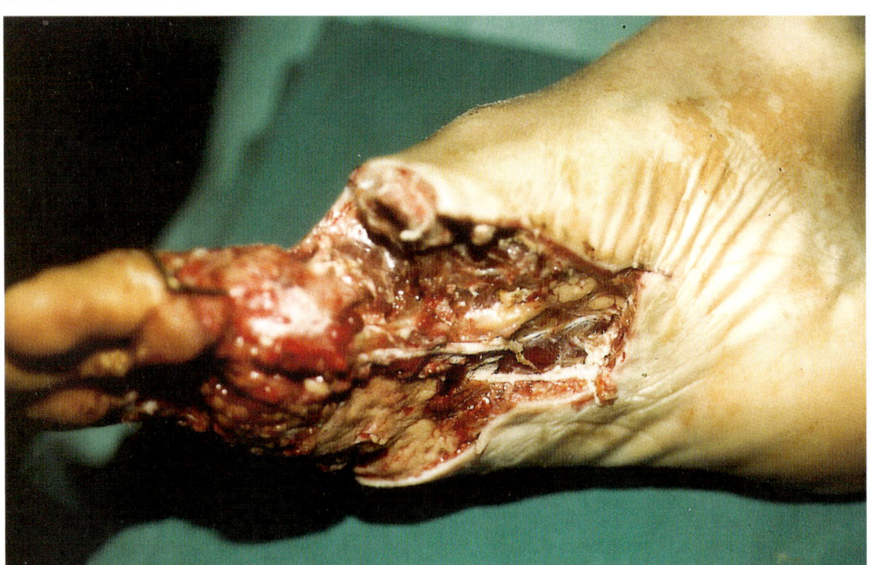

Figure 6.33c After debridement, a latissimus dorsi (muscle only) is transferred and its vessels anastomosed with the posterior tibial artery and vein. Mesh graft was used to cover the muscle.

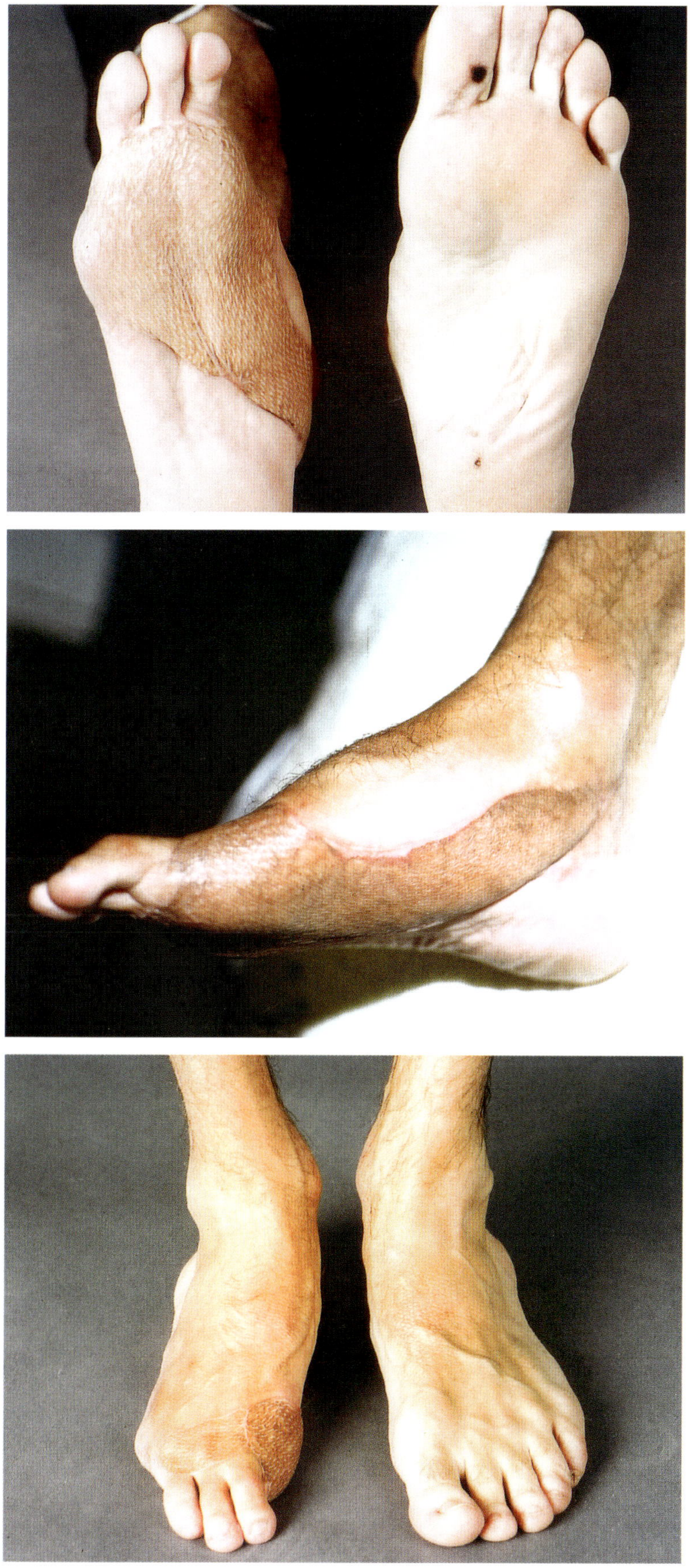

Figure 6.33d–f 2½ years after the operation. There is a good functional result and the patient walks without restriction. Most authors agree that a muscle flap in combination with a split thickness skin graft gives better functional results than a latissimus dorsi flap that is elevated with a large skin island. Shear forces affect the dermal and subdermal layer of the overlying skin island which result sometimes in postoperative ulcerations.

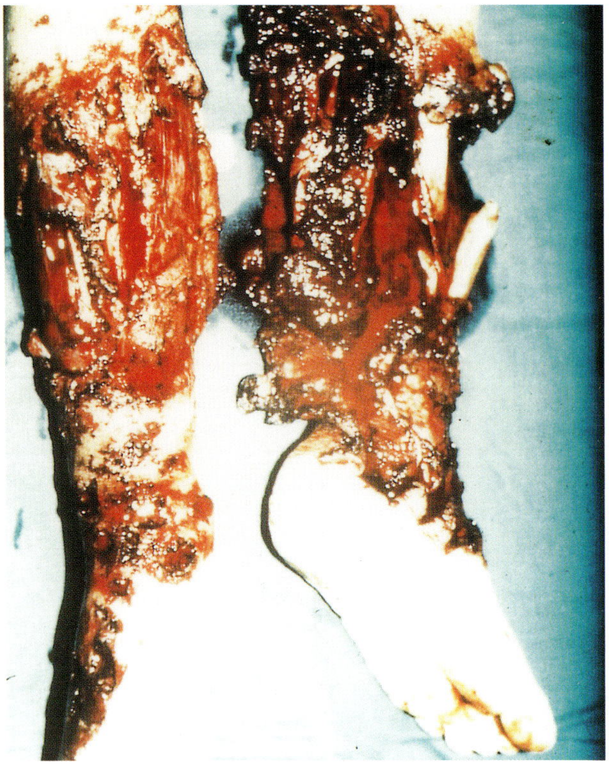

Figure 6.34a Explosion injury (grenade) of both lower legs.
– Extensive bilateral soft tissue loss
– Fourth-degree left lower leg fracture
– Third-degree right lower leg fracture
– Ischemia of left foot

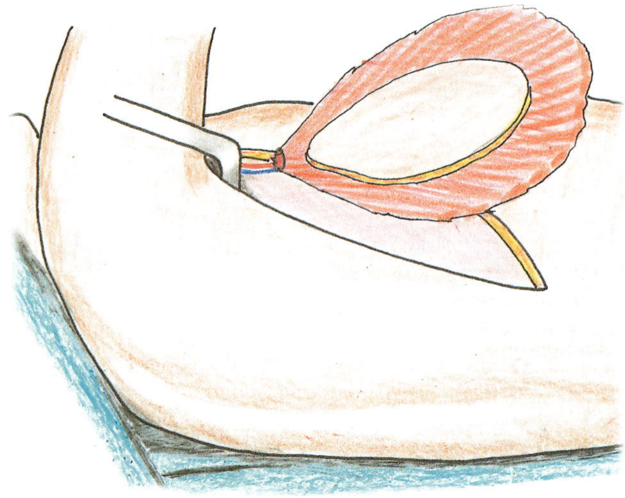

Figure 6.34b Preparation of both latissimus dorsi flaps.
In these cases the orthopedic and plastic surgeon work in partnership.
The sequence of treatment is as follows:
1) The left foot is ischemic therefore after external fixation of the fracture, immediate reconstruction of the vessels using vein grafting is essential.
2) Radical debridement
3) Accurate bone reposition (external fixations and plates)
4) Two latissimus dorsi free flaps
5) Split thickness skin grafting for coverage of defects distant from the fractures
6) If necessary osteoplasty can be performed three months postoperatively.

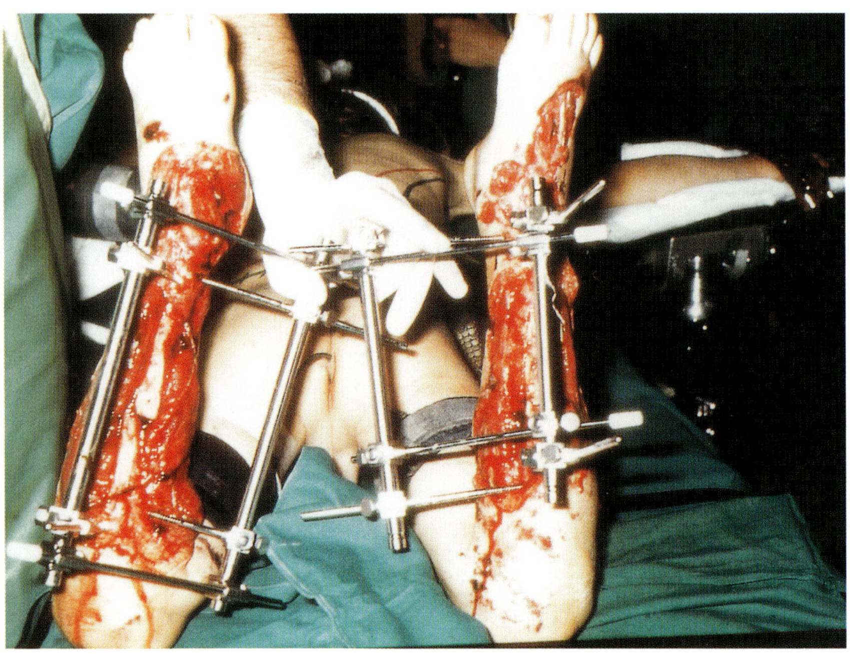

Figure 6.34c Bilateral external fixation. Vein grafting for revascularization of the left foot is performed followed by a bilateral latissimus dorsi free flap.

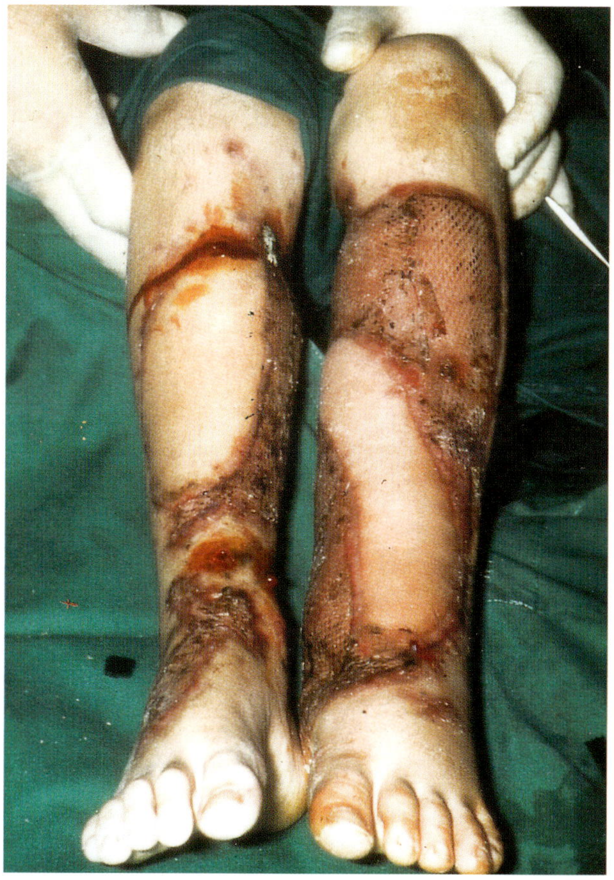

Figure 6.34d Two months postoperatively. The latissimus dorsi free flap covered the exposed fractures and the remaining defects were healed with split-thickness skin grafts. There was 3 cm shortening of the left lower leg.

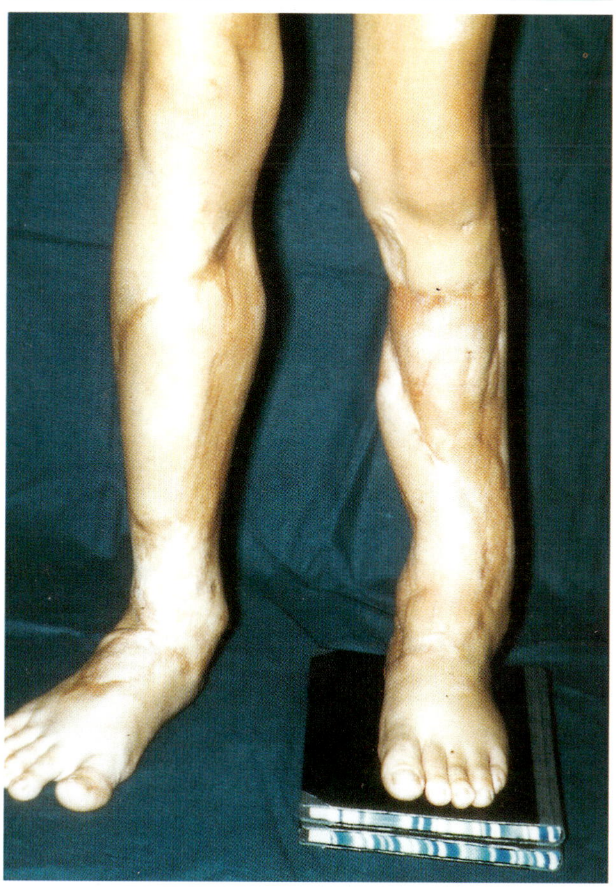

Figure 6.34e Two years postoperatively. The shortening of the left lower leg necessitated a raised shoe.

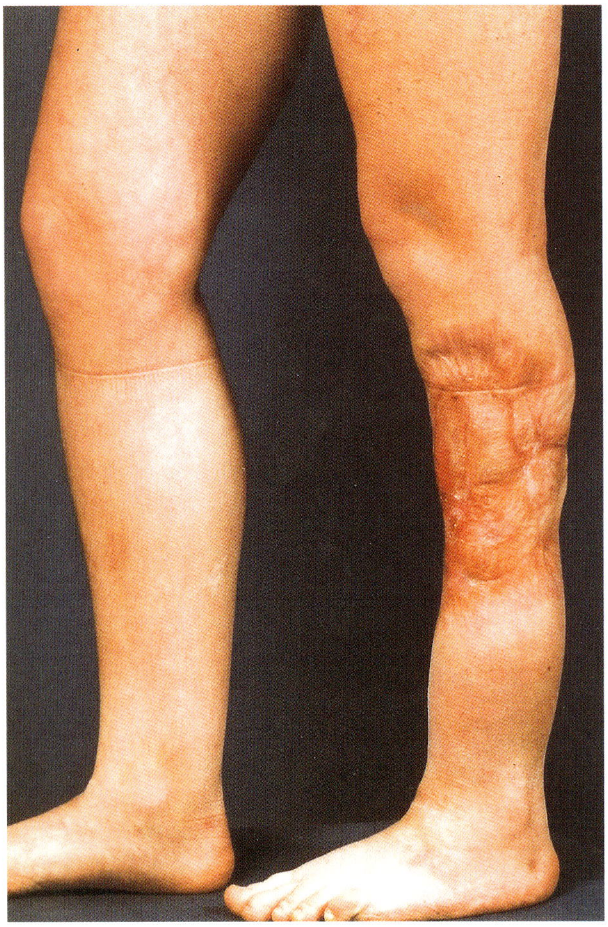

Figure 6.35a Post-traumatic soft tissue defect of the left lower leg with partial exposure of the tibial periosteum.

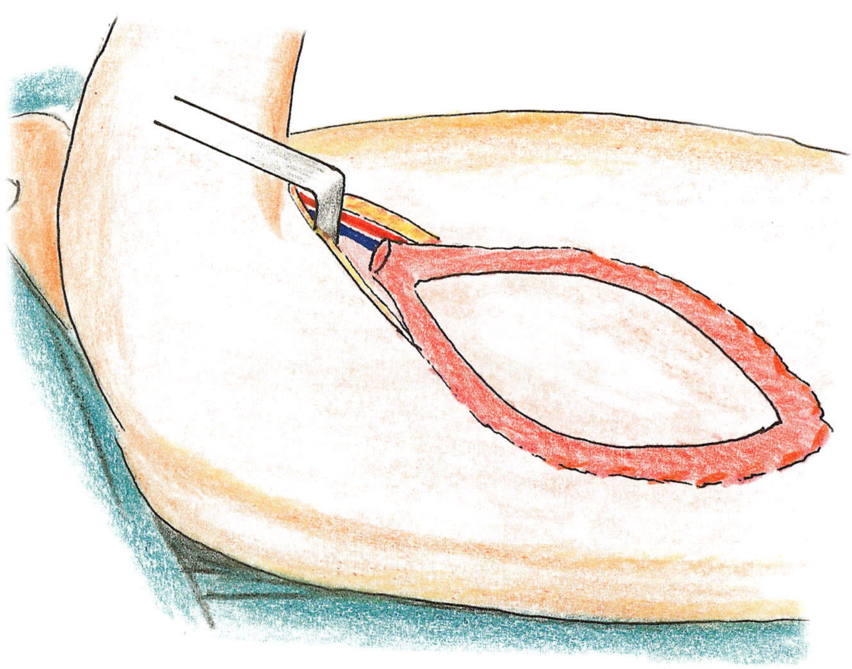

Figure 6.35b Elevation of a latissimus dorsi free flap

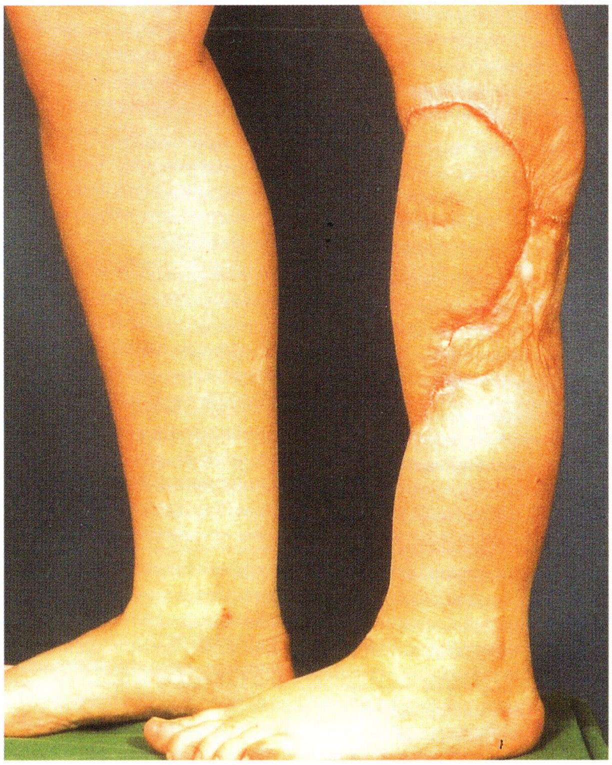

Figure 6.35c Seven months after latissimus dorsi transfer

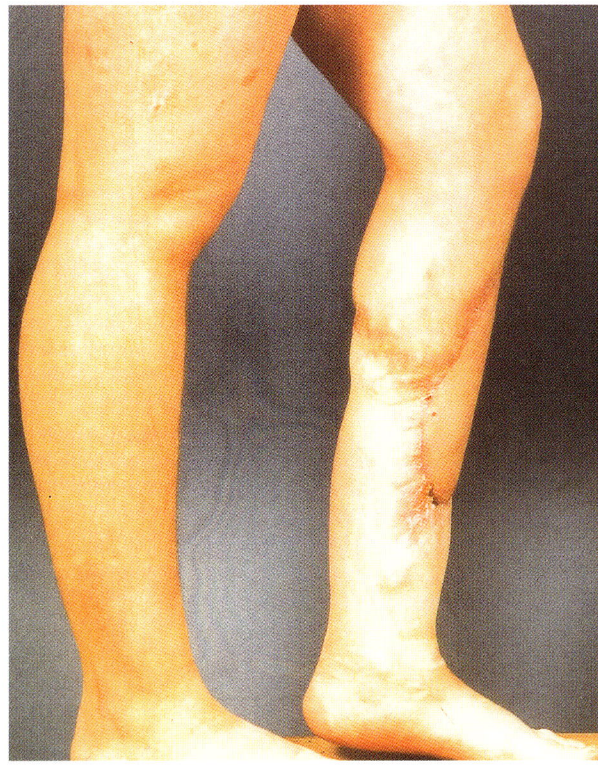

Figure 6.35d Seven months postoperatively

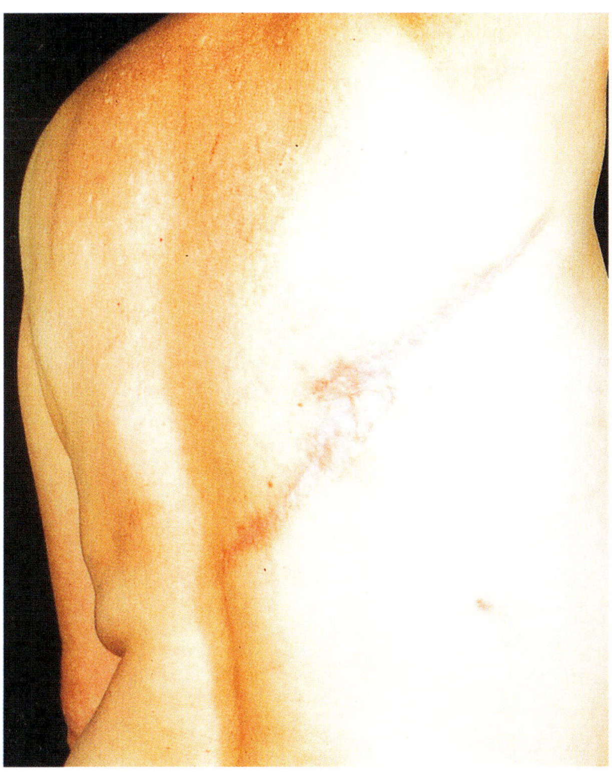

Figure 6.35e Donor site of the flap

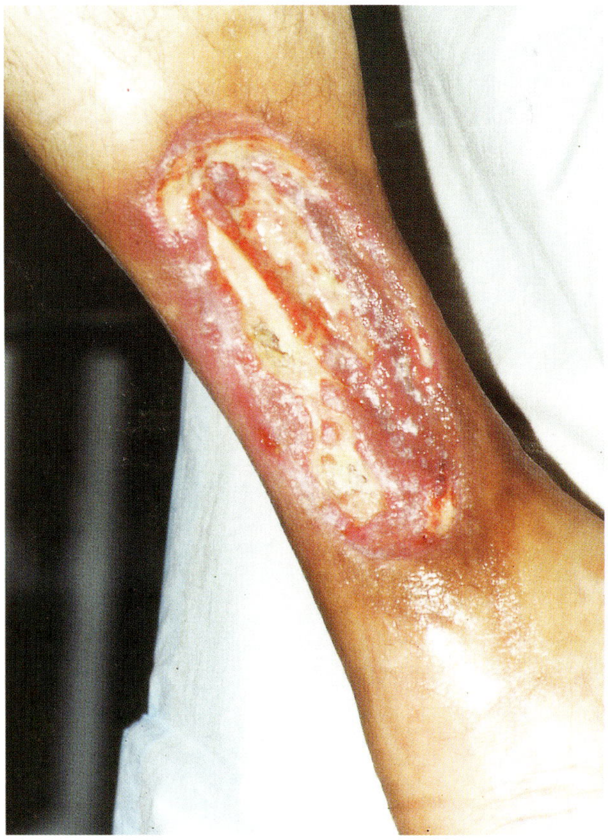

Figure 6.36a Radiation ulcer and dermatitis following treatment of a basal cell carcinoma on the right lower leg. Partial necrosis of muscles and tendons. Circular compression leads to an impaired blood flow with a hypoperfusion of the foot and constant pain. Even amputation was considered.

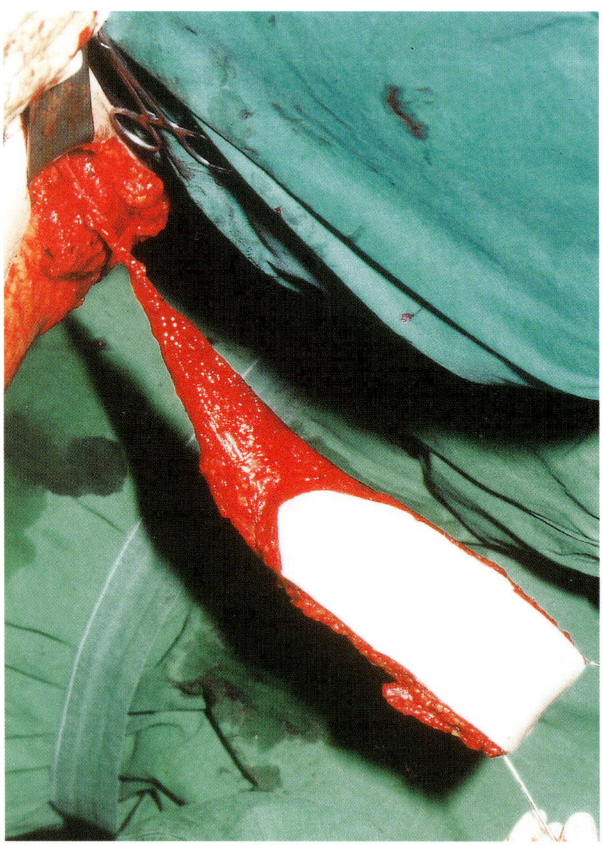

Figure 6.36b After radical debridement of all necrotic and fibrotic tissue a latissimus dorsi free flap is elevated.

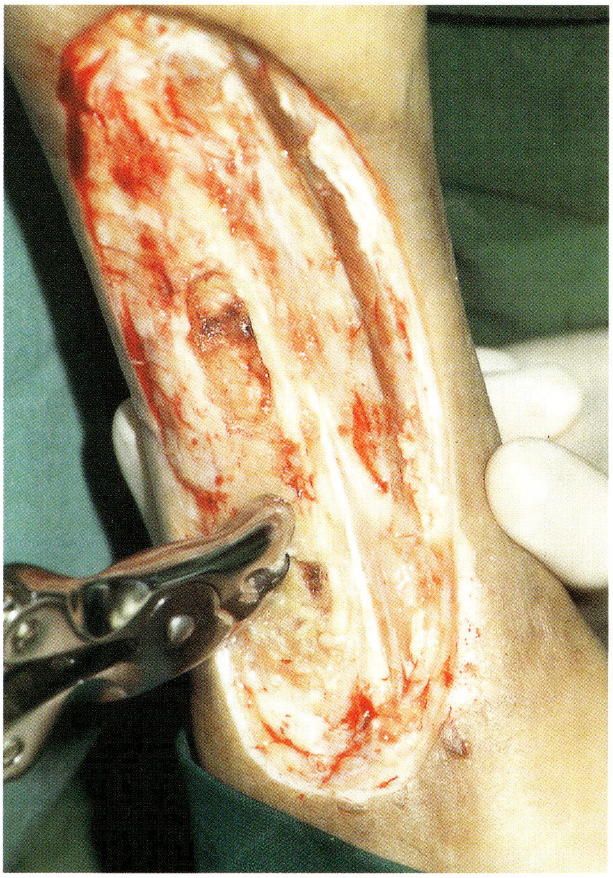

Figure 6.36c The avascular soft tissue and necrotic bone is removed.

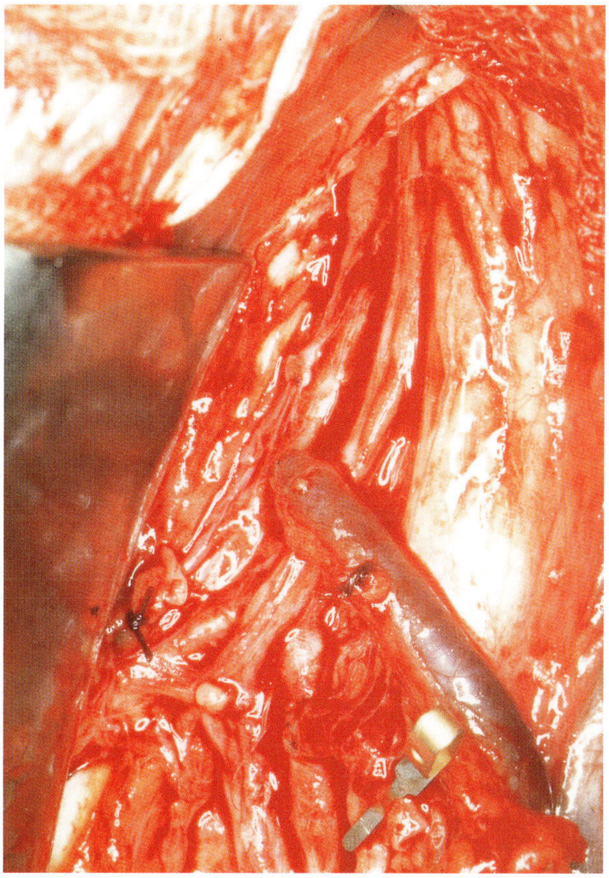

Figure 6.36e End-to-side anastomosis to the popliteal artery is performed distant from the radiation area (out of the zone of injury). Vessels in area of irradiation are not suitable for microsurgical anastomosis.

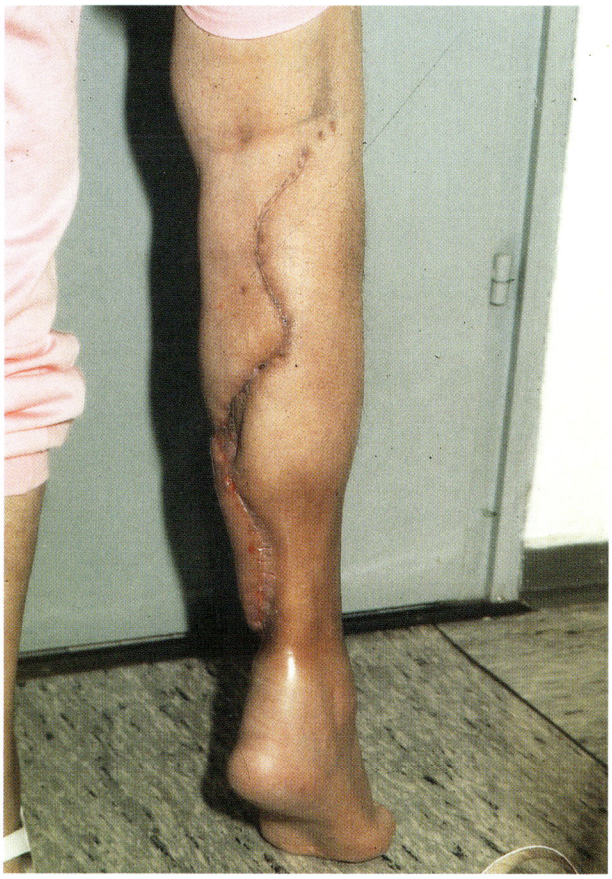

Figure 6.36d Good functional result

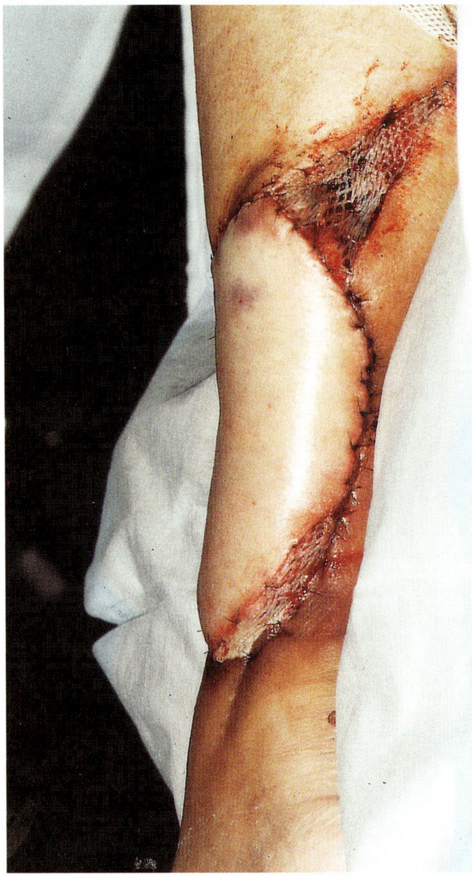

Figure 6.36f End-to-side anastomosis with the popliteal artery to avoid impairment of the perfusion of the distal lower leg. It should be performed as far proximal as possible from to the radiation area. Chronic infection and irradiation damages blood vessels and they cannot be used for the microanastomosis. The latissimus dorsi flap with its long pedicle is ideal for covering these defects.

Figure 6.36g Three months after the operation the patient is able to walk. Blood supply of the foot is improved.

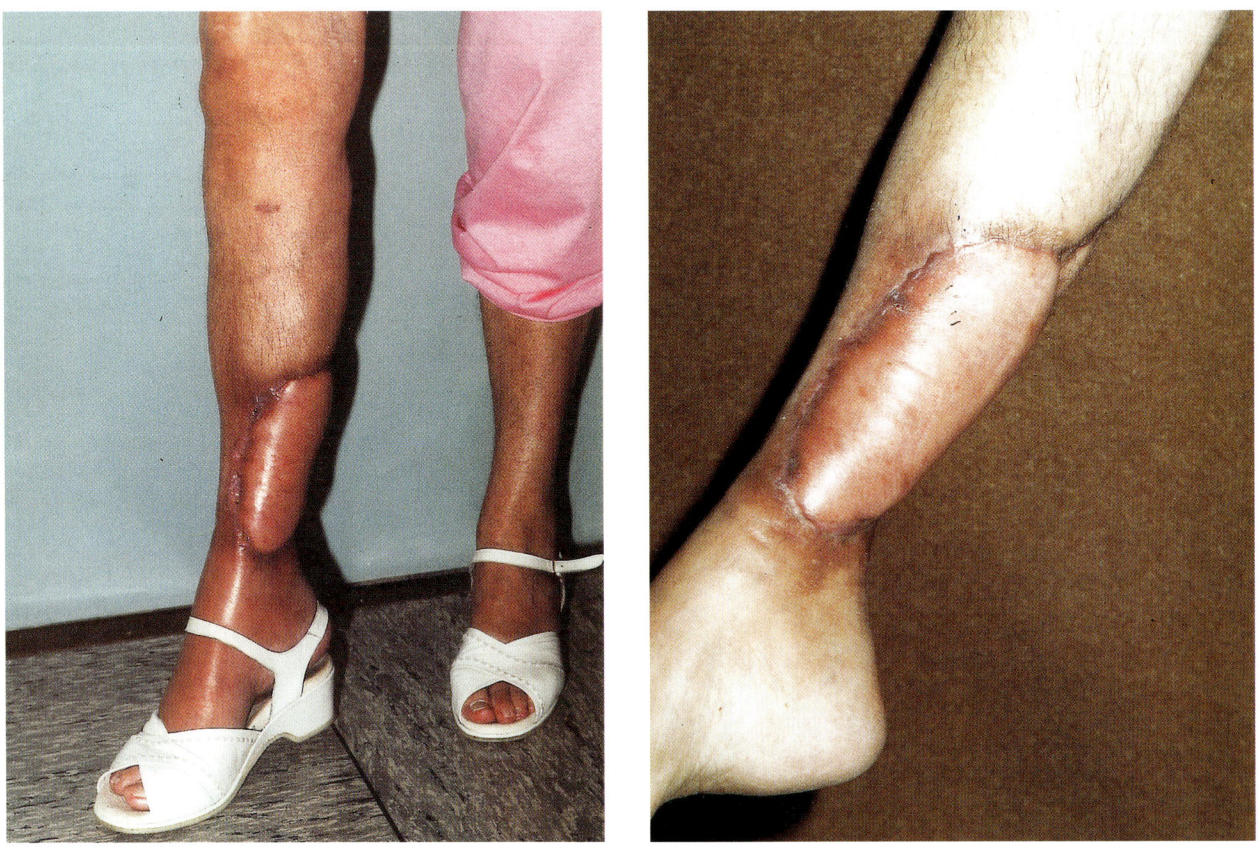

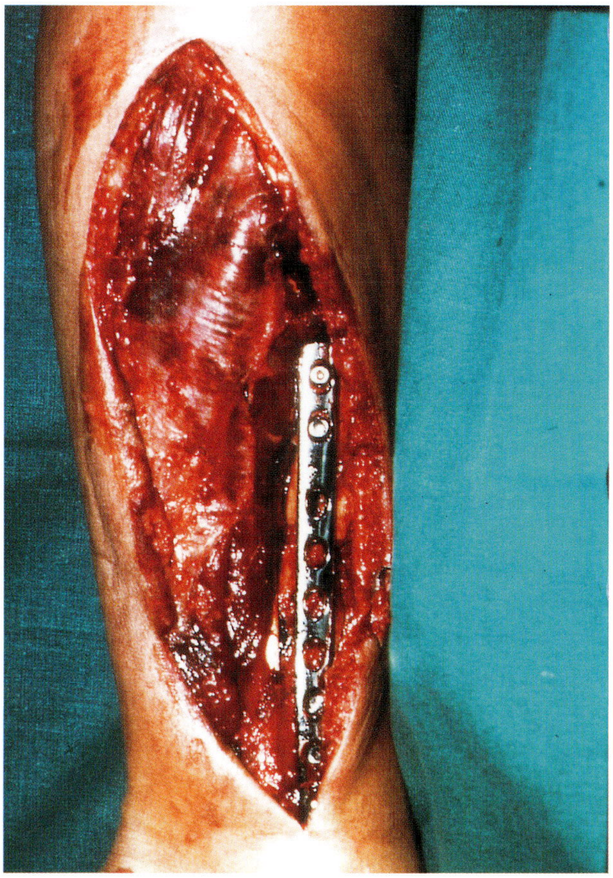

Figure 6.37a Third-degree open fracture of the lower leg with a large soft-tissue defect. Plate fixation and primary latissimus dorsi free flap to cover the defect. In this case a good cooperation between the orthopedic and plastic surgeon is important. Soft tissue coverage is essential. Primary or early-secondary defect coverage using a free flap reduces morbidity of these patients.

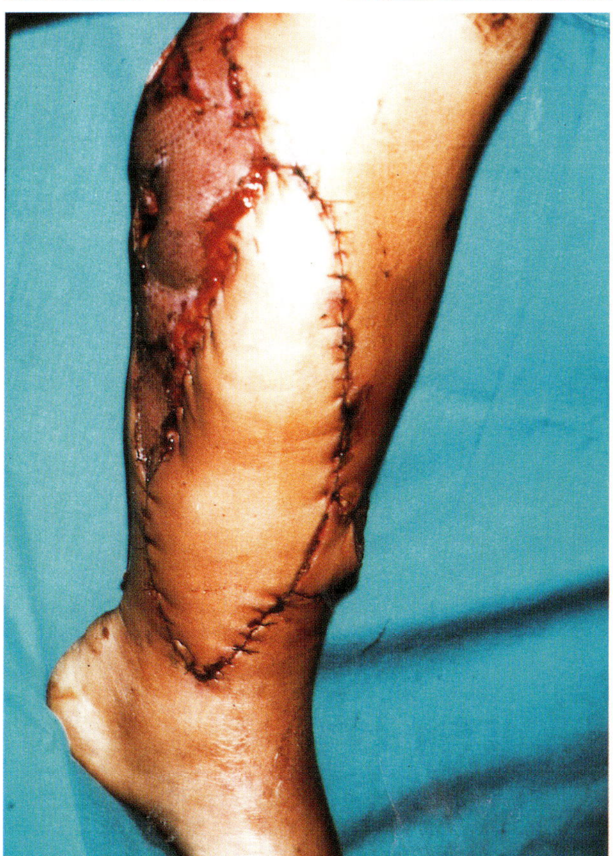

Figure 6.37b Two weeks postoperatively. Coverage of bone and osteosynthesis plate was achieved with a latissimus dorsi free flap (only one operation). The dorsal aspect was covered using a split thickness skin graft. Osteosynthesis can be performed with external fixation, plate fixation or intramedullary nailing. The risk of infection in these severe injuries can be reduced if complete reconstruction of bone and soft tissue is performed immediately or within one week after trauma (Godina 1986).

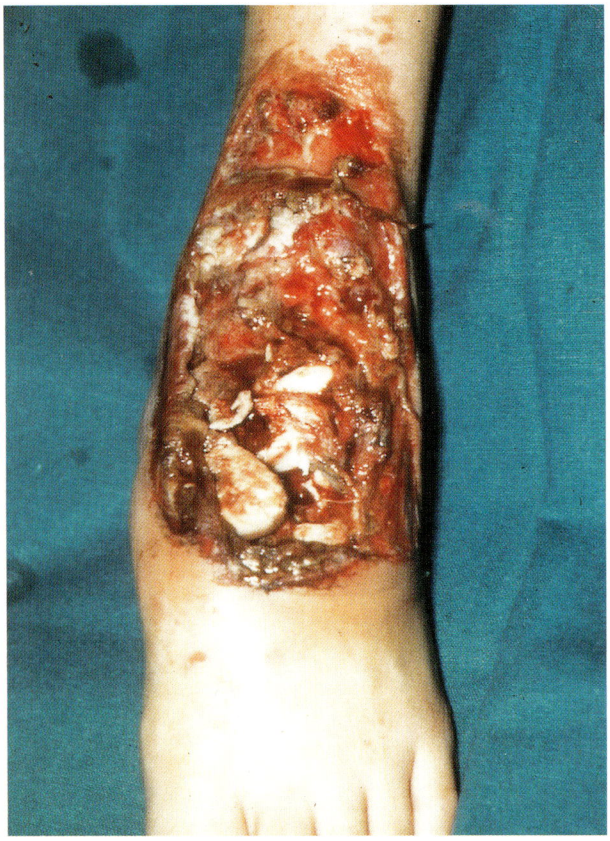

Figure 6.38a Defect after a car accident. Substantial loss of soft tissue, dorsalis pedis artery, extensor hallucis longus muscle, extensor hallucis brevis muscle, anterior tibial muscle, retinaculum, part of the talar, navicular, cuboid and cuneiforme bone and superficial peroneal nerve. The extensor digitorum communis muscle is preserved.

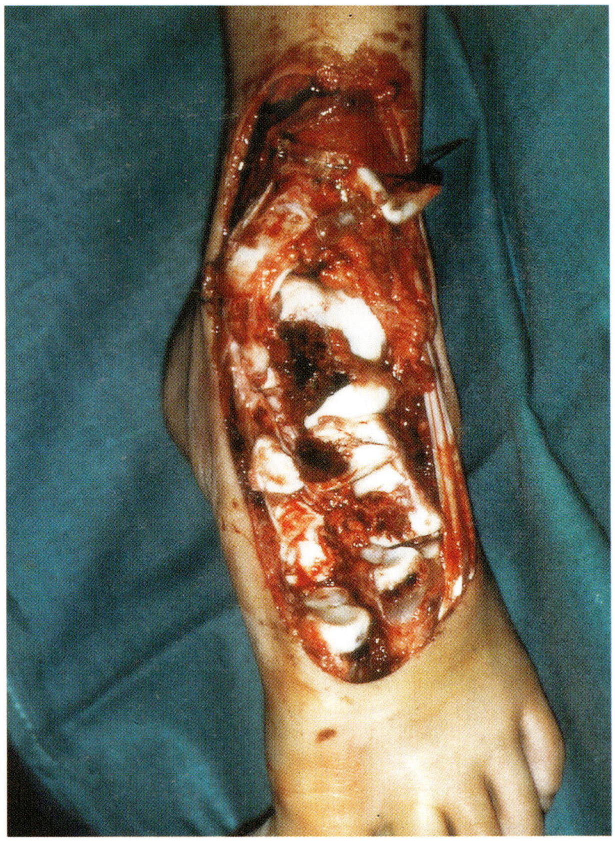

Figure 6.38b A radical primary debridement is performed including the bone.

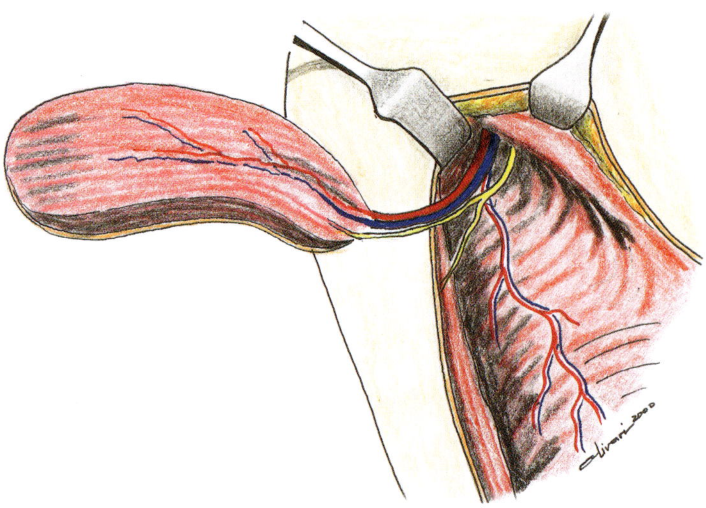

Figure 6.38c After the osteosynthesis a latissimus dorsi flap is elevated. If the operation is performed with two surgical teams the duration of surgery is considerably shortened.

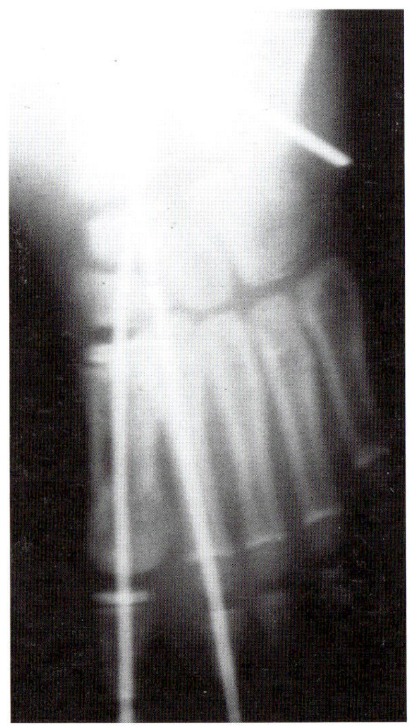

Figure 6.38d Intraoperative X-ray: Internal K-wire fixation of the bones

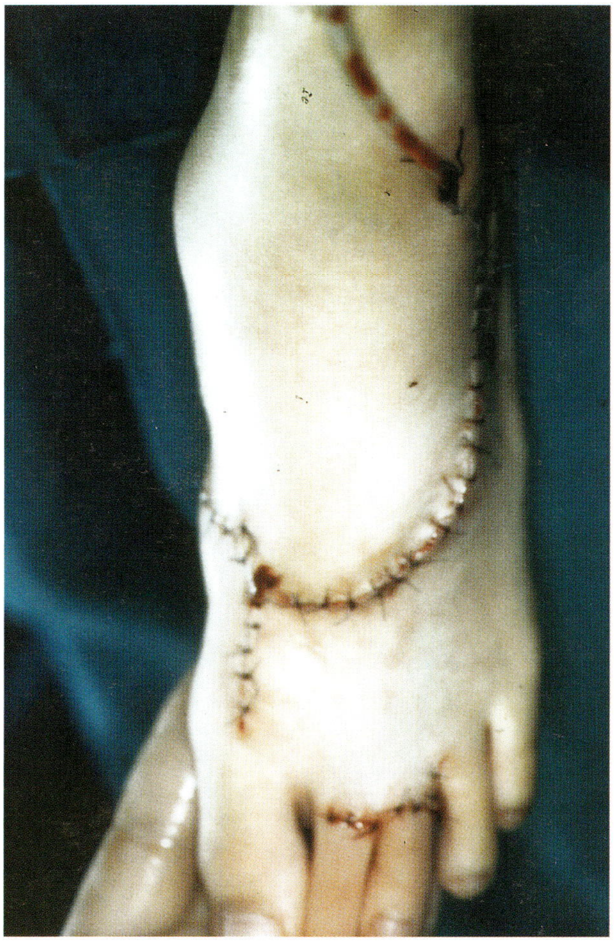

Figure 6.38e Coverage of the primary defect was achieved using a latissimus dorsi free flap and the vessels anastomosed with the anterior tibial artery and vein. Simultaneously fascia lata strips were used for reconstruction of the extensors tendons.

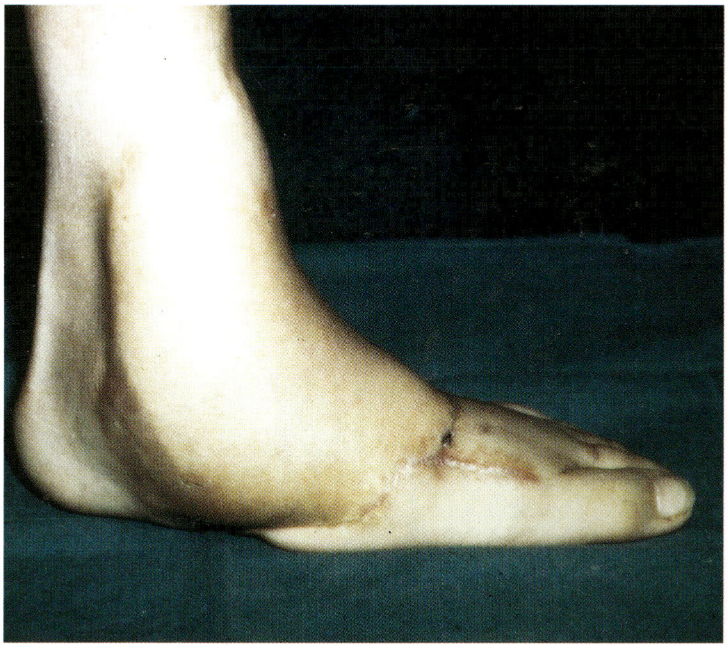

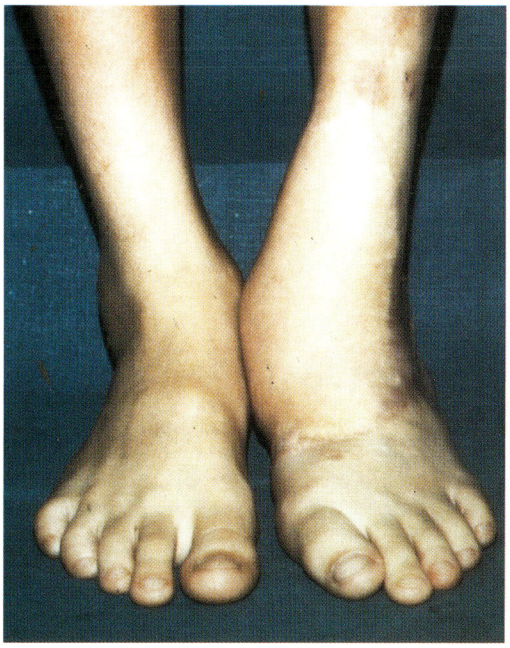

Figure 6.38f, g Two years postoperatively. Good functional result with normal weight bearing

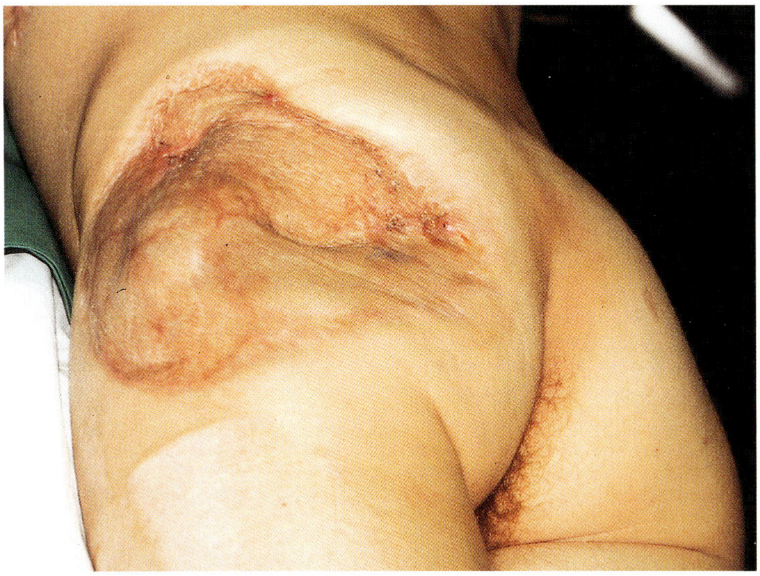

Figure 6.39a Battlefield injury (Croatia). Below knee amputation of the right lower leg. Fracture and luxation of the left femoral head in combination with an avulsion of the gluteal muscles. Primary defect was covered with split thickness skin grafting. A prosthesis was needed for reconstruction of left hip but there was inadequate soft tissue coverage in this area.

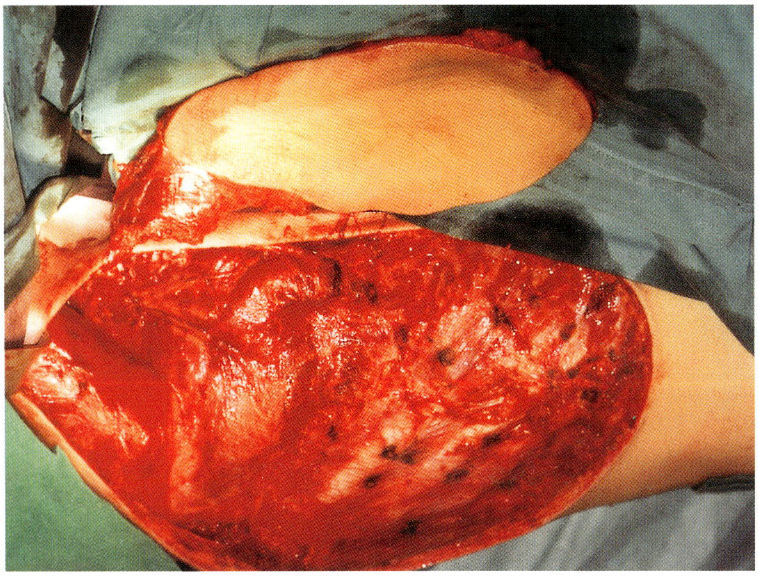

Figure 6.39b A large latissimus dorsi free flap procedure is planned for soft tissue coverage.

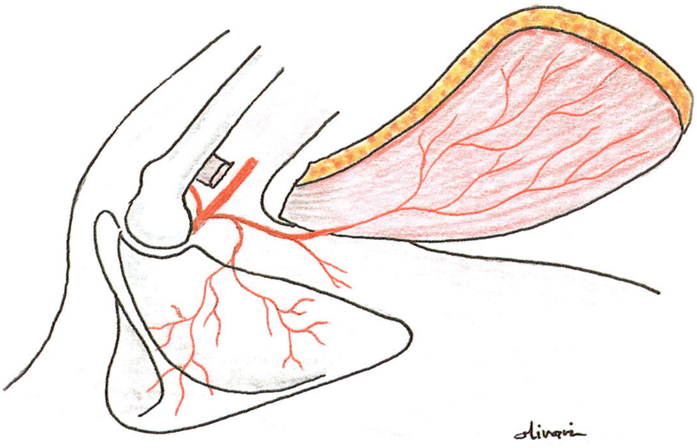

Figure 6.39c Elevation of the latissimus dorsi free flap

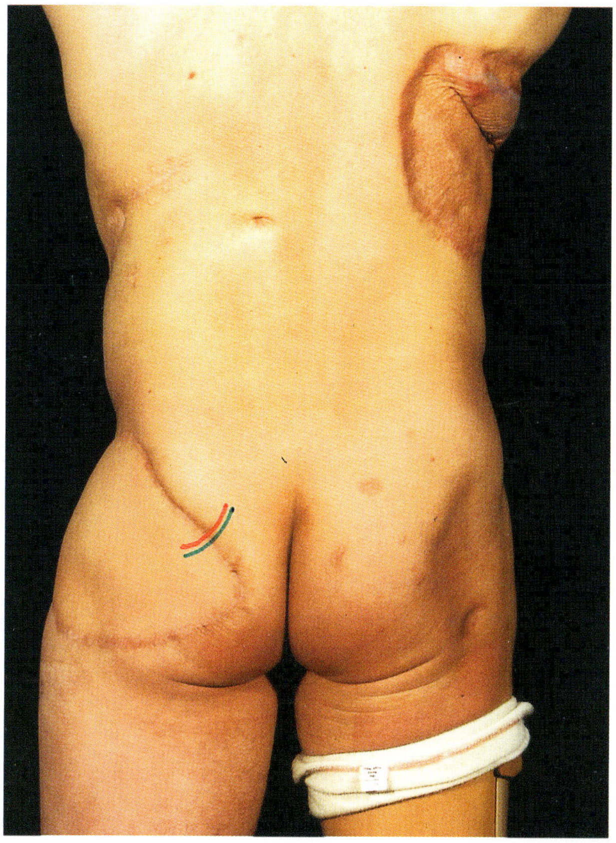

Figure 6.39d Anastomosis of the thoracodorsal artery with the superior gluteal artery. Donor site closure was performed with mesh graft.

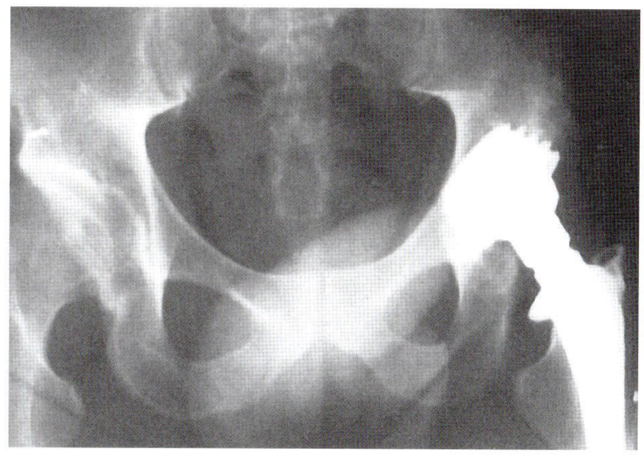

Figure 6.39e Three months after the flap procedure a hip prosthesis was implanted by the orthopedic surgeon.

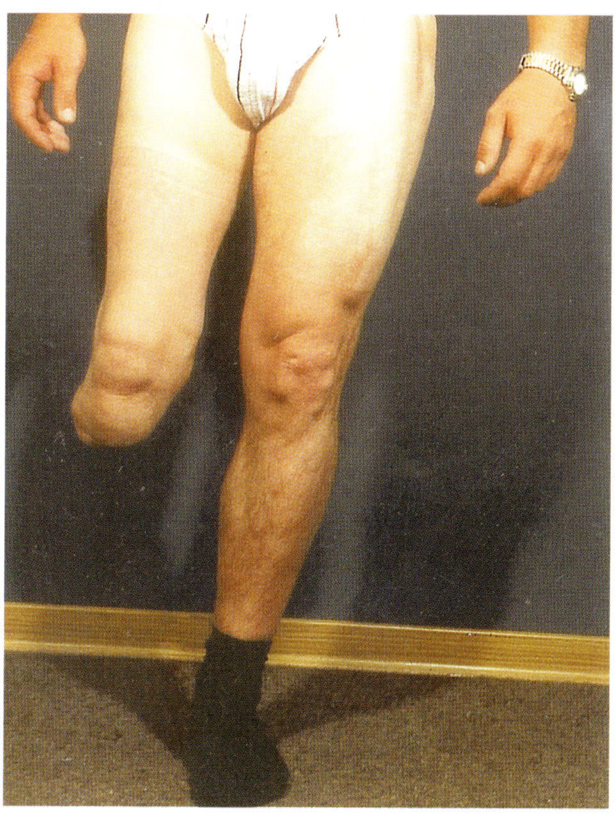

Figure 6.39f Three months after hip prosthesis there is unrestricted weight bearing.

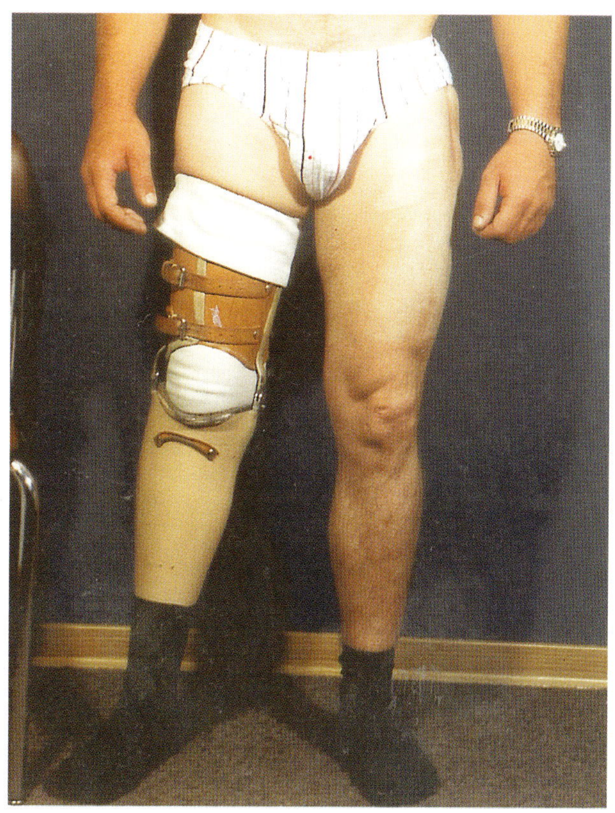

Figure 6.39g Right lower leg prosthesis was fitted and the patient is now able to walk.

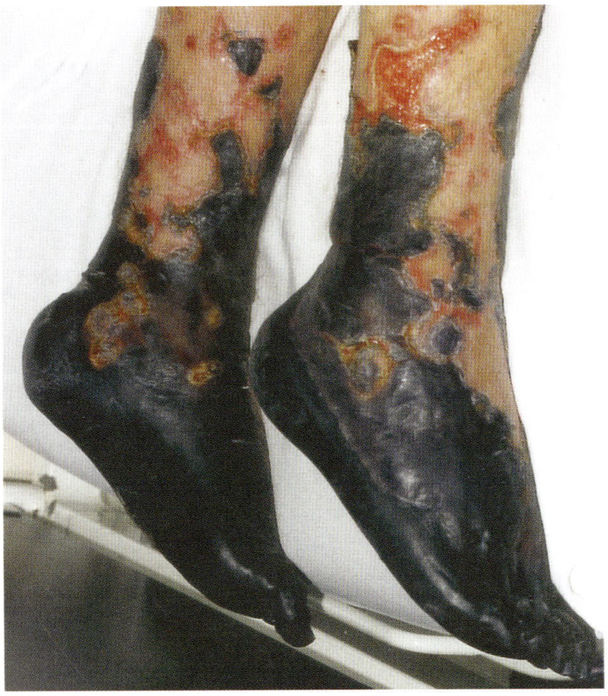

Figure 6.40a Necrosis of both feet after meningococcal septicemia. There was necrosis of the skin, almost all parts of the toes, subcutaneous tissue, dorsal and plantar muscles and tendons and the lateral and medial ankle.

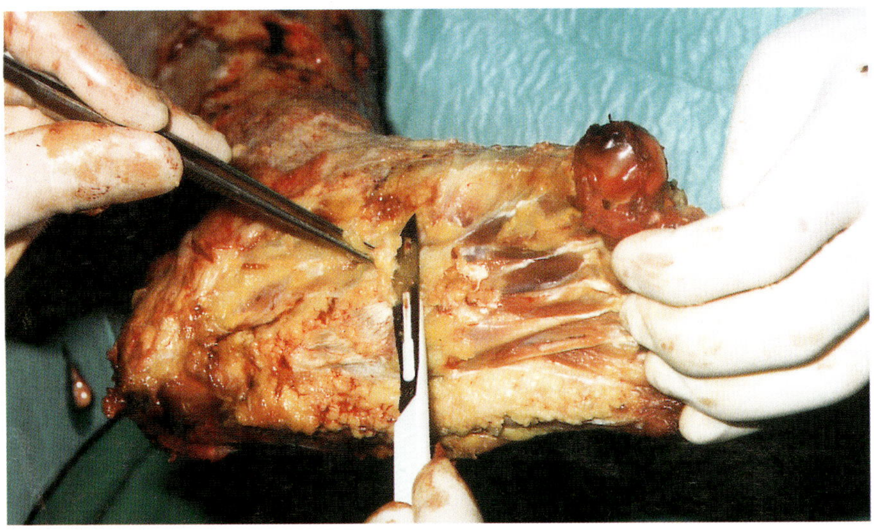

Figure 6.40b Initially radical debridement was performed. All the toes had to be amputated; skin and subcutaneous tissue were debrided up to the distal third of the lower leg. Resection of the extensor and flexor muscles, tendons including a part of the Achilles tendon.

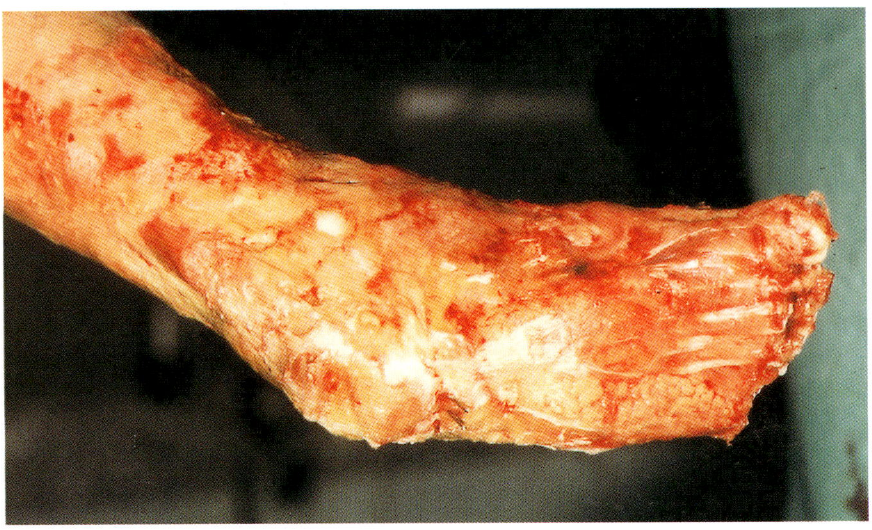

Figure 6.40c Only well perfused tissue were left

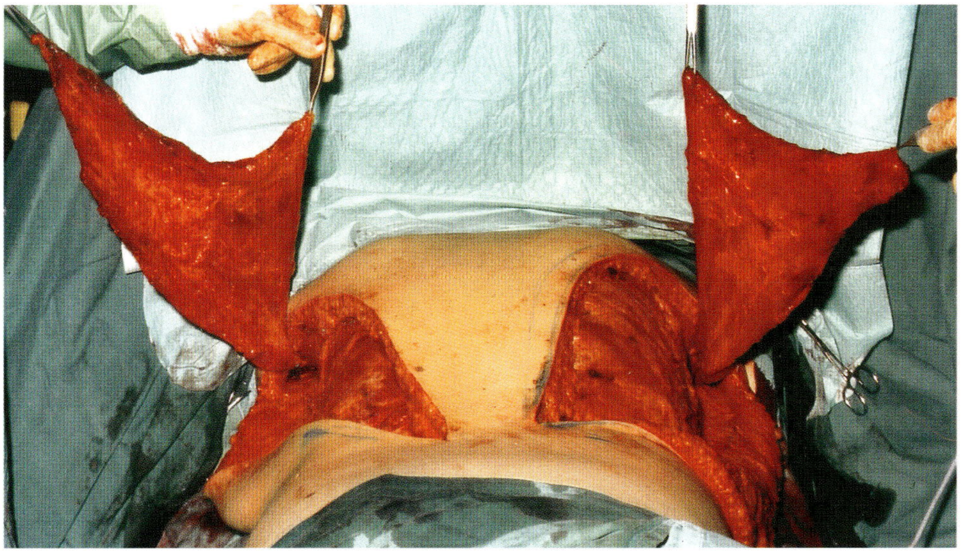

Figure 6.40d Both latissimus dorsi muscles were elevated without a skin island and separated from the humeral bone.
The thoracodorsal vessels were dissected as far proximal as possible to create a long vascular pedicle.

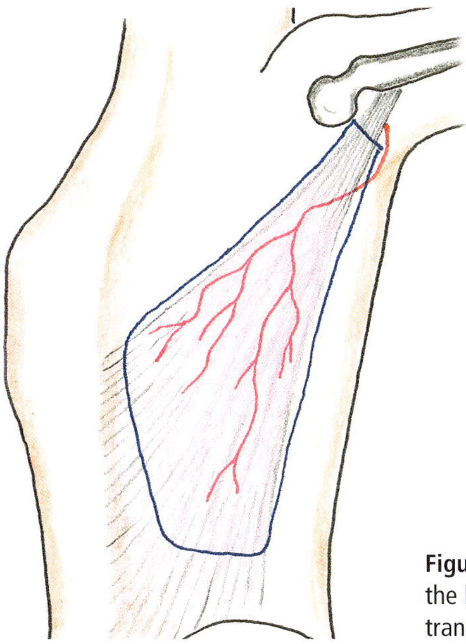

Figure 6.40e Preparation of the latissimus dorsi muscle for transplantation

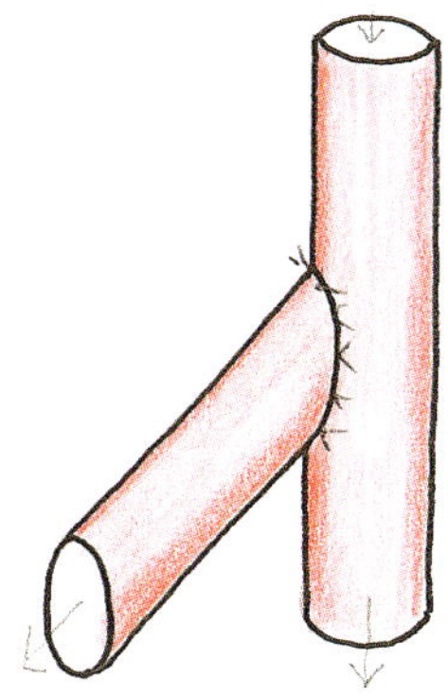

Figure 6.40g End-to-side anastomosis preserves a good perfusion of the foot.

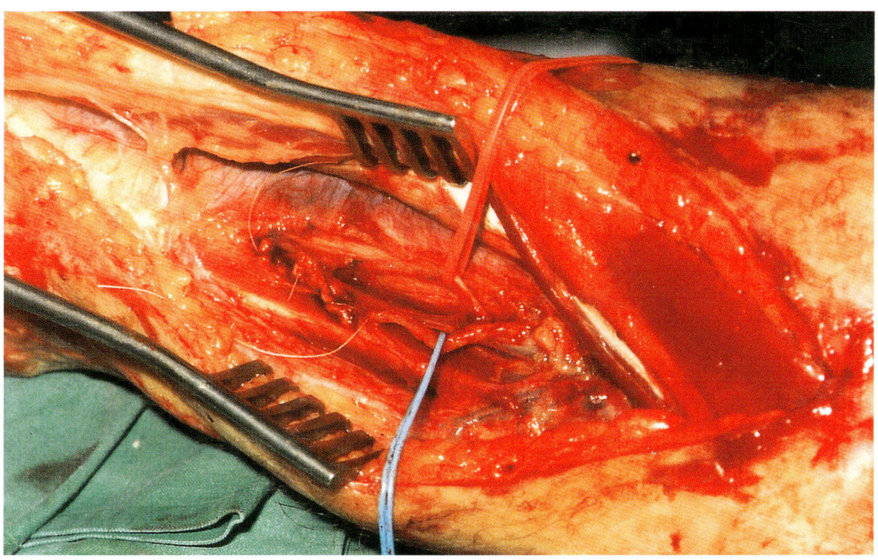

Figure 6.40f Anastomosis was performed between the thoracodorsal artery and vein and the posterior tibial vessels, end to side, in order to preserve the perfusion of the foot so the posterior tibial artery remained intact. The anastomosis was sited as proximal as possible.
One should never perform anastomosis in infected, irradiated or atrophic area.

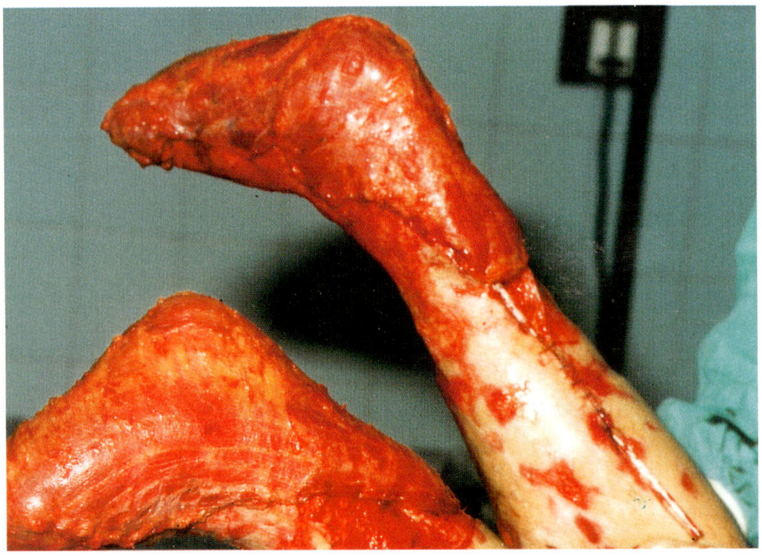

Figure 6.40h Both latissimus dorsi muscles are sufficient to cover the large defects.

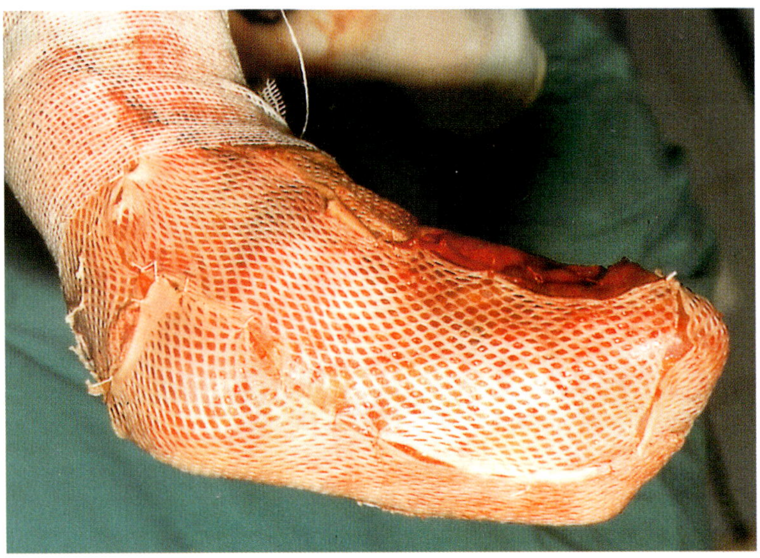

Figure 6.40i At the end of the operation both latissimus dorsi muscles were covered with meshed split thickness skin grafts and no skin island was used. The whole operation for both sides lasted 13 hours.

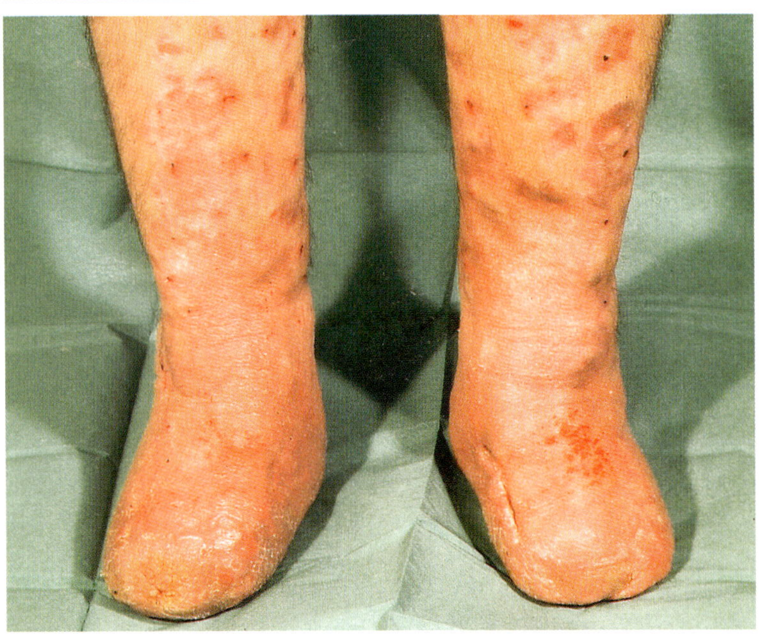

Figure 6.40j Situation three months after operation. Long-term studies of latissimus dorsi free flaps shows that are transplanted to the sole of the foot show better results if the muscle is covered with a meshed split thickness skin graft.
A well fitting orthopedic shoe is essential to prevent pressure ulcers.

Free Bone Transplantation

a) Free Vascularized Fibula Bone Transfer

The vascularized fibula bone flap is used to reconstruct larger bone defects (over 10 cm). A vascularized fibula bone graft has less resorption than to standard bone grafting.

Removal of the fibular bone causes little impairment of the function of the lower leg as long as at least 8 to 10 cm of the distal fibula remains in place to stabilize the ankle.

The transplant can be used as a composite flap if the lateral soleus muscle and the overlying skin (supplied by the peroneal artery) are included in the flap.

Blood supply is assured by the peroneal artery and the small nutrient vessels which enter the proximal and middle third of the fibula.

Perfusion of the fibula bone is much better if the periosteum and a circular muscle cuff (flexor hallucis longus muscle) are included in the transplant.

Through a lateral approach the fascia is incised and dissection is continued between the soleus and peroneus brevis muscle.

The lateral surface of the fibula is identified after the soleus muscle is dissected. The interosseus fascia is incised longitudinally on its ventral surface. After mobilization of the flexor hallucis longus muscle the peroneal artery and vein are identified.

Only in the area of the bone resection is the periosteum incised.

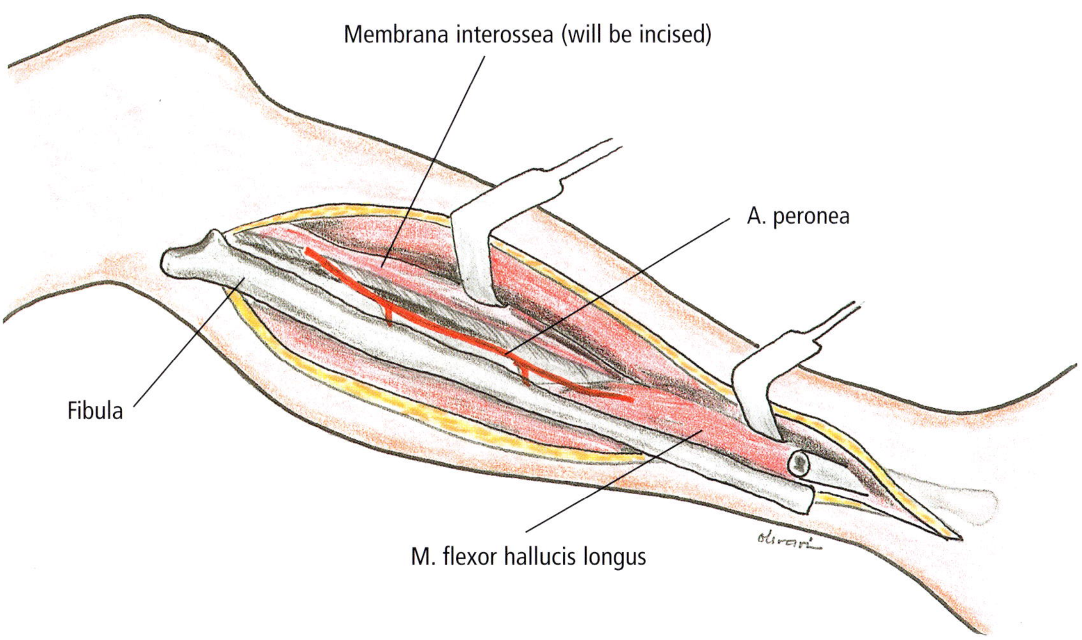

Figure 6.41 Elevation of a vascularized fibula flap. There is a better perfusion of the fibula bone if it is removed as a composite flap with a small muscle cuff consisting of parts of flexor hallucis longus. Almost the whole fibula bone including its head can be removed but at least 8 to 10 cm of the distal part of the bone have to stay in place to preserve the function of the ankle.

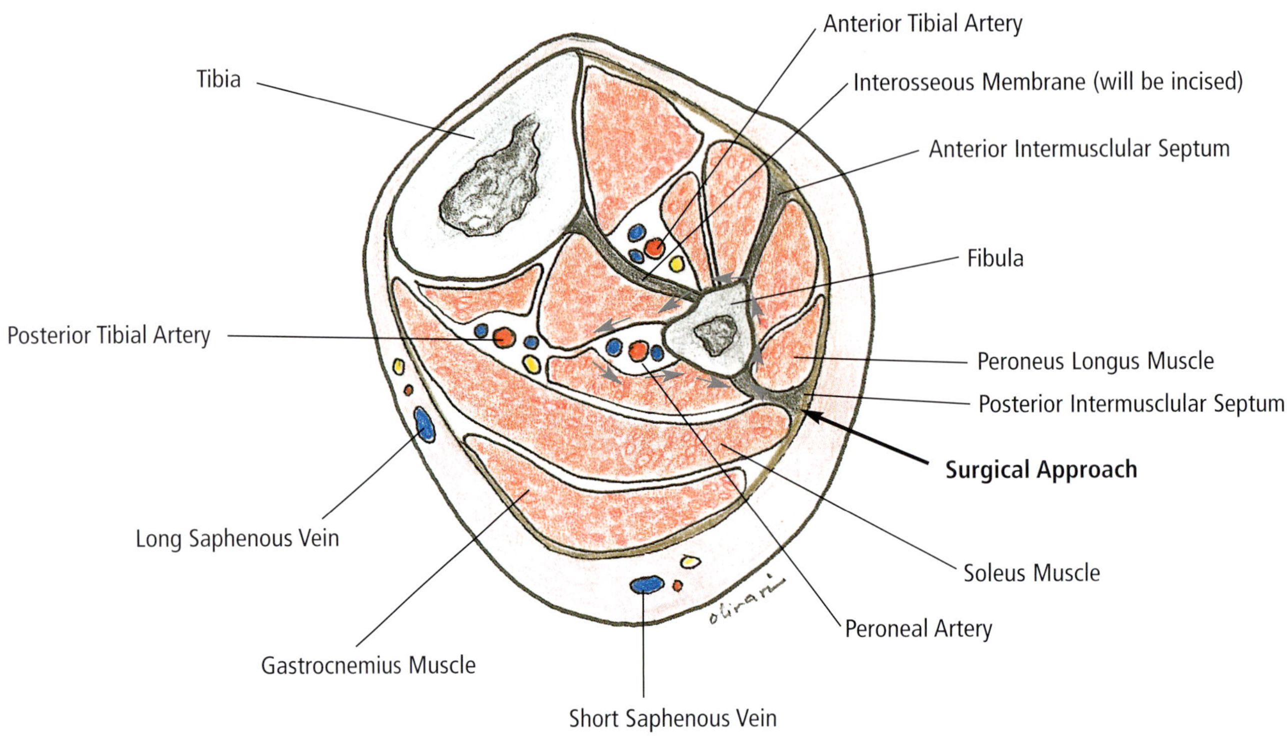

Figure 6.42a Cross section of the middle part of the lower leg for a free fibula flap (the arrow shows the surgical approach and the amount of resection).

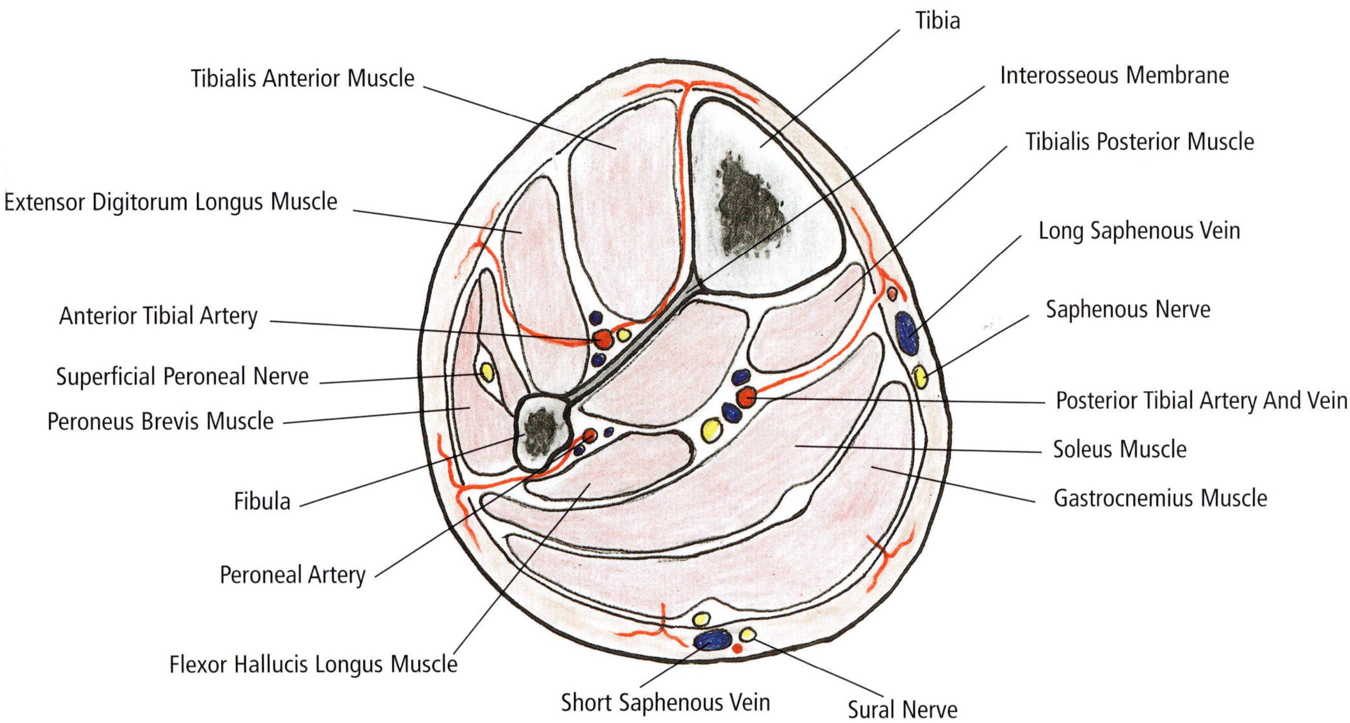

Figure 6.42b Blood supply of the skin of the lower leg

Free Fibula Transfer

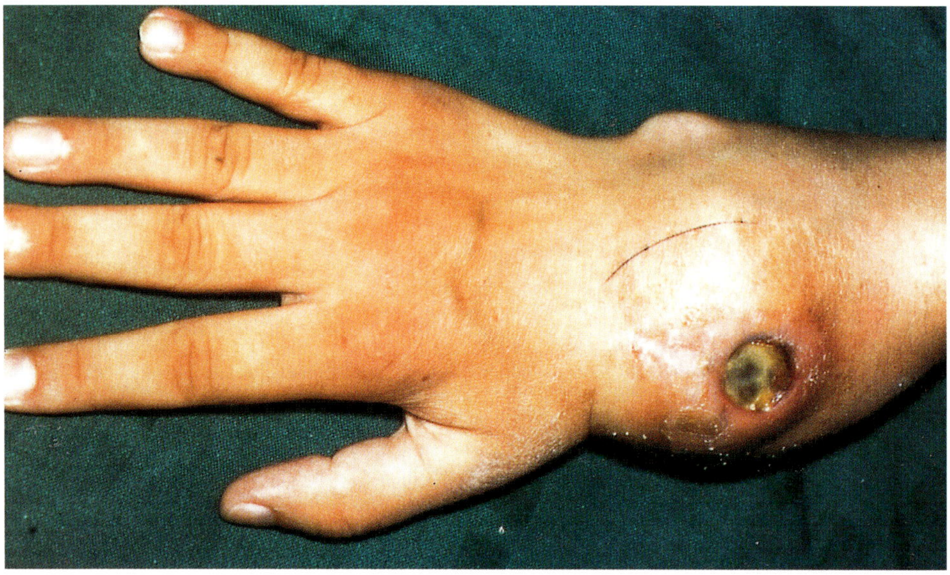

Figure 6.43a Giant cell tumor of the distal part of the radial bone

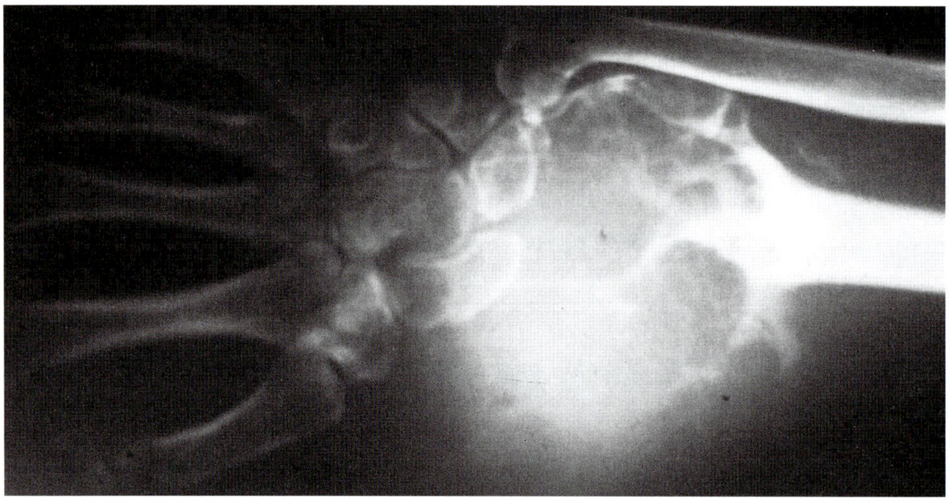

Figure 6.43b X-ray analysis shows no tumor infiltration of ulna and carpal bones

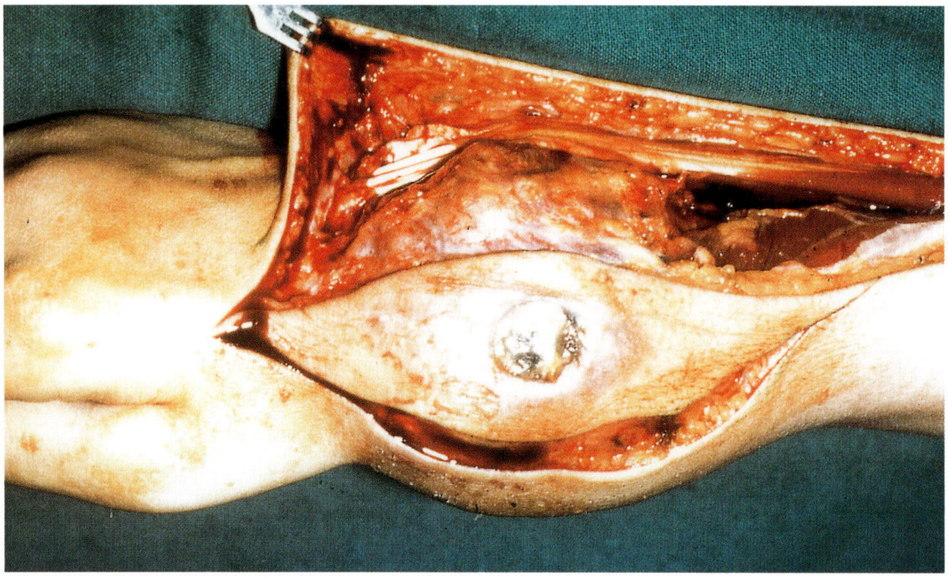

Figure 6.43c En-bloc resection of the tumor and the distal part of the radial bone

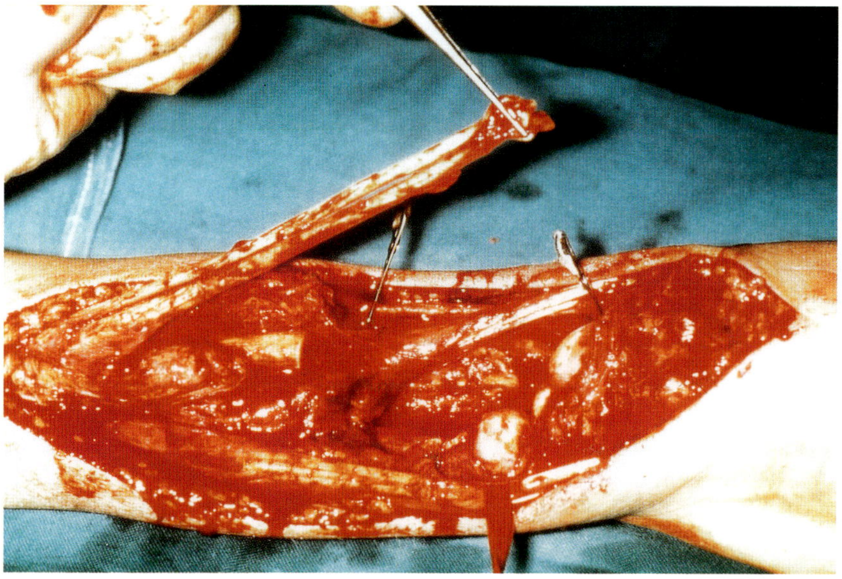

Figure 6.43d Elevation of a vascularized fibula

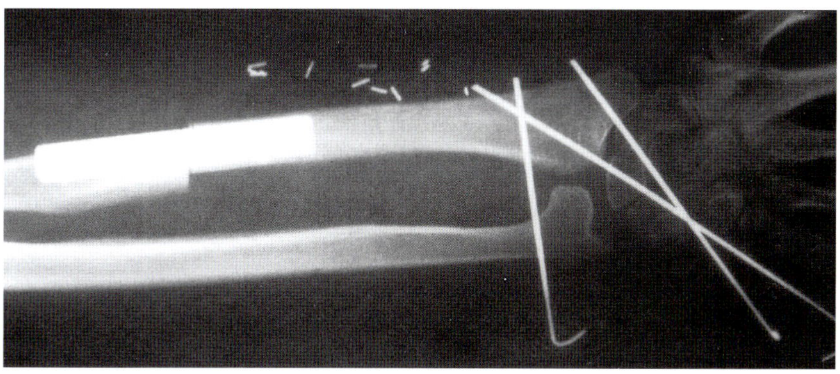

Figure 6.43e The fibula is removed from the right lower leg and fixed to the radial diaphysis using a plate. Fixation to the carpal bones and the ulna is done using K-wires. Microsurgical anastomosis is performed between the peroneal and radial artery and their concomitant veins.

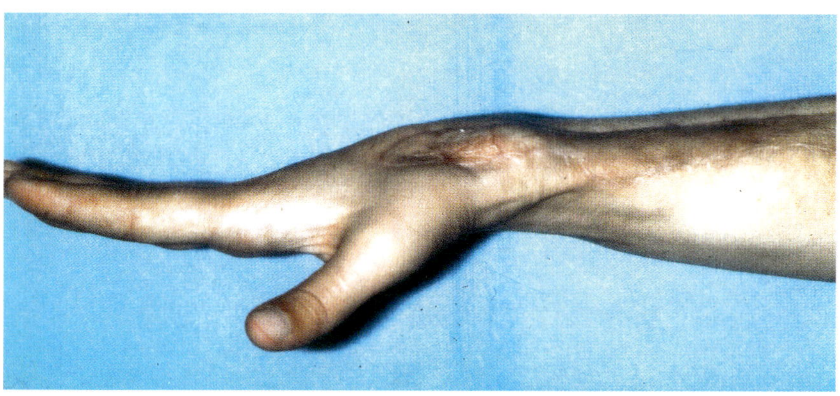

Figure 6.43f One year postoperatively

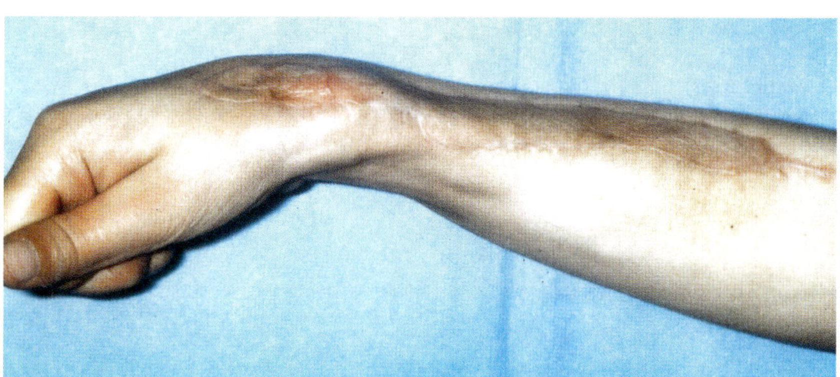

Figure 6.43g Functional result

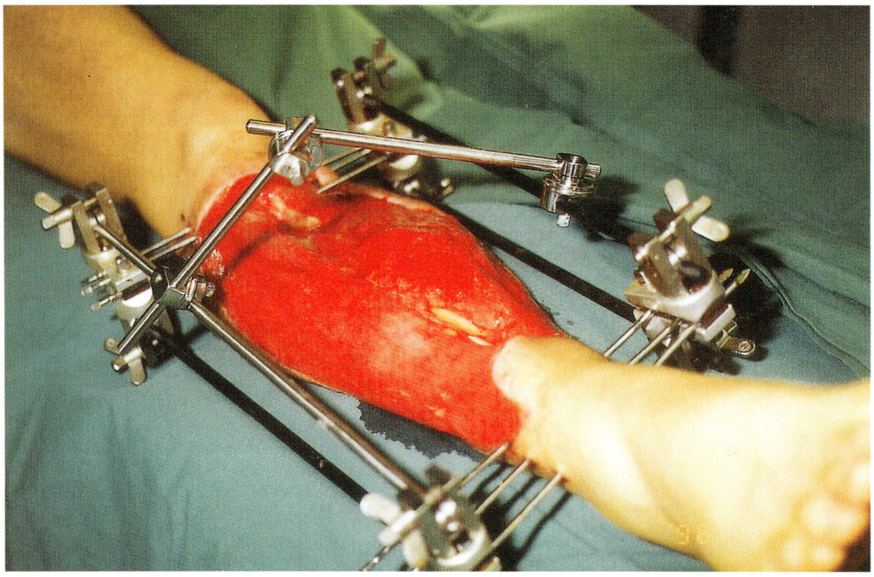

Figure 6.44a Third-degree open fracture of the right lower leg with a large soft tissue defect and a 21 cm long tibial bone defect

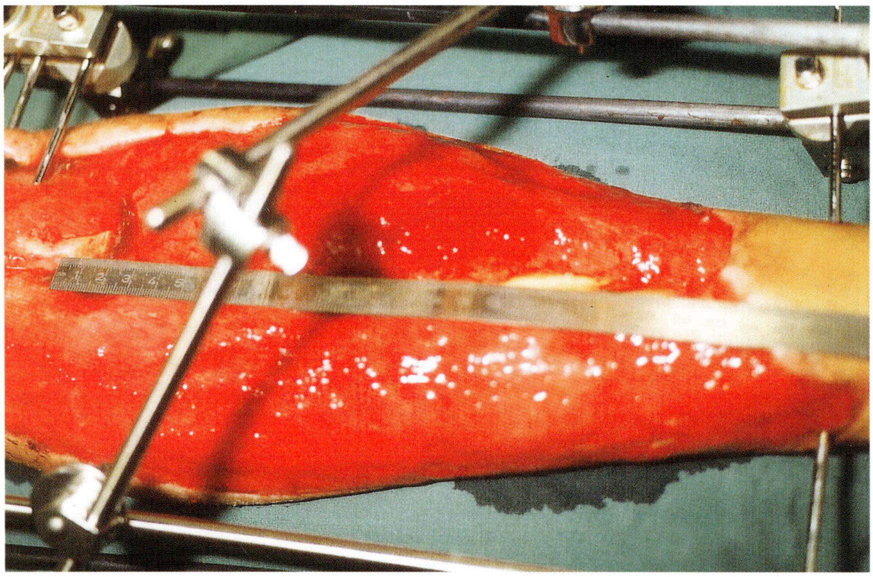

Figure 6.44b Distance of the fragments is conserved by the use of external fixation.

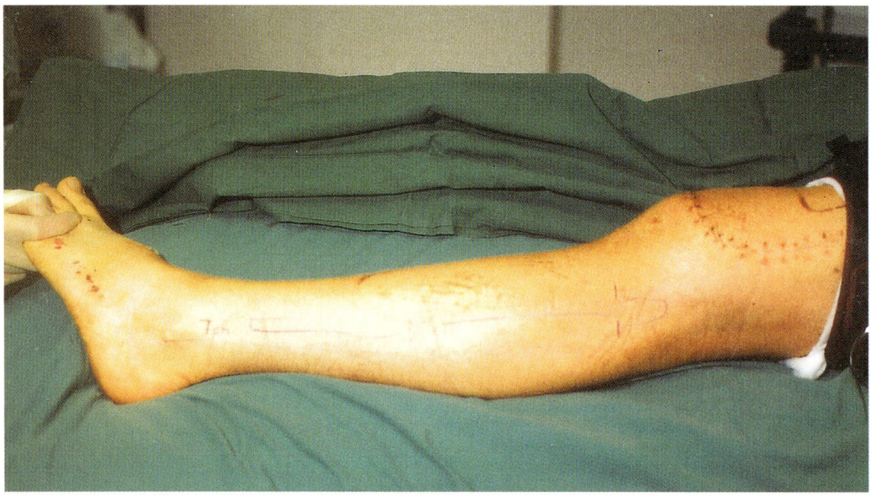

Figure 6.44c Planning of an osteomyocutaneus fibula flap from the contralateral side

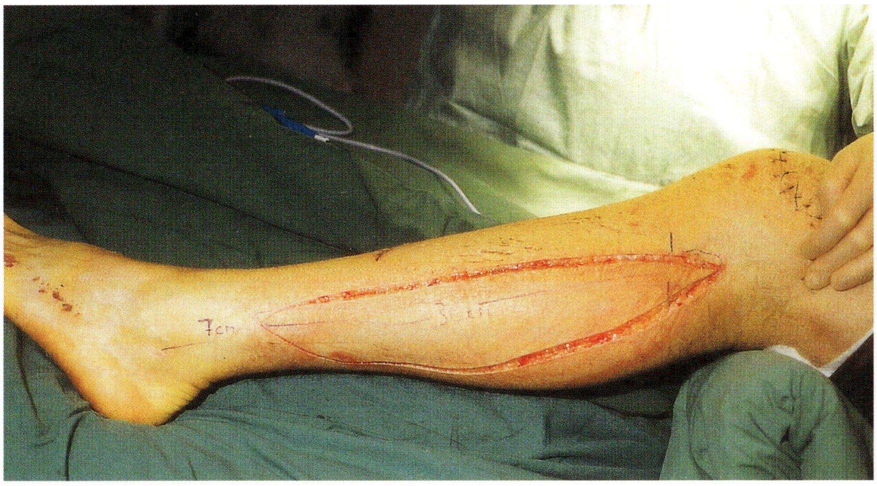

Figure 6.44d Surgical approach to elevate the osteomyocutaneus fibula flap

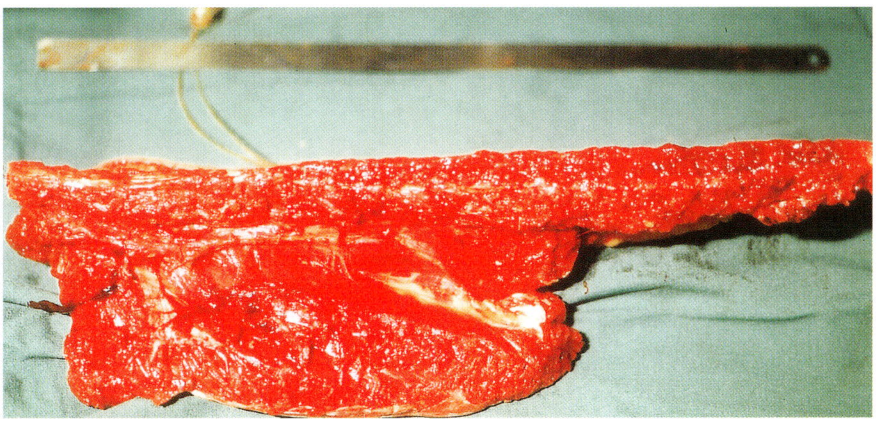

Figure 6.44e It is important to elevate the fibula in combination with a surrounding muscle cuff for a better blood supply of the bone although small branches of the peroneal artery enter the bone directly.

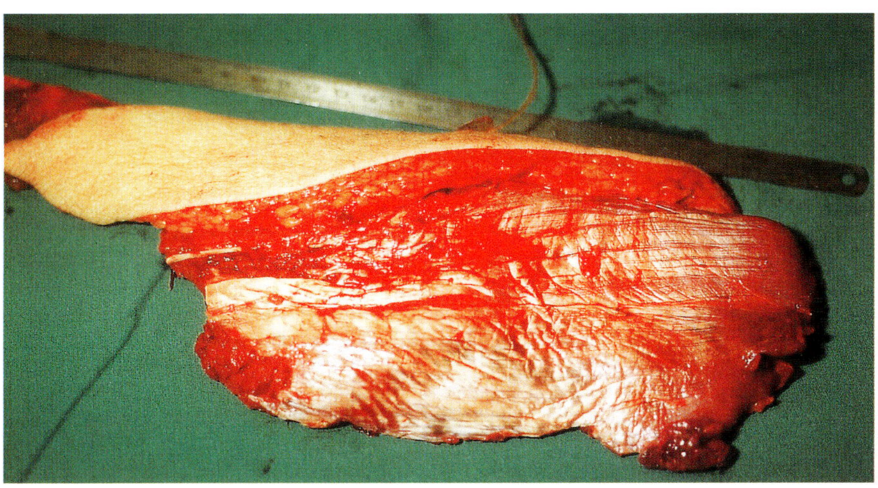

Figure 6.44f In this case the fibula transplant is elevated as an osteomyocutaneus flap including the overlying skin and the soleus, posterior tibial and flexor hallucis longus muscle to cover the defect of the right lower leg.

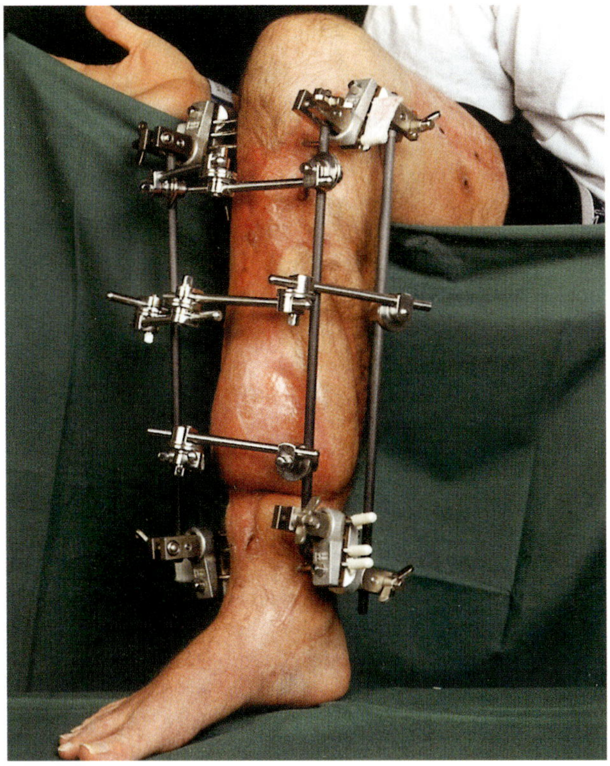

Figure 6.44g After nine months of fixation physiotherapy was initiated without weight bearing for six months. Then a gradual increase in weight bearing was allowed until full movement and weight bearing was achieved.

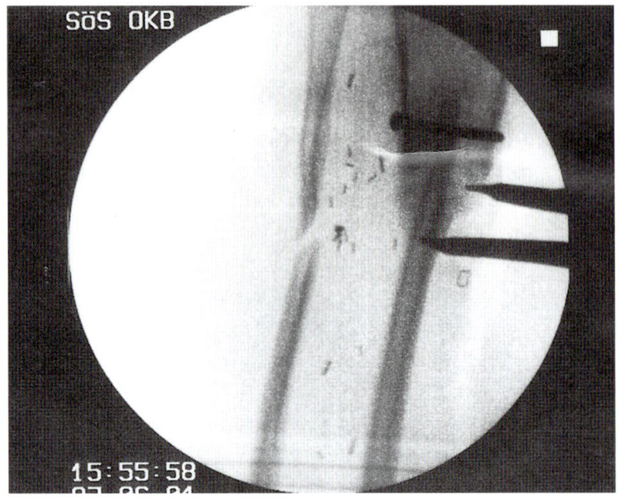

Figure 6.44h For tibia reconstruction the fibula bone was fixed into the intramedullary cavity of the tibia.

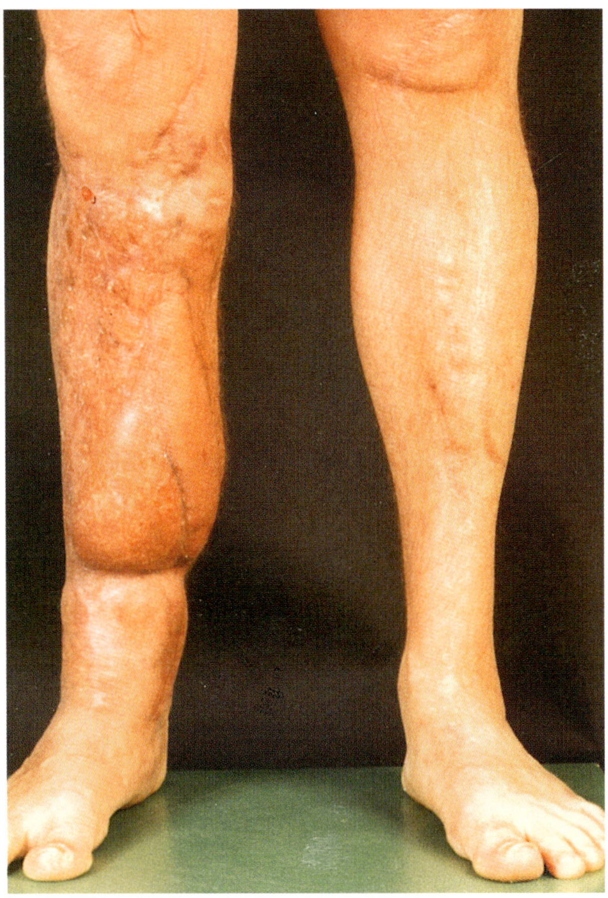

Figure 6.44i Two years postoperatively. The patient is walking with full weight bearing on the two fibula bones.

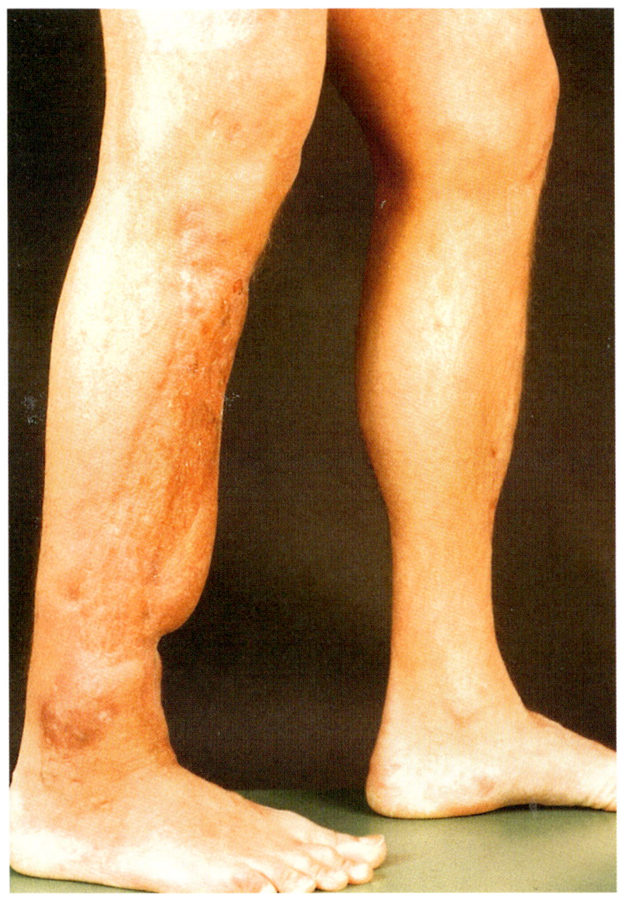

Figure 6.44j Lateral aspect two years postoperatively: Due to concerns of venous insufficiency the elevation of the fibula in combination with the soleus muscle is indicated only for difficult reconstruction of the lower leg.

Cross-Leg Flap

The cross-leg flap is the traditional method to cover defects of the lower leg and foot. It is today only used occasionally due to a long immobilization period and unstable perfusion of the flap.

There remain indications for this technically easy operative procedure in parts of the world where free flap procedures are not available. In the preoperative planning of the flap it is essential to achieve a good blood supply by including fascia.

Immobilization in a plaster cast or by external fixation should last for three to four weeks. Then the pedicle is compressed with using a soft intestinal clamp to ensure that there is a good blood supply from the recipient site. If there are any doubts immobilization can be prolonged for another week.

For coverage of defects over the Achilles tendon a donor site below the popliteal space is favoured. The donor site can be closed using a local flap and is therefore cosmetically advantageous.

Older patients or patients with varicosis or vein thrombosis are unsuitable for this procedure.

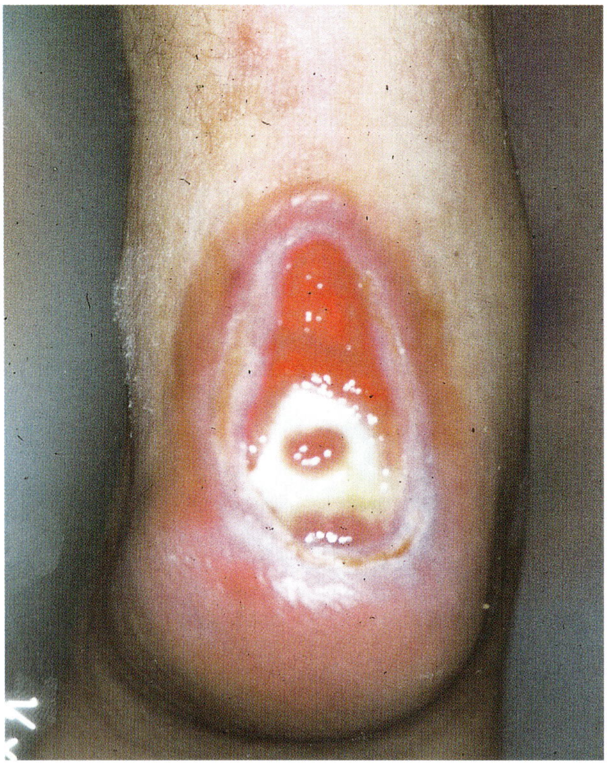

Figure 6.45a Pressure ulcer of the left heel after plaster cast immobilization. First the ulcer was excised.

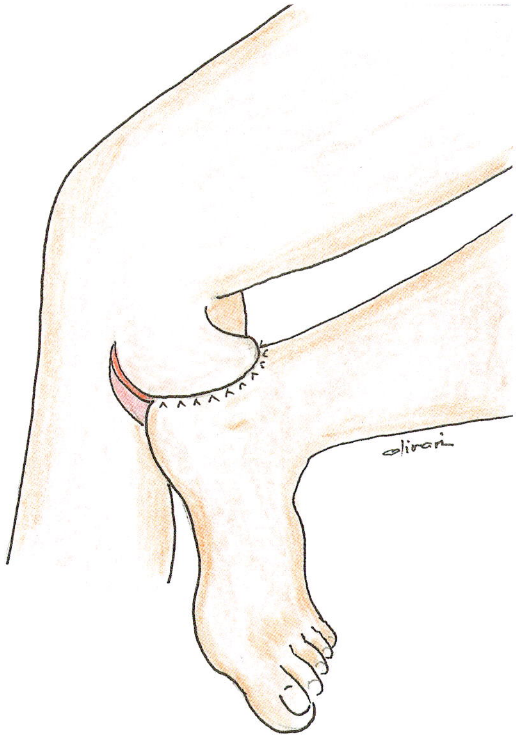

Figure 6.45b The fasciocutaneous flap is protected in this position for four weeks using external fixation.

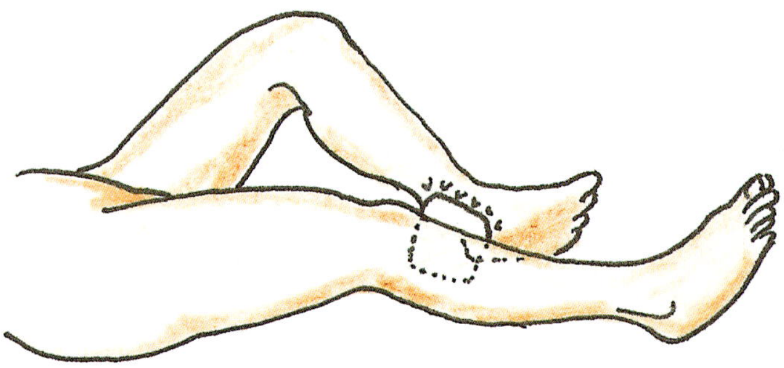

Figure 6.45c The cross-leg flap is elevated in the proximal third of the lower leg as a fasciocutaneous flap. The donor site is favoured for small defects as it can be closed primarily by local flap and skin grafting is unnecessary.

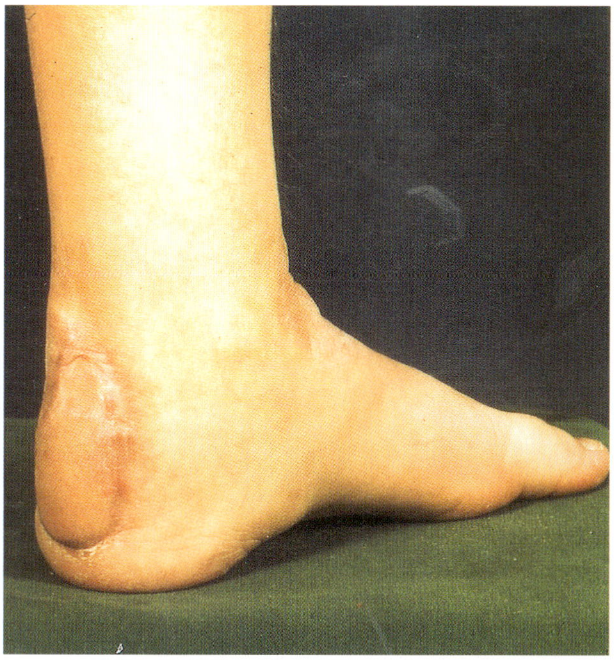

Figure 6.45d 18 months postoperatively

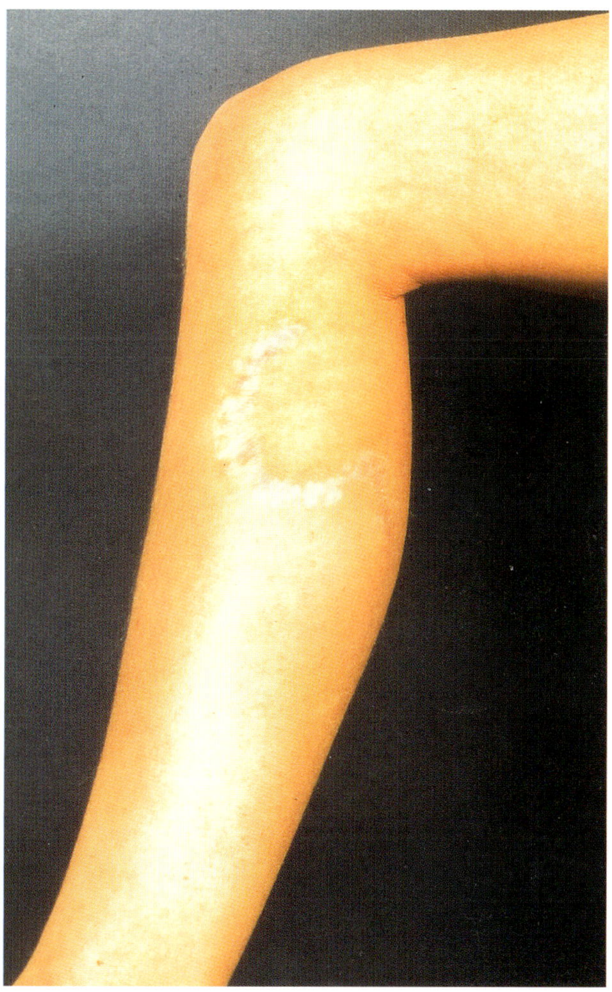

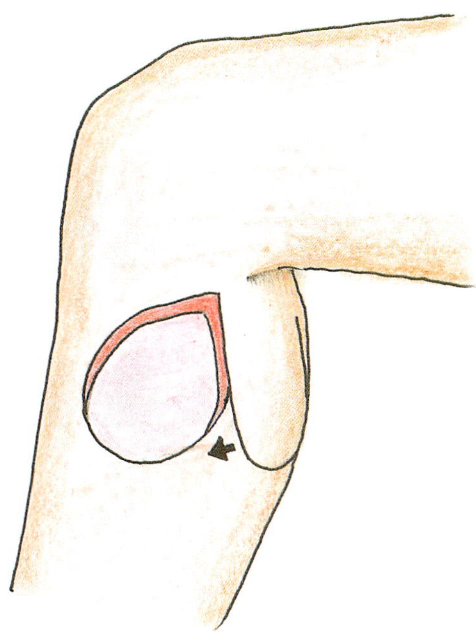

Figure 6.45e, f The donor site is closed using a local flap. A better cosmetic result is achieved than with a skin graft.

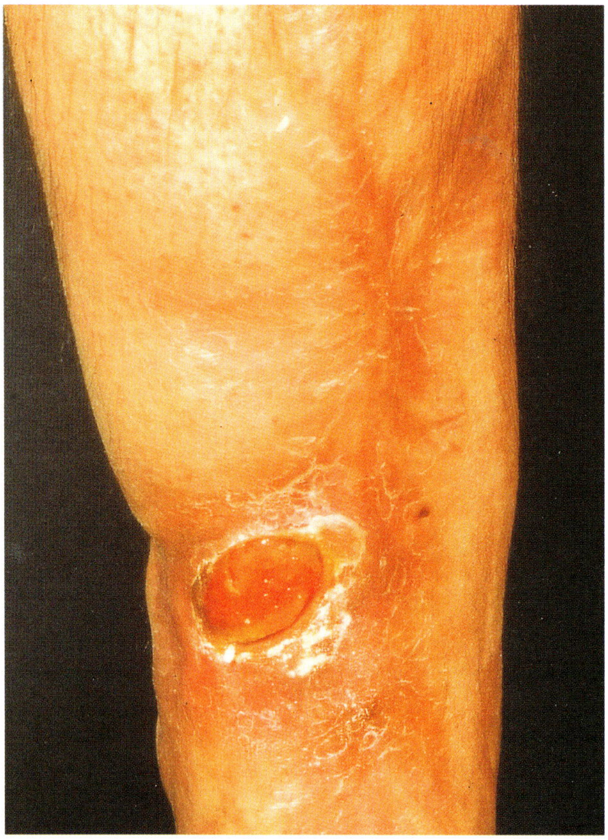

Figure 6.46a Chronic ulceration following soft tissue injury of the right lower leg

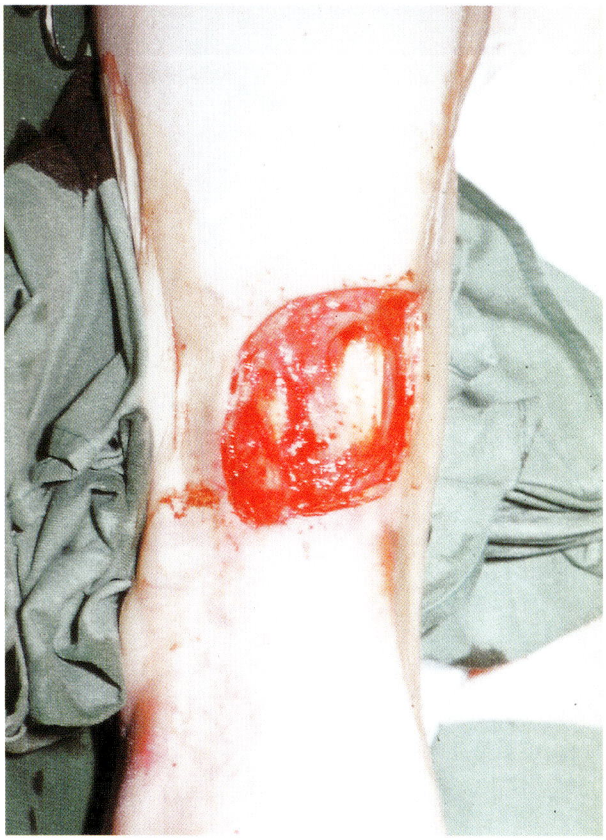

Figure 6.46b Radical debridement. The surrounding scar tissue is removed as well. The tibial bone is exposed.

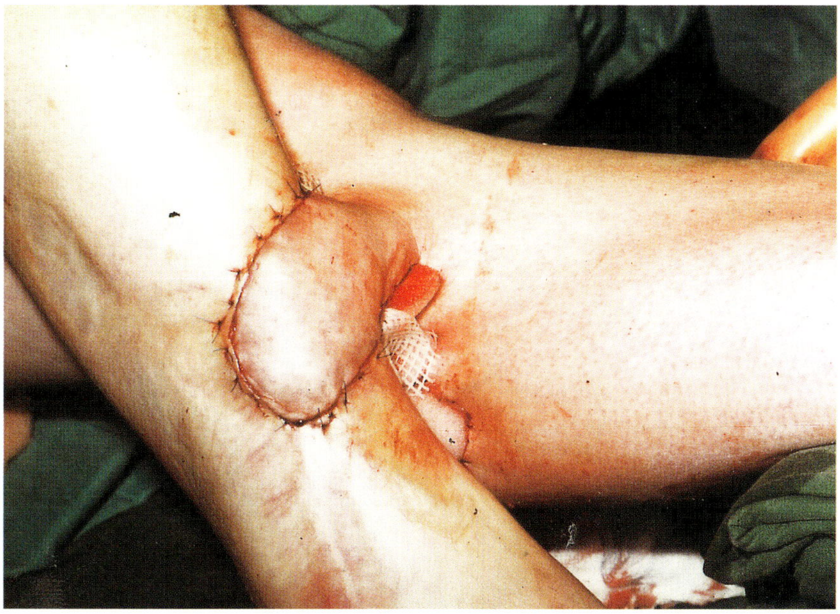

Figure 6.46c A fasciocutaneous cross-leg flap is elevated below the popliteal space. For four weeks the legs are immobilized in a relatively relaxed position. The donor side is temporary closed using a mesh graft.

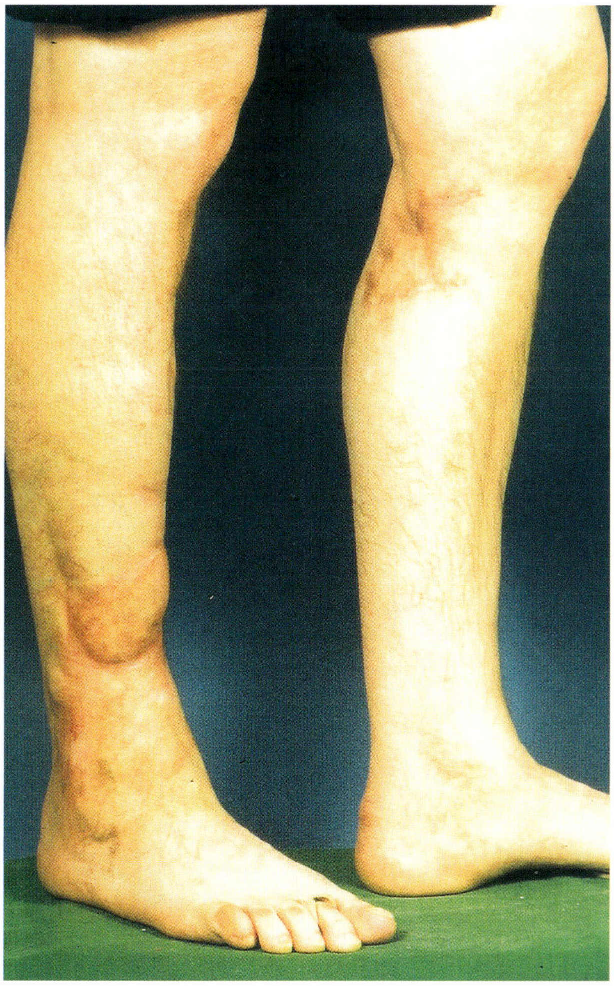

Figure 6.46d Nine months postoperatively. An inconspicuous scar results after donor side closure with a local flap.

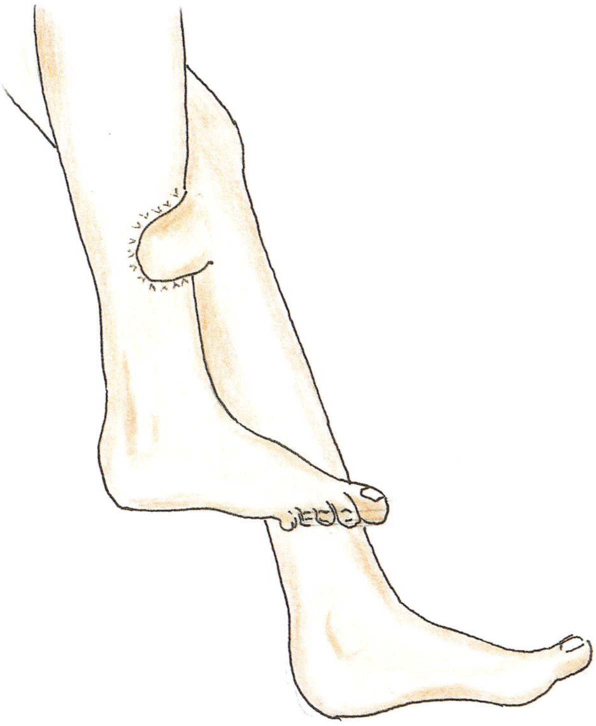

Figure 6.46e Both legs were immobilized with external fixation in this position for three to four weeks.

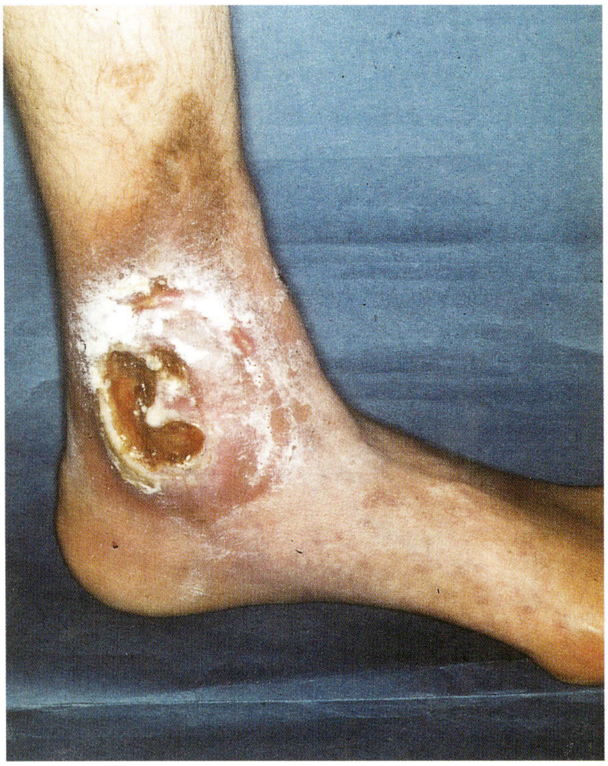

Figure 6.47a Posttraumatic ulceration of the right ankle for two years

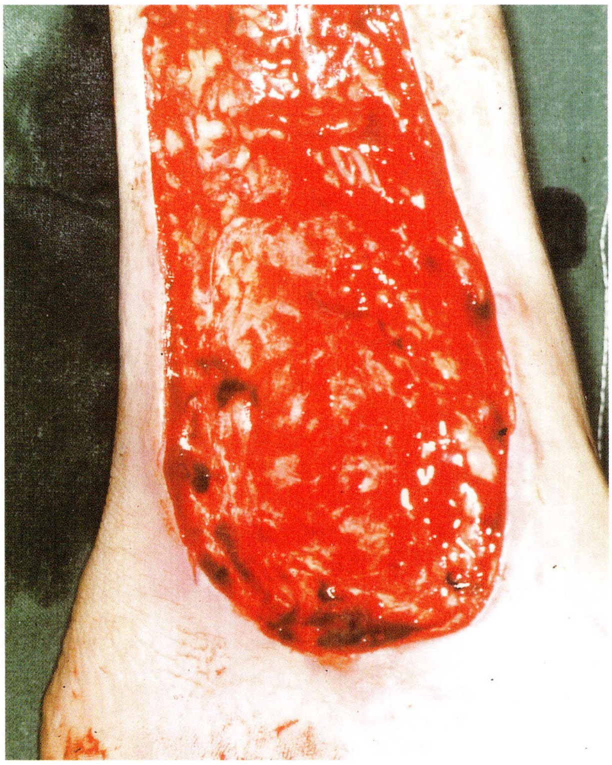

Figure 6.47b Radical debridement of the necrotic and infected tissue and the surrounding hypoperfused area

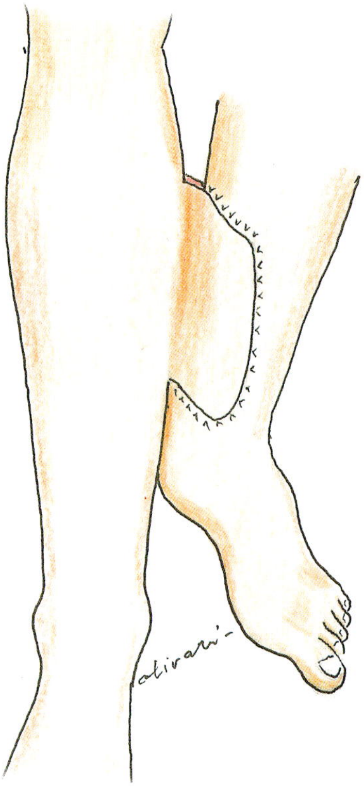

Figure 6.47c Position of the external fixation

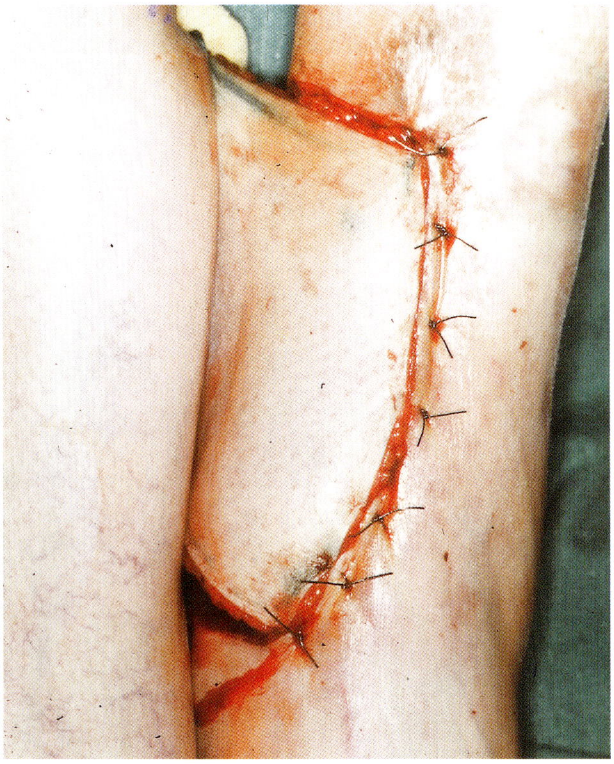

Figure 6.47d The cross-leg flap as a fasciocutaneous flap

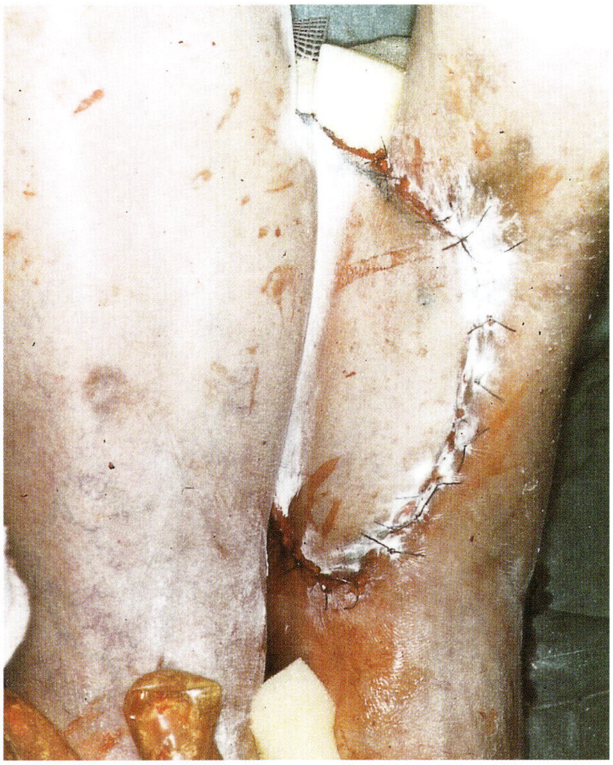

Figure 6.47e At the end of the operation. Four weeks later the pedicle is divided.

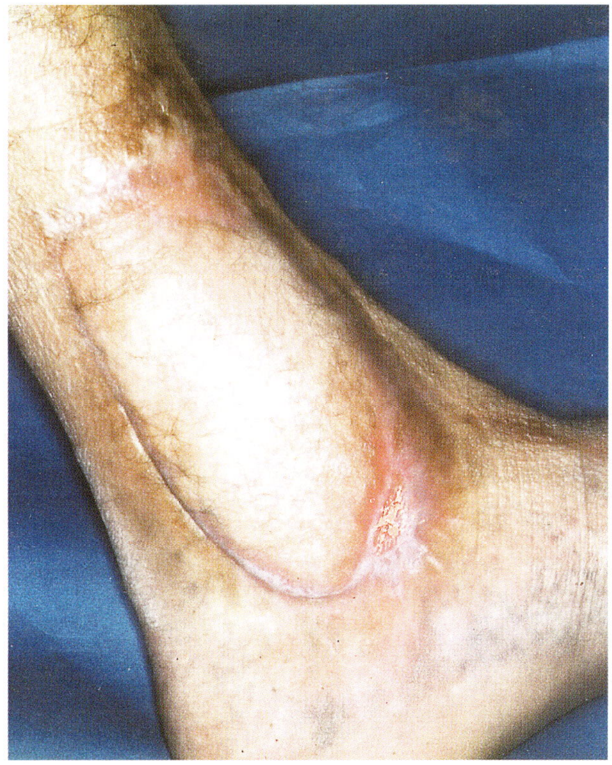

Figure 6.47f One year postoperatively. The patient wears compressive stockings for at least three months.

Expanders

The indication for the use of expansion on lower leg is limited. There is a high risk for nerve and/or blood vessel compression. Complications like infection of the implant, partial necrosis of skin or exposure of the implant occur in up to 40 % of cases. Additionally compartment syndrome can occur if tissue expansion is done too fast.

Therefore a strict monitoring of the patients after expander implantation is essential. If loss of sensation, movement or vascular impairment occurs the expander has to be deflated or removed.

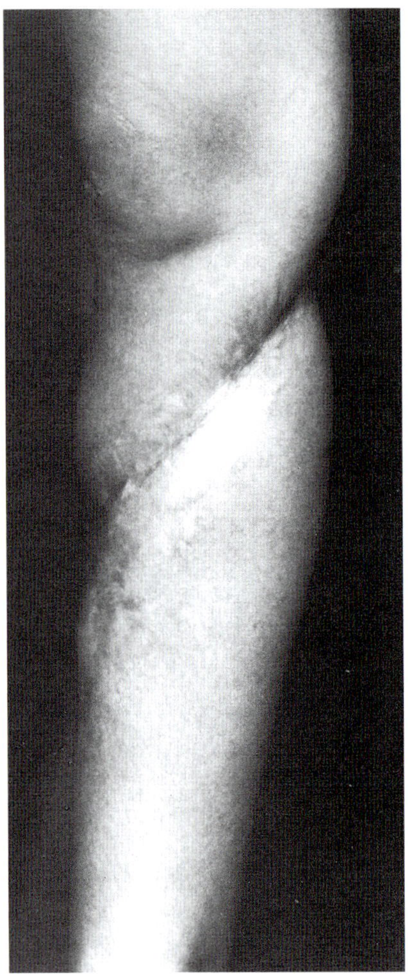

Figure 6.48a Spiral traumatic defect of the lower leg

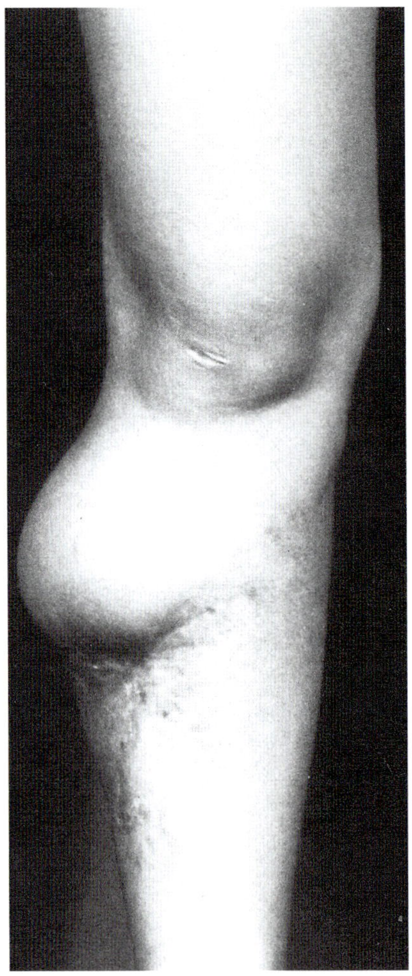

Figure 6.48b Epifascial implantation of an expansion device (350 ml) and slow filling over six weeks. The expansion device should not be implanted through a scar. The radial surgical approach should be far from the defect.

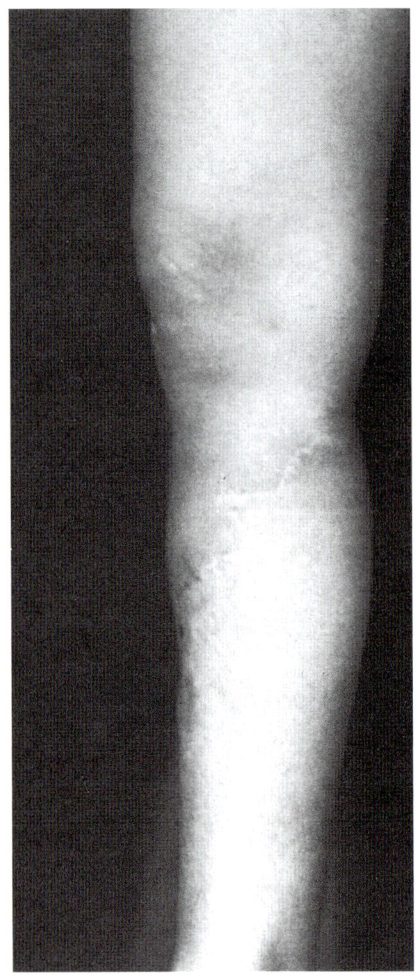

Figure 6.48c After six weeks the expander was removed and the defect was covered with the expanded healthy skin. The picture shows the result one year postoperatively.

Split-Thickness Skin Grafts

A surgeon who is expert at subtle techniques should never forget the simple methods. Skin graft is a well established method and is a convenient speedy procedure for the patient as well as for the surgeon. Often a split-thickness skin graft (mostly mesh graft) is indicated for temporary defect coverage particularly if infection is present.

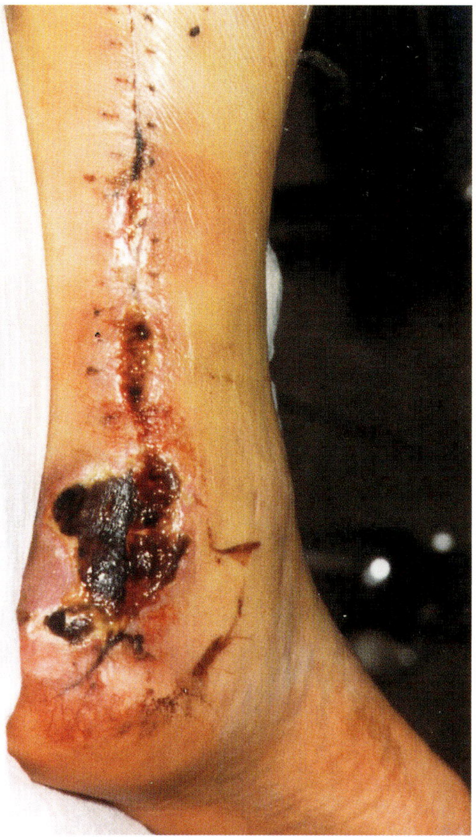

Figure 6.49a Necrosis of the left heel after osteosynthesis of the lower leg. Plan: After necrectomy the defect was covered with a meshed split-thickness skin graft. A reconstruction with a free flap was intended in the future.

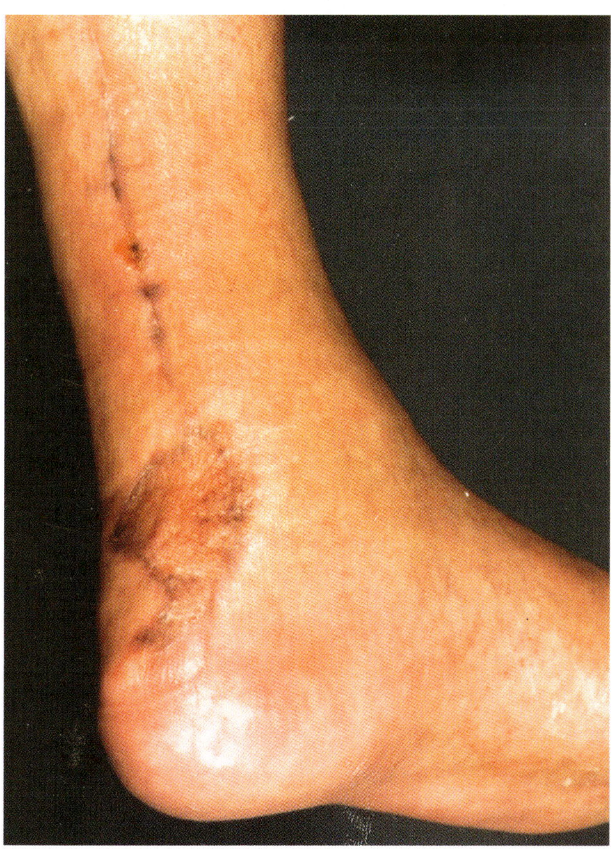

Figure 6.49b Four months postoperatively. Application of a split-thickness skin graft. Good functional result and a free flap procedure was not necessary. **Mind:** A simple procedure is often preferrable.

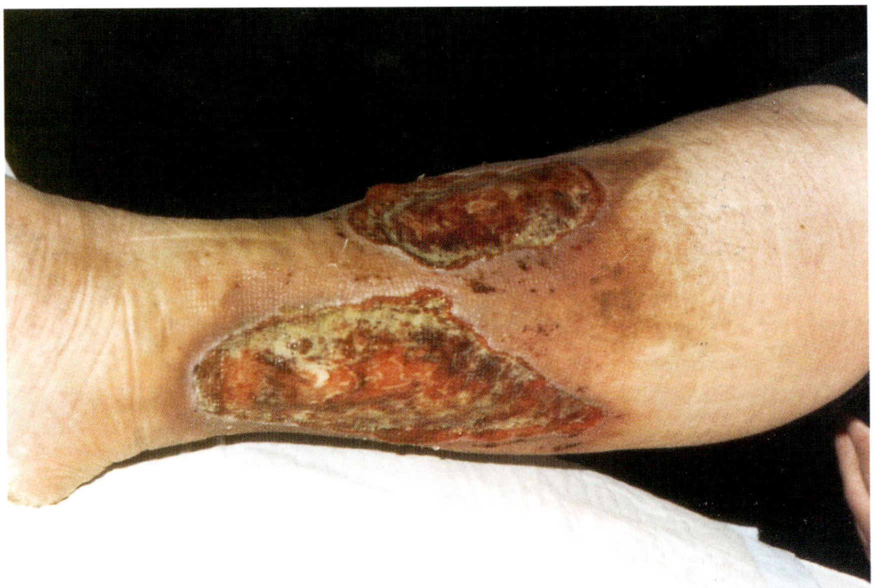

Figure 6.50a Chronic left ulcer (ulcus cruris) for two years. Prolonged infection, caused induration of the surrounding tissue and excessive edema: Dressing changes were performed twice a day for five days to clean the wound. Then a radical removal of all the dead tissue was performed until the fascial layer was reached. Meshed split-thickness skin grafting. After healing an improvement of the venous system is noted.

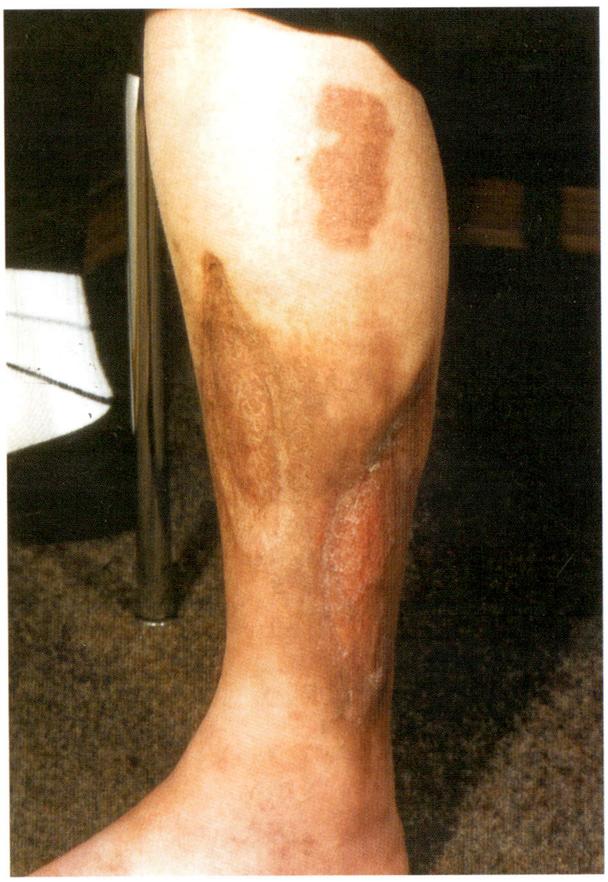

Figure 6.50b Six months postoperatively. The patient has to wear compressive stockings continuously otherwise a relapse can occur. The operation treats the symptoms rather then the basic problem. These patients need conservative treatment by a phlebologist.

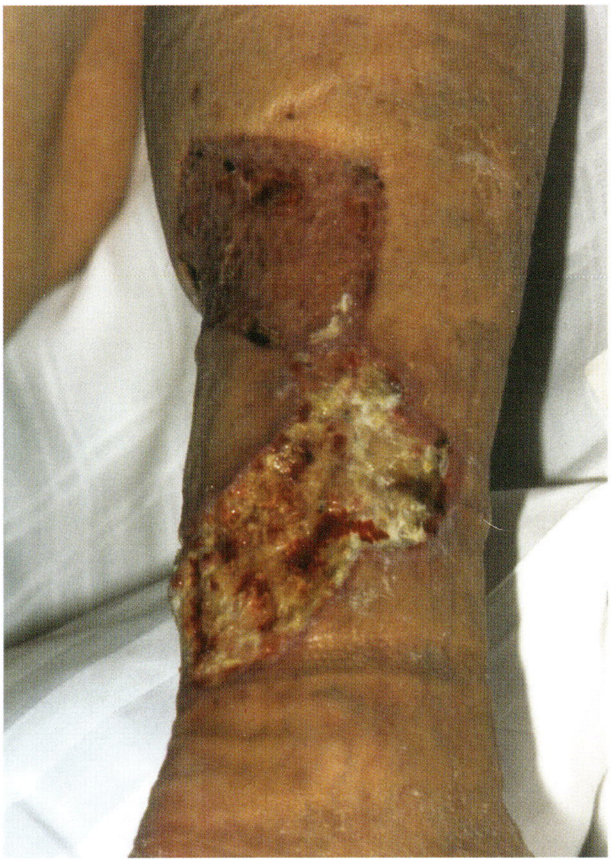

Figure 6.51a Relapse of a chronic ulcer of the right leg: An inadequate compression therapy was performed postoperatively. Operation: Necrectomy and meshed split-thickness skin grafting.

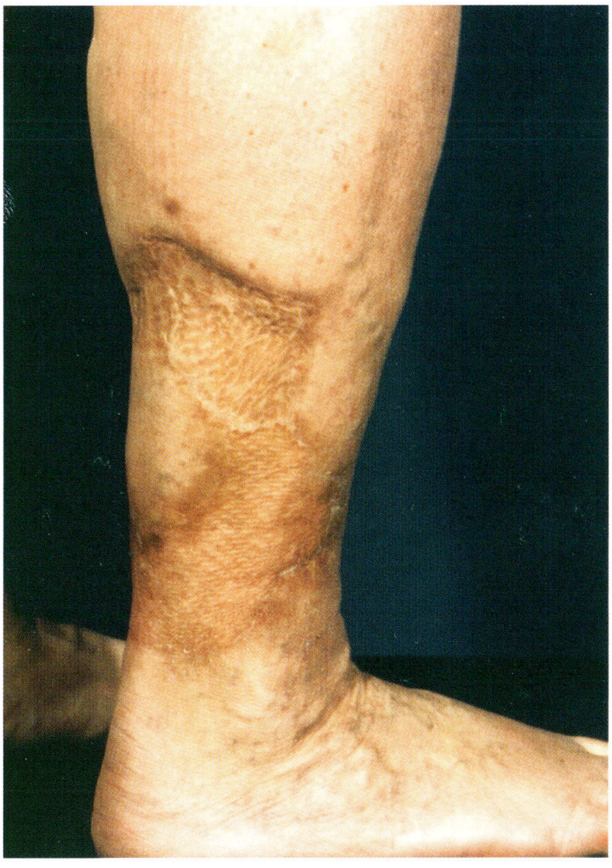

Figure 6.51b Three years postoperatively

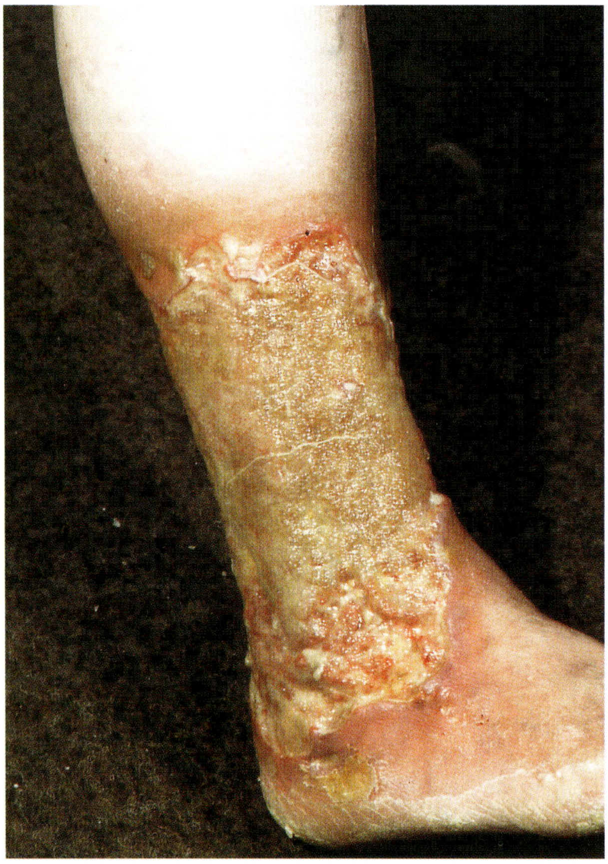

Figure 6.52a Infected "tree bark" chronic varicose ulcer.

Therapy: Twice a day the wound was washed with soap and afterwards Neomycin solution dressings were applied for one week. Excision of the whole area down to fascia was performed after one week. The defect was closed with a meshed split-thickness skin graft.

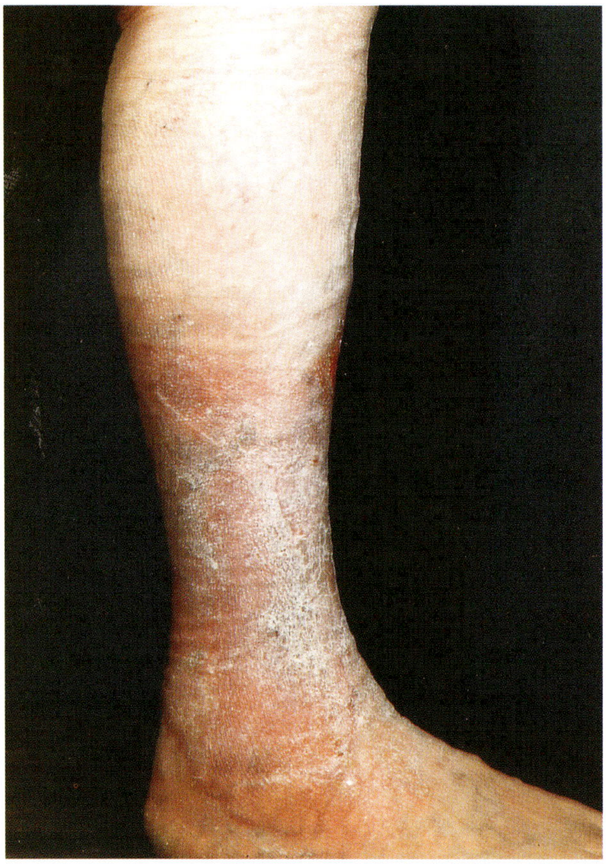

Figure 6.52b Six months postoperatively. The patient continues to wear compression stockings as otherwise there is a high incidence of relapse.

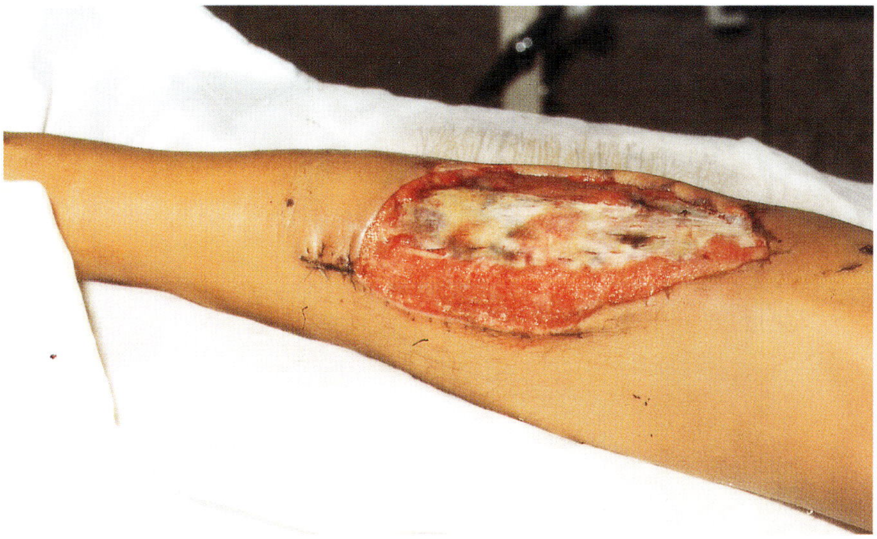

Figure 6.53a Post-traumatic skin defect on the right lower leg. Operation: Debridement, meshed split thickness skin grafting.

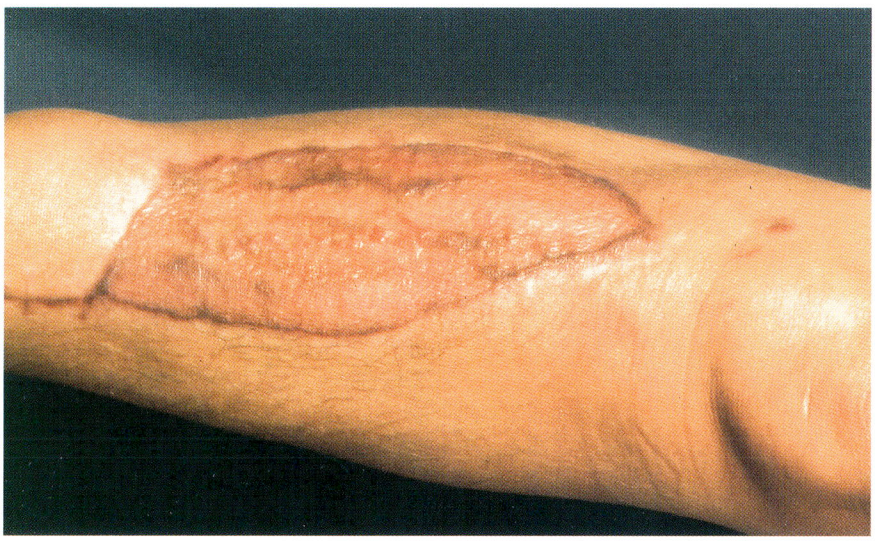

Figure 6.53b Six weeks postoperatively. The patient wears compression stockings continuously for three months.

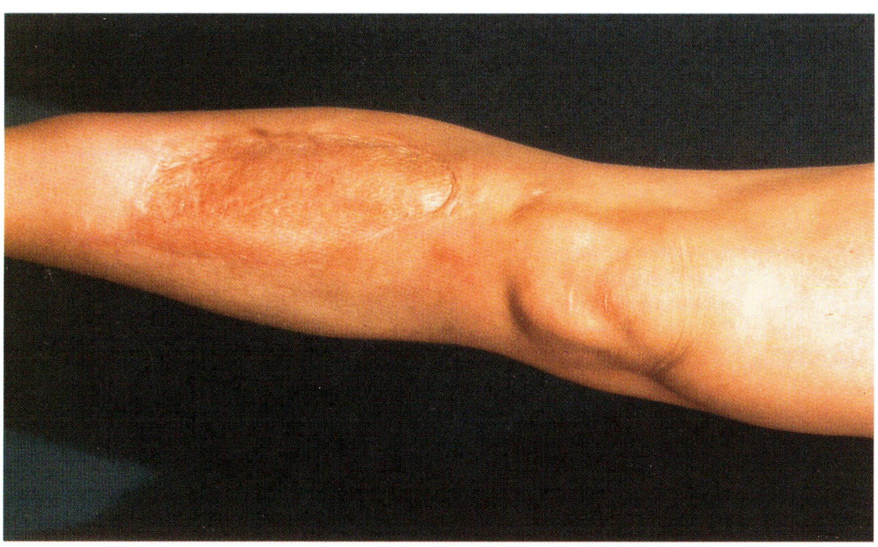

Figure 6.53c Two years postoperatively

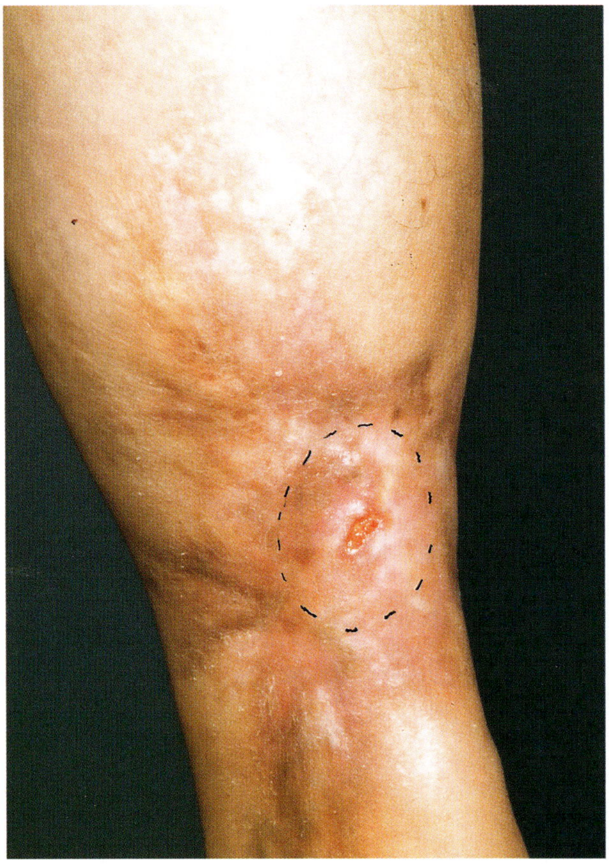

Figure 6.54a Chronic ulceration and painful scarring on the tibia. The patient refused any extensive surgery.

Remember: Sometimes simple methods are best! The ulceration and the scar tissue were excised and the defect was covered using a meshed split-thickness skin graft.

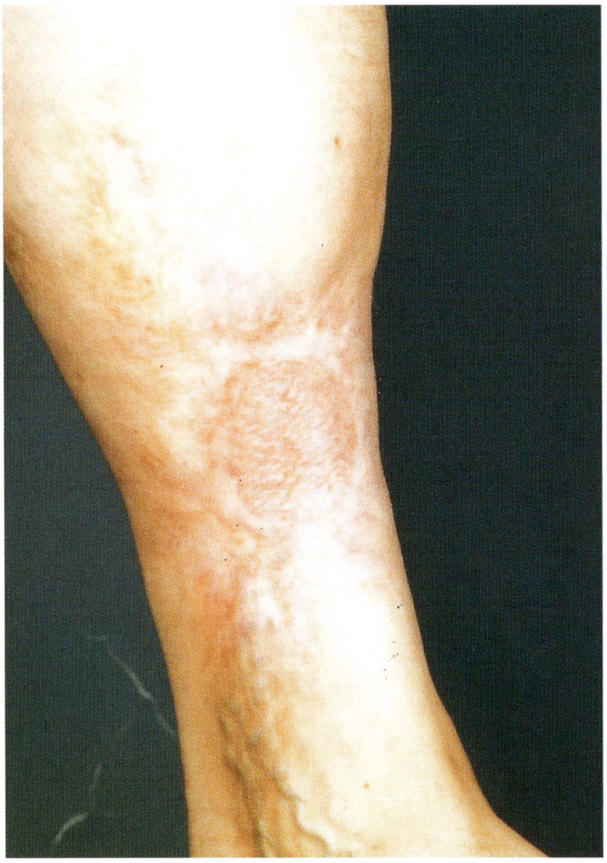

Figure 6.54b One year postoperatively. The patient has no discomfort. The perfusion of the surrounding tissue has improved after the source of infection was removed.

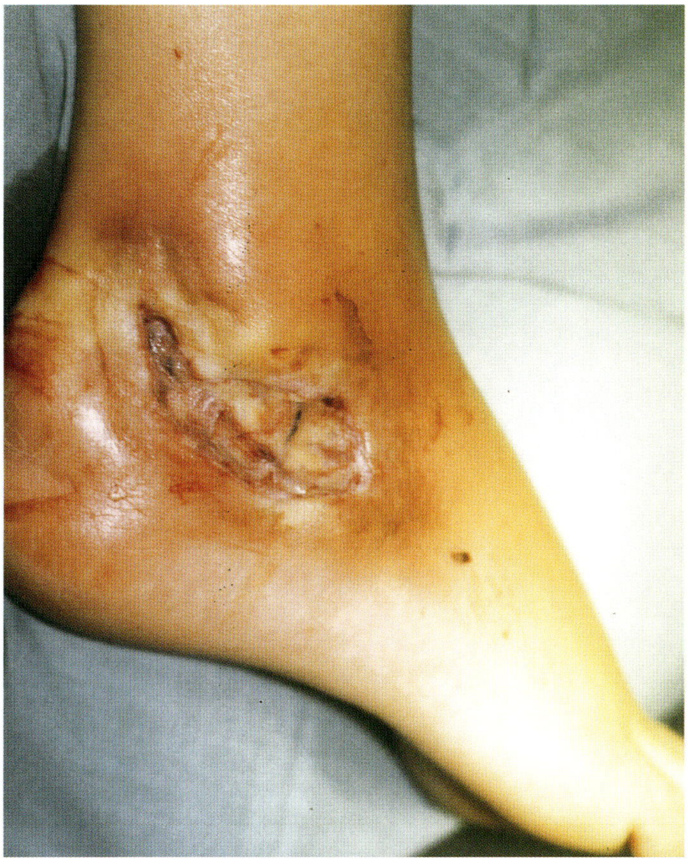

Figure 6.55a Posttraumatic ulceration combined with infection of the right foot. The infected area was excised and a temporary cover was obtained using a meshed split-thickness skin graft. It was intended to use a free radial forearm flap once the infection was controlled.

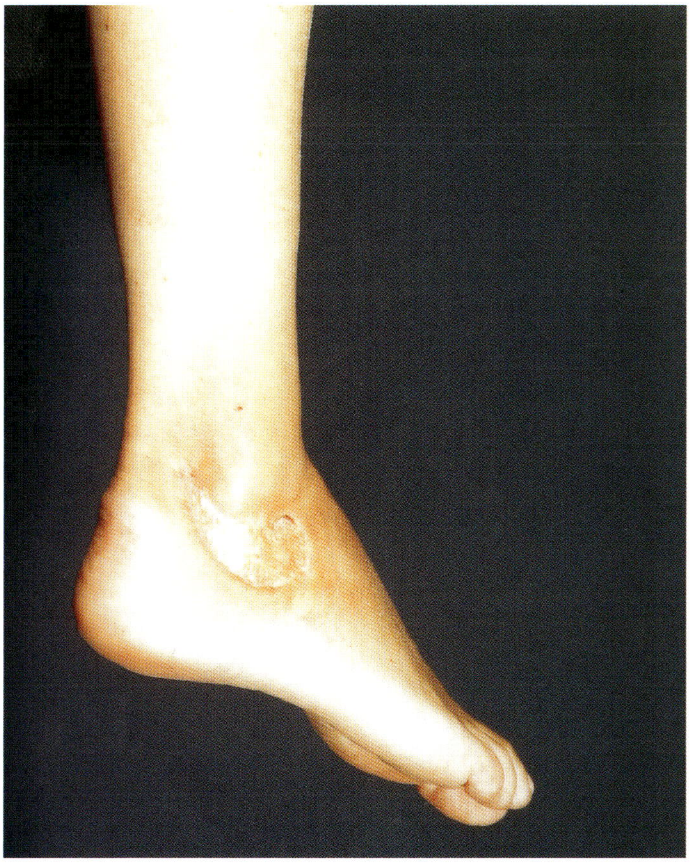

Figure 6.55b 14 months postoperatively. The patient has no discomfort and was pleased with the situation. The free radial forearm flap procedure was not necessary.

Amniotic Bands

Amniotic bands are found in every 2000–2500th newborn. It is considered to be a primary dysplasia of the subcutaneous tissue. In severe cases there is an additional dysplasia of the blood vessels and a dysgenesis of the distal extremity. Skeletal abnormalities are secondary. There are many varieties of abnormalities from single bands to strangulating cords. Single bands of the leg are rare. Often different kinds of bands of fingers and toes are combined with terminal syndactyly or intrauterine finger amputation. Amniotic bands are classified into five levels of severity (Olivari):

- Grade I
  Superficial bands with affect of skin with only minimal involvement of subcutaneous tissue.
- Grade II
  Deep bands with total loss of subcutaneous tissue to the fascia.
- Grade III
  Pressure atrophy of subcutaneous tissue and muscle, and involvement of nerves and vessels. Lymphedema and elephantiasis occur in the distal segment because of dysfunctional lymph drainage.
- Grade IV
  Enormous pressure causes green stick fractures, distal extremity segments can develop necrotic parts due to obstruction of the circulation.
- Grade V
  Intrauterine minor or, in rare cases, major amputations.

Surgical Treatment

Most authors have described the amniotic bands as scars. These cords interfere with normal growth of the affected area.

In the fetus and newborns growth takes place rapidly. So the effect of the bands is obvious. The growth of the affected part is reduced and the flow of lymph and blood diminished.

In severe cases massive edema and deformity occurs in the distal segment. The only way to eliminate such mechanical obstacle is surgical intervention. Aim of the surgical intervention in the resection of the constrictive ring, the reconstruction of skin and subcutaneous tissue. Nerves and vessels must be relieved of any pressure.

Ombredanne (1937) described multiple W-plasties, identical with "running w" as described later.

We have used multiple Z-plasties in our patients. The most important part of the operative procedure is the careful resection of the fibrous ring. In bands grade III to IV the vessels and nerves should be prepared with magnification.

Multiple Z-plasties with angles of 45 degree are planned. To obtain a good functional and aesthetic result the depth of the incision should be down to the normal skin-subcutaneous-tissue level.

Surgical treatment, especially for deep amniotic bands, needs to be early to avoid irreversible anatomical and functional changes of extremities.

a) Amniotic Bands Type I

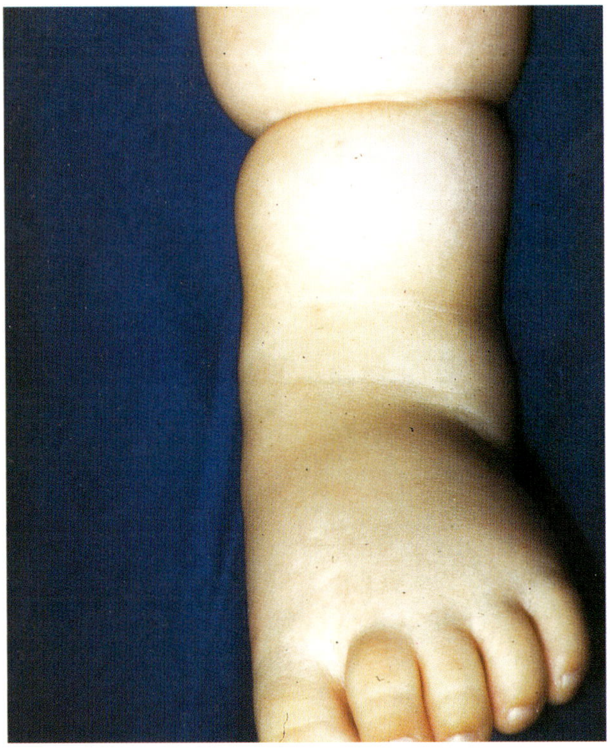

Figure 6.56a Amniotic bands type I. The skin is constricted, no lymphedema occurs, vessels and nerves are free.

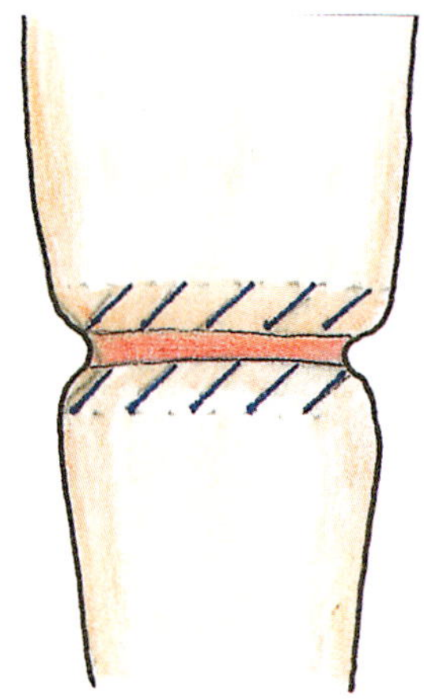

Figure 6.56b Planning of the operation. The red marked area is excised. Multiple Z-plasties reach the normal skin. **Important:** Precise coaptation of subcutaneous tissue and the skin surface is needed.

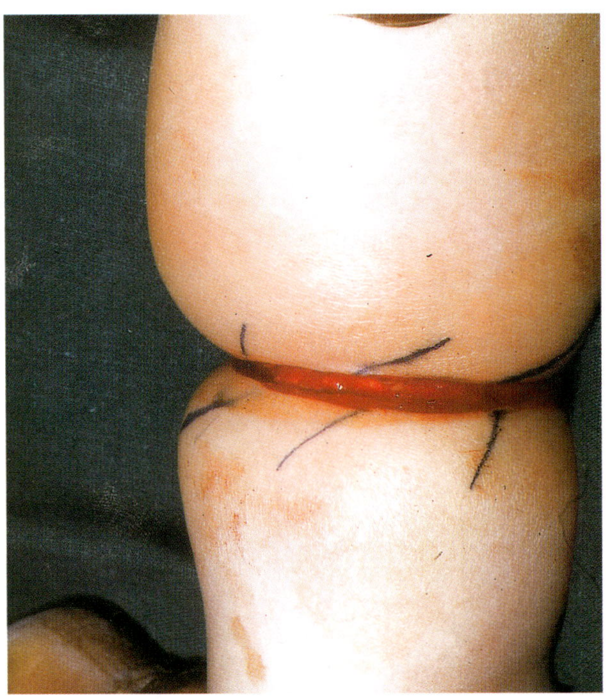

Figure 6.56c The amniotic ring has been excised. Multiple Z-plasties are planned.

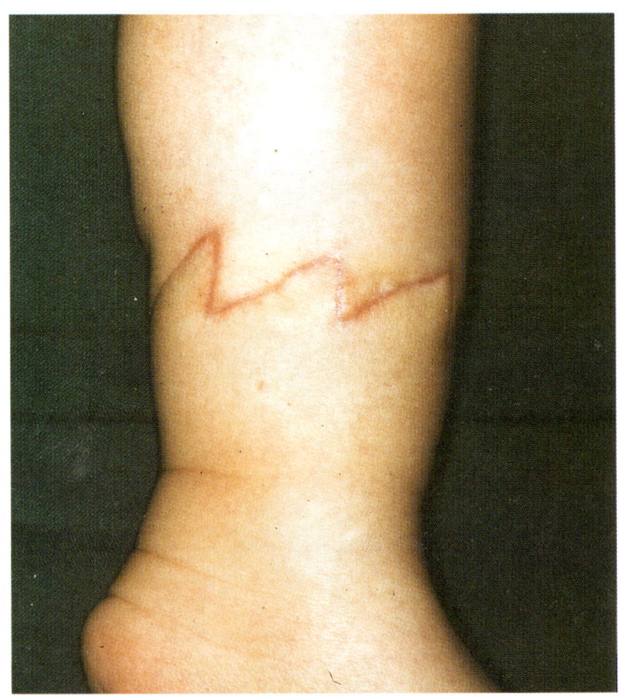

Figure 6.56d Result six weeks after the operation

b) Amniotic Bands Type II

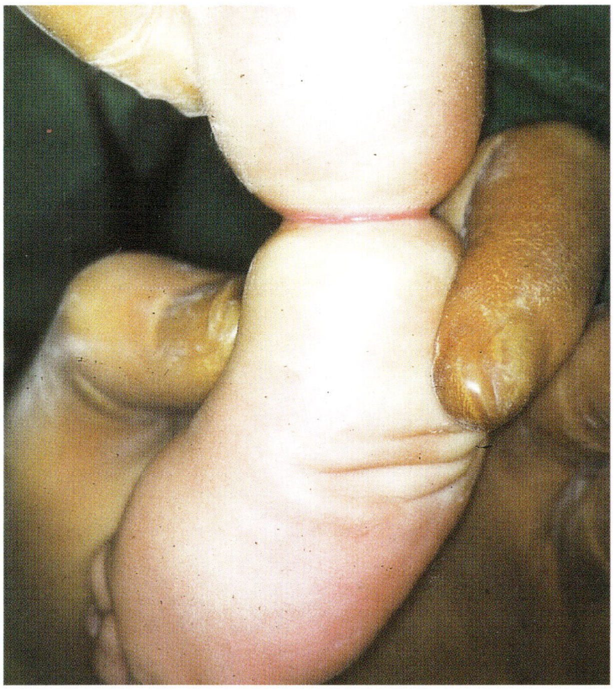

Figure 6.57a Amniotic band type II on the left. Lymphedema due to strangulation of the subcutaneous tissue. Vessels and nerves are moderately compressed.

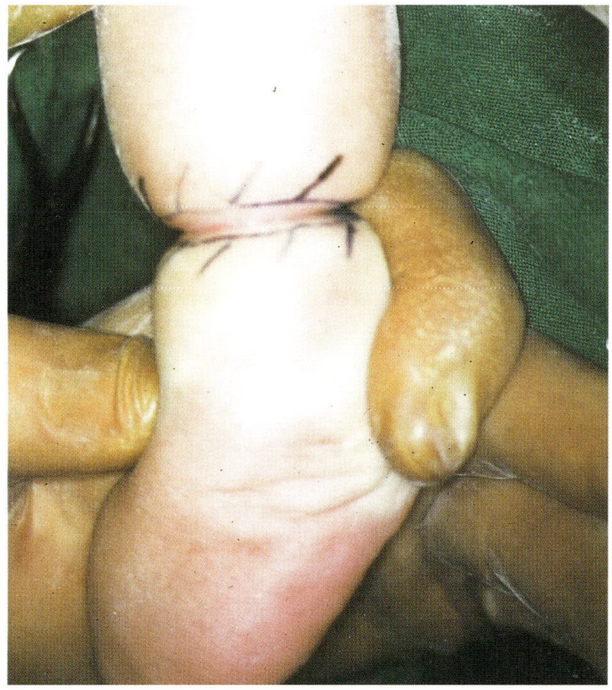

Figure 6.57b Planning of the operation: Excision of the amniotic ring, multiple Z-plasties.

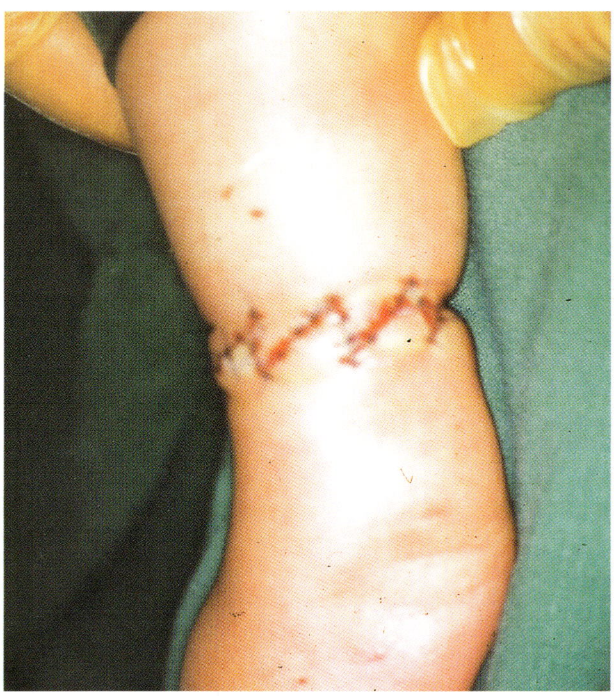

Figure 6.57c Result at the end of the operation

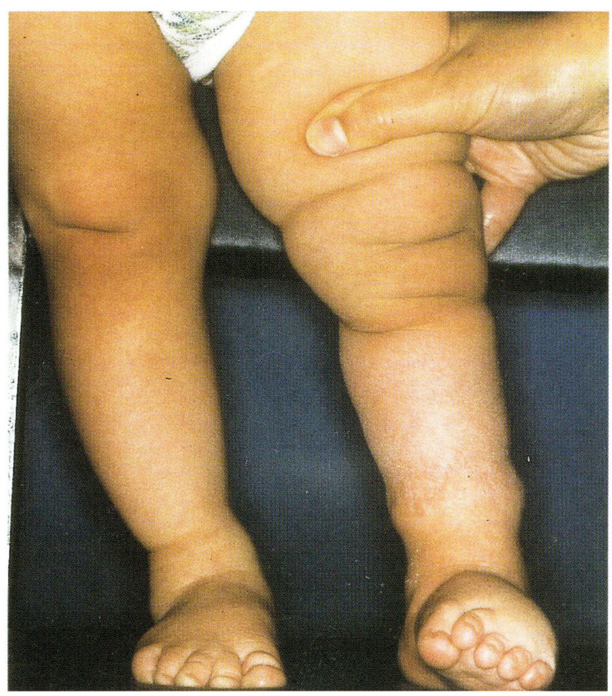

Figure 6.57d Result two years after the operation

c) Amniotic Bands Type IV

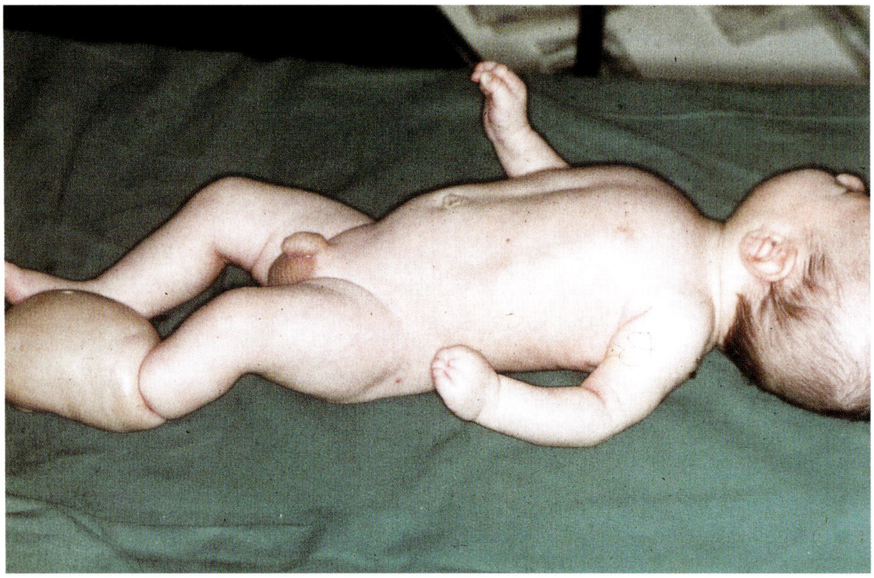

Figure 6.58a Amniotic bands Type IV of the left lower leg and of both hands with lymphedema, vessel and nerve constriction. The amniotic ring has caused a fracture of the tibia.

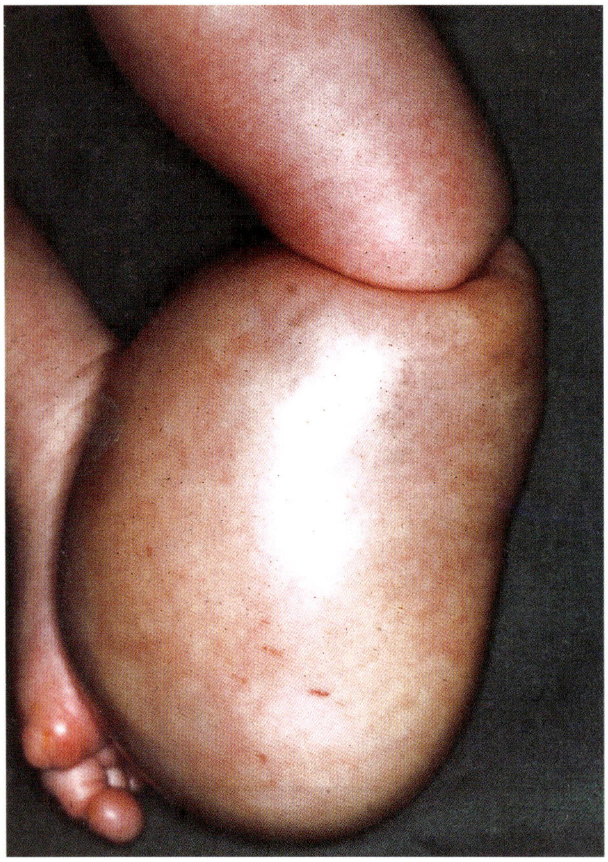

Figure 6.58b Massive lymphedema distal to the constriction. Due to diminished blood circulation a necrosis is likely to occur and requires immediate operation.

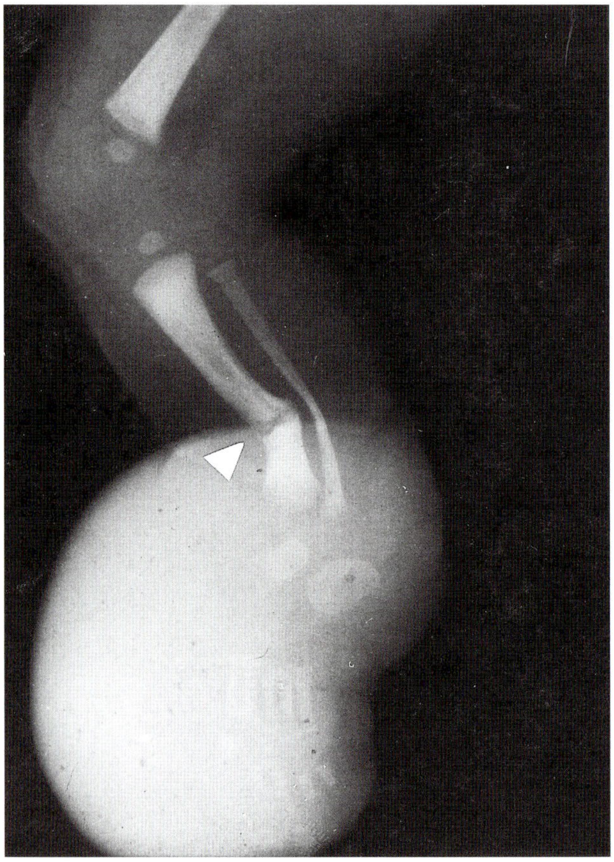

Figure 6.58c The extremely tight amniotic ring caused a green stick fracture of the tibia.

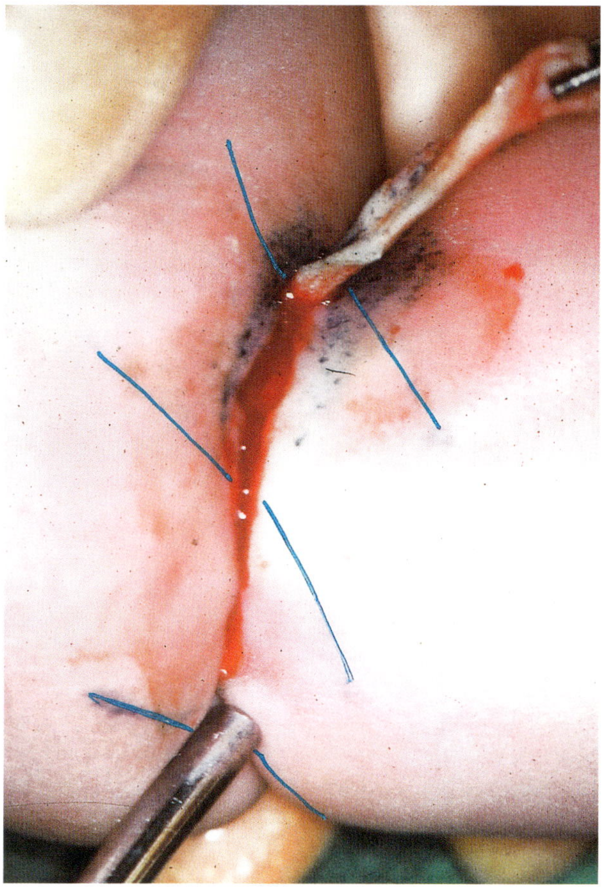

Figure 6.58d Resection of the amniotic ring is the most important part of the operation (magnification is necessary).

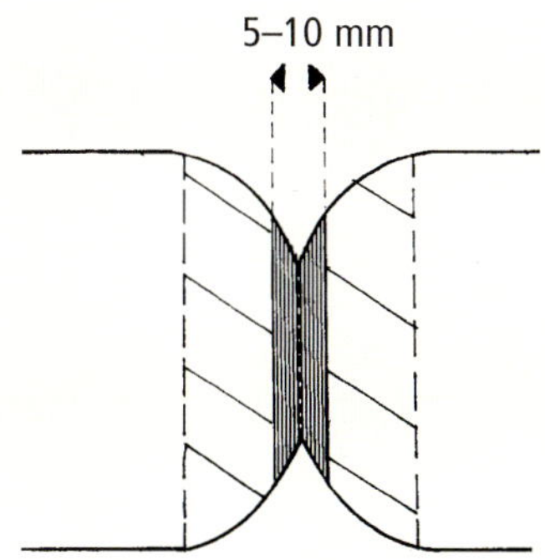

Figure 6.58e The band is excised with 1 cm margin and must include normal skin. Multiple Z-plasties are then planned in the wound edge.

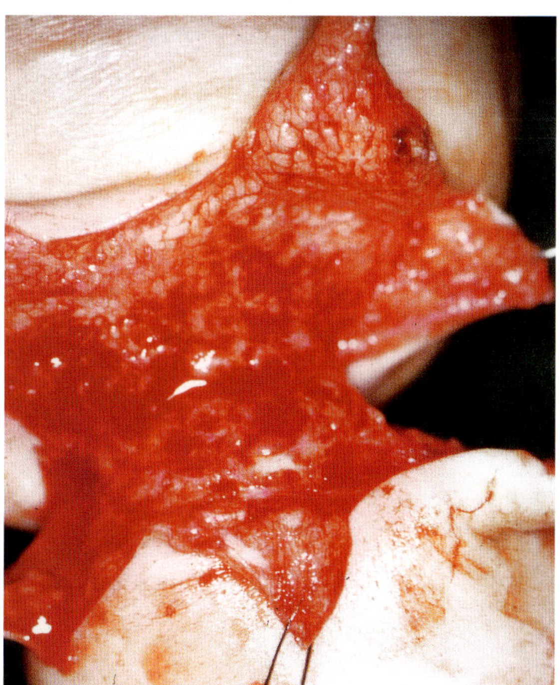

Figure 6.58f The amniotic ring has been excised. There is no longer any pressure on vessels and nerves. The skin-flaps for the Z-plasties are mobilized. To provide a normal lymph drainage a wide area of subcutaneous tissue is brought together both proximally and distally.

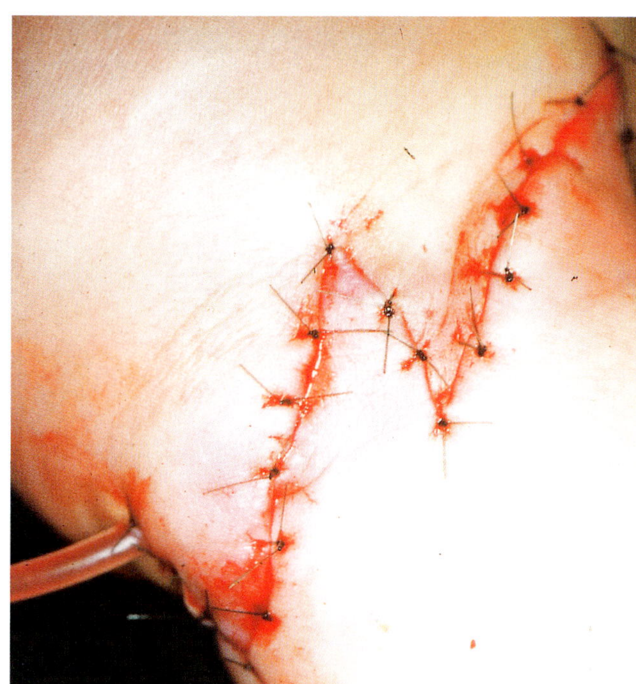

Figure 6.58g Result at the end of the operation. The skin level is equal. The subcutaneous tissue adapted. This allows a normal lymph drainage.

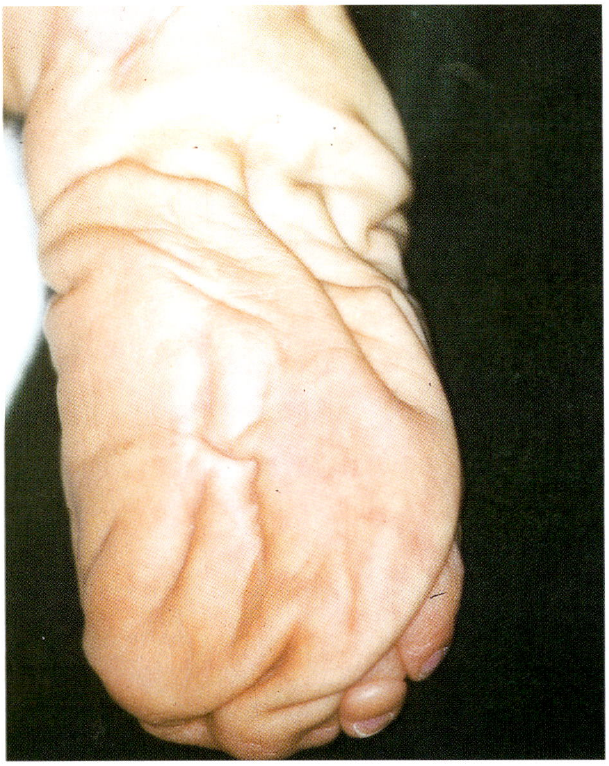

Figure 6.58h Two months after the operation the lymphedema has gone. A considerable skin excess then had to be excised.

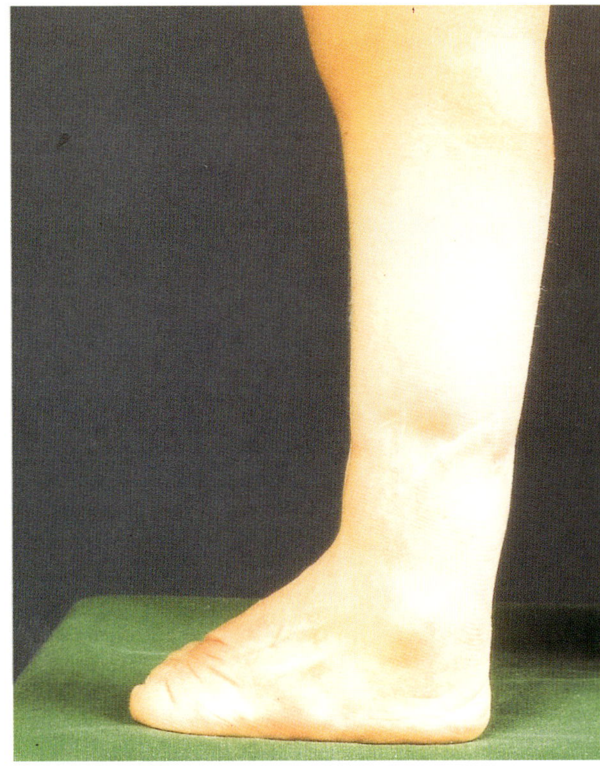

Figure 6.58i Result four years after the operation

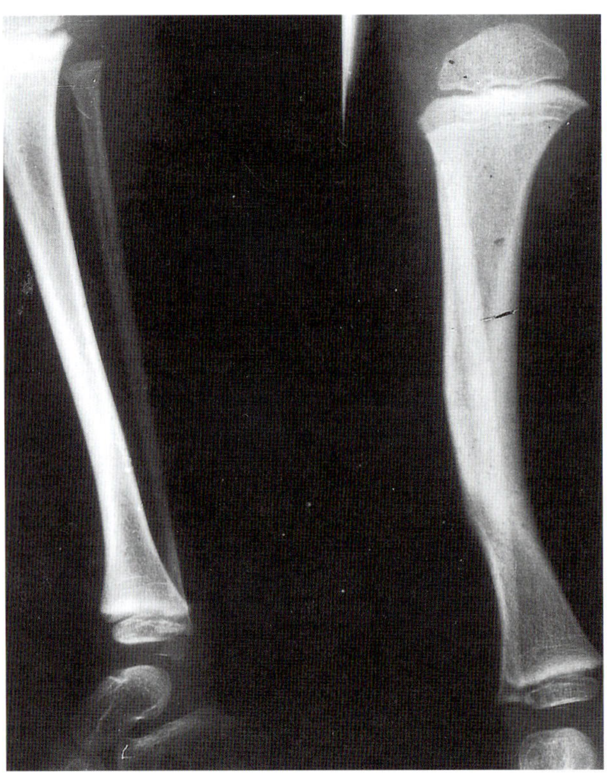

Figure 6.58j The fracture of tibia has healed spontaneously.

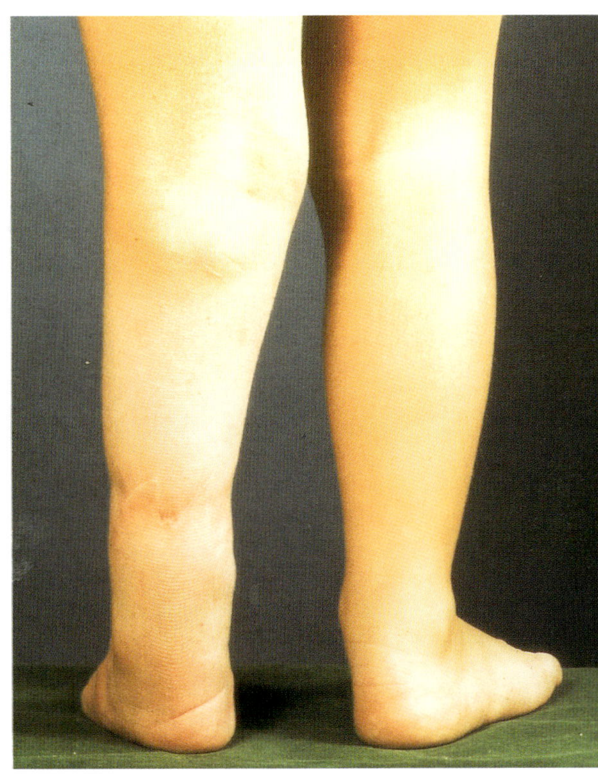

Figure 6.58k The leg has a normal length and the child is able to participate in sports.

Lymphedema (Elephantiasis)

The lymphatic system functions by draining high-molecular weight proteins from the tissues. About 20 litres of plasma protein diffuses through the capillary walls each day and are returned to the circulation via the lymphatic system [Clodius 1977]. This passage into the tissues is due to osmotic and hydrostatic pressure. The perfusion is regulated by fenestrations of different sizes in capillary wall on the arterial side.

About 90 % of the fluid is drained by the capillaries on the venous side. The remaining 10 % consist of high molecular weight protein with water osmotically linked. The protein molecules are too big to migrate back through the capillary walls, so they are transported by the lymphatic system.

The lymphatic system consists of a network of different sized vessels with valves. The combination of muscle contraction and valve function ensures the transport of lymph fluid.

Pathophysiology

If the capacity for the lymph drainage is less than the production lymph collects in the tissues.
The causes for this are as follows:

1) The production of lymphatic fluid in the periphery is normal and the lymphatic transport is reduced. High molecular proteins remain in the periphery as lymphedema.
2) The peripheral lymphatic production is higher than the transport capacity; for instance in cardiac insufficiency or renal dysfunction.
3) Inadequacy of the lymphatic valves. This is a rare occurrence. The transport of lymphatic fluid is significantly reduced. A protein-rich edema occurs and in extreme cases can result in necrosis of tissue.

Classification

Primary Lymphedema
The primary lymphedema arises without any evident cause. This is called congenital dysfunction of the lymphatic system (lymphedema congenitum).

Secondary Lymphedema
The secondary lymphedema arises due to external influence, for instance compression by tumors, intra-lymphatic growth of tumor. Trauma and tropic infections can cause lymphedema. Iatrogenic reasons are: The resection of local lymphatic nodes, vein stripping, radiation.

Therapy

A stable lymphedema is often resistant to any therapy. A complete remission by surgical intervention is not possible. The surgical task focuses on two topics:

- Improvement of the lymphatic transport
- Reduction of peripheral stasis of the lymphatic fluid
- Correction of the form

Surgical resection should be carried out sparingly and performed only by experts. Conservative treatment should be attempted first. Only if this fails should surgery be considered. Patients usually consult the doctor when a permanent lymphedema (elephantiasis) has occurred and the main part of the lymphatic system is already destroyed.

Methods like lymphovenous anastomosis and lymph-collector graft are sophisticated but do not ensure a sufficient transport of lymph fluid. An obvious stasis can be converted into a latent stasis. Initial improvement are often only temporary and sooner or later a recurrence occurs [Clodius 1977].

a) Conservative Therapy

- Diuretics
  Diuretics are of no value. Lymphedema is not caused by retention of sodium rich fluid. Diuretics eliminate water, which is osmotically linked to proteins. The proteins remain in the tissue. Fibrosis is accelerated.
- Benzopyrone
  In 80 % of all patients benzopyrone leads to a minimal reduction of the extremity diameter (0.5 cm in 10 months). It is indicated as an adjuvant therapy, but not as a single therapy.

b) Other Treatment

- Hygiene
  It is important to institute good hygienic precautions to prevent bacterial or fungal infection. If infection occurs, urgent antibacterial therapy has to be commenced.
- Manual drainage of the lymphatic fluid
  This is a highly effective therapy which gives considerably better results than operative intervention. Manual lymphatic drainage should only be performed by experts and should begin as early as possible.
- Elastic bandage
  The use of elastic socks and sleeves which are custom-made increases the tissue pressure and improves the lymphatic drainage.

c) Surgical Therapy

Surgically therapy can be used as a means to reduce the abnormal subcutaneous tissue. There are three options:

1. Resection of the altered tissue down to the deep fascia and a primary closure of the remaining skin. Shaving the epidermis off the edge and burying it below the deep fascia is said to give an additional advantage of lymph drainage [Thompson 1969].
2. Complete excision of the skin and the subcutaneous tissue down to the fascia, coverage with split-thickness skin graft or full-thickness skin graft of the excised tissue.
3. Liposuction

In severe elephantiasis excision improves the situation considerably. Unfortunately there are recurrences several years later. This method is indicated for severe elephantiasis in which all other methods fail. In spite of the tendency to recurrences the incidence of erysipelas is greatly reduced.

Using full-thickness skin grafts from the excised area provides good results. Split-thickness skin grafts have the disadvantage of scarring and constrictions in the multiple spaces between the grafts.

Liposuction leads to a reduction of the diameter of the limb, lymphatic drainage is improved and compression therapy is facilitated, but it is not a final solution for the problem. If surgery is indicated the first option is liposuction.

There is no surgical treatment with a perfect solution.

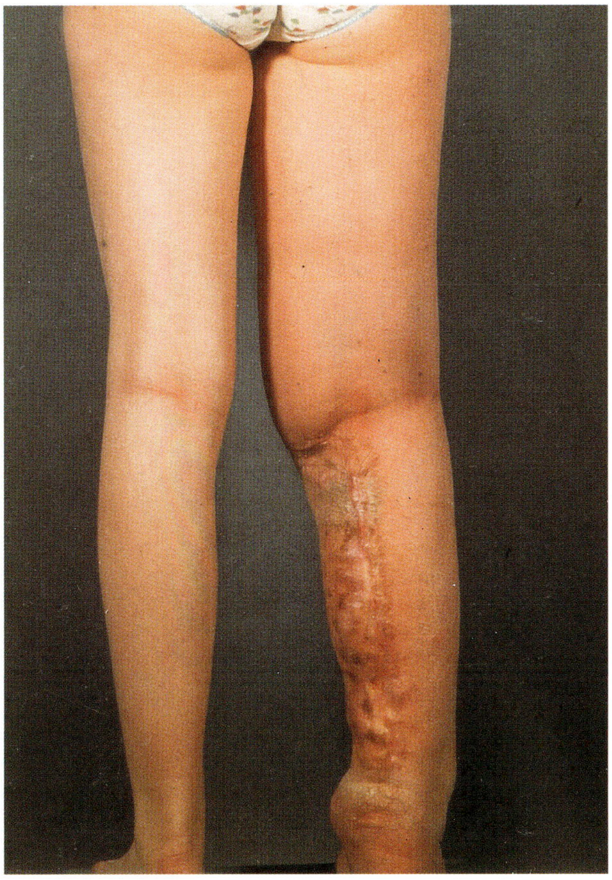

Figure 6.59a Elephanthiasis of the right leg (Result after Thompson operation – without success).

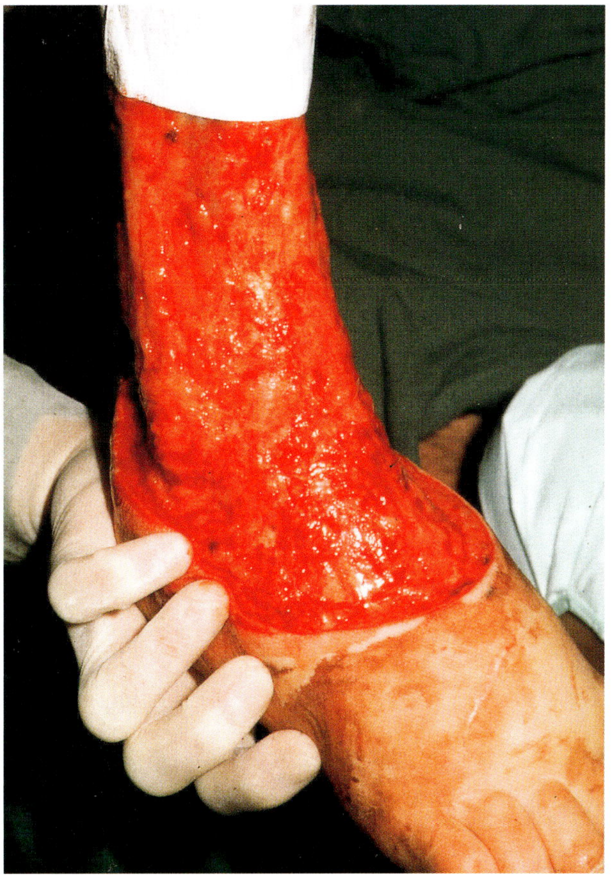

Figure 6.59b Skin, subcutaneous tissue and fat are excised down to the fascia, from knee to the dorsal foot.

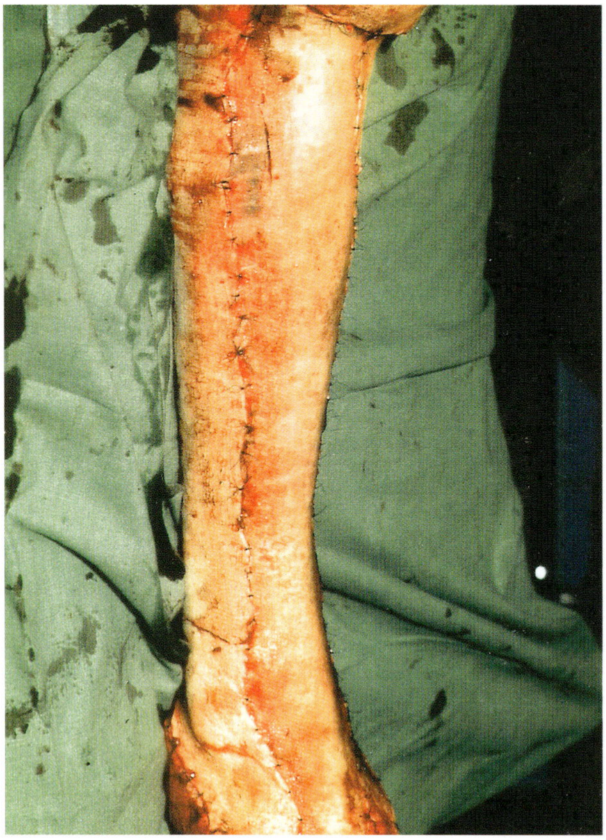

Figure 6.59c The fat of the excised skin is removed and the full thickness skin is grafted on the fascia.

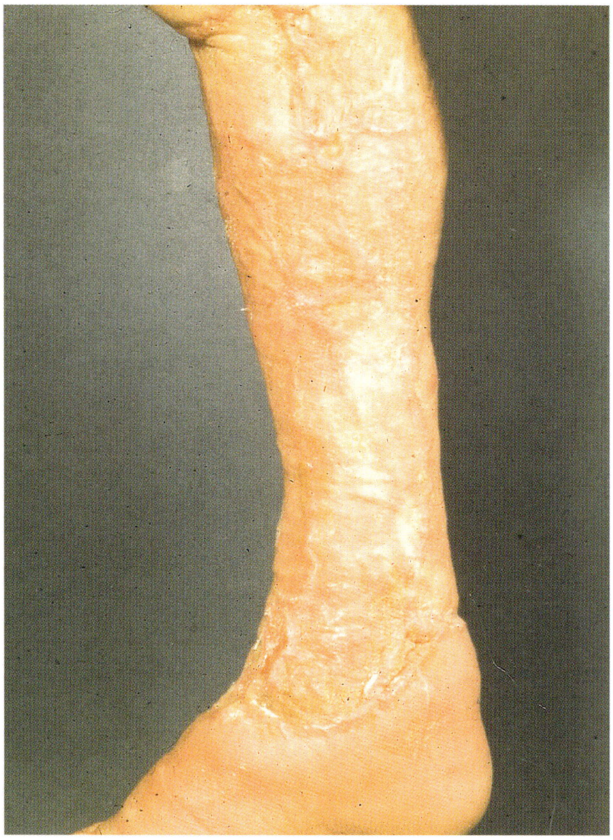

Figure 6.59d Result one year after the operation

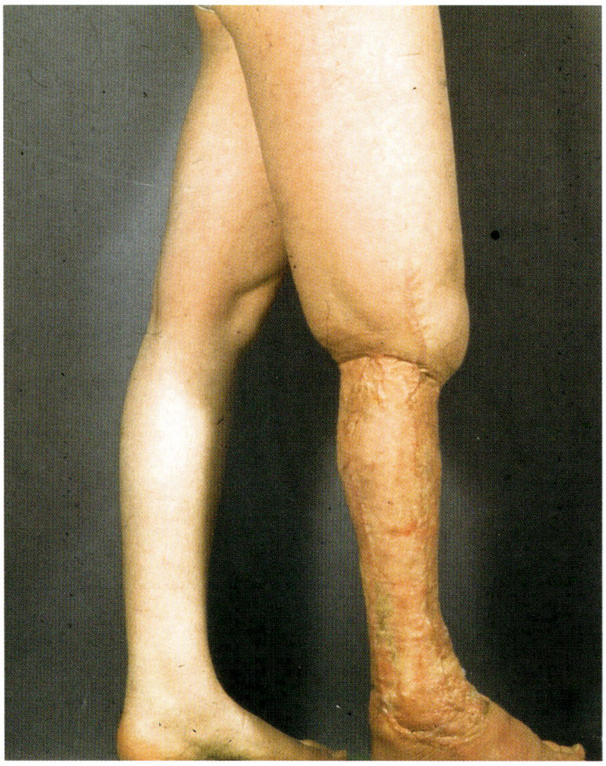

Figure 6.59e An ugly step has occurred between thigh and lower leg. It is probable that a recurrence will occur in the future.
This operation should only be used if all other options fail.

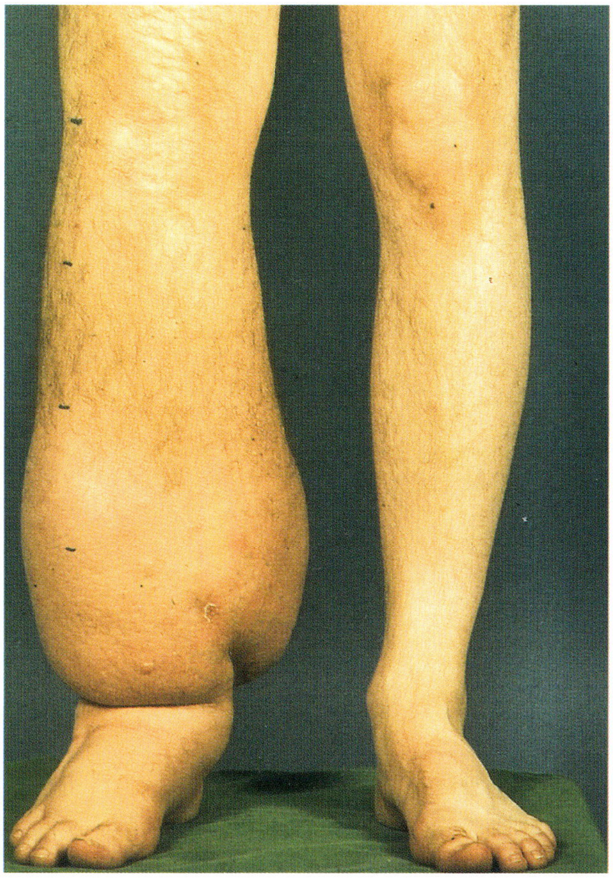

Figure 6.60a 22-year old man with elephantiasis of the right leg.

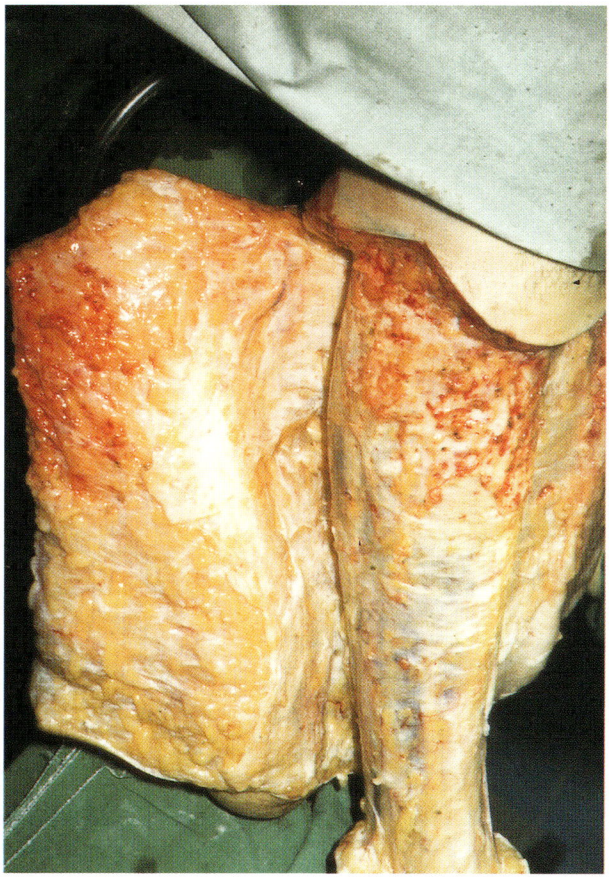

Figure 6.60b Resection of the all of the skim and subcutaneous tissue from the knee to the ankle joint

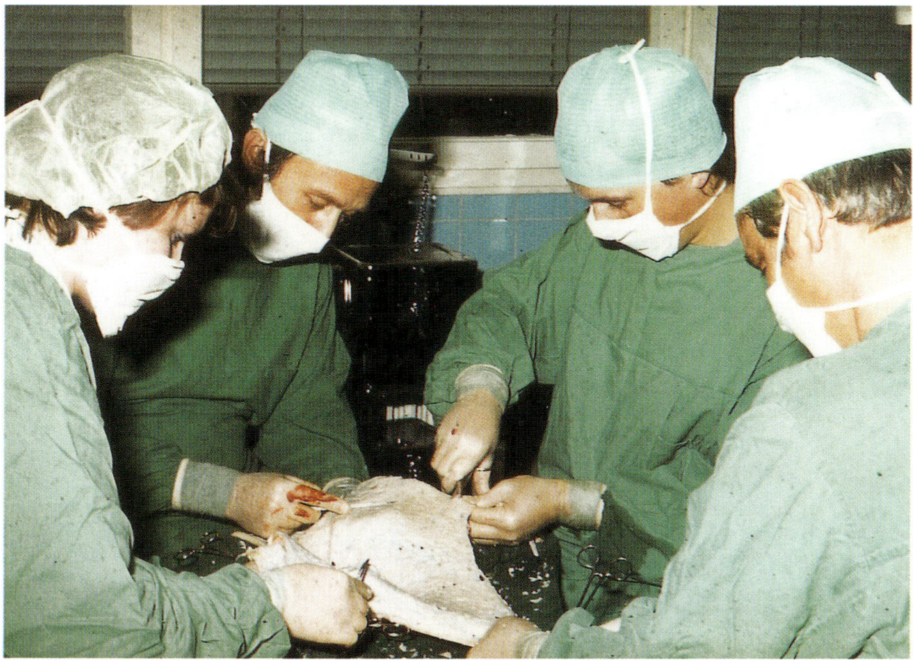

Figure 6.60c The doctors Olivari, Schuwerak and Pless are working hard to remove the fat. A full thickness skin graft remains as a unit.

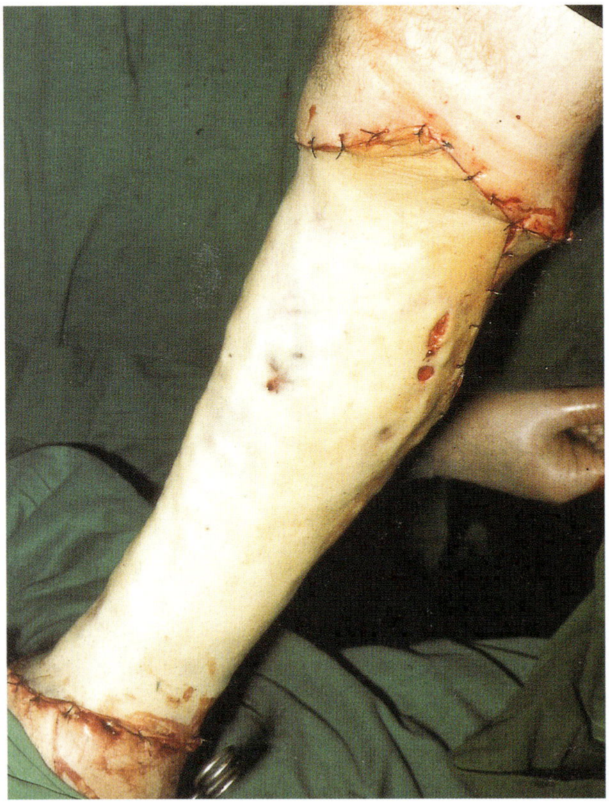

Figure 6.60d The full thickness skin is grafted on the fascia

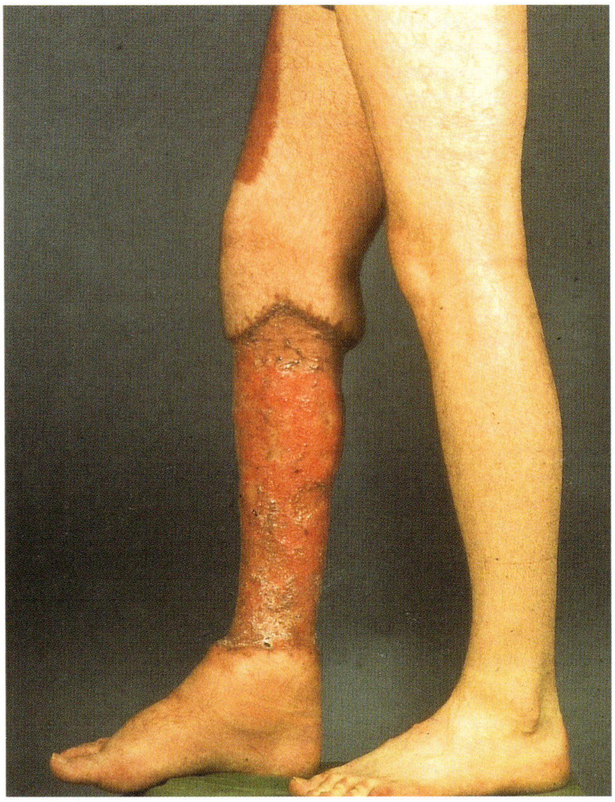

Figure 6.60e Satisfying result four months after the operation. About one year after the operation the situation deteriorates. Once again lymphedema of the tissue has occurred.

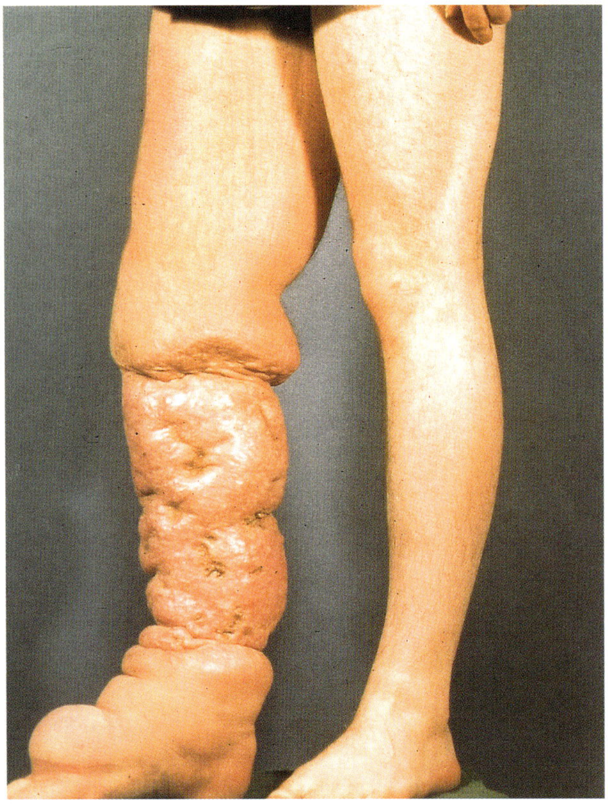

Figure 6.60f Result four years after the operation. The area of the foot is much firmer than before the operation.
The grafted part of the lower leg shows recurrent swelling.
Consequence: It is questionable whether this operation was warranted.

Principles of Replantation Surgery

Today microsurgical techniques have enabled replantations to become routine procedures. However it requires a perfect technique, regular practice and a methodical approach. Proper training in the laboratory is needed. However when replantation is not indicated the classical stump surgery is of value.

Definition

Replantation is defined as reconstruction of the circulation when the limb has been completely detached. If some insufficient residual circulation remains but reconstruction of the main vessels is needed one talks about *revascularization*.

Micro-replantation (e.g. a finger) is technically more difficult and is principally performed under microscopic magnification. Good functional results including reinnervation are to be expected. The amputated limb tolerates up to 24 hours of cold ischemia.

Macro-replantation (e.g. forearm, arm, lower leg): The amputated part contains muscle and, thus, tolerates much less ischemia. Necrosis of muscle is a consequence. Reinnervation takes about 1 mm per day. If an amputation is located in the middle of the forearm, the motor reinnervation of the hand muscles (e.g. interossei muscles) requires several months. During this time the denervated muscle becomes atrophied and reinnervation lacks a responsive muscle. The more proximal the amputation, the worse the outcome. Sensation recovers at the same speed (about 1 mm per day), but functional results are much better.

Result

After replantation a completely normal function cannot be expected. Replantation of finger can achive a good result with single operation. In more proximal replantation secondary surgery is needed to obtain a good functional result. Post operative intensive physiotherapy are important to obtain a good result.

Preoperative Treatment of the Amputated Part

a) No cleansing and no disinfection.
b) No storing in ***any*** solutions.
c) The amputated part should be wrapped in dry compresses or clean cloths.
d) Place in a water-tight plastic bag and store on ice.
e) Fast transport to a hospital with replantation team (remember to inform the replantation team).
f) In the clinic the amputate is packed sterile and placed in the fridge (+4 °C).
g) Hemostasis of the amputation stump is achieved by compression only.
No tourniquet! No clamp!

In subtotal amputation injuries in which skin bridges and/or tendons and nerves are maintained, the extremity is provided with dry dressings and a splint. Dry chilling with ice is indicated for a longer transport, in shorter transports it is not necessary.

Indication for Replantation

The indication for a replantation depends on the extent, kind of amputation, occupation and age of the patient. Though should be given to the length of the operation. Even a finger amputation needs two to four hours. When several fingers are involved the operation takes eight to 16 hours.

Hospitalization last about two to three weeks and unfitness for work about three to 18 months. These factors have to be kept in mind when indications for replantation are discussed. Replantation of the fifth finger is useless in a patient who is a manual worker. A replanted finger could hamper hand function and delay return to work for some months. Employment may be jeopardised by slow or poor workmanship. Cold intolerance may be present for over two years and interfere with the occupational rehabilitation.

Indications for Replantation

1) Thumb amputation
2) Amputation of multiple fingers
3) Metacarpal amputation
4) Hand amputation
5) Amputation of a finger in combination with injuries to multiple fingers
6) Amputation injuries in children
7) Amputation of a foot

Relative Indications for Replantation

1) Amputation of a single finger (some special occupations)
2) Single distal phalanx amputations
3) Single fingers with injured proximal interphalangeal or metacarpophalangeal joints
4) In crush amputation of the hand proximal to the wrist a heterotopic replantation (Godina) can be considered
5) Severe crush injuries to the foot

No Indications for Replantation

1) Additional life threatening injuries
2) Amputated part frozen or transported in antiseptic solutions
3) Severe crush injury of the amputated digit
4) an amputated finger tip (proximal to the nail root)
5) Non compliance of the patient
6) Severe underlying medical illness (diabetes, heart failure, arterial occlusive disease, etc.)

If the thumb has multiple amputation injuries or crush injuries an uninjured finger (e.g. third finger) is transposed into the thumb position to give a good functional result.

Types of Amputations

Clean Amputation

Clean amputations are beneficial because there are only limited injuries on amputate and stump. Replantation procedure is easy to perform and shortening of the limb is minimised. Unfortunately these injuries are rare (5 to 10 %).

Circular Saw Injuries

Circular saw injuries are more difficult because of soft tissue and bone injuries of the amputated part and stump. Nevertheless this kind of amputation is beneficial for replantation surgery. Injured structures are resected and shortening of the limb is acceptable. This is a frequent injury (40 to 60 %).

Crush and Avulsion Injury

Crush and avulsion injuries with partial skeletization of the amputation stump causes technical problems. Vein interposition to reconstruct injured vessel parts can preserve the length of the finger. Mostly these amputated parts cannot be replanted a good stump procedure is needed.

Preoperative Planning

The amputated part is cleaned with saline solution under sterile conditions.

One team prepares the amputated part and the other team the stump. If there is only one team the stump is prepared first meanwhile the amputated part is stored at +4°C until the preparation of the stump is completed.

Operation

1) All damaged tissue has to be removed. Mediolateral incisions are necessary to identify the important structures.
2) Bone is shortened to allow soft tissue to be repaired without tension. Afterwards osteosynthesis is performed. It is better to shorten the bone than to suture a structure under tension (arteries, veins, nerves).
3) Suture of the flexor tendons is performed.
4) First the arterial anastomosis. In the finger both digital arteries are repaired. At the level area of the metacarpus the superficial palmar arch is repaired. The level of the wrist or the lower arm, the radial and ulna artery are repaired. If there is too much tension on the vessel a vein graft is interposed.
5) The nerve stumps are reconstructed using epineural suture technique.
6) Extensor tendons are repaired.
7) Vein anastomosis is performed. In the area of the finger and the hand two veins should be sutured. If tension occurs a vein graft is interposed.
8) Skin closure is done with single interrupted sutures without any tension. Pressure on the veins should be avoided. To avoid postoperative edema a skin graft may be needed.

Table 6.1 Order of replantation

■ Osteosynthesis
■ Flexor tendons
■ Arteries
■ Nerves
■ Extensor tendons
■ Veins

Replantation surgery is possible due to the invention of the microscope. Most operators perform a replantation of fingers or the hand under the microscope.

If multiple finger replantations are performed the microscope is required. You can see much better and wearing magnifying glasses use for prolonged periods is uncomfortable.

Replantation of the lower arm or lower leg can be performed with magnifying glasses.

Postoperative Monitoring

1) Colour of the replanted limb (is it livid white, pink, red or purple)
2) Temperature
3) Capillary flow (test by pressure on the nail, or tensioning the skin)
4) Turgor (is there congestion, normal or empty)
5) Anastomosis control using ultrasound

Postoperative Care

Microtransplantation

1) Positioning of the replanted limb at body level or higher
2) No constrictive dressing
3) Daily dressing changes, a bloody dressing should be changes

Macrotransplantation

1) Partial necrosis of the muscles occurs due to toxic products of catabolism (myoglobin, metabolic products). The amount of muscle necrosis is dependent on the duration of ischemia. To shorten the duration of ischemia prior to the osteosynthesis a shunt could be temporarily applied (connection between the artery of the amputated part and the artery of the stump). The shunt is opened every minute.
2) Monitoring is performed in the intensive care unit.
3) To protect renal function sufficient infusion therapy is given.
4) Local control is performed as described for microreplantation.

Postoperative Treatment

Intensive physiotherapy is important. This therapy continues for several months depending on the type of injury and should be performed in a specialized centre.

Complications

1) Thrombosis (veins, arteries) due to poor technique or damage to the vessels. Treatment: Immediate revision of the anastomosis, if needed resection and vein interposition
2) Thrombosis in the periphery with necrosis. Treatment: If possible distal interposition, but necrectomy may be needed and a secondary correction performed
3) Bleeding. Therapy: Immediate exploration of the operative field and the anastomosis
4) Complete necrosis; in a crush injury the anastomosis may still be intact. Treatment: Amputation, and construction of a good stump
5) Infection. Treatment: In the case of a well perfuse replant, incision of the infected area and flushing with antibiotics (Nebacetin), amputation where there is poor perfusion.

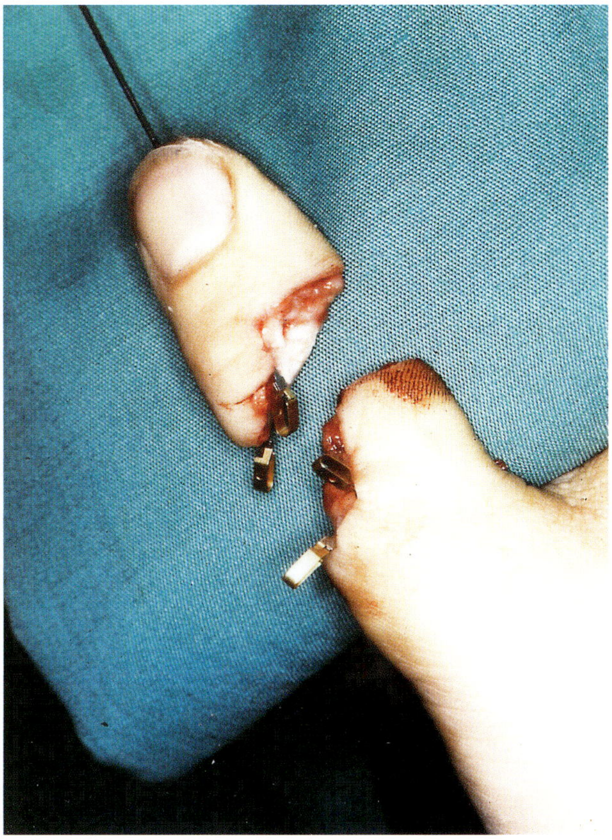

Figure 6.62a Thumb amputation with a circular saw.
Indication: Isolated thumb amputation is always an indication for replantation.

1) Injured tissue is removed from stump and amputated part
2) Bone shortening. Osteosynthesis with K-wire is performed in a functional position
3) Arterial anastomosis (only one artery was possible)
4) Flexor tendon suture
5) Suture of the nerves
6) Extensor tendon suture
7) Suture of a vein (only one vein was possible)
8) Skin suture without any tension. A split-thickness skin graft was necessary on some areas

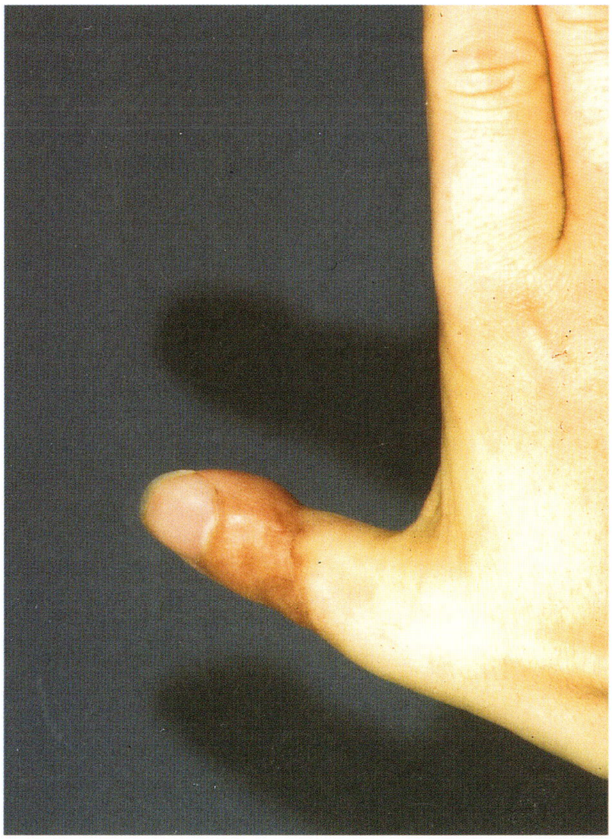

Figure 6.62b Eight months postoperatively.
The interphalangeal joint is stiff but adequate function was achieved.

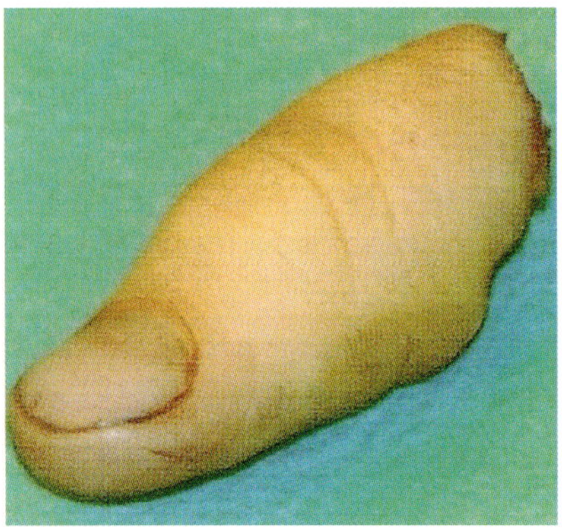

Figure 6.63a Amputation of the left thumb at the middle of the proximal phalanx with a wood splitter machine.

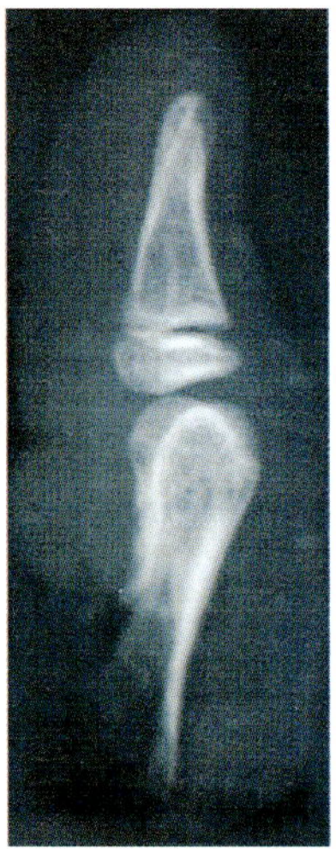

Figure 6.63b Amputated digit

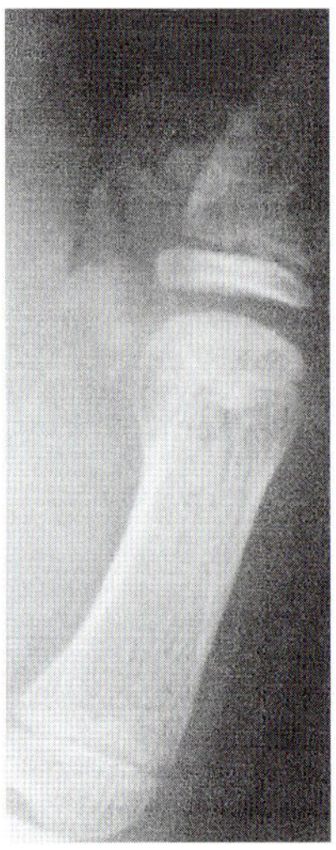

Figure6.63c Proximal stump

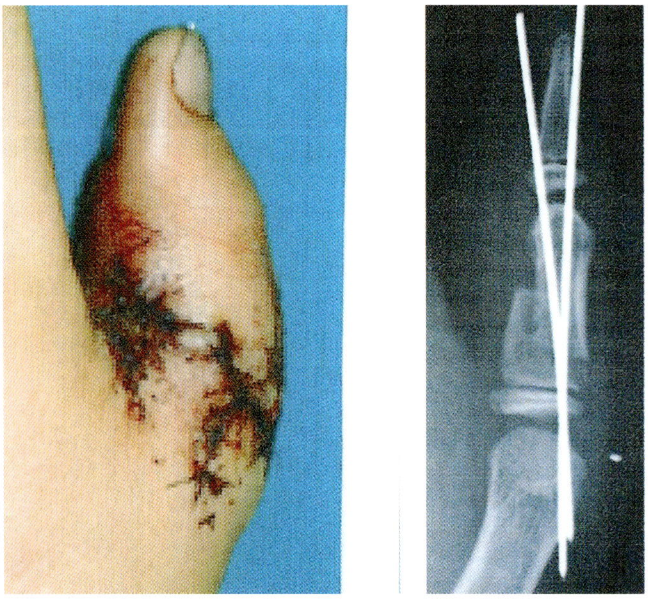

Figure 6.63d After shortening the bone internal fixation with K-wires and anastomosis of one artery and one vein. A vein graft was necessary for the vein anastomosis.

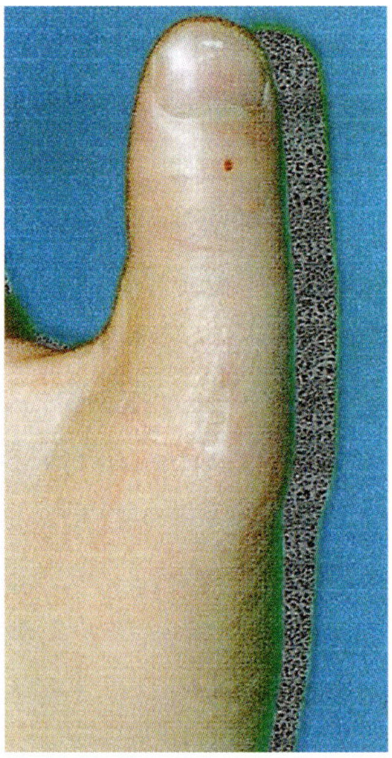

Figure 6.63e 15 months after replantation

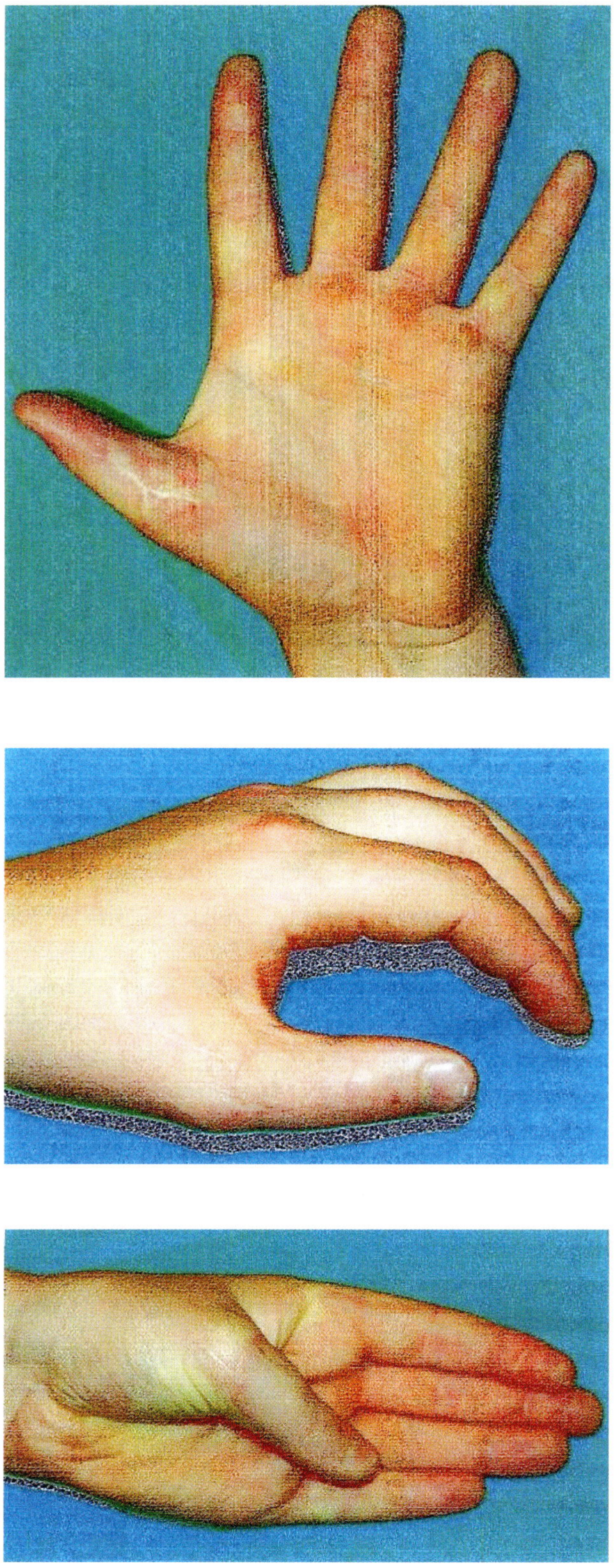

Figure 6.63f–h
Functional result 15 months after surgery

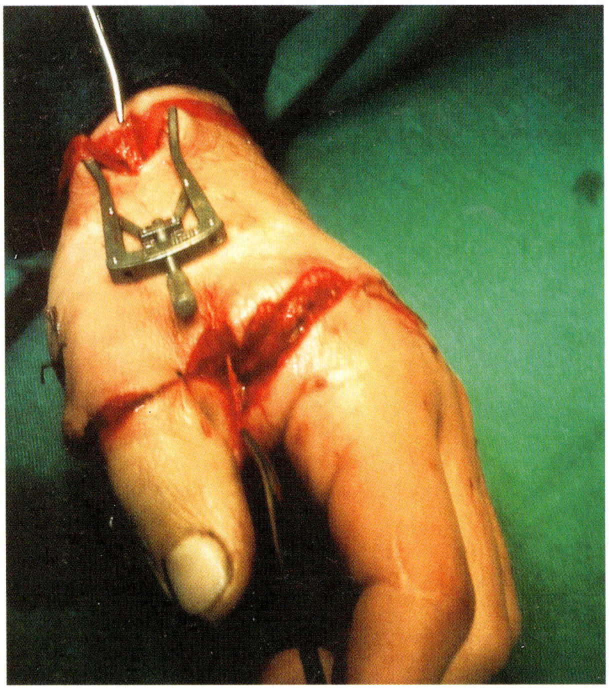

Figure 6.64a Subtotal amputation and avascular thumb. Vessels of the thumb were contused. To create a direct anastomosis a considerable shortening of the thumb would have been necessary.

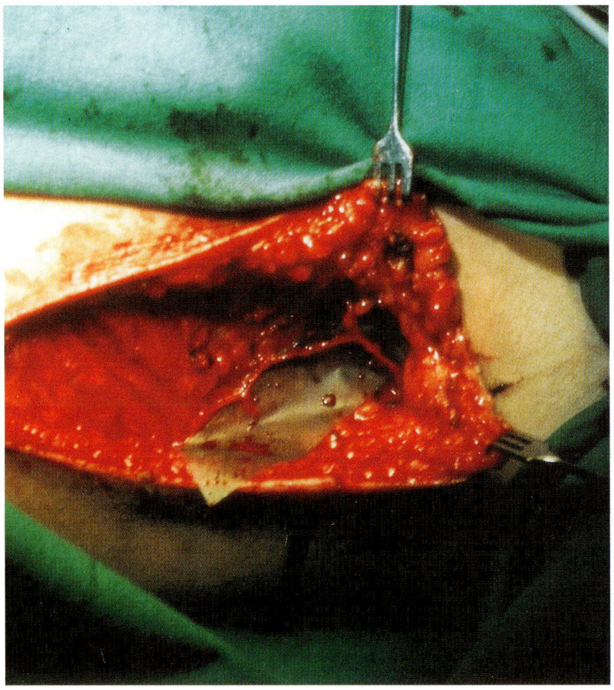

Figure 6.64b A branch from the thoracodorsal artery is taken.

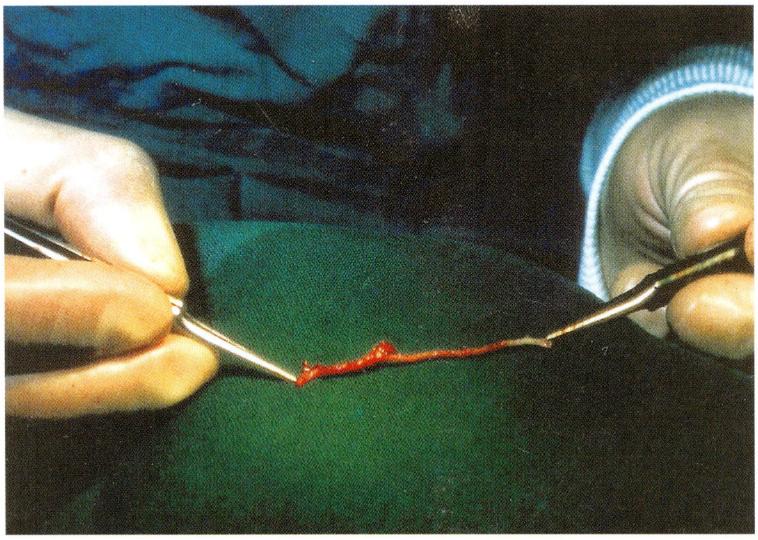

Figure 6.64c Interpositional graft

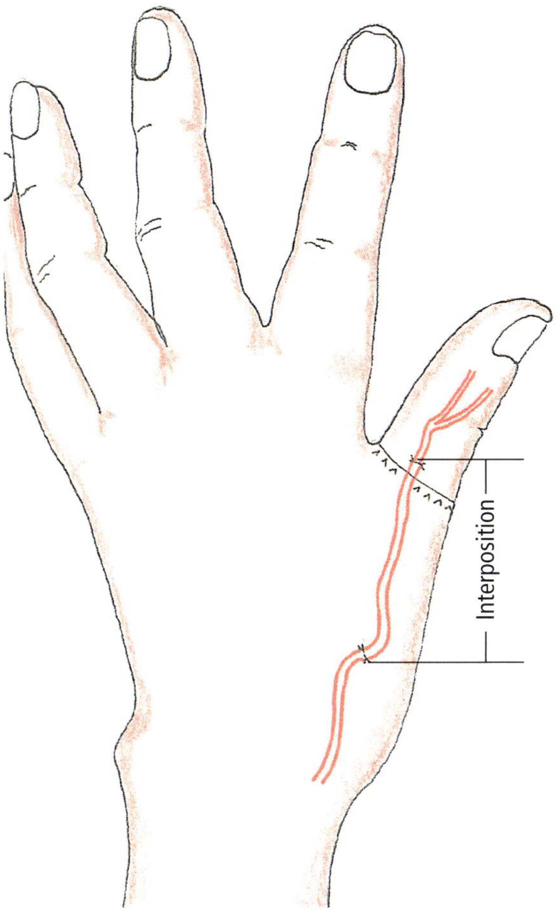

Figure 6.64d The serratus branch is interposed between the radial artery and the ulnar thumb artery without any tension.

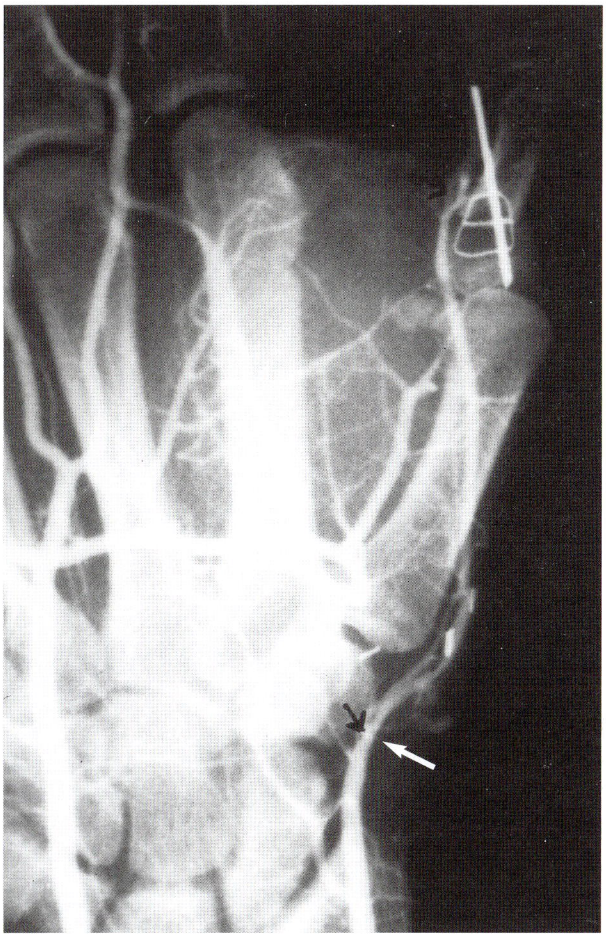

Figure 6.64e Anastomosis of the radial artery with the interpositional vessel (arrow)

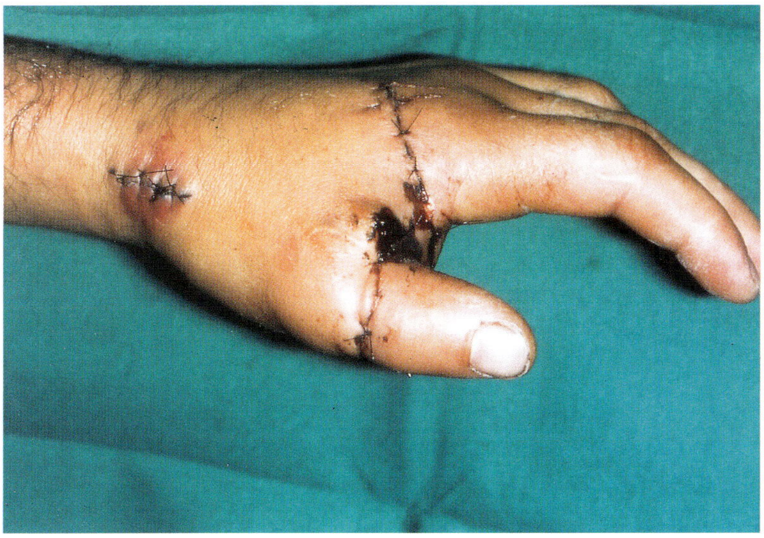

Figure 6.64f One week postoperatively

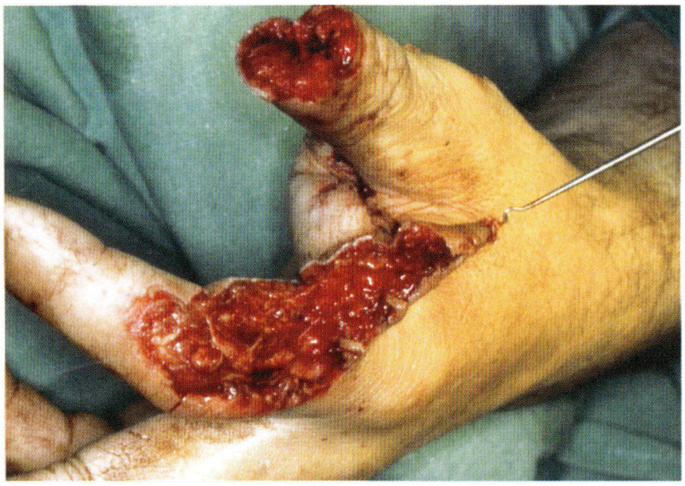

Figure 6.65a Circular saw injury: Avascular thumb

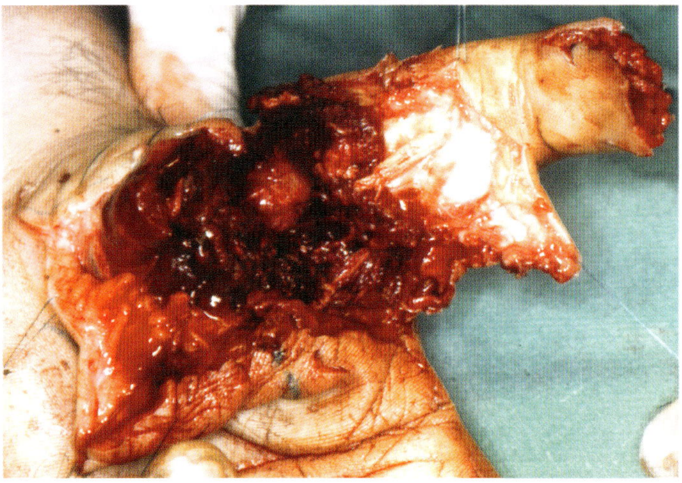

Figure 6.65b All arteries and veins are divided. Operation: Two arterial anastomoses, one vein anastomosis, one nerve anastomosis.

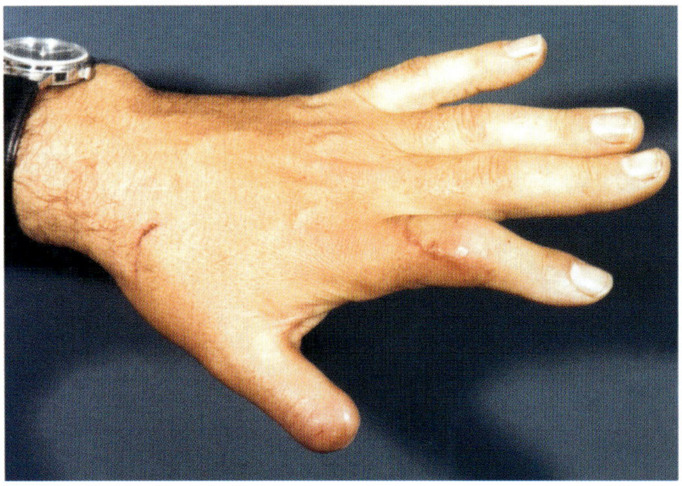

Figure 6.65c Five months after revascularization

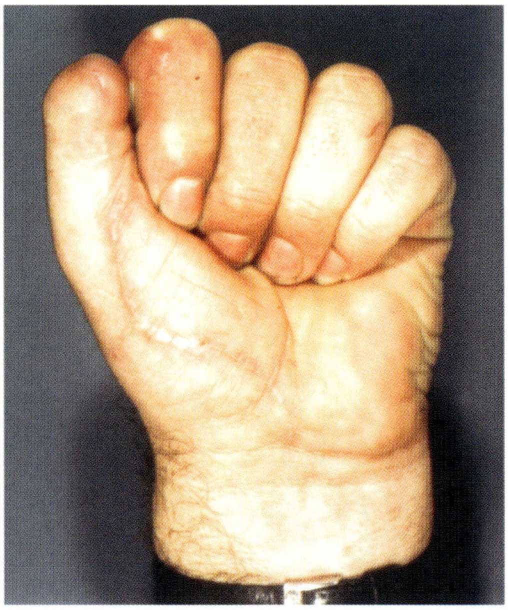

Figure 6.65d Good function five months postoperatively

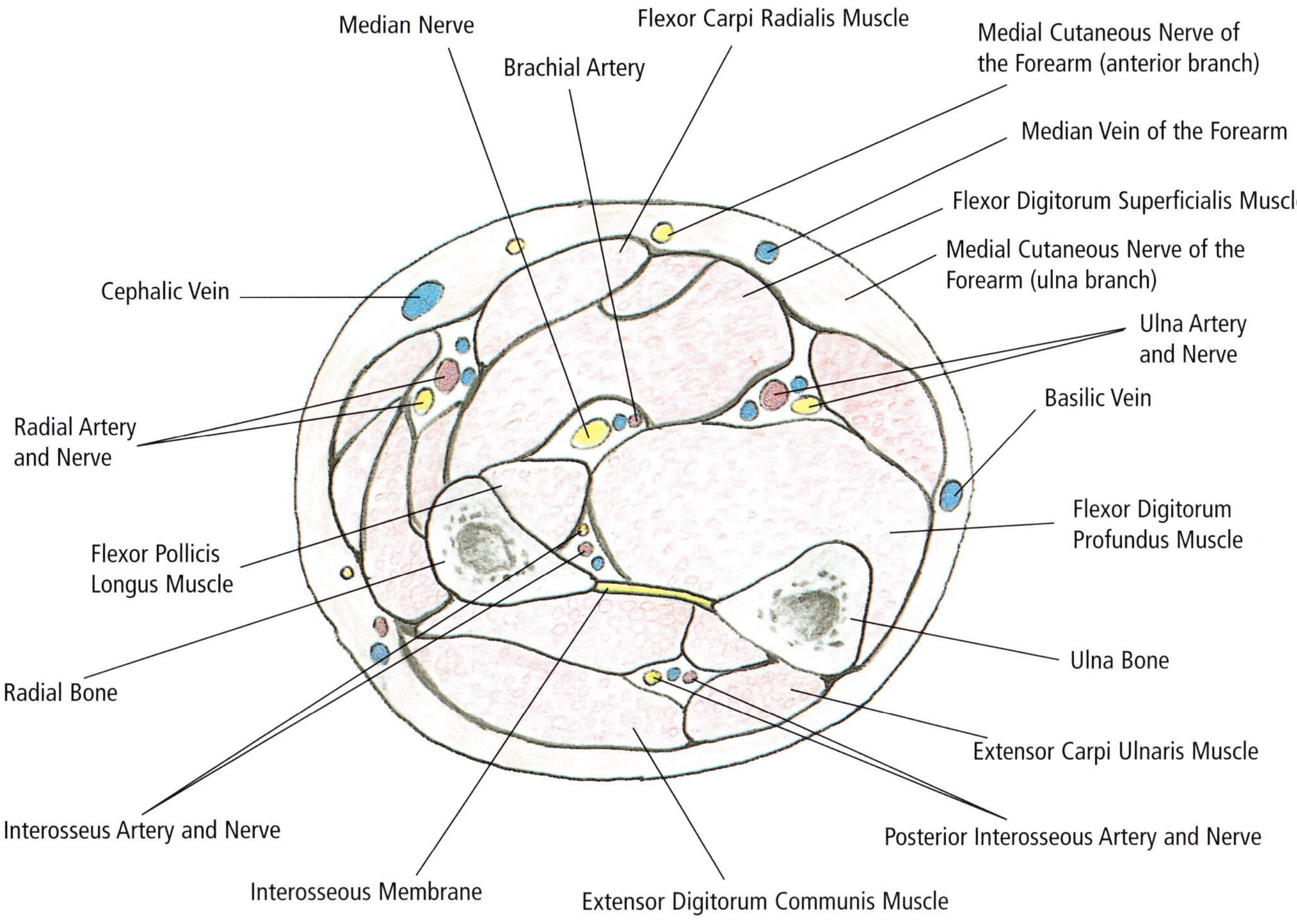

Figure 6.66a Cross section at the middle of the lower arm

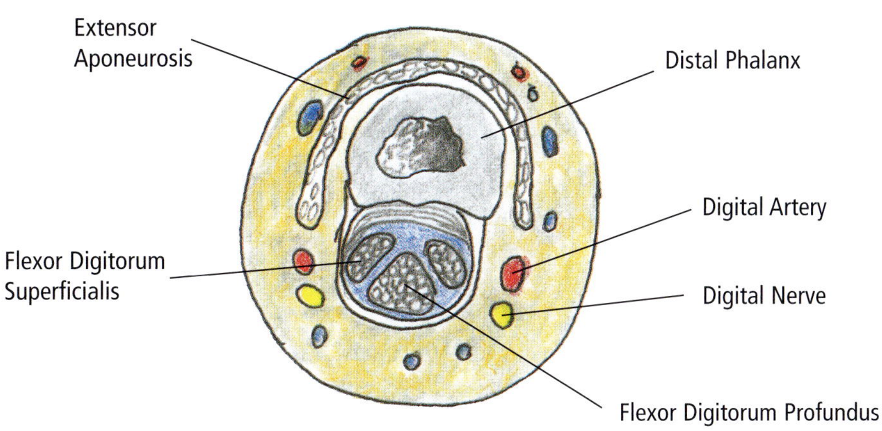

Figure 6.66b Cross section of the distal part of a finger

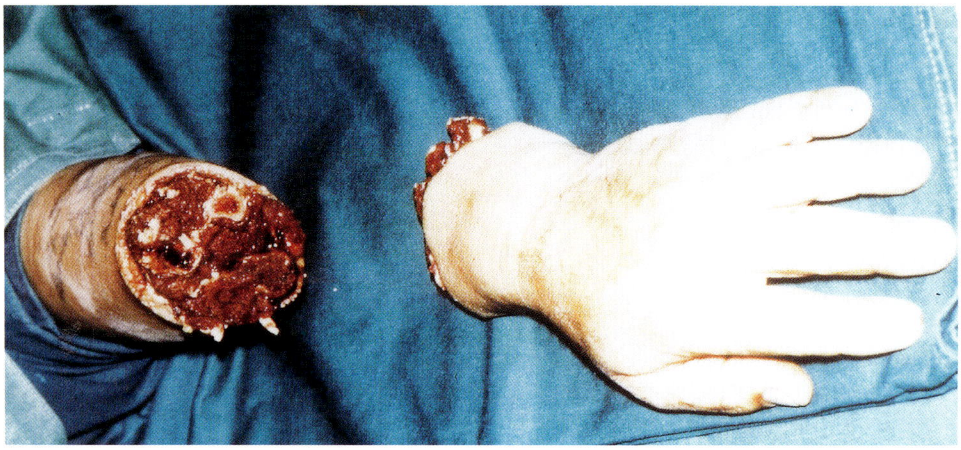

Figure 6.67a Amputation of the lower arm with a circular saw. Admission to hospital within one hour. Excessive muscle tissue damage and therefore a reduced tolerance to ischemia.

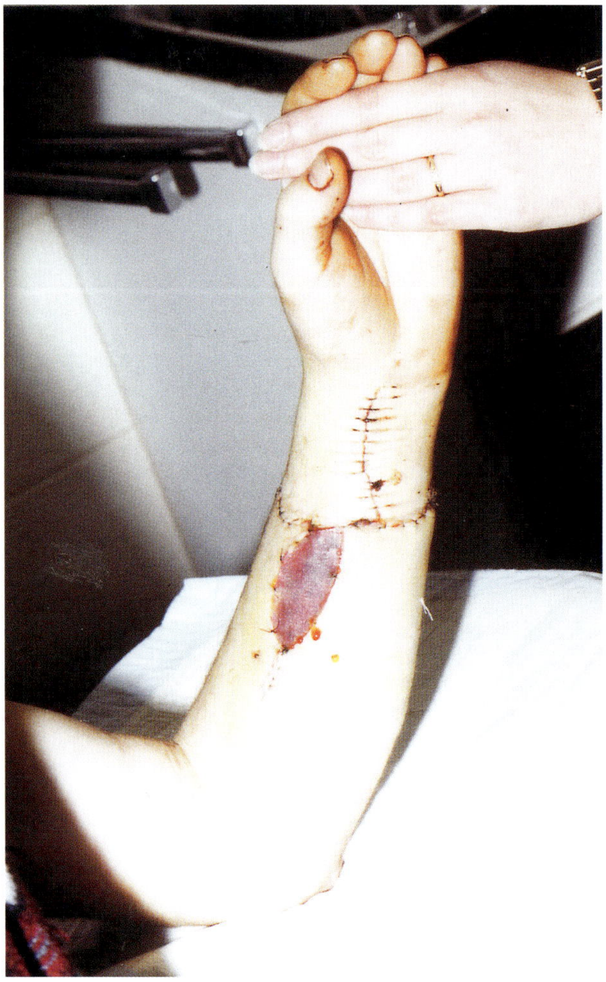

Figure 6.67c Five days after replantation

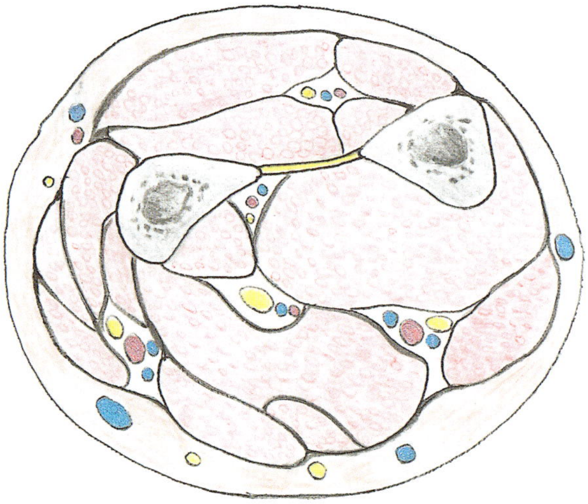

Figure 6.67b Anatomy of the distal part of the left lower arm.
Operation:
1) 5 cm shortening of both bones (10 to 15 cm is possible), osteosynthesis, removal of all crushed and contused tissue.
2) Suture of the flexor tendons
3) Anastomosis of both the radial and ulnar artery
4) Suture of the nerves (ulnar, median, radial nerve, anterior cutaneous nerve)
5) Extensor tendon suture
6) Vein anastomosis (cephalica, radial, ulna, basilic)
7) Skin closure. The proximal part is grafted with a split thickness skin graft to avoid any tension.

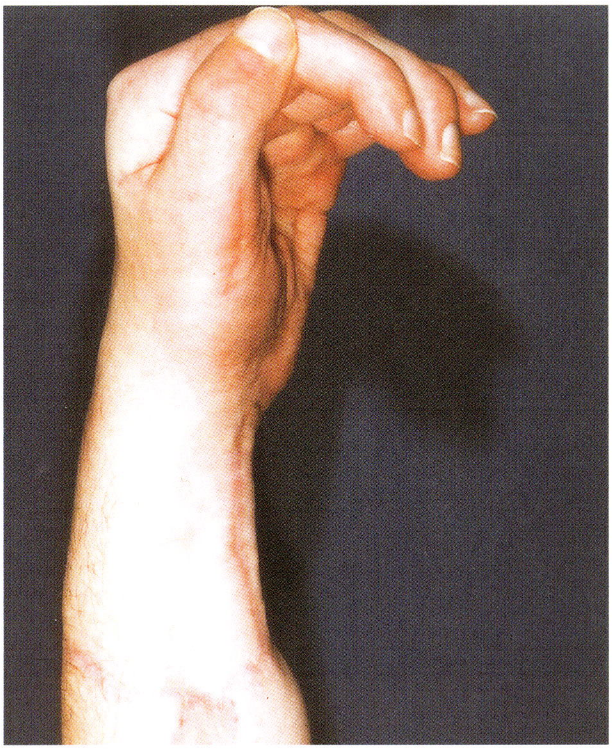

Figure 6.67d One year after replantation. Although intensive physiotherapy was performed the functional result is moderate. The re-innervation of the hand muscles (interossei and others) took for 5 to 6 months (1 mm per day – 150 mm = 5 months). Despite intensive physiotherapy muscle atrophy occurred.

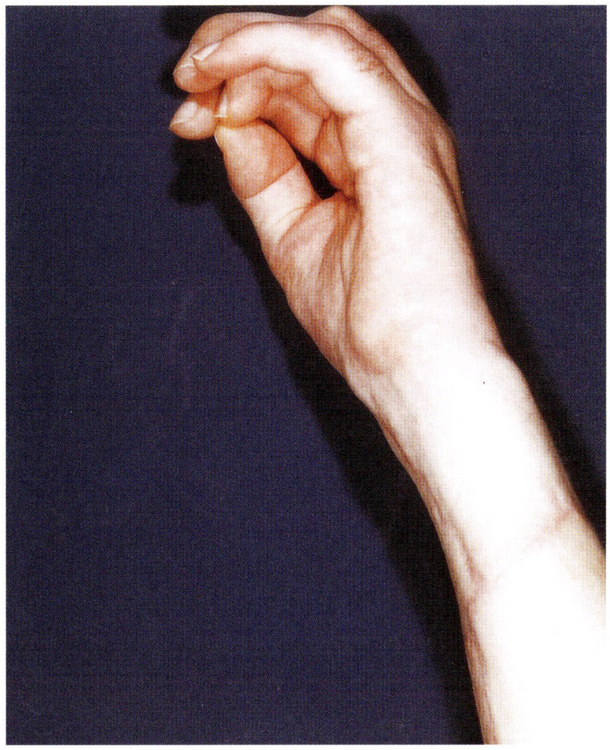

Figure 6.67e One year after replantation

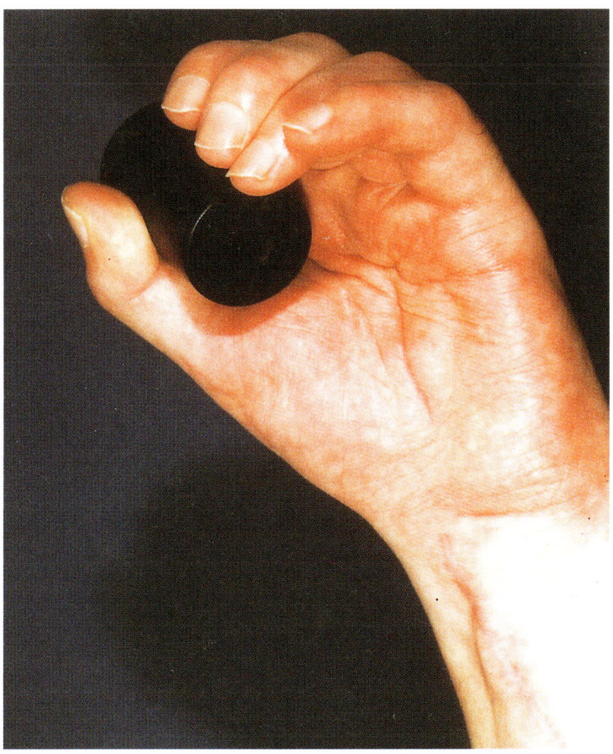

Figure 6.67f Adequate functional result

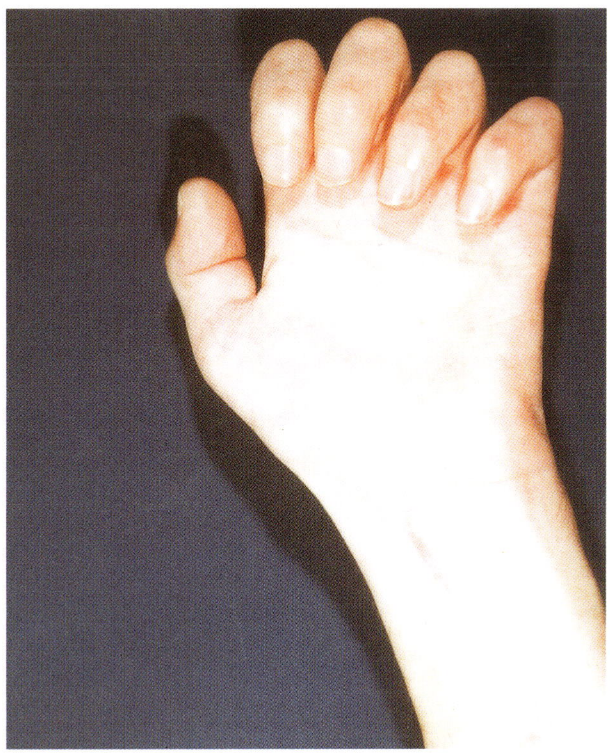

Figure 6.67g Adequate functional result

Heterotopic Replantation (Godina)

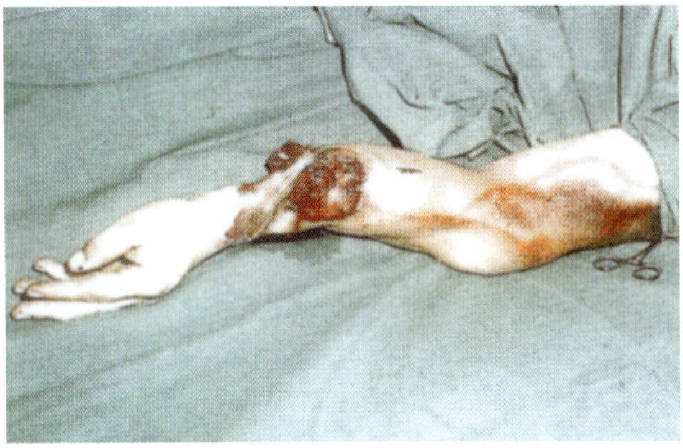

Figure 6.68a Severe crush injury of the lower third forearm. Avascular hand (case of Marko Godina)

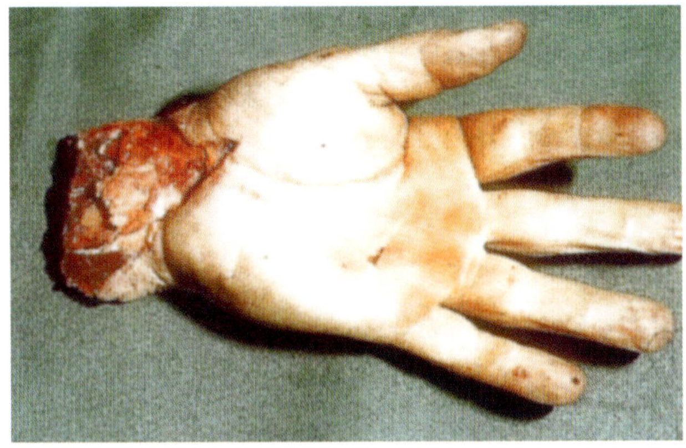

Figure 6.68b The amputated part is prepared for heterotopic replantation. A direct replantation was not possible due to the severe crush injury of the stump.

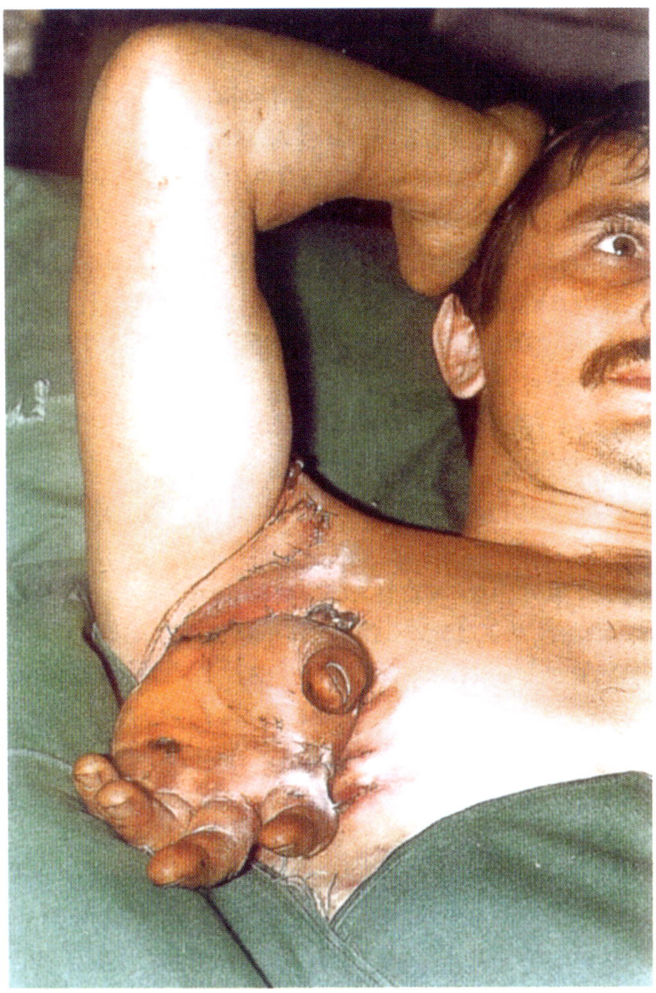

Figure 6.68c The hand is replanted to the right axilla and good healing took place.

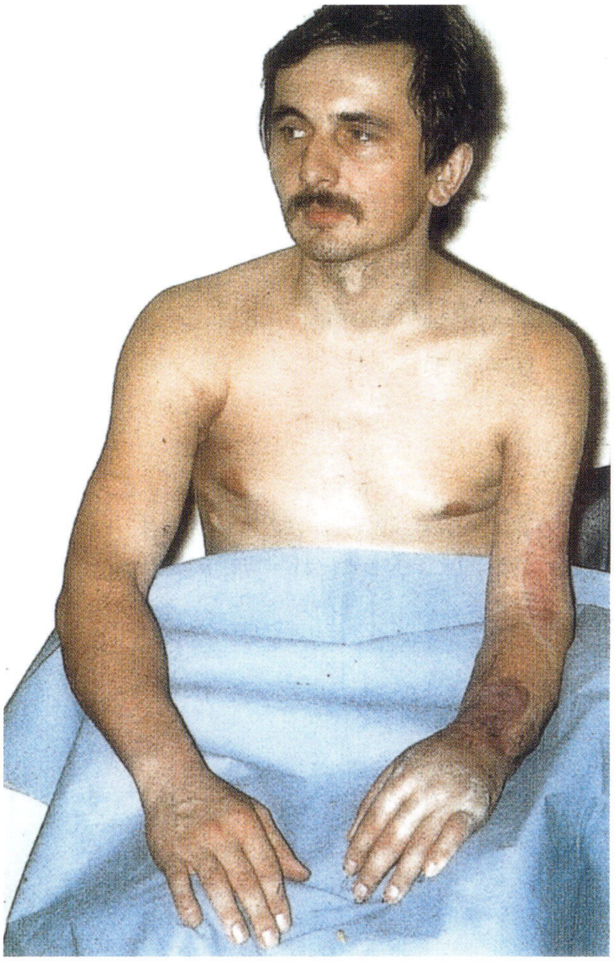

Figure 6.68d One month after the initial surgery the hand was replantation to the proper site [From: Marko Godina: A thesis. Presernova druzba (1991)].

In 1984 Marko Godina presented the first staged replantation of a hand. Due to excessive crush injury of the stump a direct replantation was impossible. Godina replanted the hand to another site using the axillary vessels for anastomosis. One month later when the stump was healed the hand was replanted to its proper position. Godina was the first surgeon to performed a temporary heterotopic replantation. He was one of the most skilled microsurgeons but sadly he was killed in a motor accident at a young age.

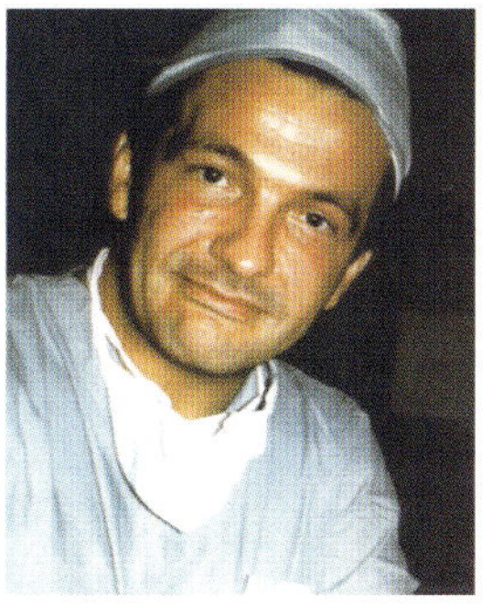

Figure 6.69 Marko Godina (1943–1986)

CHAPTER 7
Surgical Therapy of Burn Injuries

Pathophysiologic Aspects of Burn Injuries

One of the key pathophysiologic changes within the first hours after burn injury is volume loss due to capillary leakage. Numerous experimental studies have proven this pathophysiologic mechanism of volume loss into the extravascular space. Molecules up to a size of about 125 kDa can directly cross through the capillary leaks into the extravascular tissue. Burns of medium size (approx. 20–30 % TBSA) also induce a generalized increase of capillary permeability, but to a lesser extent than in the case of larger burns [Baxter 1971]. In this context, the overall fluid loss is directly proportional to the extent of injury (TBSA burned) and the burn depth. The clinical correlates to this pathophysiologic mechanism are generalized edema and – if untreated – hypovolemic shock.

The excessive loss of plasma proteins including fibrinogen into the extravascular space is evident if we look at data revealing protein concentrations in the extracellular space of approximately 3 % (3 g per 100 ml). Subsequently, oncotic mechanisms shift large fluid volumes to the extravascular proteins inducing the burn edema. The reabsorption of fluid from the extravascular space is induced synchronously with the capillary leakage, however, reabsorption within the first hours after burn injury cannot keep pace with the extravascular fluid loss. Clinical data and assessment of extracellular protein levels after extensive burn injuries have shown that protein loss within the first four days after injury doubles the normal plasma protein amount. About half of the protein volume is lost by burn wound exsudation, the other half is located in the extravascular intercellular space until it is absorbed within the first three weeks after injury.

The destruction of the capillaries and the concomitant loss of semipermeability abrogates the applicability of Starling´s principles, which are key to the maintenance of an adequate plasma volume.

During this phase, colloid fluids cannot be used effectively to maintain an acceptable oncotic pressure. For example, in burns extending 40 % or more of the total body surface area, the plasma volume drops rapidly to approximately 25 % of the regular volume.

It is known that capillary leakage induces the highest plasma loss within the first 12 hours after trauma and experimental and clinical data shows it is still significant 24 hours after burn injury. Monafo and colleagues have shown in a clinical study that a burn injury of 40 % total body surface area (TBSA) leads to a plasma loss of 4 ml per kg body weight and percent burned skin. If we take a burn victim of 70 kg body weight and a 40 % TBSA burn area, this means that the burn-induced fluid loss can be calculated at around 11.2 litres within the first 24 hours after trauma. These facts highlight the importance of aggressive volume replacement after burn injuries.

To maintain homeostasis of the protein metabolism, the physiologic response is an increase in protein synthesis, which is deranged in patients with extensive burns. In these cases, the dynamic equilibrium is shifted and more protein is lost than synthesized. The increased capillary permeability can be measured directly after trauma and reaches maximal levels at approximately three hours post burn. Later in the course of injury, the capillary permeability is reconstituted. The physiologic mechanisms normal-

This chapter is based on elementary research by Neven Olivari at the University of Cologne ('Habilitation', second post-doctoral thesis in 1975)

izing the capillary permeability are still incompletely understood. Edema formation is maximal at 48 hours after burn injury and resorption dominates the clinical situation. Serum albumin levels are used to monitor the protein status of the burn patient and albumin substitution may be used to support resorption. However, one has to keep in mind that the evidence level of albumin substitution is low, the advantages and disadvantages are discussed in literature.

The nadir of immunoglobulins such as IgG, IgM, IgA and macroglobulin α_2 can be detected four to seven days after burn injury. Serum IgG levels fall to 40 to 70 % of the baseline values. In contrast, the drop of IgM and IgA is not that accentuated, but their levels correlate proportionally with the extent and depth of the burn. About seven days after thermal injury, serum protein recovery begins and synthesis takes over consumption and loss.

Electrolytes

Extensive burn injuries induce critical electrolyte imbalances. Sodium loss from the circulating plasma stands at the forefront of clinical relevance: In general, the bodies' overall sodium supply consists of about 4200 mval (= 60 mval/kg body weight) in a 70 kg person. Ninety percent are located extracellularly and ten percent intracellularly. Normal serum sodium levels are 135–145 mval/l. Sodium is of critical importance for the maintenance of body fluid osmolarity. Pathophysiologically, the increased capillary permeability ("capillary leak") leads to fluid loss and sodium flux into the extracellular space. As a consequence, sodium and plasma volume are not only lost through burn wound secretion, but are also shifted temporarily into the interstitial space leading to edema formation. Therefore, close monitoring of serum sodium levels in burn patients is of utmost importance for the reconstitution of plasma volume and cardiac output.

A rise in the extracellular sodium concentration ultimately leads to a mild increased intracellular sodium concentration and an outflux of intracellular potassium.

Erythrocytes

Hemolysis, rigidity and shrinking of erythrocytes are typical hematological sequelae of burns. It is known that burns of 20 to 30 % TBSA lead to rapid hemolysis of approximately 10 to 20 % of the erythrocyte pool.

On the other hand, we know that erythropoesis is increased during the first four to five days after injury, but is considerably inhibited from day 15 to 17 after trauma. This is the hematologic basis for the typical burn-induced anemia [Baar 1970, Vanasek 1970].

The intracellular potassium concentration is reduced in favour of the intracellular sodium concentration.

Volume Substitution

The first steps of the specific management of burn injuries – after securing the airway and protecting the patient from hypothermia – includes cardiovascular stabilization: The burn-induced capillary leak does not allow colloidal solutions for volume substitution. That is the primary reason why the first-line volume substitution of burn patients should be established using crystalloid solutions such as Ringer`s solution or its modifications (Ringer`s lactate etc.). Based on clinical and experimental data, Baxter generated a general formula which helps to calculate the volume needs of burn patients:

4 ml crystalloid solution × kg body weight
× % TBSA burned

Using this formula, two thirds of the calculated fluid volume should be given within the first 16 hours after trauma, the remaining volume should be infused within the next eight hours.

However, nowadays, the Baxter formula is only of historical interest in burn therapy and burn-specific critical care medicine. If at all, the formula can be used preclinically when no specific monitoring is available and the patient cannot be transferred to a burn center primarily.

All monitoring options of modern critical care medicine are used to control fluid substitution of burn patients: First, continuous arterial blood pressure monitoring is essential (including the calculated mean arterial pressure, MAP), the mean arterial pressure should be kept around 70 to 80 mmHg using fluid boli and continuous infusion. Second, the central venous pressure (CVP) should be used to monitor adequate volume substitution, generally, the CVP should be kept within 5 to 12 mmHg. However, it is important to note that the use of CVP and its accuracy in reflecting the exact volume status of the patient is discussed in literature (REF). Third, hematocrit and haemoglobin levels should be used to indirectly monitor intravasal dilution and intravasal volume and efficacy of the established therapy (hematocrit 35–40 %). Last, the urine output should be monitored using Foley catheterization, depending on the clinical situation, around 100 to 150 ml per hour urine production marks the therapeutic goal. The use of silicone catheters is recommendable, they should also be equipped with a temperature probe, so that the body temperature can be monitored.

The generalized edema that is paired with aggressive volume substitution of burn patients prompted experimental studies to evaluate the use of hypertonic solutions: Monafo and Polk have already shown in the early 1970´s using experimental approaches that the survival rate of burn patients is equal with the use of hypertonic solutions compared to the standard isotonic crystalloid solutions (REF). However, clinical studies have demonstrated that hypertonic solutions are not tolerated very well by many patients. Also, assessment of cardiac output parameters have demonstrated that the pump function of patients is decreased about 40 % in burn patients that received hypertonic solutions compared to isotonic crystalloid solutions [Baxter, Moylan 1971]. The use of hypertonic solutions for burn resuscitation can therefore not be recommended.

There is general agreement about the fluid substitution of burn patients at 24 to 72 hours after injury: Within the first 24 hours after injury, the capillary leak is greatly reduced, so that the further extensive use of crystalloid solutions would only add on to exacerbate the generalized edema and lead to volume overload. Colloidal solutions can improve cardiac output within 24 to 48 hours after burn, during the resorptive phase when the generalized edema is being resorbed, the capillary integrity is reconstituted.

Due to tissue necrosis, hemolysis and disturbances of cellular transmineralization, the extracellular and consecutively the serum potassium concentration increases. Therefore, the use of potassium-free fluid solutions during the early postburn period has been advocated by some authors to avoid supraphysiologic potassium concentrations. The intensive experimental and clinical evaluation of this theory by Ahnefeld and colleagues revealed that when balanced electrolyte solutions are used to keep up sufficient kidney function, oliguria and anuria as a reason for hyperkalemia can be avoided in almost all cases.

Other Metabolic Aspects of Burn Injury

The basal metabolic rate of burn patients is markedly increased. There is a direct connection between water loss by evaporation and an increased metabolic rate. To evaporate one litre of fluid on a one square meter burned skin surface, an energy expenditure of 580 kcal is necessary. This equals a five-fold increase of energy expenditure as compared to the evaporation of one litre of fluid on unburned, normal skin. The water vapour pressure of normal, unburned skin is about 4 to 5 mmHg, whereas it increases over burned skin up to 30 to 35 mmHg. This causes the excessive consumption of oxygen, in other words energy. Barr and Jelenko showed that the fluid loss by evaporation is almost proportional to the depth and extent of the burned area. In severely burned patients, a volume loss of about 150 to 300 ml per hour and square meter burned skin surface area must therefore be anticipated by the burn surgeon.

The energy expenditure in burn patients with extensive injuries can be as high as 4000 kcal per day. The generation of the same energy equivalents under maintenance of a constant body temperature leads to lipolysis first, then protein consumption (muscle). When calorie needs are calculated, the basal metabolic expenditure has to be added to the increased calorie needs of the burn trauma state. Clinical and experimental studies have shown that energy expenditure and oxygen consumption of burn patients can be reduced, but not normalized, when the room temperature is increased to 29 to 32 °C. The borderline room temperature is 28 ± 2 °C. The catabolic protein loss and the resulting nitrogen production is reduced by increased ambient temperatures due to the lower oxygen consumption of the burn patient.

Clinical studies conducted by Campbell, Davis and Arturson included cohorts of burn patients with TBSA burns between 10 and 50 %: Patients that have been treated under room temperature of 32 °C had lower nitrogen excretion values than burn patients treated under ambient temperatures of 22 °C. These and other studies have led to the fundamental paradigm in burn care: Avoid hypothermia by passive measures.

The basic aspect of the "avoid hypothermia" concept can also be extended to the concept of early surgical excision and grafting of the burn wound: Among many advantages of this concept, the improved thermoregulation of excised and grafted burn wounds can indirectly add on to improving the disturbed metabolism of burn patients.

Microcirculation

Hypovolemia, increased viscosity and albumin loss aggravate postburn thrombocyte adhesion which culminates in platelet aggregate formation. The activation of the clotting cascade then induces erythrocyte aggregation and microthrombus generation. Endothelial damage and subsequent perivascular edema are due to mediator production and hypoxia further hamper the microcirculation. This phenomenon can be observed in inadequately or undertreated burn injuries where impaired microperfusion progresses to stasis in the affected zones and is then called sludge or "no-reflow" phenomenon. Tissue hypoxia and metabolic acidosis are key elements of the burn shock. Even though during the early postburn period no marked acidosis is detectable – due to respiratory compensation – substantial tissue acidosis is present.

Renal Function

Severe burn trauma induces suppression of kidney function or at worst acute renal failure, in particular when resuscitative therapy and volume replacement is insufficient. Hypovolemia, hypotension and hypoperfusion can in most cases be effectively managed by aggressive volume substitution, so that the glomerular filtration rate remains within the physiologic range. Experimental studies have shown that tubular resorption remains unaffected in (underresuscitated) burn injury and the glomerulo-tubular balance stays normal. Renin production is only one of the key elements of the pathogenesis of acute postburn renal failure. It is well known that inadequate resuscitation of burn patients leads to a complete stop of sodium excretion and it seems that aldosterone is among the most prominent but not the only pathogenetic factor. Serum urea levels increase substantially in this phase, the excretion, however, can be stimulated using diuretics and volume substitution. Early clinical trials have shown that volume substitution using crystalloid solutions increases the urine output and significantly lowers serum urea levels as a consequence. In this context, it is important to note that the use of diuretics during the early postburn phase cannot be recommended due to the pathomechanisms of burn injury: Diuretics will only increase the volume deficit and lower water and electrolyte excretion. In summary, the pathomechanisms of burn injury, namely the initial capillary leak and the consecutive intravasal hypovolemia and tissue edema, are the primary culprits of postburn renal dysfunction. Therefore, adequate treatment of renal dysfunction in burn patients means adequate volume substitution and tight monitoring of organ function.

Inhalation Injury

Thermal injury of the lung in the early stages and treatment is frequently difficult to recognize. All burn injuries in closed spaces and the affection of the face, nasal hair singeing and smut particles periorally and in the oral cavity are highly suspicious of concomitant inhalation injury. Short exposure more frequently affects upper airway structures such as oral cavity, pharynx, epiglottis and trachea, whereas longer exposure frequently also leads to the affection of lower airway structures such as bronchioli and alveoli. Inhalation injury is still associated with higher incidence of complications and higher mortality rate of burn victims.

The pathophysiologic picture is dominated by massive edema formation after a latency period of six to 48 hours. Edema formation is progressive and frequently accompanied by the obliteration of smaller airway structures. Pulmonary gas exchange in the alveolar region is markedly impaired by the edema. Thermal injury of the lower airway leads to injury of the bronchial epithelium and formation of pseudodiphteric lesions and necrotic parts obstruct the smaller bronchi together with sputum and exsudate. This induces obstructive emphysema, multiple atelectases and smaller bleedings. When only smaller bronchial parts are obstructed, a tracheobronchitis that is very resistant to therapy may be the clinical consequence. When large necrotic parts are dissociated into larger portions of the airway, lethal obstruction may develop.

Severe burn injury without direct inhalation trauma also affects pulmonary function: The generalized tissue edema also affects the lung and impairs gas exchange. The hypovolemia-induced loss of blood pressure in the pulmonary arteries leads to alveolar collapse in large pulmonary regions. Circulatory disorders such as precapillary constriction and microthrombus formation induce disturbances of the ventilation-perfusion-ratio. The formation of microatelectases further aggravate the hypoxemia. These disturbances as well as the primary erythrocyte damage are physiologically balanced by hyperventilation. The pCO_2 can be maintained within the physiologic range in most cases, however, blood oxygenation cannot be improved by hyperventilation. Therefore and because chest x-ray studies are frequently normal during the early postburn phase, blood gas analysis is of utmost clinical importance and is one of the key diagnostic tools in the management of ventilation disorders of burn patients.

In the case of slight indirect affection of the lung, oxygen supplementation and supportive measures such as air humidification is indicated. More severe inhalation injuries frequently necessitate intubation and ventilation. Excessive tracheobronchial edema formation are an indication for bronchodilatative pharmacotherapy, steroids may be used, but their clinical value in the treatment of inhalation injury is debated in literature. Loss of oxygen partial pressure and rise of carbon dioxide partial pressure are cardinal signs of respiratory insufficiency and are treated by manipulation of the positive end-expiratory pressure (PEEP), ventilation pressure (P insp.) and inexpiration (I:E) ratio (inversion). Pneumonia is a frequent complication after burn injury and especially in cases of inhalation trauma: Microbiological assessment of the antibiogram must lead to adapted antibiotic treatment after initial use of broad-spectrum antibiotic when no antibiogram is obtained but the clinical diagnosis is made. Supportive measures such as frequent endobronchial suction and sterile techniques in the management of these patients add on to treatment measures of postburn pulmonary complications. Physiotherapy and side-positioning, prone positioning of the burn patient – in special beds – are also important elements of respiratory management of burn patients.

Stomach

Clinically, approximately 11 % of the burn patients develop gastroduodenal ulceration within their hospital stay (curling ulcer). It is interesting that in burn patients with a TBSA burned between 20 and 40 % *and* concomitant sepsis or infection, stress ulcer formation is significantly more frequent. The curling ulcer is basically identical with stress ulcers in trauma of other cause than burn injury, however, there are some differences: Stress ulcers that have developed after other stress types than burn injury most often form in the proximal portion of the stomach along the greater curvature. The curling ulcer is most often located in the antrum and duodenum. The posttraumatic stress ulcer develops within the first 24 hours after trauma, the "burn ulcer" can develop at any time within the first four weeks after burn injury. Of course helicobacter pylori is more active under such circumstances.

It is important to note that there is no hyperproduction of gastric secretes, rather, a hypoproduction of normal gastric secretes is notable after burn injury.

Liver

The hepatic function is drastically inhibited in patients suffering from burn shock, even though the clinical symptomatology is not that obvious. The pathologic-morphologic correlate of the shock liver is mainly the hyperemia due to venous congestion, microthrombus formation of the liver vasculature and micro necroses. Disorders of hepatic function due to toxins develop under the clinical picture of hyperglycemia and glycogen depletion and lowered to abolished protein synthesis (albumin, fibrinogen, prothrombin), decreased energy generation, reduced enzyme activity and functional reduction of the reticuloendothelial system. Pathological studies reveal sepsis-induced central hepatocyte necroses, later on fatty degeneration or abscess formation.

Burn Wound Infections

Bacterial contamination of the burn wound is an almost inevitable complication of burn injuries. Even though substantial progresses have been made in burn care, problems still remain concerning burn wound infection control and therapy. The burn wound itself is not sterile, within the first three days after injury grampositive saprophytes (e.g. B. subtilis, Enterococci etc.), later on gramnegative microbes take over. Approximately from day five post injury on, the burn wound contamination becomes more and more invasive, both in terms of depth and surface extension. Burn-induced sepsis was the leading cause of deaths in about 75 % of the cases in the preantibiotic era. It is of importance to note that the burn-induced sepsis does not derive from clinically obvious burn wound infection in about 50 % of the cases. This means that blood culture sampling is of essential clinical importance when infection or sepsis is suspected. The reasons for burn wound infections are multifactorial: First, exogenous reasons like smear infection (hospital personnel, lack of sterile management principles), contact with contaminated objects, insufficient initial management of the patient (insufficient debridement etc.) and autocolonisation with cutaneous bacteria, feces etc. are among the primary ways how burn wound infections can occur. These facts underline that it is not realistic to believe that only with sterile measures, bacterial contamination of the burn patient can be avoided, it is in many cases the patient himself who is the source for bacteria that become pathogeneic under the immunocompromised situation of burn injury.

The burned skin is a good "culture media" with serous transudation and damage of essential cellular and non-cellular barriers (dermis, local immunoactive cells etc.).

The bactericidal ability of leukocytes, especially of neutrophils, is markedly impaired in extensive burns. The resistance of severely burned patients is impaired by the hypoperfusion if the liver, the massive production of bacterial toxins and the generation of cellular debris and fibrin clots. The functions of the reticuloendothelial system like phagocytosis, antibody generation and detoxification are also inhibited in burn patients. The immunoglobulin levels fall to approximately 40 to 70 % of the normal value within the first four to seven days after injury. Substitution of gamma-globulins does not increase their serum levels and does not increase the survival rate.

The following microbes are frequently isolated from burn wounds:

a) β-Hemolytic Streptococci
Appears within the first three days after trauma in the burn wound. The production of toxins, especially streptolysins, negatively affect cellular respiration in general and damage specifically myocardial structures. The secreted hyaluronidase permits the bacterial translocation into the cell. Streptococci are generally sensitive to antibiotic therapy and therefore do not pose significant clinical problems at present.

b) Staphylococcus aureus
Staphylococcus aureus is frequently isolated from burn wounds. Its pathogenicity depends on the production of necrotizing exotoxins, hemolysins, leukocidins, enterotoxins and staphylocoagulase. The virulence is abolished under a 100 % oxygen atmosphere, however, its virulence increases with anaerobic conditions. Penicillinase production is the reason for the isolation of more and more resistant strains.

c) Pseudomonas aeruginosa
Pseudomonas aeruginosa (or pyocyaneus) is a gram-negative, mobile microbe that produces pigments which lead to greenish pus coloration. The produced ferment leads to anoxic cell necrosis. In burn wounds, pseudomonas is rarely isolated within the first week after injury, most frequently it appears in the wound within the second week after burn trauma. Its toxin induces hypotension, decreased cardiac output, tissue acidosis, leukopenia and an increase of the endogenous catecholamine levels. Pseudomonas strains are more and more resistant to antibiotic therapy. It is important to note that pseudomonas is physiologically isolated from normal skin as a saprophyte, only toxically damaged skin lead to its virulence.

There are also many another germs and strains which appears in the area of burn wounds.

Simultaneous assessment of neutrophil function and bacterial counts in the burn wound have shown that septic disorders only evolve in cases of massive dysfunction of leukocyte phagocytosis. Constant bacterial influx from infected burn wounds into the bloodstream maintain the septic state of the burn patient. Usually, septicemia occurs within the second or third week after trauma. Today septic disorders and pneumonia rank first among the most frequent lethal complications of burn injury. Negative side-effects of aggressive antibiotic therapy include candidosis and fungal contamination of the burn wound, which may also become inciting agents of sepsis, which once more underlines the necessity of early surgical excision of the burn wound and reconstruction of an intact skin barrier.

Classification of Burn Trauma and Severity

In the case of flame burns or scald burns, the tissue reacts with permeability disorders at temperatures of about 50 to 70 °C. Higher temperatures induce coagulation necrosis of the affected tissue. The depth of the pathohistologic alterations is determined by the duration and the intensity (temperature) of heat exposure.

Usually, burn wounds are classified into three grades which goes back to Hildanus in the 17th century: Redness, blistering and necrosis.

Today, it is generally accepted that in modern burn care this classification is insufficient and does not comprise all aspects of injury. Blistering or bulla formation, for example, which would be classified as a second degree injury, can occur in superficial second degree burns (IIa) as well as in deep superficial (IIb) burns. Therefore, the following classification is generally used to classify burn depth:

I	Superficial burn
IIa	Superficial epidermal burn
IIb	Deep dermal burn
III	Full-thickness burn (comprising all skin layers, necrosis of cutis)

The correct diagnosis of burn depth and extent is important for the prognosis as well as for planning of the treatment.

When applying the current, modern concept of early burn wound excision and grafting, exact and fast diagnosis of the burn depth is essential. The decision, which regions of the burn wound have to be excised and grafted must be taken within the first 72 hours after injury.

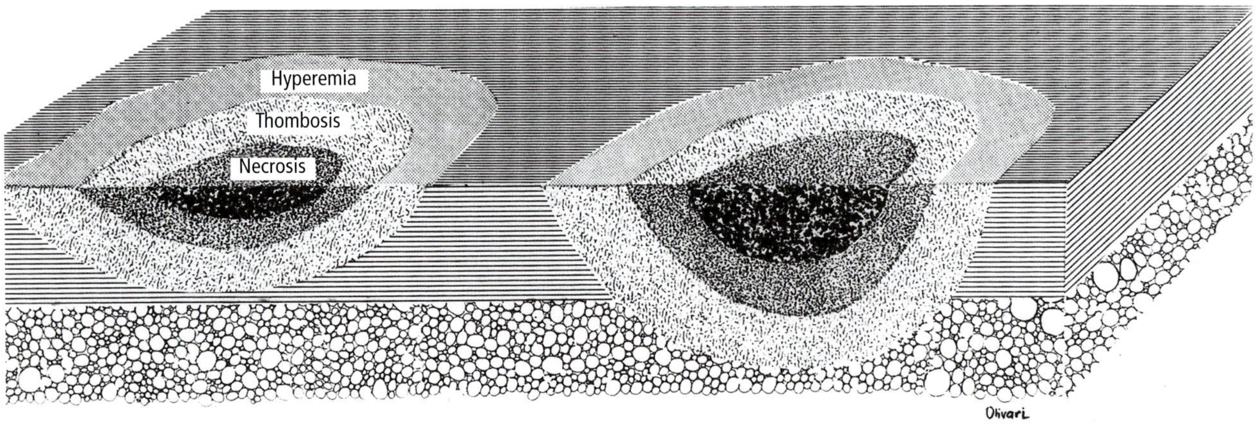

Figure 7.1a Appearance of burn wounds and correct diagnosis of burn depth: Both (left and right) burn wounds clinically appear the same, however, the injury depicted on the right is deeper.

The external appearance of burn wounds is sometimes the same in burns of different degrees. Pathohistologically, we can subdivide the following zones of the burn wound [Jackson et al. 1969]:

1. Central zone of necrosis or coagulation. The color of this zone is whitish-brown.
2. Zone of thrombosis, which is characterized by thrombotic, dilated vessels. During the first 24 hours after injury, tissue perfusion is decreased, but still intact. This is of clinical importance, since compression can induce ischemia within the first 24 hours after injury.
   Up to approximately 24 hours after injury, there is no clinical difference to the zone of hyperemia. After approximately 24 hours post burn, the perfusion is further decreased and then halted, thrombosis of all vessels and tissue necrosis occur in the zone of thrombosis.
3. Zone of hyperemia with typical vessel dilation. This zone heals spontaneously within approximately eight toten days.

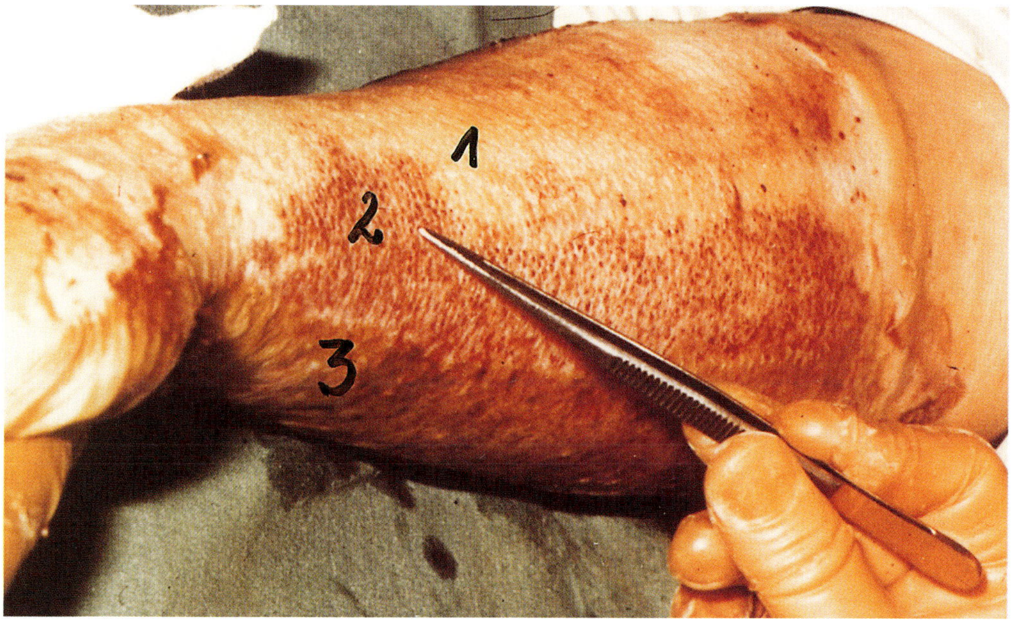

Figure 7.1b Tangential excision under ischemic conditions: 1) excised area (under tourniquet), 2) zone of thrombosis, 3) zone of necrosis.

Diagnosis of Burn Depth

Patient History, Injury Mechanism

Sunburns most often induce grade I or grade IIa injuries.

Boiling water, hot oil or short flame exposure most frequently lead to grade IIa and grade IIb injuries, depending on the duration of heat exposure. Most injuries occur at temperatures of around 65 °C (hot coffee, tea etc.)

Chemical burns most often lead to grade IIb and grade III injuries.

Flame burns or contact burns (oven, metal) should per primam rise the index of suspicion for grade III injuries.

Clinical Appearance

Epidermal burns instantly lead to erythema (grade I), the skin surface is dry. Superficial dermal burns (IIa) induce a reddish-livid skin discoloration and frequent bulla formation (blistering), which reveal a reddish base after mechanical ablation. The skin surface is wet. First and second degree burns can be assessed with compression (sterile glass spatula), an immediate ischemia is seen. This is a useful tool and a clinical proof that there is no vessel thrombosis within the examined area of the burn wound.

Grade IIb burns show a livid to whitish-yellow, wet skin surface, often, the concomitant bullae have a white, ischemic base. Under compression with a sterile glass spatula, ischemia.

Occurs frequently within the first 24 hours after injury because of the still ongoing thrombotic processes. However, at 24 to 48 hours after injury, thrombotic vessels stop the microcirculation and the glass spatula test is negative.

Third-degree burns are characterized by a white-brownish discoloration and parchment-like consistence of the skin. Furthermore, thrombotic vessels can be observed and rarely the skin surface is charred and black (sometimes classified as injury grade IV). These areas reveal a negative ischemia test.

Sensibility Testing

Explicit sensibility testing cannot be recommended for multiple reasons: First, the majority of burn patients admitted to a burn centre have already been administered pain medication, so that initial sensitivity tests may be inaccurate. Second, many patients are ventilated on admission, so no sensibility testing can be done. Third, sensibility testing using prick tests pose the risk of wound contamination and also further damage skin continuity. Generally: Superficial dermal burns are painful; deep burns are not painful.

Tangential Test Excision

In the situation of uncertainty about the correct diagnosis of the burn wound depth, the suspicious region can be "test excised" tangentially under sterile (operating room) conditions within the first 48 hours after trauma. The Weck knife should be adjusted to an excisional depth of 0.2 mm. Punctual, homogenous bleedings indicate burn wounds of the depth IIa, no further excision and grafting is usually necessary. If no bleeding occurs, this indicates deeper, grade IIb and III injuries which require excision and grafting. Our own clinical results show in a cohort of 148 burn patients that the exclusive use of this method for depth assessment of the burn wound was sufficient to indicate excision and grafting or conservative treatment, only two cases, where the indication for excision has erroneously not immediately been made, required further diagnostic assessment.

Development of Necrosis in Deep Dermal Burns (Grade IIb)

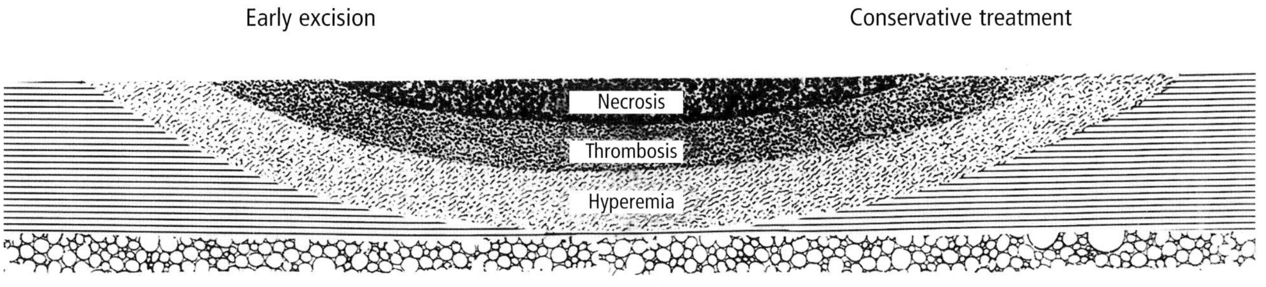

Figure 7.2a Schematic depiction of a deep dermal burn injury (IIb). The corium is still intact, but is located in the zone of hyperemia.

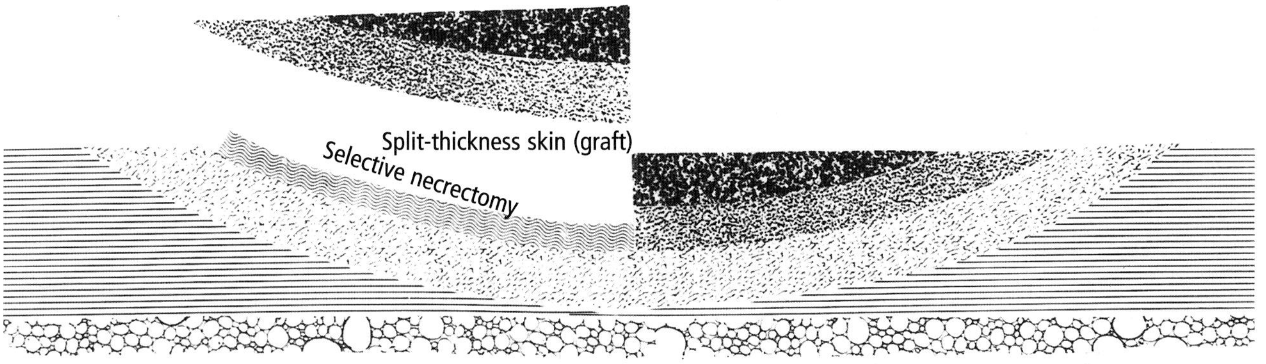

Figure 7.2b A portion of the burned area is excised on day three post injury and grafted using split-thickness skin grafts. The other portion of the burn wound is subjected to conservative treatment.

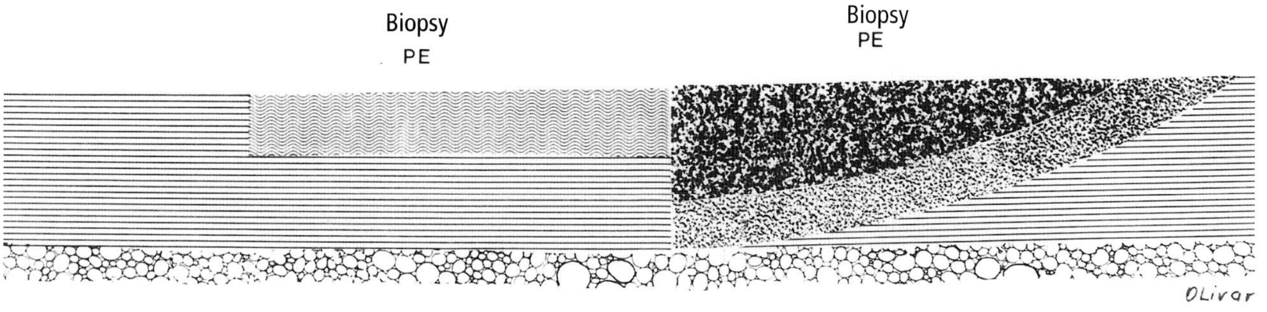

Figure 7.2c Ten days later, the excised and grafted area healed completely. The conservatively treated region progressed to deepening and necrosis of the burn wound.

Early Excision and Healing – Clinical Proof

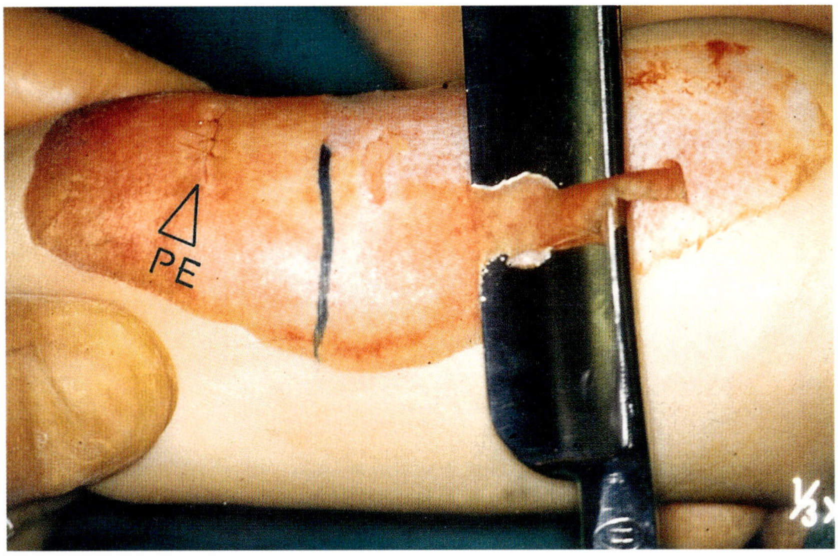

Figure 7.3a Scald burn injury three days after trauma. The right half of the burn wound is tangentially excised. Status post biopsy excision on the left side (arrow).

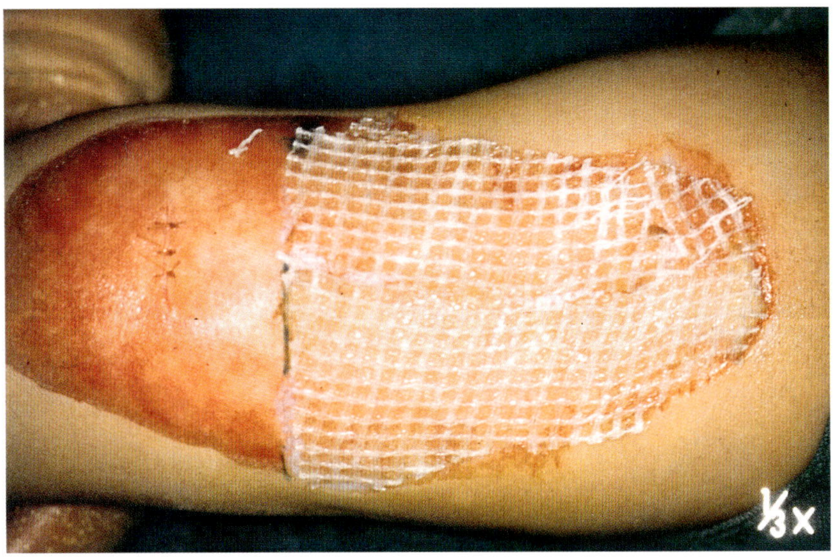

Figure 7.3b The right half of the burn wound is grafted with a split-thickness skin graft, the left portion of the wound is conservatively managed.

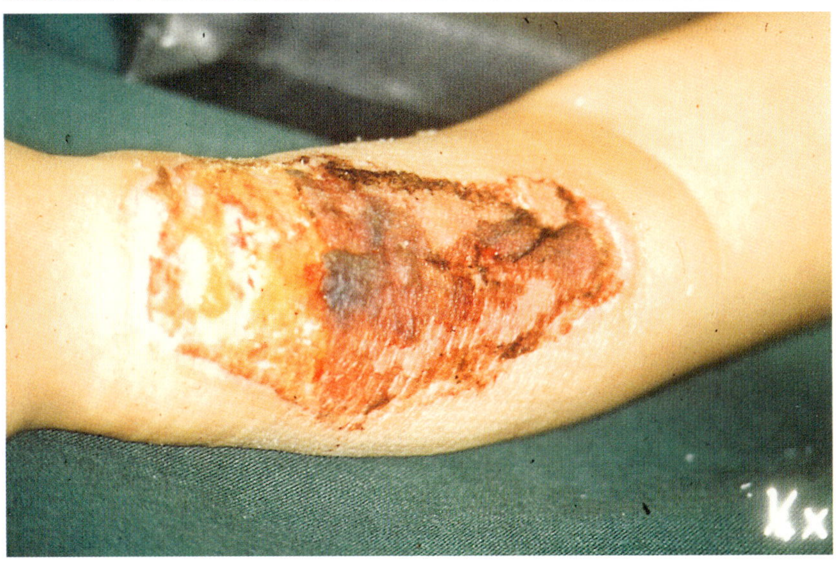

Figure 7.3c Status after 14 days. Right side: The grafts healed in very well. Left side: The tissue necrosis is substantially deeper than on day three. The wound is beginning to epitheliali-ze from the edges.

Table 7.1 Assessment of burn depth

Grade	History	Clinical Appearance	Pathologic Changes (major points)	Sensibility (pin prick)	Ischemia Test (glass spatula)	Test Excision (0.2 mm Weck knife)	Prognosis	Indication for Surgical Excision
I Epidermal burn	Sunburn	□ Erythema (reddish discoloration) □ Dry skin	Vasodilatation	Hyperalgesia	Pressure: Ischemia	Punctual bleeding	Primary healing within 5 days	No excision
IIa Superficial dermal burn	Hot fluid	□ Reddish-livid bullae with red base □ Wet skin	Epidermal necrosis	Hyperalgesia	Pressure: Ischemia	Punctual bleeding	Primary healing within 14 days – pigmentary abnormality	
IIb Deep dermal burn	□ Boiling fluid □ Hot oil □ Flame burn (short exposure)	□ Livid to white-yellowish bullae with white base □ Wet skin	Epidermal necrosis and two thirds of the cutis	Hyperalgesia, partially analgesia	No ischemia on pressure (frequently during the first 24 hours)	No bleeding	Secondary healing within 4–12 weeks – scar formation	Excision (tangential/epifascial) and grafting
III Complete loss of cutaneous structures	□ Open fire □ Contact burn □ Electrical burn	□ Brown-white □ Parchment-like □ Black	Complete necrosis of cutaneous structures coagulation	Analgesia	No ischemia on pressure	No bleeding	After three weeks rejection of the necrotic tissue debris. Epithelialization from edges of burn wound	

Determination of the Burned Skin Surface Area in Percent

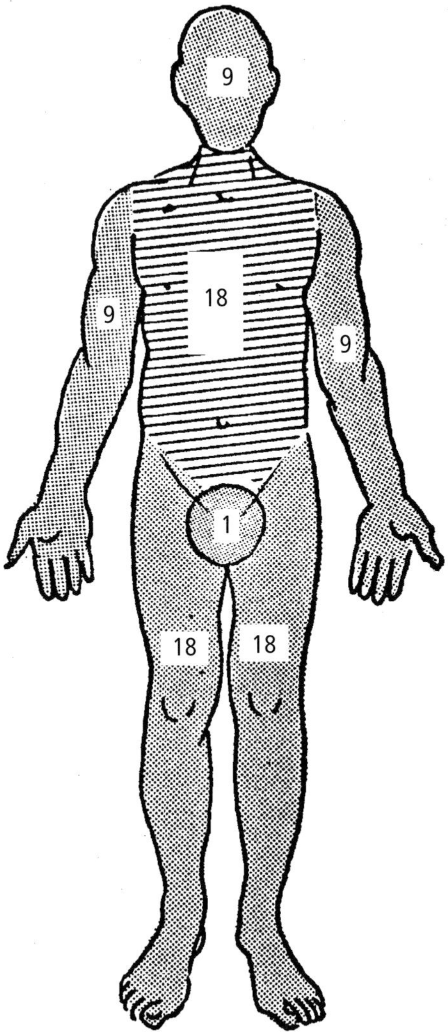

Figure 7.4a Rule of nines

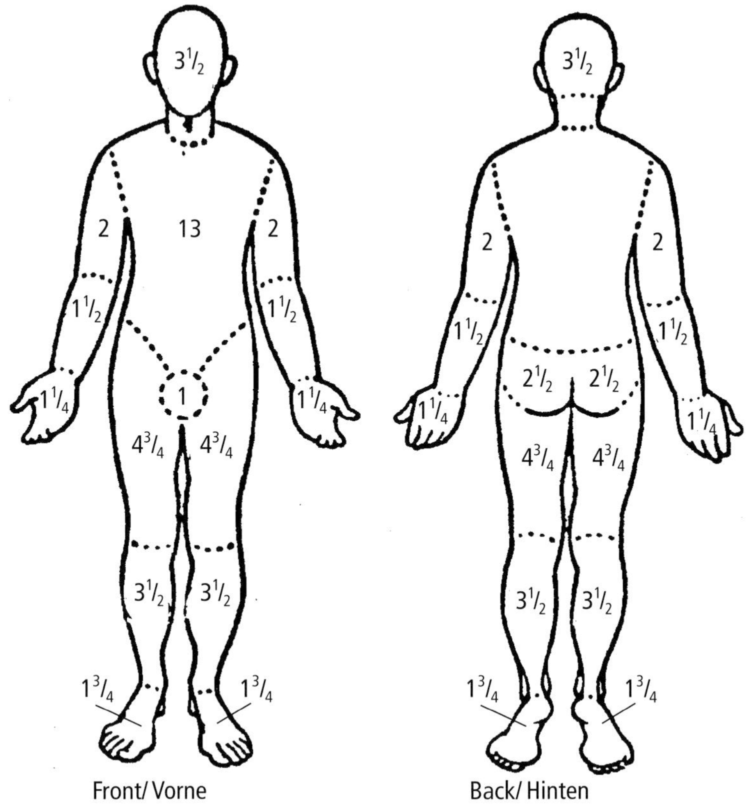

Figure 7.4b Determination according to Lund and Browder

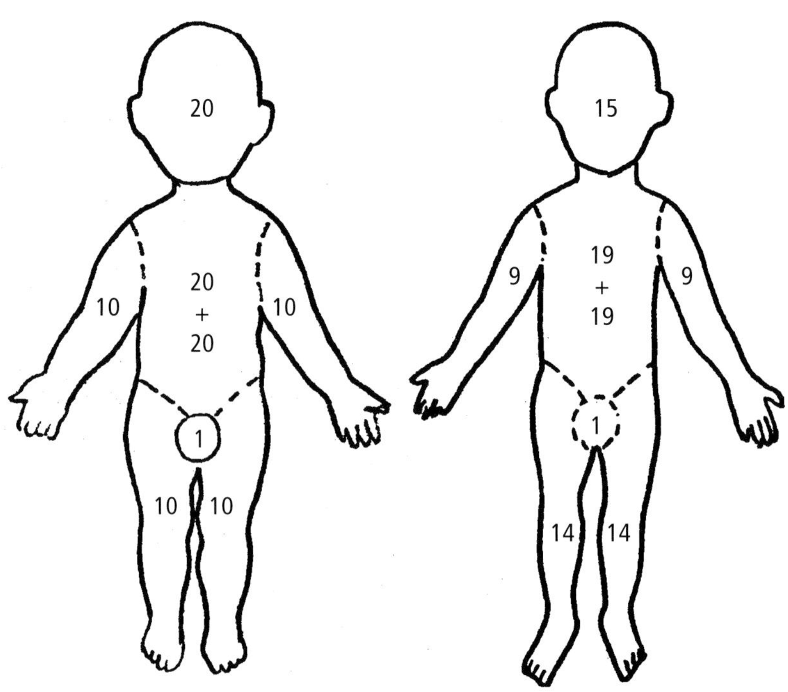

Figure 7.4c Children 1 Jahr /One year 7 Jahre / Seven years

Excision

Indication

Not only complete loss of the cutis (grade III), but also deep dermal burns (grade IIb) should be excised and grafted. In principle, no regions should be left to primary healing. The spontaneous healing of an area measuring two to three centimetres in diameter takes about four to six weeks (formation of granulation tissue). The underestimation of such areas unnecessarily prolongs the hospitalization and treatment. In general, several regions of the body do not have to be operated on immediately, and it is frequently a good decision, to wait and see which areas of the burn wound have to be operated on. This can be done for the face, the soles of the feet and the palms. In contrast, other surgeons proclaim that radical excision of the burn wound is necessary, no matter where the localization.

Timing of the Operation

Third-degree burns should be excised within the first 48 hours after trauma, if the patients' general condition allows the operation. More extensive burns with mixed depth (IIb and III) are excised around day three after trauma (principle of early excision). Up to this point of time, the burn patient should be stabilized and sufficiently resuscitated. The correct diagnosis of burn depth should also have been done at this point of time. Longer waiting up to 14 days or 21 days after injury cannot be considered standard therapy anymore. The only indication to wait longer is the fact that extensive burns comprising large body surface areas can sometimes not be excised in one session and the burn team has to wait and restabilize the patient so that the next operation can be done.

Grafting Area

The best graft bed is the freshly excised, vital wound surface. And it is irrelevant, whether the graft bed is dermis, subcutaneous fat, fascia, musculature or any other vital tissue. Even on bony structures (debrided) skin grafts can be successfully transplanted.

Planning

Burned body surface areas up to 20 % (IIb, III) are very often excised and grafted in one session. In burns of greater extent, jeopardized structures (dorsum of the hands, joint areas) are excised and grafted during the first session. Generally, the grafts are harvested before the excision is made so that the excisions can be done according to the available skin grafts (most frequently mesh grafts). The face, the dorsa of the hands, the décolleté, the dorsa of the feet and the genitals have to be transplanted with unmeshed grafts (!).

Surgical Technique

The face and the torso are excised with a hand dermatome (Weck knife, Humbey knife) which is usually set to a thickness of 0.2 to 0.5 mm until punctual bleedings are seen.

It is of utmost importance to graft on dry, non-bleeding wound surfaces only; otherwise, hematoma formation under the grafts may occur and hamper healing and graft take. By using meshed skin grafts, this risk is significantly reduced.

The tangential excision of extremity burn wounds are done under local ischemia (tourniquet). Besides the significantly reduced blood loss, one of the main advantages of this procedure is the better accuracy and the better protection of intact structures.

Brownish zones of necrosis, livid areas with thromboses and reddishly discolored tissue have to be excised. The excision of older burn wounds is done in the same fashion: Granulation tissue that has formed also needs to be excised. Granulation tissue is uncoordinatedly growing, vascularized connective tissue which can develop thick, fibrous scar plates with significant disturbance of function and aesthetic appearance. It is an ideal media for the growth of bacteria of all kinds and an entrance site for septic disorders that are difficult to treat and it is also exit site for protein-rich secretion. This fact has already been recognized in 1891 by Urban. Unfortunately, grafting on granulation tissue is still commonly done in the treatment of burn injuries.

Transplantation

Split-Thickness Skin Grafting (Usually Mesh Grafts)

After the excision of the burn wound, the grafts are positioned onto the wound. Suturing of the grafts is in most cases not necessary. Only in body regions that are frequently moving, for example axilla, neck area or shoulders, the grafts are sutured in place using atraumatic stitches or skin staples. Mesh grafts can be fixated using fibrin glue.
Most frequent sources of error:

a) *Bleeding and Hematoma Formation Under the Skin Grafts*
These complications are caused by insufficient coagulation of bleeders. In heparinized patients, hematoma formation can progressively occur due to capillary bleedings. The definitive loss of worthy grafts can be avoided, if they are inspected at the time of the first dressing change 24 hours after the excision and all coagulates and potential bleeders are removed.
b) *Insufficient Excision*
Insufficient excision of the burn wound (no punctual bleedings) precludes or substantially delays revascularization.
c) *Graft Infections*
Skin graft infections are extensively discussed in literature. Our own experience revealed that graft infections only occur in cases of insufficient excision or when the excision of the burn wound is delayed. Skin graft infections are almost inevitable when a large body surface area is burned.

Generally, mesh grafts are used. The face, hands, feet, the decolleté and the genitals are grafted with unmeshed skin grafts (sheets), because of the better functional and aesthetic results.

Homografts

In the early period after trauma, cadaver skin has the same advantages as autografts: Reduction of the bacterial load, evaporation and the plasma and electrolyte loss.

From day eight after grafting, rejection takes over and leads to complete loss of the homograft. Portions of the homografts can be integrated into the regenerating skin – these areas need to be excised (dermabrasion) and then autografted.

Sandwich Technique

In burns of large body surface areas (>40 %), portions of the auto grafted wound areas can be overlayed with cadaveric skin (homografts).

The homograft overlay protects the surface from plasma loss and infection for seven to ten days.

Combined Method

For a longer time, burn surgeons from the People Republic of China have used homografts in extensive burns: Small holes are cut into the homografts, these are "filled" with autologous skin grafts, which are fixated in place [Yang et al. 1980, 1982].

The homografts temporarily protect the excised area. In the meantime, the small autograft island heal and spread in. This method can be used in large body surface area burns.

Synthetic Skin Substitutes

Epigard or similar synthetic foils (nylon, polyurethane) can be used for temporary closure of the excised burn wound. They have the advantage of ready availability at any time.

Synthetic skin substitutes avoid plasma loss and infection. Epigard can be used for seven to ten days and even longer, until a definitive plan and method for the closure of the burn wound has been organized and the patient is stable and sufficiently resuscitated. Actually newer skin substitutes are under evaluation (Integra, Matriderm a.o.) which show an interesting progress.

In-Vitro Epidermal Cell Cultivation

This technique promises a substantial progress in burn care. The culture of epidermal cells (keratinocytes) is extensive and time-consuming (15–20 days). The keratinocyte suspension is directly applied to the excised burn wound and homografts are temporarily used in overlay technique and fixated with skin staples or sutures. Epithelialization then occurs. This epithelium is not stable, if the cell suspensions are not grafted onto dermal parts. If parts of the dermis are still viable, a definitive result can be obtained. If keratinocytes are grafted onto fascia, the grafted area remains unstable and frequently has to be skin-grafted later on.

Tangential Excision Under Ischemic Conditions (Tourniquet)

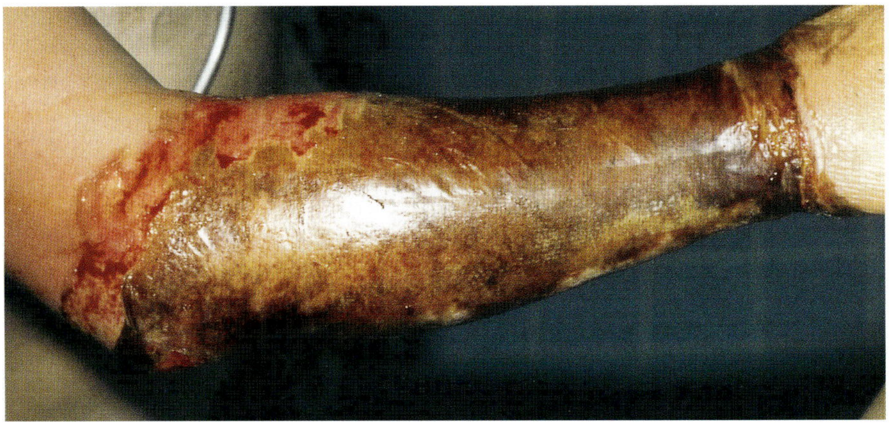

Figure 7.5a Burn injury of the right forearm, mainly third degree injury

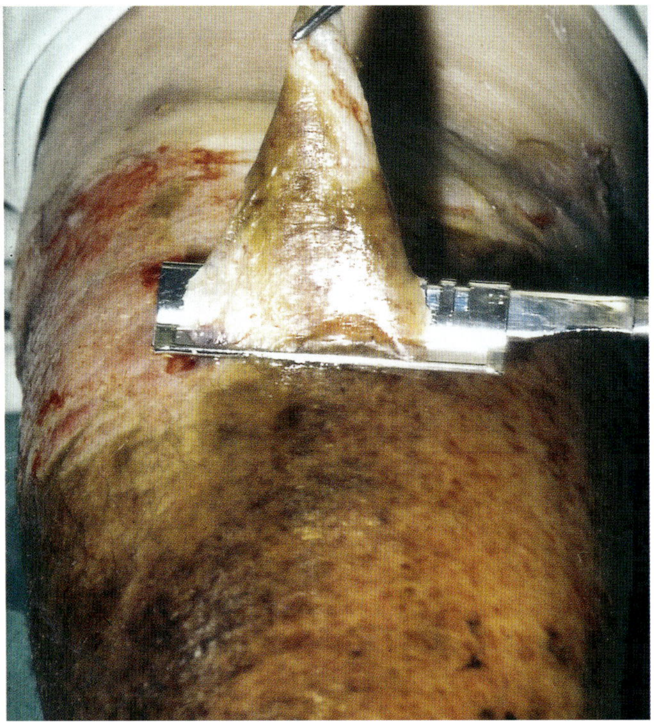

Figure 7.5b Tangential excision under ischemic conditions (tourniquet, Weck knife). This technique avoids bleedings of the extremity and facilitates the diagnosis of burn depth.

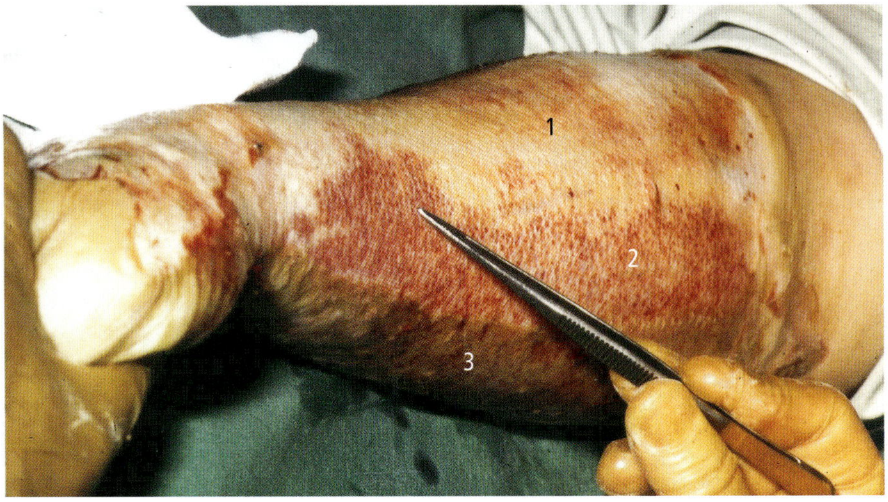

Figure 7.5c 1) Vital, healthy tissue after excision is of whitish-yellow color when excised under ischemic conditions. 2) The zone of thrombosis (blue-red) needs to be excised, otherwise the tissue necrosis progresses in depth. 3) Non-excised zone of necrosis.

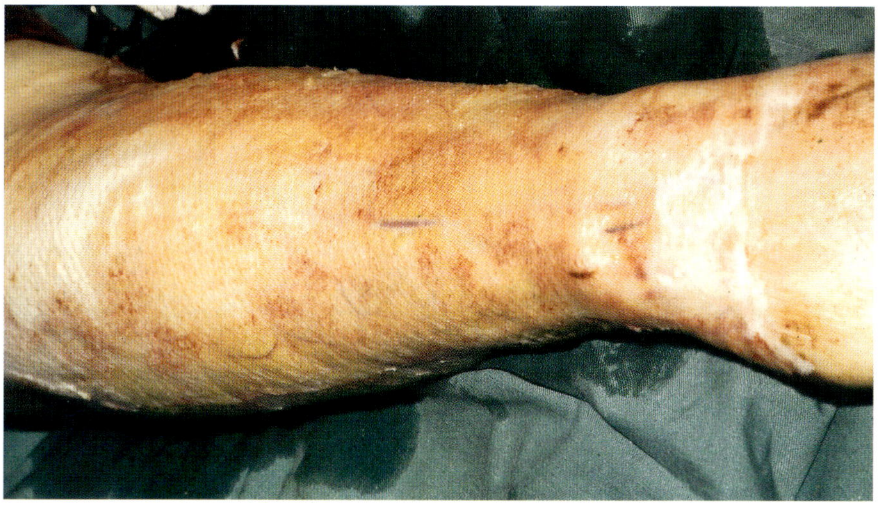

Figure 7.5d Status after complete excision (under ischemic conditions). Afterwards, skin grafts are used, compressive dressings are put in place under sterile conditions. Then the tourniquet is opened.

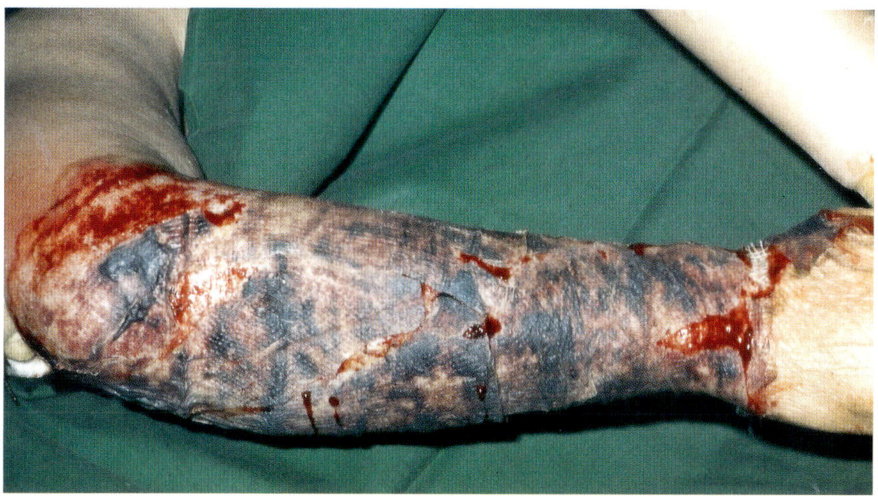

Figure 7.5e Status one day after the operation

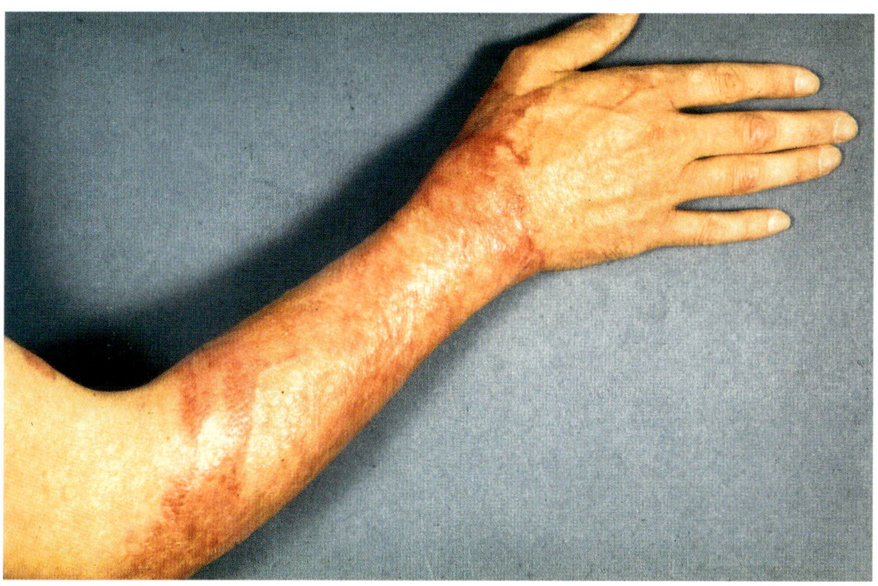

Figure 7.5f Status six months after the burn trauma

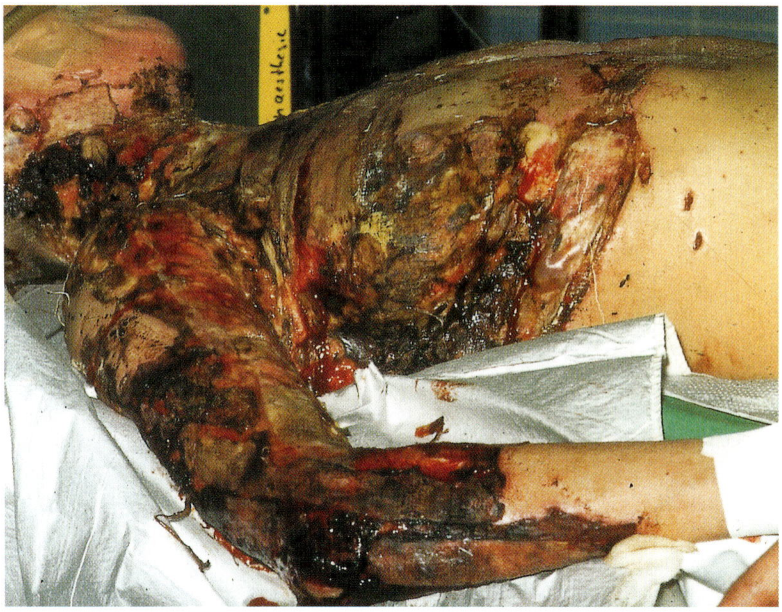

Figure 7.6a Third-degree burn (fuel spill). The burn shock was controlled at 48 hours post injury.

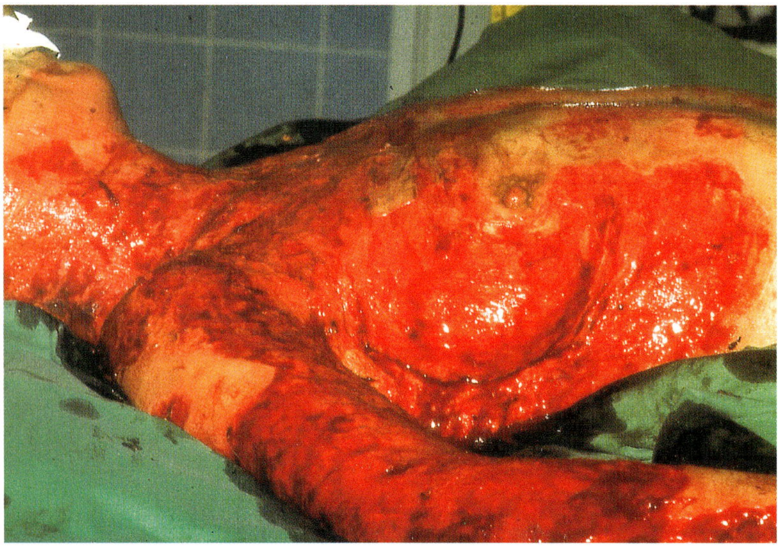

Figure 7.6b 48 hours after trauma, the burn wound is tangentially excised until punctual bleedings occurred. The blood loss is significant, which has to be anticipated and PRBC´s have to be available.

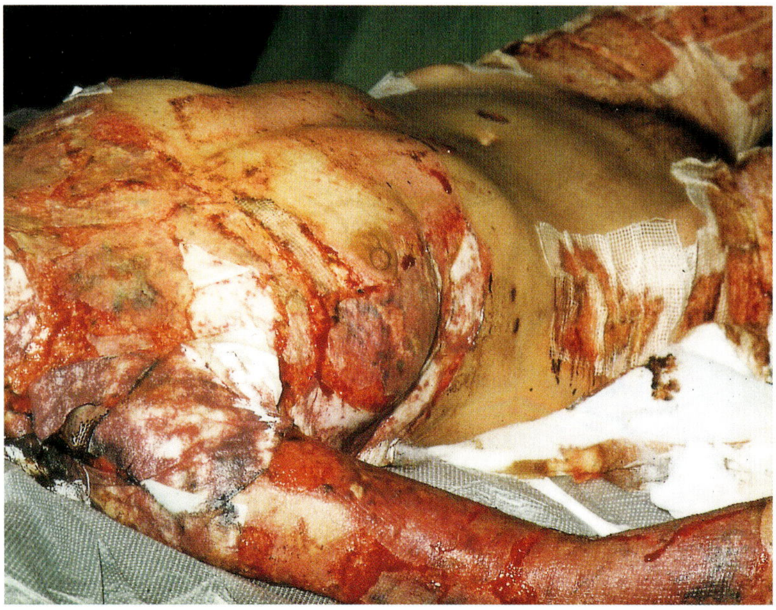

Figure 7.6c A part of the excised area is skin grafted , the other part is temporarily closed with Epigard. One week later, Epigard was removed and replaced by split-thickness skin grafts.

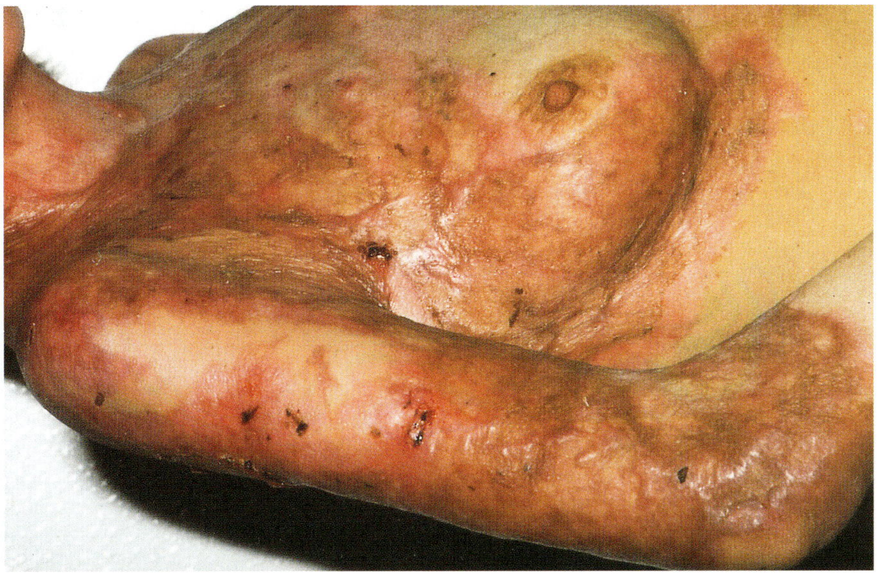

Figure 7.6d Status 14 days after the excision and 17 days after the trauma. Daily physiotherapy has been initiated from postoperative day four on.

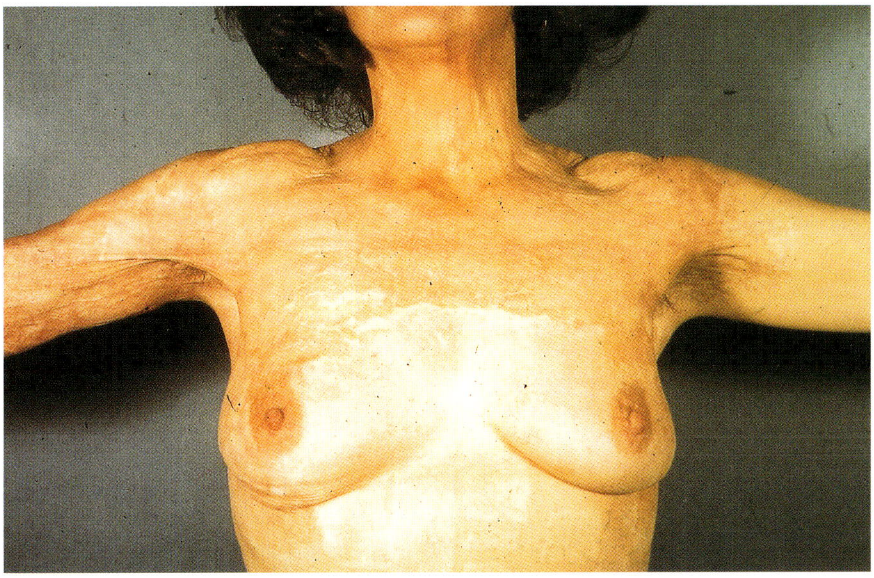

Figure 7.6e Status one year after the trauma. No other reconstructive procedures have become necessary.

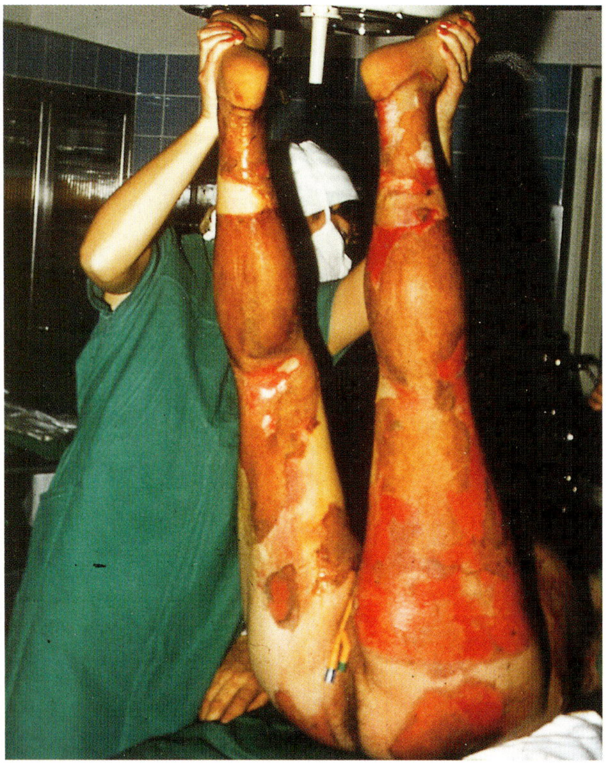

Figure 7.7a Flame burn of 45 % TBSA caused by gas explosion (35 % third degree injury and excised). Both legs, arms and the face are affected.

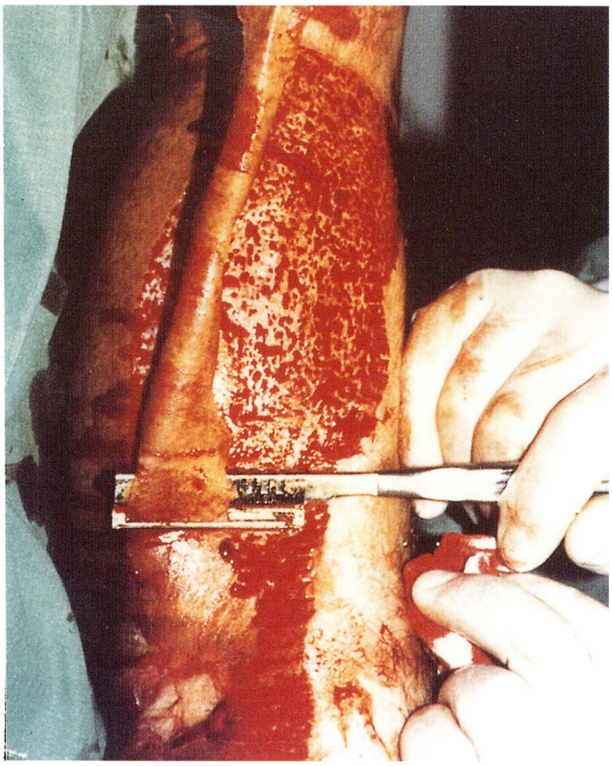

Figure 7.7b Excision to the level of punctual bleedings

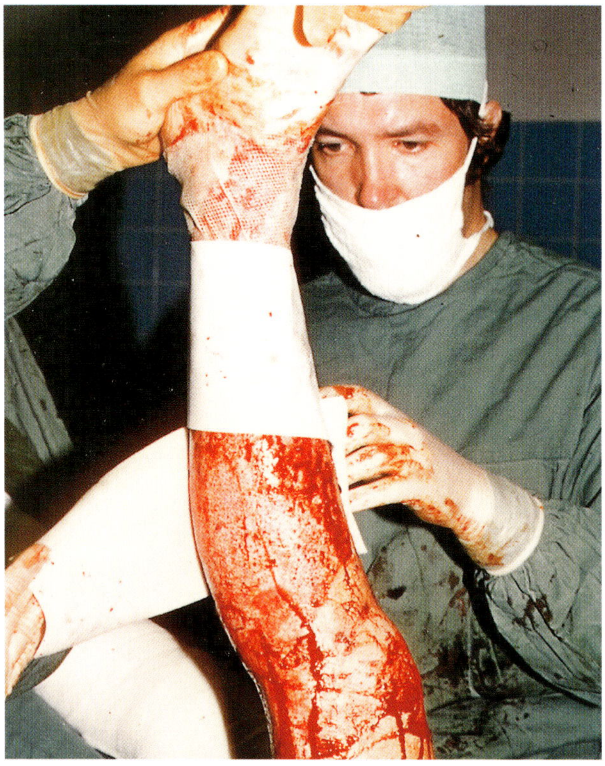

Figure 7.7c Both arms and the right leg are skin grafted, the left leg is temporarily treated with Epigard wound dressing.

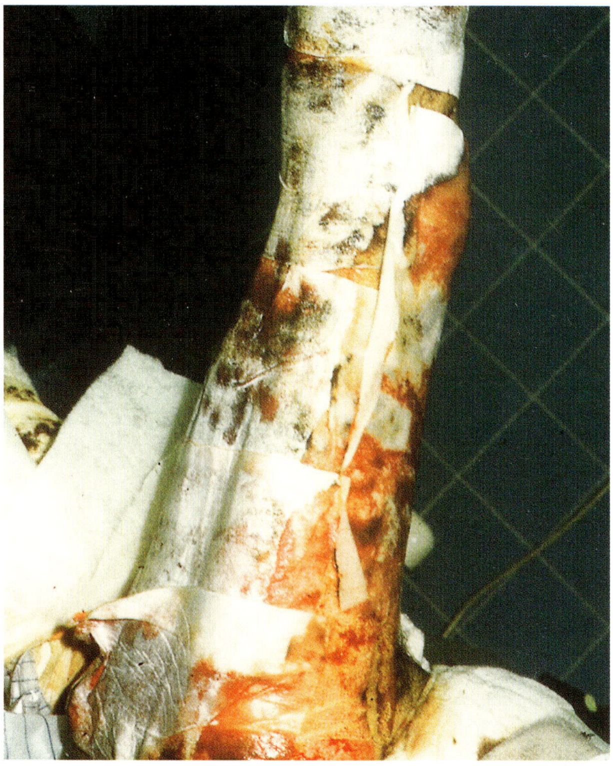

Figure 7.7d Aspect of the Epigard-treated region seven days post excision. The Epigard protects the excised area against contamination and avoids plasma loss.

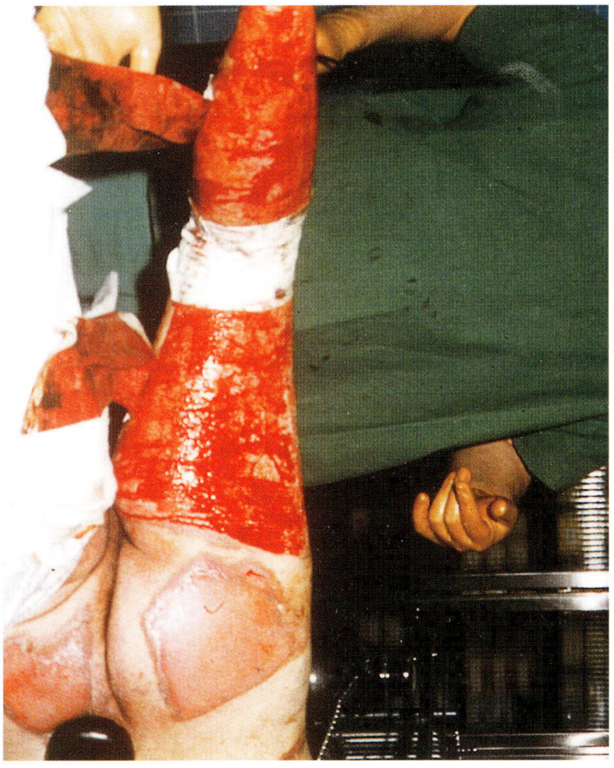

Figure 7.7e After removal of the Epigard dressing, the graft area is clean.

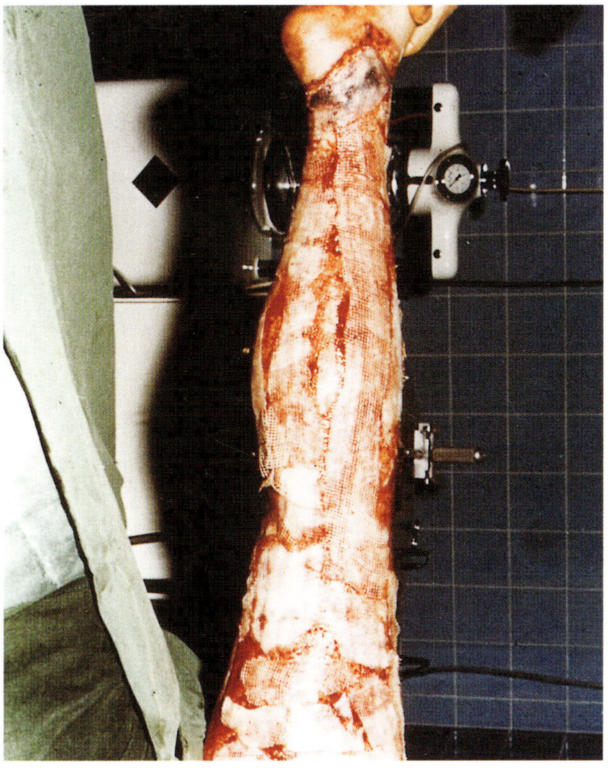

Figure 7.7f Split-thickness skin grafts

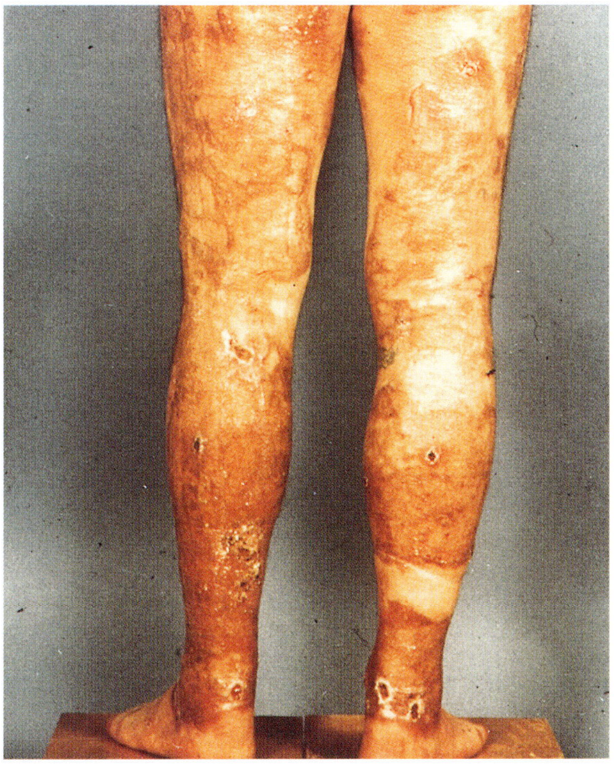

Figure 7.7g Status six weeks after trauma at the time of hospital discharge

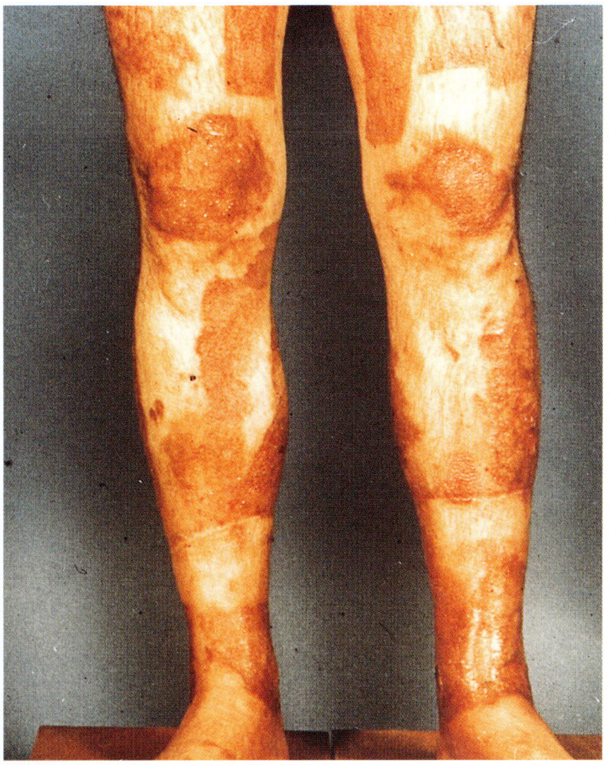

Figure 7.7h Status six weeks after the injury

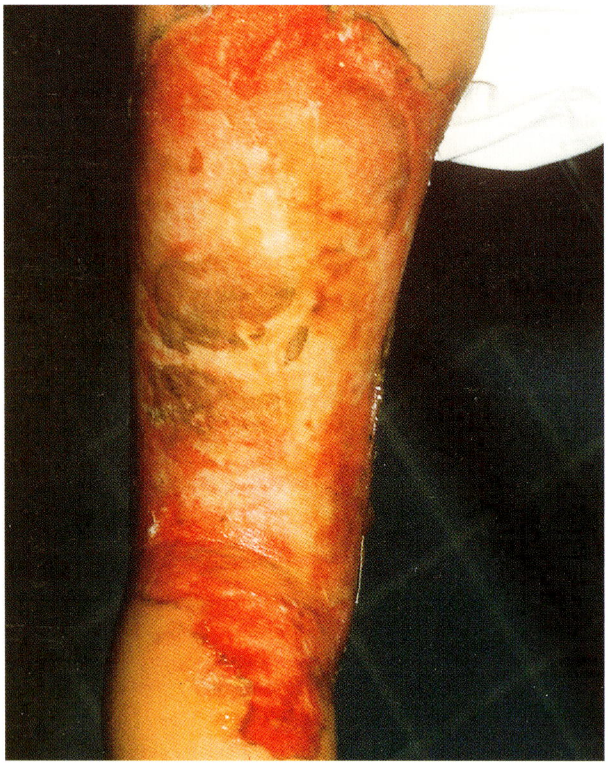

Figure 7.8a 10 % TBSA flame burn. All 10 % of the affected surface

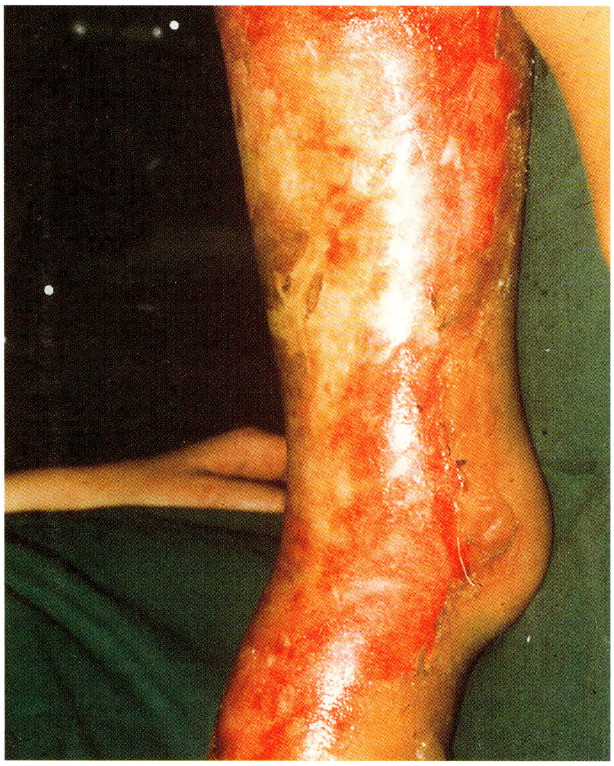

Figure 7.8b The operation was done 24 hours after the accident (burn wound excision and skin grafting).

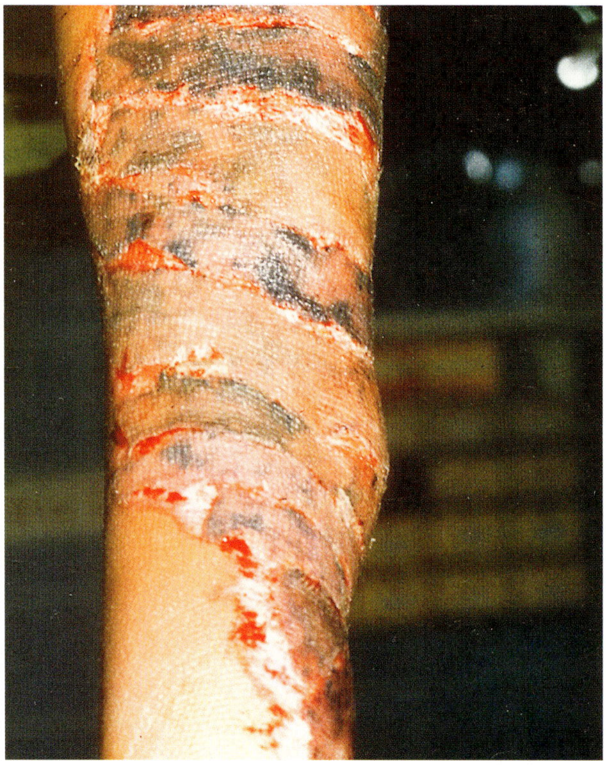

Figure 7.8c Status one day after the operation. The grafts are adherent. The patient was hospitalized for 15 days. **Important:** Transversally oriented skin grafting of the joint areas to avoid contractures!

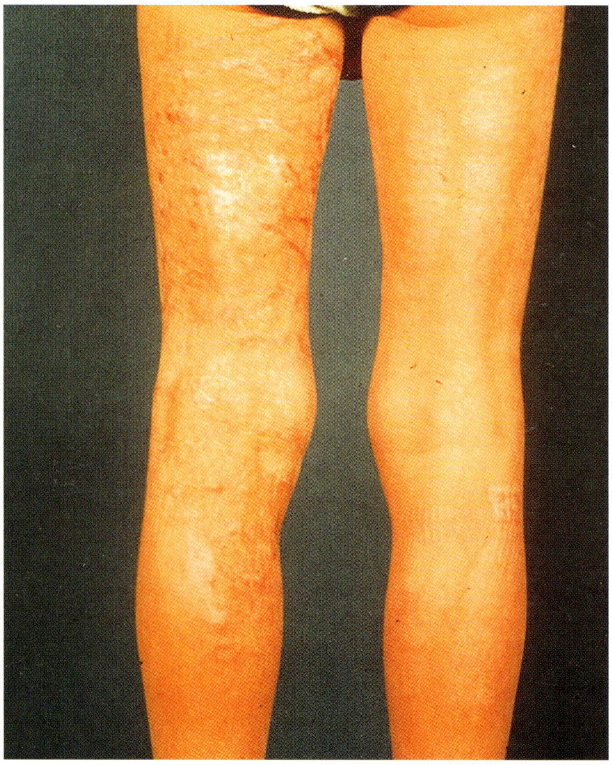

Figure 7.8d Status one year after the procedure. No contractures are evident.

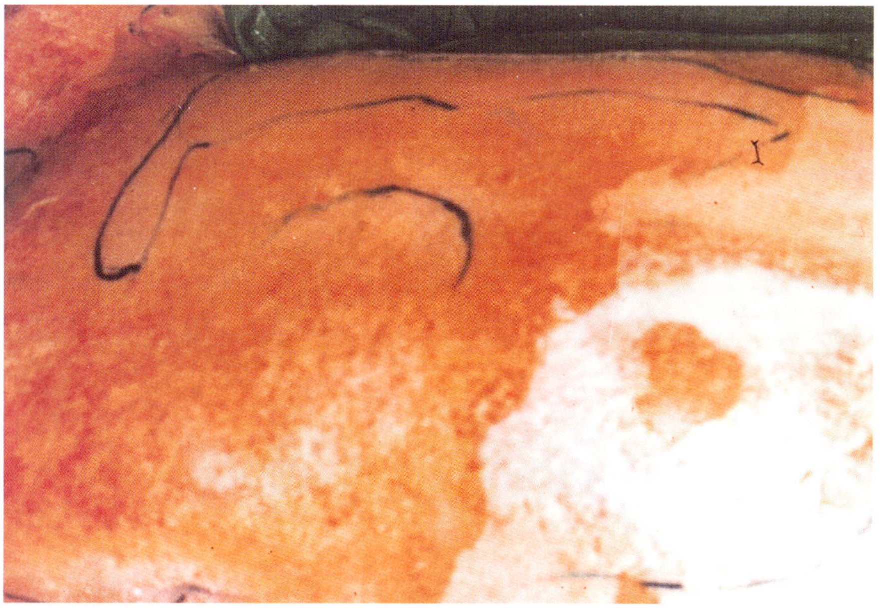

Figure 7.9a 30 % TBSA grade III flame burn induced by the inflammation of spirit (excised area 20 % TBSA). Chest, neck region and left arm are affected. The excision was done on day 4 after trauma.

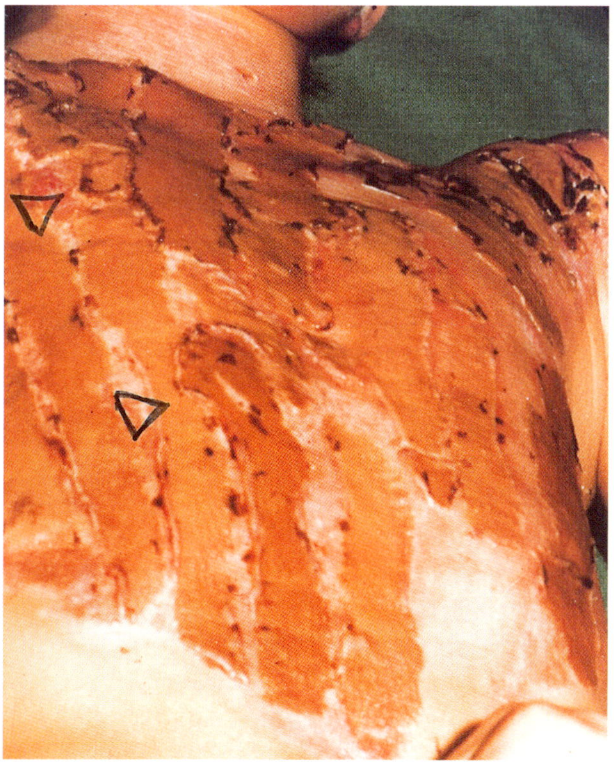

Figure 7.9b Aspect ten days after surgical excision and grafting. The nipple regions have not been grafted without gaps.

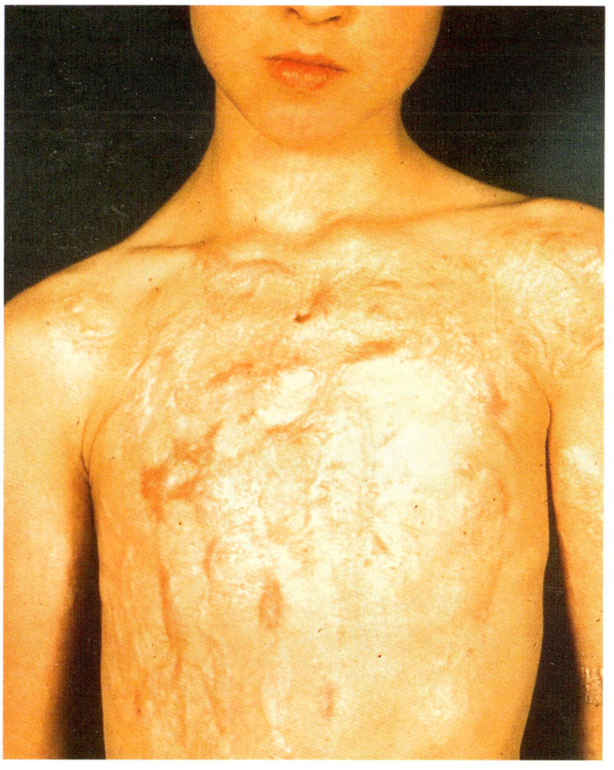

Figure 7.9c The spots that have not been grafted (gaps) show hypertrophic scar formation one year after injury.

Tangential Excision in Third-Degree Burns (Janzekovic)

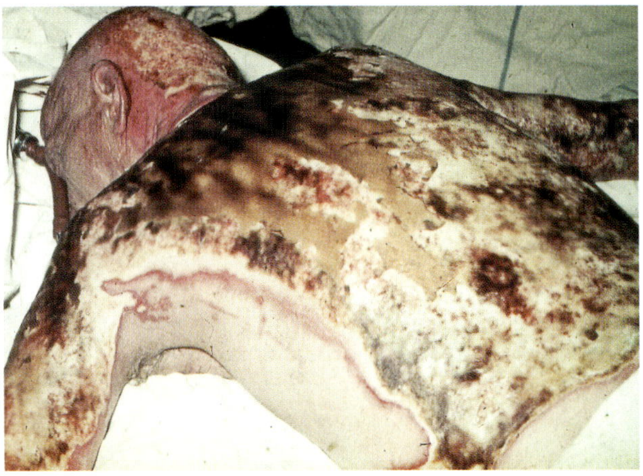

Figure 7.10a Third-degree burn comprising 32 % TBSA – the back and both upper arms – in a 63-year old patient.

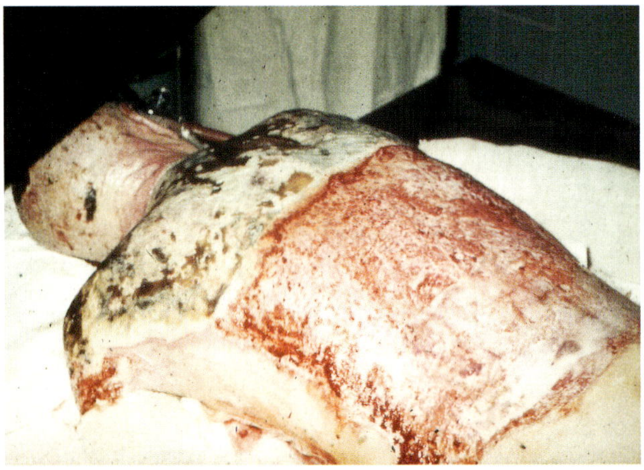

Figure 7.10b Tangential excision on post-burn day four. The excised area is grafted with split-thickness skin grafts.

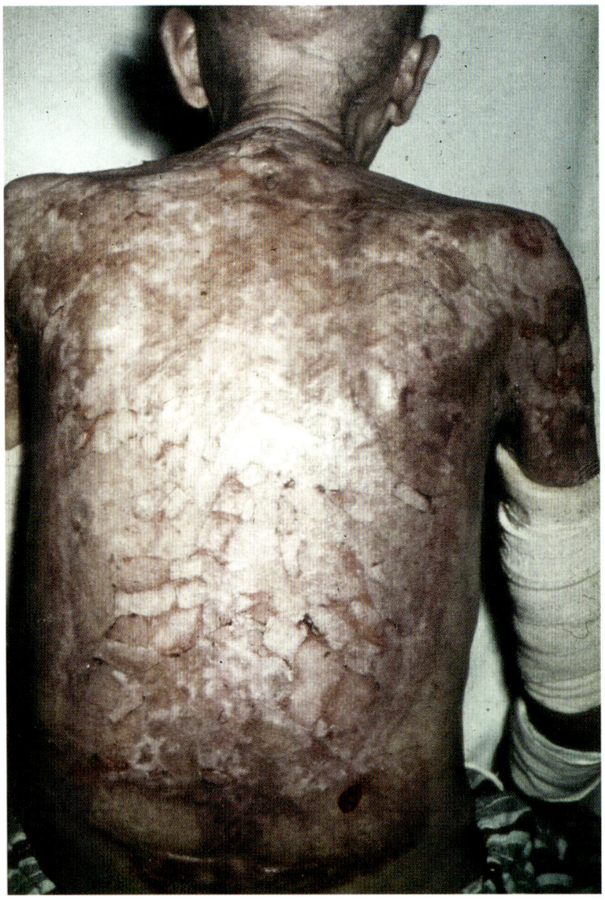

Figure 7.10c Status three months after the operation.

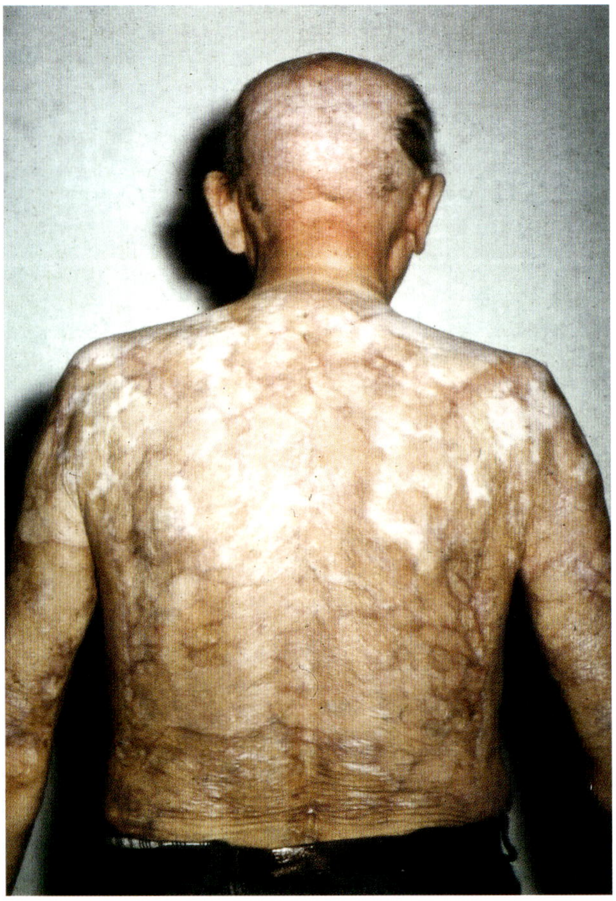

Figure 7.10d Status two years after the procedure. No hypertrophic scar formation or contractures. This result is only possible by early excision and grafting of the burn wound.

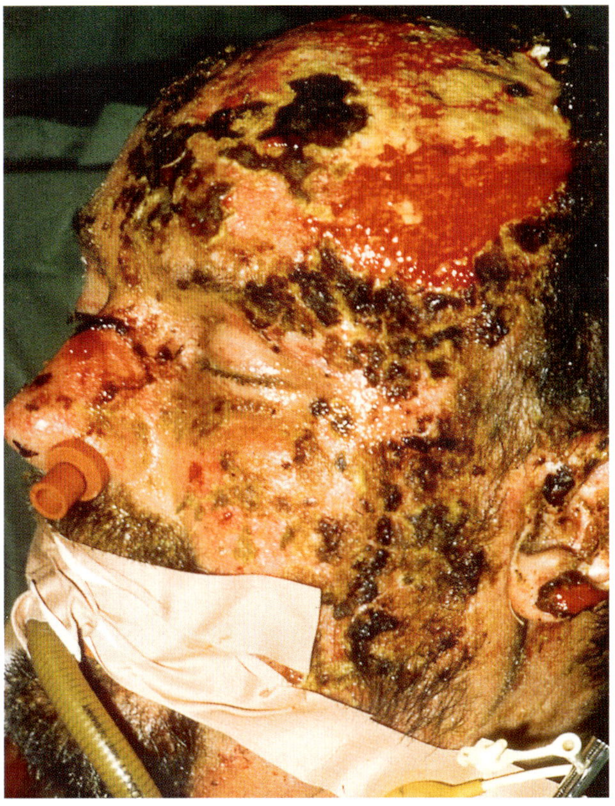

Figure 7.11a Delayed treatment of a flame burn comprising 26 % of the total body surface area (20 % TBSA excised and grafted). Admission two weeks after the burn. Signs of local and systemic infection were present at the time of admission. The face/skull, both arms and the left leg were affected.

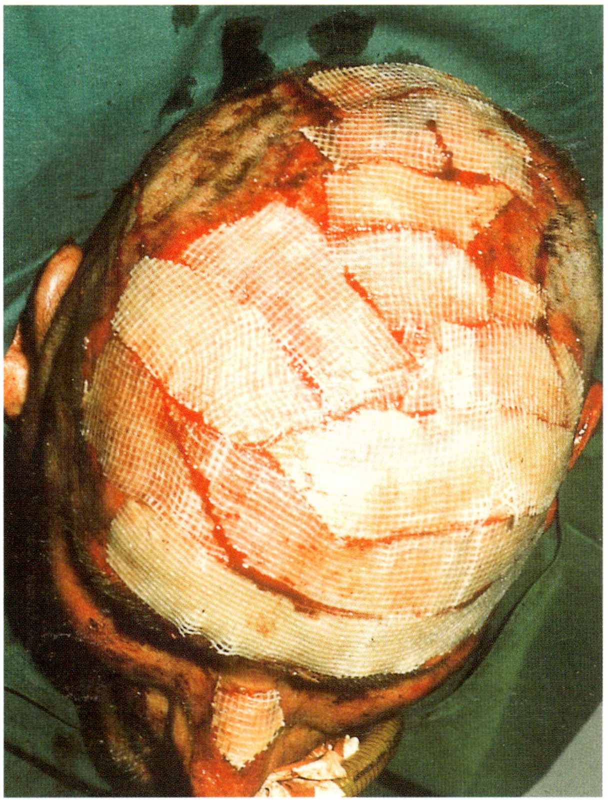

Figure 7.11b Despite the local infection, 24 hours after admission the burn wound and granulation tissue was completely excised and skin grafted using split-thickness skin grafts.

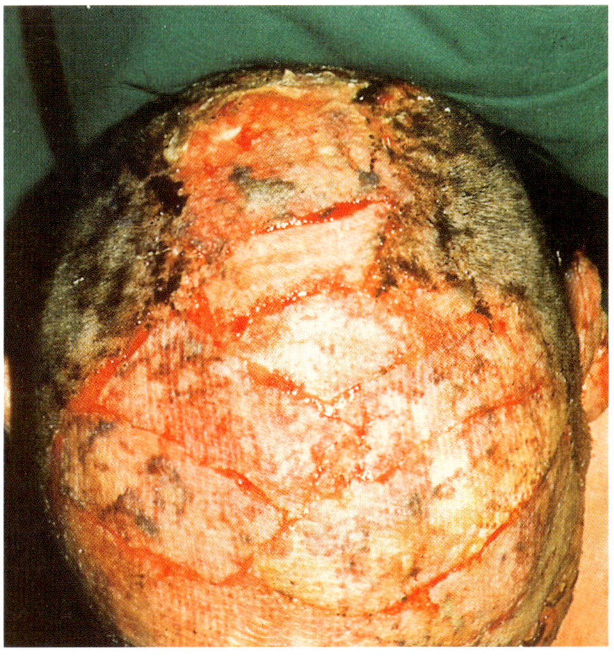

Figure 7.11c Aspect five days after excision and grafting. The wound situation is clean.

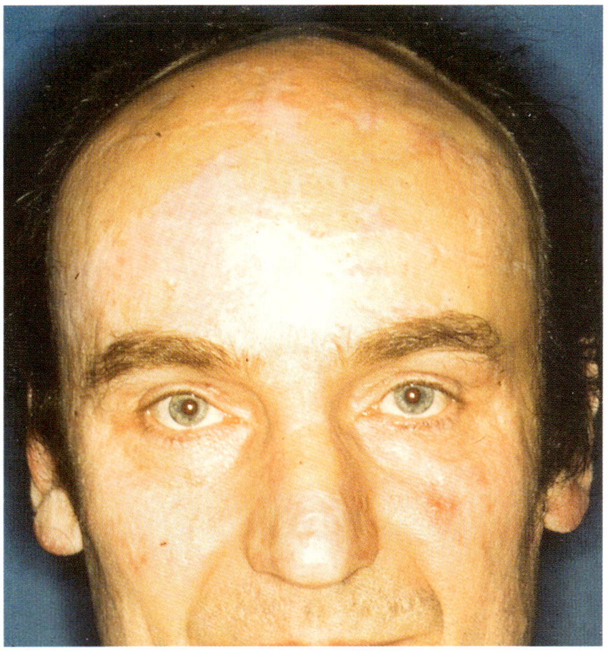

Figure 7.11d Status one year after the procedure

Delayed Treatment

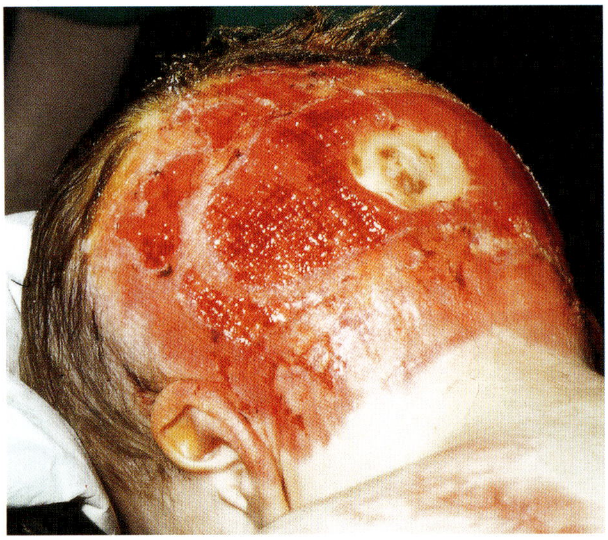

Figure 7.12a Status after third-degree burn injury to the head. The conservative treatment has been done for over three months. Osteitis of the exposed bone.

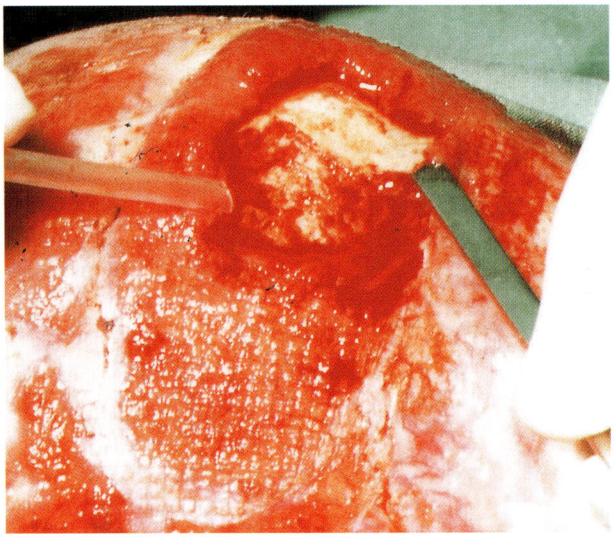

Figure 7.12b The avital bone is debrided using a chisel. The cancellous bone is still sufficiently perfused.

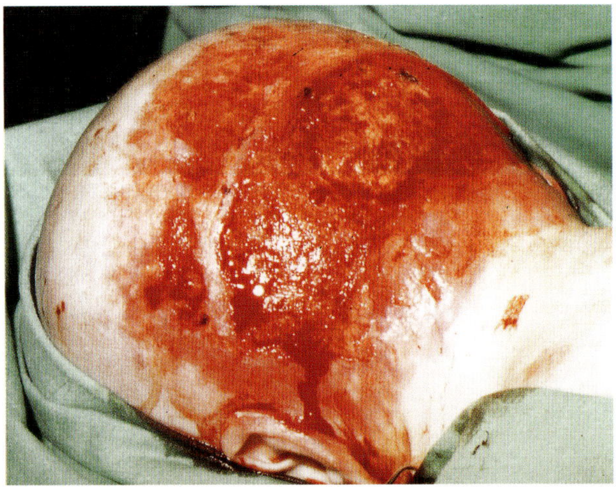

Figure 7.12c Status after complete debridement

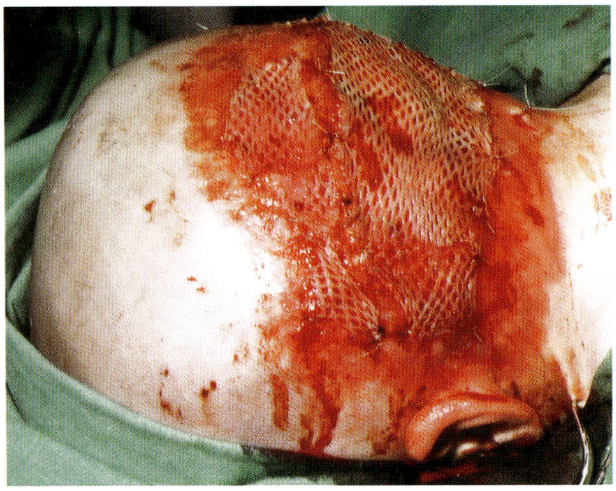

Figure 7.12d Mesh grafts are sutured in place. **Important: Mesh grafts heal in very well on cancellous bone.**

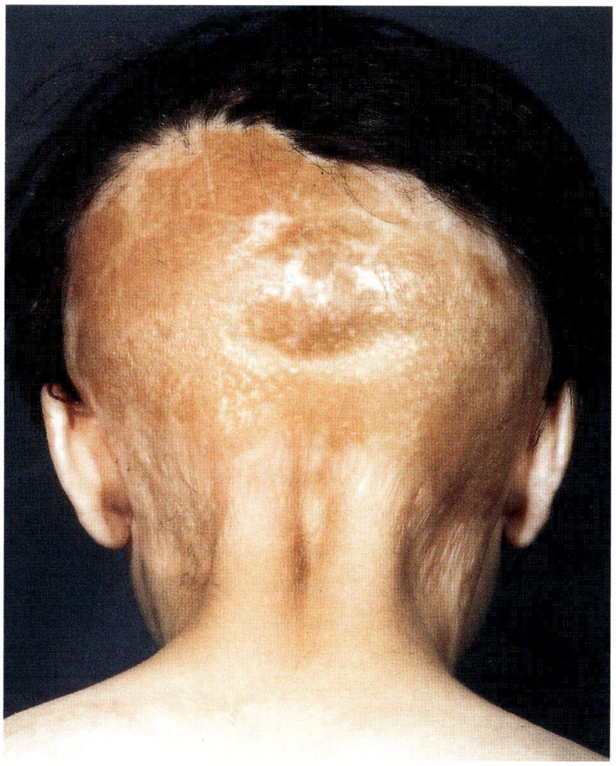

Figure 7.13a Completely healed skin grafts. After four years, the patient wanted further reconstruction.

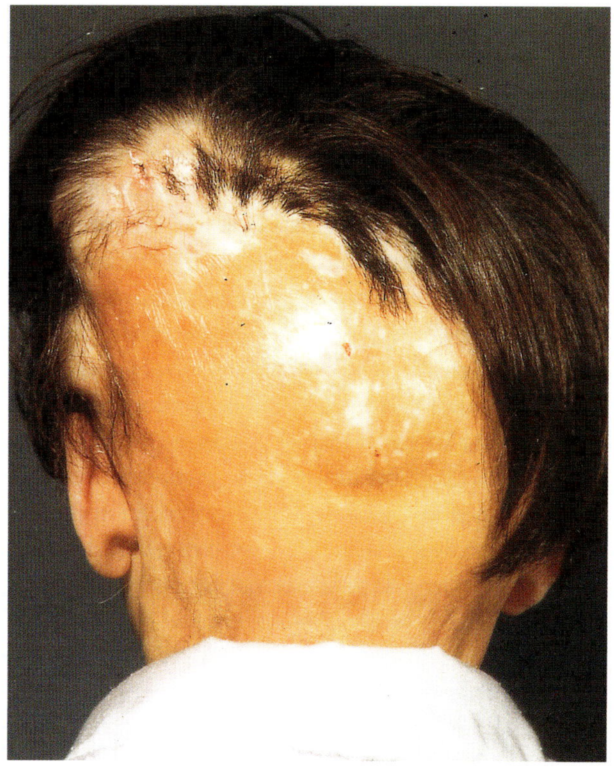

Figure 713b. A tissue expander was implanted on the left parietal side (220 ccm), another one was implanted on the right parietal side (200 ccm).

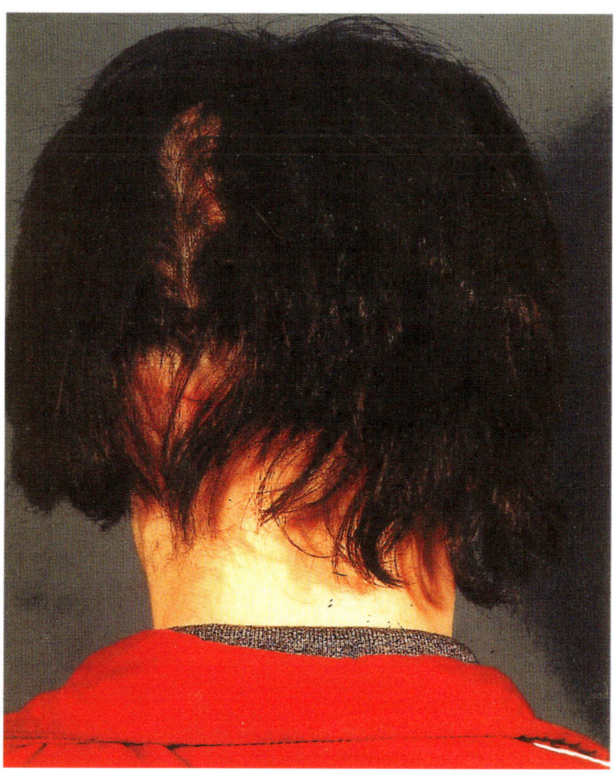

Figure 7.13c Status after two expansion procedures with implantation of two expanders each time.

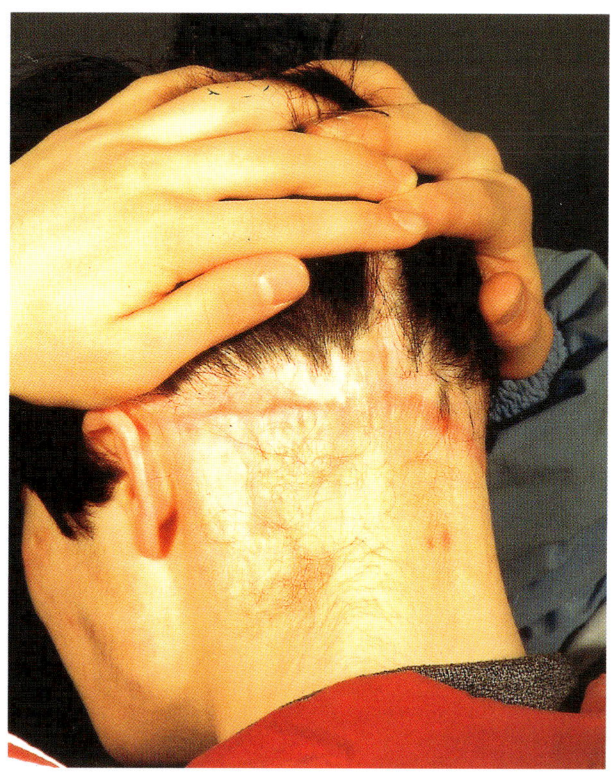

Figure 7.13d Aspect at the end of the treatment. Overall, five procedures have become necessary.

Hyperextension of the metacarpophalangeal joints further induces loss of interosseus and lumbrical muscle tone. Damage of the intermediate tract over the proximal interphalangeal joint leads to ankylosis. The flexor muscles of the hand loose an antagonist by loss of function of the dorsal aponeurosis. Adhesions of the flexor and extension tendons are the results. The latter and the increasing contraction of the atonic, atrophied muscles result in flexion of the interphalangeal joints. This is the pathogenetic basis for the development of the burn-induced "claw hand".

In addition, damage of the nail bed and matrix with deformation of the fingernails are frequently seen in hand burns. At the same time, significant dysesthesia and increased cold sensitivity very often. Scar-induced webs lead to limited and sometimes abolished finger abduction. Positive flexion testing of the interphalangeal joints reveals whitening of the skin on the dorsal side of the interphalangeal joints. This is due to the loss of elasticity. The crippling of the hand is directly proportional to burn depth and the time between the burn and the surgical treatment. The shorter this time lag, the better are the functional results. A burn-induced claw hand in the end stage can hardly be corrected even by complex and elaborate surgical interventions. The older the patient´s age, the faster is the development of the above-described state.

Whether a contracture is of dermatogenic or of arthrogenic cause is hard to recognize clinically and can often only be determined intraoperatively.

The mentioned mechanisms lead to the conclusion that an early and adequate surgical intervention with selective resection of necrotic tissue and skin under cautious preservation of vital anatomic structures and subsequent skin grafting is the treatment method of choice. The process of edema formation, fibrosis, infection, induration and contracture has to be interrupted early by surgical treatment.

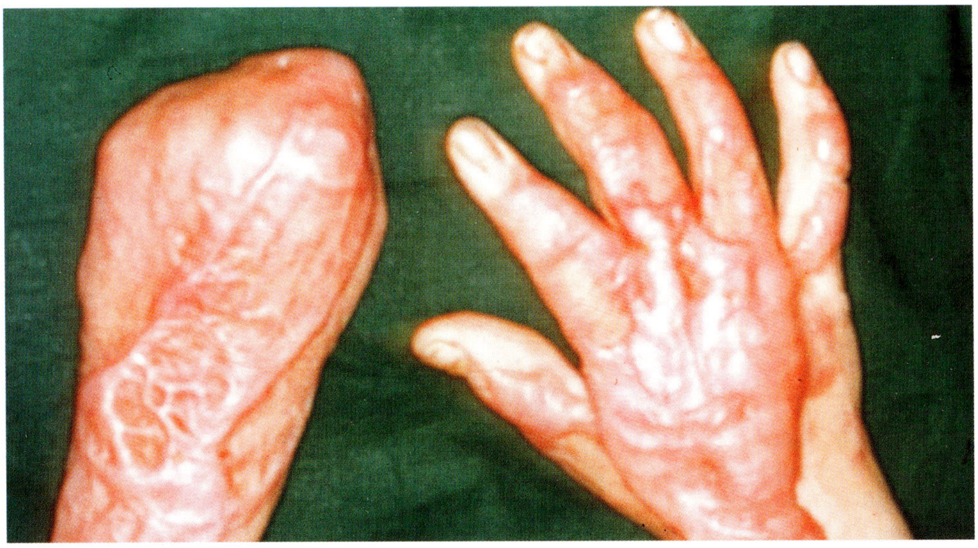

Figure 7.14c Status after burn injury in a 5-year old child. Spontaneous healing took seven months. Left: Amputation of all fingers; right: heavy contractures. No skin transfer has been made.

Treatment of the Burned Hand

First-Line Treatment

The undoubtedly best method of treatment immediately after the thermal impact is cold water treatment [Lemperle, Köhnlein 1971]. It has to be initiated directly after the insult, is best done with running water and should be maintained for about 15 to 20 minutes (not longer). Ice treatment has become obsolete, since it has been experimentally shown that the optimal temperature for cold water treatment is about 20 °C [Lemperle 1971].
After that, the hand should be kept clean and warm which can be accomplished by wrapping either in clean cloth (preclinically) or – better – in a so-called "burn pac": This is a heat-reflecting and – conserving thin foil with a temperature-reflecting surface. The transfer to a burn center is mandatory in the case of hand burns and should be done timely under aseptic conditions. The hand exam in the burn centre is done in a sterile fashion. The preclinical application of ointments, powder or other local treatment agents is not necessary and makes diagnosis and treatment only harder.
If the general condition of the patient allows for it, wound cleaning and debridement of necrotic tissue is done under (general) anesthesia. The initial cleaning is done using an antiseptic solution. Blisters have to be opened and debrided. The general opinion that blisters protect from external infection is lacking any clinical or experimental evidence. The burn-induced blisters are primarily infected in about 75 % of the cases via bacteria of the holocrine gland ducts and the hair follicles [Wenzel 1972]. The opinion, whether a burned hand has to be subjected to open or closed wound management until the time of operation, is debated in literature. All patients presented in this chapter were treated with closed wound management. The possibility of superinfection is thereby undoubtedly reduced.

After the wound debridement and cleaning, the hand dressing is done as follows:

1. Greasy Wound Gauze
   Each finger is separately wrapped, also the whole hand is wrapped.
2. Sterile, Antibiotic-Soaked Gauze Bandage
   Care has to be taken that the web spaces are padded sufficiently.
3. Synthetic Cotton
   It has the excellent feature of being able to soak up large amounts of wound secrete.
4. The last layer should be sterile gauze bandage, which is applied so that slight pressure is exerted.

The hand dressing should be changed on a daily basis, if necessary under (general) anesthesia.

Surgical Treatment

When the depth of the burn injury is determined (see chapter diagnosis of burn depth), the indication for an operative intervention is established. In the case of definitive third-degree burn injury (destruction of the entire cutis), excision and grafting is done within the first 24 hours after injury. In the case of deep dermal burns (IIb), it is impossible to determine the necessary excisional depth within the first 24 hours after injury. The microcirculation in the burned regions is partially still intact. After 24 to 48 hours, the burn area that needs to be excised is thrombotic and shows no ischemia under pressure using a glass spatula. At this time, the excision of these regions should be done.

Excision

The regions that have to be excised are marked with methylene blue, after that, a pressure tourniquet is used to achieve and maintain extremity ischemia. Basically, the excision can be done with any available hand dermatome. However, our experience shows that in hand burn injuries the excision can be done best using a small Weck knife, because larger dermatomes are uncomfortable to use especially in the finger region. Rarely, we have used a scalpel to excise smaller wound areas. The excision is done under regional ischemia in a tangential fashion until a whitish-yellow tissue layer is homogenously exposed. The excision has to be continued in depth until the damaged tissue is of reddish-livid color, otherwise the graft take on these thrombotic areas will be compromised. Under no circumstance the excision should always be done down to the level of the fascia, because the worthy subcutaneous tissue layer is then lost.

If a deep net-like corium layer can be preserved after the excision, the outcome is much better because of the better skin elasticity after the procedure. However, the excision has to be carried on down to the level of vital yellowish subcutaneous fat in the case of damage to this net-like corium layer. The common opinion that split-thickness skin grafts cannot heal in ("graft take") on fat tissue, is completely arbitrary. All split-thickness skin grafting procedures that we have done revealed uneventful split-thickness skin graft take on vital subcutaneous fat tissue. The preserved fat layer under the split-thickness skin graft results in better elasticity and lymphatic drainage. After meticulous and thorough excision of the burn wound – especially in the case of burned fingers patience has to be exercised – the split-thickness skin grafts are positioned under regional ischemia conditions. The grafts are harvested using air-driven dermatomes or hand dermatomes such as a Weck or Davis knife. The correct thickness of the harvested skin grafts can be assessed clinically very easily: They should not roll when they are laid out onto sterile gauze. The grafts have to be positioned very carefully, so that there are no ungrafted spaces between the graft sheets. In general, the space between two grafts should not measure more than 1mm, otherwise the risk of later scar formation in this gap is very high and can cause functional deficits. As one can deduce from the above-mentioned facts, split-thickness skin grafts have very rarely been sutured in place in our patients. Even though nothing can be objected against suturing in of skin grafts, it is time-consuming. If only one hand is affected, the time aspect does not matter, however, if larger body surface areas are burned that need to be excised and grafted, prolonged duration of the operation is the result.

In our experience, burn wound excision under regional ischemic conditions is the best treatment approach, because depth assessment of the excised area can be done much more reliably and the decision whether the excisional depth is sufficient, is much easier to take.

Excision Technique of Hand Burn Injuries (Grades IIb and III)

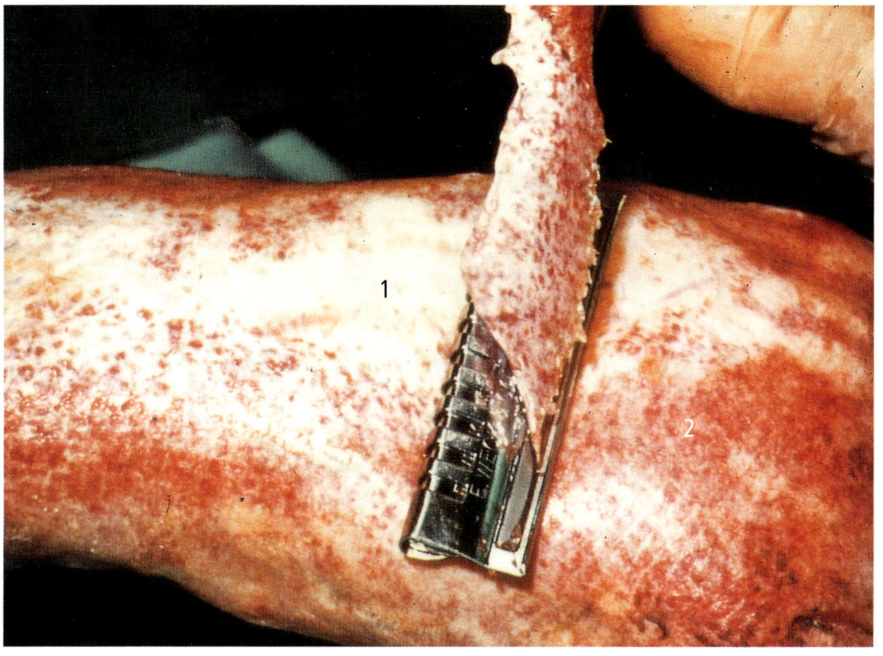

Figure 7.15a The tangential excision is done under regional ischemia (tourniquet). Vital tissue under regional ischemia has a white-yellowish appearance (1). Reddish-livid areas are usually not vital (2) (thrombotic vessels do not exsanguinate under ischemic conditions). Here, the excision was done using a Weck knife, which is especially suitable for hand burn wound excisions. Smaller necrotic areas of the web spaces can be excised with the use of a scalpel.

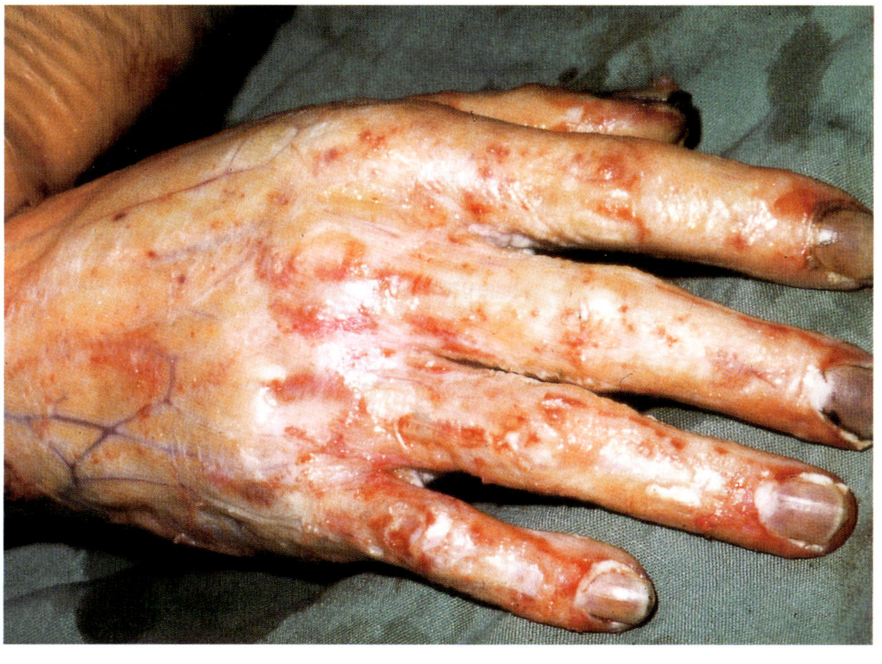

Figure 7.15b Status at the end of the burn wound excision.
The exact technique is especially important when burn wounds of the fingers are excised. If the necrotic (or thrombotic) layer is not completely removed, graft take is compromised. If the excision is carried out unnecessarily deep, tendons, nerves or blood vessels can be damaged. An even minimally conserved subcutaneous tissue layer means faster reconstitution and better function.

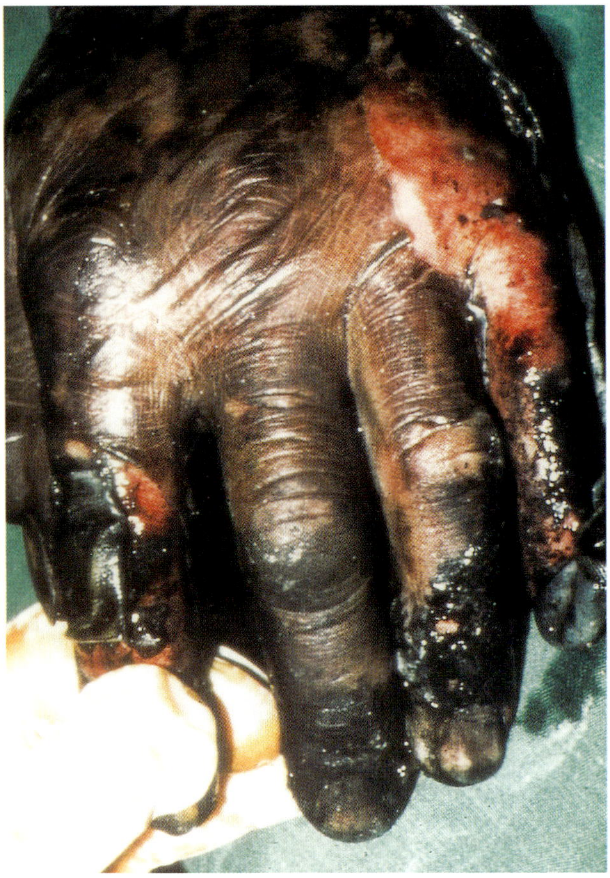

Figure 7.16a Flame burn of both hands and arms, the face and the thorax.

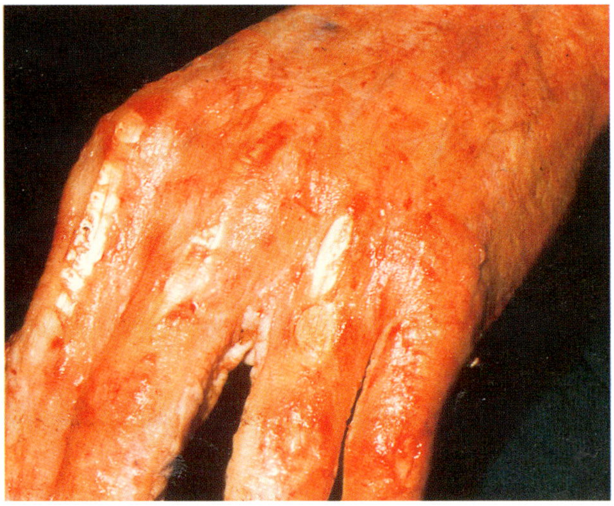

Figure 7.16b The excision was carried out under regional ischemia 24 hours after the trauma. The necrotic tissue was excised, partly down to the level of the extensor tendons.

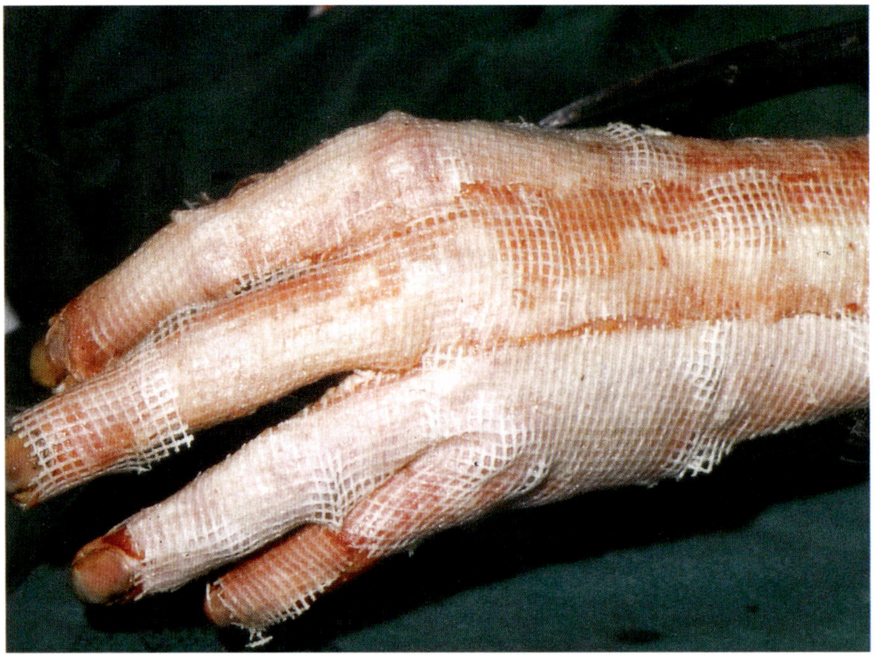

Figure 7.16c The split-thickness skin grafts are covered with fat gauze and not sutured in place.

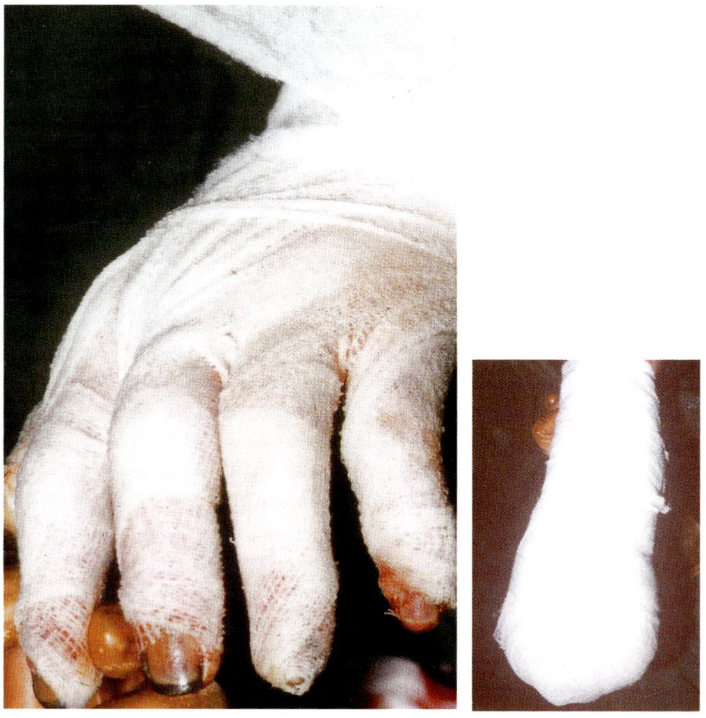

Figure 7.16d Fixation of the grafts using sterile gauze, sterile cotton and a slightly compressive dressing using sterile gauze bandage. Not until then the ischemia is lifted.

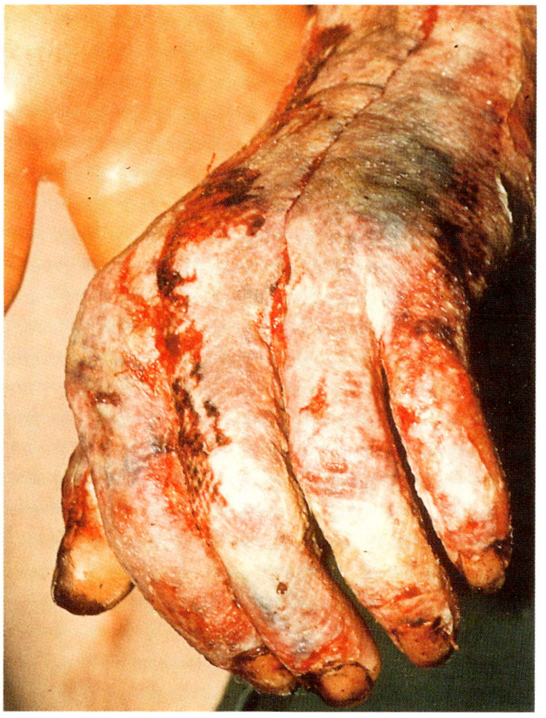

Figure 7.16e Status three days after the procedure (four days after trauma). The grafts healed in without gaps, even in the area of the extensor tendons.

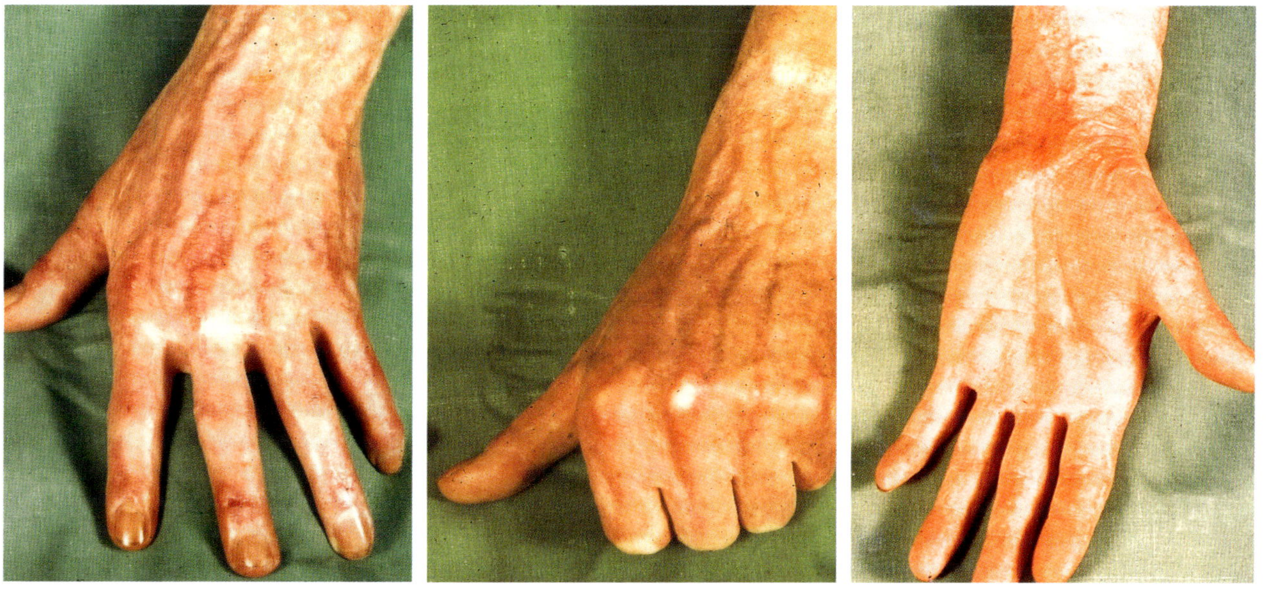

Figure 7.16f Status one year after the trauma. During the first six months insufficient elasticity, which has normalized at this time. Intensive physical therapy and consequent wearing of custom-made compressive gloves is necessary for at least three to six months after the injury.

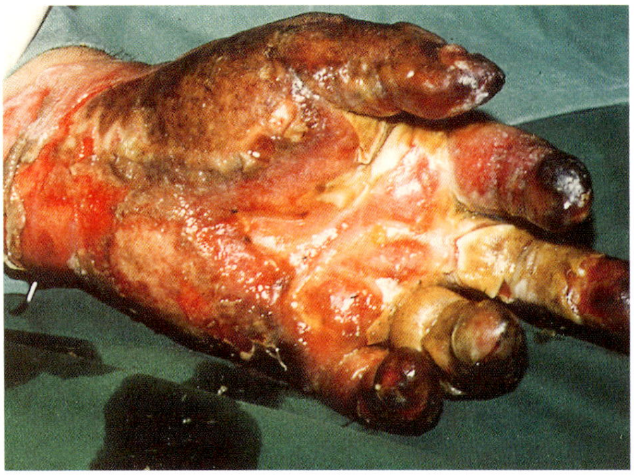

Figure 7.17a Flame burn injury comprising 45 % TBSA (35 % third-degree injury which was excised). Deep burn of the left hand.

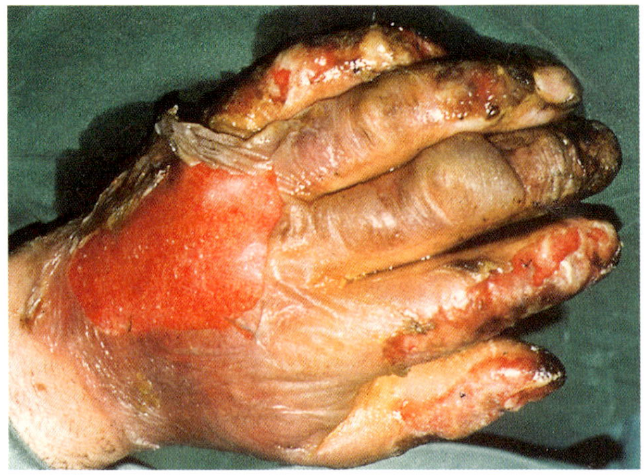

Figure 7.17b The injury was caused by petrol incineration and extended over both hands, the face and both legs.

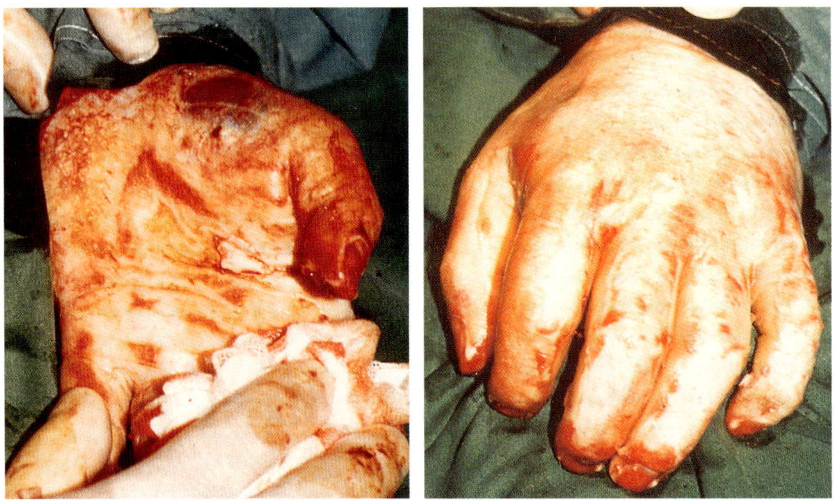

Figure 7.17c Excision 48 hours after the injury. The burn wound in the thenar region extends down to the muscle level.

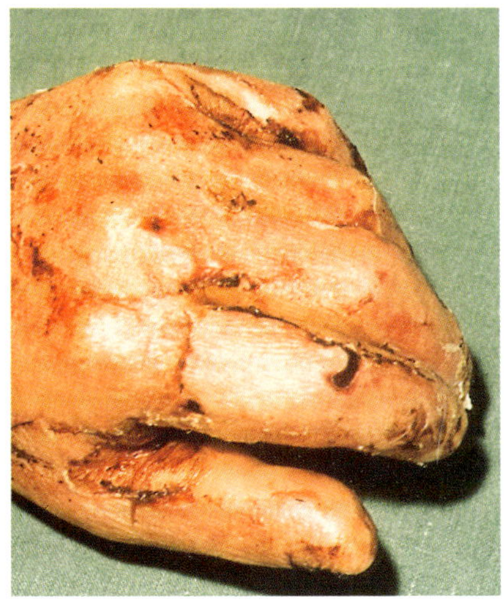

Figure 7.17d Ten days after the procedure, graft take is complete and the hands are actively moved.

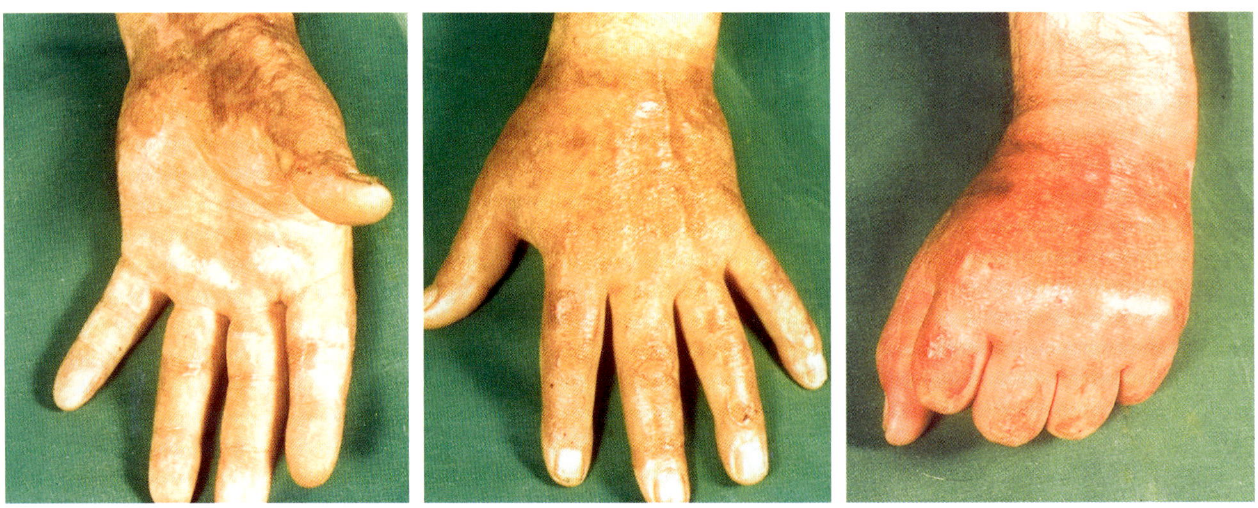

Figure 7.17e Three months after the injury, hand function is almost complete.

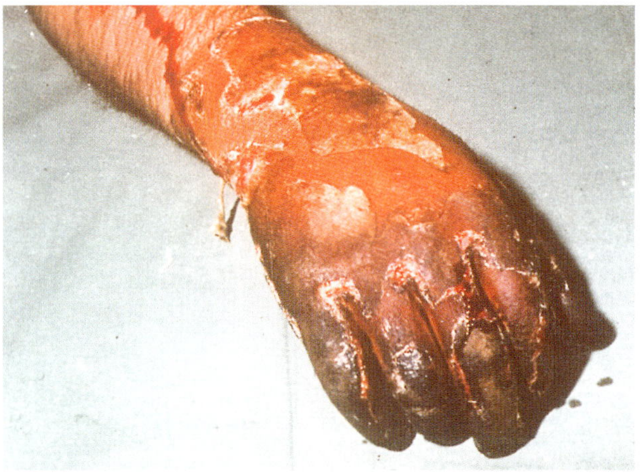

Figure 7.18a Flame burn comprising 22 % TBSA (15 % third-degree injury which was excised).

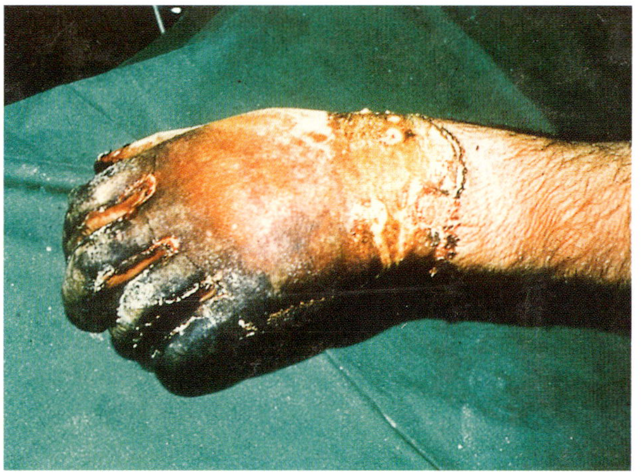

Figure 7.18b Both hands, the face and the legs are affected.

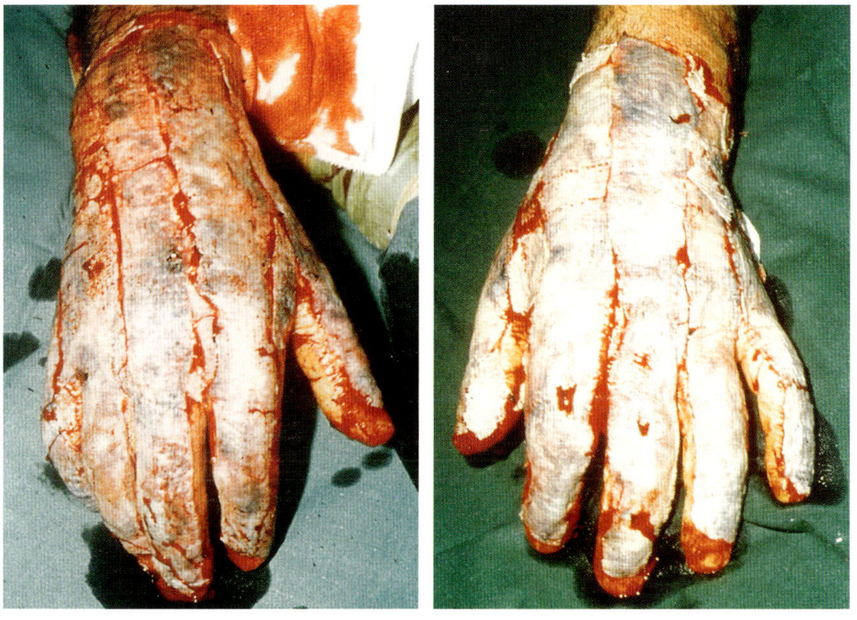

Figure 7.18c Status 24 hours after the excision, two days after the injury at the time of the first dressing change. Hematomas are cleared out and dislocated grafts are repositioned.

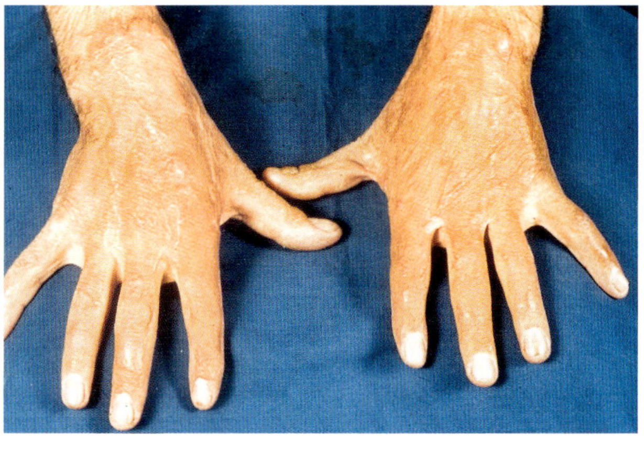

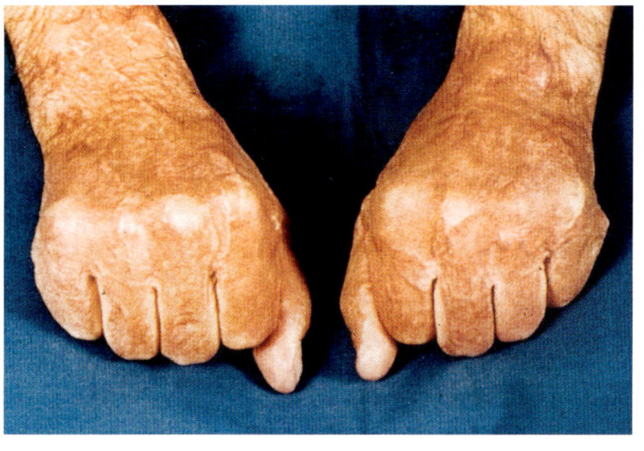

Figure 7.18d Status one year after the procedure

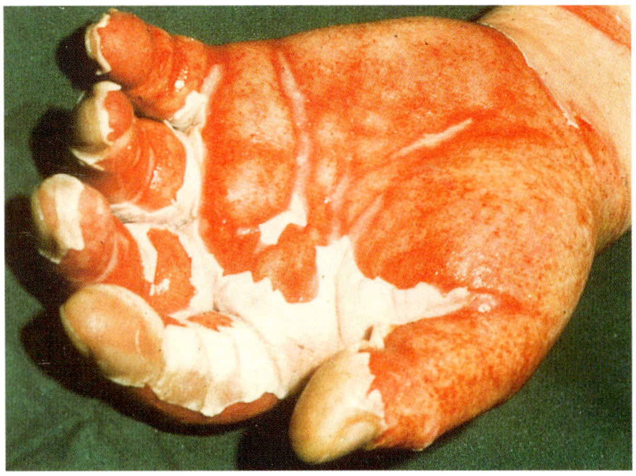

Figure 7.19a Burn injury due to explosion of the left hand.

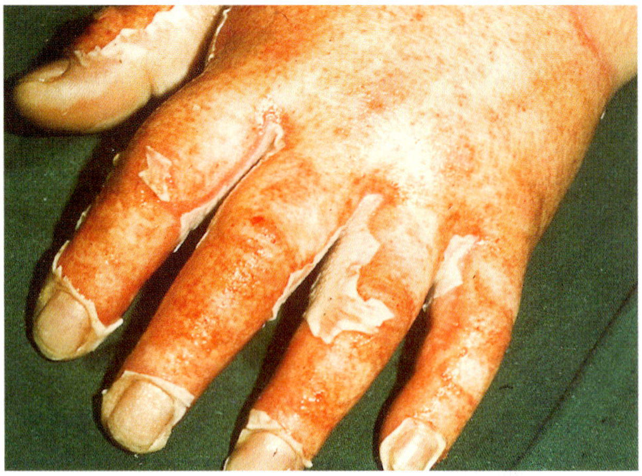

Figure 7.19b 3 % TBSA burn injury (3 % third-degree injury which was excised).

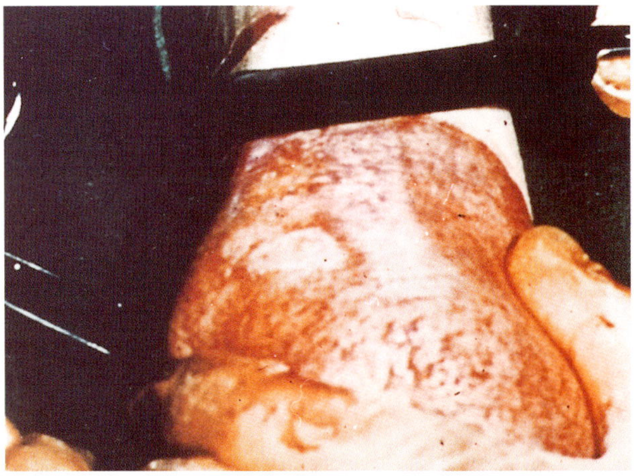

Figure 7.19c Tangential excision 24 hours after the injury

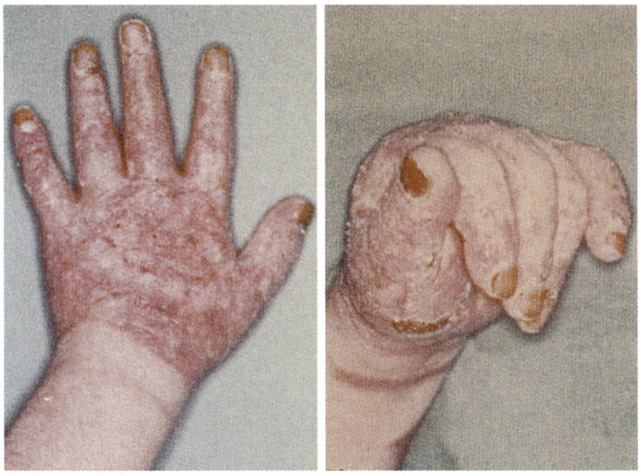

Figure 7.19d Status at the time of hospital discharge at postoperative day 12

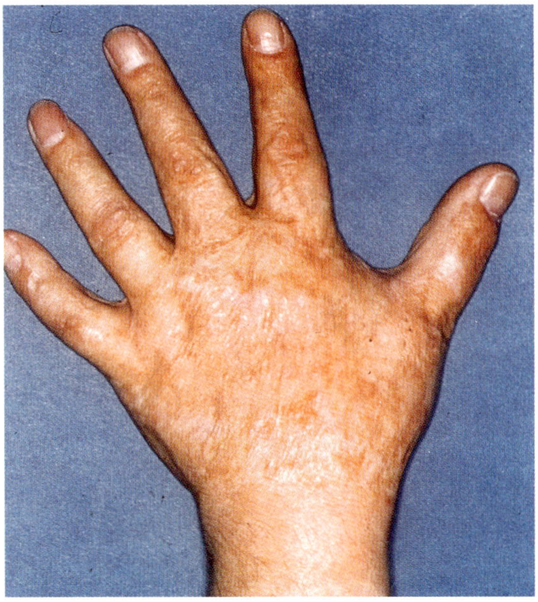

Figure 7.19e Status two years after the accident

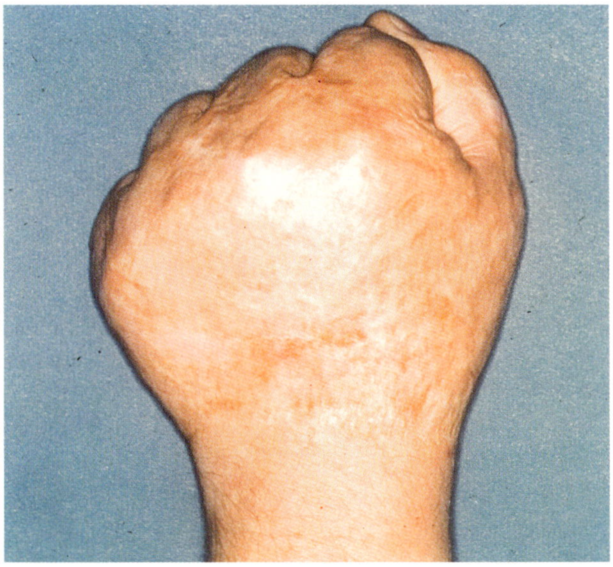

Figure 7.19f Besides slight pigment irregularities no grave sequelae of the burn trauma were observed.

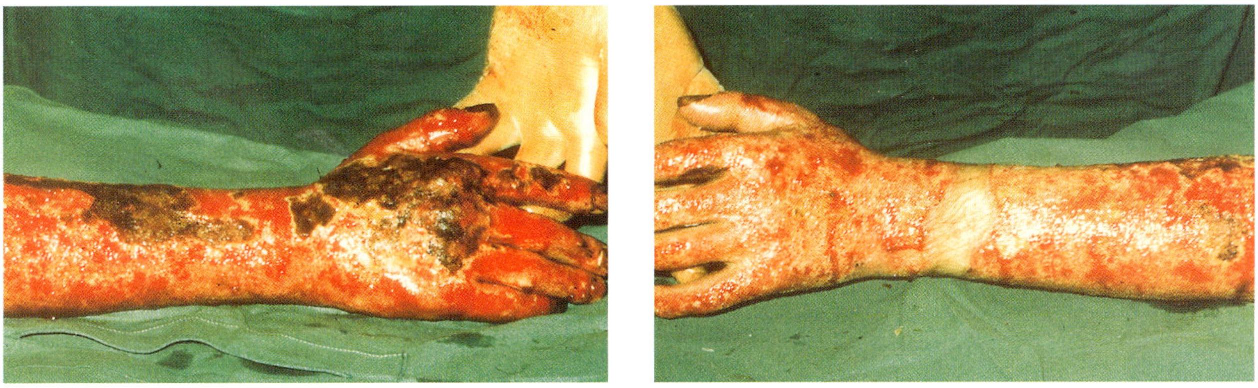

Figure 7.20a, b Burn injury comprising 26 % TBSA (20 % third-degree injury which was excised). Only the region which was covered by a watch remained unaffected. The cutis was destroyed mostly down to the level of the subcutis, the corium was only partly intact. The patient was admitted to our hospital two weeks after the injury in a septic state. The excision was immediately carried out.

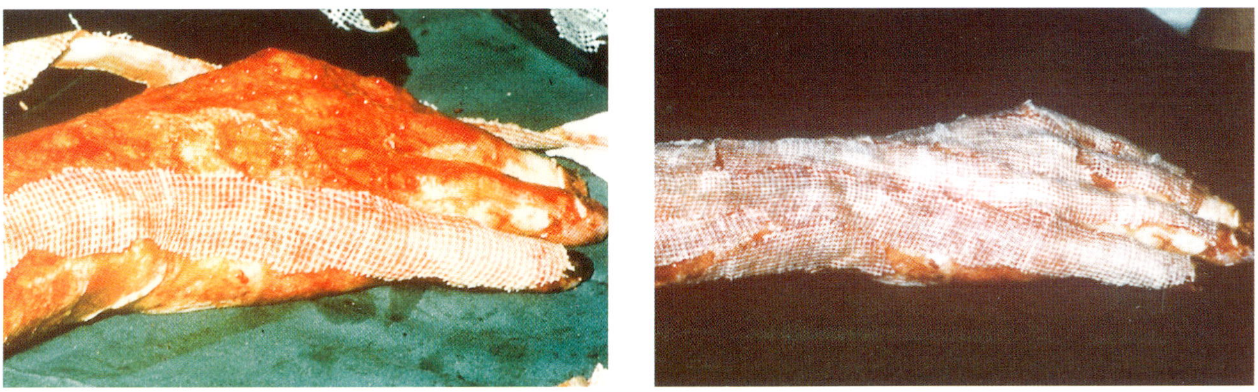

Figure 7.20c, d When positioning the grafts, it is important that they cover all joint areas of the fingers without interruption and preferably reach to the mid-side line of the fingers. Gaps between the grafts lead to secondary healing, scar tissue formation and functional deficits.

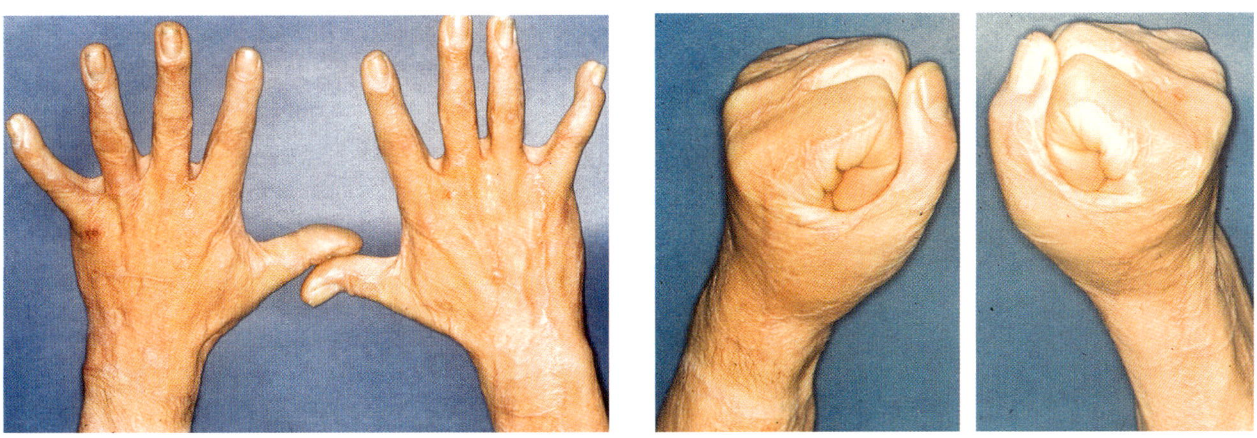

Figure 7.20e, f Status two years after the procedure. The function of the hands is almost completely reconstituted. The small gaps between the grafts are visible as light-colored bands (no scar tissue).

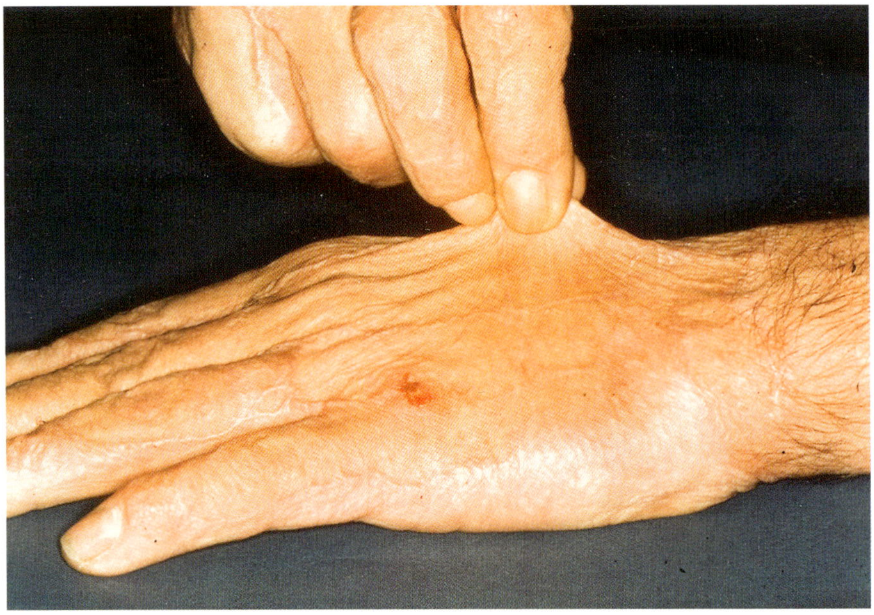

Figure 7.21a The skin elasticity within the first three months after the injury is only moderately existent, but improves within the next three months and is almost normal after one year.

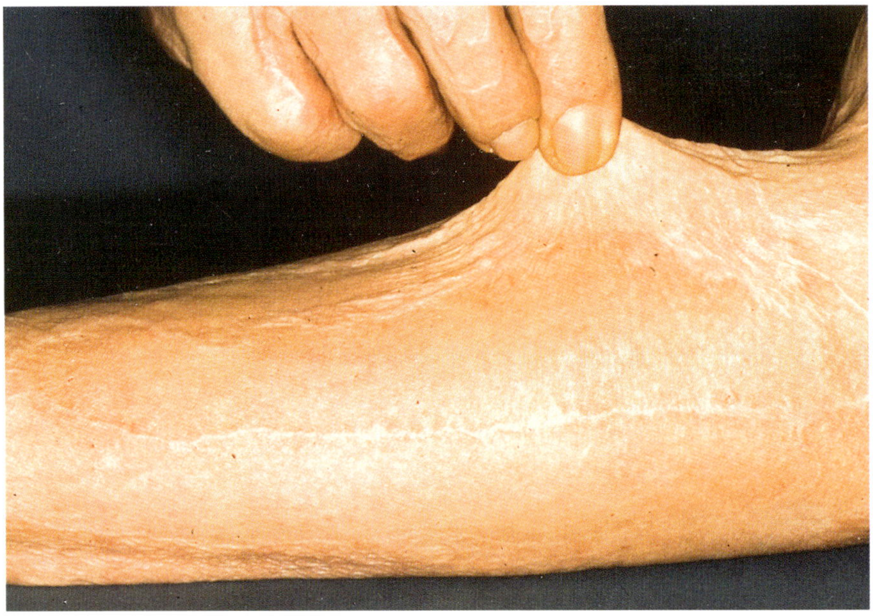

Figure 7.21b In our hospital, we prefer larger-sized grafts for economy of time. The results are equal to the use of smaller sized grafts, provided that the gaps between the grafts do not measure more than one to two millimetres. Here, the gaps are visible as elastic, light-colored bands.

Corrective Operation of the Burn-Induced "Claw Hand"

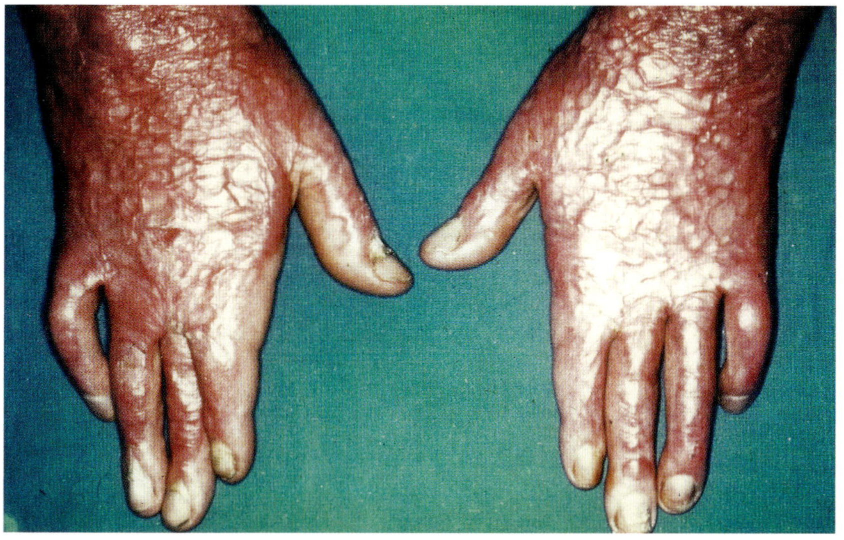

Figure 7.22a Status after IIb and IIIrd degree burn injury of both hands. Conservative treatment was done for six weeks, after that, small split-thickness skin grafts were transplanted onto the granulative tissue.
The appearance at one year after the injury is depicted.

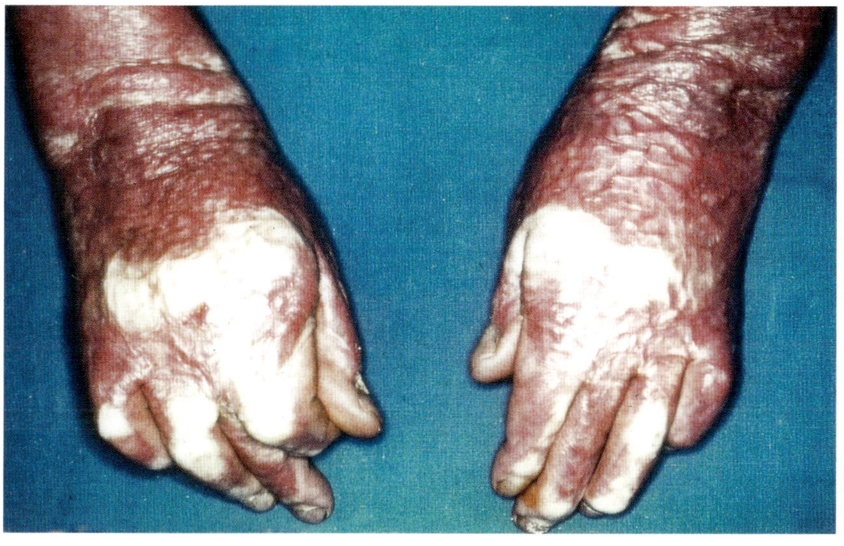

Figure 7.22b Considerable functional deficits are caused by thick scar tissue and interdigital adhesions. The left proximal and distal interphalangeal joint of the 5th finger are ankylosed. This is the typical clinical appearance of the burn-induced "claw hand".

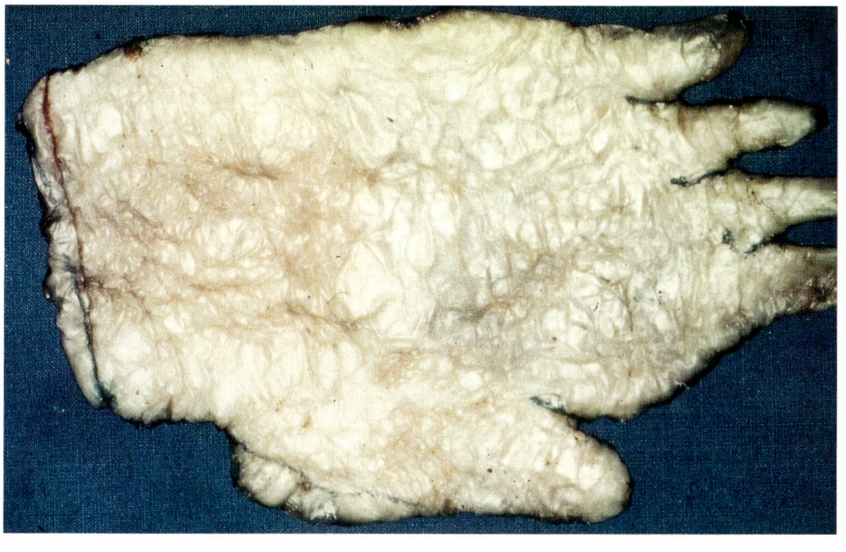

Figure 7.22c The surgical procedure included the meticulous resection of the scar plate down to the level of the subcutis.
The created wound was covered (gap-free) using split-thickness skin grafts. The functionally disturbing left 5th finger was amputated.

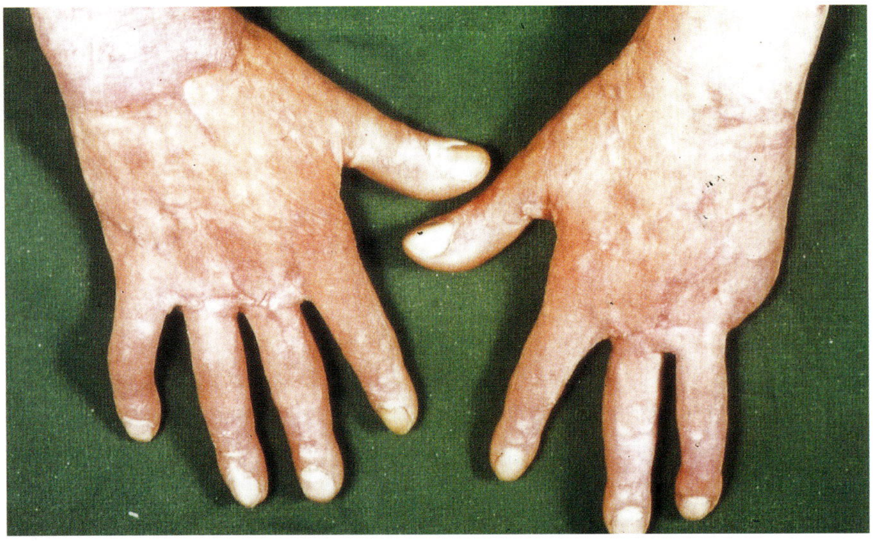

Figure 7.22d Status ten months after the procedure, six months of intensive physical therapy and wearing of custom-made compressive gloves.

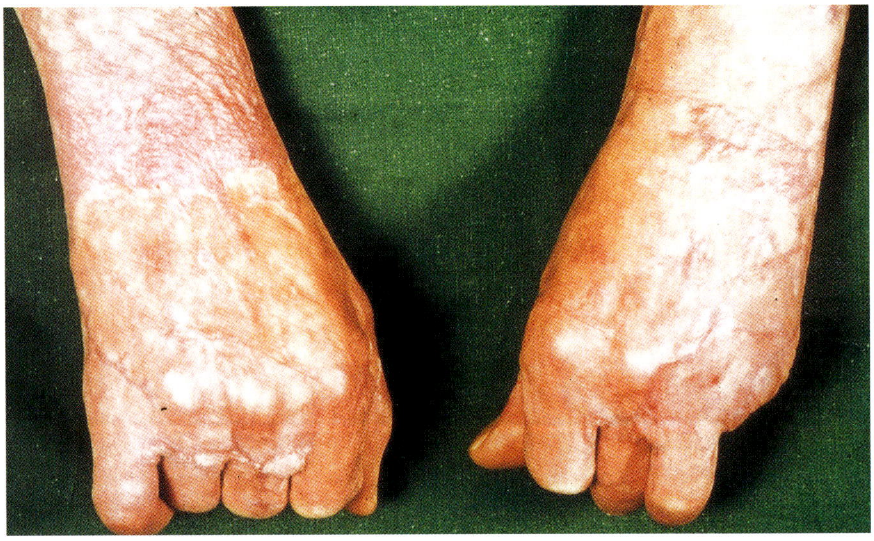

Figure 7.22e Good residual function considering the initial situation. Early excision and grafting would have resulted in significantly better hand function.

Results and Summary

In a group of 29 patients, 53 burned hands were treated by early tangential excision and split-thickness skin grafting. In 24 patients both hands were affected, whereas in five patients only one hand was thermally injured. The mean age of the patients was 26.7 years. The most frequent mechanism was flame burn (65.5 %), followed by scald injuries (13.8 %), contact burns (10.3 %) and chemical burns (7 %).

In the most cases besides the hands other regions of the body were affected, on the average 18 % of the total body surface area.

The determination of the burn extent in the hand region was done separately for the dorsal and the palmar side of the hand. The dorsum of the hand was much more often affected, namely in 69.5 % of right hand burns versus 72.9 % of the burns of left hand in contrast to the palmar side, where in 23.4 % the right hand palm and in 40 % the left hand palm was injured.

On the average, the surgical treatment was done 3.6 days after the injury except for two cases, where secondary transfer in our hospital delayed excision and grafting until posttraumatic days 13 to 15.

The mean duration of the procedures that have been conducted under regional ischemia (tourniquet) versus the operations without ischemic conditions was largely identical with an average of 52 minutes. Regional ischemia is exceptionally helpful in terms of depth accuracy and also minimization of intraoperative blood loss. Regional ischemia was used in 45 excision and grafting procedures of hand burn injuries.

The mean length of hospital stay of the surgically treated patients with hand burns was 14.4 days. Patients, who also suffered burns to other body regions than the hands had to be hospitalized for a longer time.

We can deduce the following recommendations from our clinical experience:

1. The technique of early tangential excision in combination with immediate split-thickness skin grafting of hand burn injuries yields the best functional results and early rehabilitation.
2. None of the treated hand burns developed burn wound infection. Both patients that were admitted to our hospital at posttraumatic day 13 and 15 revealed infected burn wounds, but showed primary healing after excision and grafting.
3. The functional results were good. On the average, all patients started active motion exercises between postoperative day 7 and 10. At this point of time, the patients were able to eat independently and to perform small tasks with their hands. In no case we tried to accelerate the rehabilitative way and the functional reconstitution by passive motion exercises. In the 53 operated hands, one finger had to be amputated because of infection and subsequent loss of function.
4. The moderate skin elasticity decreased within the first 6 weeks after excision and grafting, but improved slightly later on. Between six and twelve months after the intervention, all hands were completely functional and the skin elasticity was within the normal range. No keloid-like alterations were seen in our patients and the web spaces did not show abnormal scarring. The scars between the skin grafts were narrow and elastic. In all cases, the sensibility was reconstituted within six months after the surgical intervention.

Due to our clinical experience, early tangential excision and skin grafting is the best method in the treatment of severely burned hands.

References

Abbé R (1898) A new plastic operation for the relief of deformity due to harelip. Med Rec 53: 477

Acland RD (1974) Microvascular anastomosis: A device for holding stay sutures and a new vascular clamp. Surgery 75: 185–187

Acland RD (1979) Factors that influence success in microvascular surgery. In: Serafin D, Buncke HJ (eds) Microsurgical composite tissue transplantation. Mosby, St Louis, pp 78–81

Acland RD, Schusterman M, Godina M, et al (1981) The saphenous neurovascular free flap. Plast Reconstr Surg 67: 763–774

Adenis JP (1996) Efficacy of fat removal orbital decompression in Graves' ophthalmopathy. Presented at the American Academy of Ophthalmology – Annual Meeting

Ahnefeld FW, Burri C (1973) Infusionstherapie. Klin Anästhesiol 3: 156

Aiach G (2003) Atlas of rhinoplasty, 2nd edition. Quality Medical Publishing, St Louis

Alexander JW, Fisher MW (1970) Immunological determinants of pseudomonas infections of man accompanying severe burn injury. J Trauma 10: 565

Alexander JW, Wixon D (1970) Neutrophil dysfunction and sepsis in burn injury. Surg Gynecol Obstet 130: 431

Allen RJ, Treece P (1994) Deep inferior epigastric perforator flap for breast reconstruction. Ann Plast Surg 32: 32

Allgöwer M, Städtler K, Schoenenberger GA (1974) Burn sepsis and burn toxin. Ann R Coll Surg Engl 55: 226

Alpert S, Levenson SM (1970) Respiratory tract injury associated with burns. NY J Med 70: 1633

Anderl H (1973) Cross-face nerve transplant. (Chirurgia Plastica et Reconstructiva, Vol 6) Springer, Berlin, S 433

Anderl H (1973) Reconstruction of the face through cross-face nerve transplantation in facial paralysis. Chir Plastica 2: 17

Anderl H (1977) Cross-face nerve grafting-up to 12 months of seventh nerve disruption. In: Rubin LR (ed) Reanimation of the paralysed face. Mosby, St Louis, pp 241–277

Anderl H, Bauer M, Ioannovich J (1974) Erfahrungen mit der tangentialen Frühexzision dermaler Verbrennungen. Chir Praxis 18: 57

Anderson BO, Harken AH (1990) Multiple organ failure: inflammatory priming and activation sequences promote autologous tissue injury. J Trauma 30: 44–49

Anderson RG (1991) Facial nerve disorders. Select Read Plast Surg 6: 1–34

Arnez ZM, Smith RW, Eder E, Solinc M, Kersnic M (1988) Breast reconstruction by the free lower transverse rectus abdominis musculocutaneous flap. Br J Plast Surg 41: 500

Arnez ZM, Tyler MPH, Valdatta L (1994) The anatomy of the internal mammary view and their application in free TRAM breast reconstruction. Presented at the Winter Meeting of the British Association of Plastic Surgeons, London

Arnholdt H, et al (1998) Pathomorphologie des Mammakarzinoms. In: Empfehlungen zur Diagnostik, Therapie und Nachsorge Mammakarzinome. Tumorzentrum München.

Arons MS, Lynch JB, Lewis SR, Blocker TG (1965) Scar tissue carcinoma. Ann Surg 161: 170–188

Arturson G (1961) Pathophysiological aspects of the burn syndrome with special reference to liver injury and alterations of capillary permeability. Acta Chir Scand, Suppl 274: 1–135

Arturson G (1972) Effects of O-Hydroxyethyl-Rutosides (HR) on the increased microvascular permeability in experimental skin burns. Preliminary report. Acta Chir Scand 138: 111

Arturson G (1980) Pathophysiology of the burn wound. Ann Chir Gynaecol Fenn 69: 176–190

Artz CP, Thompson NJ (1968) Early excision of large areas in burns. Surgery 63: 868

Ashikari R, Park K, Huvos A, Urban J (1970) Paget's disease of the breast. Cancer 26: 680–685

Aufricht G (1943) A few hints and surgical details in rhinoplasty. Laryngoscope 53: 317

Axhausen G (1952) Technik und Ergebnisse der Spaltplastiken. Hanser, München

Baar S (1970) Plasma protein changes in mild thermal trauma. J Trauma 10: 684

Baar S, Arrowsmith DJ (1970) Thermal damage to red cells. J Clin Pathol 23: 572

Baar S, Birke G, Liljedahl SO, Plantin LO (1969) Studies on burns. X. Changes in BMR and evaporative water loss in the treatment of severe burns with warm dry air. Scand J Plast Reconstr Surg 3: 30

Bäckdahl M, Liljedahl SO (1962) Excision of deep burns. Acta Chir Scand 123: 351

Baker DC (1984) Anatomy and injuries of the facial nerve in cervicofacial rhytidectomy. In: Kaye BL, Gradinger GP (eds) Symposium on problems and complications in aesthetic plastic surgery of the face. Mosby, St Louis

Baker DC (1985) Reanimation of the paralysed face: nerve crossover, cross-face nerve grafting and muscle transfers. In: Chretien PB, et al (eds) Head and neck cancer. Decker, Philadelphia

Banic A, Boeckx W, Greulich M, et al (1995) Late results of breast reconstruction with free TRAM flaps: a prospective multicentric study. Plast Reconstr Surg 95: 1195

Barbanera M (1971) Relationship between water and heat loss from evaporation and increased metabolism in burned patients. Pathologica 63: 133

Barinka L (1977) The technique of the excisional operation for lymphedema of the lower extremity using a new instrument. In: Clodius L (ed) Lymphedema. Thieme, Stuttgart

Barnette RN, Eisenberg H (1964) Histologic grading in breast cancer. Conn Med 28: 123

Baroudi R, Lewis JR (1976) The augmentation-reduction mammaplasty. Clin Plast Surg 3: 301

Barrera A (1999) Hair transplantation: The art of micrografting & minigrafting. Quality Medical Publishing, St Louis
Barron JN (1971) The Maribor method of burns treatment. Hand 3: 179
Barrow RE, Jeschke MG, Herndon DN (2000) Early fluid resuscitation improves outcomes in severely burned children. Resuscitation 45: 91–96
Bartley GB, Fatourechi V, Kadrmas EF, et al (1996) Long-term follow-up of Graves' ophthalmopathy in an incidence cohort. Ophthalmology 103: 958–962
Basedow K von (1840) Exophthalmus durch Hypertrophie des Zellgewebes in der Augenhöhle. Wochenschr Ges Heilkd G 13: 197–204
Baudet J, Guimbertean JC, Nascimento E (1976) Successful clinical transfer of two free thoracodorsal axillary flaps. Plast Reconstr Surg 58: 680–686
Baumeister RG (1985) Five years of autogenous lymph vessel transplantation. Progress in Lymphology: Proceedings of the Tenth International Congress of Lymphology, University of Adelaide Press, Adelaide, p 250
Baumeister RGH, Siuda S (1990) Treatment of lymphedemas by microsurgical lymphatic grafting: What is proved? Plast Reconstr Surg 85: 64–74
Baxter CR (1971) Crystalloid resuscitation of burn shock. In: Polk HC Jr, Stone HH (eds) Contemporary burn management. Little, Brown and Company, Boston
Baxter CR (1974) Current status of burn research. J Trauma 14: 1
Baxter CR, Cook WA, Shires GT (1966) Serum myocardial depressant factor of burn shock. Surg Forum 17: 1–2
Ben-Hur N (1977) Primary nerve suturing of severed motor nerves in facial trauma. In: Rubin LR (ed) Reanimation of the paralyzed face. Mosby, St Louis
Berdijis ChC (1971) Pathology of irradiation. Williams & Wilkins, Baltimore
Bernard Cl, Huette Ch (1848) Précis iconographique de médicine opératoire et d'anatomie chirurgicale. Méquignon-Marvis Fils, Paris
Bernard F, Gueugniaud PY, Bertin-Maghit M, et al (1994) Prognostic significance of early cardiac index measurements in severely burned Patients. Burns 20: 529–531
Berrino P, Campora E, Santi P (1987) Postquadrantectomy breast deformities: classification and techniques of surgical correction. Plast Reconstr Surg 79: 567
Berson ML (1948) Atlas of plastic surgery. Grune & Stratton, New York
Biemer E (1986) Der freie Gewebetransfer an der unteren Extremität – eine Standortbestimmung. Chirurg 57: 141–142
Biemer E (1986) Der Fußrückenlappen (Dorsalis-pedis-Lappen). Chirurg 57: 137–139
Biemer E (1986) Indikationen für freie Lappenplastiken im Gegensatz zu alternativen Deckungsmethoden. Chirurg 57: 113–114
Biemer E, Duspiva W (1979) Rekonstruktive Mikrogefäßchirurgie. Springer, Berlin
Biemer E, Duspiva W (1980) Komplikationen bei der Replantation abgetrennter Gliedmaßen. Handchirurgie 9: 67–70
Biemer E, Jaeger K (1986) Medikamentöse Behandlung, Nachbehandlung und Sekundäreingriffe nach Unterschenkelrekonstruktion durch freien Gewebetransfer. Chirurg 57: 140
Biemer E, Steinau HU (1993) Mikrochirurgische Replantation und Gewebetransplantation. In: Heberer G, et al (Hrsg) Chirurgie und angrenzende Gebiete. Springer, Berlin, S 765–769
Billroth T (1866) Die allgemeine und chirurgische Pathologie und Therapie in 50 Vorlesungen. Reimer, Berlin, p 128
Birke G, Liljedahl SO (1972) Studies on burns. XV. Treatment with war dry air. Clinical results compared with those of earlier treatment series. Acta Chir Scand (Suppl) 422: 5
Birke G, Liljedahl SO, Olsson KE, Plantin LO (1970) Total exchange and insensible loss of water in severe burns during the first two weeks. Acta Chir Scand 136: 125
Birke G, Liljedahl SO, Plantin LO (1968) Studies on burns. IX. The distribution and losses through the wound of „I-albumin measured by hole body counting". Acta Chir Scand 134: 27
Blandford SE, Garcia FA (1953) Case report: Successful homogenous skin graft in a severe burn using an identical twin as donor. Plast Reconstr Surg 11: 31
Blocker GT (1964) Burns. In: Converse JM (ed) Reconstructive plastic surgery, vol I. Saunders, Philadelphia
Bohmert H (1975) Eine neue Methode zur Rekonstruktion der weiblichen Brust nach radikaler Mastektomie. In: Bohmert H (Hrsg) Plastische Chirurgie des Kopf- und Halsbereichs und der weiblichen Brust. Thieme, Stuttgart
Bohmert H (1982) Brustkrebs und Brustrekonstruktion. Thieme, Stuttgart
Bohmert H, Baumeister R (1987) Breast reconstruction with the transverse upper and lower rectus-flap. In: Maneksha RJ (ed) Transaction of the IX. Congress of Plastic and Reconstructive Surgery. McGraw Hill, New Delhi, p 391
Bohmert H, Gabka J (1997) Plastic and reconstructive surgery of the breast. Thieme, Stuttgart
Bohmert H, Strömbeck JO (1986) Postmastectomy reconstruction. In: Strömbeck JO, Rosato FE (eds) Surgery of the breast. Thieme, Stuttgart
Boldt J, Lenz M, Kumle B, Papsdorf M (1998) Volume replacement strategies on intensive care units: results from a postal survey. Intensive Care Med 24: 147–151
Borges P (1904) Autoplastic pour dédoublement et échange des lambeaux. Chirurgie orthopédique, Paris
Bostwick J III (2002) Plastic and reconstructive breast surgery, 2nd edition. Quality Medical Publishing, St Louis
Bostwick J III, Eaves FE III, Nahai F (1996) Endoscopic plastic surgery. Quality Medical Publishing, St Louis
Bowle J (1960) Primary Excision in third degree burns. Plast Reconstr Surg 25: 240
Bramann F von (1893) Heilung grosser Weichtheil- und Hautdefecte der Extremitäten mittelst gestielter Hautlappen aus entfernten Körpertheilen. 23. Congr Dtsch Ges Chir 626
Breslow A (1970) Thickness, cross sectional areas and depth of invasion in the prognosis of cutaneous melanoma. Ann Surg 172: 902–908
Brown HC (1973) Current concepts of burn pathology and mechanisms of deformity in the burned hand. (Symposium on practical surgery of the hand). Orthop Clin North Am 4: 987

Bruck J, Steen M, Müller S (2003) Handbuch der Verbrennungstherapie. Ecomed, Landsberg

Brugger H (1895) Die Behandlung der Gaumenspalten mit besonderer Berücksichtigung der Prothesen mit Korkkern. Sallmann, Basel Leipzig

Brunner H (1926) Surgical treatment of facial paralysis. Z Hals Nasen Ohrenheilkd 15: 379

Bruns V von (1857) Chirurgischer Atlas. Laupp, Tübingen

Buck-Gramcko D (1967) Verbrennungen der Hand in Verbindung mit ausgedehnten Verbrennungen der Körperoberfläche. Klin Med 22: 393

Bull JP, Fisher AJ (1954) A study of mortality in a burns unit. Ann Surg 139: 269

Buncke H (1983) Serratus anterior free muscle grafts for facial paralysis. Presented at the American Association for Plastic Surgery annual meeting

Buncke HJ (1975) Free toe to hand transplantation by microvascular anastomosis. In: Transactions of the sixth international congress of plastic and reconstructive surgery. Masson, Paris, p 127

Buncke HJ, Colen LB (1980) An island flap from the first web space of the foot to cover plantar ulcers. Br J Plast Surg 33: 242

Bunnell S (1927) Suture of the facial nerve within the temporal bone with a report of the first successful case. Surg Gynecol Obstet 45: 7

Burgess LPA, Goode RL (1994) Reanimation of the paralysed face. Thieme, New York, p 5–9

Burian F (1958) Proposta di una collaborazione internazionale per lo studio die problemi inerenti alla labio-palatoschisi. Minerva Chir 13: 931

Burian F (1963) Chirurgie der Lippen- und Gaumenspalten. VEB Verlag Volk und Gesundheit, Berlin

Burow AB (1856) Beschreibung einer neuen Transplantationsmethode. Peters, Berlin

Carpue JC (1816) An account of two successful operation for restorning the lost nose from the integuments of the forehead. London

Chang TS, Wang W, Hsu CY (1982) The free forearm flap. A report of 25 cases. Ann Med Singapore 11: 236–244

Chang WHJ, Gomes NH, Edelstein LM (1973) Use of lyophilised skin for donor site cover. Br J Plast Surg 26: 147

Chen ZW, Chien YC, Pao YS (1963) Salvage of the forearm following complete traumatic amputation: report of a successful case. Chin Med J 82: 632

Chen ZW, Zeng BF (1983) Replantation of the lower extremity. Clin Plast Surg 10: 103

Christ W (1961) Sekundäre plastische Deckung ausgedehnter infizierter Hautdefekte. Aesth Med 10: 7

Clark WH Jr, From L, Bernardino EA, Mihm MC Jr (1969) The histogenesis and biologic behaviour of primary human malignant melanomas of the skin. Cancer Res 29: 705–727

Clodius L (1977) The experimental basis for the surgical treatment of lymphedema. In: Clodius L (ed) Lymphedema. Thieme, Stuttgart

Clodius L, Gibson T Lymphedema. In: Rob C, Smith R (eds) Operative surgery, 3rd edition. Butterworths, London (1979)

Clodius L, Piller NB, Casley-Smith JR (1981) The problems of lymphatic microsurgery for lymphedema. Lymphology 14: 69

Cobbett JR (1969) Free digital transfer – report of a case of transfer of a great toe to replace amputated thumb. J Bone Joint Surg [Br] 51: 677–679

Conley J, Baker DC (1979) Hypoglossal-facial nerve anastomosis for reinnervation of the paralysed face. Plast Reconstr Surg 63: 63–72

Conley J, Baker DC (1983) Myths and misconceptions in the rehabilitation of facial paralysis. Plast Reconstr Surg 71: 538

Converse JM (1942) New forehead flap for nasal reconstruction. Proc R Soc Med 35: 811

Converse JM, Rapaport FT (1956) The vascularization of skin autografts and homografts. An experimental study in man. Ann Surg 143: 306

Converse JM, Wood-Smith D (1977) Techniques for the repair of defects of the lips and cheeks. In: Converse JM (ed) Reconstructive, plastic surgery. Saunders, Philadelphia, Vol III, p 1544

Conway H (1958) Muscle plastic operations for facial paralysis. Ann Surg 147: 541

Conway H, Joslin D, Rees TD, Stark RB (1952) Observations on the development of circulation in skin grafts. Plast Reconstr Surg 9: 557

Cook WA, Baxter CR, Ferrell JM Jr (1968) Pulmonary circulation after dermal burns. Vasc Surg 2: 1

Cope O, Moore FD (1947) The redistribution of body water and the fluid therapy of the burned patient. Ann Surg 126: 1010

Cormack GC, Lamberty BGH (1984) A classification of fasciocutaneous flaps according to their patterns of vascularisation. Br J Plast Surg 37: 80–87

Cormack GC, Lamberty BGH (1984) Fasciocutaneous vessels in the upper arm: application to the design of new fasciocutaneous flaps. Plast Reconstr Surg 74: 244–249

Cormack GC, Lamberty BGH (1995) The arterial anatomy of skin flaps, 2nd ed. Churchill Livingstone, Edinburgh

Cronin TD (1958) Lengthening columella by use of skin from nasal floor and alae. Plast Reconstr Surg 21: 417

Cronin TD (1966) A modification of the Tennison-type lip repair. Cleft Palate J 3: 376

Cronin TD, Gerow F (1963) Augmentation mammaplasty – A new „natural feel" prosthesis. In: Transactions of the third international congress of plastic surgeons. Excerpta Medica, New York, pp 41–49

Daniel R, Taylor GI (1973) Distant transfer of an island flap by microvascular anastomoses, a clinical technique. Plast Reconstr Surg 52: 111–116

Davies JWL, Ricketts CR, Bull JP (1962) Studies of plasm protein metabolism. I. Albumin in burned and injured patients. Clin Sci 23: 411

De Cholnoky T (1970) Augmentation mammaplasty: survey of complications in 10,941 patients by 265 surgeons. Plast Reconstr Surg 45: 573

Dellon L (1999) Free split and segmental latissimus dorsi muscle transfer in on stage for facial reanimation. Plast Reconstr Surg 103: 481–482

Delpech J (1823–1828) Chirurgie clinique de Montpellier aux observations et reflexions des traveaux de chirurgie de cette école.

Demling RH, Kramer G, Gunther R, Nerlich M (1985) Effect of non-pro-

tein colloid on post-burn edema formation in soft tissues and lung. Surgery 95: 593–602
Demling RH, Kramer G, Harms B (1984) Role of thermal injury-induced hypoproteinemia on edema formation in burned and non-burned tissue. Surgery 95: 136–144
Derganc H (1970) An uniform classification of the depth of burns. In: Matter P, Barclay TL, Konickova Z (eds) Research in burns. Huber, Bern
Deutinger M, Meissl G, Koller R, et al (1995) Results after different forms of neuromuscular reconstruction for facial palsy. In: Frey M, Giovanoli P (eds) Proceedings of the 4th international muscle symposium, Zürich, Nr 3, S 23–25
Deutschmann W, Scharnagl E (1980) Long term results in the surgical treatment of lymphedema. Surg Gynecol Obstet 125: 607–610
Dieffenbach FJ (1829) Chirurgische Erfahrungen, besonders über die Wiederherstellung zerstörter Teile menschlichen Körpers nach neuen Methoden. Enslin, Berlin
Dieffenbach FJ (1833) Ersatz der Unterlippe durch Heranziehen und seitliche Einschnitte. Operative Chirurgie Bd 1, S 419–420
Dieffenbach FJ (1833) Surgical observations on restoration of the nose. Operative Chirurgie Bd 1, S 359
Dieffenbach FJ (1845) Die operative Chirurgie. Brockhaus, Leipzig
Dittmann EM (2007) Der Chirurg Erich Lexer (1867–1937). Kaden Verlag, Heidelberg
DiVincenti FC, Curreri PW, Pruitt BA (1969) Use of mesh skin autografts in the burned patient. Plast Reconstr Surg 44: 464
Dollinger J (1911) Die Druckentlastung der Augenhöhle durch Entfernung der äußeren Orbitalwand bei hochgradigem Exophthalmus (Morbus Basedowii) und konsekutiver Hornhauterkrankung. Dtsch Med Wochenschr 37: 1888
Dreyer JT (1831) Nova blepharoplastices methodus (Dissertation). Gerold, Wien
Dries DJ, Waxman K (1991) Adequate resuscitation of burn patients may not be measured by urine output and vital signs. Crit Care Med 19: 327–329
Eade GG (1958) The relationship between granulation tissue bacteria and skin grafts in burned patients. Plast Reconstr Surg 22: 42
Edwards JM, Kinmonth JB (1969) Lymphovenous shunts in man. Br Med. J 4: 579
Ehrly AM (1971) Rheologische Probleme beim Schock. Med Welt 22: 1167
Eriksson G (1972) Regeneration of epidermis after second degree burns. Scand J Plast Reconstr Surg 6: 83
Ernst H (1980) Strahlenreaktionen – Bestrahlungsfolgen, Strahlenschäden. Diagnostik 13: 291–294
Esser JFS (1917) Studies in plastic surgery of the face. Ann Surg 65: 297
Esser JFS (1918) Die Rotation der Wange und allgemeine Bemerkungen bei chirurgischer Gesichtsplastik. Vogel, Leipzig
Esser JFS (1918) Gestielte lokale Nasenplastik mit zweizipfligen Lappen. Dtsch Z Chir 143: 385
Esser JFS (1918) Schwerer Verschluß einer Brustwandperforation. Berl Klin Wochenschr 55: 1197–1202
Evans AJ (1970) Baseline of fluid replacement during the first 48 hours. In: Research in burns. Huber, Bern
Exner K (1999) Standard Facelifting einschließlich SMAS-Straffung. In: Lemperle G (Hrsg) Ästhetische Chirurgie. Ecomed, Landsberg
Fara M (1977) The musculature of cleft lip and palate. In: Converse JM (ed) Reconstructive plastic surgery. Saunders, Philadelphia, p 2104
Fatourechi V, Bartley GB, Garrity JA, Bergstralh EJ, Michael MS, et al (1993) Transfrontal orbital decompression after failure of transantral decompression in optic neuropathy of Graves' disease. Mayo Clin Proc 68: 552–555
Fatourechi V, Garrity JA, Bartley GB, Bergstralh EJ, DeSanto LW, Gorman C (1994) Graves' ophthalmopathy – results of transantral orbital decompression performed primarily for cosmetic indications. Ophthalmology 101: 938–942
Filatow VP (1922) Plastik mit rundem Stil. Klin Monatsbl Augenheilkd 68: 124
Fisch U (1974) Facial nerve grafting. Otolaryngol Clin North Am 7: 517
Fisch U (1976) Cross-face grafting in facial paralysis. Arch Otorhinolaryngol 102: 453–457
Fisher B, Bauer M, Margolese R, et al (1985) Five year results of a randomized clinical trial comparing total mastectomy and segmental mastectomy with or without radiation in the treatment of breast cancer. N Engl J Med 312: 665–673
Fisher B, Redmond C, Fisher E, et al (1985) Ten-year results of a randomised clinical trial comparing radical mastectomy and total mastectomy with or without radiation. N Engl J Med 312: 574–681
Fisher B, Slack NH, Bross IDJ (1969) Cancer of the breast: Size of neoplasm and prognosis. Cancer 24: 1071
Fisher ER, Gregorio R, Fisher B (1976) Prognostic significance of histopathology. In: Stoll BA (ed) Risk factors in breast cancer. Heinemann, London
Fisher JC (1992) The silicone controversy – When will science prevail? N Engl J Med 326: 1996
Fogh-Andersen P (1982) Ätiologie und Epidemiologie der Lippen-Kiefer-Gaumenspalten. In: Pfeifer G (Hrsg) Lippen-Kiefer-Gaumenspalten. Thieme, Stuttgart, p 13
Földi M (1983) Lymphedema. In: Földi M, Casley-Smith JR (eds) Lymphangiology. Schattauer, Stuttgart
Freilinger G (1975) A new technique to correct facial paralysis. Plast Reconstr Surg 56: 44
Freilinger G, Gruber H, Happak W, Pechmann U (1987) Surgical anatomy of the mimic muscle system and the facial nerve: Ineportance for reconstructive and aesthetic surgery. Plast Reconstr Surg 80: 686–690
Freilinger G, Holle J, Carlson BM (1981) Muscle transplantation. Springer, Wien
Frey M (1989) Die freie, funktionelle Muskeltransplantation mit mikroneurovaskulären Anastomosen – Die Entwicklung zur standardisierten Operationsmethode. Wiener Klin Wochenschr 101: 57–62
Frey M (1999) Smile reconstruction using the gracilis muscle. Op Tech Plast Reconstr Surg 6: 180–189
Frey M (1999) Three-dimensional video analysis of facial movements: a new

method to assess the quantity and quality of the smile. Plast Reconstr Surg 104: 2031–2039

Friedman RJ, Argenta LC, Anderson R (1985) Deep inferior epigastric free flap for breast reconstruction after radical mastectomy. Plast Reconstr Surg 76: 455

Fritze HE, Reich OFG (1845) Die plastischen Operationen, in ihrem weitesten Umfange dargestellt und durch Abbildungen erläutert. Hirschwald, Berlin

Fujino T, Harashina T, Aoyagi R (1975) Reconstruction for aplasia of the breast and pectoral region by microvascular transfer of a free flap from the buttock. Plast Reconstr Surg 56: 178

Gabka C, et al (1998) Sofortrekonstruktion nach modifizierter radikaler Mastektomie. In: Empfehlungen zur Diagnostik, Therapie und Nachsorge Mammakarzinome. Tumorzentrum München

Gabka HJ (1964) Hasenscharte und Wolfsrachen, 2. Aufl. de Gruyter, Berlin

Garré C (1888) Über die histologischen Vorgänge bei der Anheilung der Thiersch'schen Transplantationen. Bruns Beitr Klin Chir 4: 625

Garrity JA, Saggau DD, Gorman CA, Bartley GB, Fatourechi V, Hardwig PW, Dyer JA (1992) Torsional diplopia after transantral orbital decompression and extraocular muscle surgery associated with Graves' orbitopathy. Am J Ophthalmol 113: 363–373

Gary-Bobo A, Fuentes JM (1983) Long-term follow-up report on cross-facial nerve grafting in the treatment of facial paralysis. Br J Plast Surg 36: 48–50

Geldmacher J, Brug E (1973) Arbeitsunfall und Handverletzung. Münch Med Wochenschr 115: 1211

Georgiade N (1970) Plastic surgery and burns. Surg Gynecol Obstet 130: 311

Germann G, Barthold U, Janshoff G, Steinau HU (1992) The impact of inhalation trauma, risk factors and concomitant diseases on the precision of burn scores. Proc Am Burns Assoc 202

Germann G, Hartmann B (1996) Thermische und chemische Verletzungen. In: Durst J (Hrsg) Traumatologische Praxis. Schattauer, Stuttgart, S 621–638

Germann G., Steinau U (1995) Aktuelle Aspekte der Verbrennungsbehandlung. Zentralbl Chir 118: 290–302

Gershon-Cohen J (1967) Self-examination and detection of early breast cancer. Pa Med 70: 75

Gershon-Cohen J, Berger SM, Kockstein HS (1963) Roentgenography of breast cancer moderating concept of „biologic predeterminism". Cancer 16: 961

Ghormley RK, Overton LM (1935) The surgical treatment of severe forms of lymphedema (elephantiasis) of the extremities: a study of end results. Surg Gynecol Obstet 61

Gibson T, Medawar PB (1942) The fate of skin homografts in man. J Anat 77: 299

Gibson T, Tough JS (1954) The surgical correction of chronic lymphedema of the legs. Br J Plast Surg 7: 195

Gilbert A, Teot L (1982) The free subscapular flap. Plast Reconstr Surg 69: 601–604

Gillies HD (1934) Experience with fascia lata grafts in the operative treatment of facial paralysis. Proc R Soc Med 27: 1372

Gillies HD (1937) Up and down flap, Vol 3. Appleton, New York, p 762

Gillies HD, Fry WK (1921) A new principle in the surgical treatment of congenital cleft palate and its mechanical counterpart. Br Med J I: 335

Girdner JJ (1881) Skin grafting with grafts taken from the dead subject. Med Record NY 20: 119

Gluck Th (1921) Über Osteoplastik. Arch Klin Chir 117: 22–29

Godina M (1979) Preferential use of end-to-side arterial anastomoses in free flap transfers. Plast Reconstr Surg 64: 673–682

Godina M (1980) The saphenous and cubital flaps. Presented at Reconstructive Surgery: An in-depth course in microvascular and peripheral microneurosurgery. October 1980, New York

Godina M (1981) Medial arm flap. Symposium on reconstructive microsurgery. Albert Einstein Institute, New York

Godina M (1986) Early microsurgical reconstruction of complex trauma. Plast Reconstr Surg 78: 285–292

Godina M (1986) Early microsurgical reconstruction of complex trauma of the extremities. Clin Plast Surg 13: 619

Godina M, Bajec J, Eder E (1978) Freie Transplantation vom Latissimus dorsi Lappen. Summaries of 9. Tagung der Vereinigung der Deutschen Plastischen Chirurgen, 2

Goldmann EE (1894) Über das Schicksal der nach dem Verfahren von Thiersch verpflanzten Hautstückchen. Bruns Beitr Klin Chir 11: 229

Goodstein LD (1961) Intellectual impairment in children with cleft palates. J Speech Hear Res 4: 287–294

Graefe CF (1818) Rhinoplastik oder die Kunst, den Verlust der Nase organisch zu ersetzen. Berlin

Graves RJ (1835) Clinical lectures. London Med Surg J 7: 516–517

Grimm A, Kopp J, Bach AD, Kneser U, et al (2004) „Life before limb" – Indikation und Kontraindikation der Replantation. CHAZ 5: 315–324

Grisotti A, Veronesi U (1992) Reconstruction of the radiated partial mastectomy defect with autogenous tissues (discussion). Plast Reconstr Surg 90: 866

Grotting JC (1995) Reoperative aesthetic and reconstructive plastic surgery. Quality Medical Publishing, St Louis

Guelinckx PJ, Sinsel NK (1996) Muscle transplantation for reconstruction of the smile after facial paralysis past, present, and future. Microsurgery 17: 391–401

Haab O (1904) Atlas und Grundriss der Lehre von den Augenoperationen. Lehmanns, München

Haab O (1910) Atlas der äusserlich sichtbaren Erkrankungen des Auges, nebst Grundriss ihrer Pathologie und Therapie. Lehmanns, München

Hackett ME, Batchelor JR (1970) The HL-A system and its importance for skin grafting in burned patients. In: Matter P, Barclay TL, Konickova Z (eds) Research in burns. Huber, Bern

Hagedorn W (1892) Die Operation der Hasenscharte mit Zickzack-Naht. Zentralbl Chir 19: 281–285

Hagerty RF, Smith W (1958) The nasolabial cheek flap. Am Surg 24: 506

Hakelius L (1979) Free muscle grafting. Clin Plast Surg 6: 301

Halsted WS (1907) The results of radical operations for the cure of cancer of the breast. Ann Surg 46: 1–19

Hamra ST (1992) Composite rhytidectomy. Plast Reconstr Surg 90: 1–22

Hamra ST (1993) Composite rhytidectomy. Quality Medical Publishing, St Louis

Hargest TS, Rittenbury MS, Artz CP (1964) Early removal of burns by air blasting. Surg Forum 20: 74

Harii K (1979) Microneurovascular free muscle transplantation for reanimation of facial paralysis. Clin Plast Surg 6: 361–375

Harii K (1979) Microvascular free tissue transfers. World J Surg 3: 29–42, 124–126

Harii K, Asato H, Yoshimura K, Sugawara Y, Nakatsuka T, Ueda K (1998) One-stage transfer of the latissimus dorsi muscle for reanimation of a paralysed face: a new alternative. Plast Reconstr Surg 102: 941–951

Harii K, Ohmori K, Torii S (1976) Free gracilis muscle transplantation with microneurovascular anastomoses for the treatment of facial paralysis. Plast Reconstr Surg 57: 133–143

Harii K, Ohmori K, Torii SS, et al (1975) Free groin skin flaps. Br J Plast Surg 28: 225

Harii K, Ohmori, K, Ohmori, S (1974) Successful clinical transfer of ten free flaps by microvascular anastomoses. Plast Reconstr Surg 53: 259–270

Harris JR, Hellmann JS, Henderson IC, Kinne D (1987) Breast diseases. Lippincott, Philadelphia

Harrison D, Morgan DG (1981) The instep island flap to resurface plantar defects. Br J Plast Surg 34: 315

Harrison DH (1985) The pectoralis minor vascularized muscle graft for the treatment of unilateral facial palsy. Plast Reconstr Surg 75: 206

Hartrampf CR, Bennet GK (1987) Autogenous tissue reconstruction in the mastectomy patient. A critical review of 300 patients. Ann Surg 205: 508

Hartrampf CR, Noel RT, Drazan LL, Elliot LF, Bennet GK, Beegle PH (1994) Rubens's fat pad for breast reconstruction: a peri-iliac soft tissue free flap. Plast Reconstr Surg 93: 402

Hartrampf CR, Scheflan M, Black PW (1982) Breast reconstruction with a transverse abdominal island flap. Plast Reconstr Surg 69: 216

Haug (1894) Eine einfache neue plastische Methode zur Rücklagerung hochgradig abstehender Ohrmuscheln. Dtsch Med Wochenschr S 776

Held L (1961) Die chirurgische Behandlung der Röntgen-Ulcera. Chirurg 32: 363

Herden HN (1974) Pathophysiologie und Allgemeinbehandlung der Verbrennungskrankheit. Prakt Anaesth 9: 43

Hergenroeder F (1938) Results of surgical therapy for elephantiasis of the lower extremity. Total excision of the skin of the lower leg, defect closure by Thiersch grafts. Vestn Khir 55: 603

Heufelder AE (1996) Endokrine Orbitopathie – Aktueller Stand der Pathophysiologie und Therapie. Arzneimitteltherapie 5: 138–143

Heufelder AE, Smith TJ, Gorman CA, Bahns RS (1991) Increased induction of HLA-DR by interferon gamma in cultured fibroblasts derived from patients with Graves' ophthalmopathy and pretibial dermopathy. J Clin Endocrinol Metab 73: 307–313

Hill LH, Nahai F, Vasconez LO (1978) The tensor fascia lata myocutaneous free flap. Plast Reconstr Surg 61: 517–522

Ho LC, Lai MF, Kennedy PJ (1983) Microlymphatic bypass in the treatment of obstructive lymphedema of the arm: case report of a new technique. Br J Plast Surg 36: 350

Holle J (1994) Plastische Operationen im Bereich der Ohrmuschel. In: Krupp S (Hrsg) Plastische Chirurgie. Ecomed, Landsberg

Holle J, Mandl H, Krepler R (1982) Überbrückung eines Lymphgefäßdefektes mittels Veneninterposition. Handchirurgie 14: 83–86

Holle J, Pierini A (1983) Breast reconstruction by a turn-over flap of the external oblique ab dominis muscle and double Z-plasty of the abdominal skin. In: Transaction of the VII International Congress on Plastic and Reconstructive Surgery, p 592

Holm C, Melcer B, Hörbrand F, Henckel von Donnersmarck G, Mühlbauer W (2000) The relationship between oxygen delivery and oxygen consumption during fluid resuscitation of burn-related shock. J Burn Care Rehabil 21: 147–154

Holmström H (1979) The free abdominoplasty flap and its use in breast reconstruction. Scand J Plast Reconstr Surg 13: 423–432

Hopewell JW (1980) The importance of vascular damage in the development of late radiation effects in normal times. In: Meyn RE, Withers HR (eds) Radiation biology in cancer research. Raven Press, New York

House JW, Brackman DE (1985) Facial nerve grading system. Otolaryngol Head Neck Surg 93: 144–147

Huang GK, Hu RQ, Liu ZZ, Suen YL, Lan TD, Pan GP (1985) Microlymphaticovenous anastomosis in the treatment of lower limb obstructive lymphedema. Analysis of 91 cases. Plast Reconstr Surg 76: 671–685

Hughes GB (1982) Electroneurography: objective prognostic assessment of facial paralysis. Am J Otol 4: 73

Illingworth RS, Birch CB (1956) The intelligence of children with cleft palate. Arch Dis Childh 31: 300–302

Ingianni G, Holzmann Th (1985) Klinische Erfahrungen in der Anwendung von lymphovenösen Anastomosen beim sekundären Lymphödem. Handchirurgie 17: 43–46

International Union Against Cancer – UICC (1974) TNM – Classification of malignant tumors, 2nd edn, Geneva

Irwin OC, Chen HP (1943) Speech sound developments during the first years of life, a review of the literature. J Speech Disord 8: 109–121

Jackson DMG (1969) Second thoughts on the burn wound. J Trauma 9: 839

Jackson DMG, Stone PA (1972) Tangential excision and grafting of burns. Br J Plast Surg 258: 416

Jackson DMG, Topley E, Cason JS, Lowbury EJL (1960) Primary excision on grafting of large burns. Ann Surg 152: 167

Jackson IT (1997) Local flap reconstruction of defects after excision of nonmelanoma skin cancer. Clin Plast Surg 24: 747–767

Jackson IT (2002) Local flaps in head and neck reconstruction. Quality Medical Publishing, St Louis

Jackson IT (2003) The keystone design perforator island flap in reconstructive surgery (Comment). Aust NZ J Surg 73: 261

Jacobson J, Suarez EL (1960) Microsurgery in anastomosis of small vessels. Surg Forum 11: 243–251

Jaeger K (1986) Präoperative Vorbereitungen und Voruntersuchungen beim freien Gewebetransfer zur Unter-

schenkelrekonstruktion. Chirurg 57: 115–117

Jänicke F, et al (1998) Prognosefaktoren beim Mammakarzinom. In: Empfehlungen zur Diagnostik, Therapie und Nachsorge Mammakarzinome. Tumorzentrum München.

Janzekovic Z (1968) Consistent application of generally adopted surgical principles in the treatment of the burn wound. In: Derganc M (ed) Present clinical aspects of burns: a symposium. Mariborski Tisk, Maribor

Janzekovic Z (1968) The dermal burn. In: Derganc M (ed) Present clinical aspects of burns: a symposium. Mariborski Tisk, Maribor

Janzekovic Z (1970) A new concept in the early excision and immediate grafting of burns. J Trauma 10: 1103–1108

Johnson HA (1967) Reconstruction of hand surface defects. Int Surg 48: 221-228

Jordan (1895) Über den plastischen Ersatz der Augenlider. Dtsch Med Wochenschr 45: 477

Joseph J (1898) Über die operative Verkleinerung einer Nase (Rhinomiosis). Berl Klin Wochenschr 40

Joseph J (1904) Intranasale Nasenhöckerabtragung. Berl Klin Wochenschr 24 und Verhandlungen der Berliner Medizinischen Gesellschaft, Sitzung 1. Juni 1904

Joseph J (1907) Beiträge zur Rhinoplastik. Berl Klin Wochenschr 16

Joseph J (1912) Plastische Keilhebung bei Doggennasen. Korrektive Nasen- und Ohrenplastik. In: Katz L, Preysing H, Blumenfeld F (Hrsg) Handbuch der speziellen Chirurgie des Ohres und der oberen Luftwege. Bd. 1 / 2. Hälfte. C Kabitzsch, Würzburg

Joseph J (1931) Nasenplastik und sonstige Gesichtsplastik nebst einem Anhang über Mammachirurgie. C Kabitzsch/ JA Barth, Leipzig [reprinted by Kaden Verlag, Heidelberg, 2004]

Jungengel M (1890/1891) Die Hauttransplantation nach Thiersch. Verhandl Physikal Med Ges Würzburg 25

Juri J (1975) Use of parieto-occipital flaps in surgical treatment of baldness. Plast Reconstr Surg 55: 456

Kahaly G, Otto E, Förster G, Gansen K, Olivari N, Beyer J, Hansen Ch (1998) T-cells and orbital tissue in endocrine orbitopathy. Exp Clin Endocrinol Diabetes 104: 79–83

Kaplan EN, Minami RT, Wu G (1974) Palatopharyngeal incompetence. In: Saad MN, Lichtveld P (eds) Reviews in plastic surgery. Excerpta Medica, American Elsevier, Amsterdam New York, p 223

Karapandzic M (1990) Innervated musculocutaneous lip and cheek flaps. In: Grabbs's encyclopedia of flaps. Little, Brown Co, Boston, S 691–670

Kausch W (1904) Beiträge zu den plastischen Operationen. Fingerbeuger- und Fingerstreckerplastik, Ersatz der Fingerkuppe, Nasenplastik aus der Zehe, Penishaut- und Scrotumplastik. Arch Klin Chir 74: 495–532

Keller GS, Hucherson R (1997) Endoscopic forehead and brow lift. In: Hurley (ed) Endoscopic facial plastic surgery. Mosby-Year Book, St Louis, pp 49–81

Kister S, Haagensen C (1970) Paget's disease of the breast. Am J Surg 119: 606–609

Klinke O (1914) Die operativen Erfolge bei der Behandlung des Morbus Basedowii. Karger, Berlin

Klose H (1929) Die Chirurgie der Basedowschen Krankheit. Enke, Stuttgart

Koberg W (1971) System der Rehabilitation von Patienten mit Lippen-Kiefer-Gaumenspalten. Westdeutscher Verlag, Opladen

König F (1914) Über Nasenplastik. Bruns Beitr Klin Chir S 94

Körte W (1903) Ein Fall von Nervenpfropfung des Nervus facialis auf den Nervus hypoglossus. Dtsch Med Wochenschr 17: 293

Koshima I, Moriguchi T, Soeda S, Hamanaka T, Ohta S (1994) Free rectus femoris muscle transfer for one-stage reconstruction of established facial paralysis. Plast Reconstr Surg 94: 421–428

Koshima I, Soeda S (1989) Inferior epigastric artery skin flaps without rectus abdominis muscle. Br J Plast Surg 42: 645–648

Kraske H (1923) Die Operation der atrophischen und hypertrophischen Hängebrust. Münch Med Wochenschr S 70

Krause F (1893) Über die Transplantation grosser ungestielter Hautlappen. Verh Dtsch Ges Chir 22: 46

Kriens O (1967) Anatomische Untersuchungen am gespaltenen weichen Gaumen. Beitrag als Grundlage der Veloplastik. (Chirurgia Plastica et Reconstructiva, Vol 4), Springer, Berlin, S 14

Krizek TJ, Tani T, Despez JD, Kilhn CL (1965) Experimental transplantation of composite grafts by microsurgical vascular anastomoses. Plast Reconstr Surg 36: 538–543

Krönlein RU (1889) Zur Pathologie und operativen Behandlung der Dermoidcysten der Orbita. Beitr Klin Chir 4: 149–163

Krupp S, Assé N'Dri H (1989) Transfer of lower orbicularis muscle flap for lower lip incontinence. Eur J Plast Surg 12: 51–55

Krupp S, Nigst H (1967) Tiefgreifende Verbrennungen der Hände. Klin Med 22: 396

Kubik S (1980) Drainagemöglichkeiten der Lymphterritorien nach Verletzung peripherer Kollektoren und nach Lymphadenektomie. Folia Angiol Berlin 28: 228

Kühn Th, Bembenek A, Büchels HK, et al (2004) Konsensus der Deutschen Gesellschaft für Senologie: Sentinel-Node-Biopsie beim Mammakarzinom. CHAZ 5: 29–34

Labat L (1833) De la rhinoplastie et de la rhinoraphie soit dans les cas d'absence congénitale ou d'enlevement accidental de la partie dorsale du nez. Méd Phys 24: 619

Lamberty BGH, Cormack GC (1983) The anticubital fasciocutaneous flap. Br J Plast Surg 36: 428–432

Lamke LO, Liljedahl SO (1971) Evaporative water loss from burns, grafts and donor sites. Scand J Plast Reconstr Surg 5: 17

Langenbeck BRK von (1859) Beiträge zur Osteoplastik. Dtsch Klinik Nr. 48

Langenbeck BRK von (1861) Operation der angeborenen totalen Spaltung des harten Gaumens nach einer neuen Methode. Dtsch Klinik 13: 231

Larson DL, Abston S, Evans EB, Dobrokovsky M, Linares HA (1971) Techniques for decreasing scar formation and contractures in the burned patient. J Trauma 11: 807

Lassus C (1970) A technique for breast reduction. Int Surg 53: 69–72 (1970)

Lassus C (1981) New refinements in vertical mammaplasty. Chir Plastica 6: 81–86

Lassus C (1987) Breast reduction: evolution of a technique – a single vertical scar. Aesth Plast Surg 11: 107

Lawrence JC, Carney SA (1973) Tangential excision of burns: Studies on the metabolic activitiy of the recipient areas for skin grafts. Br J Plast Surg 26: 93

Le Mesurier AB (1949) A method of cutting and suturing the lip in the treatment of complete unilateral clefts. Plast Reconstr Surg 4: 1–12 (1949)

Leape LL (1970) Initial changes in burns: tissue changes in burned and unburned skin of rhesus monkeys. J Trauma 10: 488

Lee YC (1972) Early heterografting of partial-thickness burns. J Trauma 12: 818

Lehnhardt M, Homann HH, Druecke D, Steinau HU (2003) Liposuktion – kein Problem? Chirurg 74: 808–814

Lehnhardt M, Palka P, Homann HH, Druecke D, Steinau HU (2004) Majorkomplikationen und Todesfälle nach kosmetischer Liposuktion. CHAZ 5: 25–28

Lejour M (1994) Vertical mammaplasty and liposuction of the breast. Quality Medical Publishing, St Louis

Lemperle G (1991) Plastische Mammachirurgie. Springer, Heidelberg

Lemperle G (Hrsg) Ästhetische Chirurgie. Ecomed, Landsberg

Lemperle G, Köhnlein HE, Kannen W (1971) Die Kaltwasserbehandlung frischer Verbrennungen. Langenbecks Arch Chir (Kongressber) 329: 898

Lemperle G, Radu D (1981) Die plastisch-chirurgische Deckung von Strahlenulzera im Thorax- und Beckenbereich. Langenbecks Arch Chir 355: 187–192

Lexer E (1906) Der plastische Ersatz des Septum cutaneum. Dtsch Z Chir 81: 560

Lexer E (1919/1924) Die freien Transplantationen. 2 Bde. (Neue Deutsche Chirurgie, 26a/b). Enke, Stuttgart

Lexer E (1920) Wiederherstellungschirurgie. Barth, Leipzig

Lexer E (1925) Kosmetische Operationen der Nase. In: Denker H, Kahler O (Hrsg) Handbuch der Hals-, Nasen-, Ohrenheilkunde. Springer, Berlin

Lexer E, Eden R (1911) Über die chirurgische Behandlung der peripheren Fazialisparese. Beitr Klin Chir 73: 116

Lily NR (1971) Reinnervation of a free skin autograft. Acta Chir Acad Sci Hung 12: 237

Limberg AA (1946) Eine neue, mathematisch fundierte Methode zur Planung lokalplastischer Operationen der Körperfläche. VEB Fischer, Jena

Lister GD, Gibson T (1972) Closure of rhomboid skin defects: the flaps of Limberg and Dufourmentel. Br J Plast Surg 25: 300

Lister GD, Kalisman M, Tsu-Min Tsai (1983) Reconstruction of the hand with free microneurovascular toe-to-hand transfer: experience with 54 toe transfers. Plast Reconstr Surg 71: 284–372

Loew D, Meng K (1974) Blutchemische Veränderungen und Mortalität beim standardisierten Verbrennungschock der Ratte. Langenbecks Arch Chir 335: 321

Loew D, Meng K (1974) Untersuchungen über das akute Nierenversagen beim Verbrühungsschock der Ratte. Langenbecks Arch Chir 335: 295

Loyal D (1934) The return of sensation to transplanted skin. Surg Gynecol Obstet 59: 533

MacCarroll HR (1938) The regeneration of sensation in transplanted skin. Ann Surg 108: 309

MacCarty CS, Kenefick TP, McConahey WM, Kearns TP (1970) Ophthalmopathy of Graves' disease treated by removal of roof, lateral walls, and lateral sphenoid ridge: reviews of 46 cases. Mayo Clin Proc 45: 488–493

MacCoy F (1949) The value of homografts. Plast Reconstr Surg 4: 389

MacMillan BG (1958) Early excision of more than 25 % of body surface in the extensive burned patient. Arch Surg 77: 369

Manchot C (1889) Die Hautarterien des menschlichen Körpers. Vogel, Leipzig

Mandl H (1981) Experimentelle Untersuchungen zur mikrochirurgischen Rekonstruktion von Lymphgefässdefekten. Z Plast Chir 5: 70

Mandl H, Kokoschka EM, Konrad K, Pehamberger H, Scharnagl E, Waclawiczek W (1984) Melanome der Haut. In: Fasching W (Hrsg) ACO-Manual der Chirurgischen Krebs-Therapie. Facultas, Wien, S 127–133

Mandry (1908) Rhinoplastik mit direkter Einpflanzung eines Hautperiostknochenlappens aus der Schlüsselbeinschultergegend. Beitr Klin Chir 77

Manktelow RT (1984) Free muscle transplantation for facial paralysis. Clin Plast Surg 11: 215

Manktelow RT (1985) Mikrovaskuläre Wiederherstellungschirurgie. Anatomie, Anwendung und chirurgische Technik. Springer, Berlin

Mantkelow RT, Zuker RM (1999) Cross-facial nerve graft-the long and short graft: the first stage for microneurovascular muscle transfer. Op Tech Plast Reconstr Surg 6: 174–179

Marchac D (1987) Craniofacial surgery. Springer, Berlin

Marchac D, Ascherman J, Arnaud E (1997) Fibrin glue fixation in forehaead endoscopy: evaluation of our experience with 206 cases. Plast Reconstr Surg 100: 704–714

Maris F, Jurkovic P, Kohut P, Suchanek KA (1963) Re-innervation of free and flap skin grafts. Acta Chir Plastica 5: 57

Mathes S, Vasconez LO, McCraw JH (1974) Myocutaneous transposition flaps for coverage of lower extremity defects. Anatomical considerations. Surg Clin North Am 54: 1337–1352

Mathes SJ, Nahai F (1979) Clinical atlas of muscle and musculocutaneous flaps. Mosby, St Louis

Mathes SJ, Nahai F (1982) Clinical applications for muscle and musculocutaneous flaps. Mosby, St Louis

Mathes SJ, Nahai F (1996) Reconstructive surgery: principles, anatomy & technique. Quality Medical Publishing, St Louis

Matthews D (1967) Burns. In: Andina F (ed) Reconstructive surgery of thermal injuries and other subjects. Excerpta medica Foundation

Matton G (1996) Orbital decompression by en bloc resection of the lateral wall and floor. In: Van der Meulen JC, Gruss JS (eds) Ocular plastic surgery. Mosby-Wolfe, London, pp 117–122

May JW Jr, Chait LA, Cohen BE, O'Brien BM (1977) Free neurovascular flap from the first web of the foot

in hand reconstruction. J Hand Surg 2: 387
May M (1986) Microanatomy and pathophysiology of the facial nerve. In: May M (ed) The facial nerve. Thieme, New York, pp 63–74
May M, Podvinec M, Ulrich J, et al (1986) Idiopathic (Bell's) palsy, herpes zoster cephalicus and other facial nerve disorders of viral origin. In: May M (ed) The facial nerve. Thieme, New York, pp 365–399
Mayou BJ, Watson JS, Harrison DH, Parry CBW (1981) Free microvascular and microneural transfer of the extensor digitorum brevis muscle for the treatment of unilateral facial palsy. Br J Plast Surg 34: 362–366
McDivitt RW, Farrow JH, Stewart FW (1967) Breast carcinoma arising in solitary fibroadenomas. Surg Gynecol Obstet 125: 572–576
McDivitt RW, Holleb AI, Foote FW Jr (1968) Prior breast disease in patients treated for papillary carcinoma. Arch Pathol 85: 117–124
McEvitt WG (1971) The incidence of persistent rhinolalia following cleft palate repair. Plast Reconstr Surg 47: 258–261
McGrath MH, Burkhardt BR (1984) The safety and efficacy of breast implants for augmentation mammaplasty. Plast Reconstr Surg 74: 550
McGraw JB, Dibble DG (1977) Experimental definition of independent myocutaneous vascular territories. Plast Reconstr Surg 60: 341
McGregor IA (1955) The vascularisation of homografts of human skin. Br J Plast Surg 7: 331
McGregor IA (1957) The theoretical basis of the Z-plasty. Br J Plast Surg 4: 256
McGregor IA (1966) The tongue flaps in lip surgery. Br J Plast Surg 19: 252
McGregor IA (1983) The extended deep inferior epigastric flap: a clinical technique. Discussion. Plast Reconstr Surg 72: 765
McGregor IA, Jackson IT (1972) The groin flap. Br J Plast Surg 25: 3–16
McGregor IA, Morgan RG (1973) Axial and random pattern flaps. Br J Plast Surg 26: 202
McKissock PK (1976) Reduction mammaplasty by the vertical bipedicle flap. Plast Reconstr Surg 49: 245
McLaughlin CR (1950) Epiphora in facial paralysis. Br J Plast Surg 3: 87
McLaughlin CR (1953) Surgical support in permanent facial paralysis. Plast Reconstr Surg 11: 302
McMinn RMH (1960) The cellular anatomy of experimental wound healing. Ann R Coll Surg 26: 245
Medgyesi S, Olsen G (1969) On X-ray burns and irradiated skin. In: Müller FE Wallace AB: Verbrennungskrankheit. Schattauer, Stuttgart
Meng K, Loew D (1974) Mikropunktionsversuche über die Ursachen des akuten Nierenversagens beim experimentellen Verbrennungsschock. Langenbecks Arch Chir 333: 245
Miehlke A (1958) Über die Topographie des Faserverlaufes in Facialisstamm. Arch Ohren Nas Kehlk 171: 340
Millard DR (1958) A radical rotation in single harelip. Am J Surg 95: 1318
Millard DR (1971) Outline for surgery of complete unilateral cleft lip. In: Transactions 5th International Congress Plast Reconstr Surgery. Butterworth, Australia
Millard DR Jr (1996) A rhinoplasty tetralogy: corrective, secondary, congenital, reconstructive. Little Brown and Co, Boston
Miller JG, Bunting P, Burd DAR, Edwards JD (1994) Early cardiorespiratory patterns in patients with major burns and pulmonary insufficiency. Burns 20: 542–546
Millesi H (1977) Technique of free nerve grafting in the face. In: Rubin LR (ed) Reanimation of the paralyzed face. Mosby, St Louis
Millesi H (1979) Nerve suture and grafting to restore the extratemporal facial nerve. Clin Plast Surg 6: 333
Milroy FJ, Anson BJ, McAfee DK (1960) The rectus abdoninus muscle and the epigastric arteries. Surg Gynecol Obstet 110: 293
Mödder G (1996) Der Schilddrüsenpatient. Medical Trends Verlag, Solingen
Monafo WW (1971) Hypertonic sodium solutions for the treatment of burn shock. In: Polk HC Jr, Stone HH (eds) Contemporary burn management. Little, Brown and Co, Boston
Moncrief JA (1966) Effects of various fluid regimens and pharmacologic agents on the circulatory hemodynamics of the immediate postburn period. Ann Surg 164: 723
Moncrief JA (1973) Burns. N Engl J Med 288: 444
Moncrief JA, Switzer WE, Rose LR (1964) Primary excision and grafting in the treatment of third degree burns of the dorsum of the hand. Plast Reconstr Surg 33: 305
Monks GH (1950) Restoration of lower eyelid by a new method. Boston Med Surg J 139: 385
Morel-Fatio D, Lalardrie JP (1964) Palliative surgical treatment of facial paralysis. The palpebral spring. Plast Reconstr Surg 33: 446
Morestin H (1914) De la correction des flexions permanentes de doigts consecutives aux panaris et aux phlegmones de la palme de la main. Rev Chir 50: 1
Mourits MP, Koornneef L, Wiersinga WM, Prummel MF, Berghout A, van der Gaag R (1989) Clinical criteria for the assessment of disease activity in Graves' ophthalmopathy: a novel approach. Br J Ophthalmol 73: 639–644
Moy RL (1998) Denervation techniques for facial rejuvenation. Dermatol Surg 24: 1168–1245
Mühlbauer W, Olbrisch RR (1977) The latissimus dorsi myocutaneous flap for breast reconstruction. Chir Plastica 4: 27–34
Mühlbauer WD (1977) Five years' experience with lid magnet implantation for paretic lagophthalmos. Klin Monatsbl Augenheilkd 171: 938
Müller FE (1966) Grenzen der Behandlungsmöglichkeit und Mortalität schwerer Verbrennungen. Hefte Unfallheilkd 87: 121
Müller W, Allgöwer M, Städtler K, Burkhart F, Schönenberger GA (1974) Specific impairment of host defense for pseudomonas infection in mice by a burn toxin derived from thermally altered human skin. Res Exp Med (Berl) 162: 153
Mutter TD (1842) Cases of deformity from burns, relived by operation. Am J Med Sci 4: 66–80
Naffziger HC (1931) Progressive exophthalmos following thyroidectomy: its pathology and treatment. Ann Surg 94: 582–586
Nahai F (1992) Inferior gluteus maximus musculocutaneous flap for breast

reconstruction. Perspectives Plast Surg 6: 65
Nahai F, Silverston JS, Hill HL, et al (1978) The tensor fascia lata musculocutaneous flap. Ann Plast Surg 1: 372–379
Napier JR (1952) The return of pain sensibility in full thickness skin grafts. Brain 75: 147
Nassif TM, Vidal L, Baudet J (1982) The parascapular flap: A new cutaneous microsurgical free flap. Plast Reconstr Surg 69: 591–600
Nedwich A, Sokolic IH, Foreman J, Howard JM (1964) Histochemical observations of second degree burns. J Trauma 4: 269
New GB (1928) Total rhinoplasty. JAMA 91: 380
New GB (1945) Sickle flap for nasal reconstruction. Surg Gynecol Obstet 80: 597
Nielubowicz J, Olzewski W (1966) Surgical lymphovenous shunts for decompression of secondary lymphedema. J Cardiovasc Surg, Special issue, Amsterdam, pp 384–386
Niermann W (1979) Umbauvorgänge am transplantierten Knochen im Kieferbogenbereich. 10. Jahrestagung, Vereinigung Dtsch Plast Chirurgen, Düsseldorf
Niermann W (1980) Sekundäre operative Rehabilitationsmöglichkeiten nach LKG-Operation. Z Plast Chir 4: 11–20
Niermann W, Goyer K (1981) Die Intelligenzleistung bei Spaltträgern. Z Plast Chir 5: 218–227
Nigst H (1955) Die Chirurgie der peripheren Nerven. Thieme, Stuttgart
Nygaard B, Specht L (1998) Transitory blindness after retrobulbar irradiation of Graves' ophthalmopathy. Lancet 351: 725–726
O'Brien BM (1985) Microlymphatic surgery in the treatment of lymphedema. Progress in lymphology: Proceedings of the Tenth International Congress of Lymphology, University of Adelaide Press, Adelaide, p 235
O'Brien BM, Franklin JD, Morrison WA (1980) Cross-facial nerve grafts and microneurovascular free muscle transfer for long established facial palsy. Br J Plast Surg 33: 202–210
O'Brien BM, Hayhurst JW (1973) Metalized microsutures and a new micro needle holder. Plast Reconstr Surg 52: 673–676
O'Brien BM, McLeod AM, Hayhurst JW, Morrison WA (1973) Successful transfer of a large island flap from the groin to the foot by microvascular anastomoses. Plast Reconstr Surg 52: 271–278
O'Brien BMcC, Mellow CG, Khazanchi RK, Dvir E, Kumar V, Pederson WC (1990) Long-term result after microlymphaticovenous anastomosis for the treatment of obstructive lymphedema. Plast Reconstr Surg 85: 562–572
Oestrup LT, Fredrickson JM (1974) Distant transfer of a free living bone graft by microvascular anastomoses. Plast Reconstr Surg 54: 274–289
Ogura JH, Walsh TE (1962) The transantral orbital decompression operation for progressive exophthalmos. Otolaryngol Clin North Am 13: 29–37
Ohmori K, Harii K (1976) Free dorsalis pedis sensory flap to the hand, with microvascular anastomosis. Plast Reconstr Surg 58: 546–553
Ohmori K, Sekiguchi J, Ohmori S (1979) Total rhinoplasty with a free osteocutaneous flap. Plast Reconstr Surg 63: 387–394
Olivari N (1969) Verschiebeschwenkplastik bei Deckung von Hautdefekten bzw. Dekubitalulzera. (Chirurgia plastica et reconstructiva, Bd 6). Springer, Berlin, S 209–217
Olivari N (1972) Lateral subperiostal osteotomy using the rhinotome. Chir Plastica 1: 261–264
Olivari N (1973) Die Behandlung der Hämangiome im Kindesalter – Chirurgische Therapie. Z Allgemeinmed 49: 60
Olivari N (1973) Narbenbildung nach Verbrennungen durch frühzeitige Nekrektomie und Transplantation zu vermindern. Medical Tribune 52: 15
Olivari N (1975) Die selektive Frühexzision bei Verbrennungen und ihre Bedeutung für die Vorbeugung von Verbrennungskomplikationen. In: Höhler H (Hrsg) Plastische und Wiederherstellungschirurgie. Schattauer, Stuttgart
Olivari N (1976) Chirurgische Frühbehandlung der Verbrennungen. Habilitationsschrift, Universität Köln
Olivari N (1976) The latissimus dorsi flap. Br J Plast Surg 29: 126–128
Olivari N (1979) Use of thirty latissimus dorsi flaps. Plast Reconstr Surg 64: 654
Olivari N (1980) Der Latissimus-dorsi-Lappen und Brustrekonstruktion nach Ablatio und Bestrahlung. In: Bohmert H (Hrsg) Brustkrebs und Brustrekonstruktion. Thieme, Stuttgart
Olivari N (1980) Der Latissimus-Lappen (myocutaner Lappen). Chirurg 51: 166–174
Olivari N (1980) The latissimus dorsi flap: experience with 51 operations. Acta Chir Belg 2: 111–114
Olivari N (1984) Deckung von Thoraxwanddefekten mit dem Latissimus-dorsi-Lappen. In: Lemperle G, Koslowski L (Hrsg) Chirurgie der Strahlenfolgen. Urban & Schwarzenberg, München, S 91–101
Olivari N (1988) Transpalpebrale Dekompressionsoperation bei endokriner Orbitopathie (Exophthalmus). Wien Med Wochenschr 18: 452–455
Olivari N (1991) Transpalpebral decompression of endocrine ophthalmopathy (Graves' disease) by removal of intraorbital fat: experience with 147 operations over 5 years. Plast Reconstr Surg 87: 627–641
Olivari N (1992) Transpalpebral orbital decompression. In: Blodi FC, Mackensen G, Neubauer H (eds) Surgical ophthalmology 2. Springer, Berlin, pp 662–665
Olivari N (2001) Endokrine Orbitopathie – Chirurgische Therapie. Kaden Verlag, Heidelberg [englische Version: Olivari N (2001) Endocrine ophthalmopathy. Surgical treatment. Kaden Verlag, Heidelberg]
Olivari N, Niermann W (1980) Die Abhängigkeit der Lippenform von der Schnittführung bei Lippen-Kiefer-Gaumenspalten. Z Plast Chir 4: 3–10
Olivari N, Noever G (1994) Brustrekonstruktion mit dem Latissimus-Lappen. In: Krupp S (Hrsg) Plastische Chirurgie. Ecomed, Landsberg, VI-4.2, S 1–12
Olivari N, Petrovici V (1978) Chirurgische Behandlung der Schnürringe im Unterschenkelbereich. Z Plast Chir 2: 169–180
Olivari N, Pless H (1975) Strahlenschäden der Haut und ihre chirurgische

Behandlung. In: Höhler H (Hrsg) Plastische und Wiederherstellungschirurgie. Schattauer, Stuttgart

Olivari N, Reismann B, Bayer HW (1973) Die operative Behandlung des infizierten „Sacraldermoids". Bruns Beitr Klin Chir 220: 306–312

Olivari N, Schrudde J (1973) Defektdeckung im Rumpfbereich. Vortrag, Symposium „Die Bedeutung der Plastischen und Wiederherstellungschirurgie im berufsgenossenschaftlichen Heilverfahren", Mainz

Olivari N, Schrudde J, Wahle H (1972) The surgical treatment of bedsores in paraplegics. Plast Reconstr Surg 50: 477

Olivari N, Toennissen J, Schrudde J, Petrovici V (1979) Ersatzoperationen bei Facialisparese. Z Plast Chir 3: 147–158

Ombrédanne L (1937) Maladie amniotique. In: Ombrédanne L, Mathieu P (eds) Traité de chirurgie orthopédique, vol 1. Masson, Paris

Orticochea M (1968) Construction of a dynamic muscle sphincter in cleft palates. Plast Reconstr Surg 41: 323

Padron JG (1992) Peritenon and senile lips. Plastic surgery, Vol II, pp 531–532. Excerpta Medica, Elsevier, Amsterdam

Paré A (1575) Les oeuvres. Avec les figures et portraits tant de l'anatomie que des instruments de chirurgie et de plusieurs monstres. Gabriel Buon, Paris

Parry CH (1825) Collections from the unpublished medical writings, vol. 2. Underwoods, London, p 11

Payr E (1908) Die Osteoplastik mittels eines in einem Brustwandlappen befindlichen Rippenstückes. Zentralbl Chir

Payr E (1934) Gelenksteifen und Gelenkplastik. Springer, Berlin

Pearson RW (1965) Response of human epidermis to graded thermal stress. Arch Environm Health (Chicago) 11: 498

Pehamberger H (1993) Malignes Melanom: State of the art. Österr Ärztez 11: 40–44

Pennington DG (1980) The rectus abdominis myocutaneous free flap. Br J Plast Surg 33: 277

Peters EO (1836) De blepharoplastice (Dissertation). Staritz, Leipzig

Petroff MA, Goode RL, Levet Y (1992) Gore-Tex implants: applications in facial paralysis rehabilitation and soft-tissue augmentation. Laryngoscope 102: 1185–1189

Peyster RG, Ginsberg F, Silber JH, Adler LP (1986) Exophthalmos caused by excessive fat. CT volumetric analysis and fifferential diagnosis. AJR 146: 459–464

Pfannenstiel P, Hotze LA, Saller B (1997) Schilddrüsen-Krankheiten. Henning, Berlin

Pfarr B, Burri C (1973) Der Elektrolythaushalt in der Verbrennungskrankheit. Klin Anästhesiologie 3: 156

Pfolsprundt H von [Pfolspeundt/Pfalzpaint] (1868) Buch der Bündth-Ertznei. 1460. (Hrsg von H Haeser, A Middeldorpf). Reimer, Berlin

Pierer H (1967) Die Versorgung früh- und spätinfizierter drittgradiger Verbrennungen der Hand. Klin Med (Wien) 22: 408

Ponten B (1965) Versorgung von Verbrennungen. In: Gohrbandt E, Gabka J (Hrsg) Handbuch der Plastischen Chirurgie 2, Kapitel 16, 1–43. de Gruyter, Berlin

Ponten B (1981) The fasciocutaneous flap: ists use in soft tissue defects of the lower leg. Br J Plast Surg 34: 215–221

Pruitt BA Jr, Mason AD Jr, Moncrief JA (1971) Hemodynamic changes in the early posthum patient: the influence of fluid administration and of a vasodilatior. J Trauma 11: 36

Prummel MF, Mourits MP, Blank L, Berghout A, Koornneef L, Wiersinga WM (1993) Randomised double-blind trial of prednisone versus radiotherapy in Graves' ophthalmopathy. Lancet 342: 949–954

Purpura F (1908) Tansini method for the cure of cancer of the breast. Lancet I: 634

Radovan C (1982) Breast reconstruction after mastectomy using the temporary expander. Plast Reconstr Surg 69: 195–208

Rappaport I, Pepino AT, Dietrick W (1970) Early use of xenografts as a biological dressing in burn trauma. Am J Surg 120: 144

Reverdin JL (1870) Greffe épidemique. Expérience faite dans dans le service de M. le docteur Guyon à l'hôpital Necker. Gaz Des Hôp Nr. 4

Reverdin JL (1872) De la greffe épidermique. Arch Gén Méd 19: 276, 555, 703

Rhoads JE, McMillan BG, Law EJ (1973) The use of tissue-matched meshed homografts in the treatment of massivae burns. Rev Surg 30: 451

Ridolfi RL, Rosen PP, Port A, Kinne D, Mike V (1977) Medullary carcinoma of the breast: a clinicopathologic study with 10 year follow-up. Cancer 40: 1365–1385

Rintala A (1967) Radiation cancer. Scand J Plast Reconstr Surg I: 5–11

Rogers BO (1959) Historical development of free skin grafting. Surg Clin North Am 39: 289

Rosenthal W (1916) Über die muskuläre Neurotisation bei Fazialisparese. Zentralbl Chir 43: 489

Rubin LR, Bongiovi J (1971) Human skin – antibacterial in vitro. J Surg Res 11: 321

Rubin LR, Lee GW, Simpson RL (1986) Reanimation of the long-standing partila facial paralysis. Plast Reconstr Surg 77: 41–44

Sachs M (2002) Historisches Chirurgenlexikon. (Geschichte der operativen Chirurgie in 5 Bänden, Band 3). Kaden Verlag, Heidelberg

Salisbury RE, Loveless S, Silverstein P, Wilmore DW (1973) Postburn edema of the upper extremity evaluation of present treatment. J Trauma 13: 857

Samii M (1977) Rehabilitation of the face by VIIth nerve substitution (panel discussion no. 6). In: Fisch U (ed) Facial nerve surgery. Aesculapius, Birmingham, AL

Sanvenero-Roselli G (1955) Verschluss von Gaumenspalten unter Verwendung von Pharynxlappen. Fortschr Kiefer-Gesichtschir 1: 65–69

Sanvenero-Rosselli G (1931) Chirurgia plastica des naso. Pozzi, p 148

Sarrazin D, Le M, Rouesse J, et al (1984) Conservative treatment versus mastectomy in breast cancer tumors with mascroscopic diameter of 20 millimetres or less. Cancer 53: 1209–1213

Scaramella LF (1970) Preliminary report on facial nerve anastomosis. Second International Symposium on Facial nerve Surgery, Osaka, Japan

Scea SM, Caulfield B, Burke JF (1973) Microvascular ultrastructure in thermal injury. Microvasc Res 5: 87

Scharnagl E, Smola MG, Hellbom AB, Pierer G, Hoflehner H (1991) Narbenkarzinom: Beobachtungen und Ergebnisse in 23 Fällen. Langenbecks Arch Chir 376: 341–345

Scherer E (1976, 1980) Strahlentherapie. Springer, Berlin

Schiller WR, Bay RC, Garren RL, Parker I, Sagraves SG (1997) Hyperdynamic resuscitation improve survival in patients with life-threatening burns. J Burn Care Rehabil 18: 10–16

Schink W (1960) Handchirurgischer Ratgeber. Springer, Berlin

Schmid E (1952) Über neue Wege in der plastischen Chirurgie der Nase. Beitr Klin Chir 184: 385

Schmid E (1982) Spätergebnisse nach primärer Osteoplastik. In: Pfeifer (Hrsg) Lippen-Kiefer-Gaumenspalten. Thieme, Stuttgart, p 93

Schmidt A, Gay B (1972) Zur Behandlung frischer Verbrennungen an den Händen. Zentralbl Chir 97: 609

Schneider WJ, Hill HL, Brown RG (1977) Latissimus dorsi myocutaneous flap for breast reconstruction. Br J Plast Surg 30: 277

Schnettler R, Steinau HU; Hrsg (2004) Septische Knochenchirurgie. Thieme, Stuttgart

Schönenberger GA, Städtler K (1974) Verbrennungskrankheit – Toxinwirkung oder Infektionsfolge. Chirurg 45: 20

Schreus HAT (1963) Zur operativen Behandlung von Röntgen-Spätschäden. Arch Klin Exp Derm 110: 89

Schrudde J (1957) Primary osteoplasty for clefts of the lip, palate and jaw. Br J Plast Surg 18: 183–187

Schrudde J (1963) Die Deckung von Hautdefekten durch gestielte Lappenplastik. Ästh Med 5: 166

Schrudde J, Petrovici V (1981) Use of slide-swing plasty in closing defects: a clinical study based on 1308 cases. Plast Reconstr Surg 67: 167

Schultz-Ehrenberg U (1980) Der Strahlenschaden aus dermatologischer Sicht. Diagnostik 13: 298–300

Seckel BR (199) Facial danger zones: avoiding nerve injury in facial plastic surgery. Quality Medical Publishing, St Louis

Sédillot C (1846) Traité de médicine opératoire, p 650

Seiffert A (1936) Die Operationen an Nase, Mund und Hals. C Kabitzsch, Leipzig

Serafin D, Smith DH (1979) Composite tissue transplantation in soft tissue reconstruction of the lower extremity. In: Serafin D, Buncke HJ (eds) Microsurgical composite tissue transplantation. Mosby, St Louis, pp 743–771

Serafin D, Voci V, Georgiane N (1982) Microsurgical composite tissue transplantation: Indications and technical considerations in breast reconstruction following mastectomy. Plast Reconstr Surg 70: 24

Sewall EC (1936) Operative control of progressive exophthalmos. Arch Otolaryngol 24: 621–624

Shaw DT, Payne RL (1946) One stage tubed abdominal flaps. Surg Gynecol Obstet 83: 205

Shaw HJ (1980) Transantral orbital decompression for endocrine exophthalmos – an appraisal. J Laryngol Otol 94: 1151–1163

Shaw MH, Fell SR (1948) Columella reconstruction. Br J Plast Surg 2: 111

Shaw WW (1983) Breast reconstruction by superior gluteal microvascular free flaps without silicone implants. Plast Reconstr Surg 72: 490–515

Sheen JH (1997) Aesthetic rhinoplasty. Quality Medical Publishing, St Louis

Sherpukhovskaja KE (1963) Neurotization of a free skin flap grafted on the face. Exp Chir Anaesth 2: 48

Skoog T (1963) A technique of breast reduction, transposition of the nipple on a cutaneous vascular pedicle. Acta Chir Scand 126: 453

Skoog T (1963) The surgical treatment of burns. Acta Chir Scand, Suppl 305: 1

Skoog T (1974) Plastic surgery, new methods and refinements. Thieme, Stuttgart/Almqvist & Wiksell, Stockholm

Smith JA, Gamez-Araujo JJ, Gallager HS, et al (1977) Carcinoma of the breast: analyses of total tymph node involvement versus level of metastases. Cancer 39: 527

Smith JW (1971) A new technique of facial reanimation. Transactions 5th International Congress Plast Reconstr Surgery. Butterworth, Australia

Smith PJ (1973) The vascular basis of axial pattern flaps. Br J Plast Surg 26: 150–157

Snyder WM, Bowles BM, McMillan BG (1970) The use of expansion meshed grafts in the acute and reconstructive management of thermal injury: a clinical evaluation. J Trauma 10: 740

Song R, Gao Y, Song Y, Yu Y, Song Y (1982) The forearm flap. Clin Plast Surg 9: 21–26

Song R, Song Y, Yu Y, Song Y (1982) The upper arm free flap. Clin Plast Surg 9: 27–35

Stark B, Olivari N (1993) Treatment of exophthalmos by orbital fat removal. Clin Plast Surg 20: 285–289

Stark B, Olivari N (1996) Management of thyroid orbitopathy by removal of orbital fat: a long-term follow-up study. Eur J Plast Surg 19: 1–6

Stark B, Olivari N (1996) Orbital decompression by removal of orbital fat. In: Van der Meulen JC, Gruss JS (eds) Ocular plastic surgery. Mosby-Wolfe, London New York, pp 123–130

Steinau HU (1986) Der mikrovaskuläre Latissimus-dorsi-Transfer. Chirurg 57: 126–133

Steinau HU, Askenazy L, Biemer E, Gradinger J (1991) Bilateraler Armverlust bei Starkstromverbrennung im Kindesalter: Stumpfkonstruktion durch Gewebeexpansion und Fibulatransfer. Chirurg 62: 426–429

Steinau HU, Biemer E (1990) Stand der Replantationsindikation und Grenzen in der Handchirurgie. Langenbecks Arch Chir Suppl II (Kongressber)

Steinau HU, Biemer E, Feller AM, Hörl HW (1988) Primärversorgung und sekundäre Wiederherstellungschirurgie der schweren kombinierten Handverletzung. Chirurg 59: 740–748

Steinau HU, Feller AM, Hörl HW, Kunisch M, Klein B, Biemer E (1989) Zur Problematik posttraumatischer Fersenweichteildefekte. Chirurg 60: 287–294

Steinau HU, Germann G (1991) Plastisch-rekonstruktive Mikrochirurgie zur posttraumatischen Infektionsprophylaxe und -therapie. Chirurg 62: 852–860

Steinau HU, Germann G, Büttemeyer R, Hussmann J, Hebebrand D (1993) Zur Wiederherstellungschirurgie kniegelenksnaher Amputationsstümpfe. Unfallchirurgie 19: 272–277

Steinau HU, Hebebrand D, Vogt PM, Peter FW, Tosson R (1997) Plastische Rekonstruktion von Thoraxwanddefekten. Chirurg 68: 461–468

Steinau HU, Hussmann J, Hebebrand D (1993) Rekonstruktionsmöglichkeiten nach erweiterter Resektion maligner Weichteilgeschwülste. Chirurg 64: 517–526

Stock W, Wolf K (1986) Der Radialis-Lappen. Chirurg 57: 134–136

Stone PA, Lawrence JC (1973) Healing of tangentially excised and grafted burns in man. Br J Plast Surg 26: 20

Stör O (1952) Die Verbrennungskrankheit und ihre Behandlung. Enke, Stuttgart

Stranc M, West M (1988) A four-wall orbital decompression for dysthyroid orbitopathy. J Neurosurg 68: 671–677

Stranc MF, Labandter H, Roy A (1975) A review of 196 tube pedicles. Br J Plast Surg 28: 54–69

Stransky E (1899) Sensibilitätsuntersuchungen an transplantierten Hautstückchen. Wien Klin Wochenschr 12: 815

Strauch B, Fox M (1989) VY bipedicle flap for resurfacing the nasal supratip region. Plast Reconstr Surg 83: 899–903

Strömbeck JO (1983) Reduction mammaplasty: some observations and reflections. Aesth Plast Surg 7: 249

Strömbeck, JO (1960) Mammaplasty: report of a new technique based on the two pedicle procedure. Br J Plast Surg 13: 79

Sushruta: Bericht über den ersten Nasenersatz um 1000 vor Christi Geburt. [Sushruta S: Sushruta Samhita. Calcutta, Bose (1907–1916)]

Szymanowsky (1865) Die Operationen an der Oberfläche des menschlichen Körpers. Kiew

Tagliacozzi G (1597) De curtorum chirurgia per insitionem. Gaspare Bindoni, Venedig

Tanner JC, Vandeput J, Olley JF (1964) The mesh skin graft. Plast Reconstr Surg 34: 287

Tansini I (1896) Nuovo processo per l'amputazione della mammella per cancre. Reforma Medica 12: 3–16

Taylor GI, Corlett RJ, Boyd JB (1983) The extended deep inferior epigastric flap: a clinical technique. Plast Reconstr Surg 72: 751–764

Taylor GI, Corlett RJ, Boyd JB (1984) The versatile deep inferior epigastric (inferior rectus abdominis) flap. Br J Plast Surg 73: 330–350

Taylor GI, Daniel RK (1975) The anatomy of several free flap donor sites. Plast Reconstr Surg 56: 243

Taylor GI, Miller GD, Ham FJ (1975) The free vascularized bone graft: a clinical extension of microvascular techniques. Plast Reconstr Surg 55: 533–544

Taylor GI, Razaboni RM (1992) Michel Salmon anatomic studies. Quality Medical Publishing, St Louis

Taylor GI, Townsend P, Corlett RJ (1979) Superiority of the deep circumflex iliac vessel as the supply for free groin flaps: clinical study. Plast Reconstr Surg 64: 745–758

Taylor PH, Moncrief JA, Pugsley LQ, Switzer WE (1962) The management of extensively burned patients by staged excision. Surg Gynecol Obstet 115: 347

Tennison CW (1952) The repair of the unilateral cleft lip by the stencil method. Plast Reconstr Surg 9: 115–120

Teraski PI, Cannon JA, Longmire WD (1960) Antibody response to homografts. Plast Reconstr Surg 25: 415

Terzis J (1987) Microreconstruction of nerve injuries. Saunders, Philadelphia

Terzis JK (1989) Pectoralis minor: a unique muscle for correction of facial palsy. Plast Reconstr Surg 83: 767–776

Terzis JK, Noah ME (1997) Analysis of 100 cases of free-muscle transplantation for facial paralysis. Plast Reconstr Surg 99: 1905–1921

Tessier P (1969) Expansion chirurgical de l'orbite. Ann Chir Plast 14: 207–214

Tessier P (1989) Le lifting facial sous-perioste. Ann Chir Plast Esth 34: 193

Thames HD, Withers HR, Peters LJ, Fletcher GH (1982) Changes in early and late radiation responses with altered dose fractionation: implications for dose-survival relationships. Int J Radiat Oncol Biol Phys 8: 219–226

Thiersch C (1876) Über die feineren anatomischen Veränderungen bei Anheilung von Haut auf Granulationen. Arch Klin Chir 17: 318

Thiersch C (1886) Über Hautverpflanzung. Verh Dtsch Ges Chir 15: 17–32

Thiersch K (1874/1886) Über die feineren anatomischen Veränderungen der Haut auf Granulationen. Dtsch Ges Chir, Bd 2: 73. Zentralbl Chir 24: 17–18

Thompson N (1969) The surgical treatment of advanced postmastectomy lymphedema of the upper limb. With the late results of treatment by the buried dermis flap operation. Scand J Plast Surg 3: 54

Thompson N (1971) Autogenous free grafts of skeletal muscle. A preliminary experimental and clinical study. Plast Reconstr Surg 48: 11

Thompson N, Gustavson EH (1976) The use of neuromuscular free autografts with microneural anastomosis to restore to the paralysed angle of the mouth in cases of unilateral facial paralysis. Chir Plastica 3: 165–174

Tilkorn H, Drepper H, Ehring F (1984) Indikationen für die plastisch-chirurgische Versorgung von Strahlenfolgen an der Haut. In: Lemperle G, Koslowski L (Hrsg) Chirurgie der Strahlenfolgen. Urban & Schwarzenberg, München

Tolhurst DE (1980) Skin and bone: The use of muscle flaps to cover exposed bone. Br J Plast Surg 33: 99–114 (1980)

Tolhurst DE, Bos KE (1982) Free revascularized muscle grafts and facial palsy. Plast Reconstr Surg 69: 760

Tolhurst DE, Haeseker B, Zeeman RJ (1983) The development of the fasciocutaneous flap and its clinical application. Plast Reconstr Surg 72: 597–605

Trott KR, Kummermehr J (1983) Strahlenwirkungen auf die Haut. In: Scherer E, Heuck F (Hrsg) Handbuch der Medizinischen Radiologie, Bd XX, 1. Springer, Berlin

Tubiana R, Baux S, Kenesi C (1967) A propos de 300 brulures thermiques récentes des mains. Ann Chir 21: 1387

Tumorzentrum München (1996) Empfehlungen zur Diagnostik, Therapie und Nachsorge – Mammakarzinome

Veau V (1941) Division palatine. Masson, Paris

Vedung S, Hakelius L, Stalberg E (1984) Cross-face nerve grafting followed by free muscle transplantation in young patients with long-standing facial paralysis. Reanimation of the cheek and the angle of the mouth. Scand J Plast Reconstr Surg 18: 201–208

Veronesi U, Banfi A, Salvatori B, et al (1990) Conservative surgery is the treatment of choice in small breast cancer: long term results of a randomised trial. Eur J Cancer 26: 668–670

Veronesi U, Saccozzi S, del Veccio M, et al (1981) Comparino radical mastectomy with quadrantectomy, axillary dissection and radiotherapy in patients with smal cancer of the breast. N Engl J Med 305: 6–11

Vogt PM, Eichhorn-Sens J (2002) Fettabsaugung – Möglichkeiten und Risiken des populärsten ästhetischen Eingriffs. Plastische Chirurgie 2: 69–74

Walsh TE, Ogura JH (1957) Transantral orbital decompression for malignant exophthalmos. Laryngoscope 67: 544–568

Warden GD (1996) Fluid resuscitation and early management. In: Herndon DN (ed) Total burn care. Saunders, London, p. 53

Weber EG, Steckenmesser R (1982) Die Behandlung des chronischen Lymphödems unter Verwendung von Silikonschläuchen nach der Methode von Schrudde. Z Lymphol. 6: 103

Wei W, Zuoliang Q, Xiaoxi L, Chuan Y, et al (1999) Free split and segmental latissimus dorsi muscle transfer in one stage for facial reanimation. Plast Reconstr Surg 103: 473–480

Weiland AJ, Villarreal-Rios A, Kleinert HE, et al (1977) Replantation of digits and hands: Analysis of surgical techniques and functional results in 71 patients with 86 replantations. J Hand Surg 2: 1–12

Werner SC (1969) Classification of the eye changes of Graves' disease. J Clin Endocrinol Metab 29: 982–984

Whitson TC, Allen BD (1971) Management of the burned hand. J Trauma 11: 606

Whittaker AH (1953) Treatment on burn by excision and immediate skin grafting. Am J Surg 85: 411

Willis AM (1925) The value of debridement in the treatment of burns. JAMA 84: 655

Wilm M (1901) Studien zur Pathologie der Verbrennung. Mitt Grenzgeb Med Chir 8: 393

Wilson RD (1971) Thermoregulatory failure of the burn scar. J Trauma 11: 518

Withers HR, Thames HD, Flow BL, Mason KA, Hussey DH (1978) The relationship of acute and late skin injury in 2 and 5 fractions/week X-ray therapy. Int J Radiat Oncol Biol Phys 4: 595–601

Wolfe JR (1875) A new method for performing plastic operations. Br Med J II: 360–369

Wolfe JR (1876) A new method of performing plastic operations. Med Times Gaz 1: 608

Wolfe SA (1979) Modified three-wall orbital expansion to correct persistent exophthalmos or exorbitism. J Plast Reconstr Surg 64: 448–455

Wood-Smith D (1973) Encircling Silastic band for paralysis of the orbicularis oculi muscle. Presented at the Society of Ophthalmic Plastic Surgeons, Dallas, TX

Wrede L (1933) Die Operationen am Nervus facialis, chirurgische Operationslehre, Bd I. Barth, Leipzig

Zarem HA, Pandya NJ (1974) Biological assay for a vasoactive factor in serum from human burn victims. J Trauma 14: 409

Zeis E (1863) Die Literatur und Geschichte der Plastischen Chirurgie. Engelmann, Leipzig

Zoltan J (1972) Transplantationslehre. In: Handbuch der plastischen Chirurgie. De Gruyter, Berlin

Index

Neven Olivari was born in 1932 in Gradac, Dalmatia, Croatia. After high school he studied medicine at the University of Zagreb and qualified as medical doctor in1958. His resident year was at University Clinic Rijeka. In 1960 was appointed as a junior registrar in the surgical department of the Dreifaltigkeits Hospital in Lippstadt, Germany (Head: Dr. Schroeder). In May 1964 he moved to the surgical department of the University Clinic of Cologne (Professor Schink), and he was able to work in the Department for Plastic Surgery (Professor Schrudde). In 1970 Neven Olivari was appointed as a consultant plastic surgeon in the independent Clinic for Plastic Surgery of the University of Cologne (Head: Professor Schrudde), where he remained until 1982. During this time Neven Olivari published numerous scientific papers. In 1974 he developed the Latissimus dorsi Flap and 1975 presented it at The Royal College of Surgeons in London. He wrote a thesis on plastic surgery in 1977 and was appointed as Professor of Plastic Surgery at University Clinic of Cologne in1982. From 1982–1997 he was head of the department for plastic surgery at the Dreifaltigkeits Hospital, Wesseling. During the time in Wesseling he published numerous scientific papers and contributions to books. 1982 he received the scientific award of the Association of the Plastic Surgeons of Germany for the rediscover and development of the Latissimus dorsi flaps. 1990–1993 he was President of the Association of the German Plastic Surgeons (he had served in many official capacities on the executive committee from 1978–1997). In 1991 his paper "Transpalpebral decompression of endocrine ophthalmopathy (Grave's disease) by removal of intraorbital fat: experience with 147 operations in 5 years" was named as the best clinical paper in *Journal of Plastic and Reconstructive Surgery*. He was awarded

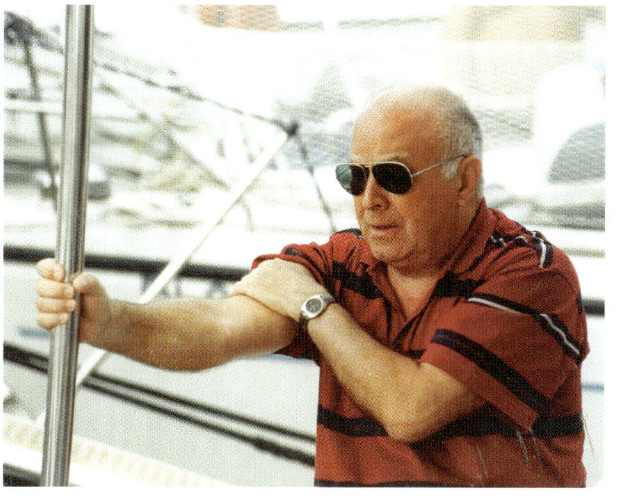

Order of Merit, First Class, by the German Federal President Roman Herzog in 1998 for services in development of plastic surgery in Germany. His book "Endocrine ophthalmopathy, surgical treatment" was published 2001. In this book he described his new method of orbital decompression. Neven Olivari is an Honorary Member of the German Association of Plastic Surgeons, a Member of the Croatian Academy of Medical Sciences and a Honorary Member of the British Association of Plastic Surgeons and several another Scientific Associations. He is a frequent speaker on national and international congresses and an irreverent critic, on plastic surgery topics. He respects authorities that speak from well founded knowledge and experience. The colleagues, who show only beautiful results and don't discuss complications, are anathema to him. He is happy to give his opinion loud and clear. His hobbies are tennis, piano playing, painting and navigating in the Dalmatian Archipelago. Neven Olivari is married to Anna Maria, has two sons, Alexander and Nicolas as well as three grandchildren, Lina Maria, Ella Brigitte and Karlo.

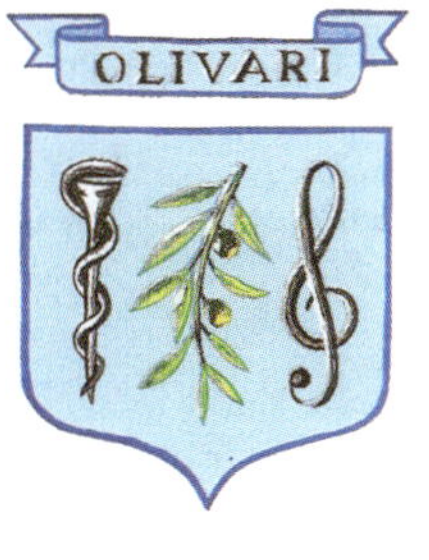

Neven Olivari

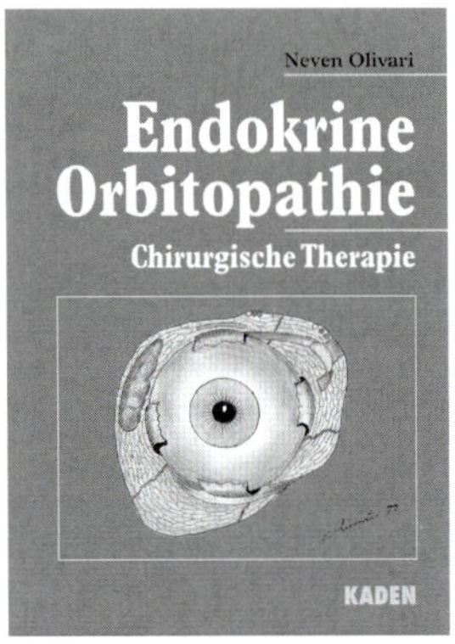

Endokrine Orbitopathie – Chirurgische Therapie

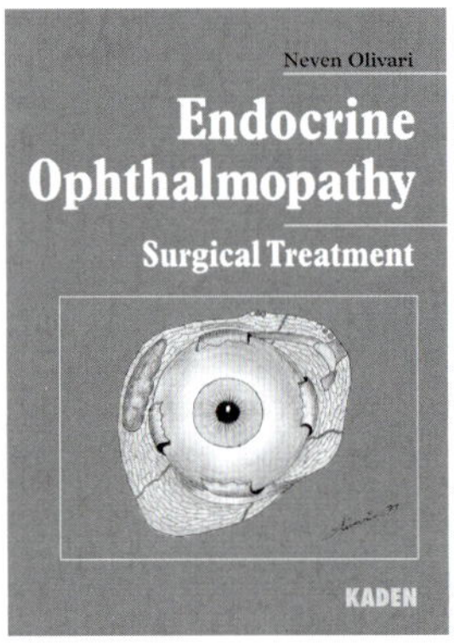

Endocrine Ophthalmopathy – Surgical Treatment

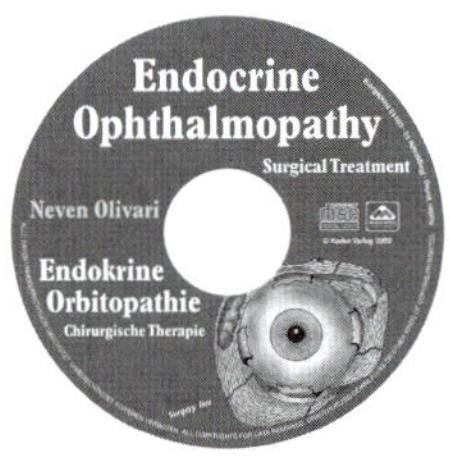

Inklusive Video-CD

41 Minuten Live-OP!
Von Prof. Olivari, mit der im Buch beschriebenen Technik.

From the Preface by Ian T. Jackson

… The method described by Neven Olivari, and so beautifully presented in this book, is logical. Unfortunately, when it is presented or demonstrated by Neven Olivari, it seems simple to execute. However, at that point we are watching or listening to a master surgeon with a huge amount of experience in all aspects of plastic surgery but particularly in the orbit, demonstrating a technique which he has pioneered and developed over many years. …

Atlasformat 21 x 29,7 cm; Gebunden
XVI, 144 Seiten; 31 Tabellen; 250 Abbildungen (davon 162 in Farbe)
ISBN 3-922777-30-9 (Deutsche Ausgabe), 2001
ISBN 3-922777-35-X (English Edition), 2001

Dr. Reinhard Kaden Verlag GmbH & Co. KG
Ringstraße 19 · 69115 Heidelberg · Telefon (06221) 1377610 · Telefax (06221) 6599590
www.kaden-verlag.de